ESSENCE OF
ANESTHESIA
PRACTICE

—

Michael F. Roizen, M.D.
Professor and Chairman
Department of Anesthesia and Critical Care
Professor of Medicine
The University of Chicago
Chicago, Illinois

Lee A. Fleisher, M.D.
Assistant Professor
Department of Anesthesiology and Critical Care Medicine
Joint Appointment in Medicine (Cardiology)
Johns Hopkins University School of Medicine
Baltimore, Maryland

W.B. SAUNDERS COMPANY
A Division of Harcourt Brace & Company
Philadelphia • London • Toronto • Montreal • Sydney • Tokyo

W.B. SAUNDERS COMPANY
A Division of Harcourt Brace & Company

The Curtis Center
Independence Square West
Philadelphia, Pennsylvania 19106

Library of Congress Cataloging-in-Publication Data

Essence of anesthesia practice / [edited by] Michael F. Roizen, Lee A.
    Fleisher. — 1st ed.

p.   cm.

ISBN 0–7216–5972–1

1. Anesthesia—Handbooks, manuals, etc.   I. Roizen, Michael F.
    II. Fleisher, Lee A.
    [DNLM: 1. Anesthesia handbooks.   2. Anesthetics—handbooks.
    WO 39 E78 1997]

RD82.2.E87 1997   617.9'6—dc20

DNLM/DLC   96–24185

Essence of Anesthesia Practice   ISBN 0–7216–5972–1

Printed in the United States of America

Last digit is the print number: 9   8   7   6   5   4   3   2   1

ESSENCE OF
ANESTHESIA PRACTICE

DEDICATIONS

Dedication from Lee A. Fleisher:
To my wife, Renee—For her loving support; and to my children,
Jessica and Matthew, for their inspiration.

Dedication from Michael F. Roizen:
To Nancy, Jeffrey, and Jennifer—Whose support, sacrifices, and
love make even writing and editing at home fun; and to the
members of The Department of Anesthesia and Critical Care at
The University of Chicago, who allowed the time and sacrificed
their own interests to the production of this work, and who make
work fun.

From Lee and Mike—To the many colleagues who took time to
share their expertise, and to future patients who, we hope, will
benefit because their care is being delivered by someone who is able
to efficiently review the perioperative implications of the patho-
physiology of their diseases, drug therapies, procedures, and test
abnormalities.

Lee A. Fleisher, M.D.
Michael F. Roizen, M.D.

Contributors

Tamara H. Abbas, M.D.
Department of Anesthesiology, Providence Hospital, Washington, D.C.
Succinylcholine

Theresa K. Abboud, M.D.
Professor of Anesthesiology, University of Southern California School of Medicine, Los Angeles, California
Eclampsia

Erzat I. Abouleish, M.D.
Professor, Department of Anesthesiology and Obstetrics, The University of Texas, Houston, Health Science Center, Houston, Texas
Cephalopelvic Disproportion (CPD)

Jerome H. Abrams, M.D.
Associate Professor, Department of Surgery, University of Minnesota Medical School, Minneapolis, Minnesota
Nutritional Support

Anil Aggarwal, M.D.
Associate Professor, Department of Anesthesiology, Medical College of Wisconsin, Milwaukee, Wisconsin
Dobutamine

Charles Ahere, M.D.
Assistant Professor, University of Mississippi Medical Center, Jackson, Mississippi
Sleep Apnea, Obstructive

David B. Albert, M.D.
Director of Ambulatory Anesthesia, Hospital for Joint Diseases, New York, New York
Osteoporosis

Richard D. Alessi, Jr., M.D.
Assistant Professor, The University of Chicago, Pritzker School of Medicine, Chicago, Illinois
Blalock-Taussig (BT) Shunt

Hassan H. Ali, M.D.
Professor of Anaesthesia, Harvard Medical School, Boston, Massachusetts
Physostigmine Salicylate (Eserine, Antilirium)
Pyridostigmine Bromide

John C. Alverdy, M.D., F.A.C.S.
Associate Professor of Surgery, The University of Chicago Hospitals, Chicago, Illinois
Gastric Bypass Stapling for Morbid Obesity

John R. Ammon, M.D.
Senior Lecturer, Department of Anesthesiology, University of Arizona, Tucson, Arizona
Diabetic Ketoacidosis (DKA)
Hyperosmolar Nonketotic Coma

Jeffrey L. Apfelbaum, M.D.
Professor and Vice-Chair, Department of Anesthesia and Critical Care, The University of Chicago, Chicago, Illinois
Propofol

Marvin L. Appel, M.D., Ph.D.
Assistant Professor, Department of Anesthesiology, Johns Hopkins Hospital, Baltimore, Maryland
Cardiopulmonary Bypass

James F. Arens, M.D.
Professor, Department of Anesthesiology, The University of Texas Medical Branch, Galveston, Texas
Pulmonary Atresia

James Armstrong, M.D.
University of Ottawa, Heart Institute, Ottawa, Ontario, Canada
Treacher Collins Syndrome

Solomon Aronson, M.D.
Associate Professor and Director of Cardiovascular Anesthesia, Department of Anesthesia and Critical Care, The University of Chicago, Chicago, Illinois
Myxoma
Renal Function Testing

Takashi Asai, M.D.
Research Associate, Kansai Medical University, Osaka, Japan
Constipation

Rajakumari V. Asrani, M.D.
Clinical Professor of Anesthesiology, University of California, Irvine, Medical Center, Orange, California VA Medical Center, Long Beach, California
Trigeminal Neuralgia (Tic Douloureux)

John L. Atlee, M.D.
Professor of Anesthesiology, Medical College of Wisconsin, Milwaukee, Wisconsin
Atrial Flutter
AV and Bifascicular Heart Block
Sick Sinus Syndrome (SSS)
Supraventricular Tachycardia (Tachyarrhythmias)
Ventricular Pre-excitation
Ventricular Tachyarrhythmias

Catherine R. Bachman, M.D.
Assistant Professor of Anesthesia and Critical Care, The University of Chicago, Chicago, Illinois
Rett Syndrome

Douglas Bacon, M.D.
Assistant Professor of Anesthesiology, State University of New York at Buffalo, School of Medicine and Biomedical Sciences, Buffalo, New York
Sarcoma

Jeffrey M. Baden, M.D.
Professor, Department of Anesthesia, Stanford University School of Medicine, Stanford, California
Hepatic Encephalopathy

Andrew D. Badley, M.D.
Instructor in Medicine, Mayo Clinic and Foundation, Rochester, Minnesota
Cytomegalovirus Infection

Peter L. Bailey, M.D.
Associate Professor, University of Utah Health Sciences Center, Salt Lake City, Utah
Nonsteroidal Anti-Inflammatory Drugs (NSAIDs)

Kristy Z. Baker, M.D.
Assistant Professor of Anesthesiology, Columbia University College of Physicians and Surgeons, New York, New York
Transsphenoidal Surgery

Jeffrey R. Balser, M.D., Ph.D.
Assistant Professor of Anesthesiology and Critical Care Medicine, Johns Hopkins University School of Medicine, Baltimore, Maryland
Paroxysmal Atrial Tachycardia
Wolff-Parkinson-White (WPW) Syndrome

Anis S. Baraka, M.D.
Professor and Chairman, Department of Anesthesiology, American University of Beirut Medical School, Beirut, Lebanon
Echinococcosis

Paul G. Barash, M.D.
Professor, Department of Anesthesiology, Yale University School of Medicine, New Haven, Connecticut
Aortic Regurgitation

Jean-François Baron, M.D.
Hôpital Broussais, Paris, France
Congestive Heart Failure

Deborah M. Barron, M.D.
Clinical Instructor, Harvard Medical School, Boston, Massachusetts
Liver Transplantation

Richard R. Bartkowski, M.D., Ph.D.
Professor of Anesthesiology, Jefferson Medical College, Thomas Jefferson University, Philadelphia, Pennsylvania
Urticaria, Cold

Christopher D. Beatie, M.D.
Assistant Clinical Professor of Anesthesiology, University of California, Los Angeles, School of Medicine, Los Angeles, California
Aspirin (Acetylsalicylic Acid)
Oral Hypoglycemics
ESWL (Extracorporeal Shock Wave Lithotripsy)

Charles Beattie, M.D., Ph.D.
Professor and Chairman, Department of Anesthesiology, Vanderbilt University School of Medicine, Nashville, Tennessee
Abdominal Aortic Aneurysm Repair

Robert F. Bedford, M.D.
Clinical Professor, Department of Anesthesiology, University of Virginia School of Medicine, Charlottesville, Virginia
Supratentorial Brain Tumors

Joel Bennett, M.D.
Assistant Professor of Anesthesiology, Medical College of Pennsylvania and Hahnemann University, Philadephia, Pennsylvania
Coagulopathy—Intrinsic Pathway

David L. Berger, M.D.
Clinical Assistant Professor, Stanford University School of Medicine, Stanford, California
Mitral Valve Replacement

M. Lawrence Berman, M.D.
Professor of Anesthesiology and Associate Professor of Pharmacology, Vanderbilt University School of Medicine, Nashville, Tennessee
Hashimoto's Thyroiditis

Ralph L. Bernstein, M.D.
Professor of Clinical Anesthesiology, New York University School of Medicine, New York, New York
Scoliosis and Kyphosis
Surgery for Scoliosis and Kyphosis

Wendy K. Bernstein, M.D.
Physician, Department of Anesthesia and Critical Care, Johns Hopkins University School of Medicine, Baltimore, Maryland
Splenectomy

Arnold J. Berry, M.D.
Professor of Anesthesiology, Emory University School of Medicine, Atlanta, Georgia
Hepatitis B
Hepatitis C

Frederic A. Berry, M.D.
Professor of Anesthesiology and Pediatrics, University of Virginia Health Sciences Center, Charlottesville, Virginia
Foreign Body Aspiration

Brian K. Bevacqua, M.D.
Assistant Professor of Anesthesiology, Case Western Reserve School of Medicine, Cleveland, Ohio
Diphtheria

Wendy B. Binstock, M.D.
Assistant Professor, Department of Anesthesia and Critical Care, Department of Pediatrics, The University of Chicago, Chicago, Illinois
Omphalocele Surgery

David J. Birnbach, M.D.
Assistant Professor of Anesthesiology and Obstetrics and Gynecology, Columbia University College of Physicians and Surgeons, New York, New York
HELLP Syndrome

Bruno Bissonette, M.D.
Associate Professor, University of Toronto, Faculty of Medicine, Toronto, Ontario, Canada
Opitz-Frias Syndrome (The G Syndrome)

Timothy M. Bittenbinder, M.D.
Assistant Professor, Texas A&M University College of Medicine, Texas A&M Health Science Center, Temple, Texas
Geriatric Surgery

Matthew L. Black, M.D.
Physician, Department of Anesthesia and Critical Care, The University of Chicago, Chicago, Illinois
Propofol

Jordan L. Blinder, M.D.
Assistant Professor of Anesthesiology, Tufts University School of Medicine, Boston, Massachusetts
Appendicitis, Acute

Robert H. Bode, Jr., M.D.
Clinical Instructor in Anaesthesia, Harvard Medical School, Boston, Massachusetts
Amputation, Lower Extremity

Thomas F. Boerner, M.D.
Assistant Professor of Anesthesiology and Critical Care Medicine, University of Pittsburgh School of Medicine, Pittsburgh, Pennsylvania
Tetracyclines

Cecil O. Borel, M.D.
Associate Professor of Anesthesiology, Associate Professor of Neurosurgery, Duke University School of Medicine, Durham, North Carolina
Myasthenia Gravis

Gregory H. Botz, M.D.
Associate in the Department of Anesthesiology, Duke University School of Medicine, Durham, North Carolina
Cardiomyopathy, Alcoholic
Cardiomyopathy, Ischemic

Charles D. Boucek, M.D.
Clinical Associate Professor of Anesthesiolgoy and Internal Medicine, University of Pittsburgh School of Medicine, Pittsburgh, Pennsylvania
Bone Marrow Transplantation (Harvest Procedure)

Denis L. Bourke, M.D.
Associate Professor of Anesthesiology, University of Maryland School of Medicine, Baltimore, Maryland
Transurethral Resection of Bladder Tumor
Ureteral Stent Placement

Gwendolyn L. Boyd, M.D.
Professor, Department of Anesthesiology, University of Alabama at Birmingham School of Medicine, Birmingham, Alabama
Brain Death

Floyd S. Brauer, M.D.
Professor and Chair, Department of Anesthesiology, Loma Linda University School of Medicine, Loma Linda, California
Carotid Sinus Syndrome (CSS)

Michelle Braunfeld, M.D.
Assistant Clinical Professor, University of California, Los Angeles, School of Medicine, Los Angeles, California
Diarrhea, Acute and Chronic
Drug Overdose—Rat Poison (Warfarin Toxicity)
Hypercalcemia

Candidad Bravo-Fernandez, M.D.
Staff Anesthesiologist and Assistant Pain Clinic Director, Anesthesia and Pain Center of Akron, Crystal Clinic Surgery Center, Akron, Ohio
Amputation, Above-Knee (AKA)

Peter H. Breen, M.D.
Assistant Professor in Residence, Department of Anesthesiology, University of California, Irvine, College of Medicine, Orange, California
Carbon Monoxide (CO) Poisoning
Cyanide Poisoning

Michael J. Breslow, M.D.
Associate Professor, Departments of Anesthesiology and Critical Care Medicine, Johns Hopkins University School of Medicine, Baltimore, Maryland
Paroxysmal Atrial Tachycardia

Jay B. Brodsky, M.D.
Professor, Department of Anesthesiology, Stanford University School of Medicine, Stanford, California
Guillain-Barré Syndrome

Burnell R. Brown, Jr., M.D., Ph.D.*
Former Professor and Chair, Department of Anesthesiology, University of Arizona College of Medicine, Tuscon, Arizona
Multiple Endocrine Neoplasia (MEN) Types I and II

Eli Brown, M.D.
Professor and Chairman Emeritus, Department of Anesthesiology, Wayne State University School of Medicine, Detroit, Michigan
Parathyroidectomy

Morris Brown, M.D.
Professor and Chair, Department of Anesthesiology, Wayne State University School of Medicine, Detroit, Michigan
Atrial Flutter

---

* Deceased.

Sorin J. Brull, M.D.
Associate Professor of Anesthesiology, Yale University School of Medicine, New Haven, Connecticut
Cholecystectomy, Laparoscopic
Cholecystectomy, Open

Claude Brunson, M.D.
Assistant Professor, Department of Anesthesiology, University of Mississippi School of Medicine, Jackson, Mississippi
Sleep Apnea, Obstructive

David Bui, M.D.
Clinical Assistant Professor of Anesthesiology, State University of New York at Buffalo School of Medicine and Biomedical Sciences, Buffalo, New York
IgA Deficiency

Michelle Burnett, M.D.
Assistant Professor, Department of Anesthesia, Georgetown University School of Medicine, Washington, D.C.
Eisenmenger's Syndrome

John Butterworth, M.D.
Associate Professor and Vice-Chairman for Research, Department of Anesthesia, The Bowman Gray School of Medicine of Wake Forest University, Winston-Salem, North Carolina
Hypothyroidism

James E. Caldwell, M.B.Ch.B.
Associate Professor of Anesthesia, University of California, San Francisco, School of Medicine, San Francisco, California
Vecuronium

Jerry M. Calkins, M.D.
Professor of Clinical Anesthesiology, University of Arizona College of Medicine, Tucson, Arizona
Gonorrhea
Reflex Sympathetic Dystrophy (Complex Peripheral Pain Syndrome)

Enrico Camporesi, M.D.
Professor and Chairman, Department of Anesthesiology, State University of New York and Syracuse Health Science Center, Syracuse, New York
Burn Injury—Flame

Roy D. Cane, M.B., B.Ch.
Professor of Anesthesiology and Surgery, University of South Florida College of Medicine, Tampa, Florida
Tetanus

Lisa A. Caramico, M.D.
Assistant Professor of Anesthesiology, Yale University School of Medicine, New Haven, Connecticut
Shy-Drager Disease

Helmut F. Cascorbi, M.D.
Professor and Chairman, Department of Anesthesiology, Case Western Reserve University School of Medicine, Cleveland, Ohio
Chloramphenicol (Chloromycetin)

Henry Casson, M.D.
Associate Professor, Anesthesiology, Oregon Health Science University, Portland, Oregon
Tetralogy of Fallot (TOF), Correction of

Charles B. Cauldwell, M.D., Ph.D.
Associate Professor, Department of Anesthesiology, Wayne State University School of Medicine, Detroit, Michigan
Pierre Robin Syndrome

Andrei Cernea, M.D.
Staff Anesthesiologist, Providence Hospital, Washington, D.C.
Cleft Palate
Cleft Lip Repair

Bernard R. Chaitman, M.D.
Professor of Medicine, St. Louis University School of Medicine, St. Louis, Missouri
Exercise Stress Testing

Susan Chan, M.D.
Assistant Clinical Professor, University of California, Los Angeles, School of Medicine, Los Angeles, California
Laparoscopy, Gynecologic

Bobby Su-Pen Chang, M.D.
Assistant Professor of Anesthesiology, Cornell University Medical College, New York, New York
Mycoplasma pneumoniae Infection

Ronald P. Chavez, M.D.
Assistant Professor of Anesthesia and Critical Care, The University of Chicago, Chicago, Illinois
Pregnancy: Maternal Physiology
Vitamin K Deficiency

Eugene Y. Cheng, M.D.
Associate Professor of Anesthesiology and Medicine and Director of Critical Care Medicine, Department of Anesthesiology, Medical College of Wisconsin, Milwaukee, Wisconsin
Herpes—Type I

Albert T. Cheung, M.D.
Assistant Professor, Department of Anesthesia, University of Pennsylvania School of Medicine, Philadelphia, Pennsylvania
Mitral Stenosis
Mitral Valve Prolapse

Daniel Chou, M.D.
Rockville, Maryland
Endoscopic Sinus Surgery (ESS)

Rose Christopherson, M.D., Ph.D.
Assistant Professor of Anesthesiology, Johns Hopkins University School of Medicine, Baltimore, Maryland
Bypass Graft Procedure—Infrainguinal

Noel Lee Chun, M.D.
Assistant Clinical Professor of Anesthesiology, University of California, Los Angeles, School of Medicine, Los Angeles, California
Burn Injury—Chemical
Radical Neck Dissection
Rotator Cuff Surgery

Richard Clark, M.D.
Professor, Departments of Anesthesiology and Obstetrics/Gynecology, University of Arkansas College of Medicine, Little Rock, Arkansas
Diabetes, Type III (Gestational Diabetes Mellitus)

Dennis W. Coalson, M.D.
Assistant Professor, Department of Anesthesia and Critical Care, The University of Chicago, Chicago, Illinois
Kidney Transplantation
Pancreas Transplantation

Neal H. Cohen, M.D.
Professor, Anesthesia and Medicine, and Vice-Chairman, Department of Anesthesia, University of California, San Francisco, School of Medicine, San Francisco, California
Pneumocystis carinii Pneumonia (PCP)

Stephan J. Cohn, M.D.
Assistant Professor, Department of Anesthesia and Critical Care, The University of Chicago, Chicago, Illinois
Raynaud's Phenomenon

Daniel J. Cole, M.D., Ph.D.
Associate Professor of Anesthesiology, Loma Linda University School of Medicine, Loma Linda, California
Amyotrophic Lateral Sclerosis (ALS)

Lydia A. Conlay, M.D., Ph.D.
Associate Professor of Anesthesia, Harvard Medical School, Boston, Massachusetts
Cholelithiasis

Aisling Conran, M.D.
Physician, The University of Chicago, Chicago, Illinois
Hepatitis—Halothane

Richard I. Cook, M.D.
Assistant Professor, Department of Anesthesia and Critical Care, The University of Chicago, Chicago, Illinois
Duchenne Muscular Dystrophy (Pseudohypertrophic Muscular Dystrophy)
Adriamycin (Doxorubicin), Daunorubicin (Cerubidine)

Thomas Corbridge, M.D.
Assistant Professor of Medicine, Physical Medicine, and Rehabilitation, Northwestern University Medical School, Chicago, Illinois
Asthma, Acute

Randall C. Cork, M.D., Ph.D.
Professor and Chair, Department of Anesthesiology, Louisiana State University Medical Center, Shreveport, Louisiana
Intraoperative Recall

Martin G. Cascio, M.D.
Assistant Professor of Anesthesiology and Critical Care Medicine, University of Pittsburgh School of Medicine, Pittsburgh, Pennsylvania
Labor—Peripheral Blocks

Vincent S. Cowell, M.D.
Instructor in Anesthesiology, Medical College of Pennsylvania/Hahnemann University, Philadelphia, Pennsylvania
Breast Cancer
Hemophilia

Paula A. Craigo, M.D.
Assistant Professor, Department of Anesthesia and Critical Care, The University of Chicago, Chicago, Illinois
Aspiration, Perioperative: Prevention and Management
Pneumonectomy

Roy F. Cucchiara, M.D.
Professor and Chairman, Department of Anesthesiology, University of Florida College of Medicine, Gainesville, Florida
Central Neurogenic Hyperventilation

David J. Cullen, M.D.
Clinical Professor of Anesthesiology, Tufts University School of Medicine, Boston, Massachusetts
Delirium (Postanesthetic)

Anthony J. Cunningham, M.D.
Professor of Anaesthesia, Royal College of Surgeons in Ireland, Dublin, Ireland
AV Graft for Hemodialysis

S. I. Dagher, M.D.
Pain Fellow, Texas Tech University Health Sciences Center and University Medical Center, Lubbock, Texas
Headache—Migraine

Nicola D'Attellis, M.D.
Attending Physician, Hospital Broussais, Paris, France
Congestive Heart Failure

Paul J. Dauchot, M.D.
Professor of Anesthesiology, Case Western Reserve University School of Medicine, Cleveland, Ohio
Dilated Cardiomyopathies (DCMs)

Peter J. Davis, M.D.
Professor of Anesthesia and Pediatrics, University of Pittsburgh School of Medicine, Pittsburgh, Pennsylvania
Gastroschisis Surgery

Richard F. Davis, M.D.
Professor of Anesthesiology, Oregon Health Sciences University, Portland, Oregon
Buerger's Disease; Thromboangiitis Obliterans (TAO)

Bhaskar Deb, M.D.
Assistant Professor of Anesthesiology and Critical Care, Temple University School of Medicine, Philadelphia, Pennsylvania
Multisystem Organ Failure, Lung Dysfunction in

Ellise Delphin, M.D.
Associate Professor of Clinical Anesthesiology, Columbia University College of Physicians and Surgeons, New York, New York
Antithrombin III Deficiency

Dawn P. Desiderio, M.D.
Associate Professor, Department of Anesthesiology, Cornell University Medical College, New York, New York
Esophageal Cancer

Stanley Deutsch, M.D., Ph.D.
Professor of Anesthesiology, George Washington University School of Medicine and Health Sciences, Washington, D.C.
Diverticulosis

Stephen F. Dierdorf, M.D.
Professor of Anesthesia, Indiana University School of Medicine, Indianapolis, Indiana
Rheumatoid Arthritis

Jeffrey Dodd-o, M.D.
Assistant Professor, Department of Anesthesiology and Critical Care Medicine and Department of Surgery, Johns Hopkins Hospital, Baltimore, Maryland
Ulcerative Colitis, Chronic

Barbara A. Dodson, M.D.
Associate Professor, Department of Anesthesia, University of California, San Francisco, School of Medicine, San Francisco, California
Cerebral Arteriovenous Malformations (AVMs)
Depression—Unipolar
Seizure Surgery

Karen B. Domino, M.D.
Associate Professor of Anesthesiology, University of Washington School of Medicine, Seattle, Washington
Silicosis

John V. Donlon, Jr., M.D.
Associate Clinical Professor of Anaesthesia, Harvard Medical School, Boston, Massachusetts
Glaucoma—Closed Angle
Glaucoma—Open Angle

Joseph Dooley, M.D.
Associate Resident, University of Rochester School of Medicine and Dentistry, Rochester, New York
Intracranial Hypertension (ICH)

Todd Dorman, M.D.
Assistant Professor, Department of Anesthesiology and Critical Care Medicine and Department of Surgery, Johns Hopkins Medical Institutions, Baltimore, Maryland
Deep Vein Thrombosis

Thomas J. Ebert, M.D.
Professor of Anesthesiology, Adjunct Professor of Physiology, Medical College of Wisconsin, Milwaukee, Wisconsin
Familial Dysautonomia (Riley-Day Syndrome)
Autonomic Function

Paul D. Eckenbrecht, M.D.
Associate Professor of Anesthesiology, University of South Carolina School of Medicine, Columbia, South Carolina
Implantable Cardioverter-Defibrillators (ICDs)—Implantation
Implantable Cardioverter-Defibrillators (ICDs)—Management

Talmage D. Egan, M.D.
Assistant Professor, Department of Anesthesiology, University of Utah School of Medicine, Salt Lake City, Utah
Cigarette Smoking Cessation

Nadir El-Gamal, M.D.
Assistant Professor of Anesthesiology, Alexandria University, Alexandria, Egypt
Eye Enucleation
Retinal Buckle Surgery

John Peder Erickson, M.D.
Assistant Clinical Professor, Departments of Anesthesia and Critical Care and Pediatrics, The University of Chicago, Chicago, Illinois
Pyloric Stenosis Repair

Lucinda L. Everett, M.D.
Associate Professor, Medical College of Virginia/Virginia Commonwealth University, Richmond, Virginia
Inguinal Herniorrhaphy

Jane Eyrich, M.D.
Associate Professor, Department of Anesthesiology, Louisiana State University School of Medicine, New Orleans, Louisiana
Gastrinoma

Nauder Faraday, M.D.
Assistant Professor, Department of Anesthesiology and Critical Care Medicine, Johns Hopkins University School of Medicine, Baltimore, Maryland
Thrombocytopenia

Thomas W. Feeley, M.D.
Professor of Anesthesia, Stanford University School of Medicine, Stanford, California
Multisystem Organ Failure, Lung Dysfunction in

James J. Fehr, M.D.
Fellow, Department of Anesthesiology and Critical Care Medicine, Johns Hopkins Hospital, Baltimore, Maryland
Mucopolysaccharidoses

James M. Feld, M.D.
Assistant Professor of Anesthesiology, University of Illinois College of Medicine, Chicago, Illinois
Hypomagnesemia

Kenneth Fickling, M.D.
University of Rochester School of Medicine and Dentistry, Rochester, New York
Myringotomy and Tympanostomy

Leonard Firestone, M.D.
Professor and Chair, Department of Anesthesiology and Critical Care Medicine, University of Pittsburgh School of Medicine, Pittsburgh, Pennsylvania
Heart Transplant (Adult)
Heart Transplant (Pediatric)

Susan Firestone, M.D.
Associate Professor of Anesthesiology and Critical Care Medicine, University of Pittsburgh School of Medicine, Pittsburgh, Pennsylvania
Heart Transplant (Pediatric)

Stephen P. Fischer, M.D.
Assistant Professor of Anesthesiology, Stanford University School of Medicine, Stanford, California
Addison's Disease
Conn's Syndrome

Dennis M. Fisher, M.D.
Professor of Anesthesia and Pediatrics, University of California, San Francisco, School of Medicine, San Francisco, California
Edrophonium
Neostigmine

Lee A. Fleisher, M.D.
Assistant Professor, Department of Anesthesiology and Critical Care, Joint Appointment in Medicine (Cardiology), Johns Hopkins University School of Medicine, Baltimore, Maryland
Angina, Chronic Stable
Varicella Zoster
Radical Prostatectomy (Retropubic)
Splenectomy
Nitroglycerin
Dipyridamole Thallium Imaging

Pierre Foëx, M.D.
Nuffield Professor, Nuffield Department of Anaesthetics, University of Oxford, Radcliffe Infirmary, Oxford, England
Hypertension

Joseph Foss, M.D.
Assistant Professor, Department of Anesthesiology and Critical Care, The University of Chicago, Chicago, Illinois
Arteritis, Takayasu's
Cisplatin

James Foster, M.B.B.S., F.R.C.P.C.
Attending Physician, Department of Anesthesiology, State University of New York at Buffalo, Buffalo, New York
Rickettsial Diseases/Q Fever

Nancy K. France, M.D.
Associate Professor, Medical College of Wisconsin, Milwaukee, Wisconsin
Arnold-Chiari Syndrome

David Francisco, M.D.
Resident in Anesthesiology, University of Rochester School of Medicine and Dentistry, Rochester, New York
Thalassemia

Steven M. Frank, M.D.
Assistant Professor, Department of Anesthesiology and Critical Care Medicine, Johns Hopkins University School of Medicine, Baltimore, Maryland
Liver Resection

Edward J. Frink, Jr., M.D.
Associate Professor of Anesthesiology, The University of Arizona Health Sciences Center, Tucson, Arizona
Multiple Endocrine Neoplasia (MEN) Types I and II
Liver Function Tests

William Furman, M.D.
Associate Professor, Department of Anesthesia and Critical Care, The University of Chicago, Chicago, Illinois
Emphysema

Robert Gaiser, M.D.
Assistant Professor of Anesthesia, University of Pennsylvania School of Medicine, Philadelphia, Pennsylvania
Split-Thickness Skin Graft

T. James Gallagher, M.D.
Professor of Anesthesiology and Surgery and Chief of Critical Care Medicine, University of Florida College of Medicine, Gainesville, Florida
Respiratory Distress Syndrome

David R. Gambling, F.R.C.P.C.
Associate Clinical Professor of Anesthesiology, University of California, San Diego, School of Medicine, San Diego, California
Hypermagnesemia

Jeremy M. Geiduschek, M.D.
Assistant Professor, Department of Anesthesiology, University of Washington School of Medicine, Seattle, Washington
Kearns-Sayre Syndrome

Simon Gelman, M.D., Ph.D.
Leroy D. Vandam/Benjamin G. Covino Professor of Anaesthesia, Harvard Medical School, Boston, Massachusetts
Liver Transplantation

Ghaleb A. Ghani, M.D.
Associate Professor of Anesthesiology, Emory University School of Medicine, Atlanta, Georgia
Glomus Jugulare Tumors

Charles P. Gibbs, M.D.
Professor and Chair, Department of Anesthesiology, University of Colorado School of Medicine, Denver, Colorado
Abruptio Placentae

Kevin J. Gingrich, M.D.
Assistant Professor of Anesthesiology, Pharmacology, and Physiology, University of Rochester School of Medicine and Dentistry, Rochester, New York
Intracranial Hypertension (ICH)

D. David Glass, M.D.
Professor of Medicine and Anesthesiology, and Chair, Department of Anesthesiology, Dartmouth Medical School, Hanover, New Hampshire
Disseminated Intravascular Coagulation (DIC)

Stanley Glowacki, M.D.
Assistant Professor, Department of Anesthesiology, Medical College of Pennsylvania and Hahnemann University, Philadelphia, Pennsylvania
Advanced Cardiac Life Support (ACLS)

Barbara S. Gold, M.D.
Assistant Professor of Anesthesiology, University of Minnesota Medical School, Minneapolis, Minnesota
HIV Testing

Glenn S. Goldsher, M.D.
Anesthesiologist, Saint Francis Hospital of Evanston, Evanston, Illinois
Procaine (Novocain)

Randolph B. Gorman, M.D.
Staff Anesthesiologist, Greater Baltimore Medical Center, Towson, Maryland
Abdominoperineal Resection

Alexander W. Gotta, M.D.
Professor of Anesthesiology, State University of New York Health Science Center at Brooklyn, Brooklyn, New York
Trauma

Alexandru Gottlieb, M.D.
Associate Professor, Ohio State University College of Medicine, Columbus, Ohio
Bypass—Femoral-Femoral

Nishon G. Goudsouzian, M.D.
Associate Professor of Anaesthesia, Harvard Medical School, Boston, Massachusetts
Atropine

George Graf, M.D.
Clinical Assistant Professor, Department of Anesthesiology, University of California, Los Angeles, School of Medicine, Los Angeles, California
Diabetes Insipidus

Brent A. Graham, M.D.
Assistant Professor of Anesthesia and Critical Care, The University of Chicago, Chicago, Illinois
ECMO (Extracorporeal Membrane Oxygenation)

Gilbert J. Grant, M.D.
Assistant Professor of Anesthesiology, New York University School of Medicine, New York, New York
Tubal Ligation

Nikolaus Gravenstein, M.D.
Professor and Executive Associate Chairman, University of Florida College of Medicine, Gainesville, Florida
Diuretics

William J. Greeley, M.D.
Associate Professor of Anesthesiology and Pediatrics, Duke University Medical Center, Durham, North Carolina
Marfan's Syndrome
Total Anomalous Pulmonary Venous Return, Correction of

James A. Greenberg, M.D.
Assistant Professor of Anesthesiology and Pediatrics, University of Pittsburgh School of Medicine, Pittsburgh, Pennsylvania
Down Syndrome

George A. Gregory, M.D.
Professor of Anesthesia and Pediatrics, University of California, San Francisco, School of Medicine, San Francisco, California
Patent Ductus Arteriosus

Alan W. Grogono, M.D.
Chairman and Merryl and Sam Israel Professor, Department of Anesthesiology, Tulane University School of Medicine, New Orleans, Louisiana
Acidosis, Lactic/Metabolic

Brett B. Gutsche, M.D.
Professor of Anesthesia, Professor of Obstetrics and Gynecology, University of Pennsylvania Medical Center, Philadelphia, Pennsylvania
Magnesium Sulfate

J. Michael Haering, M.D.
Instructor in Anaesthesia, Harvard Medical School, Boston, Massachusetts
Cardiomyopathy, Hypertrophic (HCM)

Jonathan D. Halevy, M.D.
Attending Anesthesiologist, Wills Eye Hospital, Philadelphia, Pennsylvania
Burr Hole

Jesse Hall, M.D.
Professor of Medicine, Anesthesia, and Critical Care, The University of Chicago, Chicago, Illinois
Adult Respiratory Distress Syndrome (ARDS)
Asthma, Acute

Long K. Han, M.D.
Assistant Professor of Anesthesia and Critical Care, The University of Chicago, Chicago, Illinois
Atrial Septal Defect—Ostium Primum
Atrial Septal Defect—Ostium Secundum

Mark Hanna, M.D.
Physician, Department of Anesthesia and Critical Care, The University of Chicago, Chicago, Illinois
Diabetes, Type II

Raafat S. Hannallah, M.D.
Professor of Anesthesiology and Pediatrics, George Washington University Medical Center, Washington, D.C.
Anhidrosis (Congenital Anhidrotic Ectodermal Dysplasia)
Carnitine Deficiency

C. William Hanson III, M.D.
Assistant Professor of Anesthesia, Surgery, and Internal Medicine, University of Pennsylvania School of Medicine, Philadelphia, Pennsylvania
Bronchitis, Chronic

Charles Hantler, M.D.
Professor, University of Texas Health Science Center at San Antonio, San Antonio, Texas
Adrenal Insufficiency, Acute or Secondary

Andrew P. Harris, M.D., M.H.S.
Associate Professor, Department of Anesthesiology and Critical Care Medicine, Johns Hopkins University School of Medicine, Baltimore, Maryland
Cesarean Section, Planned

Stephen N. Harris, M.D.
Assistant Professor of Anesthesiology, Yale University School of Medicine, New Haven, Connecticut
Pericarditis, Constrictive

Martin Hautkappe, M.D.
Physician, Department of Anesthesiology, University of Munich, Munich, Germany
Capsaicin

John K. Hayes, Ph.D.
Research Assistant Professor, University of Utah College of Medicine, Salt Lake City, Utah
Hypernatremia
Hyponatremia

Stephen O. Heard, M.D.
Associate Professor of Anesthesiology and Surgery, University of Massachusetts Medical Center, Worcester, Massachusetts
TMJ Arthroscopy

James E. Heavner, D.V.M., Ph.D.
Professor, Anesthesiology and Physiology, Texas Tech University Health Sciences Center, Lubbock, Texas
Dibucaine Number

Eugenie Heitmiller, M.D.
Associate Professor, Department of Anesthesiology and Critical Care Medicine, Johns Hopkins University School of Medicine, Baltimore, Maryland
Patent Ductus Arteriosus, Ligation of

Mark Helfaer, M.D.
Associate Professor of Anesthesiology and Critical Care Medicine and Pediatrics, Johns Hopkins University School of Medicine, Baltimore, Maryland
Friedreich's Ataxia

Ian A. Herrick, M.D., F.R.C.P.C.
Associate Professor, Department of Anesthesia, University of Western Ontario, London, Ontario, Canada
Occlusive Cerebrovascular Disease

Michael S. Higgins, M.D.
Assistant Professor, Vanderbilt University School of Medicine, Nashville, Tennessee
Ileostomy

Roberta Hines, M.D.
Chairman and Professor of Anesthesia and Critical Care, Department of Anesthesia, Yale University School of Medicine, New Haven, Connecticut
Beta-Adrenergic Receptor Antagonists (Blockers)

Irving A. Hirsch, M.D.
Assistant Clinical Professor, Case Western Reserve University School of Medicine, Cleveland, Ohio
Hyperkalemia
Hypokalemia

Michael Ho, M.D.
Assistant Professor of Anesthesiology, Baylor University School of Medicine, Houston, Texas
Conversion Disorder
Schizophrenia

Charles W. Hogue, Jr., M.D.
Assistant Professor of Anesthesiology, Washington University School of Medicine, St. Louis, Missouri
Chagas' Disease
Atrial Septal Defect, Repair of

Kenneth J. Holroyd, M.D.
Assistant Professor of Anesthesiology, Johns Hopkins University School of Medicine, Baltimore, Maryland
Amyloidosis

William Hope, M.D., Ph.D.
Instructor of Anesthesiology, Medical College of Wisconsin, Milwaukee, Wisconsin
Familial Dysautonomia (Riley-Day Syndrome)

Phillippe Housmans, M.D.
Associate Professor of Anesthesiology, Mayo Medical School, Rochester, Minnesota
Procainamide

Wendy Howard, M.D.
Instructor, Department of Anesthesiology, State University of New York Health Science Center at Syracuse, Syracuse, New York
Burn Injury—Flame

Simon J. Howell, M.D.
Consultant, Nuffield Department of Anaesthetics, University of Oxford, Radcliffe Infirmary, Oxford, England
Hypertension

Michael B. Howie, M.D.
Professor and Vice Chair, Department of Anesthesiology, The Ohio State University Medical Center, Columbus, Ohio
Quinidine

John M. Huffman, M.D.
Assistant Professor of Anesthesiology, George Washington University Medical Center, Washington, D.C.
Drug Abuse—Lysergic Acid Diethylamide (LSD)

Cindy Hughes, M.D.
Associate Professor of Anesthesiology, Albany Medical College, Albany, New York
Ventricular Septal Defect, Repair of

Catherine Huraux, M.D.
Research Fellow, Emory University School of Medicine, Atlanta, Georgia
Anticoagulation, Preoperative

Fumito Ichinose, M.D.
Assistant Professor of Anesthesia, Tokyo Women's Medical College, Tokyo, Japan
Cholelithiasis

Lorna L. Im, M.D.
Physician, Department of Anesthesia and Critical Care, University of Chicago Hospitals, Chicago, Illinois
Trimethaphan

Shiroh Isono, M.D.
Assistant Professor, Department of Anesthesiology, Chiba University School of Medicine, Chiba, Japan
Swallowing Disorders

Eric Jacobsohn, M.B.Ch.B., F.R.C.P.C.
Assistant Professor of Anesthesia and Critical Care, The University of Chicago, Chicago, Illinois
Ephedrine
Epinephrine
Isoproterenol (Isuprel)
Lithium Carbonate

Subhash Jain, M.D.
Associate Professor of Anesthesiology, Cornell University Medical Center, New York, New York
Leukemia

Uday Jain, M.D., Ph.D.
Assistant Professor of Anesthesia, University of California, San Francisco, School of Medicine, San Francisco, California
Hypercholesterolism
Hypertriglyceridemia
Lipidemias

Karen Jaranowski, M.D.
Department of Anesthesiology, University of Rochester Medical Center, Rochester, New York
Strabismus Surgery

Roger A. Johns, M.D.
Professor of Anesthesiology, University of Virginia School of Medicine, Charlottesville, Virginia
Bretylium Tosylate

Madelyn Kahana, M.D.
Associate Professor, Department of Anesthesia and Critical Care Medicine and Department of Pediatrics, The University of Chicago, Chicago, Illinois
Meningomyelocele Repair
Spinal Fusion

Zeev N. Kain, M.D.
Assistant Professor of Anesthesiology and Pediatrics, Yale University School of Medicine, New Haven, Connecticut
Neurofibromatosis
Cocaine

Surinder K. Kaller, M.D.
Professor, Medical College of Virginia/Virginia Commonwealth University, Richmond, Virginia
Inguinal Herniorrhaphy

Helen W. Karl, M.D.
Associate Professor, Department of Anesthesiology, University of Washington School of Medicine, Seattle, Washington
Tonsillectomy and Adenoidectomy

Jeffrey Katz, M.D.
Professor and Chairman, Department of Anesthesiology, The University of Texas Medical School, Houston, Texas
Encephalopathy, Hypertensive

Jeffrey A. Katz, M.D.
Professor of Clinical Anesthesia, University of California, San Francisco, School of Medicine, San Francisco, California
Candidiasis
Pemphigus

Shubjeet Kaur, M.D.
Assistant Professor of Anesthesiology, University of Massachusetts Medical Center, Worcester, Massachusetts
Cromolyn Sodium

Nancy B. Kenepp, M.D.
Associate Professor of Anesthesiology, Temple University School of Medicine, Philadelphia, Pennsylvania
Epidermolysis Bullosa

Mary A. Keyes, M.D.
Associate Professor of Clinical Anesthesia, University of California, Los Angeles, School of Medicine, Los Angeles, California
Anemia of Infancy
Bronchopulmonary Dysplasia (BPD)
Reye's Syndrome

Woo Chan Kim, M.D.
Physician, Department of Anesthesia and Critical Care, The University of Chicago, Chicago, Illinois
Herpes—Type II

Jerome M. Klafta, M.D.
Assistant Professor, Department of Anesthesia and Critical Care, The University of Chicago Pritzker School of Medicine, Chicago, Illinois
Blebs and Bullae

P. Allan Klock, Jr., M.D.
Assistant Professor, Department of Anesthesia and Critical Care, The University of Chicago, Chicago, Illinois
Amniotic Fluid Embolism
Terbutaline

Arthur J. Klowden, M.D.
Assistant Professor, Rush Medical College of Rush University, Chicago, Illinois
Myotonia Dystrophica (Myotonic Dystrophy, Steinert's Disease)

Paul R. Knight III, M.D., Ph.D.
Professor and Chairman, Department of Anesthesiology, State University of New York at Buffalo, Buffalo, New York
IgA Deficiency
Immune Suppression
Rickettsial Diseases/Q Fever
Rocky Mountain Spotted Fever

Donald D. Koblin, M.D., Ph.D.
Professor of Anesthesia, University of California, San Francisco, School of Medicine, San Francisco, California
Vitamin B$_{12}$/Folate Deficiency
Fluoxetine (Prozac)
Haloperidol (Haldol)

W. Andrew Kofke, M.D.
Professor, Departments of Anesthesiology and Critical Care Medicine and Neurological Surgery, University of Pittsburgh, Pittsburgh, Pennsylvania
Seizures—Epilepsy

Anne C. Kolker, M.D.
Assistant Professor, Department of Anesthesiology, Cornell University Medical College, New York, New York
Esophageal Cancer

Vincent J. Kopp, M.D., F.A.A.P.
Assistant Professor of Anesthesiology and Pediatrics, Adjunct Assistant Professor of Social Medicine, University of North Carolina at Chapel Hill School of Medicine, Chapel Hill, North Carolina
Pertussis (Whooping Cough)

Ronald P. Kufner, M.D.
Instructor, Department of Anesthesiology, Mayo Medical School, Rochester, Minnesota
Subphrenic Abscess

Vandana Kulkarni, M.D.
Assistant Professor of Anesthesia and Critical Care, The University of Chicago, Chicago, Illinois
Phenytoin

C. Dean Kurth, M.D.
Assistant Professor, Departments of Anesthesia, Pediatrics, and Physiology, University of Pennsylvania School of Medicine, Philadelphia, Pennsylvania
Cleft Palate Repair

Carol L. Lake, M.D.
Professor of Anesthesiology, University of California, Davis, School of Medicine, Davis, California
Double Aortic Arch
Endocardial Cushion Defect

George Lampe, M.D.
Staff Physician, Good Samaritan Hospital, San Jose, California
Cushing's Syndrome

Ira S. Landsman, M.D.
Assistant Professor of Anesthesiology and Critical Care Medicine and Pediatrics, University of Pittsburgh School of Medicine, Pittsburgh, Pennsylvania
Acetaminophen

William L. Lanier, M.D.
Professor of Anesthesiology, Mayo Clinic and Mayo Medical School, Rochester, Minnesota
Hyperglycemia

Lawrence O. Larson, M.D.
Assistant Professor of Anesthesiology, Wayne Sate University School of Medicine, Detroit, Michigan
Lesch-Nyhan Syndrome

Jonathan G. Latour, M.D.
Assistant Professor, Department of Anesthesiology, University of Missouri School of Medicine, Columbia, Missouri
Aortic Valve Replacement

John P. Lawrence, M.D.
Physician, Department of Anesthesia and Critical Care, The University of Chicago, Chicago, Illinois
Folic Acid

David Eric Lees, M.D.
Professor and Chairman, Department of Anesthesia, Georgetown University Medical Center, Washington, D.C.
Dementia
Do Not Resuscitate (DNR) Orders

George S. Leisure, M.D.
Assistant Professor of Anesthesiology, University of Virginia Health Sciences Center, Charlottesville, Virginia
Bleomycin Sulfate Toxicity
Bretylium Tosylate

William A. Lell, M.D.
Professor of Anesthesiology, Division of Cardiothoracic Anesthesia, The University of Alabama at Birmingham School of Medicine, Birmingham, Alabama
Bronchiolitis Obliterans

Mark J. Lema, M.D., Ph.D.
Associate Professor and Vice Chairman for Academic Affairs, Department of Anesthesiology, State University of New York at Buffalo, School of Medicine and Biomedical Sciences, Buffalo, New York
Alkylating Agents
Bleomycin

Harry J.M. Lemmers, M.D.
Assistant Professor of Anesthesia, Stanford University School of Medicine, Stanford, California
Benzodiazepines (Midazolam, Lorazepam, Diazepam)

W. Casey Lenox, M.D.
Assistant Professor, Johns Hopkins University School of Medicine, Baltimore, Maryland
Orchiopexy

Jacqueline M. Leung, M.D.
Associate Professor of Anesthesia, University of California, San Francisco, School of Medicine, San Francisco, California
Atherosclerotic Disease
Peripheral Vascular Disease

Jerrold H. Levy, M.D.
Professor of Anesthesiology, Emory University School of Medicine, Atlanta, Georgia
Allergy
Anticoagulation, Preoperative

Lance Lichtor, M.D.
Professor and Associate Chair, Department of Anesthesia and Critical Care, and Professor of Pediatrics, The University of Chicago, Chicago, Illinois
Pyloric Stenosis Repair

Kevin C. Limp, M.D.
Assistant Professor, Department of Anesthesiology and Critical Care Medicine, Johns Hopkins University School of Medicine, Baltimore, Maryland
Colostomy

Karen S. Lindeman, M.D.
Associate Professor, Department of Anesthesia and Critical Care Medicine, Johns Hopkins University School of Medicine, Baltimore, Maryland
Placenta Previa

Ronald S. Litman, D.O.
Assistant Professor of Anesthesiology and Pediatrics, University of Rochester School of Medicine and Dentistry, Rochester, New York
Klippel-Feil Syndrome
Thalassemia
Strabismus Surgery
Testicular Torsion Surgery

Maywin Liu, M.D.
Assistant Professor, Department of Anesthesia, University of Pennsylvania School of Medicine, Philadelphia, Pennsylvania
Autonomic Hyperreflexia

Terrence H. Liu, M.D.
Research Fellow, Critical Care Department of Surgery, University of Minnesota Hospitals and Clinics, Minneapolis, Minnesota
Nutritional Support

Wen Shin Liu, M.D.
Professor of Anesthesiology, Northeastern Ohio Universities College of Medicine, Rootstown, Ohio
Prostate Cancer

Aaron Lloyd, M.D.
Resident, Department of Anesthesiology, Johns Hopkins University School of Medicine, Baltimore, Maryland
Ventriculoperitoneal Shunt

Martin J. London, M.D.
Associate Professor of Anesthesiology, University of Colorado Health Sciences Center, Denver, Colorado
Diagnostic 12-Lead ECG

Sandra V. Lowe, M.D.
Assistant Professor of Anesthesiology and Pediadrics, Department of Pediatric Critical Care and Anesthesiology, Vanderbilt University School of Medicine, Nashville, Tennessee
Achondroplasia—Dwarfism

Edward Lowenstein, M.D.
Professor of Anaesthesia, Harvard Medical School, Boston, Massachusetts
Cardiomyopathy, Hypertrophic (HCM)

Jeffrey K. Lu, M.D.
Assistant Professor, University of Utah Medical School, Salt Lake City, Utah
Phenothiazines

Phil D. Lumb, M.D.
Professor and Chair, Department of Anesthesiology, Albany Medical College, Albany, New York
Lyme Disease

Carl Lynch III, M.D., Ph.D.
Professor of Anesthesiology, University of Virginia Medical Center, Charlottesville, Virginia
Bleomycin Sulfate Toxicity
Pacemaker Implantation for Sick Sinus Syndrome

Anne Marie Lynn, M.D.
Professor, Anesthesiology and Pediatrics, University of Washington School of Medicine, Seattle, Washington
Jeune Syndrome (Asphyxiating Thoracic Dystrophy)

Tesuji Makita, M.D.
Research Fellow, Emory University School of Medicine, Atlanta, Georgia
Allergy

Vinod Malhotra, M.D.
Associate Professor, Department of Anesthesiology, Cornell University Medical College, New York, New York
Nephrectomy / Radical Nephrectomy

Andrew M. Malinow, M.D.
Associate Professor of Anesthesiology, University of Maryland School of Medicine, Baltimore, Maryland
Preeclampsia

Dennis Mangano, M.D., Ph.D.
Professor, University of California, San Francisco, School of Medicine, San Francisco, California
Myocardial Ischemia (MIsch)

Srinivas Mantha, M.D.
Associate Professor, Nizam's Institute of Medical Sciences, Hyderabad, India
Hyperparathyroidism
Malnutrition

Jonathan B. Mark, M.D.
Associate Professor of Anesthesiology and Assistant Professor of Medicine, Duke University Medical Center, Durham, North Carolina
Cardiomyopathy, Alcoholic
Cardiomyopathy, Ischemic

H. Michael Marsh, M.B.
Chair, Department of Anesthesiology, Henry Ford Hospital, Detroit, Michigan
Bronchiectasis
Methemoglobinemia

Jackie Martin, M.D.
Associate Professor, Johns Hopkins University School of Medicine, Baltimore, Maryland
Subclavian Steal Syndrome

J.A. Jeevendra Martyn, M.D.
Professor, Harvard Medical School, Boston, Massachusetts
Burn Injury—Electrical
Sulfonamides

Douglas Martz, M.D.
Assistant Professor of Anesthesiology, University of Maryland Hospital, Baltimore, Maryland
Narcolepsy

Gertie F. Marx, M.D.
Professor, Albert Einstein College of Medicine, Bronx, New York
Cesarean Section—Emergent

M. Jane Matjasko, M.D.
Professor and Chair, Department of Anesthesiology, University of Maryland School of Medicine, Baltimore, Maryland
Encephalitis

Richard S. Matteo, M.D.
Professor of Clinical Anesthesiology, Columbia University College of Physicians and Surgeons, New York, New York
Dimethyltubocurarine (d-Tubocurarine, dTc)

John P. McCarren, M.D.
Clinical Associate Professor of Anesthesia, University of California, San Diego, Hospital and Medical Center, La Jolla, California
Cancer—Bronchial

William A. McDade, M.D.
Assistant Professor, Department of Anesthesia and Critical Care, The University of Chicago, Chicago, Illinois
Sickle Cell Disease

Kathryn E. McGoldrick, M.D.
Professor of Anesthesiology, Yale University School of Medicine, New Haven, Connecticut
Blowout Orbital Fracture
Cataract ± IOL

Brian J. McGrath, M.D.
Associate Professor of Anesthesiology, University of Maryland, Baltimore, Maryland
Fat Embolism

Charles H. McLeskey, M.D.
Professor and Chairman, Department of Anesthesiology, Texas A&M University Health Science Center, Temple, Texas
Geriatric Surgery

Thomas M. McLoughlin, Jr., M.D.
Assistant Professor of Anesthesiology, Uniformed Services University of the Health Sciences, Bethesda, Maryland
Coagulopathy—Factor IX Deficiency
Von Willebrand's Disease

Robert McPherson, M.D.
Associate Professor, Department of Anesthesiology and Critical Care Medicine, The Johns Hopkins Medical Institute, Baltimore, Maryland
Craniotomy

William L. Meadow, M.D.
Associate Professor, Department of Pediatrics, The University of Chicago, Chicago, Illinois
Apnea of the Newborn

Robert G. Merin, M.D.
Professor of Anesthesiology, Medical College of Georgia School of Medicine, Augusta, Georgia
Coronary Artery Spasm (CAS)
Digitalis

William T. Merritt, M.D.
Associate Professor, Division of Critical Care Anesthesia, Johns Hopkins University School of Medicine, Baltimore, Maryland
Jaundice

Scott Metzger, M.D.
Fellow, Department of Pain Medicine, Johns Hopkins University of Medicine, Baltimore, Maryland
Alcohol Abuse

Leslie Newberg Milde, M.D.
Professor of Anesthesiology, Mayo Medical School, Rochester, Minnesota
Carbamazepine

Edward D. Miller, Jr., M.D.
Professor and Chairman, Department of Anesthesiology, Johns Hopkins University School of Medicine, Baltimore, Maryland
Hypertension, Uncontrolled, with Cardiomyopathy

Ronald Miller, M.D.
Professor and Chairman, Department of Anesthesia, University of California, San Francisco, School of Medicine, San Francisco, California
Vecuronium

Marek A. Mirski, M.D., Ph.D.
Associate Professor of Surgery and Medicine, University of Hawaii John A. Burns School of Medicine, Honolulu, Hawaii
Seizures—Grand Mal (Tonic-Clonic)
Seizures—Petit Mal Absence

Scott Mittman, M.D., Ph.D.
Assistant Professor, Department of Anesthesiology and Critical Care Medicine, Johns Hopkins University School of Medicine, Baltimore, Maryland
Carpal Tunnel Syndrome

Terri G. Monk, M.D.
Associate Professor, Department of Anesthesiology, Washington University School of Medicine, St. Louis, Missouri
Urinary Lithiasis

Richard E. Moon, M.D.
Associate Professor of Anesthesiology, Duke University Medical Center, Durham, North Carolina
Gas Embolism
Carbon Monoxide (CO) Poisoning

Laurel E. Moore, M.D.
Assistant Professor, Department of Anesthesiology, Johns Hopkins University School of Medicine, Baltimore, Maryland
Anterior Cervical Fusion
Electroconvulsive Therapy (ECT)

Roger A. Moore, M.D.
Associate Professor, University of Pennsylvania School of Medicine, Philadelphia, Pennsylvania
Anomalous Pulmonary Venous Drainage
Cancer—Lung Parenchyma

Jeffrey P. Morray, M.D.
Professor of Anesthesiology and Pediatrics, University of Washington School of Medicine, Seattle, Washington
Truncus Arteriosus

Jonathan Moss, M.D., Ph.D.
Professor and Vice Chairman for Research, Department of Anesthesia and Critical Care, The University of Chicago, Chicago, Illinois
Anaphylaxis
Syndrome X

John R. Moyers, M.D.
Professor, Department of Anesthesia, University of Iowa College of Medicine, Iowa City, Iowa
Mesothelioma

Robert A. Mueller, M.D., Ph.D.
Professor of Anesthesiology and Pharmacology, University of North Carolina at Chapel Hill School of Medicine, Chapel Hill, North Carolina
Amphetamines

Jesse J. Muir, M.D.
Assistant Professor of Anesthesia, Mayo Clinic—Scottsdale, Scottsdale, Arizona
Insulinoma

John M. Murkin, M.D.
Professor of Anaesthesia, University of Western Ontario, London, Ontario, Canada
Thyroid Supplements

Michael L. Nahrwold, M.D.
Professor of Anesthesiology, Indiana University School of Medicine, Indianapolis, Indiana
Hyperparathyroidism

Rosa M. Navarro, M.D.
Physician, Department of Anesthesia and Critical Care, The University of Chicago, Chicago, Illinois
Herpes—Type II

Stephen P. Nebbia, M.D.
Clinical Assistant Professor of Anesthesiology, State University of New York at Buffalo, Buffalo, New York
Sarcoma

Philippa Newfield, M.D.
Attending Anesthesiologist, California Pacific Medical Center, San Francisco, California
Syndrome of Inappropriate Antidiuretic Hormone Secretion (SIADH)

Susan Craig Nicolson, M.D.
Associate Professor of Anesthesia, University of Pennsylvania School of Medicine, Philadelphia, Pennsylvania
Tricuspid Atresia

Joan M. Niehoff, M.D.
Instructor, Washington University School of Medicine, St. Louis, Missouri
Diaphragmatic Hernia (Congenital)

Dolores Njoku, M.D.
Instructor, Department of Anesthesiology and Critical Care Medicine, Johns Hopkins University School of Medicine, Baltimore, Maryland
Subclavian Steal Syndrome

Mary J. Njoku, M.D.
Assistant Professor of Anesthesiology and Critical Care, University of Maryland School of Medicine, Baltimore, Maryland
Encephalitis

Edward Norris, M.D.
Assistant Professor, Department of Anesthesiology and Critical Care Medicine, Johns Hopkins University School of Medicine, Baltimore, Maryland
Whipple Procedure

Mark C. Norris, M.D.
Professor of Anesthesiology, Jefferson Medical College, Thomas Jefferson University, Philadelphia, Pennsylvania
Retained Placenta, Removal of

Michael Nugent, M.D.
Professor and Chairman, Department of Anesthesiology, Medical College of Ohio, Toledo, Ohio
Coarctation of the Aorta

Ramon Nunez-Hernandez, M.D.
Assistant Professor, Department of Anesthesia and Critical Care, The University of Chicago Hospitals, Chicago, Illinois
Alpha$_2$-Adrenergic Agonists

Daniel Nyhan, M.D.
Associate Professor of Anesthesiology, Johns Hopkins University School of Medicine, Baltimore, Maryland
Single (Including Common) Ventricle

Dorene A. O'Hara, M.D., M.S.E.
Assistant Professor of Anesthesia and Director of Research, Robert Wood Johnson Medical School, New Brunswick, New Jersey
Transurethral Resection of Prostate

Irene B. Ottara, M.D.
Lecturer, Department of Anesthesia, University of Pennyslvania School of Medicine, Philadelphia, Pennsylvania
Transposition of the Great Vessels (TGV), Repair of

David Olson, M.D.
Physician, Pulmonary and Critical Care, The University of Chicago, Chicago, Illinois
Adult Respiratory Distress Syndrome (ARDS)

Nancy E. Oriol, M.D.
Assistant Professor, Harvard Medical School, Boston, Massachusetts
Vaginal Delivery, Normal

Maureen M. O'Rourke, M.D.
Assistant Professor, University of Pennsylvania School of Medicine, Philadelphia, Pennsylvania
Botulism
Kartagener's Syndrome

Andreas M. Ostermeier, M.D.
Physician, Department of Anesthesiology, University of Munich, Munich, Germany
Sleep Apnea, Central and Mixed

Andranik Ovassapian, M.D.
Professor of Anesthesiology, Northwestern University Medical School, Chicago, Illinois
Bronchoscopy, Fiberoptic
Bronchoscopy, Rigid
Laryngoscopy

Kent Ozkum, M.D.
Staff Anesthesiologist, Providence Hospital, Washington, D.C.
Monoamine Oxidase Inhibitors; Reversible Inhibitors of Monoamine Oxidase

Richard J. Palahniuk, M.D.
Professor and Head, Department of Anesthesiology, University of Minnesota, Minneapolis, Minnesota
Anemia—Hemolytic
Pregnancy, Intra-abdominal

Susan K. Palmer, M.D.
Professor of Anesthesiology, University of Colorado School of Medicine, Denver, Colorado
Pregnancy-Induced Hypertension

Barbara Palmisano, M.D.
Associate Professor of Clinical Anesthesiology and Pediatrics, Medical College of Wisconsin, Milwaukee, Wisconsin
Cri du Chat Syndrome (5p– Syndrome)

Sally C. Palmon, M.D.
Instructor, Johns Hopkins Hospital, Baltimore, Maryland
Lumbar Laminectomy

Robert K. Parker, D.O.
Assistant Professor of Anesthesiology, Obstetrics, and Gynecology, Tufts University School of Medicine, Boston, Massachusetts
Hysterectomy, Vaginal

Jonathan L. Parmet, M.D.
Assistant Professor of Anesthesiology, Medical College of Pennsylvania/Hahnemann University, Philadelphia, Pennsylvania
Joint Replacement Cementing (Methylmethacrylate Cementing)

L. Reuven Pasternack, M.D., M.P.H.
Associate Professor of Anesthesiology, Johns Hopkins University School of Medicine, Baltimore, Maryland
Chest X-ray

Todd Patterson, D.O.
Assistant Professor, Department of Anesthesia and Critical Care, The University of Chicago, Chicago, Illinois
Protamine

Ronald W. Pauldine, M.D.
Baltimore, Maryland
Esophagectomy

Carlos V. Paya, M.D., Ph.D.
Associate Professor of Medicine, Mayo Clinic and Foundation, Rochester, Minnesota
Cytomegalovirus Infection

Ronald G. Pearl, M.D., Ph.D.
Associate Professor, Stanford University School of Medicine, Stanford, California
Pulmonary Embolism

Michael Peck, M.D.
Department of Anesthesiology, George Washington University Medical Center, Washington, D.C.
Endoscopic Sinus Surgery (ESS)

Azriel Perel, M.D.
Chairman and Associate Professor, Department of Anesthesia and Intensive Care, Sackler School of Medicine, Tel Aviv University, Tel Aviv, Israel
Mastocytosis

Edelberto Perez, M.D.
Assistant Professor, Rush Medical College of Rush University, Chicago, Illinois
Ventricular Tachycardia
Phenylephrine (Neo-Synephrine)

Charise T. Petrovitch, M.D.
Chair and Director, Department of Anesthesia, Providence Hospital, Washington, D.C.
Warfarin (Coumadin)

Patricia H. Petrozza, M.D.
Associate Professor, The Department of Anesthesia, Bowman Gray School of Medicine of Wake Forest University, Winston-Salem, North Carolina
Brain Cortex Resection (for Epilepsy)

Beverly K. Philip, M.D.
Associate Professor of Anaesthesia, Harvard Medical School, Boston, Massachusetts
Lidocaine

Rose Marie Phillip, M.D.
Instructor in Anesthesiology, State University of New York Health Sciences Center at Brooklyn College of Medicine, Brooklyn, New York
Pregnancy Testing

Evan G. Pivalizza, M.D.
Assistant Professor, Department of Anesthesiology, University of Texas Medical School at Houston, Houston, Texas
Purpura, Immune Thrombocytopenic (ITP)
Purpura, Thrombotic Thrombocytopenic (TTP)

Susan L. Polk, M.D., M.S.Ed.
Associate Professor of Clinical Anesthesia and Critical Care, Associate Chair for Education, The University of Chicago, Chicago, Illinois
Morbid Obesity
Pickwickian Syndrome

Kamla K. Prasad, M.D.
Attending Anesthesiologist, Fair Oaks Hospital, Fairfax, Virginia
Hereditary Hemorrhagic Telangiectasia (Osler-Weber-Rendu Disease)
Multiple Myeloma
Waldenström's Macroglobulinemia

Margaret G. Pratila, M.D.
Associate Professor of Clinical Anesthesiology, Cornell University Medical College, New York, New York
Chemotherapeutic Agents

Vasilios Pratilas, M.D.
Associate Professor of Clinical Anesthesiology, Mount Sinai School of Medicine of the City University of New York, New York, New York
Chemotherapeutic Agents

Hugh L. Preas II, M.D.
Clinical Instructor of Anesthesiology, University of Maryland School of Medicine, Baltimore, Maryland
Histiocytosis

Johnathan L. Pregler, M.D.
Assistant Clinical Professor, Department of Anesthesiology, University of California, Los Angeles, School of Medicine, Los Angeles, California
Hepatitis, Alcoholic
Hypopituitarism
Rifampin

Richard C. Prielipp, M.D.
Associate Professor, Department of Anesthesia and Critical Care Medicine, The Bowman Gray School of Medicine of Wake Forest University, Winston-Salem, North Carolina
Dopamine

Donald S. Prough, M.D.
Professor and Chairman, Department of Anesthesiology, The University of Texas Medical Branch, Galveston, Texas
Renal Failure, Chronic

Khether E. Raby, M.D.
Assistant Professor of Clinical Medicine, Boston University School of Medicine, Boston, Massachusetts
Holter Monitoring for Silent Ischemia

G.B. Racz, M.D.
Professor and Chairman, Department of Anesthesiology, Texas Tech University Health Sciences Center, Lubbock, Texas
Headache—Migraine

Bronwyn R. Rae, M.B., F.A.N.C.Z.A.
Instructor in Anesthesia, Northwestern University Medical School, Chicago, Illinois
Congenital Methemoglobinemia

Chandra Ramamoorthy, F.F.A.R.C.S.
Assistant Professor, Department of Anesthesiology, University of Washington School of Medicine, Seattle, Washington
Truncus Arteriosus

Sivam Ramanathan, M.D.
Professor of Anesthesiology and Critical Care Medicine, University of Pittsburgh School of Medicine, Pittsburgh, Pennsylvania
Labor—Peripheral Blocks

Ira J. Rampil, M.D.
Associate Professor of Anesthesia, University of California, San Francisco, School of Medicine, San Francisco, California
Pituitary Tumors
Laser Surgery of Airway

James G. Ramsay, M.D.
Associate Professor of Anesthesiology, Emory University School of Medicine, Atlanta, Georgia
Aortic Valve Replacement

P.D. Randolph, Ph.D.
Clinical Assistant Professor, Department of Anesthesiology, Texas Tech University Health Sciences Center, Lubbock, Texas
Headache—Migraine

Earl S. Ransom, M.D.
Assistant Professor of Anesthesiology, University of North Carolina at Chapel Hill School of Medicine, Chapel Hill, North Carolina
Amphetamines

Russell C. Raphaely, M.D.
Professor of Anesthesia and Pediatrics, University of Pennsylvania School of Medicine, Philadelphia, Pennsylvania
Botulism
Kartagener's Syndrome

Athos J. Rassias, M.D.
Assistant Professor of Anesthesiology, Dartmouth Medical School, Hanover, New Hampshire
Disseminated Intravascular Coagulation (DIC)

David L. Reich, M.D.
Associate Professor of Anesthesiology, Mt. Sinai School of Medicine of the City University of New York, New York, New York
Ventricular Septal Defect, Congenital
Ventricular Septal Rupture (Defect) Post Myocardial Infarction

Laurence S. Reisner, M.D.
Professor and Acting Chair, Department of Anesthesiology, University of California Medical Center, San Diego, California
Bupivacaine

J.G. Reves, M.D.
Professor and Chairman, Department of Anesthesiology, and Director, The Duke Heart Center, Duke University Medical Center, Durham, North Carolina
Coronary Artery Disease (Left Main and Non–Left Main Disease)

Christine Rinder, M.D.
Associate Professor of Anesthesiology and Laboratory Medicine, Yale University School of Medicine, New Haven, Connecticut
Complement Deficiency
Transfusion-Related Acute Lung Injury

Brian J. Robinson, Ph.D.
Post-doctoral Fellow, Medical College of Wisconsin, Milwaukee, Wisconsin
Autonomic Function

David M. Robinson, M.D.
Assistant Professor, Department of Anesthesiology, Medical College of Pennsylvania and Hahnemann University, Philadelphia, Pennsylvania
Systemic Lupus Erythematosus

Peter Rock, M.D.
Professor of Anesthesiology, Medicine, and Surgery, Washington University School of Medicine, St. Louis, Missouri
Flow-Volume Loops
Spirometry

Michael F. Roizen, M.D.
Professor and Chair, Department of Anesthesia and Critical Care, Professor of Medicine, The University of Chicago, Chicago, Illinois
Diabetes, Type I (Insulin Requiring)
Diabetes, Type II
Hyperthyroidism
Myocardial Ischemia (MIsch)
Pheochromocytoma
Sickle Cell Trait
Sleep Apnea, Central and Mixed
Sleep Apnea, Obstructive
Adrenalectomy for Pheochromocytoma
Thyroidectomy for Hyperthyroidism
Total Hip Arthroplasty
Cimetidine
Phenoxybenzamine
Propylthiouracil—Antithyroid Drugs

Duane K. Rorie, M.D.
Professor and Chair, Department of Anesthesiology, Mayo Medical School, Rochester, Minnesota
Subphrenic Abscess

Joseph Rosa III, M.D.
Assistant Clinical Professor of Anesthesiology, University of California, Los Angeles, School of Medicine, Los Angeles, California
Ectopic Pregnancy
Appendectomy

Robert J. Rose, M.D.
Associate Professor of Anesthesiology, Dartmouth Medical School, Hanover, New Hampshire
Bulimia

David A. Rosen, M.D.
Professor of Anesthesia and Pediatrics, West Virginia University School of Medicine, Morgantown, West Virginia
Intestinal Obstruction
Intussuscepted Bowel Repair

Kathleen R. Rosen, M.D.
Associate Professor of Anesthesia and Pediatrics, West Virginia University School of Medicine, Morgantown, West Virginia
Intestinal Obstruction
Intussuscepted Bowel Repair

Michael Rosen, F.R.C.A., C.B.E.
Formerly, Professor in Anesthetics, University of Wales College of Medicine, Cardiff, Wales
Constipation

Stanley H. Rosenbaum, M.D.
Professor of Anesthesiology, Medicine, and Surgery, Yale University School of Medicine, New Haven, Connecticut
Carcinoid Syndrome

Andrew D. Rosenberg, M.D.
Clinical Instructor, Department of Anesthesiology, New York University School of Medicine, New York, New York
Cervical Disk Disease (Cervical Spine Disease)
Sarcoidosis

Andrew L. Rosenberg, M.D.
Department of Anesthesiology and Critical Care Medicine, George Washington University School of Medicine and Health Sciences, Washington, D.C.
Myocardial Contusion

Henry Rosenberg, M.D.
Professor and Chairman, Department of Anesthesiology, Medical College of Pennsylvania and Hahnemann University, Philadelphia, Pennsylvania
Malignant Hyperthermia and Other Anesthetic-Induced Myodystrophies (AIMs)

Jeffrey Rosenberg, M.D., Ph.D.
Assistant Professor, Department of Anesthesiology and Critical Care Medicine, Johns Hopkins University School of Medicine, Baltimore, Maryland
Mediastinal Masses

Meg A. Rosenblatt, M.D.
Assistant Professor, Department of Anesthesiology, The Mount Sinai School of Medicine of the City University of New York, New York, New York
Jehovah's Witness Patient

William H. Rosenblatt, M.D.
Assistant Professor of Anesthesiology, Yale University School of Medicine, New Haven, Connecticut
Bladder Cancer

Myer H. Rosenthal, M.D.
Professor of Anesthesia, Stanford University School of Medicine, Stanford, California
Septic Hyperdynamic Shock; Systemic Inflammatory Response Syndrome (SIRS)

Steven Roth, M.D.
Associate Professor, Department of Anesthesia and Critical Care, The University of Chicago, Chicago, Illinois
Postoperative Encephalopathy—Metabolic
OKT3 (Muromonab-CD3)

Judith Ruiz-Lachica, M.D.
Department of Anesthesia, The University of Chicago, Chicago, Illinois
Uterine Rupture

Winnie Y. Ruo, M.D.
Assistant Professor, Department of Anesthesia and Critical Care, The University of Chicago, Chicago, Illinois
Drug Overdose—Propylene Glycol
Tetralogy of Fallot

Stephen M. Rupp, M.D.
Associate Clinical Professor, University of Washington School of Medicine, Seattle, Washington
Pituitary Resection—Transsphenoidal Approach
Metocurine Iodide (Metubine)
Pancuronium Bromide

Renata Rusa, M.D.
Neuroanesthesia Fellow, Johns Hopkins University School of Medicine, Baltimore, Maryland
Cerebrovascular Transient Ischemic Attack (TIA)

Garfield B. Russell, M.D.
Associate Professor, Department of Anesthesia, The Pennsylvania State University College of Medicine, Hershey, Pennsylvania
Herniated Nucleus Pulposus

W. John Russell, M.D.
Associate Professor, University of Adelaide, Adelaide, South Australia, Australia
Familial Periodic Paralysis (Hyperkalemic)
Familial Periodic Paralysis (Hypokalemic)

Thomas Ryan, M.D.
Director of Echocardiography, Duke University Medical Center, Durham, North Carolina
Dobutamine Stress Echocardiography

Lloyd R. Saberski, M.D.
Associate Professor of Anesthesiology, Yale University School of Medicine, New Haven, Connecticut
Reflex Sympathetic Dystrophy (Complex Peripheral Pain Syndrome)

M. Ramez Salem, M.D.
Chairman, Department of Anesthesiology, Illinois Masonic Medical Center, Chicago, Illinois
Bilirubinemia of the Newborn

Mukesh C. Sama, M.D.
Instructor in Anesthesia, Harvard Medical School, Boston, Massachusetts
Vaginal Delivery, Normal

Kevin V. Sanborn, M.D.
Associate Professor of Clinical Anesthesiology, Columbia University College of Physicians and Surgeons, New York, New York
ORIF of Hip

Ted J. Sanford, Jr., M.D.
Associate Chair for Education and Clinical Professor of Anesthesiology, The University of Michigan Medical School, Ann Arbor, Michigan
Hypoxemia

John J. Savanese, M.D.
Professor and Chair of Anesthesiology, Cornell University Medical College, New York, New York
Atracurium (Tracrium)
Cis-Atracurium (Nimbex [51W89]; Cis-Atracurium Besylate)
Mivacurium

Paul D. Schanbacher, M.D.
Department of Anesthesiology, Illinois Masonic Medical Center, Chicago, Illinois
Bilirubinemia of the Newborn

Randall M. Schell, M.D.
Assistant Professor of Anesthesiology, Loma Linda University School of Medicine, Loma Linda, California
Carotid Sinus Syndrome (CSS)

Armin Schubert, M.D.
Associate Professor, The Cleveland Clinic Health Sciences Campus of Ohio State University, Cleveland, Ohio
Multiple Sclerosis
Cerebral AVM Repair

Scott R. Schulman, M.D.
Assistant Professor of Anesthesiology and Pediatrics, Division of Pediatric Anesthesia and Critical Care Medicine, Duke University Medical Center, Durham, North Carolina
Marfan's Syndrome

Alan Jay Schwartz, M.D., M.S. Ed.
Professor of Anesthesiology and Pharmacology, Medical College of Pennsylvania and Hahnemann University, Philadelphia, Pennsylvania
Advanced Cardiac Life Support (ACLS)
Transposition of Great Vessels (TGV), Repair of

Jeffrey J. Schwartz, M.D.
Associate Clinical Professor, Department of Anesthesiology, Yale University School of Medicine, New Haven, Connecticut
Pancreatitis, Acute
Pancreatitis, Chronic

John F. Schweiss, M.D.
Professor of Anesthesiology, Associate Professor of Pediatrics, and Professor of Surgery, St. Louis University School of Medicine, St. Louis, Missouri
Central Venous Oxygen

Joseph L. Seltzer, M.D.
Professor and Chairman of Anesthesiology, Jefferson Medical College, Thomas Jefferson University, Philadelphia, Pennsylvania
Autoimmune Disease—Cold

Daniel I. Sessler, M.D.
Professor and Vice-Chair, Department of Anesthesia and Intensive Care, University of Vienna; Associate Professor and Director, Thermoregulation Research, University of California, San Francisco, California
Hypothermia, Mild (Core Temperature 34–36°C)

Navil Sethna, M.D., Ch.B.
Assistant Professor of Anaesthesia, Harvard Medical School, Boston, Massachusetts
Prader-Willi Syndrome

Ferne B. Sevarino, M.D.
Associate Professor of Anesthesiology, Yale University School of Medicine, New Haven, Connecticut
Total Abdominal Hysterectomy

Paul W. Shabaz, M.D.
Instructor, Department of Anesthesiology, University of Rochester Medical Center, Rochester, New York
Placenta Previa

Michael D. Sharpe, M.D.
Associate Professor, Department of Anaesthesia, University of Western Ontario, London, Ontario, Canada
Parkinson's Disease (Paralysis Agitans)

Nigel E. Sharrock, M.B., Ch.B.
Assistant Clinical Professor in Anesthesia, Cornell University Medical College, New York, New York
Knee Arthroscopy

Joanne Shay, M.D.
Assistant Professor of Anesthesiology, George Washington University School of Medicine and Health Sciences, Washington, D.C.
Anemia, Aplastic

John G. Shutack, D.O.
Associate Professor of Anesthesiology, Medical College of Pennsylvania and Hahnemann University, Philadelphia, Pennsylvania
Malignant Hyperthermia (MH) and Other Anesthetic-Induced Myodystrophies (AIMs)

Frederick E. Sieber, M.D.
Associate Professor, Johns Hopkins Hospital, Baltimore, Maryland
Cerebral Aneurysm Clipping

Daniel Siker, M.D.
Staff Anesthesiologist, Cleveland Clinic Foundation, Cleveland, Ohio
Cherubism
Treacher Collins Syndrome

J. Christopher Sill, M.D.
Associate Professor, Mayo Medical School and Mayo Clinic, Rochester, Minnesota
Tissue Plasminogen Activator

Brett A. Simon, M.D., Ph.D.
Assistant Professor, Department of Anesthesiology and Critical Care Medicine, Johns Hopkins University School of Medicine, Baltimore, Maryland
Lung Volume Reduction Surgery (Pneumoplasty)

Raymond S. Sinatra, M.D., Ph.D.
Professor of Anesthesiology, Director, Acute Pain Service, Yale University School of Medicine, New Haven, Connecticut
Labor—Epidural Block

Robert N. Sladen, M.D.
Associate Professor of Anesthesiology and Surgery, Duke University Medical Center, Durham, North Carolina
Renal Failure, Acute (ARF)

Douglas S. Snyder, M.D.
Assistant Professor, Department of Anesthesiology and Critical Care Medicine, Johns Hopkins University School of Medicine, Baltimore, Maryland
Herniorrhaphy

Sophia Socaris, M.D.
Associate Professor of Surgery and Anesthesiology, Albany Medical College, Albany, New York
Lyme Disease

Martin D. Sokoll, M.D.
Professor, Department of Anesthesiology, University of Iowa College of Medicine, Iowa City, Iowa
Gold (Auranofin, Aurothioglucose, Aurothiomalate)

James M. Sonner, M.D.
Assistant Professor of Anesthesia, University of California, San Francisco, School of Medicine, San Francisco, California
Candidiasis
Pemphigus

Michael Sopher, M.D.
Assistant Clinical Professor, Department of Anesthesiology, UCLA Medical Center, Los Angeles, California
Pericarditis, Acute

Donat R. Spahn, M.D.
Professor of Anesthesiology, Department of Anesthesiology, University Hospital, Zurich, Switzerland
Anemia—Chronic Disease

Bruce D. Spiess, M.D.
Associate Professor, Department of Anesthesiology, University of Washington School of Medicine, Seattle, Washington
Pericardial Effusion

Peter S. Staats, M.D.
Assistant Professor; Director, Division of Pain Medicine, Department of Anesthesiology and Critical Care Medicine, Johns Hopkins University School of Medicine, Baltimore, Maryland
Spasmodic Torticollis

Theodore H. Stanley, M.D.
Professor, Department of Anesthesiology, University of Utah Health Sciences Center, Salt Lake City, Utah
Phenothiazines

Donald R. Stanski, M.D., Ph.D.
Professor and Chair, Department of Anesthesia, Stanford University, Stanford, California
Benzodiazepines (Midazolam, Lorazepam, Diazepam)

Stanley W. Stead, M.D.
Associate Professor of Anesthesiology, University of California, Los Angeles, School of Medicine, Los Angeles, California
Blindness
Circumcision
Prilocaine
Tetracaine

Randy H. Steadman, M.D.
Assistant Clinical Professor, Department of Anesthesiology, University of California, Los Angeles, School of Medicine, Los Angeles, California
Ventricular Fibrillation
Carcinoid, Excision of
Bicarbonate Sodium

Linda Stehling, M.D.
Vice President, Medical Affairs, Blood Systems, Inc., Scottsdale, Arizona
Blood Components

Keith L. Stein, M.D.
Physician Executive Consultant, APM, Inc., New York, New York
Mitral Regurgitation

Wendell C. Stevens, M.D.
Professor of Anesthesiology, Oregon Health Sciences University School of Medicine, Portland, Oregon
Tetralogy of Fallot (TOF), Correction of

Kevin Stierer, M.D.
Clinical Assistant Professor, Department of Anesthesiology, Uniformed Services University of Health Sciences, Bethesda, Maryland
Bowel Resection

Tracy Stierer, M.D.
Assistant Professor, Department of Anesthesiology and Critical Care Medicine, Johns Hopkins Hospital, Baltimore, Maryland
Oral Contraceptives

Bryant W. Stolp, M.D., Ph.D.
Assistant Professor, Department of Anesthesiology, Duke University Medical Center, Durham, North Carolina
Carbon Monoxide (CO) Poisoning
Gas Embolism

John K. Stone, Jr., M.D., Ph.D.
Associate Professor, Department of Anesthesia, The Pennsylvania State University College of Medicine, Hershey, Pennsylvania
Riboflavin (Vitamin B_2)
Vitamin B_{12} (Cyanocobalamin)

David F. Stowe, M.D., Ph.D.
Professor of Anesthesiology and Physiology, Cardiovascular Research Center, Medical College of Wisconsin, Milwaukee, Wisconsin
Serotonin: Agonists, Antagonists, and Reuptake Inhibitors

Scott C. Streckenbach, M.D.
Instructor in Anaesthesia, Harvard Medical School, Boston, Massachusetts
Mycoplasma pneumoniae Infection

Theodore W. Striker, M.D.
Professor of Anesthesia and Pediatrics, and Vice Chairman, Department of Anesthesia, University of Cincinnati College of Medicine, Cincinnati, Ohio
Cystic Fibrosis

Cheri A. Sulek, M.D.
Assistant Professor of Anesthesiology, University of Florida College of Medicine, Gainesville, Florida
Central Neurogenic Hyperventilation

Tommy Symreng, M.D., Ph.D.
Staff Anesthesiologist, Department of Anesthesiology, Welborn Baptist Hospital, Evansville, Indiana
Steroids

Zuhayr A. Tabbarah, M.D.
Associate Clinical Professor of Medicine (Infectious Diseases), American University of Beirut Medical School, Beirut, Lebanon
Echinococcosis

Darrell Tanelian, M.D.
Associate Professor, Department of Anesthesiology and Pain Management, University of Texas Southwestern Medical Center, Dallas, Texas
Lidocaine

Rene Tempelhoff, M.D.
Associate Professor of Anesthesiology and Neurological Surgery, Washington University School of Medicine, St. Louis, Missouri
Seizures—Intractable

John E. Tetzlaff, M.D.
Associate Professor of Anesthesiology, Ohio State University–Cleveland Clinic Center for Health Science, Cleveland, Ohio
Ankylosing Spondylitis
Degenerative Disk Disease

Stephen J. Thomas, M.D.
Professor and Vice Chair, Department of Anesthesiology, New York Hospital–Cornell Medical Center, New York, New York
Aortic Stenosis

Alisa C. Thome, M.D.
Associate Professor of Clinical Anesthesia, Cornell University Medical College, New York, New York
Lymphomas
Thyroid Neoplasms

Daniel M. Thys, M.D.
Professor, Department of Anesthesiology, Columbia University College of Physicians and Surgeons, New York, New York
Norepinephrine
Coronary Artery Bypass Graft
Transesophageal Echocardiography (TEE)

Joseph R. Tobin, M.D.
Associate Professor of Anesthesia and Pediatrics, Bowman Gray School of Medicine of Wake Forest University, Winston-Salem, North Carolina
Hydrocephalus

Michael Tobin, M.D.
Assistant Professor of Anesthesia, Northwestern University Medical School, Chicago, Illinois
Tracheoesophageal Fistula Repair

I. David Todres, M.D.
Associate Professor in Anaesthesia (Paediatrics), Harvard Medical School, Boston, Massachusetts
Necrotizing Enterocolitis

Alan S. Tonnesen, M.D.
Professor of Anesthesiology, University of Texas Medical School at Houston, Houston, Texas
Hypophosphatemia

Thomas J. Toung, M.D.
Associate Professor, Department of Anesthesiology, Johns Hopkins University School of Medicine, Baltimore, Maryland
Craniotomy—Sitting Position
Venous Air Embolism

Karen Traber, M.D.
Assistant Professor, Department of Anesthesiology, University of Pennsylvania School of Medicine, Philadelphia, Pennsylvania
Tuberculosis (TB)

Mark F. Trankina, M.D.
Assistant Professor, Department of Anesthesiology, University of Florida College of Medicine, Gainesville, Florida
Pacemaker

Kevin K. Tremper, M.D., Ph.D.
Professor and Chair, Department of Anesthesiology, University of Michigan Medical Center, Ann Arbor, Michigan
Cigarette Smoking

Kenneth J. Tuman, M.D.
The Max S. Sadove, MD, Professor of Anesthesiology, Department of Anesthesiology, Rush Medical College, Chicago, Illinois
Ventricular Tachycardia
Phenylephrine (Neo-Synephrine)

Avery Tung, M.D.
Assistant Professor, Department of Anesthesia and Critical Care, The University of Chicago, Chicago, Illinois
Necrotizing Fasciitis
Aminophylline

Herman Turndorf, M.D.
Professor and Chairman, Department of Anesthesiology, New York University School of Medicine, New York, New York
Pituitary Tumor, Excision of

Rebecca Twersky, M.D.
Associate Professor of Anesthesiology; Director, Division of Ambulatory Anesthesia, State University of New York Health Science Center at Brooklyn, Brooklyn, New York
Pregnancy Testing

Donald C. Tyler, M.D.
Associate Professor, Anesthesiology and Pediatrics, University of Washington School of Medicine, Seattle, Washington
Hirschsprung's Disease
Otitis Media

Nolan Tzou, M.D.
Fellow, Pain Management, Department of Anesthesiology and Critical Care Medicine, Memorial Sloan-Kettering Cancer Center, New York, New York
Leukemia

John A. Ulatowski, M.D., Ph.D.
Assistant Professor, Department of Anesthesiology, Johns Hopkins University School of Medicine, Baltimore, Maryland
Transverse Myelitis

Michael Urban, M.D., Ph.D.
Assistant Clinical Professor of Anesthesiology, Cornell University Medical College, New York, New York
Total Knee Arthroplasty

Carole Vannier, M.D.
Assistant Professor of Anesthesiology and Critical Care Medicine, Johns Hopkins University School of Medicine, Baltimore, Maryland
Intra-aortic Balloon Counterpulsation (IABP)

R. Lee Wagner, M.D.
Clinical Assistant Professor of Anesthesiology, University of California, San Diego, School of Medicine, La Jolla, California
Hyperaldosteronism (Secondary)

Garry V. Walker, M.D.
Assistant Professor of Anesthesiology, Vanderbilt University School of Medicine, Nashville, Tennessee
Abdominal Aortic Aneurysm Repair

Russell T. Wall III, M.D.
Professor of Anesthesiology, Georgetown University School of Medicine, Washington, D.C.
Acromegaly
Anorexia Nervosa

David C. Warltier, M.D., Ph.D.
Professor and Vice Chairman, Department of Anesthesiology, Medical College of Wisconsin, Milwaukee, Wisconsin
Dobutamine

Lucy Waskell, M.D., Ph.D.
Professor, Department of Anesthesia, University of California, San Francisco, School of Medicine, San Francisco, California
Penicillins

W. David Watkins, M.D., Ph.D.
Professor and Vice Chairman, Department of Anesthesiology and Critical Care Medicine, University of Pittsburgh Medical Center, Pittsburgh, Pennsylvania
Tetracyclines

Eileen Watson, M.D.
Department of Anesthesiology, State University of New York at Buffalo, Buffalo, New York
Rocky Mountain Spotted Fever

Walter L. Way, M.D.
Professor Emeritus of Anesthesia/Pharmacology, University of California, San Francisco, School of Medicine, San Francisco, California
Allopurinol

Michael Webb, M.D.
Department of Anesthesiology and Critical Care Medicine, Johns Hopkins Hospital, Baltimore, Maryland
Gastrectomy

Denise J. Wedel, M.D.
Professor of Anesthesiology, Mayo Medical School, Rochester, Minnesota
Osteoarthritis

Herbert D. Weintraub, M.D.
Professor of Anesthesiology, George Washington University School of Medicine and Health Sciences, Washington, D.C.
Drug Abuse—Lysergic Acid Diethylamide (LSD)

Charles Weissman, M.D.
Professor of Clinical Anesthesiology and Clinical Medicine, Columbia University College of Physicians and Surgeons, New York, New York
Encephalopathy, Metabolic
Encephalopathy, Postanoxic
Protein C Deficiency

Paul F. White, M.D., Ph.D.
Professor and McDermott Chair of Anesthesiology, Department of Anesthesiology and Pain Management, University of Texas Southwestern Medical Center, Dallas, Texas
Etomidate (Amidate)
Ketamine

John P. Williams, M.D.
Associate Professor of Anesthesiology, University of California, Los Angeles, School of Medicine, Los Angeles, California
Pericarditis, Acute

Roger S. Wilson, M.D.
Professor of Anesthesiology, Cornell University Medical College, New York, New York
V/Q Scan (Split Lung Function)

Bernard Wittels, M.D., Ph.D.
Assistant Professor of Clinical Anesthesia and Critical Care, The University of Chicago, Chicago, Illinois
GIFT Procedure

David Wlody, M.D.
Clinical Associate Professor of Anesthesia; Director, Obstetric Anesthesia, State University of New York Health Science Center at Brooklyn, Brooklyn, New York
Hysteroscopy

David H. Wong, M.D., Pharm.D.
Associate Clinical Professor of Anesthesiology, University of California, Irvine, College of Medicine, Orange, California
Cryptococcus Infection

K.C. Wong, M.D., Ph.D.
Professor and Chairman, Department of Anesthesiology, University of Utah College of Medicine, Salt Lake City, Utah
Cigarette Smoking Cessation
Hypernatremia
Hyponatremia

Margaret Wood, M.D.
E.M. Papper Professor and Chairman, Department of Anesthesiology, Columbia University College of Physicians and Surgeons, New York, New York
Scopolamine (L-Hyoscine)

Evelina Worwag, M.D.
Assistant Professor; Co-Director, Pain Management Center, The University of Chicago, Chicago, Illinois
Glossopharyngeal Neuralgia

Peter M.C. Wright, M.D.
Senior Lecturer, Department of Anaesthesia, University of Newcastle upon Tyne, United Kingdom
Edrophonium
Neostigmine

Ron Yaniv, M.D.
Clinical Instructor, Dermatology, Sackler School of Medicine, Tel-Aviv University, Tel-Aviv, Israel
Mastocytosis

Kelvin Yee, M.D.
Assistant Professor, Department of Anesthesiology and Critical Care Medicine, Johns Hopkins University School of Medicine, Baltimore, Maryland
Crohn's Disease

Christopher C. Young, M.D.
Assistant Professor, Department of Anesthesia, Duke University School of Medicine, Durham, North Carolina
Thoracic Aortic Repair

Christopher J. Young, M.D.
Assistant Professor, Department of Anesthesia and Critical Care, The University of Chicago, Chicago, Illinois
Nicotine (Tobacco, Cigarettes, Snuff), Nicotine Replacement Therapies (Nicorette [Gum], Nicoderm [Patch])

Marie L. Young, M.D.
Associate Professor of Anesthesia, University of Pennsylvania Medical Center, Philadelphia, Pennsylvania
Infratentorial Tumors

John A. Youngberg, M.D.
Professor of Anesthesiology; Director, Cardiac Anesthesia, Tulane University Medical Center School of Medicine, New Orleans, Louisiana
Carotid Endarterectomy

James P. Zacny, Ph.D.
Assistant Professor, Department of Anesthesia and Critical Care, Department of Psychiatry, The University of Chicago, Chicago, Illinois
Marijuana
Nicotine
Phencyclidine (PCP)

James R. Zaidan, M.D.
Professor of Anesthesiology, Emory University School of Medicine, Atlanta, Georgia
Mobitz I (Second Degree Atrioventricular Block)
Mobitz II (Second Degree Atrioventricular Block)

Paul Zanaboni, M.D.
Cardiac Anesthesia Fellow, Johns Hopkins University School of Medicine, Baltimore, Maryland
Cor Pulmonale

Warren M. Zapol, M.D.
Reginald Jenney Professor of Anaesthesia, Harvard Medical School, Boston, Massachusetts
Nitric Oxide, Inhaled

William Zimmermann, M.D.
Assistant Professor, Department of Anesthesia and Critical Care, The University of Chicago, Chicago, Illinois
Parkinson's Disease (Paralysis Agitans)

Ross H. Zoll, M.D., Ph.D.
Chief of Anesthesia, Providence Hospital, Holyoke, Massachusetts
Cardioversion

Howard Alan Zucker, M.D.
Assistant Professor of Pediatrics and Anesthesiology, Columbia University College of Physicians and Surgeons, New York, New York
Aortopulmonary Window

Rhonda Zuckerman, M.D.
Assistant Professor, Department of Anesthesiology and Critical Care Medicine, Johns Hopkins University School of Medicine, Baltimore, Maryland
Pregnant Surgical Patient

Maurice S. Zwass, M.D.
Associate Professor of Anesthesia and Pediatrics, University of California, San Francisco, School of Medicine, San Francisco, California
Croup (Laryngotracheal Bronchitis)
Epiglottitis

Foreword

Michael Roizen and Lee Fleisher have ingeniously encapsulated information important for any anesthesia consultant. Having been their associates at The University of California, San Francisco, and at Yale before they accepted their present positions at The University of Chicago and The Johns Hopkins University, we respect their clinical judgments, the fruit of years of experience in the practice of anesthesia. This book reflects the innovative yet comprehensive approach that they often take. They are no ivory tower practitioners—they work "in the trenches." We think that they have succeeded well in summarizing the pertinent aspects of the disease process, as well as the procedures, drugs, and tests that are considered before a patient is anesthetized. Succinctly, each chapter points the reader toward optimal care of a patient, by exploring the pathophysiology of a disease process and the management appropriate to specific conditions, clinical situations, and drug interactions. The intent is to help the physician rapidly and comprehensively plan perioperative management.

This is not a how-to-do-it book or "recipes" for perioperative care. Rather, it suggests that the pathophysiology of a disease or the physiologic imbalance caused by an operation should influence our thinking about therapeutic options. It offers a method for setting priorities to facilitate exemplary performance as a consultant in anesthesia. *Essence of Anesthesia Practice* will prove useful not only to anesthesiologists but also to our colleagues in other specialties who interface with the surgical patient.

The editors are to be congratulated for succeeding in developing an innovative clinical and educational format to serve both novice residents and experienced practitioners.

PAUL G. BARASH, M.D.
New Haven, CT

RONALD D. MILLER, M.D.
San Francisco, CA

It was in 1986 that the idea of a one-page summary of the pathophysiology of diseases and their implications for anesthesia was conceived. Drs. Cherise T. Petrovitch and Michael F. Roizen were formulating questions at that time to assess whether candidates for Board certification could qualify as consultants. That an anesthesiologist can deliver anesthesia safely for the majority of patients is assessed by the Board's multiple-choice test and the Clinical Competence Committee in their training program. But as a consultant, the anesthesiologist must be able to convey an understanding that many diseases cause pathophysiologic disturbances that may affect perioperative management. Awareness of those disturbances and an ability to integrate that knowledge in clinical care to minimize their consequences separates the merely good anesthetic practitioner from the master practitioner or consultant.

We thought that the implications of disease, chronic drug therapy, procedures, and abnormalities on diagnostic tests for perioperative care could be most easily understood and remembered if they were summarized on one page. The summaries presented in this book review the pathophysiologic implications of specific diseases, including suggestions for evaluation of patients, the effective medications for the disease, the implications of anesthesia for operative procedures, and the pathophysiologic implications of a diagnostic test abnormality. These summaries are not substitutes for textbooks of medical specialties but are offered as brief overviews of the essentials to be reviewed in caring for the patient.

The book is divided into four sections: Diseases, Procedures, Drugs, and Tests. In all sections, each topic is outlined on a single page divided into three sections.

The top section presents an overview of information about a disease, chronic drug therapy, procedure, or test. This section lists the etiology of the condition, indications, and usual treatments. For diseases or procedures, perioperative risk and potential problems during the perioperative period are outlined. The objective is to assist the practitioner in choosing topics to discuss with a patient in the preanesthetic interview and tailoring an anesthetic plan to reduce risk. Indications for drugs and tests and alternative treatments or procedures are also suggested. An ICD-9-CM code has been included for diseases and the primary underlying pathology for many operations. Since a wide range of codes can be ascribed to particular conditions, we have included the most common ICD-9-CM codes; these codes can help the practitioner locate the most applicable one for each individual patient but are not meant to be definitive.

The middle section is arranged in table format. The table outlines the effects of a procedure, disease, drug therapy, or test implication on an organ system. The contributors have identified aspects from a patient's history and physical examination that can be used to diagnose each effect. Finally, tests that may be used to further assess the probability of morbidity are suggested. These tests should be performed only if indicated by a patient's history or physical examination. Such tests are by no means intended to be part of every evaluation nor are they the only laboratory tests to be considered.

The bottom section is devoted to perioperative implications. Again, the pathophysiologic approach is emphasized for management. Finally, there is a subsection on anticipated problems and concerns during the postoperative period.

Publication of *Essence of Anesthesia Practice* required assistance from many individuals. We especially acknowledge the efforts of Dr. Charise Petrovitch; Lewis Reines, President of W.B. Saunders, who took a personal interest in the project; and John Cooke, Evelyn Adler, Constance Burton, Linda R. Garber, and Joan Slowinski of W.B. Saunders, for translating our ideas into a workable text. Our secretaries, Kelle Martin, Elaine Lowery, and Annette Y. Hargrave worked with a combination of over 600 contributors and manuscripts. While all of us try to ensure brevity, accuracy, consistency of style (both of us edited each summary page at least twice), and freedom from typographical errors, we are sure that some errors have eluded us. We hope you will write or e-mail us (mrzz@midway.uchicago.edu *or* lfleishe@welchlink.welch.jhu.edu) so that should future printings or editions be warranted, we may correct our errors. If you notice an omission from any of the four sections, we would appreciate having the omission called to our attention. Further, although we tried to prepare the summaries in a format ready for electronic media, most people do not yet have screens big enough to show the full page. We believe that will soon be corrected.

Although Dr. Petrovitch's family and other obligations forced her to drop out of working on this project, we, Drs. Roizen and Fleisher, and the contributors have tried to convey in this work the essence of the pathophysiologic implications of acute or chronic conditions, drug therapies, procedures, and test abnormalities. *Essence of Anesthesia Practice* is not intended to be a "cookbook" of anesthesiology. While some people with expertise in one area were approached to write or contribute a page on the conditions that they know most about, some initially refused, saying that they did not want to be involved in a "cookbook." Most later accepted after we further explained the concept to them. This book and each summary is anything but a "cookbook"; in fact, it is close to the opposite. It assumes that the practitioner knows how to deliver anesthesia. It is intended to highlight concisely the pathophysiologic derangements and perioperative implications of diseases, procedures, drugs, and test abnormalities in an ordered fashion. This book was designed for the novice and consultant alike to help each one function better. We believe that our patients have already benefited from the work done on this book. We hope that you will feel that you and your patients have benefited also.

MICHAEL F. ROIZEN, M.D.

LEE A. FLEISHER, M.D.

Contents

Section II
PROCEDURES

Section III
DRUGS

Section IV
TESTS

List of Abbreviations

SYMBOLS

~	approximately
↑	increase
↓	decrease
°C	degrees centigrade
°F	degrees Fahrenheit
1°	primary
2°	secondary

A

α rb	alpha adrenergic receptor blocking agent
AAA	abdominal aortic aneurysm
Abd	abdomen, abdominal
ABG	arterial blood gas
Abn	abnormal
ACE	angiotensin converting enzyme
ACE rb	angiotensin II receptor inhibitor
ACG	angle closure glaucoma
ACh	acetylcholine
AChE	acetylcholinesterase
ACT	active clotting/coagulation time
ACTH	adrenocorticotropic hormone
ADH	antidiuretic hormone
AFib	atrial fibrillation
AKA	above-knee amputation
Alk phos	alkaline phosphatase
ALT	alanine aminotransferase
Alv	alveolar
ANA	antinuclear antibody
Angio	angiogram
ANS	autonomic nervous system
ant	anterior
AP	anterior-posterior, action potential
APTT	activated partial thromboplastin time
ARDS	adult respiratory distress syndrome
art	arterial
AS	aortic stenosis
ASA	acetylsalicylic acid; Adams-Stokes attack, American Society of Anesthesiologists
ASAP	as soon as possible
ASCVD	atherosclerotic cardiovascular disease
ASD	atrial septal defect
AST	aspartate aminotransferase
ATN	acute tubular necrosis
ATP	adenosine triphosphate
Au	gold
AV	atrioventricular
AVM	arteriovenous malformation
AVR	aortic valve replacement

B

β rb	beta adrenergic receptor blocking agent
BBB	bundle branch block, blood-brain barrier
BCNU	nitrosourea (carmustine)
bilat	bilateral
BKA	below-knee amputation
BLS	basic life support
BMI	body mass index
BMR	basal metabolic rate
BO	bronchiolitis obliterans
BP	blood pressure
BPD	bronchopulmonary dysplasia
BS	breath sounds
BSA	body surface area
BT	bleeding time
BUN	blood urea nitrogen

C

C-section	cesarean section
CA	cancer
ca.	about (L., circa)
Ca^{2+}	calcium
Ca rb	calcium channel receptor blocking agent
CABG	coronary artery bypass graft
CAD	coronary artery disease
cAMP	cyclic adenosine monophosphate
CAS	coronary artery spasm
cath	catheter
CBC	complete blood count
CBF	cerebral blood flow
CCNU	nitrosourea (lomustine)
cGMP	cyclic guanosine monophosphate
CHB	complete heart block
ChE	cholinesterase
ChemoRx	chemotherapy
CHF	congestive heart failure
CK	creatine kinase
CMRO	cerebral metabolic rate of oxygen
CNS	central nervous system
CO	cardiac output, carbon monoxide
Coag	coagulation
COHg	carboxyhemoglobin
COMT	catechol-o-methyltransferase
conc	concentrated
concn	concentration
COPD	chronic obstructive pulmonary disease
CPAP	continuous positive airway pressure

CPB	cardiopulmonary bypass		FVC	forced vital capacity
CPD	cephalopelvic disproportion		Fx	fracture
CPK	creatine phosphokinase			
CPP	cerebral perfusion pressure		**G**	
CPZ	chlorpromazine			
Cr	creatinine		GA	general anesthesia
Cryo	cryoprecipitate		G-CSF	granulocyte colony stimulating factor
CSF	cerebrospinal fluid		GER	gastroesophageal reflux
CSM	carotid sinus massage		GFR	glomerular filtration rate
CSS	carotid sinus syndrome		GH	growth hormone
CT	computed tomography		GI	gastrointestinal
CTX	cyclophosphamide (Cytoxan)		GIFT	gamete intrafallopian transfer
CV	cardiovascular		Gn-RH	gonadotropin-releasing hormone
CVA	cerebrovascular accident		G6PD	glucose-6-phosphate dehydrogenase
CVD	cerebrovascular disease		GU	genitourinary
CVP	central venous pressure		GVHD	graft vs. host disease
CXR	chest x-ray			

D

D_5	dextrose 5% in water		**H**	
DIC	disseminated intravascular coagulation		H_2	histamine
Dig	digoxin		hCG	human gonadotropic hormone
DJD	degenerative joint disease		HCO_2	bicarbonate
DKA	diabetic ketoacidosis		Hct	hematocrit
DM	diabetes mellitus		HDL	high-density lipoprotein
DNR	do not resuscitate		He	helium
DOE	dyspnea on exertion		HEENT	head, eyes, ears, nose, throat
DTIC	dacarbazine		HEME	hematology
DTR	deep tendon reflex		Hg	mercury
DTs	delirium tremens		Hgb	hemoglobin
DVT	deep vein thrombosis		HN_2	nitrogen mustard
Dx	diagnosis		HR	heart rate
			ht	height
			5-HT	5-hydroxytryptamine
E			Htn	hypertension
			Hx	history
EBL	estimated blood loss			
ECG	electrocardiogram		**I**	
ECHO	echocardiogram			
ECT	electroconvulsive therapy		IABP	intra-aortic balloon pump
ED_{50}	median effective dose		IBS	irritable bowel syndrome
EF	ejection fraction		ICD	implantable cardioverter-defibrillator
EMG	electromyography		ICP	intracranial pressure
ENDO	endocrine		ICU	intensive care unit
esp	especially		IDDM	insulin-dependent diabetes mellitus
ESR	erythrocyte sedimentation rate		IFN	interferon
ESRD	end-stage renal disease		Ig	immunoglobulin
ET	endotracheal		IGF	insulin-like growth factor
ETOH	ethanol		IHD	ischemic heart disease
ETT	exercise tolerance test, endotracheal tube		IHSS	idiopathic hypertrophic subaortic stenosis
ext	exterior		IL	interleukin
			inf	inferior
			INR	International Normalization Ratio
F			intox	intoxication
			I/O	input/output
FBS	fasting blood sugar		IOP	intraocular pressure
FEV	forced expiratory volume		IRMA	immunoradiosorbent assay
FFA	free fatty acid		IV	intravenous
FFP	fresh frozen plasma		IVC	inferior vena cava
FHR	fetal heart rate		IVP	intravenous pyelogram
FIO_2	fractional inspired oxygen			
FRC	functional residual capacity		**J**	
freq	frequent			
FSH	follicle stimulating hormone		JV	jugular vein
FSP	fibrin split products		JVD	jugular venous distention

K

K^+	potassium
KUB	kidney, ureter, bladder

L

LAD	left anterior descending (coronary artery)
LAP	left atrial pressure
lat	lateral
LBBB	left bundle branch block
LDH	lactate dehydrogenase
LDL	low-density lipoprotein
LES	lower esophageal sphincter
LFT	liver function test
LH	luteinizing hormone
LLQ	left lower quadrant
LMA	laryngeal mask airway
LMW	low molecular weight
LOC	loss of consciousness; level of consciousness
LPO	left posterior oblique
LR	lactated Ringer's [solution]
L→R	left to right
LUQ	left upper quadrant
LV	left ventricle
LVEDP	left ventricular end-diastolic pressure
LVEF	left ventricular ejection fraction
LVET	left ventricular ejection time
LVF	left ventricular failure
LVH	left ventricular hypertrophy
Lytes	electrolytes

M

MABP	mean arterial blood pressure
MAC	minimum alveolar concentration
MAO	monoamine oxidase
MAP	mean arterial pressure
MEN	multiple endocrine neoplasia
MEP	motor/multimodality evoked potential
metab	metabolism
metHb	methemoglobin
Mg^{2+}	magnesium
MI	myocardial infarction
min	minimum, minimal, minute
MS	musculoskeletal (in tables), mental status, multiple sclerosis
MUGA	multiple gated acquisition
MVP	mitral valve prolapse
MW	molecular weight

N

N	nitrogen
n.	nerve
Na^+	sodium
NCV	nerve conduction velocity
neg	negative
NEURO	neurologic
NG	nasogastric
NIDDM	non–insulin-dependent diabetes mellitus
NIF	negative inspiratory force
NM	neuromuscular
NMB	neuromuscular blockade

NMJ	neuromuscular junction
nml	normal
NMS	neuroleptic malignant syndrome
NO	nitric oxide
N_2O	dinitrogen monoxide (nitrous oxide)
no.	number
N/S	normal saline
NSAID	nonsteroidal anti-inflammatory drug
NSR	normal sinus rhythm
NTG	nitroglycerin
N/V	nausea/vomiting

O

O_2	oxygen
OA	osteoarthritis
OB/GYN	obstetrics and gynecology
OD	overdose
O/P	output
OR	operating room
Osm	osmole, osmolality
OTC	over-the-counter

P

P	phosphorus
PA	pulmonary artery
PAC	premature atrial contraction
PACU	postanesthesia care unit
PAF	platelet activating factor
L-PAM	melphalan (Alkeran)
PAP	pulmonary artery pressure
PAT	paroxysmal atrial tachycardia
PCA	patient-controlled analgesia
PCR	polymerase chain reaction
PCWP	pulmonary capillary wedge pressure
PDA	patent ductus arteriosus
PE	physical examination, pulmonary embolism
PEEP	positive end-expiratory pressure
PEF	peak expiratory flow
PET	positron emission tomography
PFT	pulmonary function test
pharm	pharmacy, pharmaceutical
PID	pelvic inflammatory disease
Plt	platelet
PMN	polymorphonuclear leukocyte
PND	paroxysmal nocturnal dyspnea
PNS	peripheral nervous system
PO_2	oxygen partial pressure
ppm	parts per million
PPV	positive pressure ventilation
PRBCs	packed red blood cells
preg	pregnant
prep	preparation
PT	prothrombin time
PTCA	percutaneous transluminal coronary angioplasty
PTH	parathyroid hormone
PTT	activated partial thromboplastin time
PUD	peptic ulcer disease
PULM	pulmonary
PVC	premature ventricular contraction
PVD	peripheral vascular disease
PVR	pulmonary vascular resistance

Q

QRS	Q wave, R wave, S wave

R

R→L	right to left
RA	rheumatoid arthritis
RAE	right atrial enlargement
RAH	right atrial hypertrophy
RAO	right anterior oblique
RAP	right atrial pressure
RBBB	right bundle branch block
RBC	red blood cell
RDS	respiratory distress syndrome
RESP	respiratory
RHD	rheumatic heart disease
RIA	radioimmunoassay
ROM	range of motion
ROS	review of systems
RSD	reflex sympathetic dystrophy
RTA	renal tubule acidosis
RUQ	right upper quadrant
RV	right ventricle
RVH	right ventricular hypertrophy
Rx	therapy, treatment

S

SA	sinoatrial
SAH	subarachnoid hemorrhage
Sat	saturation
sc	subcutaneous
SEP	sensory evoked potential
SG	specific gravity
SIADH	syndrome of inappropriate secretion of antidiuretic hormone
SIDS	sudden infant death syndrome
SLE	systemic lupus erythematosus
SNS	sympathetic nervous system
SOB	shortness of breath
SPECT	single-photon emission computed tomography
SSEP	somatosensory evoked potential
SSS	sick sinus syndrome
Stz	streptozocin
SVC	superior vena cava
SVR	systemic vascular resistance
SVT	supraventricular tachycardia
Sx	signs and symptoms

T

T	temperature
$T_{1/2}$	half-life
TB	tuberculosis
T&C	type and crossmatch
TCA	tricyclic antidepressant
TEE	transesophageal echocardiography
TEF	transesophageal fistula
TENS	transcutaneous electrical nerve stimulation
TGV	transposition of great vessels
THR	total hip replacement
TIA	transient ischemic attack
TKR	total knee replacement
TLC	total lung capacity/compliance
TMJ	temporomandibular joint
TMP/SMX	trimethoprim/sulfamethoxazole
TNF	tumor necrosis factor
TOF	train-of-4, tetralogy of Fallot
t-PA	tissue plasminogen activator
TPN	total parenteral nutrition
TSH	thyroid stimulating hormone
TURP	transurethral prostatic resection
TV	tidal volume

U

UA	urinalysis
UGI	upper gastrointestinal
UO	urine output
URI	upper respiratory tract infection
UROL	urology
US	ultrasound
UTI	urinary tract infection

V

VC	vital capacity
VFib	ventricular fibrillation
vit	vitamin
vol	volume
V/Q	ventilation-perfusion
VS	vital signs
vs.	versus
VSD	ventricular septal defect
VTach	ventricular tachycardia

W

WBC	white blood cell
WNL	within normal limits
WPW	Wolff-Parkinson-White syndrome
wt	weight

XYZ

Xe	xenon
XS	excessive
y	year

SECTION I

DISEASES

ABRUPTIO PLACENTAE

Charles P. Gibbs, M.D.

RISK

- People within US: ~1% of the 4 million pregnancies/y
- Race with highest prevalence: ?
- Increased prevalence with cocaine use, trauma, increased age and parity, smoking, premature rupture of membranes, and prior abruptio

PERIOPERATIVE RISKS

- Maternal: Antepartum and postpartum hemorrhage; DIC
- Fetal: Hypoxia due to maternal hypotension and/or decreased area for placental exchange

WORRY ABOUT

- Concealed hemorrhage behind the placenta that does not manifest as vaginal bleeding — may be considerable
- Fetal distress

- Postpartum hemorrhage refractory to usual oxytocic agents
- Need for cesarean hysterectomy

OVERVIEW

- Along with placenta previa, a major cause of antepartum hemorrhage and maternal mortality
- Perinatal mortality also high: 30–40%
- Abruptio placentae is the most common cause of DIC in pregnant patients; 20% with clinically significant abruption develop clotting defects.
  – DIC probably due to release of thromboplastin by damaged tissues at abruption site
  – Postpartum hemorrhage correlates directly with severity of coagulopathy.
  – FSP may inhibit ability of uterus to contract, leading to more blood loss.

ICD-9-CM Code: 641.2

ETIOLOGY

- Etiology unknown
- HTN; smoking, cocaine use, trauma, increased age and parity, premature rupture of membranes, and history of previous abruption are predisposing factors

USUAL TREATMENT

- Maintenance of volume status and fetal surveillance
- If fetus premature and hemorrhage not great, careful observation would be appropriate to allow for fetal growth.
- If at term and volume status OK, labor with vaginal delivery optimal.
- If hemorrhage continues and/or fetal distress occurs, C-section is necessary.

ASSESSMENT POINTS

SYSTEM	EFFECT	ASSESSMENT BY HX	PE	TEST
CV	Hemorrhage	Vaginal bleeding and abdominal pain	Vaginal bleeding and firm, tender uterus; hypotension, tachycardia, low CVP and wedge pressures, decreased UO	Hematocrit
HEME	Hypovolemia, acute anemia,	Bleeding diathesis	Hypotension, tachycardia, bleeding from puncture sites, easy bruisability	Hgb, Hct, clotting evaluation that includes platelets, fibrinogen, and FSP
RENAL	Oliguria and/or acute renal failure	UO	Signs of hypovolemia	Urinalysis to include specific gravity and sodium excretion, possibly in addition to central hemodynamic monitoring values
UTERUS/ VAGINA	Abruption Hemorrhage	Painful vaginal bleeding	Tender, firm uterus. Vaginal bleeding may be < CV signs and symptoms indicate (concealed hemorrhage).	Hct and hemodynamic monitoring values
FETUS	Fetal distress and/or demise	Presence or absence of fetal movement	Fetal movement, heart rate	Electronic fetal monitoring

Key Reference: Mayer DC, Spielman FJ: Antepartum and postpartum hemorrhage. *In* Chestnut DH (ed): Obstetric Anesthesia: Principles and Practice. St. Louis, Mosby, 1994, pp 699–721.

PERIOPERATIVE IMPLICATIONS — FOR LABOR AND VAGINAL DELIVERY

Preinduction/Induction/Maintenance

- Optimize CV status and evaluate coag system.
- Epidural analgesia appropriate if volume status can be maintained and if hemorrhage controllable
- Technique not different from that for normal labor and vaginal delivery except that the smallest effective doses should be utilized
- Electronic fetal monitoring essential
- CV monitoring appropriate for volume and bleeding status

PERIOPERATIVE IMPLICATIONS — FOR CESAREAN SECTION

- Optimization of CV and fetal status, usually by means of appropriate volume replacement

Monitoring

- All cases will require electronic fetal monitoring.
- UO
- Hct and clotting studies as above

- Consider CVP and/or PA catheter depending upon severity of hemorrhage; decreased UO not responsive to simple fluid challenges.

Preinduction/Induction

General Anesthesia: Probably required for massive hemorrhage and/or acute fetal distress
- Aspiration prophylaxis
- Rapid-sequence induction with cricoid pressure
- Consider ketamine and large-bore lines.

Maintenance

- Watch for continued hemorrhage after delivery of infant. Uterus may not respond to usual tocolytic agents.
  – Oxytocin 20–40 mU in 1 L of balanced salt solution
  – Methergine 0.2% mg IM; NOT in the presence of HTN
  – Prostaglandin 250 µg IM or intramyometrial
  – Hypogastric artery ligation
  – Cesarean hysterectomy

Extubation

- Awake extubation required
Regional Anesthesia: In the absence of severe hemorrhage and/or acute fetal distress
- Aspiration prophylaxis

- Optimize volume status
- Epidural preferred over spinal because can raise level *slowly*
- Treat hypotension early and vigorously

Postoperative Period

- Patient needs to be in an appropriately staffed and equipped recovery/SICU area.
- Be alert for continuing uterine hemorrhage and/or development of coagulopathy.
- Continue intraoperative monitoring.

ANTICIPATED PROBLEMS/CONCERNS

- Amount of bleeding may be considerably greater than what is evident per vagina. A significant amount of blood can be trapped behind the abrupted placenta.
- Be alert to the need for immediate C-section for fetal distress and/or dramatic increase in hemorrhage.
- Best therapy for DIC is removal of the placenta by C-section or vaginal delivery.
- Hemorrhage may continue post partum from an atonic uterus that is refractory to the usual oxytocic agents.
- C-section hysterectomy may be necessary — may be accompanied by large blood loss.

ACHONDROPLASIA — DWARFISM
Sandra V. Lowe, M.D.

RISK

- People within USA: 1 million
- 28/1 million in Northern Ireland
- 1:26,000 live births
- Most common type of dwarfism

PERIOPERATIVE RISKS

- Foramen magnum and cervical spine stenosis. Small rib cage, abnormal spinal curvatures may impair respiratory function
- Persistent thoracolumbar kyphosis can compress the spinal cord

WORRY ABOUT

- Paresthesia or paraplegia
- Cauda equina syndrome
- Small intervertebral foramina can cause compression of individual nerve root

OVERVIEW

- Results from failure in development and premature fusion of bones, which ossify in cartilage. Short arms and legs, trident hands, prominent frontal region with bridge of nose depression
- Small, flat chest; lumbar lordosis. Vertebrae of skull base fuse prematurely; foramen magnum is small and funnel-shaped
- Lateral diameter of spinal cord is narrowed
- Compression of neural tissue by bone can occur at three levels: foramen magnum, thoracolumbar, and lumbar spine
- Trunk length, intelligence, and life span are normal
- Mean adult height is 52 inches in males, 48 inches in females
- Mean adult weight is 120 lbs (55 kg) for males and 100 lbs (45 kg) for women
- Obesity is often present in both sexes

ICD-9-CM Code: 756.4

ETIOLOGY

- Autosomal dominant skeletal dysplasia primarily of endochondral bone
- >80% are new mutations: children born to parents of average height
- Achondroplastic parent has 50% chance of an affected child
- Both achondroplastic parents have 75% penetrance
- Homozygous form is usually fatal within first few weeks of life from respiratory insufficiency

USUAL TREATMENT

- Myringotomy and tube placement, suboccipital craniectomy, various orthopedic procedures, laminectomy, ventricular-peritoneal shunts, C-section, tracheostomy

ASSESSMENT POINTS

SYSTEM	EFFECT	ASSESSMENT BY HX	PE	TEST
HEENT	Choanal stenosis Prominent forehead and mandible Flattened midface with saddle nose Hearing loss from chronic otitis media Long narrow mouth with high-arched palate		Nasopharyngoscopy Limited head extension	Flexion/extension neck films
CV	Pulmonary artery hyperplasia Right ventricular hypertrophy RV strain			ECG CXR ECHO
RESP	Restrictive disease from constrictive thoracic cage Encroachment of upper airways Hypoxemia, hypercapnia	Apnea with cyanotic spells Loud snoring Recurrent pneumonia Cyanotic episodes/apnea		ECG ABGs
GI	Obesity	Reflux symptoms		
ENDO	Rule out other causes for growth failure			Growth hormone assay
CNS	Hyperreflexia, sustained clonus Hypertonia, paresis, asymmetry of movement or strength, abnormal plantar response Obstructive sleep apnea	Pyramidal signs Paresis Snoring, restless sleep Enuresis Daytime somnolence	Increased lateral ventricular size Increased extracerebral CSF Small foramen magnum Craniocervical stenosis Absent posterior subarachnoid space	Axial head CT SSEPs Polysomnography
PNS	Atropine fever	Increased sweating		
MS	Decrease in overall limb length Hyperlordosis Rhizomelia Kyphoscoliosis		Kyphosis of thoracolumbar spine Proximal segments of limbs shorter than distal segments	Bone scan Bone x-ray

Key Reference: Berkowitz I, Raja S, Bender K, Kopits S: Dwarfs: Pathophysiology and anesthetic implications. Anesthesiology 1990; 73:739–759.

PERIOPERATIVE IMPLICATIONS

Preoperative Preparation

- Consider metoclopramide/ranitidine in obesity
- Assess respiratory, CV, CNS status
- Assess airway and assume C-spine stenosis

Monitoring

- Difficult IV access
- Respiratory status may require arterial line
- SSEP for spinal cord procedures

Airway

- Difficult mask fit
- No guidelines for endotracheal tube size and length
- Difficult direct laryngoscopy
- Avoid hyperextension or hyperflexion
- Consider awake fiberoptic intubation
- Laryngeal mask airway

Induction

- General anesthesia with controlled airway
- Conduction anesthesia may cause neurologic impairment

Maintenance

- Controlled ventilation
- Consider SSEP in spinal surgery

Postoperative Period

- Respiratory insufficiency
- Pain control
- ICU monitoring

ANTICIPATED PROBLEMS/CONCERNS

- Increased incidence of SIDS
- Postop ventilation
- Neurologic impairment

ACIDOSIS — LACTIC/METABOLIC

Alan W. Grogono, M.D.

RISK

- Incidence requiring surgery in US: unknown
- Gender/race predilection: unknown

PERIOPERATIVE RISKS

- Contributes to cardiovascular instability
- Inhibits local anesthetic solution uptake
- Diminishes effect of morphine and meperidine by decreasing availability of lipophilic, uncharged base
- ↑ Extracellular potassium

WORRY ABOUT

- ↓ Effect of vasopressors, inotropes, and vasodilators
- ↓ Oxygen uptake in lung by ↓ affinity for hemoglobin

OVERVIEW

- All body acids are "metabolic" except CO_2
- A pH that is more acidic than appropriate for PCO_2
- Cell membranes enclose 70% of body water; transfer of respiratory acid (CO_2) is rapid, but transfer of polar, ionized substances (e.g., metabolic acids) is slow
- Extracellular [H^+], 40 nmol/L, pH 7.4 is one quarter of the intracellular 160 nmol/L, pH 6.8; this gradient favors H^+ elimination from cell; counterbalanced by intracellular potential of –60 mV, which attracts H^+ into cell

ICD-9-CM Codes: 276.2 (acidosis; metabolic, mixed, or lactic); 276.4 (mixed acid-base disorder); 250.1 (diabetic ketoacidosis)

ETIOLOGY

- Accumulation of nonrespirable acids (e.g., lactic, pyruvic, ketoacids) at a rate too great for correction by renal elimination or hepatic metabolism

USUAL TREATMENT

- Treat the underlying disease because neutralizing metabolic acid does not cure diabetes, ischemia, etc.
- Bicarbonate therapy (e.g., 1 mEq/L) may be indicated during resuscitation or with some other cause of CV instability

ASSESSMENT POINTS

Measurement: Several techniques have been used to estimate a metabolic abnormality, e.g., the *standard pH* and the *standard bicarbonate,* both measured at normal body temperature and PCO_2 = 40 mm Hg; today, two techniques are in widespread use.

Base Excess (BE): BE is normally 0; blood base (total base) is about 48 mmol/L, depending mostly on Hgb concentration; changes are termed *excess* or *deficit. "This patient has a base excess of minus 10"* means *"this patient has a metabolic acid excess (acidosis) of plus 10 mEq/L."* Base excess estimates amount of treatment required to fully neutralize metabolic acidosis (or alkalosis).

Bicarbonate: In acid-base determinations the concentration (in mEq/L) of the bicarbonate ion (HCO_3^-) is a calculated value derived from PCO_2 and pH. Both respiratory and metabolic components affect bicarbonate level; it cannot, therefore, be an ideal measure of either. In practice, changes in bicarbonate ion concentration may be used as a rough guide to metabolic change.

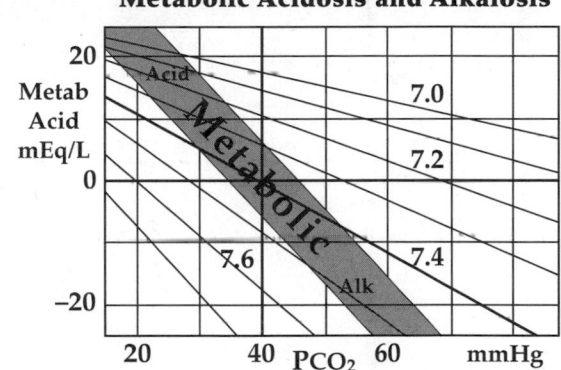

Metabolic Acidosis and Alkalosis

Characteristic Compensation: The figure illustrates that metabolic disturbances are usually accompanied by a characteristic degree of respiratory compensation. In practice, the pH lies halfway between no respiratory compensation (PCO_2 = 40 mmHg) and complete compensation (pH = 7.4).

Treatable Volume: Extracellular fluid is 20% of body weight (e.g., 14 L). For therapy, treatable space is calculated as 30% (e.g., 21 L) because some equilibration occurs between intra- and extracellular fluid; treatable volume, therefore, tends to appear to be somewhat greater. In addition, further change may occur during the period of therapy, because the body may be either correcting the abnormality or making it worse.

Bicarbonate Therapy: This may be indicated when metabolic acidosis accompanies difficulty in resuscitating an individual or in maintaining cardiovascular stability. A typical dose of bicarbonate is 1 mEq/kg of body weight followed by repeated blood gas analysis. Bicarbonate's effect can be anticipated by calculating the dose that would be required for complete correction: **dose (mEq) = 0.3 × wt (kg) × BE (mEq/L).** This dose would return the metabolic disturbance to about 0. This full dose is rarely recommended. It is customary to either give a small standard dose (1 mEq/L) and to reevaluate, or to give about half the calculated dose and then expect about half the effect.

Key Reference: Grogono AW: Fundamentals of Acid Base Balance. American Society of Anesthesiologists, refresher course lecture 154, 1994.

PERIOPERATIVE IMPLICATIONS

- Correction of acid-base balance becomes more critical in patients with compromised cardiovascular stability:
  - in myocardial ischemia
  - following cardiopulmonary bypass
  - following any prolonged cardiac arrest
- Metabolic acidosis may also be a compensatory mechanism for chronic hyperventilation (e.g., in hyperventilation syndrome), or as an adaptive response to high-altitude exposure for many days. This compensatory metabolic response rarely requires therapy.

ANTICIPATED PROBLEMS/CONCERNS

- Caution when administering bicarbonate: give only when clinically required, and then give small dose
- Bicarbonate initially injected into plasma volume (3 L) instead of into the calculated treatable space (21 L)
- Bicarbonate converted to CO_2 and has to be eliminated; each 100 mEq yields ~2.24 L of CO_2, which has to be exhaled (~10 min of normal production)
- CO_2 enters cells freely, unlike bicarbonate ions that have been administered

- Bicarbonate ions are accompanied by sodium ions, which increase osmolality of extracellular fluid; with other Rx, such as IV glucose, hyperosmolality may cause coma; in neonates, rapid bicarbonate infusion may distort vascular structures and result in intracranial hemorrhage
- After recovery, when the body has dealt with metabolic acidosis, bicarbonate Rx leaves residual metabolic alkalosis, hypernatremia, and hyperosmolality

ACROMEGALY

Russell T. Wall III, M.D.

RISK

- People within USA:
  - Prevalence is 40/million; incidence is 3/million/y.
  - Occurs with equal frequency in men and women and most frequently 4th and 5th decades of life

PERIOPERATIVE RISKS

- Common conditions increasing perioperative risk include airway abnormalities, cardiovascular dysfunction (HTN), respiratory impairment (obstructive sleep apnea), endocrine abnormalities (hyperglycemia)

WORRY ABOUT

- Difficulty in or inability to ventilate/intubate
- Extent of cardiovascular disease
- Postop airway obstruction

OVERVIEW

- Acromegaly is an endocrinopathy resulting from excess secretion of growth hormone, usually from pituitary gland, characterized by enlargement of extremities of skeleton (nose, jaw, fingers, toes).

ICD-9-CM Code: 253.0

ETIOLOGY

- >99% of cases result from primary pituitary adenoma

USUAL TREATMENT

- Surgery — primary therapy
  - Transsphenoidal pituitary microsurgery vs. transcranial; transsphenoidal more common, with less morbidity. Smaller tumors (<10 mm diameter) yield probable cure.
- Pituitary radiation — reserved for persistent postsurgical disease
- Medical — adjunctive therapy or for nonsurgical candidates
  - Dopamine agonists — bromocriptine
  - Somatostatin analogue — octreotide

ASSESSMENT POINTS

SYSTEM	EFFECT	ASSESSMENT BY HX	PE	TEST
HEENT	Bone and soft tissue overgrowth of head and neck	TMJ arthritis Hoarseness	Enlarged frontal, nasal bones Macroglossia Prognathism Vocal cord thickening Subglottic narrowing	Indirect laryngoscopy Lateral neck x-rays CT of neck
CV	PVD LV dysfunction (?cardiomyopathy)	HTN CHF Dysrhythmias	HTN CHF Dysrhythmias Cardiomegaly	CXR ECG ECHO
RESP	Airway soft tissue overgrowth	Obstructive sleep apnea	Kyphoscoliosis	PFTs (if indicated)
RENAL	↑ (GI) Ca^{2+} absorption ↑ Intravascular volume	Urolithiasis	↑ Total body Na^+, plasma vol	
ENDO	↑ BMR	Heat intolerance	Hyperhidrosis	To diagnose acromegaly: ↑ 24 hr GH levels ↑ serum IGF I Oral glucose tolerance test (GH levels do not ↓)
	Hyperprolactinemia	↓ Libido, impotence Menstrual abnormalities		
	Hyperthyroidism (3–7%) Glucose intolerance (30–45%) (10–20% overt DM) Hypertriglyceridemia (20–45%)		Goiter	Thyroid function Glucose
CNS	Pituitary mass effect	Hypersomnolence Visual field defects		CT MRI
PNS	Carpal tunnel syndrome	Paresthesias	Median nerve compression	EMG, NCVs
MS	Bone and soft tissue overgrowth Osteoporosis	Arthralgias/arthritis (knees, hips, shoulders, LS spine)	Enlarged hands and feet	X-rays
	Myopathy	Fatigue, weakness	Muscle weakness	

Key Reference: Katz J, Benumof JL, Kadis LB (eds): Anesthesia and Uncommon Diseases, 3rd ed. Philadelphia, WB Saunders, 1990, pp. 264, 300.

PERIOPERATIVE IMPLICATIONS

Preoperative Preparation

- Optimize hemodynamics — BP control, no CHF

Monitoring

- Pulse oximeter may be difficult to fit (large fingers, toes); if A-line, brachial or femoral preferable

Airway

- Large masks, airways, blades available.
- Consider awake fiberoptic endotracheal intubation.

Induction

- If GA, anticipate airway obstruction.

Maintenance

- For transsphenoidal approach — surgical use of cocaine.
- If preop pneumoencephalography, do not use nitrous oxide.

Extubation

- Anticipate airway obstruction.

Adjuvants

- If myopathy, cautious use of muscle relaxants.

- If sleep apnea, cautious use of narcotics.
- If peripheral neuropathy, document prior to regional.

Postoperative Period

- Diabetes insipidus <5% of patients
- CSF rhinorrhea <5% of patients
- Anterior pituitary insufficiency (ACTH , TSH, gonadotropins)
- Meningitis, sinusitis, hematoma, cranial nerve palsy <1% each

ANTICIPATED PROBLEMS/CONCERNS

- Airway management
- Hemodynamic stability

ADDISON'S DISEASE

Stephen P. Fischer, M.D.

RISK

- People within USA: 1 per 100,000
- Race/gender predominance: none

PERIOPERATIVE RISKS

- Increased risk of circulatory collapse 2° to inability to respond to stress
- Postop instability may be > than intraoperative

WORRY ABOUT

- Addisonian crisis
- ↓ Response to circulating catecholamines
- Severe hypotension with ↓ SVR and ↓ LV stroke index
- Cardiac conduction abnormalities, including hyperkalemic arrest
- Volume status/electrolyte imbalance

OVERVIEW

- Primary adrenal insufficiency with cortex destruction
- Glucocorticoid/mineralocorticoid deficiency (especially if bilateral)
- Perioperative stress increased with magnitude of surgery
- Dx by ACTH stimulation test
- Clinical Sx usually insidious over months
- Proper treatment should result in normal life expectancy if no associated diseases

ICD-9-CM Code: 255.4

ETIOLOGY

- Autoimmune destruction of adrenal cortex (80% of nonexogenous steroid–induced cases)
- Associated with Hashimoto's, TB, sepsis, adrenal hemorrhage (anticoagulants)
- Congenital adrenal hyperplasia (rare); autosomal recessive
- Associated with suppression of adrenocortical function due to exogenous steroids

USUAL TREATMENT

- Surgical excision of adrenal gland(s)
- Glucocorticoid/mineralocorticoid replacement

ASSESSMENT POINTS

SYSTEM	EFFECT	ASSESSMENT BY HX	PE	TEST
HEENT	Severe dental caries	Pain, loose teeth	Teeth for structural stability	
CV	Hypotension/hypovolemia Cardiopenia ↓ Response to catecholamines Arrhythmias if ↑ K+	Orthostatic Sx		BP change on standing CXR ECG, K+
RESP	Possible resp muscle weakness	Exercise tolerance	2-flight walk	
GI	Dehydration/hypovolemia Abdominal pain/cramping	Nausea/emesis/diarrhea Orthostatic Sx		Na+, Cl–, K+ BP change on standing
RENAL	Azotemia			BUN/Cr
ENDO	↓ Na+, ↓ Cl–, ↓ glucose, ↑ K+			Na+, Cl–, K+, glucose
HEME	Hemoconcentration Lymphocytosis/eosinophilia			CBC
CNS		Nervous/mental irritability		
MS	Muscle weakness Weight loss	Fatigue Anorexia	Strength (ability) to rise from chair without using hands	K+ Albumin

Key Reference: Roizen MF: *In* Miller RD (ed): Anesthesia, 4th ed. New York, Churchill Livingstone, 1994, pp 916–922.

PERIOPERATIVE IMPLICATIONS

Preoperative Preparation

- Correct hypovolemia, hyperkalemia, hyponatremia, hypoglycemia
- Stress steroid coverage: up to 300 mg/d hydrocortisone/70 kg body wt
- For mineralocorticoid treatment: 0.05–0.1 mg PO fludrocortisone
- Benzodiazepine premed OK

Monitoring

- Consider arterial and pulmonary artery catheterization if cardiac filling pressures indicated/major surgery

Airway

- No change from usual

Induction

- No specific anesthesia regimen superior

Maintenance

- May not see changes in HR despite ↓ SVR
- Check electrolytes, glucose intraoperatively

Extubation

- Prolonged emergence possible

Adjuvants

- Avoid etomidate: causes adrenal suppression
- Myocardial sensitivity to drugs (narcotics/barbiturates)
- Muscle weakness/wt loss may require a reduced muscle relaxant dose

Postoperative Period

- CXR for pneumothorax if adrenalectomy: up to 20% postop
- ↑ Pancreatitis with left adrenalectomy
- Perioperative steroids may ↓ wound healing, ↑ infections, ↑ stress ulcers, ↑ glucose intolerance, ↑ BP
- Postop stress greater than intraop

ANTICIPATED PROBLEMS/CONCERNS

- Addisonian crisis/circulatory collapse both intra- and postop. Consider ICU observation postop.
- Cardiac arrhythmias with hyperkalemia

ADRENAL INSUFFICIENCY, ACUTE OR SECONDARY

Charles B. Hantler, M.D.

RISK

- Risk of adrenal insufficiency 1/4000–1/10,000 (if steroids used in prior year)
- With steroids >20 mg/day (cortisol equivalent), >7–14 d within 1 y
- Clinical signs worse with stress, such as trauma, surgery, or infection

PERIOPERATIVE RISKS

- Increases cardiovascular instability, fever, CHF, electrolyte abnormalities
- High cardiac output failure with signs of tissue hypoperfusion
- Often evidence of systemic vasodilation with decreased reactivity to vasopressors

WORRY ABOUT

- GI; N/V; dehydration and risk of aspiration
- Anemia, neutropenia with androgen deficiency: rare
- CV response; ↓ SVR, ? cardiac reserve, and ↓ vascular responsiveness to maintain perfusion pressure; steroids necessary for blood vessel responsiveness to catecholamines

- Hyperkalemia with/without hyponatremia; usually aldosterone deficiency; cardiac conduction abnormalities

OVERVIEW

- Adrenal insufficiency due to exogenous steroid administration leads to inadequate production of glucocorticoids (cortisol), mineralocorticoids (aldosterone), and androgens
- May present without symptoms until stress
- Chronic adrenal insufficiency from use of steroids in prior year may manifest as weakness, fatigue, nausea, emesis, weight loss, and a variety of psychiatric disturbances
- Inadequate mineralocorticoid production can cause hyperkalemia, hyponatremia, and metabolic acidosis, with or without signs of dehydration
- Inadequate glucocorticoid production may cause signs of hemodynamic instability (hypotension) during stress
- Abdominal trauma and/or sepsis may cause signs of adrenal corticoid insufficiency, which resolve within hours of steroid administration
- Anecdotal evidence exists of restoration of circulatory function (e.g., normalization of car-

diac output and SVR) following steroid administration in cases of trauma, and of possible synthetic glucocorticoid–induced adrenal suppression that resolved with the intraoperative administration of synthetic glucocorticoid

ICD-9-CM Code: 255.4
See also Addison's Disease (in Diseases section)

ETIOLOGY

- Inadequate replacement of synthetic glucocorticoids
- Renin deficiency (hypoaldosterone) rare

USUAL THERAPY

- Normal conditions: 12–15 mg/m² of hydrocortisone replacement daily
- Minor stress (minor surgery): 50–75 mg or about 2× normal production for 1–2 days postoperatively
- Major stress (major trauma, major surgery): 150–200 mg of hydrocortisone per day 2–3 days postoperatively, followed by taper to usual dose
- Aldosterone deficiency (manifested by abnormalities in Na⁺/K⁺ or dehydration): fludrocortisone (Florinef), 50–200 µg/day

ASSESSMENT POINTS

SYSTEM	EFFECT	ASSESSMENT BY HX	PE	TEST
CV	Dehydration Hypotension High-output failure	Postural symptoms Fatigue Wt loss, Hx of surgery on adrenals, pituitary	Low BP, postural drop Signs of dehydration	Hct(?), BUN/Cr, adrenal, ACTH stimulation, insulin tolerance, metyrapone test
RESP	CHF (high or low output)	DOE, SOB	S₃, rales	CXR
GI	Dehydration, nausea, emesis	Appetite Hx of emesis	See CV	Lytes
HEME	Anemia Neutropenia			Hct WBC
CNS	Depression, confusion, psychosis			Reverses with replacement
MS	Weakness, potentiation of neuromuscular blockage			Nerve stimulator

Key Reference: Werbel SS, Ober KP: Acute adrenal insufficiency: Endocrinology Metab Clin North Am 1993; 22:303–328.

PERIOPERATIVE IMPLICATIONS

Preoperative Preparation

- Consider perioperative steroid coverage if benfits outweigh risks if high index of suspicion of adrenal depression (e.g., supraphysiologic doses of steroids for >1 wk within last year)
- Correct electrolyte abnormalities, hypoglycemia, and dehydration prior to elective surgery
- Fludrocortisone with resistant aldosterone (K⁺ and Na⁺) abnormalities; glucose for hypoglycemia

Monitoring

- ECG for signs of abnormal conduction (QRS duration, u waves)
- Consider CVP, PCWP, or TEE if fluid/electrolyte abnormalities

Airway

- None

Premedication/Induction

- Consider volume status with regard to hydration and choice of agents

Maintenance

- No hemodynamic instability: follow electrolytes and glucose as needed
- Hemodynamic instability (hypotension):
  – R/O other causes, then consider hydrocortisone hemisuccinate, 25–100 mg IV then 100 mg q 12–24 h for 2–3 days
  – Fluid resuscitation as needed

Extubation

- Possible potentiation of nondepolarizing muscle relaxants with use of high-dose steroids; ensure adequate muscle relaxant reversal

Adjuvants

- Glucose, fluids, careful monitoring of temperature to avoid hyperthermia

Postoperative Period

- Stress steroids poss required several days postop
- High steroid doses may be assoc with ↓ wound healing and immunodepression with infection risk
- Consider prolonged steroid coverage if severe stress continues (e.g., severe trauma with multiple operations)
- Mineralocorticoid administration as needed; usually glucocorticoids have significant mineralocorticoid action

ANTICIPATED PROBLEMS/CONCERNS

- Severe resistant hypotension, hyperthermia, and CNS abnormalities, such as confusion, coma, lethargy, may occur intraoperatively or postoperatively and may be unpredictable
- Syndrome may occur in severely traumatized patients without history of steroid use, with clinical picture of sepsis and associated abnormalities in adrenal function; Rx is lifesaving

ADULT RESPIRATORY DISTRESS SYNDROME (ARDS)

David Olson, M.D.
Jesse Hall, M.D.

RISK

- In US: approximately 5 cases per 100,000 population per year; many predisposing conditions occur in perioperative setting (e.g., aspiration, hemorrhagic shock, sepsis) and have incidence of acute lung injury as predictably high as 30–40%
- Racial predominance: None
- Mortality ranges widely, 25–75%, determined largely by predisposing conditions (e.g., highest when associated with sepsis or aspiration, lowest when associated with tocolytic Rx or other easily reversed conditions)

PERIOPERATIVE RISKS

- Profound hypoxemia following any ↓ in cardiac output (intraoperative fluid shift, ↑ PEEP, myocardial depression) due to mixed venous O_2 desaturation in presence of large intrapulmonary shunt
- ↑ FIO_2 requirements and worsened shunt due to dependent lung atelectasis, large intraoperative fluid requirements

WORRY ABOUT

- Inability of standard operating room ventilators to deliver minute ventilation and inspiratory pressures often required
- Maintaining required PEEP during manual bag ventilation and patient transport
- Minimizing fluid administration to avoid edemagenesis on one hand, and inadequate cardiac output, and hence oxygen delivery, on the other

OVERVIEW

- Defined as acute onset of lung dysfunction with PaO_2/FIO_2 ≤200 mmHg (regardless of PEEP level), 3–4 quadrant infiltrates on CXR, PCWP ≤18 when measured, or no clinical evidence of left atrial hypertension
- Within 72 h of clearly identifiable clinical predisposition: sepsis syndrome, aspiration, hypertransfusion during shock resuscitation, pancreatitis, near-drowning, or following pneumonia, DIC, CNS injury, inhaled toxins, cardiopulmonary bypass, air or fat embolism, opiate or other drug overdose
- Differentiated from focal pulmonary processes (e.g., lobar pneumonia) because standard Rx for ARDS (e.g., PEEP) may worsen gas exchange in focal disease
- Clinically useful to distinguish two phases: exudative (first 7–10 days with pulmonary capillary leak and proliferative (10 days to several weeks); exudative phase, reduce edemagenesis and lung injury; proliferative phase ARDS: abnormal deposition and fibrosis with increased dead space fraction, predisposition to zone 1 lung, high minute ventilation requirements, less PEEP, and high FIO_2 dependency, and more fixed pulmonary hypertension
- Mortality from ARDS results primarily from predisposing injury, sepsis from superinfection, or multi-system organ failure (MSOF)

ICD-9-CM Code: 518.81 (with respiratory failure)

ETIOLOGY

- Two mechanisms: direct parenchymal cell injury (e.g., aspiration) or indirect injury resulting from a systemic inflammatory response (e.g., sepsis) producing a derangement of lung microvascular permeability resulting in extensive alveolar and interstitial edema, with subsequent development of fibrin and collagen deposition characterizing the proliferative phase

USUAL TREATMENT

- Respiratory: mechanical ventilation using least degree of PEEP to provide O_2 saturation of ≥90% on nontoxic FIO_2 (≤0.6); maintain transpulmonary pressures (≈ plateau pressure) at ≤35 cm H_2O by employing permissive hypercapnia through use of low tidal volumes (6–8 ml/kg) and correction of respiratory acidosis <7.15 with bicarbonate; other ventilator strategies or pharmacologic interventions (nitric oxide, surfactant) may be useful as salvage therapy
- Circulatory: reduce edemagenesis through fluid restriction or judicious diuretic or inotrope therapy; correct anemia (Hct = 30–35); ↓ oxygen demands by sedation, paralysis, fever reduction; late (proliferative) ARDS may require higher filling pressures to overcome increased dead space and zone 1 lung
- Diagnosis and treatment of underlying condition and prevention of complications (superinfection, barotrauma, GI bleeding, protein-calorie malnutrition, MSOF)

ASSESSMENT POINTS

SYSTEM	EFFECT	ASSESSMENT BY HX	PE	TEST
CV	↓ CO	Hypotension, hypoxemia, ↓ mental status, urine output	Cool extremities, narrow pulse pressure	PA catheter, MvO_2 sat, urine electrolytes
	Pulm HTN		↑ P_2, RV heave, peripheral edema	PA catheter, ECHO
RESP	Barotrauma	Hypotension, hypoxemia, ↑ Paw	Absent breath sounds, tracheal deviation	CXR
	Pneumonia	Fever, ↑ WBC/bandemia, purulent tracheal aspirate	Focal rales, hyperdynamic circulation	CXR, blood and sputum culture Bronchoscopy
GI	Hemorrhage	↓ Hct	Melena, bloody NG output	Guaiac stool, esophagogastroduodenoscopy
GU	↓ Function	↓ CO, urine output Nephrotoxic drugs, multisystem organ failure		Cr Urine electrolytes
MS	Prolonged weakness	Pharmacologic paralysis	Diffuse myopathy	Electromyography, muscle biopsy

PERIOPERATIVE IMPLICATIONS

Preoperative Preparation

- Reevaluate least PEEP required to maintain adequate arterial saturation
- Have proper ventilator available in OR to meet patient's minute ventilation and airway pressure demands
- Correct hypovolemia, fluid overload
- Consider use of mechanical ventilation during transport
- Meticulous attention to aseptic technique

Monitoring

- PA catheter, particularly in exudative phase, when fluid shifts can produce marked hypoxemia

- TEE may be useful in estimating adequate cardiac filling and cardiac output

Airway

- Loss of PEEP during ET tube disconnect, even for a few seconds, can produce profound hypoxemia that may take many minutes or hours to reverse

Preinduction/Induction

- Expect worsening shunt with loss of hypoxemic pulmonary vasoconstriction and/or V/Q mismatch with increased FIO_2 requirements intraoperatively

Maintenance

- Maintain appropriate LV filling pressures to avoid worsening edema with excessive fluid administration or increased dead space and diminished cardiac output with inadequate fluid administration
- Maintain adequate circulating hemoglobin

Postoperative Period

- Close monitoring of volume status, PEEP requirements
- Reduce FIO_2 to nontoxic levels as soon as possible

ANTICIPATED PROBLEMS/CONCERNS

- Maintaining adequate oxygenation on nontoxic FIO_2 requires vigilant attention to volume status
- Vigilance to complications of mechanical ventilation (O_2 toxicity, barotrauma, ↓ CO, pneumonia)
- Superinfection, MSOF associated with worse prognosis

ALCOHOL ABUSE

Scott Metzger, M.D.

RISK

- People within US: 15 million
- Alcoholic physicians in US: 22,000
- Third leading cause of death and disability
- Male gender and family Hx major risk factors

PERIOPERATIVE RISKS

- Severe malnutrition as significant as ethanol-induced end-organ injury
- Risk of HTN, stroke, diabetes, GI disease
- Liver most severely affected organ
- Dilated cardiomyopathy
- Withdrawal symptoms can themselves be life-threatening

WORRY ABOUT

- Concomitant use of amphetamines, cocaine, diazepam
- Chronic smoking and COPD
- Vasopressor effect of ethanol or its withdrawal may cause HTN
- Avoid all medications with ETOH, including skin prep solutions
- Withdrawal symptoms

OVERVIEW

- Large number of individuals have the disease characterized by addiction (compulsion and craving despite consequences) to alcohol
- Clinical syndromes related to direct effect of ethanol and secondary adaptive response to excess ETOH exposure

- Ethanol rapidly absorbed and metabolized
- Hepatic dysfunction usually takes 10–15 y to develop
- Cirrhosis may develop after 1 or more acute episodes

ICD-9-CM Code: 303.0 (acute)

ETIOLOGY

- Unknown: has environmental, genetic, and psychosocial components

USUAL TREATMENT

- Recovery involves almost all of the following:
  - disulfiram (Antabuse): acetaldehyde dehydrogenase inhibitor
  - Alcoholics Anonymous
  - psychiatric counseling

ASSESSMENT POINTS

SYSTEM	EFFECT	ASSESSMENT BY HX	PE	TEST
CV	Cardiomyopathy Arrhythmias Hypertension	Orthopnea, nocturnal urination, coughing, and leg swelling	Dyspnea BP lying and standby HR	ECG, ECHO Electrolytes
GI	Erosive gastritis	Hx of bleeding		Upper endoscopy, stool guaiac
	Hepatic cirrhosis Acute hepatitis	Easily bruised Anorexia, N/V	Ascites, jaundice Hepatomegaly, "spider" angiomas	LFTs LFTs
	Pancreatitis Fatty liver		Abd pain Abd pain, hepatomegaly	Serum amylase Mg^{2+}; K^+
ENDO	Gynecomastia, testicular atrophy, irregular menses			
HEME	Leukopenia, anemia, thrombocytopenia			CBC with differential
CNS	Wernicke's syndrome Korsakoff's syndrome Peripheral polyneuropathy Cerebellar degeneration	Amnesia, impaired reasoning	Sixth nerve palsy, ataxia CNS exam Distal numbness and paresthesias Unsteady gait	MRI or CT scan

Key Reference: Lieber CS: Medical disorders of alcoholism. N Engl J Med 1995; 333:1058–1065.

PERIOPERATIVE IMPLICATIONS

Preoperative Preparation

- Gastric prophylaxis
- Blood ETOH and toxicology screen if indicated

Monitoring

- Routine
- Consider invasive monitors for severe cardiomyopathy and hepatic dysfunction

Airway

- Consider full stomach in acute intoxication

Preinduction/Induction

- Consider long-acting benzodiazepine or barbiturate
- Anesthetic doses increased in chronic disease

- Decreased dose in acute intoxication
- Rapid sequence in acute intoxication
- Consider Rx of nutritional/metabolic deficiencies

Maintenance

- Requirements vary by age, general health, nutrition and hydration states, concomitant disease

Extubation

- Ensure return of airway reflexes

Postoperative Period

- Provide adequate analgesia in PACU
- Anxiety can worsen withdrawal symptoms
- Withdrawal syndrome may develop within 6–8 h; treat with IV ETOH, ß-adrenergic agonist, α_2-adrenergic agonist, benzodiazepines

- DTs develop in 5% of patients in withdrawal
- 10% mortality secondary to hypotension, arrhythmias; treat with diazepam, ß-adrenergic agonist

Adjuvants

- Long-term consumption of ETOH impairs hepatic metabolism
- Short-term consumption inhibits drug metabolism
- Polyneuropathy a relative contraindication to regional anesthesia
- Consider clonidine patch perioperatively

ANTICIPATED PROBLEMS/CONCERNS

- Recognition and treatment of withdrawal important, as significant mortality occurs if inadequately treated

ALLERGY

Tesuji Makita, M.D.
Jerrold H. Levy, M.D.

RISK

- 5% of adults in USA are allergic to one or more drugs.
- The incidence of perioperative anaphylaxis is 1:4500, with a mortality of 6%.
- Females > males (1.6:1)

PERIOPERATIVE RISKS

- Intensity of Sx variable: from an isolated cutaneous eruption to CV collapse and death
- CV, cutaneous, respiratory systems are mostly involved
- Increased morbidity and hospitalization time if intensive care required

WORRY ABOUT

- Patient's Hx: Knowledge of prior allergic event leads to avoiding drugs or other components involved.
- Hypotension, bronchospasm, and swelling may become life-threatening events.

OVERVIEW

- IgE anaphylaxis (type I immediate hypersensitivity reaction): Adverse response of host; mediated by antibodies: the antigen bridges with two IgE on the surface of basophils and mast cells; can be reproduced if foreign substance reinjected.
- Anaphylactoid reaction or histamine release: describes a clinically indistinguishable syndrome, probably involving similar mediators but not mediated by IgE antibody and not necessarily requiring previous exposure to the inciting substance, associated with vancomycin, benzylisoquilinium-derived muscle relaxants.

ICD-9-CM Codes: 995.3 (allergic reaction); 477.0–477.9 (inhaled allergen)
See also Anaphylaxis.

ETIOLOGY

- Clinical history of allergy or perianesthetic allergic reaction considered to put patient at increased risk for a reaction, from neuromuscular blocking agents, induction agents.

USUAL TREATMENT

- "Preventive therapy" with corticosteroids and antihistamines is of unproven value.
- Severe allergic therapy: Stop antigen; maintain the airway with 100% O_2 and intubate if necessary; discontinue all anesthetic drugs; volume expansion; epinephrine (5–10 µg IV boluses as starting doses and titrate upward); antihistamines; ß$_2$-sympathomimetic if bronchospasm; phosphodiesterase inhibitors for RV dysfunction, airway evaluation prior to extubation; ICU observation.

ASSESSMENT POINTS

SYSTEM	EFFECT	PE	TEST
CV	Hypotension Tachycardia, dysrhythmias Pulmonary hypertension Cardiac arrest	BP	ECG PA pressure
RESP	Dyspnea, sneezing Coughing, wheezing Laryngeal edema Fulminant pulmonary edema Acute respiratory failure	Chest exam	CXR PA catheter End tidal CO_2 ABG
SKIN	Urticaria, flushing Perioral, periorbital edema	Skin exam	

Key Reference: Levy JH: Anaphylactic Reactions in Anesthesia and Intensive Care, 2nd ed. Boston, Butterworth-Heinemann, 1992.

PERIOPERATIVE IMPLICATIONS

Preoperative Preparation

- Prick tests, intradermal testing: anesthetic drugs (muscle relaxant)
- Most of the allergic reactions are unexpected. In case of established allergy, those drugs or latex should be strictly avoided.

Monitoring

- Routine if major anaphylaxis occurs, consider pulmonary and radial arterial catheterization to guide therapeutic interventions.

Airway

- None, except specific care for the asthmatic patient

Preinduction/Induction/Maintenance/Extubation

- Slow injection of drugs. Avoid histamine-releasing drugs in high-risk patients.

ANTICIPATED PROBLEMS/CONCERNS

- Consider for each patient who has a perioperative allergic reaction evaluation 1 mo after with skin testing, antigen-specific IgE level dosage (radioallergosorbent test, ELISA).
- Latex allergy incidence is increasing and Hx has to be evoked at the preanesthetic evaluation.

AMNIOTIC FLUID EMBOLISM

P. Allan Klock, Jr., M.D.

RISK

- Prevalence: 0.8 to 5 cases/100,000 live births

PERIOPERATIVE RISKS

- Amniotic fluid embolism accounts for approximately 9% of maternal deaths in USA
- Mortality is approximately 86%

WORRY ABOUT

- Hypoxia
- Cardiopulmonary collapse
- Right heart failure
- DIC—occurs in nearly all survivors of the initial catastrophic event
- Hemorrhage—40% of amniotic fluid embolism-associated deaths are due to hemorrhage.

OVERVIEW

- Amniotic fluid going to central circulation
- There are three necessary conditions:
  - amniotomy (rent in the membranes)
  - laceration of endocervical or uterine vessels
  - pressure gradient (intrauterine pressure > CVP or uterine venous pressure)
- Although not a common disease of pregnancy amniotic fluid embolism has a significant impact on health care providers because it is usually fatal and often presents without warning.

ICD-9-CM Code: 673.1

ETIOLOGY

- Postulated mechanism of action: Powerful contractions force amniotic fluid into the maternal circulation through a defect in the fetal membranes, placenta, or elsewhere.

- Risk factors: Advanced maternal age; multiparity (88% of patients with amniotic fluid embolism are multiparas); meconium (present in 75% of cases); cervical laceration (present in 50% of cases); intrauterine fetal demise (present in 40% of cases); very strong, frequent, or "tetanic" contractions; sudden fetal expulsion; uterine rupture; choramnionitis; macrosomia.

USUAL TREATMENT

- Treatment is usually supportive.
- Case reports of successful treatment with cardiopulmonary bypass and thrombectomy
- Employ left uterine displacement to prevent aortocaval compression.
- Stop oxytocin infusion if present.
- Cardiopulmonary resuscitation (100% O_2 with PEEP)
- Pressors and inotropes will often be required.
- Delivery of fetus as soon as is practical; may require operative or cesarean delivery.
- Replacement of clotting factors if patient develops DIC.

ASSESSMENT POINTS

SYSTEM	EFFECT	ASSESSMENT BY HX	PE	TEST
CV	Tachycardia Hypotension			
RESP	Hypoxia Pulmonary edema	Dyspnea	Tachypnea Cyanosis Frothy pink sputum	Pulse oximetry Aspirate blood from the PA or renal artery Stain the buffy coat for cells and mucin
GI		Nausea	Vomiting	
HEME	DIC		Excessive bleeding Thrombolysis (bleeding from IV sites)	PT, PTT, plt, fibrinogen, FSP
CNS		Anxiety	Convulsions Shivering Sweating	

Key Reference: Sperry K: Amniotic fluid embolism. JAMA 1986; 255:2183–2186.

PERIOPERATIVE IMPLICATIONS

- Usually this disease presents as sudden CV collapse.

Preoperative Preparation

- Maximize maternal oxygen delivery.
- Place several large-bore IVs.
- Notify blood bank of anticipated coagulopathy and crossmatch for several units of packed RBCs and FFP.
- Consider preparing for cardiopulmonary bypass if an option.

Monitoring

- If suspected, consider PA catheter to aspirate blood, hemodynamic management.

Maintenance

- Usually resuscitative with support of breathing and circulation
- Case reports of use of CPB

Extubation

- If survive, remain intubated until stable.

ANTICIPATED PROBLEMS/CONCERNS

- Not all sudden deaths during the peripartum period are due to amniotic fluid embolism. The pathologic diagnosis is quite specific (finding hair, mucin, or nucleated squamous cells in the maternal circulation), but its sensitivity is unknown.
- The emotional impact on caregivers can be tremendous. One should confirm the pathologic diagnosis and share the results of the postmortem examination with those who helped care for the deceased. While surgeons and anesthesiologists occasionally witness an intraoperative death, labor and delivery nurses are not accustomed to having their patients die. Psychologic counseling may be helpful for those who have difficulty after the event.

AMYLOIDOSIS

Kenneth J. Holroyd, M.D.

RISK
- People within USA: 50,000
- Race with highest prevalence: unknown

PERIOPERATIVE RISKS
- Increased risk of perioperative renal failure, CHF; bleeding from coagulopathy
- Autonomic neuropathy

WORRY ABOUT
- Signs of CHF
- Decreasing urine output

OVERVIEW
- Extracellular deposition of amyloid type proteins
- Congo red stain of tissue reveals green birefringence in a polarizing microscope
- Associated end-stage renal, myocardial, and neuropathic disease
- Best diagnosed by subcutaneous abdominal fat pad aspirate or rectal biopsy

ICD-9-CM Code: 277.3

ETIOLOGY
- Both acquired and hereditary forms exist.
- Major risk factors for acquired disease: multiple myeloma, chronic infectious or inflammatory disease (osteomyelitis, rheumatoid arthritis)
- Hereditary forms very rare

USUAL TREATMENT
- Acquired: treat underlying disease
- Hereditary: colchicine, liver transplantation

ASSESSMENT POINTS

SYSTEM	EFFECT	ASSESSMENT BY HX	PE	TEST
HEENT	Macroglossia Tracheal stenosis	Enlarged tongue Dyspnea	Macroglossia Stridor	CT scan Flow-volume loop
CV	Restrictive myopathy LV and RV dysfunction Conduction abnormalities	Exercise tolerance Dyspnea Syncope	S_3 Bradycardia	ECHO ECG
RESP	CHF Lung nodules	Cough Chest wall pain	Rales	CXR
GI	Autonomic dysfunction	Wt loss Diarrhea		Biopsy
HEME	Factor X deficiency	Bruising	Periorbital bruises	Factor X assay
RENAL	Decreased renal perfusion Nephrotic syndrome			BUN/Cr Urine
CNS	Autonomic neuropathy	Inability to sweat; hoarseness; early satiety; postural dizziness	Orthostasis	Biopsy

Key Reference: Mizutani AR, Ward CF: Amyloidosis associated bleeding diatheses in the surgical patient. Can J Anaesth 1990; 37:910–912.

PERIOPERATIVE IMPLICATIONS

Preoperative Preparation
- Optimize treatment of heart failure.
- Avoid dehydration (renal failure).

Monitoring
- Consider PA catheter for large fluid shift operations or patients with severe LV dysfunction.

Airway
- Macroglossia or tracheal stenosis
- Increased risk of bleeding into airway from capillary fragility and possible coagulopathy

Preinduction/Induction
- May develop reduced CO and hypotension
- Coagulopathy may contraindicate regional anesthesia

Maintenance
- No agent or technique shown superior
- Maintain adequate urine output

Extubation
- Patient fully awake to minimize risk of reintubation
- Caution with nasal airway—may cause hemorrhage

Postoperative Period
- Close monitoring of CV and renal status
- Consider ICU setting for postop care

Adjuvants
- Avoid digoxin—not usually helpful in treating amyloid CHF, associated with increased arrhythmias

ANTICIPATED PROBLEMS/CONCERNS
- Difficult airway
- CHF
- Hypotension
- Renal failure

AMYOTROPHIC LATERAL SCLEROSIS (ALS) Daniel J. Cole, M.D.

RISK

- Annual incidence: 0.8–1.5:100,000
- Prevalence: 4–6:100,000
- Age (most common) at onset: 55–60 y
- Male:female incidence: 1.5:1
- Minimal racial/geographic variation: decreased incidence African-Americans (?). Increased prevalence in Guam and regions of Japan.

PERIOPERATIVE RISKS

- Aspiration
- Respiratory failure
- Infection

WORRY ABOUT

- Hyperkalemia after succinylcholine
- Prolonged response to nondepolarizing muscle relaxants
- Respiratory failure postoperatively

OVERVIEW

- A degenerative process causing upper and lower motor neuron death with denervation and atrophy of corresponding muscle fibers. If condition is limited to motor cortex, disease is termed primary lateral sclerosis; with limitation to brainstem nuclei, pseudobulbar palsy; with limitation to spinal cord, progressive muscular atrophy. Typically, extraocular muscles, bowel/bladder sphincters, sensory system, movement coordination, intellect remain intact. ALS may be associated with malignant tumors.
- Laboratory aids in diagnosis:
  - ↑ serum creatinine kinase in ~⅔ of patients
  - ↓ compound muscle action potential
  - EMG evidence of denervation with reinnervation
  - abnormal evoked responses
- Progressive course leading to death within 3–5 y (50% of cases)

ICD-9-CM Code: 335.20

ETIOLOGY

- Genetic predisposition in <5% of cases (autosomal dominant gene). Other hypotheses include:
  - Autoimmune factors, excitotoxins, viral factors, exogenous toxins, other neurotransmitters/neuropeptides

USUAL TREATMENT

- Supportive care:
  - Psychosocial support, exercise, baclofen for spasticity, antihistamines/anticholinergics for sialorrhea, pyridostigmine sometimes increases strength
  - Tube feedings if difficulty swallowing
  - Chest physiotherapy, bronchodilators, and mechanical ventilation

ASSESSMENT POINTS

SYSTEM	EFFECT	ASSESSMENT BY HX	PE	TEST
HEENT	Dysfunction of pharyngeal muscles, dysphagia, dysarthria, sialorrhea	Dysphagia, dysarthria, sialorrhea	Gag reflex	
CV	Vagal dysfunction		Tachycardia	
RESP	Respiratory impairment from muscle weakness and diaphragm paralysis; susceptible to infection and aspiration	Dyspnea, restlessness, fatigue, lethargy, apnea, regurgitation, cough, fever, sputum	↓ Breath sounds and excursion, wheezing	CXR (to rule out current infection) PFTs (optional) ABG
GI	Poor nutrition	Caloric intake Infection		Serum albumin/transferrin Skin test anergy
ENDO	Abnormal glucose/Ca^{2+} metabolism, thyroid dysfunction, B_{12} and hexosaminidase A deficiency, dysproteinemia, vasculitis, ganglioside antibodies			Hyperglycemia Hypercalcemia Fractures on x-ray
CNS	Motor cell loss in cortex, brain stem, spinal cord	Dysarthria, dysphagia, labile emotional expression, dementia (<5% of cases)		Abnormal evoked responses
MS	Loss of large myelinated fibers in ventral roots with abnormalities of the motor end-plate	Muscle weakness and atrophy	Spasticity Fasciculations Hyperreflexia	↑ Serum creatinine kinase, ↓ muscle action potential, denervation with evidence of reinnervation on EMG, abnormal evoked responses

Key Reference: Swash M, Schwartz MS: What do we really know about amyotrophic lateral sclerosis? J Neurol Sci 1992; 113:4–16.

PERIOPERATIVE IMPLICATIONS

Preoperative Preparation

- Maximize respiratory status. Treat any superimposed respiratory condition.
- Become familar with communication difficulties.

Monitoring

- Routine

Airway

- Management of secretions

Induction

- Local or regional anesthesia if possible.
- If general anesthetic necessary, avoid succinylcholine (hyperkalemic response) and expect an exaggerated response and response duration to nondepolarizing muscle relaxants.
- May be susceptible to aspiration

Maintenance

- No technique shown to be superior (in theory, local or regional technique preferable).

Extubation

- Low risk for postop mechanical ventilation if peak inspiratory pressure >30cm H_2O, vital capacity >1.5 L, and no concurrent problems.
- Moderate risk for postop mechanical ventilation if peak inspiratory pressure 20–30cm H_2O, vital capacity 1.0–1.5 L, or mild hypercarbia.
- High risk for postop mechanical ventilation if peak inspiratory pressure <20cm H_2O, vital capacity <1.0 L, hypercarbic, hypoxic, or a concurrent problem.

Adjuvants

- Avoid succinylcholine (hyperkalemic response)
- Pyridostigmine to ↑ muscle strength

Postoperative Period

- Monitor for respiratory failure or complications.
- Pain management may be critical for return of baseline motor function.
- Glucose management
- Communication difficulties

ANTICIPATED PROBLEMS/CONCERNS

- Respiratory insufficiency with potential requirement for prolonged mechanical ventilation. Treat concurrent conditions (e.g., pneumonia) that may exacerbate respiratory status.
- Aspiration from weak pharyngeal muscles. Extubate when patient completely awake with full return of baseline muscle function.
- Prolonged response to nondepolarizing muscle relaxants.
- Hyperkalemic response to succinylcholine.

ANAPHYLAXIS

Jonathan Moss, M.D., Ph.D.

RISK

- Approximately 1 in 5000 anesthetic procedures
- Females outnumber males 3:1.
- No prospective data to suggest an increased risk of generalized allergy, although Hx of atopy is overrepresented in several series of life-threatening anaphylaxis to anesthetic agents.

PERIOPERATIVE RISKS

- Significant risks of life-threatening airway compromise, CV collapse, and bronchospasm—particularly severe in patients on ß blockers

WORRY ABOUT

- Patients with pre-existing ASCVD tolerate CV sequelae poorly
- Patients with Hx of allergy to anesthetics. Antibodies to muscle relaxants may persist for >25 y.

OVERVIEW

- The body's response to what is perceived to be a foreign substance.
- Although itching, cutaneous manifestations, and a feeling of doom are present in the awake patient, CV collapse is the most common and serious presentation under general anesthesia.
- Bronchospasm occurs in <50% of life-threatening cases of anaphylaxis.
- Usually occurs during induction of anesthesia and within 10 min of drug administration

ICD-9-CM: 995.0

ETIOLOGY

- IgE binds to mast cells and causes a degranulation, releasing many vasoactive substances, including histamine. Although patients may not have been exposed to anesthetics, there may be common epitopes between cosmetics and myorelaxants.
- Risk factors for latex allergy include meningomyelocele and other congenital defects.
- Is most commonly associated with administration of muscle relaxants, particularly succinylcholine. Can be caused by all muscle relaxants, even those that do not release histamine chemically.
- The second most common cause appears to be latex allergy.
- Rarely due to opiates or local anesthetics

USUAL TREATMENT

- IV fluids (put in large-bore IV), often to 7 L in adults
- Epinephrine even in the face of significant tachycardia
- O_2 and supportive measures
- Possible H_1 and H_2 antagonists

ASSESSMENT POINTS

SYSTEM	EFFECT	ASSESSMENT BY HX	PE	TEST
HEENT	Head and neck swelling and potential glottic edema	Will occur suddenly	Swelling	Clinically obvious
CV	↑ HR; ↓ BP and SVR; ↑ ectopy; change in PR interval; coronary vasospasm		Hypotension, tachycardia	ECG may reveal PVCs or change in PR interval; CV collapse may ensue
RESP	Bronchospasm		Wheezing	↑ Peak insp pressure; ↓ O_2 saturation
SKIN	Urticaria or other cutaneous manifestations; generalized edema with fluid leakage		Body rash	Not needed CVP or PA pressures or TEE

Key Reference: Alessi R, Moss J: A clinician's guide to allergy and anesthesia. Semin Anesth 1993; 12:211–221.

PERIOPERATIVE IMPLICATIONS

Monitoring

- It is important to distinguish from drug effects or mechanical problems.
- CV collapse with or without associated bronchospasm or cutaneous manifestations during induction, but without evidence of mechanical problems, suggest anaphylaxis.
- Prophylactic H_1 and H_2 antagonists may attenuate the severity, although not the incidence.
- The airway may swell, making intubation very difficult.

Induction

- Reactions usually occur during induction. Give antibiotics in the preop holding area rather than during induction.

Maintenance

- Perpetuation of reaction can occur, particularly if due to latex.
- Significant cross-reactivity between myorelaxants (approaching 80%)
- Avoid all muscle relaxants if necessary to proceed with the operation.

Extubation

- Stable from a cardiorespiratory viewpoint
- Assess for airway edema

Adjuvants

- Epinephrine is drug of choice in true anaphylaxis, even in the face of tachycardia

Postoperative Period

- Blood should be drawn for possible tryptase levels. Although histamine measurements during the acute event can assist in Dx, they can be difficult to perform. Tryptase can be drawn up to 2 h afterward and may reveal an important pattern. Skin testing may be done several weeks after initial event to assess etiologic agent.

ANTICIPATED PROBLEMS/CONCERNS

- Advise patients exactly what drugs they have received.

ANEMIA — APLASTIC

Joanne Shay, M.D.

RISK

- 2,000 new cases/y in USA
- 1.1 per million up to age 9 y
- Southeast Asia and South Africa have 10–20 × higher incidence
- Within USA, related to agricultural areas or petrochemical industry and chemical exposures

PERIOPERATVE RISKS

- Infection
- Hemorrhage
- LV dysfunction due to high output state and fluid overload

WORRY ABOUT

- Sepsis
- Co-existing congenital anomalies, especially renal and cardiac
- Concomitant GI and intracranial hemorrhage
- Difficulty cross-matching blood products after previous multiple transfusions

OVERVIEW

- Self-perpetuating disorder resulting in pancytopenia due to a congenital or acquired loss of hemopoietic pluripotent stem cells
- Fanconi anemia is congenital familial marrow hypoplasia associated with mental retardation, kidney, spleen, and skeletal hypoplasia
- Estren-Dameshek anemia is inherited marrow hypoplasia without physical abnormalities
- Pathophysiology: reduction or dysfunction of pluripotent stem cells or their microenvironment from toxic or immunologic causes
- Prognosis for long-term survival has increased to 40–75% in those treated with antilymphocyte serum and 60–80% in those treated with bone marrow transplantation (BMT)
- Two forms of drug-induced aplastic anemia possible:
  - hypersensitivity: not related to dose or duration
  - "reversible" reaction: often resolves with discontinuation; severity proportional to dosage

ICD-9-CM Code: 284.9

ETIOLOGY

- 50–75% of cases idiopathic
- Fanconi anemia demonstrates autosomal recessive inheritance with heterozygote frequency of 1 in 300,000–600,000 in USA
- Drug-induced: chloramphenicol, NSAIDs, antiepileptics, gold and sulfa group–containing compounds
- Environmental toxins including aromatic hydrocarbons (benzene, naphthalene, toluene), pesticides (DDT, indane), and radiation
- Infectious causes include hepatitis C, CMV, EBV, HIV, TB, and toxoplasmosis
- Sequelae of other processes such as pancreatitis, pregnancy, and lupus erythematosus

USUAL TREATMENT

- Patients < 55 y are managed with HLA-matched BMT; patients die from complications related to BMT, such as GVHD or sepsis
- Patients > 55 y or those unable to find HLA-matched donor receive immunosuppression and immunomodulation Rx including ATG, cyclosporine, steroids, androgens, and G-CSF

ASSESSMENT POINTS

SYSTEM	EFFECT	ASSESSMENT BY HX	PE	TEST
HEENT	Epistaxis			CBC, differential, Plt
	Oral/mucosal friability		Stomatitis	PT, PTT
	Sinusitis	Headache		CT scan
RESP	Pulmonary embolism	Dyspnea	Tachypnea	CXR, V/Q scan
	Pneumonia		Lung field	CT scan
	Interstitial pneumonitis		consolidation	ABG, bronchoscopy
	Pulmonary edema		Wheezing	± bronchoalveolar lavage, biopsy
CV	LV failure	Dyspnea	Tachycardia, S₃	ECG
	ASD/VSD	Lethargy	Displaced posterior MI	Echocardiography
GI	GI bleeding	N/V, diarrhea	Acute abdomen	Endoscopy, bleeding scan
	GI GVHD	Melena	Hypoactive bowel sounds	Selective angiography
	Hepatic veno-occlusive		Jaundice	Albumin, transferrin
	disease			LFT, liver biopsy
CNS	Microcephaly			
	Meningitis	Irritability, lethargy	Meningismus	Lumbar puncture after coagu-
	Intracranial hemorrhage	Headache, seizures	Papilledema	lopathy treated, head CT, MRI
HEME	Pancytopenia	Bleeding gums, infections	Petechiae	CBC, differential
	Leukemia	Easy bruisability	Retinal hemorrhage	Reticulocyte count,
	Paroxysmal nocturnal	Fatigue	Pallor	BM biopsy
	hemoglobinuria			Ham's test
METABOL	Electrolyte abnormalities	Long-term hyperalimentation		Electrolytes
	Glucose intolerance			Ca²⁺, Mg²⁺, phosphate,
	Hypoproteinemia	GI GVHD		albumin, transferrin

Key Reference: Fickhoffen, et al: Treatment of aplastic anemia with ATG and methylprednisolone with or without cyclosporine. N Engl J Med 1991; 324:1297–1304.

PERIOPERATIVE IMPLICATIONS

Preoperative Preparation

- Reverse isolation precautions
- Timing and adequacy of blood product administration and availability
- Severe neutropenia, coexisting congenital heart disease (HD) may warrant prophylactic antimicrobial therapy
- Preoperative sedation, but IM and rectal routes should be avoided
- Concomitant steroid therapy and necessity of "stress" doses should be considered

Monitoring

- Arterial line if indicated
- Consider CVP or PA catheter as indicated
- Urine output for new-onset hemoglobinuria as first sign of transfusion reaction

Airway

- Avoidance of nasal manipulation
- Use extreme caution with friable oral and pharyngeal mucosal surfaces

Preinduction/Induction

- May exhibit hypotension and excessive fluid requirements to maintain adequate cardiac output
- Central neuraxial blockade contraindicated in ongoing thrombocytopenia requiring transfusion
- Peripheral neural blockade may be approached cautiously if coagulation status is judged adequate

Maintenance

- PEEP assures adequate tissue oxygenation at lower FIO₂ as hyperoxia depresses normal erythropoietin synthesis and marrow function
- Nitrous oxide depresses bone marrow function even after brief exposure; best to use O₂-air mixture
- Normothermia promotes coagulation

- Chronically anemic patients may tolerate lower Hct; however, adequacy of tissue oxygenation must be addressed if CV decompensation ensues
- Avoid induced hypotension in anemic patients

Extubation

- Period with greatest O₂ demands

Postoperative Period

- Continued monitoring of coagulation status
- Transfusion requirements > normal
- Increased susceptibility to infection
- Pain management improves pulmonary toilet

ANTICIPATED PROBLEMS/CONCERNS

- Age of RBC in patients with aplastic anemia is older than usual, with lower 2,3-DPG levels inside cells resulting in increased O₂ binding by Hb (shift to the right of O₂Hb dissociation curve) and decreased delivery of oxygen to tissues for same SaO₂

ANEMIA — CHRONIC DISEASE

Donat R. Spahn, M.D.

RISK

- People within USA: ~10%
- Race with highest prevalence: African-Americans
- Gender with higher prevalence: Age <55 y: F 8–15%, M 3–5%. Age >55 y: progressively increasing in both sexes; at age ≥ 80 years: F 9–20%, M 15–40%.

PERIOPERATIVE RISKS

- Related to underlying disorders
- Anemia per se not an additional risk as long as minimal Hgb level and compensatory mechanisms maintained in perioperative period
- Minimal Hgb level is individual; in general, this level is not higher than the preop Hgb level in chronic anemia.

WORRY ABOUT

- Underlying diseases and their perioperative complications
- Compensatory mechanisms aimed at maintaining O_2 delivery to tissue despite low Hgb and arterial O_2 content

OVERVIEW

- WHO definition of anemia: Children 6 mo–6 y: Hgb <11 g/dl; 6–14 y: Hgb <12 g/dl; nonpregnant females: Hgb <12 g/dl; pregnant females: Hgb <11 g/dl; males: Hgb <13 g/dl.
- Chronic anemia may itself be a disease but more often is secondary manifestation of another primary disorder (see Etiology).
- Symptoms of anemia depend on the underlying disease, severity and chronicity (time of development) of anemia, adequacy of compensatory mechanisms, and secondary manifestation of anemic state, e.g., angina pectoris, intermittent claudication, and transient cerebral ischemia due to local obstructive vascular disease.

ICD-9-CM Code: 285.9 (nonspecific)

ETIOLOGY

- Chronic blood loss, particularly in GI tract
- Iron, folic acid, cobalamin deficiencies
- Due to other primary disorders, e.g., chronic infections, malignancies, chronic renal failure, endocrine failure such as hypothyroidism
- Hemolytic anemia
- Aplastic anemia

USUAL TREATMENT

- Treatment of underlying disease
- Iron, folic acid, cobalamin supplementation
- Human recombinant erythropoietin
- Rarely, allogeneic blood transfusion

ASSESSMENT POINTS

SYSTEM	EFFECT	ASSESSMENT BY HX	PE	TEST
CV	Hyperdynamic circulation Myocardial ischemia CHF	Palpitation Pounding pulse Angina Sx, dyspnea Exercise intolerance	Tachycardia Wide pulse pressure	ECG Exercise ECG
RESP		Dyspnea		
GI	Chronic blood loss Hypoperfusion	Blood in stool Angina equivalent (pain, nausea, indigestion)		Occult blood in stool See CV
HEME	Hgb below WHO definition level (see Overview)	↓ Exercise tolerance		Hgb
RENAL	Chronic renal failure	Decreased urine output Dialysis	Shunt	Cr K^+
CNS	Decreased cerebral O_2 delivery	Dizziness Headache Transient cerebral ischemia		
MS	Low exercise capacity	Fatigability		

Key Reference: Roizen MF: Anesthetic implication of concurrent diseases. *In* Miller RD (ed): Anesthesia. New York, Churchill Livingstone, 1994, pp 903–1014.

PERIOPERATIVE IMPLICATIONS

Preoperative Preparation

- None

Monitoring

- T
- UO
- CVP, Hgb, electrolytes
- ST segment analysis in patients with signs of CAD
- PA catheter for large fluid shifts or patients with signs of LV dysfunction or advanced renal failure
- ABG in patients with severe anemia

Airway

- None

Preinduction/Induction

- Prehydrate liberally if CV status will tolerate.
- Avoid marked reduction in CO.
- Choose drugs according to renal function.

Maintenance

- Aim at high Pao_2.
- Avoid hyperventilation or acute alkalosis.
- Aim at high CO.
- Avoid hypovolemia.
- Keep the patient warm.
- Maintain Hgb above critical level. This level is individual, not above preop Hgb.

Extubation

- Keep patient warm.
- Maintain high Pao_2.
- In patients with CAD, this is the period of greatest risk for ischemia.

Postoperative Period

- Keep patient warm, prevent shivering.
- Maintain high Pao_2.

Adjuvants

- According to underlying disorder

ANTICIPATED PROBLEMS/CONCERNS

- Myocardial ischemia/infarction or CHF in patients with concomitant CAD
- Deterioration of renal function in patients with moderate renal failure
- Prolonged effects of drugs in patients with impaired renal and/or hepatic function

ANEMIA — HEMOLYTIC

Richard J. Palahniuk, M.D.

RISK

- Up to 1% of USA population
- Highest prevalence in African-Americans (sickle cell disease, G6PD deficiency)

PERIOPERATIVE RISKS

- Increased risk of tissue hypoxia intra-operatively
- May have pre-existing renal or hepatic dysfunction

WORRY ABOUT

- Maximizing FIO_2
- Maintaining adequate alveolar ventilation
- Maintaining normal body T unless hypothermia is intended

OVERVIEW

- Hemolytic anemias occur from a variety of causes with a variety of perianesthetic implications.
- Patients with previous splenectomy may be at increased risk of perioperative infection.
- Acute hemolytic crises require a different therapeutic approach from that for chronic slow hemolysis.

ICD-9-CM Code: 283.9

ETIOLOGY

- Acquired hemolytic anemias
  – hypersplenism, immune hemolysis, microangiopathic hemolytic anemia, infection (malaria), paroxysmal nocturnal hematuria, spur cell anemia
- Hereditary hemolytic anemias
  – membrane defects (spherocytosis), enzyme defects (G6PD deficiency, pyruvate kinase deficiency), thalassemias, hemoglobinopathies (sickle cell disease)

USUAL TREATMENT

- None
- Some disorders respond to splenectomy.
- Cholecystectomy may be indicated if cholelithiasis is a problem.
- Repeated transfusion may be necessary in some disorders.
- Erythropoietin prior to operation can be considered even if only 3 d

ASSESSMENT POINTS

SYSTEM	EFFECT	ASSESSMENT BY HX	PE	TEST
GI	Acute hemolytic crisis	Abdominal pain	Splenomegaly Hepatomegaly	
HEME	Hemolytic anemia			Hgb Reticulocyte count Peripheral blood smear Serum haptoglobin ^{51}Cr RBC half-life

Key Reference: Ballas SK: The pathophysiology of hemolytic anemias. Tranfus Med Rev 1990; 4:236–256.

PREOPERATIVE IMPLICATIONS

Preoperative Preparation

- Preop transfusion should be utilized judiciously, usually after consultation with a hematologist. Erythropoietin is often prescribed even if only 3 d preoperatively.
- Acute drops in Hgb to <8 g/dl and chronic reductions to below 6 g/dl should be considered for preop packed cell transfusion.

Monitoring

- Core T
- Consider arterial line and PA catheter for cases with even a modest risk of blood loss.

Airway

- None

Preinduction/Induction

- Maintain supplemental FIO_2, adequate alveolar ventilation
- No agent or technique specifically indicated or contraindicated

Extubation

- Routine

Postoperative Period

- Maintain supplemental oxygen

Adjuvants

- None

ANTICIPATED PROBLEMS/CONCERNS

- Inadequte tissue O_2 delivery if SaO_2 falls, blood loss occurs, or cardiac output falls.
- Variation in oxygenation, acid-base balance, and/or body T may promote hemolysis in some disorders.

ANEMIA OF INFANCY

Mary A. Keyes, M.D.

RISK

• Occurs in all infants but with variable severity

PERIOPERATIVE RISKS

• Well tolerated by healthy, term infant. In preterm infant, may be associated with episodes of apnea, bradycardia, tachycardia, lactic acidosis.

WORRY ABOUT

• Surgery requiring blood transfusion with physiologic anemia (9–12 wk of age)
• Episodes of apnea/bradycardia that are more severe the lower the hemoglobin in preterm infants

OVERVIEW

• Normal physiologic response to extrauterine life. Nadir at 9th–12th wk and is 9.5 to 11 g/dl.
• In preterm infant, nadir at 4–8 wk and may decrease to 8 g/dl.

ETIOLOGY

• Hypoxic intrauterine environment ↑ erythropoietin levels. With the sudden rise in arterial O_2 saturation following birth, erythropoietin levels abruptly fall, and do not rise for several wk.
• Survival of neonatal erythrocytes is shorter than that of adult's.
• Rapid increase in blood volume that accompanies rapid gain leads to hemodilution.

USUAL TREATMENT

• No treatment necessary in term infant
• Preterm infants with episodes of apnea and bradycardia, tachycardia, lactic acidosis may benefit from RBC transfusion.

ASSESSMENT POINTS (applies to preterm infants only)

SYSTEM	EFFECT	ASSESSMENT BY HX	PE	TEST
CV	Tachycardia	None	Tachycardia	±ECG
RESP	Apnea/bradycardia	# episodes/d		

Key Reference: O'Brien RT, Pearson HA: Physiologic anemia of the newborn infant. J Pediatr 1971; 79:132–138.

PERIOPERATIVE IMPLICATIONS

Preoperative Preparation
• Timing of elective blood-losing surgery depending on Hgb levels

Monitoring
• Routine

Airway
• None

Preinduction/Induction
• Routine

Extubation
• If apnea and bradycardia, extubation may be delayed until any drugs given during anesthesia are eliminated.

Adjuvants
• Spinal anesthesia, when appropriate, may be beneficial in preterm infant.

Postoperative Care
• Consider monitoring preterm infant for apnea and bradycardia for 24 h.

ANTICIPATED PROBLEMS/CONCERNS

• Anemia is significant risk factor for postop apnea in preterm infant undergoing surgery and anesthesia

ANGINA, CHRONIC STABLE

Lee A. Fleisher, M.D.

RISK

- People within USA: 3 million
- Race with highest prevalence: ?
- African-Americans have highest death rates

PERIOPERATIVE RISKS

- Increased risk of perioperative MI and death varies, depending on study (3–12%)
- Risk of LV dysfunction, hypotension, myocardial infarction

WORRY ABOUT

- Increasing frequency of symptoms
- Signs of LV dysfunction with ischemia
- Silent myocardial ischemia

OVERVIEW

- Chronic stable angina identifies patients at risk for developing myocardial ischemia and MI
- Angina is present in <25% of episodes of myocardial ischemia
- Symptoms should be stable for previous 60 d for "stable" diagnosis
- Can result from:
  - Inadequacy of myocardial oyxgen supply in patients with critical coronary artery stenosis
  - Coronary vasospasm
  - Inadequacy of myocardial oxygen supply 2° to increased demand from ventricular hypertrophy
  - Endothelial cell–mediated vasoconstriction

ICD-9-CM Code: 413

ETIOLOGY

- Acquired disease with genetic predisposition
- Patients with diabetes have higher incidence of CAD, frequently silent
- Other risk factors include HTN, hyperlipidemia, advanced age, tobacco use, homocystinemia

USUAL TREATMENT

- Medical therapy—β adrenergic receptor antagonist, Ca^{2+} channel antagonists, nitrates, aspirin, folate, lipid-reducing agents
- Angioplasty
- CABG

ASSESSMENT POINTS

SYSTEM	EFFECT	ASSESSMENT BY HX	PE	TEST
CV	Myocardial ischemia LV dysfunction	Angina Sx Angina-equivalent Sx Dyspnea Exercise tolerance	Displaced posterior MI S_3	ECG Exercise ECG Exercise radionuclide scintigraphy Pharmacologic stress testing ECHO Coronary angiography
RESP	CHF	Dyspnea; nighttime cough Orthopnea Chest tightness	S_3 Rales Wheezing	CXR
GI		Angina-equivalent Sx – LUQ pain – Nausea, indigestion		See CV Assessment
RENAL	↓ Renal perfusion	↑ UO at night		Cr
CNS	Syncope	Syncope with chest pain		Exercise stress test
MS		Angina-equivalent Sx – Arm pain/neck pain		See CV Assessment

Key Reference: Fleisher LA, Barash PG: Preoperative cardiac evaluation for noncardiac surgery: A functional approach. Anesth Analg 1992; 74:568–598.

PERIOPERATIVE IMPLICATIONS

Preoperative Preparation

- Preop β adrenergic receptor antagonist associated with a lower incidence of myocardial ischemia

Monitoring

- ST segment analysis
- PA catheter for large fluid shift operations or patients with signs of LV dysfunction
- TEE most sensitive, but technical issues of real-time interpretation

Airway

- None

Preinduction/Induction

- May develop reduced CO and hypotension with ischemia
- Avoid tachycardia, hypotension

Maintenance

- Myocardial ischemia may manifest as:
  - CV instability
  - Intraoperative myocardial ischemia
  - Reduced CO, increased PCWP
- No one agent or technique shown superior
- Maintain normothermia, adequate hematocrit (≥ 28%)

Extubation

- Period at greatest risk for developing ischemia
- CABG patients frequently left intubated until warm

Postoperative Period

- Pain management may be critical
- Epidural analgesia may be beneficial

Adjuvants

- β adrenergic receptor antagonist, nitroglycerin, calcium channel blockers

ANTICIPATED PROBLEMS/CONCERNS

- Patients with angina who develop dyspnea on exertion are at greatest risk for developing perioperative cardiac complications.
- Exercise tolerance may be the best predictor of perioperative risk. Patients with a good exercise tolerance may not require further evaluation.

ANHIDROSIS (CONGENITAL ANHIDROTIC ECTODERMAL DYSPLASIA)

Raafat S. Hannallah, M.D.

RISK

- Rare

PERIOPERATIVE RISKS

- Impaired thermoregulation (risk of hyperthermia in infants)
- Postop chest infections

WORRY ABOUT

- Impaired thermoregulation

OVERVIEW

- Absent sebaceous and sweat glands; heat loss by evaporation is impaired.
- Absent mucous glands from respiratory tract and esophagus; frequent respiratory infections
- Partial or complete absence of teeth
- Hypotrichosis (absent hair)
- Characteristic facies: prominent supraorbital ridges, depressed bridge and root of nose, large deformed ears, thick lips, underdeveloped maxilla and mandible

ICD-9-CM Code: 705.0

ETIOLOGY

- Sex-linked recessive disorder
- Full expression only in males; carrier females may be mildly affected.

USUAL TREATMENT

- Protect from risks of hyperpyrexia due to infection, hot weather, vigorous exercise

ASSESSMENT POINTS

SYSTEM	EFFECT	ASSESSMENT BY HX	TEST
HEENT	Airway anomalies	Snoring Difficult breathing	
RESP	Decreased mucus	Repeated infections	
OPHTHAL	Decreased lacrimation	Dryness, ulceration	
METAB	Hyperpyrexia		Record/monitor T

Key Reference: Smith GB, Shribman AJ: Anaesthesia and severe skin disease. Anaesthesia 1984; 39:443–455.

PERIOPERATIVE IMPLICATIONS

Preoperative Preparation

- Avoid anticholinergic premedication

Monitoring

- Routine
- T

Airway

- Awkward mask fit
- Laryngoscopy and intubation may be difficult.

Maintenance

- Regional anesthesia may be preferable when possible.
- Warm and humidify anesthetic gases.

Extubation

- Vigorous postop chest physiotherapy

Adjuvants

- Protect eyes with tape and ophthalmic ointment (lacrimation is reduced).

ANTICIPATED PROBLEMS/CONCERNS

- Difficult airway (mask and/or intubation)
- Hyperthermia
- Postop chest infections

ANKYLOSING SPONDYLITIS

John E. Tetzlaff, M.D.

RISK

- 1:2000 incidence in Caucasians, rare in non-Caucasians
- M:F 10:1; more severe in males
- 18–50% incidence in Native Americans

PERIOPERATIVE RISKS

- Difficult airway, atlantoaxial instability
- "Bamboo spine" with potential for fracture during airway manipulation
- Rigid chest with difficult ventilation, myocarditis, myocardial conduction defects

WORRY ABOUT

- Inability to intubate, spine fracture, arrhythmia, inability to ventilate

OVERVIEW

- An arthritic process, seronegative for rheumatoid factor, that attacks ligamentous attachments of the spinal column
- Characterized by low back pain, sacroiliitis, multiplane rigidity of spine, chest stiffness, uveitis, and insidious onset at <40 y of age
- Autosomal dominant and strongly prevalent among first-degree relatives.

ICD-9-CM Code: 720.00

ETIOLOGY

- Etiology unknown
- Genetic transmission led to discovery of a genetic marker, HLA-B27
- Infectious origin speculated; one species of *Klebsiella* reported to be associated with some cases

USUAL TREATMENT

- Symptomatic, with exercise, NSAIDs, immunosuppression can be tried in severe cases.
- Wedge osteotomy is a drastic surgical intervention.

ASSESSMENT POINTS

SYSTEM	EFFECT	ASSESSMENT BY HX	PE	TEST
HEENT	Uveitis TMJ arthritis, arytenoid deviation	Visual disturbance Limited mouth opening, jaw pain, voice abnormality	Funduscopic exam Airway exam, indirect laryngoscopy	Fiberoptic nasopharyngoscopy
CV	Cardiomyopathy, conduction defects	SOB, chest pain, palpitation	Distant heart sounds, rales, arrhythmia	ECG, CXR, ECHO
RESP	Pleuritic inflammation, chest rigidity	Chest pain, limited exercise tolerance	Decreased breath sounds, chest excursion	Pulmonary function tests, CXR
GI	IBS	Abdominal pain, bowel dysfunction	Abdominal pain	
GU	Chronic prostatitis	Pain with urination	Rectal exam	
CNS	Atlantoaxial subluxation, occult spine fracture	Long tract signs, sphincter abnormality; sometimes no symptoms	Basic neurologic exam	Cervical spine x-ray with flexion-extension
PNS	Radiculopathy	Radiating pain in extremities	ROM of the extremity	EMG (medicolegal use)
MS	Back pain, sacroiliitis, joint ankylosis, kyphosis ("chin on chest"), "bamboo spine," spondylodiskitis	Review of skeletal function	Spine, skeleton	Radiologic studies

Key Reference: Calin A: Ankylosing spondylitis. *In* Kelly WN, Harris ED Jr, Ruddy S, Sledge CB (eds): Textbook of Rheumatology, 3rd ed. Philadelphia, WB Saunders, 1989.

PERIOPERATIVE IMPLICATIONS

Preoperative Preparation

- Airway evaluation, pulmonary function assessment; consider positioning difficulties. Anti-sialagogue for awake intubation

Monitoring

- ST segment analysis; pulmonary artery catheter if severe myocardial dysfunction.

Airway

- Inability to intubate possible, owing to cervical spine fusion, distortion. Fiberoptic intubation may be necessary. Cervical spine instability possible. Spine fracture possible with airway manipulation. Occult spine fracture may already be present.

Induction

- If general anesthesia, any approach acceptable. If limited cardiac reserves, avoid depressants of myocardial contractility. If regional, skeletal abnormality can make the block difficult to perform, and response to injection is unpredictable. If local anesthetic toxicity, airway management can be difficult.

Maintenance

- With positive pressure ventilation, decrease tidal volume and increase rate.

Extubation

- Awake is preferable

Adjuvants

- None

Postoperative

- Comfortable position, pain control without airway embarrassment

ANTICIPATED PROBLEMS/CONCERNS

- Airway Control
  - The extreme distortion of the spine, especially the neck, may make intubating trachea and ventilating patient very difficult
  - Any airway compromise or depression of ventilation can result in catastrophe
  - Depression of ventilation with opiate analgesics can be dangerous.
- Pulmonary Function
  - Owing to abnormal mechanics of the thorax and neck, the ability to ensure normal oxygenation during surgery and in the postop period can be a potential problem.
- Regional Anesthesia
  - Placement of spinal, epidural, or caudal block could be technically very difficult. Action of local anesthetics in the central axis could be unpredictable.

ANOMALOUS PULMONARY VENOUS DRAINAGE

Roger A. Moore, M.D.

RISK

- 1% of all congenital heart defects
- Complete (total anomalous pulmonary venous drainage [TAPVD]) or partial (partial anomalous pulmonary venous drainage [PAPVD]) exists when pulmonary veins drain into the venous circulation.
- 4:1 male-female ratio in infradiaphragmatic type

PERIOPERATIVE RISKS

- Rapid CV deterioration secondary to acidosis
- Sudden pulmonary HTN and right heart failure during hypoventilation
- Mortality: 2–20% depending on preop status

WORRY ABOUT

- Air bubbles entering the venous circuit

- Polycythemic hyperviscosity attack with
  - perioperative dehydration
  - cold OR environment

OVERVIEW

- Incompatible with life unless an ASD allows R→L shunting of blood. TAPVD patients with small ASDs are more critically ill. Some cyanosis, usually with O_2 saturations of 85–95%
- Increased flow through pulmonary vascular beds, resulting in pulmonary HTN
- Four types of TAPVD:
  - Supracardiac—pulmonary veins connect to the left innominate vein via an anomalous "vertical vein" or connect to right SVC via an anomalous "short connecting vein," or connect to the left SVC (45%).
  - Cardiac—pulmonary veins drain into coronary sinus or directly into the right atrium (23%).

- Infracardiac—pulmonary veins drain into IVC, portal veins, hepatic veins, or ductus venosus (21%).
- Mixed—combined supracardiac, cardiac, and infracardiac connections (11%)

ICD-9-CM Code: 747.41

ETIOLOGY

- Embryologic atresia or malformation of the common pulmonary venous system resulting in persistence of abnormal connections

USUAL TREATMENT

- Severe TAPVD with little systemic shunt needs immediate cardiac correction after birth. Most children with TAPVD require cardiac correction before 1 y of age.
- Cardiac correction of PAPVD may be postponed into childhood.

ASSESSMENT POINTS

SYSTEM	EFFECT	ASSESSMENT BY HX	PE	TEST
HEENT	Hypoxemia	Snoring	Airway class	
CV	CHF Hypoxemia	Decreased activity level Dyspnea	Rales Cyanosis	ECG—RVH, RAH ECHO; catheterization Cardiac consultation
	Monitoring problems	Anomalous peripheral vessels	Pulses and blood pressures in all 4 extremities	
RESP	Hypoxemia	Bronchospasm Shortness of breath Pulmonary edema	Wheezing Tachypnea	CXR Granular lung fields
HEME	Sludging DIC	Polycythemia Bleeding or bruising	Clubbing Bruises	Hg PT, PTT, bleeding time
CNS		Previous stroke	Complete neurologic evaluation	CT scan if neurologic findings
MS		Feeding difficulty Failure to thrive	Ht, wt, head circumference	Plot of growth curves

Key Reference: Lake CL: Anomalies of systemic and pulmonary venous return. *In* Lake CL (ed): Pediatric Anesthesia, 2d ed. Norwalk, CT, Appleton & Lange, 1993, pp 281–294.

PERIOPERATIVE IMPLICATIONS

Preoperative Preparation

- Desired hemodynamics: Preload—normal (CVP 10—12 mmHg); afterload—low; PVR—normal; HR—normal to high; contractility—normal.
- Liberal oral fluids preoperatively
- Avoid heavy premedication
- Subacute bacterial endocarditis prophylaxis

Monitoring

- Absolute air bubble precautions
- Arterial catheter
- CVP catheters
- Capnography and pulse oximetry for respiratory trends
- ECG and T

Airway

- Associated congenital syndromes with airway anomalies
- Cricoid ring limiting diameter of airway

- Primary need to maintain airway and avoid increased $PaCO_2$.

Induction

- If IV in place use fentanyl or ketamine with pancuronium or vecuronium.
- If no IV
  - if unstable, ketamine IM
  - if stable, slow inhalational induction with halothane (avoid high halothane levels) until IV placed
- Actively avoid hypoventilation and agents that produce myocardial depression.

Maintenance

- Positive pressure ventilation usually improves oxygenation.
- Use narcotics in conjunction with inhalational agents as tolerated.
- Avoid nitrous oxide.
- Use high FIO_2.
- Capnographic end tidal CO_2 will not accurately reflect $PaCO_2$.
- Avoid hypothermia

Extubation

- Do not attempt deep or early extubation.
- Prior to extubation assess adequacy of ventilation with inspiratory pressures of at least –20 mmHg and adequate tidal volumes.

Postoperative Period

- Close monitoring of ventilation and pulse oximetry
- Active warming with avoidance of shivering
- Be prepared for immediate reintubation.

Adjuvants

- Inotropic support with dopamine or dobutamine

ANTICIPATED PROBLEMS/CONCERNS

- If pulmonary hypertensive crisis occurs
  - hyperventilate
  - 100% inspired oxygen
  - consider prostaglandin E_1, tolazoline, amrinone, or isoproterenol

ANOREXIA NERVOSA

Russell T. Wall III, M.D.

RISK

- Primarily in white adolescent females from middle- or upper-class families
- 0.4–1.5/100,000 population
- Age of onset from prepuberty to mid-20s

PERIOPERATIVE RISKS

- Predisposing conditions include cardiovascular dysfunction (bradycardia, hypotension), acid-base abnormalities (both acidosis and alkalosis are possible), lyte abnormalities ($\downarrow$ K$^+$, $\downarrow$ Mg^{2+}, $\downarrow$ Ca^{2+}, $\downarrow$ P), hematologic abnormalities ($\downarrow$ Hgb, $\downarrow$ WBC, $\downarrow$ fibrinogen, $\downarrow$ Plt), hypothermia, delayed gastric emptying, and renal dysfunction (prerenal azotemia).

WORRY ABOUT

- Degree of malnutrition (excess protein depletion = impaired cellular function)
- Greater weight loss = greater risk

OVERVIEW

- Anorexia nervosa
  - obsessive fear of being fat
  - radical restriction of caloric intake
  - wt loss ≥15% of ideal wt
  - risk of death high if wt loss ≥35% of ideal weight
- Bulimia
  - obsessive fear of being fat
  - irresistible urge to overeat
  - wt control by vomiting, diuretic and laxative use
  - wt loss less than in anorexia

ICD-9-CM Code: 307.1

ETIOLOGY

- Unknown
- Possibly hypothalamic dysfunction or psychiatric cause

USUAL TREATMENT

- No specific treatment
- Therapies offered
  - psychotherapy
  - behavior modification
  - antidepressants
  - nutritional (1500–2500 calories/d, metoclopramide or bethanechol for gastric emptying, benzodiazepine before meals)
  - relaxation exercises
- If severe: hospitalization, with tube feedings or hyperalimentation

ASSESSMENT POINTS

SYSTEM	EFFECT	ASSESSMENT BY HX	PE	TEST

CV	$\downarrow$ Response to SNS
	Hypovolemia
	LV dysfunction
	  $\downarrow$ LV wall thickness
	  $\downarrow$ LV cavity size
	  MV prolapse
	Cardiomyopathy
	Conduction abnormalities
		CHF symptoms	Bradycardia
			Hypotension (<70 mmHg systolic)
			CHF
			
			Murmur
			
			Dysrhythmias (ventricular tachydysrhythmias, A-V blocks)
				CXR
				ECHO
				
				ECG

RESP	Aspiration pneumonia	Vomiting	Bradypnea (<15/min)	CXR
GI	Delayed gastric emptying Esophagitis, esophageal/gastric rupture	Constipation Vomiting		
RENAL	Prerenal azotemia Acid-base abnormalities Lyte abnormalities $\downarrow$ K$^+$, $\downarrow$ Ca^{2+}, $\downarrow$ Mg^{2+}, $\downarrow$ P, Cl$^-$ Impaired concentrating ability Hypoalbuminemia	Starvation Vomiting Diuretics Polyuria	Muscle weakness Edema	BUN 60–70 mg/dl ABG Serum lytes
ENDO	$\downarrow$ BMR Hypothermia (<96.6°F rectally) Depressed immune function Abn glucose tolerance	Amenorrhea	Vasoconstriction	Serum glucose
CNS	Brain atrophy Depression Diabetes insipidus	Starvation Illicit drug, alcohol use		
MS	Osteoporosis		Peripheral edema	

Key Reference: Katz J, Benumof L, Kadis LB (eds): Anesthesia and Uncommon Diseases, 3rd ed. Philadelphia, WB Saunders, 1990, pp 503–504.

PERIOPERATIVE IMPLICATIONS

Preoperative Preparation

- Delay elective surgery until patient is medically stable
- Optimize hemodynamics, acid-base status, lytes
- Consider metoclopramide to promote gastric emptying

Monitoring

- ABGs, lytes
- A-line, CVP, PA catheters may be indicated

Airway

- Induction
  - consider rapid-sequence induction
  - cautious dosing because of possible LV dysfunction and hypovolemia

Maintenance

- Aggressively avoid hypothermia
- Probably avoid halothane (dysrhythmias)
- Cautious use of potent inhalation agents
- Excess fluids may precipitate pulmonary edema

Extubation

- Consider awake extubation

Adjuvants

- Cautious use of muscle relaxants ($\downarrow$ muscle mass, lyte and acid-base abnormalities)

ANTICIPATED PROBLEMS/CONCERNS

- Temperature control
- Hemodynamic stability
- Acid-base and lyte management

ANTICOAGULATION, PREOPERATIVE

Catherine Huraux, M.D.
Jerrold H. Levy, M.D.

RISK

- Pts with mechanical heart valves, atrial fibrillation, pulmonary embolism, recent venous thrombosis
- Oral anticoagulant therapy may → potential risks in elective or emergency surgery
- Other populations are pts who receive heparin IV before vascular or cardiac surgery and pts undergoing cardiac surgery with extracorporeal circulation

PERIOPERATIVE RISKS

- Balance between risk of bleeding vs thromboembolic complication is major periop risk
- Risk increases with major and emergency vs elective surgery

WORRY ABOUT

- Excessive allogeneic transfusions, either to correct effects of warfarin or for risk of excessive bleeding
- In pts with valvular heart disease, concomitant hepatic dysfunction due to HF may produce abnormal PT and/or thrombocytopenia
- Can be associated with heparin therapy due to acute administration or prolonged use (7–10 d)
- Use of protamine to reverse heparin after bypass may lead to CV dysfunction and anaphylactoid reactions

OVERVIEW/PHARMACOLOGY

Heparin (Standard Unfractionated)

- For preventive therapy and acute management, binds to antithrombin III and factor X to inhibit their effects
- Variability in response to heparin depends on
  - Prep of heparin administered
  - Individual characteristics of pts
  - Duration of therapy (due to ↓ antithrombin III levels)
- Duration of action depends on dose and method of administration
  - 100U/kg: $T_{\frac{1}{2}}$ 56 min
  - IV: 60 min
  - 400U/kg: $T_{\frac{1}{2}}$ tripled
  - Subcutaneous: 3 h
- Depolymerized in endothelial cells
- Eliminated in urine
- Heparin resistance (many proteins neutralize anticoagulant therapy; prolonged therapy can lower antithrombin III levels)
- Monitoring of the anticoagulant effect: PTT

Heparin (LMW)

- $T_{\frac{1}{2}}$ 4–7 h
- Higher and more predictable bioavailability: 100%
- Removed by renal filtration

Warfarin

- Oral anticoagulant
- Member of the coumarin family
- Vit K antagonist causing inactivation of factors II, VII, IX, X and anticoagulants C, S
- Used for thromboembolic complication prevention
- Peak plasma concentration reached 1–4 h after ingestion
- $T_{\frac{1}{2}}$: 36–42 h
- International normalization ratio (INR) required: 2–3
- Stop for surgery and replace with heparin

Warfarin Reversal Treatment

- Vit K: 10–20 mg PO, IM, or IV; IV form potentially associated with anaphylactoid reactions
- Normalization of INR within 24 h
- Fresh frozen plasma starting with 2 U

Heparin Reversal Treatment

- Protamine reversal according to the ratio heparin:protamine 1:1.3 (or start with 50–100 mg and check the ACT)
- Monitoring: ACT in cardiac surgery

ASSESSMENT POINTS

SYSTEM	EFFECT	ASSESSMENT BY HX
ENDO	Risk of protamine reactions is 10- to 30-fold higher in diabetics receiving protamine-containing insulin	History of insulin use

Key Reference: Onishchuk JL, Carlsson C: Epidural hematoma associated with epidural anesthesia: Complications of anticoagulant therapy. Anesthesiology, 1992; 77:1221.

PERIOPERATIVE IMPLICATIONS

Preoperative Preparation

- Elective surgery/warfarin therapy
  - Stop warfarin 5 d before surgery
  - Replace with heparin in checking/INR, PTT, platelet count
  - Stop heparin 60–90 min before surgery
- Reversal for emergency surgery
  - Warfarin therapy can be acutely reversed with FFP, and heparin therapy can be reversed with protamine
- Consider avoiding regional anesthesia
- Approach anticoagulation reversal cautiously in the anticoagulated patient

Postoperative Period

- Restart heparin therapy immediately after surgery (PTT, platelet count, blood cell count, bleeding)

ANTICIPATED PROBLEMS/CONCERNS

- Introduction of epidural or spinal anesthesia requires minimum 60–120 min between stopping and restarting heparinization; consider removing catheter at least 120 min after stopping heparinization and complete restoration of normal clotting time

ANTITHROMBIN III DEFICIENCY

Ellise Delphin, M.D.

RISK

- Incidence in US: 1 in 2,000–1 in 5,000 (may be higher)
- Race with highest prevalence: Caucasian

PERIOPERATIVE RISKS

- Risk of postoperative thromboembolic phenomena; 40–70% most common (in descending order): deep vein thrombosis, pulmonary embolus, mesenteric thrombosis, highest risk in those with antithrombin III (AT III) levels <50% of normal
- Heparin resistance is common

WORRY ABOUT

- Hypercoagulable state perioperatively
- Thrombus formation on indwelling catheters

- Pulmonary emboli or DVT with immobility
- Mesenteric, inferior vena caval, or CNS thrombosis
- Withdrawal of warfarin sodium preoperatively, as patients may be heparin-resistant

OVERVIEW

- AT III is an α_2-globulin capable of inactivation of thrombin and factor x_a in blood; AT III deficiency results in an unusual susceptibility to thromboembolic disease
- Heparin resistance may be problematic during surgery
- Massive thromboembolism can occur perioperatively with AT III levels <50%

ICD-9-CM Code: 286.5

ETIOLOGY

- Genetic: reduced AT III synthesis inherited as an autosomal dominant trait, manifests as thromboembolism in late teens to early 30s
- Acquired: secondary to consumption of AT III due to massive thromboembolic disease, disseminated intravascular coagulation, renal disease with proteinuria (esp nephrotic syndrome), chronic liver disease, prolonged heparin therapy, increased protein catabolism
- Conflicting data about role of oral contraceptive use, pregnancy, and CAD

USUAL TREATMENT

- Medical therapy: sodium warfarin or combination of oral anticoagulants and platelet suppression (aspirin or dipyridamole)
- Perioperatively: fresh frozen plasma, cryoprecipitate, AT III concentrate, heparin; heparin resistance can be treated with FFP

ASSESSMENT POINTS

SYSTEM	EFFECT	ASSESSMENT BY HX	PE	TEST
CV	CAD		Angina, dyspnea	ECG, CXR Angiography
PERIPHERAL VASC	DVT Arterial occlusion		Gangrene, absent pulses	
RESP	Pulmonary embolus	Dyspnea Exercise tolerance decreased	SOB	CXR V/Q scan
GI	Mesenteric artery/vein occlusion	Abdominal pain	Rectal bleeding	
	Decreased AT III	Chronic liver disease symptoms	Jaundice, hepatomegaly	Serum albumin, AT III level
HEME	Bleeding and thrombosis	DIC	Petechiae, purpura, thrombosis	FDP, PT, PTT, AP II, AT III level
GU	Decreased albumin and AT III levels	Nephrotic syndrome, proteinuria	Edema	Urinalysis, serum albumin
CNS	CVA	Sudden onset, Hx of other embolic disease	Seizure, loss of vision, loss of motor function	CT scan, angiogram

Key Reference: Bick RL: Clinical revelance of antithrombin III. Semin Thromb Hemost 1982; 8:276–287.

PERIOPERATIVE IMPLICATIONS

Preoperative Preparation

- Assess whether congential or acquired; if acquired, treat primary disease if possible
- Stop oral anticoagulation and substitute FFP or AT III concentrate to bring AT III level to 70–80% normal
- Heparin to provide PTT of 40–60 sec

Monitoring

- Careful attention to temperature
- Volume status, respiratory variables
- PTT, AT III levels

Airway

- None

Induction

- None

Maintenance

- Maintain normothermia to avoid hyperviscosity
- Maintain intravascular volume
- IV heparin effect should be monitored
- Careful evaluations of hypotension or change in ET CO_2

Adjuvants

- No special concerns with adjuvant agents

Postoperative Period

- Consider ICU for monitoring
- Continue anticoagulation
- Early mobilization
- Remove indwelling catheters as soon as possible
- Oral anticoagulation might be reintroduced ASAP

ANTICIPATED PROBLEMS

- Embolic phenomena can occur intraoperatively
- Monitoring lines may be foci for thrombus formation
- Perioperative thromboembolic events major concern; continuous anticoagulation is required, as is operative prophylaxis with FFP and heparin

AORTIC REGURGITATION

Paul G. Barash, M.D.

RISK

- 100,000 aortic valve operations/y
- Gender predominance: male > female, 3:1
- Racial predominance: none known

PERIOPERATIVE RISKS

- Left ventricular failure
- Right ventricular failure
- Subendocardial ischemia
- Splanchnic ischemia

WORRY ABOUT

- Aspiration pneumonitis (acute aortic regurgitation [AR])
- Avoid hypertension, which ↑ AR and ↓ cardiac output
- Avoid bradycardia, which ↑ AR and ↓ cardiac output

OVERVIEW

- Long latency period between onset of hemodynamic changes and symptoms (~20–30 y)
- Myocardial ischemia uncommon
- Abdominal pain manifestation of splanchnic ischemia

ICD-9-CM Code: 424.1

ETIOLOGY

- Damage to leaflets
- Aortic root dilatation
- Loss of commissural support

TREATMENT

- Medical: digoxin, diuretic, vasodilator
- Surgical: prosthetic valve

ASSESSMENT POINTS

SYSTEM	EFFECT	ASSESSMENT BY HX	PE	TEST
CV	Aortic valve dysfunction		High-pitched, early diastolic, decrescendo blowing murmur Mid-diastolic low-pitched murmur (Austin Flint) Widened arterial pulse pressure (water-hammer) To and fro bobbing of head (de Musset's sign)	CXR ECHO
	LV dysfunction	Dyspnea with exercise Nocturnal dyspnea	Displaced posterior MI S_3	ECG CXR ECHO Cardiac catheterization
RESP	CHF	Dyspnea Nocturnal dyspnea	Rales S_3	CXR
GI	Splanchnic ischemia	Abdominal pain	Distended abdomen	

Key Reference: Braunwald E: Valvular heart disease. *In* Braunwald E (ed): Heart Disease: A Textbook of Cardiovascular Medicine, 4th ed. Philadelphia, WB Saunders, 1992, pp 1043–1053.

PERIOPERATIVE IMPLICATIONS

Preoperative Preparation

- Consider optimizing LV performance with vasodilators, inotropes, and diuretic
- Avoid reduction in aortic diastolic pressure
- Emergent procedures (acute AR) "full stomach" precautions

Monitoring

- Arterial catheter
- ECG leads II/V5 and ST-segment analysis
- Consider PA catheter or TEE

Preinduction/Induction

- Elective: consider narcotic induction with inhalation supplement (0.25–50% MAC); nondepolarizing muscle relaxant devoid of bradycardic effects.
- Emergency (acute AR with aortic dissection): consider rapid-sequence technique with ketamine, etomidate, or low-dose narcotic plus amnestic agent

- ↓ Aortic diastolic pressure ↓ coronary perfusion pressure and may lead to subendocardial ischemia
- Bradycardia and HTN ↑ regurgitant fraction and ↓ cardiac output

Maintenance

- During period until institution of cardiopulmonary bypass, consider maintaining LV function with minimum of anesthetic interventions
- PCWP may underestimate LVEDP due to premature closure of mitral valve
- PCWP may overestimate LVEDP in patients with combined AR and MR

Extubation

- Consider extubation for patients undergoing valve replacement in ICU after respiratory and hemodynamic criteria are met

Postoperative Period

- Consider augmenting preload to maintain and preserve filling volume of still-dilated, hypertrophic LV

- Inotropic support may be required to maintain CO if inadequate intraoperative myocardial preservation
- Evaluation for neurologic injuries 2° to embolism during valve replacement

ANTICIPATED PROBLEMS/CONCERNS

- Prolonged Trendelenburg position poorly tolerated during PAC insertion
- Intra-aortic balloon counterpulsation contraindicated before valve replacement
- Atrial fibrillation or other supraventricular tachycardias poorly tolerated and require aggressive treatment
- Retrograde cardioplegia (not anterograde) may be required for myocardial protection
- Associated diseases may present difficult intubation, e.g., rheumatoid arthritis, Marfan's syndrome, trauma (acute aortic dissection)

AORTIC STENOSIS

Stephen J. Thomas, M.D.

RISK

- Bicuspid aortic valve in 1% of population; 5–15% may become stenotic
- Isolated aortic stenosis 3× more common in men

PERIOPERATIVE RISKS

- Increased risk of perioperative MI following noncardiac surgery if stenosis is severe
- ↑ Risk of CNS dysfunction following aortic valve replacement if, in addition to the valve itself, the aorta is heavily calcified

WORRY ABOUT

- If patient is symptomatic, probably needs AVR prior to noncardiac surgery
- Differentiate systolic dysfunction (impaired contractility) from diastolic dysfunction (reduced ventricular compliance); diastolic change is common, but true contractile failure occurs only late in the disease

OVERVIEW

- Chronic obstruction to left ventricular outflow due to LVH
- LVH results in
  - Reduced ventricular compliance; ventricular filling pressures (VFPs) ↑ ; small ↑ in ventricular volume are associated with wide swings in VFP
  - Potential myocardial ischemia; ↑ muscle mass requires increased basal flow; coronary reserve ↓ ; O_2 supply may be compromised by low aortic diastolic pressure combined with elevated LVEDP
  - Stroke volume is preserved

ICD-9-CM Code: 424.1

ETIOLOGY

- In patients <60 y, AS develops on a congenitally deformed valve—usually bicuspid
- Patients >60 y usually have calcific degeneration of a previously normal valve

USUAL TREATMENT

- Careful follow-up after murmur noted; usually with Doppler ECHO
- Aortic valve replacement following onset of symptoms
- From onset of angina, syncope, or CHF, 50% mortality at < 5, 3, and 2 y without surgical treatment

ASSESSMENT POINTS

SYSTEM	EFFECT	ASSESSMENT BY HX	PE	TEST
CV	Progression of stenosis	Symptoms (angina, dyspnea) appear	Murmur; S_4 gallop	Doppler ECHO for valve gradient
	Myocardial ischemia	Angina		ECG, coronary angiography
	LV dysfunction	Dyspnea, fatigue	S_3 gallop	CXR, ECHO
	Arrhythmias	Palpitations, syncope		ECG, ? Holter
	Syncope	Exertional arrhythmias		ECG, Holter
CNS	Stroke, syncope	Stroke, ± residua	Neuro exam Carotid bruit	Carotid Doppler

Key Reference: Jackson JM, Thomas SJ: Valvular heart disease. *In* Kaplan JA (ed): Cardiac Anesthesia, 3rd ed. Philadelphia, WB Saunders, 1993, ch 20.

PERIOPERATIVE IMPLICATIONS

Preoperative Preparation

- Continue antiarrhythmic drugs
- In prosthetic aortic valve, evaluate for anticoagulation status, risk of endocarditis

Monitoring

- ECG: ST-segment analysis ideal; may be difficult due to pre-existing changes of LVH
- Arterial line helpful to continuously follow arterial pressure
- PA catheter much less helpful; wide swings in filling pressure may lead to overtreatment
- TEE: not usually necessary, but can easily differentiate systolic from diastolic failure

Preinduction/Induction

- Avoid tachycardia, hypotension
- Because of sensitivity to volume depletion (low-compliance ventricle doesn't fill) and hypotension (poor coronary filling), hemodynamic changes should be either prevented or identified early and managed appropriately

Maintenance

- Fear of myocardial depression often overstated: contractility usually well preserved; however, volatile anesthetics associated with junctional rhythm, which ↓ stroke volume, cardiac output, and BP
- Bradycardia can cause hypotension; thick ventricle of limited distensibility, and excessively prolonging diastole does not improve ventricular filling

Extubation

- Period of potential ischemia

Postoperative Period

- Adequate pain relief helps to prevent undesirable tachycardia.

ANTICIPATED PROBLEMS/CONCERNS

- Prevent potential hemodynamic spiral of hypovolemia, hypotension, and tachycardia by careful attention to fluid requirements, pain relief, resolution of any sympathetic block
- Development of supraventricular arrhythmias, including AFib, deleterious; early identification and treatment can be crucial

APNEA OF THE NEWBORN

William L. Meadow, M.D., Ph.D.

RISK
- Full-term infants with neurologic disorders
- Premature infants, ± neurologic disorders

PERIOPERATIVE RISKS
- More prone to apnea during local or epidural anesthesia
- More prone to apnea postoperatively

WORRY ABOUT
- Unexpected apnea in recovery room
- Unexpected apnea in hours after outpatient procedures
- Unexpected apnea on ward hours after inpatient procedures

OVERVIEW
- Apnea in term infant never "physiologic"
- Apnea in preterm infants may signal CNS disorder or developmental immaturity
- Sudden onset of apnea in any infant may also reflect sepsis or hypoglycemia
- Relationship to subsequent SIDS unclear
- Utility of pneumogram screening controversial
- Indications for home apnea monitoring controversial

ICD-9-CM Code: 770.8

ETIOLOGY
- Term or preterm infants:
  - CNS disorders (seizures, bleeds, structural changes)
  - Systemic disorders (hypoglycemia, sepsis, GE reflux)
- Preterm infants:
  - Same as term infants
  - If full evaluation is negative, "physiologic" apnea of prematurity diagnosed

USUAL TREATMENT
- Theophylline
- Oxygen
- Transfusion
- CPAP

ASSESSMENT POINTS

SYSTEM	EFFECT	ASSESSMENT BY HX	PE	TEST
CV	Congenital heart disease leads to desaturation; PDA may cause CHF	Congenital heart disease, PGE_1 treatment	Murmur; cyanosis	Cardiac ECHO
RESP	Children with bronchopulmonary dysplasia may be prone to apnea	Hx of hyaline membrane disease or other parenchymal lung disorder	Abnormal pulmonary compliance or O_2 requirement	CXR; ABG; O_2 Sat
GI	GE reflux may cause vagal overload	Hx of reflux	None obvious	pH study; barium swallow
CNS	Seizures may cause apnea; structural abnormalities may create ineffective respiratory drive	Hx of seizures or change in neurologic development	Exam for seizures or neurologic change	EEG, head ultrasound; CT; MRI

Key Reference: Marchal F, et al: Neonatal apnea and apneic syndromes. Clin Perinatol 1987; 14:3.

PERIOPERATIVE IMPLICATIONS

Monitoring
- Routine

Airway
- Not usually a problem; obstructive apnea may occur but is rare
- Bronchospasm may occur in infants with bronchopulmonary dysplasia

Maintenance
- Usually no problem during procedure; vigilance required postoperatively

Extubation
- Watch for intermittent inadequate respiratory effort for hours

Adjuvants
- No special concerns

ANTICIPATED PROBLEMS/CONCERNS
- Perioperatively not complex; vigilance regarding care and assessment in postoperative period

APPENDICITIS, ACUTE

Jordan L. Blinder, M.D.

RISK

- Incidence 6–7% of population
- Highest in 2nd and 3rd decades
- Usual male:female ratio is 1:1, but there is a 2:1 male predominance from age 15–25 y.
- Most common extrauterine surgical emergency during gestation, occurring in 1:2000 deliveries

PERIOPERATIVE RISKS

- Mortality: <1% for nonperforated, 2% for perforated
- Risks increase with perforation and peritonitis.
- Risk of sepsis if perforated
- Fetal mortality range: 2.0–8.5% overall but as high as 35% in perforation with peritonitis.

WORRY ABOUT

- Aspiration of gastric contents
- Development of septic shock
- Antibiotic coverage
- Conversion to more extensive intra-abdominal surgery, e.g., for obstruction
- Carcinoid of the appendix

OVERVIEW

- The most common acute surgical condition of the abdomen
- Physical signs vary depending upon anatomic location and stage of disease.
- Over 50% of deaths from appendicitis are in patients over age 60 y, although this group represents only 10% of patients with appendicitis; concomitant disease, late diagnosis contribute.
- Mild dehydration and fever are common, but significant electrolyte disturbance and symptomatic dehydration are rare.

ICD-9-CM Code: 540.9

ETIOLOGY

- Obstruction of the appendiceal lumen by enlarged lymphoid tissue or fecalith
- Bacterial proliferation and fluid accumulation produce distention of hollow viscus with increased intraluminal pressure, leading to bacterial invasion of mucosal layer.
- Gangrenous infarction and eventual perforation may result in frank peritonitis.

USUAL TREATMENT

- Surgical appendectomy via classic McBurney incision or lower midline laparotomy; laparoscopic appendectomy has been advocated.
- For ruptured appendix with frank periappendiceal abscess, high-dose antibiotics followed by elective appendectomy at 6–12 wk is an option.

ASSESSMENT POINTS

SYSTEM	EFFECT	ASSESSMENT BY HX	PE	TEST
CV	Tachycardia	Review hospital record	Resting pulse Orthostatic signs	
RESP	V/Q mismatch, including MVO_2	Dyspnea Tachypnea	Splinting Observation	Pulse oximetry
GI	Ileus	Anorexia Vomiting	Abdominal auscultation	Electrolytes (if protracted)
	Perforation		Rebound tenderness Guarding	Upright CXR (rarely needed)
RENAL	Dehydration	Oliguria	Skin turgor	Urine specific gravity (rarely needed)
			Orthostatic signs	BUN/Cr (rarely needed)
CNS	Somnolence/ Confusion	Rule out sepsis	Mental status exam	WBC

Key Reference: Ortega AE, Hunter JG, Peters JH, et al: A prospective, randomized comparison of laparoscopic appendectomy with open appendectomy: Am J Surg 1995; 169: 208–213.

PERIOPERATIVE IMPLICATIONS

- Replace fluid and electrolyte deficits.
- Antibiotic coverage
- Aspiration prophylaxis: nonparticulate antacid and H_2 blocker
- Metoclopramide avoided if obstruction suspected.

Monitoring

- Routine

Airway

- Assess for rapid-sequence induction vs. awake intubation; assume full stomach.
- Secure airway with cuffed endotracheal tube.
- Laryngeal mask airway is contraindicated.

Induction

- Minimal depressant premedication
- Intravenous rapid-sequence induction
- Anticipate hypotension due to hypovolemia/peripheral vasodilation in early sepsis.
- Consider spinal anesthetic in exceptional circumstances.

Maintenance

- Requires profound skeletal muscle relaxation for dissection followed by fast recovery for brief closure.
- Intermediate-duration nondepolarizing relaxant or succinylcholine infusion for shorter cases
- Analgesic requirements for somatic pain not great once offending organ is removed

Extubation

- Assure that patient is awake and responsive.
- Assure full return of neuromuscular function.
- Vomiting common

Postoperative Period

- PCA a cost-effective option

Adjuvants

- Antibiotic interaction with nondepolarizers; "recurarization" rare
- Recrudescence of fever in postop period is common.

ANTICIPATED PROBLEMS/CONCERNS

- Concern for aspiration
- Need for intense muscle relaxation and rapid wound closure, along with potential interaction of muscle relaxants with antibiotics, increases likelihood of incomplete reversal of NMB.

ARNOLD-CHIARI SYNDROME

Nancy K. France, M.D.

RISK

- Most common anomaly involving cerebellum
- Present in all children with myelomeningocele
- Frequently asymptomatic
- >50% of those who require treatment will present before 3 mo of age
- In older children and adults commonly associated with syringomyelia

PERIOPERATIVE RISKS

- Most common causes of perioperative death are respiratory failure, meningitis, and ventriculitides
- Swallowing difficulties cause pooling of oral secretions; GER
- Gag reflex may be diminished or absent
- Mortality increased in those who rapidly progress to vocal cord paralysis, arm weakness, or cardiorespiratory arrest
- Potential air embolism during posterior fossa surgery

WORRY ABOUT

- Bulbar symptoms preop; these may influence postop airway management
- Procedure performed prone with the neck in flexion; extreme head flexion can cause brainstem compression
- Abnormal responses to hypoxia and hypercarbia because of cranial nerve and brainstem dysfunction; may persist after surgery
- Prone to apneic episodes

OVERVIEW

- Malformation characterized by caudal displacement of lower brainstem portions
- Results in frequent brainstem compression and complete obstruction of foramina of Luschka and Magendie→progressive hydrocephalus and dilation of cervical central canal (hydromelia)
- Multiple cranial n. defects (6,7,9–12)
- Presenting Sx: vocal cord paralysis with stridor and respiratory distress, apnea, ↓ gag reflex, abn swallowing and pulmonary aspiration, opisthotonos, cranial nerve deficits and upper arm weakness

ICD-9-CM Code: 741.0

ETIOLOGY

- Complex developmental anomaly appears early in life
- Associated with myelomeningocele
- Malformation consists of elongation of cerebellar vermis that results in herniation of caudal vermis and choroid plexus through the foramen magnum with kinking of medulla and upper cervical cord
- Medullary or cervical cord compression can occur

USUAL TREATMENT

- Surgical therapy: posterior fossa decompression with upper cervical laminectomy and opening of the dura to decompress the herniated cerebellar tongue and cervical cord; may include plugging obex and myelotomy

ASSESSMENT POINTS

SYSTEM	EFFECT	ASSESSMENT BY HX	PE	TEST
HEENT	Brainstem compression Cranial n. deficit	Vocal cord paralysis	Stridor, resp distress	O_2 desaturation
CV	Brainstem compression		BP instability, HTN	
RESP	Brainstem compression Cranial n. deficit	Swallowing difficulties ↓ Gag reflex	↑ Secretions Aspiration pneumonitis	CXR
RENAL	Dehydration		↓ Skin turgor	↓ UO, ↑ urine SG
GI	GE reflux			
CNS	Associated myelomeningocele, hydrocephalus	Possible ↑ ICP Central sleep apnea	Lower extremity paresis/paralysis Lyte imbalance and contraction of intravascular volume	
MS	Cervical cord compression		Upper extremity weakness and sensory changes	

Key Reference: McLeod ME, Creighton RE: Anesthesia for pediatric neurological and neuromuscular diseases. J Child Neurol 1986; 1:189–197.

PERIOPERATIVE IMPLICATIONS

Preoperative Preparation

- Preop atropine to decrease secretions
- Pulmonary infection due to recurrent aspiration; occasionally preop intubation and ventilation required
- Prone position for procedures in the posterior cranial fossa or upper cervical spine

Monitoring

- Precordial Doppler, ETN_2, or transesophageal ECHO to detect air embolism
- Occasionally, SEP

Airway

- Nasal ET tube may be better secured for prone position and postop airway control

- Extreme neck flexion may cause endobronchial intubation or brainstem compression
- Extreme head extension drives brainstem downward

Preinduction/Induction

- Preoxygenation, rapid sequence IV induction; preserve CPP, avoid ICP elevation, provide adequate depth of anesthesia
  or
  mask induction with volatile agent; mask PEEP diminishes stridor
- Prone: pad face; eyes free of compression

Maintenance

- Any anesthetic technique; frequent choice is fentanyl/isoflurane and a nondepolarizing muscle relaxant

- Controlled ventilation
- ICP reduced by hyperventilation ($PaCO_2$ 25–28 mmHg), mannitol, furosemide

Extubation

- Endotracheal tube postop if vocal cord paresis and depressed gag reflex remain

Postoperative Period

- Stridor frequently improved; pts require close monitoring for several days post surgery

ANTICIPATED PROBLEMS/CONCERNS

- Some with vocal cord paralysis and diminished gag reflex may require tracheostomy and gastrostomy.

ARTERITIS, TAKAYASU'S

Joseph F. Foss, M.D.

Joseph F. Foss, M.D.

RISK

- People within USA: rare (<< 24:100,000)
- Appears in adolescence
- Race and sex prevalence: Asian; females > males

PERIOPERATIVE RISKS

- Acute laryngeal edema seen in related syndromes (polyarteritis nodosa and temporal arteritis)
- Difficult arterial access
- Major organ ischemia or thromboembolism

WORRY ABOUT

- Pulmonary vasculitis in 50% of patients, resulting in pulmonary hypertension
- Renal function
- High cardiac afterload
- Hyperextension of neck may compromise cerebral blood flow

OVERVIEW

- Chronic occlusive panarteritis of medium and large vessels, including pulmonary vasculature
- Renal artery involvement induces neurovascular hypertension (most frequent cause of hypertension in Asian children)
- Pulmonary dysfunction may be present

ICD-9-CM Code: 446.7

ETIOLOGY

- Immune-complex mechanism is hypothesized

USUAL TREATMENT

- Steroids
- Immunomodulators and methotrexate are being studied
- PTCA for treatment of stenosis
- Platelet inhibitors or anticoagulants as adjuncts to decrease thromboembolic risk
- ACE inhibitors for hypertension

ASSESSMENT POINTS

SYSTEM	EFFECT	ASSESSMENT BY HX	PE	TEST
HEENT	Head pain	Head pain	Pain on pressure of inflamed artery	Biopsy of affected artery
CV	Multiple occlusions of peripheral arteries Ischemic heart disease (ostial occlusion) Cardiac valve dysfunction (aortic regurgitation) Cardiac conduction defects Hypertension (2° to renal artery occlusion) in 50% of patients	Angina	Diminished peripheral pulses Murmur Hypertension	ECHO
RESP	Pulmonary hypertension Hypoxemia 2° to V/Q mismatching			Arterial hypoxemia
HEME	Elevated ESR Anemia Elevated immunoglobulins			ESR Hct, Hgb
RENAL	Renal artery stenosis		Hypertension	BUN/Cr
CNS	Cerebral ischemia or infarction 2° to carotid involvement CVAs in 15% of patients	Vertigo Visual disturbances Syncope, seizures	Carotid or subclavian bruits Ocular changes	
MS	Ankylosing spondylitis Rheumatoid arthritis	Pain in head Pain in joints		

Key Reference: Stoelting RK, Dierdorf SF: Anaesthesia and Co-existing Disease, 3rd ed. New York, Churchill Livingstone, pp 123–124.

PERIOPERATIVE IMPLICATIONS

Preoperative Preparation

- Routine

Monitoring

- Noninvasive BP and pulse oximeters may be ineffective
- Arterial access may require cut-down
- Pulmonary artery catheter may be useful, but placement may fail in up to 50% of cases

Airway

- Avoid extension of neck in symptomatic patient

Induction

- Routine

Maintenance

- Maintain intraoperative BP within range usually seen for patient; hypotension may be associated with higher risk of ischemia or thrombosis of major organs
- Sympathomimetics may be used to maintain BP while correcting underlying causes of hypotension
- Avoid low CO_2 due to hyperventilation and use agents that maintain cerebral blood flow, especially with carotid involvement

Extubation

- Routine

Adjuvants

- Perioperative steroid replacement may be indicated

Postoperative Period

- Routine

ANTICIPATED PROBLEMS/CONCERNS

- Postoperative cardiorespiratory failure due to pulmonary hypertension
- Adrenal deficiency state if steroid supplementation or replacement doesn't occur in steroid-dependent patient
- Acute airway edema from disease

ASPIRATION, PERIOPERATIVE: PREVENTION AND MANAGEMENT

Paula A. Craigo, M.D.

RISK

- Risk of significant aspiration: 1.36 to 15 per 10,000 anesthetized patients
- Mortality: 0.2 to 0.3 per 10,000
- Loss of protective reflexes and sphincter function
- Obstructed or abnormal GI motility
- Increased GI contents
- Trauma, emergency/night surgery, pregnancy

PERIOPERATIVE RISKS

- Mortality after aspiration: 5%; higher if ASA >2

WORRY ABOUT

- 20% of patients who aspirated had no risk factor; 66% had difficult intubation
- Rapid-sequence induction in cardiac patients leads to tachycardia, hypertension, hypotension

OVERVIEW

- Significant aspiration has no definitive treatment and is best prevented
- Four major aspiration syndromes: airway obstruction by particulate matter, drowning, chemical pneumonitis, infectious pneumonia
- Consider aspiration in differential diagnosis of bronchospasm with hypoxemia

ICD-9-CM Codes: 997.3 (aspiration pneumonia after procedure); 668.0 (aspiration, peripartum)

ETIOLOGY

- Loss of protective reflexes: sedation, neuromuscular disorders/relaxants, altered mental status, reflux
- Obstructed or abnormal motility: achalasia, gastroparesis, pain, opioids
- Increased GI contents: bleeding, obstruction, feeds
- Other: difficult airway, pregnancy, obesity, emergency surgery

USUAL TREATMENT

- Suctioning: bronchoscopy if obstructing particles
- Lavage, steroids not helpful; surfactant investigational
- Empiric antibiotics may confuse cultures: consider if compromised patient, fulminant course, high bacterial load

ASSESSMENT POINTS

SYSTEM	EFFECT	ASSESSMENT BY HX	PE	TEST
HEENT (airway)	Awake intubation in difficult airway	Hx difficult airway, head and neck surgery/radiation, diabetes	Airway exam Palm or prayer signs	X-rays, CT scan, OR records as available
CV	Rapid-sequence intubation may lead to ischemia with tachycardia, hyper/hypotension; myocardial depression	Anginal Sx, exercise intolerance, Hx CHF, CAD Age, sex, risk factors	S_3, rales, displaced PMI	ECG, ECHO in selected patients
RESP	Rapid-sequence intubation may lead to bronchospasm	Hx pulmonary disease, wheezing with URI, smoking	Wheezing, prolonged expiratory phase	CXR
GI	Abnormal sphincters, motility, acidity	Hx peptic ulcer disease, reflux Sx, diabetes, scleroderma		
NM	↑ ICP leads to vomiting; depressed protective reflexes; muscle weakness		Neurologic exam	

Key Reference: Kallar SK, Everett LL: Potential risks and preventive measures for pulmonary aspiration: New concepts in preoperative fasting guidelines. Anesth Analg 1993; 77:171–182.

PERIOPERATIVE IMPLICATIONS

Preoperative Preparation

- NPO status
  - Traditionally, nonemergent patients NPO for >6 h, liquids and solids
  - Currently, clear liquids up to 2 or 3 h preoperatively in healthy elective surgery patients
- Prophylaxis in selected patients:
  - ↑ gastric pH: antacid, H_2 blockers, proton pump inhibition
  - ↓ GI contents: metoclopramide, NG suction

Monitoring

- Routine

Airway

- Protect airway with endotracheal tube
- Awake intubation in difficult airway
- Laryngeal mask airway not protective against aspiration

Preinduction/Induction

- Denitrogenation with 100% O_2
- Check optimal patient position, table height, drugs and tools available, suction at hand
- Rapid-sequence induction; cricoid pressure on until endotracheal tube placement assured by ET CO_2
- Highest risk during induction prior to placement of ETT

Maintenance

- Care with level of sedation during sedation/regional cases

Extubation

- Return of muscular strength/coordination/consciousness enough to protect airway if emesis occurs

Postoperative Period

- 50% of aspirations occur postoperatively
- If chemical pneumonitis occurs, initial postoperative CXR may be normal, proceeding to "white-out" in a few to 24 h
- PEEP redistributes lung water, improves oxygenation; higher PEEP may ↓ cardiac output and ventilation
- Maintaining low filling pressures may limit lung fluid accumulation, worsen negative effects of PEEP

Adjuvants

- Muscle relaxants
- Regional drugs
- Reversal agents
- Drug interactions

ANTICIPATED PROBLEMS/CONCERNS

- Careful identification of risk factors, airway quality, cardiac reserve
- Risk of aspiration must be weighed against quality of airway and cardiopulmonary effects of induction/intubation

ASTHMA, ACUTE

Thomas Corbridge, M.D.
Jesse Hall, M.D.

RISK

- 12 million in USA
- Race with highest prevalence: African Americans have higher asthma-related mortality rates than Caucasians
- Increased severity in adult females
- Greater in atopic individuals

PERIOPERATIVE RISKS

- Increased risk of exacerbation and barotrauma
- Risk may be related to degree of preop control.

WORRY ABOUT

- Endotracheal tube–induced bronchospasm
- Excessive lung hyperinflation during mechanical ventilation
- Medication side effects, including hypokalemia (β_2-adrenergic agonists)
- Adrenal insufficiency in prior oral corticosteroid users

OVERVIEW

- Characterized by bronchial wall inflammation, airway hyperreactivity, and variable degrees of reversible airflow obstruction resulting in wheeze, dyspnea, and cough
- Airflow obstruction results from airway inflammation, intraluminal mucus, and bronchoconstriction.
- Airflow obstruction and possible loss of lung elastance cause lung hyperinflation.
- Attacks may be sudden or slowly progressive.

ICD-9-CM Code: 493.9

ETIOLOGY

- Genetic predisposition; atopic individuals at risk
- Childhood exposure to tobacco smoke, allergens, or bronchial wall infection may increase risk of developing asthma later in life.
- May result from occupational exposures (e.g., grain dust, plastics, latex)
- Attacks usually triggered by respiratory tract infections or noncompliance

USUAL TREATMENT

- Medical therapy
  – First-line drugs: oxygen, inhaled albuterol, systemic corticosteroids. Subcutaneous epinephrine or terbutaline for patients unable to take inhaled drugs or not responding adequately to inhaled Rx. Terbutaline preferred in pregnant patients.
  – Second-line drugs: ipratropium bromide, theophylline (role in acute asthma controversial), helium/oxygen
- Mechanical ventilation: Endotracheal intubation is indicated for cardiopulmonary arrest, near-arrest, coma, or obtundation, or continued in those already undergoing anesthesia with endotracheal intubation.

ASSESSMENT POINTS

SYSTEM	EFFECT	ASSESSMENT BY HX	PE	TEST
HEENT	Sinusitis, nasal polyposis	Nasal congestion, post nasal drip, headaches, decreased sense of smell	Nasal mucosal erythema or edema, nasal polyps, granular pharyngitis	Sinus CT or sinus x-ray
CV	Tachyarrhythmias, possible pulmonary hypertension	Palpitations, Heart rate	Tachycardia, irregular rhythm, loud P_2	ECG ECHO
RESP	Airflow obstruction Decreased lung elastance, hyperinflation, hypoxemia, hypercapnia Variations in peak flow	Dyspnea, cough, wheeze, chest tightness, nighttime awakenings, exercise-induced symptoms Peak flow diary	Prolonged I:E, decreased breath sounds, wheezes Pulsus paradoxus	Pulmonary function tests, CXR, ABG
ENDO	Steroid-induced hyperglycemia, adrenal insufficiency (prior <1 y steroid users)	Polyuria, polydipsia, weakness	Hypotension in adrenal insufficiency	Glucose, electrolytes, cortisol, ACTH stimulation test
MS	Steroid myopathy, steroid-paralytic myopathy	Difficulty climbing stairs or rising from chair Difficulty weaning from mechanical ventilation	Proximal muscle weakness in steroid myopathy Possible quadriplegia in steroid-paralytic myopathy	Cybex testing, measurement of inspiratory muscle force, CPK, EMG, muscle biopsy

Key Reference: Corbridge T, Hall J: The assessment and management of adults with status asthmaticus. Am J Resp Crit Care Med 1995, 151:1296–1316.

PERIOPERATIVE IMPLICATIONS

Preoperative Preparation

- Assess degree of preoperative control.
- Optimize medical treatment (acute attacks require systemic corticosteroids and more frequent inhaled β-agonists).
- In intubated patients, avoid ventilator-induced lung hyperinflation.
- Assess risk of adrenal insufficiency.

Monitoring

- Airway peak-to-plateau gradient (as determined by an inspiratory pause) is a useful measure of airway resistance.
- Plateau pressure (Pplat), a measure of lung hyperinflation, may be best predictor of complications of hypotension and barotrauma. Peak pressure does not predict complications.
- Consider keeping Pplat <30 cm H_2O by prolonging expiratory time (e.g., ↓ minute ventilation and/or ↑ inspiratory flow; use square flow waveform).

Airway

- Large oral tubes to ↓ airway resistance and aid mucus clearance. Nasal intubation may be preferred in awake patients. Problems with nasal tubes include need for smaller tube and high incidence of polyps and sinusitis.

Induction

- Postintubation hypotension may result from lung hyperinflation, hypovolemia, and sedation/paralysis. Significant lung hyperinflation mimics tension pneumothorax. A trial of hypoventilation improves cardiopulmonary status within 30–60 sec in former. Volume challenge is indicated for hypotensive patients.

Maintenance

- Rising peak-to-plateau pressure gradient suggests ↑ airway resistance.
- Rising Pplat suggests worsening lung hyperinflation.
- Consider keeping Pplat <30 cm H_2O by prolonging expiratory time. May need to accept hypercapnia.

Extubation

- May precipitate exacerbation. Inhaled β-agonists may be needed more frequently post extubation.

Adjuvants

- Muscle relaxants + systemic corticosteroids may cause acute myopathy.
- Ketamine, isoflurane, and enflurane are bronchodilators.

Postoperative Period

- Observe for asthma exacerbation.

ANTICIPATED PROBLEMS/CONCERNS

- Hypokalemia
- Lung hyperinflation resulting in hypotension or pneumothorax
- ↑ Risk of tension pneumothorax. Clinical features of lung hyperinflation mimic tension pneumothorax. If hypoventilation does not quickly achieve cardiopulmonary stability, consider chest tube placement.

ATHEROSCLEROTIC DISEASE

Jacqueline M. Leung, M.D.

RISK

- Prevalence: 2,000,000 persons in US
- 56,000,000 persons have some form of cardiovascular disease

PERIOPERATIVE RISKS

- CAD ↑ the risk of developing postoperative myocardial ischemia
- Presence of CAD in vascular surgical patients increases operative and long-term mortality

WORRY ABOUT

- ↑ Risk of perioperative myocardial ischemia and perioperative cardiac complications
- ↑ Risk of CVA not evident after nonvascular surgery
- Aortic dissection in cases of aneurysm requiring emergency surgery

OVERVIEW

- Thickening and hardening of the medium-sized and large arteries accounts for large proportion of heart attacks and cases of ischemic heart disease
- Also leads to strokes, peripheral vascular disease, and aneurysm of lower abdominal aorta
- Blood vessels affected include coronary, carotid, basilar, and vertebral arteries, as well as aorta and iliac arteries

ICD-9-CM Code: 414.0 (atherosclerotic heart disease)

ETIOLOGY

- Multifactorial
- Risk factors: hyperlipidemia, HTN, cigarette smoking, male sex, diabetes mellitus

USUAL TREATMENT

- Primary prevention includes modification of risk factors, esp in high-risk individuals, and prophylaxis with aspirin
- Atherosclerotic heart disease: anti-anginal Rx is employed for symptomatic persons; other treatment includes angioplasty and CABG surgery
- Carotid artery disease: carotid endarterectomy
- Other cerebral vascular insufficiency: extracranial-intracranial bypass sometimes performed
- Peripheral vascular insufficiency: angioplasty or revascularization of lower extremities
- Abdominal aortic aneurysm: abdominal aortic aneurysmectomy

ASSESSMENT POINTS

SYSTEM	EFFECT	ASSESSMENT BY HX	PE	TEST
CV	Hypertension Coronary artery stenoses MI	Usually asymptomatic Angina, may be asymptomatic	Normal if treated S_3 and/or S_4 Cardiomegaly	Vital signs ECG ECG exercise treadmill Pharmacologic stress test, coronary angiography, ECHO, radionuclide studies
	Ventricular dysfunction	Exercise intolerance Sx of heart failure	S_3 and/or S_4 Cardiomegaly	Determine LV ejection fraction and function by ECHO, radionuclide studies
RESP	COPD (many are smokers)	Dyspnea on exertion	Decreased breath sounds, prolonged expiration, wheezes	ABG PFTs (if indicated)
CNS	Cerebral vascular insufficiency Cerebral infarct	TIAs Syncope Strokes	Carotid bruits Focal neurologic deficits	Doppler or angiogram (if indicated)
PERIPHERAL ARTERIES	Occlusive lesions Abdominal aortic aneurysm	Claudication Abdominal pain, may be asymptomatic	Decreased pulses Pulsatile abdominal mass	Angiogram (if indicated) Aortogram (if indicated) MRI (if indicated)

Key Reference: Leung J, et al: Management of patients with coronary artery disease. Semin Anesth 1990; 9:258–269.

PERIOPERATIVE IMPLICATIONS

Preoperative Preparation

- Stabilize cardiac Sx medically
- Continue anti-anginal Rx
- Attention to and stabilization of co-existent diseases

Monitoring

- Cardiovascular
  - ECG with appropriate lead placement, ST-trending
  - Consider CVP or PA catheterization to monitor preload, esp in patients with Hx of CHF
  - Consider TEE, esp in patients with uninterpretable ECG (e.g., ventricular pacemaker or LBBB)
- Cerebrovascular
  - In carotid endarterectomy, measurement of stump pressure, EEG, and SEPs have been used
  - CSF pressure monitoring and drainage in thoracoabdominal aneurysmectomy

Airway

- None

Preinduction/Induction

- Preventing tachycardia (use of short-acting β-blockers desirable)
- Treat BP changes aggressively

Maintenance

- No one anesthetic agent or technique superior, maintaining HR at low level and hemodynamic stability more important
- For peripheral vascular surgery, regional anesthesia in combination with postop epidural analgesia may ↓ incidence of graft thrombosis (see also Peripheral Vascular Disease)
- For carotid endarterectomy, maintaining cerebral perfusion pressure important goal
- For abdominal aortic surgery, optimizing loading conditions, detecting and treating myocardial ischemia and ventricular dysfunction are important, particularly during and after aortic clamping

Extubation

- Same concerns as during induction
- Rapid awakening to allow neurological assessment after carotid endarterectomy

Adjuvants

- β-blocking agents and other antihypertensives useful in hyperdynamic situations
- Prophylactic nitroglycerin and calcium-channel blockers to treat myocardial ischemia not conclusively proven effective
- Caution in use of vasoconstrictors, such as α-adrenergic agonists, to ↑ BP in cases of heart failure

ANTICIPATED PROBLEMS/CONCERNS

- Postoperative myocardial ischemia and other cardiac complications
- Graft occlusion (with peripheral revascularization procedures)
- Heart failure (with a history of CHF)
- Paraplegia, particularly after surgery for thoracoabdominal aneurysms
- Renal dysfunction in cases of aortic surgery

ATRIAL FIBRILLATION

RISK

- Affects 1% of those >60 y
- 0.4% of adult population
- Racial predominance: none

PERIOPERATIVE RISKS

- Rapid ventricular response in CHF
- Myocardial ischemia
- Embolization

WORRY ABOUT

- ↓ Cardiac output
- Myocardial ischemia
- Embolization

OVERVIEW

- Develops over 2 decades in 2% of patients >30 y
- Related to left atrial size, underlying heart disease, and abnormal electrophysiology
- Incidence ↑ with age
- Most affected people have underlying cardiac disease

ICD-9-CM Code: 427.31

ETIOLOGY

- CAD
- Rheumatic heart disease
- Cardiomyopathy
- Mitral stenosis
- Hypertensive CV disease
- Pericarditis
- Hypoxia
- Heart failure
- Pulmonary emboli
- Hyperthyroidism
- Subarachnoid hemorrhage
- Sarcoidosis/amyloidosis
- Idiopathic

TREATMENT

- Cardioversion for hemodynamic instability
- Digitalis
- ß rb's
- Calcium antagonists
- Quinidine (with digitalis)

ASSESSMENT POINTS

SYSTEM	EFFECT	ASSESSMENT BY HX	PE	TEST
CV	CHF Angina Stroke	Palpitations Chest pain Dyspnea Orthopnea	Variation in intensity of 1st heart sound; absence of A waves in jugular venous pulse; irregularly irregular ventricular rhythm	ECHO (if indicated)
RESP	CHF Pulm embolism	Dyspnea Orthopnea Chest pain Tachypnea	S_3 Rales Wheezing	CXR V/Q scan (if suspicion of pulmonary embolism)
GI	Ischemic bowel from low flow or embolization	Abdominal pain	Acute abdomen	ABGs/electrolytes
RENAL	↓ Renal perfusion	↓ Urine output		BUN/Cr
CNS	Syncope, lightheadedness, fatigue, dizziness	Stroke	Neurologic deficit	Head CT
MS		Anginal equivalent		See CV

Key Reference: Falk RH, Podrid PJ (eds): Atrial Fibrillation: Mechanism and Management. New York, Raven Press, 1992.

PERIOPERATIVE IMPLICATIONS

Preoperative Preparation

- Search for precipitating causes
- Control ventricular response or convert to normal sinus rhythm if unstable

Monitoring

- ECG with S-T segment analysis
- PA line in patients with low cardiac output

Airway

- None

Preinduction/Induction

- Avoid excessive sympathetic stimulation
- Maintain oxygenation/ventilation

Maintenance

- Monitor oxygenation, maintain normocarbia
- Control ventricular response

Extubation

- Avoid excessive sympathetic stimulation

Adjuvants

- Digitalis: little effect of anesthetic agents
- Ca^{2+} antagonists: can ↓ AV conduction; can ↑ NM blockade
- ß rb agents: can cause ↓ AV conduction
- Quinidine (with digitalis): ↑ NM blockade

Postoperative Period

- Maintain adequate analgesia

ANTICIPATED PROBLEMS/CONCERNS

- Rapid ventricular response may result in significant fall in cardiac output
- DC cardioversion establishes sinus rhythm in >90%

ATRIAL FLUTTER

John L. Atlee, M.D.

RISK

- Atrial flutter (AFlut) and atrial fibrillation (AFib) occur in 1% and 12% of hospitalized patients, respectively
- 5–10% of persons > 75 y have AFib w/o risk factors
- Risk factors: CAD, COPD, hypertension, cardiomyopathies
- No apparent race or gender predilection

PERIOPERATIVE RISKS

- Circulatory insufficiency or ischemia from slow or rapid HR in patients with CAD
- Cerebral, coronary, or systemic embolism from left atrial mural thrombus

WORRY ABOUT

- Associated disease, especially adequacy of CV and pulmonary function
- Ventricular rates > 200 bpm with quinidine, amiodarone, vagolytics, ß-agonists
- AFlut or AFib with Wolff-Parkinson-White or Lown-Ganong-Levine syndromes

OVERVIEW

- AFlut and AFib are reentry atrial tachyarrhythmias associated with structural heart disease
- Type I AFlut: regular atrial rates 240–340 bpm with fixed (often 2:1) AV conduction
- Type II AFlut: regular atrial rates 350–450 bpm with variable or fixed AV conduction
- AFib: disorganized atrial activity and "irregularly irregular" ventricular response (100–200 bpm)
- Differential: type I AFlut is, and type II AFlut and AFib are not, pace-terminable
- Risk of stroke in patients with nonvalvular AFib is 5–7× greater than in those without

ICD-9-CM Codes: 427.31 (AFib); 427.32 (AFlut)

ETIOLOGY

- AFlut and AFib are acquired, with no specific cause beside pulmonary or structural heart disease
- Associated with chronic pulmonary disease, valvular and rheumatic heart disease, CAD, postcardiac surgery, hyperthyroidism, pericarditis-myocarditis, and chronic alcoholism

USUAL TREATMENT

- Drugs to reduce ventricular rate, convert AFlut and AFib to sinus rhythm, or prevent recurrences
- Systemic anticoagulation with warfarin or heparin
- Pacing for chronic AFib with too slow V rate; DC cardioversion (acute AFlut and AFib).

ASSESSMENT POINTS

SYSTEM	EFFECT	ASSESSMENT BY HX	PE	TEST
CV	AFlut–AFib	Palpitations, dizziness, weakness, lethargy	Irregular pulse, pulse deficit, S_1–S_2 intensity vary S_3, rales, wheezes	ECG, Holter monitoring, electrophysiologic studies
	LV function	CHF, exercise intolerance		ECHO, exercise ECG, MRI, cardiac catheter
	CAD severity	Sx of angina		Stress ECG, dipyridamole scintigraphy, angiography
RESP	CHF, COPD	Dyspnea, orthopnea cough	S_3, rales, wheezes	CXR; pulmonary function testing
GI	↓ Perfusion	GI distress, diarrhea		
RENAL	↓ Perfusion	Polyuria (nocturnal)		BUN/Cr
CNS	Ischemia or stroke	Syncope, mental changes, paresis/paralysis, dementia	Neurologic or mental deficits	See CV assessment

Key Reference: Atlee JL: Arrhythmias and Pacemakers. Philadelphia, WB Saunders, 1996.

PERIOPERATIVE IMPLICATIONS

Preoperative Preparation

- Adequate ventricular rate control (80–100 bpm) with digitalis or β-blockers
- Treat CHF if present; otherwise, optimize cardiopulmonary function
- If acute onset AFlut–AFib (≤ 3 days), consider cardioversion, anticoagulation

Monitoring

- ECG with ST–T trending and strip-chart recorder for documentation of new arrhythmias
- Direct arterial and PA catheter monitoring if needed for BP instability, LV dysfunction
- SpO_2 with rapid (neonatal) response capability

Induction

- LV dysfunction and AFlut–AFib increase risk of severe hypotension during induction with agents such as thiopental or propofol
- Desflurane, ketamine, and pancuronium may accelerate ventricular rate with AFlut–AFib

Maintenance

- Expect ↑ circulatory instability and less tolerance of large fluid shifts or blood loss
- No anesthetic drugs are especially contraindicated; caution with drugs that speed conduction

Extubation

- Possibly at ↑ risk for thromboembolism with hyperdynamic circulatory state
- Use drugs/means to reduce/avoid effects of airway stimulation and hyperdynamic circulation

Adjuvants

- Sympathomimetic or antimuscarinic drugs may accelerate ventricular rate
- Best drugs to control ventricular rate are β-blockers or edrophonium (5–10 mg × 2).
- Anticoagulation indicated for most patients as soon as risk of perioperative surgical bleeding is reduced to a reasonable level

Postoperative Period

- Patients who develop AFib after CABG surgery have more strokes than those in sinus rhythm

ANTICIPATED PROBLEMS/CONCERNS

- Patients with acute or chronic AFlut or AFib appear at ↑ risk of embolic stroke
- Dangerous acceleration of ventricular rate to > 300 bpm with Wolff-Parkinson-White or Lown-Ganong-Levine syndrome

ATRIAL SEPTAL DEFECT — OSTIUM PRIMUM

Long K. Han, M.D.

RISK

- People within USA: 60,000 with ostium primum ASD (30% of ASDs)
- Gender prevalence: female > male, 2:1
- ↑ Incidence in high altitude
- ↑ Incidence in Down syndrome

PERIOPERATIVE RISKS

- Perioperative mortality rate: 1%
- Late in course, associated with atrial dysrhythmias and CHF with L→R shunt
- ↑ Risk of atrial dysrthymias, heart block, and air embolus with surgical repair

WORRY ABOUT

- Risk of infectious endocarditis and air embolization with IV access

OVERVIEW

- Failure of inferior septum to close—usually an endocardial cushion defect associated with mitral and tricuspid valve abnormalities
- Usually asymptomatic early in life
- L→R shunt causes ↑ pulmonary blood flow
- Late in course: CHF and shunt reversal
- Frequently associated with tricuspid regurgitation and/or mitral regurgitation
- Life expectancy without repair ~40 y
- Diagnosis by ECHO

ICD-9-CM Code: 745.61

ETIOLOGY

- Failure of septum primum to fuse with endocardial cushion to close ostium primum

USUAL TREATMENT

- Digitalis and diuretics for child with CHF
- Antiarrhythmics occasionally needed for atrial dysrhythmias
- Surgery indicated when Qp:Qs ratio ≥ 1.5:1, if ASD >25 mm diameter, if anomalous pulmonary venous return, if CHF, if significant cardiomegaly

ASSESSMENT POINTS

SYSTEM	EFFECT	ASSESSMENT BY HX	PE	TEST
HEENT	Difficult intubation	Down syndrome	Down syndrome facies	
CV	Atrial dysrhythmias	Palpitation SOB, frequent fatigue Cyanosis (rare)	Irregular rate and rhythm	ECG (RVH, LAD) ECHO
	Right-sided heart failure L→R shunting (rare) Hypertrophic RA and RV		Right heart enlargement Loud S$_1$, fixed S$_2$, and crescendo-decrescendo systolic murmur	Angiography Dye dilution study
RESP	↑ Pulmonary blood flow ↑ PVR	SOB Frequent URIs	Rales, wheezing	CXR
GI	Hepatic dysfunction if severe CHF	Jaundice	Hepatomegaly	LFTs, PT
CNS	Embolic stroke from chronic AFib	Various neurologic changes		Head CT, cardiac ECHO if emboli suspected
MS			Enlarged left costal cartilage	
RENAL	Renal dysfunction if severe CHF			Cr, BUN

Key Reference: Kamban J: Atrial septal defects. *In* Kamban J (ed): Cardiac Anesthesia for Infants and Children. St Louis, Mosby–Year Book, 1994, pp 182–192.

PERIOPERATIVE IMPLICATIONS

Preoperative Medications

- Narcotics and anticholinergics
- Antibiotic prophylaxis
- Continue digoxin if used for rate control

Monitoring

- Routine monitors, arterial line, CVP; TEE helpful in assessing anatomy before CPB; check for air and residual shunting after CPB; central and peripheral temperature monitoring

Induction

- IV induction theoretically slowed by L→R shunt; inhalational induction not significantly affected

Maintenance

- Avoid nitrous oxide to minimize size of air bubbles; any other techniques appropriate; watch for shunt reversal with hypothermia, hypercarbia, hypoxemia

Extubation

- Usually mechanically ventilated at end of any operative procedure, especially if heart block is present

Adjuvants

- Watch for dysrhythmia from hypokalemia if patient is on digoxin and diuretics

Postoperative Period

- Adequate analgesia for sternotomy or thoracotomy pain; pacemakers available for transient heart block

ANTICIPATED PROBLEMS/CONCERNS

- Air emboli with vascular access
- Dysrhythmia
- Heart failure
- Heart block after CPB
- Sternal infection (rare)
- Endocarditis (rare)

ATRIAL SEPTAL DEFECT — OSTIUM SECUNDUM

Long K. Han, M.D.

RISK

• People within USA: 140,000 with ostium secundum ASD (70% of ASDs)
• Gender prevalence: female > male, 2:1
• Familial incidence: significant if associated with P-R prolongation or forearm and hand abnormalities (Holt-Oram syndrome)
• ↑ Incidence in high altitude

PERIOPERATIVE RISKS

• Perioperative mortality rate: 1%
• Late in course, associated with atrial dysrhythmias and CHF with L→R shunt
• ↑ Risk of atrial dysrthymias, heart block (rare), and air embolus with surgical repair

WORRY ABOUT

• Risk of infectious endocarditis and air embolization with IV access

OVERVIEW

• Failure of closure of midseptal fossa ovalis
• Usually asymptomatic early in life
• L→R shunt causes ↑ pulmonary blood flow
• Late in course: CHF and shunt reversal
• Life expectancy without repair ~40 y
• 15% incidence of associated noncardiac anomalies
• Diagnosis by ECHO

ICD-9-CM Code: 745.5

ETIOLOGY

• Failure of septum secundum to fuse with septum primum to form interatrial septum

USUAL TREATMENT

• Digitalis and diuretics for child with CHF
• Antiarrhythmics occasionally needed for atrial dysrhythmias
• Surgery or transcatheter closure is indicated when Qp:Qs ratio equals or exceeds 1.5:1
• Surgery also indicated if ASD >25 mm diameter or if anomalous pulmonary venous return is present

ASSESSMENT POINTS

SYSTEM	EFFECT	ASSESSMENT BY HX	PE	TEST
CV	Atrial dysrhythmias Right-sided heart failure L→R shunting	Palpitation SOB, DOE	Irregular rate and rhythm Right heart enlargement Loud S_1, fixed S_2, and crescendo-decrescendo systolic murmur	Echocardiogram Angiography Dye dilution study
RESP	↑ Pulmonary blood flow ↑ PVR	SOB Frequent URIs	Rales, wheezing	CXR
GI	Hepatic dysfunction if severe CHF	Jaundice	Hepatomegaly	LFTs, PT
RENAL	Renal dysfunction if severe CHF			Cr, BUN
CNS	Embolic stroke from chronic AFib	Various changes		Head CT, cardiac ECHO if suspected emboli
MS			Holt-Oram syndrome Large left costal cartilage	

Key Reference: Kamban J: Atrial septal defects. *In* Kamban J (ed): Cardiac Anesthesia for Infants and Children. St Louis, Mosby–Year Book, 1994, pp 182–192.

PERIOPERATIVE IMPLICATIONS

Preoperative Medications

• Narcotics and anticholinergics
• Antibiotic prophylaxis
• Continue digoxin if used for rate control

Monitoring

• Routine monitors, arterial line, CVP; TEE helpful in assessing anatomy before CPB, and check for air, and residual shunting after CPB; central and peripheral temperature monitoring

Induction

• IV induction theoretically slowed by L→R shunt; inhalational induction not significantly affected

Maintenance

• Avoid nitrous oxide to minimize size of air bubbles; any other techniques appropriate; watch for shunt reversal with hypothermia, hypercarbia, hypoxemia

Extubation

• Controversial; usually can be extubated at the end of case if hemodynamically stable

Adjuvants

• Watch for dysrhythmia from hypokalemia if patient is on digoxin and diuretics

Postoperative Period

• Adequate analgesia for sternotomy or thoracotomy pain

ANTICIPATED PROBLEMS/CONCERNS

• Air emboli with vascular access
• Dysrhythmia
• Heart failure
• Heart block after CPB (rare)
• Sternal infection (rare)
• Endocarditis (rare)

AUTOIMMUNE DISEASE — COLD

Joseph L. Seltzer, M.D.

RISK

- Rare
- Autoimmune hemolytic anemias occur in 1 of 80,000 persons; of these, 17.3% are due to cold antibodies.

PERIOPERATIVE RISKS

- Acute hemolysis due to cold
- Hemoglobinemia
- Hemoglobinuria
- Rarely, vascular occlusion

WORRY ABOUT

- Cooling to 28–31°C will cause hemolysis.
- These temperatures can be reached in extremities in the OR or during cardiopulmonary bypass.

OVERVIEW

- In two circumstances antibodies will react in the cold to produce hemolysis:
  – IgG antibodies associated with mononucleosis, *Mycoplasma* pneumonia
  – IgM antibodies are found in the idiopathic form of the disease and in lymphoproliferative disease.
- Hemolysis usually occurs at temperatures below 31°C.

ICD-9-CM Code: 283.0

ETIOLOGY

- Idiopathic
- Lymphoid malignancy
- Infections: *Mycoplasma* pneumonia, mononucleosis

USUAL TREATMENT

- Keep warm, folic acid
- For severe cases, chlorambucil or cyclophosphamide
- Plasmapheresis
- Prednisone

ASSESSMENT POINTS

SYSTEM	EFFECT	PE	TEST
HEME	Mild to moderate anemia	Hgb	
			Blood bank antiglobulin tests
GU	Hemoglobinuria		

Key Reference: Gilliland BC: Autoimmune hemolytic anemia. *In* Rossi EC, Simon TL, Moss GS (eds): Principles of Transfusion Medicine. Baltimore, Williams & Wilkins, 1991, pp 99–112.

PERIOPERATIVE IMPLICATIONS

Perioperative Preparation

- Routine

Monitoring

- Temperature
- Urine output

Maintenance

- Keep warm, including extremities
- Normothermic cardiopulmonary bypass
- No preferred agent or technique

ANTICIPATED PROBLEMS/CONCERNS

- Hemolysis if temperature falls
- Renal dysfunction due to hemoglobinuria

AUTONOMIC HYPERREFLEXIA

Maywin Liu, M.D.

RISK

- Those with spinal cord transection at T7 or above have a 65–85% risk of developing autonomic hyperreflexia (AH) following resolution of spinal shock.
- Develops 2–3 wk after initial injury
- ↓ Risk with lower transections

PERIOPERATIVE RISKS

- Severe HTN and bradycardia with stimulation below level of transection. Placement of a Foley catheter a common trigger.
- May have accompanying unstable neck
- Muscle spasms during closure of abd wounds can cause evisceration of abd contents.

WORRY ABOUT

- AH in postop period

- Severe bradycardia due to postop inability to void or defecate

OVERVIEW

- AH can cause severe HTN and bradycardia →arrhythmias, pulmonary edema, CV collapse, cerebral hemorrhage, seizures, and subsequent death.
- Common triggers are hot and cold stimuli, surgery, manipulation of a hollow viscus.
- Any stimulus below the level of transection can trigger AH.
- Pathophysiology is unopposed reflex sympathetic activity. Normally sympathetic activity is modulated by inhibitory impulses from supraspinal centers. With a transected cord, inhibitory impulses cannot travel below transection.

ICD-9-CM Code: 344.61

ETIOLOGY

- Most common cause is trauma.
- Can be from infectious or oncologic causes.

USUAL TREATMENT

- Can decrease or prevent by use of neuraxial blockade (spinal >> epidural).
- When signs of AH are evident, administer ganglionic blockers (trimethaphan), direct vasodilators (nitroprusside), or α-antagonists (phentolamine) or GA or a spinal.
- Centrally acting hypotensive agents, e.g., clonidine, are *not* effective.
- Tachyarrhythmias may be treated with ß-blockers in combination with antihypertensives.

ASSESSMENT POINTS

SYSTEM	EFFECT	ASSESSMENT BY HX	PE	TEST
HEENT	Possible facial/skull Fx, unstable neck, presence of halo device	Facial trauma/pain Neck pain Discuss with neurosurgeons	Facial swelling or bruising	C-spine x-rays, ? head CT
CV	May have orthostatic hypotension; loss of compensatory CV reflexes; bradycardia, heart blocks with lesions above T4	Chest pain	Tachycardia, bradycardia	CXR EKG CVP TEE
RESP	Possible Fx ribs/pulm contusions/PTX; impaired cough reflex, pulm infections, hypoxemia with high transections	SOB, pain on inspiration Unequal BS bilat	Pain on palpation	CXR ABG
GI	Possible full stomach from GI atonicity (chronic)			
RENAL	Possible UTI; renal stones, renal failure			UA; BUN/Cr
ENDO	May have ACTH deficiency			
CNS	Bowel and bladder dysfuction May have thermoregulation problems with high lesions May have chronic pain	Incontinence	Hyperreflexic below transection Babinski sign present	
PNS	Insensate below level of transection		Demarcation on sensory exam	
MS	Paralysis, muscle atrophy below level of transection, osteoporosis Muscle spasms	Paraplegia or quadriplegia	Muscle atrophy	

Key Reference: Amzallog M: Autonomic hyperreflexia. Int Clin Anesth 1993; 31:87–102.

PERIOPERATIVE IMPLICATIONS

Preoperative Preparation

- Assess adequate CV and resp function, volume status.
- Nifedipine can be used for prophylaxis given 30 min prior to a procedure likely to trigger AH.

Monitoring

- Consider intra-arterial catheter
- Consider CVP/SG if vol changes expected and if poor cardiac reserve (esp with high lesions) and/or renal problems.

Airway

- May require fiberoptic intubation

Induction

- Use nondepolarizing muscle relaxant. Succinylcholine can cause severe hyperkalemia, especially in injuries <6 mo old.
- Consider nitroprusside prior to induction.

Maintenance

- GA with a volatile agent may be better than N_2O/narcotics for prevention/treatment of AH.

Regional Anesthesia

- Spinals highly effective in preventing AH during surgery.
- Difficult to assess height of a neuraxial block because of sensory deficits below transection.

Extubation

- May be difficult to extubate with high transection owing to resp impairment

•Adjuvants

- Require muscle relaxation for muscle spasticity despite para/quadriplegia

Postoperative Period

- AH can occur during recovery from anesthesia
- With severe HTN and difficulty in awakening, possibility of cerebral bleed.

ANTICIPATED PROBLEMS/CONCERNS

- AH occurring with placement of Foley (esp if done before anesthesia).
- Hyperkalemia with use of succinylcholine because of increased number of receptors in muscles below level of transection

AV AND BIFASCICULAR HEART BLOCK

John L. Atlee, M.D.

RISK

- Idiopathic, progressive fibrosis of the atrioventricular (AV) conducting system and MI are most common causes
- Acquired complete AV heart block (3° AVHB) occurs after age 60 y; 60% male
- Congenital 3° AVHB occurs in 1 in 15,000–25,000 live births; 60% female

PERIOPERATIVE RISKS

- Circulatory compromise due to bradycardia and escape rhythms with advanced 2° and 3° AVHB
- Unlikely progression of lesser AVHB or bifascicular heart block to high-degree AVHB

WORRY ABOUT

- Status of associated CV disease, especially coronary, congenital, or other heart disease
- If patient has pacemaker, indication(s) for device and its perioperative malfunction
- Adverse effects of chronotropic drugs used to treat bradycardia due to heart block

OVERVIEW

- Fascicular block: left anterior/posterior fascicles (LAFB, LPFB); right bundle branch block (RBBB)
- Bifascicular heart block (BFHB): LBBB or RBBB + LAFB or RBBB + LPFB.
- No studies show ↑ risk of BFHB progressing to high-degree AVHB during surgery
- Anesthetic drugs may transiently increase ratio of dropped beats (6:5 → 4:3) with type I, 2° AVHB
- Possibility that anesthetic or adjuvants may slow or enhance instability of escape rhythms

ICD-9-CM Codes: 426.10 (AV heart block); 426.53 (bifascicular heart block)

ETIOLOGY

- AVHB: congenital or acquired; BFHB: familial tendency
- 1°, 2°, and 3° AVHB occur in 9%, 5%, and 7% of patients with acute MI, respectively
- 3° AVHB develops in 12% of patients with inferior MI and 2% with anterior MI
- Valve (aortic > mitral) or congenital heart surgery (1° ASD, AV canal, VSD, Ebstein's anomaly)
- Few patients with normal PR and LBBB progress to 3° AVHB; 6 to 30% with other BFHB do
- Patients with preexisting BBB or FHB have a 12% (LBBB) to ~ 40% (RBBB + LAFB/LPFB) risk of progression to 3° AVHB during acute MI

USUAL TREATMENT

- Chronotropes (atropine, ephedrine, isoproterenol) to speed conduction or increase escape rate
- Temporary or permanent pacing to treat symptomatic or disadvantageous bradycardia

ASSESSMENT POINTS

SYSTEM	EFFECT	ASSESSMENT BY HX	PE	TEST
CV	Bradycardia, escape beats, or rhythms	Dizziness, syncope (2° rare, advanced 2° or 3° common), fatigue, weakness, lethargy, exercise intolerance, CHF, palpitations, angina rare with high 2° or 3° AVHB, mental status changes, no symptoms	Slow, full pulse with high-degree AVHB, S₁, and variation in pulse amplitude with variable atrial filling, cannon A waves	ECG, Holter monitor, cardiac evoked potential studies, exercise testing
	Heart disease	Angina, symptoms of CHF	Edema, ascites, liver enlargement, rales	ECHO, scintigraphy, MRI, coronary angiograms
	Pacemaker	Sx of arrhythmias suggest pacemaker malfunction	If inhibited, magnet or vagal maneuvers to ascertain function	Pacemaker system analyzer/programmer
RESP	COPD	Dyspnea, cough	Rhonchi, wheezes	CXR
GI	↓ Perfusion	GI distress, diarrhea		
RENAL	↓ Perfusion	Polyuria		BUN/Cr
CNS	Ischemia/stroke	Syncope, dementia, mental status changes, paralysis	Neurologic or mental deficits	See CV assessment

Key Reference: Atlee JL: Arrhythmias and Pacemakers. Philadelphia, WB Saunders, 1996.

PERIOPERATIVE IMPLICATIONS

Preoperative Preparation

- With AVHB-BFHB and symptomatic bradycardia, prophylactic perioperative pacing indicated
- BFHB without symptomatic bradycardia or acute MI not indication for temporary/permanent pacing.
- For pacemaker patients, check function and inactivate or reprogram device if electrocautery to be used
- Transport of patient with temporary pacer: caution handling leads; have chronotropes available

Monitoring

- ECG and strip-chart recorder
- Consider direct arterial and PA catheter monitoring
- Arterial pulse waveform (oximetric, direct) if patient has permanent or temporary pacer

Induction/Maintenance/Extubation

- Have chronotropes available in case of unexpected bradycardia or pacemaker malfunction
- Be prepared for pacemaker malfunction (e.g., inappropriate inhibition or triggering of output) due to sensed electromagnetic interference (EMI) or myopotentials

Adjuvants

- Atropine has little effect on lower escape pacemakers; direct acting ß-adrenergic agonists more reliable

Postoperative Period

- Check for proper pacemaker function following surgery or exposure to EMI

ANTICIPATED PROBLEMS/CONCERNS

- For patients with pacemakers: what is intended device function, does it function as intended, and what is potential for perioperative malfunction?
- Chronotropes used to treat bradycardia may be ineffective or cause paroxysmal tachycardia

BILIRUBINEMIA OF THE NEWBORN

Paul D. Schanbacher, M.D.
M. Ramez Salem, M.D.

RISK

- 3–7% of newborns have physiologic jaundice
- Low birth weight, premature neonates, breast fed, maternal diabetes ↑ incidence
- East Asian, Native American, and population in some areas of Greece have ↑ bilirubin levels
- Perinatal events: delayed cord clamping, delivery by vacuum extraction/forceps, breech delivery, oxytocin, maternal bupivacaine analgesia, cephalohematoma, bruising, Rh/ABO incompatibility

PERIOPERATIVE RISKS

- Must consider pathophysiologic conditions present in premature or low birth weight infants, e.g., RDS, sepsis
- ↑ Risk for CNS injury with high levels of unconjugated bilirubin, e.g., >20–25 mg/dl or lower values in ill preterm neonate

WORRY ABOUT

- Factors that increase blood-brain barrier permeability to unconjugated bilirubin: hypoxia, hypercarbia, acidosis, hyperosmolality, HTN, seizure activity, sepsis
- Increasing free fraction of bilirubin from drugs, e.g., sulfonamides, moxalactam, radiocontrast dye
- Surgically induced increases in heme degradation, e.g., hematoma absorption
- Liver dysfunction
- Hemolytic anemia

OVERVIEW

- Unconjugated hyperbilirubinemia is a CNS toxin; however, kernicterus occurs in only a small fraction of hyperbilirubinemic neonates—usually in sick newborns.
- Difficult to predict at what bilirubin level injury occurs or which newborn will suffer neurologic damage for a given bilirubin value
- Probable safe bilirubin level in the full term <25 mg/dl
- Probable safe bilirubin level in the preterm <15 mg/dl
- Hemolysis and other coexisting illness lower threshold and above values for CNS toxicity
- Clinical features of hyperbilirubinemia are lethargy, anorexia, nausea, vomiting, icteric skin and sclera.
- Clinical features of kernicturus (very rare):
  - *Acute:* Opisthotonic posturing, muscle rigidity, seizure, oculogyric crisis
  - *Chronic:* Sensorineural hearing loss, choreoathetoid cerebral palsy, dysarthria, dysphagia, autonomic dysfunction, hyperactivity, ↓ intellectual development

ICD-9-CM Code: 774.

ETIOLOGY

- Multifactorial: genetic, maternal and perinatal events, inborn errors of metabolism
- Besides "physiologic jaundice," hemolytic disease, intestinal obstruction, and sepsis are common causes of unconjugated hyperbilirubinemia
- ↑ Bilirubin load, ↓ glucuronyltransferase activity, and ↑ enterohepatic circulation of bilirubin are common factors.

USUAL TREATMENT

- Phototherapy for moderate hyperbilirubinemia
- Exchange blood transfusion for more severe levels of serum bilirubin (e.g., bilirubin concentration >20–25 mg/dl in a healthy full-term neonate; lower values for premature infants or infants with hemolysis, sepsis, and other coexisting illnesses and rapidly rising bilirubin levels).
- Heme oxygenase inhibitors and phenobarbital—rarely used

ASSESSMENT POINTS

SYSTEM	EFFECT	ASSESSMENT BY HX	PE	TEST
RESP	Pleural effusions possible			CXR
HEME	Hemolysis	Rh/ABO maternal-fetal incompatibility	Anemia, possible hepatosplenomegaly, hyperbilirubinemia	Peripheral blood smear Direct Coombs' test Reticulocyte count
CNS	Bilirubin toxic to CNS cells		Abnormal posture, tonicity, and reflexes	

Key Reference: Avery GB: Neonatology, 4th ed. Philadelphia, JB Lippincott, 1994, pp 630–725.

PERIOPERATIVE IMPLICATIONS

Preoperative Preparation

- Active efforts to lower bilirubin levels
- Address coexisting disease states
- Consider atropine 0.1 mg IV to help prevent bradycardia

Monitoring

- Arterial blood sampling may be indicated.

Airway

- Neonatal airway concerns

Induction

- Maintain normal hemodynamics

Maintenance

- No one agent or technique preferred
- Few data reflecting effects of anesthetic agents on bilirubin levels
- Adjust for FIO_2 to SaO_2 90–95%
- Supplemental glucose and calcium
- Maintain normothermia

Extubation

- Maintain intubation if infant ill or premature or for extensive surgical procedure

Adjuvants

- Chloral hydrate and pancuronium associated with hyperbilirubinemia
- Maternal epidural bupivacaine associated with neonatal jaundice

Postoperative Period

- Apnea/bradycardia possible
- Monitor bilirubin levels

ANTICIPATED PROBLEMS/CONCERNS

- Small ill premature neonates with hyperbilirubinemia are at particular risk for kernicterus. Perioperative phototherapy and/or exchange blood transfusion needed to reduce bilirubin load.
- Dual concern: Avoid factors known to increase blood-brain barrier permeability and treat associated neonatal diseases.

BLADDER CANCER

William H. Rosenblatt, M.D.

RISK

- Primary risk factor is smoking
- Incidence 0.7/1000
- M:F 4:1, white > African-Americans
- Aged 60–85 y
- Quitting smoking decreases risk over time (normal in 5–8 y).

PERIOPERATIVE RISKS

- Risk varies based on surgical procedure and coexisting disease
- Chemotherapy: pulmonary fibrosis, renal and cardiac dysfunction
- Fatty infiltration of liver in those with poor nutritional status
- Protein-calorie malnutrition: due to cancer metabolism and anorexia: anemia, hypo-albuminemia

WORRY ABOUT

- Significant blood loss
- Hyperextension of lumbar spine/pelvis and compression of iliac veins results in reduced venous return of blood volume.
- Monitoring of UO difficult after ligation/division of ureters

OVERVIEW

- Transitional cell cancer generally systemic disease at time of Dx—60% will die of metastatic complications.
- Patients are typically elderly with long Hx of smoking, thereby promoting concurrent disease: COPD, lung CA, atherosclerosis, angina, CAD, CHF, HTN.
- Chemotherapy/radiation therapy may be used preoperatively, thus complicating perioperative period.

ICD-9-CM Code: 188.9

ETIOLOGY

- Exposure to aromatic amines (arylamines): β-naphthylamine in cigarette smoke causes bladder cancer in mice.
- Work-related exposure: β-naphthylamine and benzene in the manufacture of rubber products, arylamines in synthetic textile and hair dyes, paint pigments.
- Drivers of diesel trucks
- "Slow acetylators" (homozygous, autosomal recessive) may be at higher risk—*N*-acetyltransferase may detoxify aromatic amines.

USUAL TREATMENT

- Chemotherapy
  – doxorubicin/bleomycin/cyclophosphamide/cisplatin/methotrexate/5-fluorouracil/vinblastine/teniposide
- Radiation therapy
- Radical surgery

ASSESSMENT POINTS

SYSTEM	EFFECT	ASSESSMENT BY HX	PE	TEST
CV	Doxorubicin (Adriamycin) toxicity: cardiomyopathy	>550mg/m², prior or concurrent mediastinal radiation therapy	CHF	Endomyocardial biopsy, serial ECHO; radionuclide angiography, DL_{CO} ECG
	5-Fluorouracil: myocardial ischemia (rare)	Angina		ECG
	Cyclophosphamide: pericarditis with effusion	CHF	CHF	ECHO
RESP	Smoking-related injury	Cough, sputum, infections	Wheezes, rhonchi, barrel chest	CXR PFT
	Bleomycin or cyclophosphamide toxicity: pulmonary fibrosis Methotrexate: inflammation	>500 mg (bleo), cough, dyspnea	Rales, fever Pulm edema, effusions, infiltrates	CXR CXR
RENAL	Cisplatin: ATN	Occurs 3–5 d after course		BUN, Cr, proteinuria, hyperuricemia
	Methotrexate: renal failure			Hematuria, proteinuria
HEPATIC	Methotrexate: fibrosis			SGPT
CNS	Methotrexate: encephalopathy	Confusion somnolence, ataxia, tremors, focal signs		

Key Reference: Walther PJ: Combined treatment approaches in regionally advanced bladder cancer. Urol Clin North Am 1992; 19:761–774.

PREOPERATIVE IMPLICATIONS

Preoperative Preparation

- Rehydration after bowel prep.

Monitoring

- Renal perfusion difficult to judge after division of ureters: consider CVP or PA catheter or TEE.
- Consider aterial catheter.

Anesthesia Technique

- Consider combined general-epidural anesthesia to treat postop incisional pain and reduce blood loss and fluid requirements.

Induction

- May be volume depleted from bladder prep

Maintenance

- Avoid high concentrations of oxygen in the face of pulmonary fibrosis.
- Consider avoiding N_2O (bowel surgery)
- Maximize efforts to prevent hypothermia.

Postoperative Considerations

- Consider overnight ventilation if long procedure, significant blood loss/fluid resuscitation. Epidural catheter can optimize pulmonary toilet and recovery.
- Fluid shifts occur during first 48 h.
- EBL: TURBT (200 ml) cystectomy: 500–1000 ml
- Pain score: 7–9 (Cystectomy)

BLEBS AND BULLAE

Jerome M. Klafta, M.D.

RISK

- Smokers with COPD
- Male predominance, 3:1

PERIOPERATIVE RISKS

- Concurrent COPD
- Pulmonary hypertension and RV failure

WORRY ABOUT

- Expiratory obstruction and air trapping
- Deadspace ventilation
- Expansion of bullae
- Rupture of bullae leading to tension pneumothorax

OVERVIEW

- Destruction of lung parenchyma with resultant formation of air-filled, thin-walled space within lung
- Walls of bullae may be connective tissue septae, compressed lung, or pleura
- "Bleb" connotes subpleural collection of air within layers of visceral pleura due to ruptured alveoli

ICD-9-CM Code: 492.0 (emphysematous bleb)

ETIOLOGY

- Usually emphysematous in origin
- Minority familial and occur in younger patients
- Air cysts similar but have epithelial lining

USUAL TREATMENT

- Surgical resection of 1 or more bullae (bullectomy) done for ↑ SOB or recurrent pneumothorax
- Bullectomy performed via thoracoscopic, thoracotomy, or median sternotomy approach and may involve laser ablation

ASSESSMENT POINTS

SYSTEM	EFFECT	ASSESSMENT BY HX	PE	TEST
CV	CAD, pulmonary hypertension, RV failure	Angina, DOE	Signs of RV failure (palpable PA, peripheral edema)	ECG, stress test, ECHO
RESP	Expiratory obstruction, air trapping V/Q mismatch Hypoxia, hypercarbia Pneumothorax	Exercise tolerance Cough	Pursed-lip breathing	CXR, ABG, chest CT, V/Q scan
ENDO	Possible steroid use			Glucose
MS	Barrel-chested			

Key Reference: Benumof JL: Anesthesia for Thoracic Surgery, 2nd ed. Philadelphia, WB Saunders, 1995, pp 542–548.

PERIOPERATIVE IMPLICATIONS

Preoperative Preparation

- Control of bronchospasm
- Treatment of concurrent infection

Monitoring

- Consider arterial catheter (for frequent ABGs and rapid identification of hemodynamic embarrassment if tension pneumothorax develops)
- Consider precordial stethoscope over hemithorax at risk (if feasible)

Airway

- Double-lumen endotracheal tube extremely useful for differential treatment

Induction

- Keep airway pressures low
- Consider spontaneously breathing induction if Hx of pneumothorax

Maintenance

- Keep airway pressures low
- Have high index of suspicion for tension pneumothorax and plan for treatment (needle or tube thoracostomy)
- Avoid nitrous oxide, which can lead to expansion of poorly ventilated bullae
- Have contingency plan for development of bronchopleurocutaneous fistula: a pressure-cycled, high inspiratory flow ventilator (e.g., Siemens Servo 900C)
- Consider regional anesthetic

Extubation

- May require postoperative ventilation
- Continued avoidance of high airway pressures ("fighting the ventilator")

ANTICIPATED PROBLEMS/CONCERNS

- Underlying lung disease with hypoxia, hypercarbia, dyspnea
- Rupture of bullae leading to bronchopleurofistula or tension pneumothorax

BLEOMYCIN SULFATE TOXICITY

George S. Leisure, M.D.
Carl Lynch III, M.D., Ph.D.

RISK

- Antineoplastic agent used in treatment of germ cell tumors of testes, lymphomas, and squamous cell carcinomas of head and neck
- May also be used by intracavitary injection as sclerosing agent to control pleural effusions caused by metastatic tumors

PERIOPERATIVE RISKS

- Postoperative hypoxemia and potentially lethal ARDS, possibly related to vigorous fluid administration or high inspired oxygen concentrations

WORRY ABOUT

- Development of interstitial pneumonitis leading to pulmonary fibrosis
- Possible relationship between intraoperative hyperoxia and postoperative pulmonary complications
- Development of acute chest pain syndrome suggestive of pleuropericarditis during continuous infusion of bleomycin

OVERVIEW/PHARMACOLOGY

- Antineoplastic antibiotic produced by *Streptomyces verticillus*
- Believed to cause DNA scission by intercalating between DNA base pairs, especially guanine and cytosine; may also inhibit incorporation of thymidine into DNA
- Concentrated primarily in lungs, skin, kidneys, peritoneum, and lymphatics
- Administered by IV, IM, or SC injection; intra-arterial and intrapleural administration also employed
- Cleared principally by renal excretion; 60–70% of parenterally administered dose is excreted in urine as active drug; terminal plasma half-life ~2 h
- In patients with Cr clearances of < 35 mL/min, terminal plasma half-life of drug is inversely related to Cr clearance

ICD-9-CM Code: E930.7 (therapeutic bleomycin)

ETIOLOGY

- Nonlethal pulmonary fibrosis may occur in 10–30% of those who have received bleomycin
- Pulmonary toxicity may ↑ with total dose >450–500 mg; fatal pulmonary toxicity has occurred with a total dose of < 63 mg
- Pulmonary toxicity may be potentiated by advanced age, chest irradiation, administration of additional chemotherapeutic agents (especially cyclophosphamide), and smoking

DRUG EFFECTS

SYSTEM	EFFECT	ASSESSMENT BY HX	PE	TEST
CV	Chest pain syndrome Rare vascular toxicities such as MI, CVA, cerebral arteritis			ECG
RESP	Pulmonary fibrosis	Cough, dyspnea	Fine rales	CXR; O_2 Sat, ? PFTs
GI	Nausea, vomiting			
METAB	Febrile reactions Anaphylactoid reactions		BP/HR	
MUCOCUTAN	Hyperesthesia of skin Urticaria, swelling Hyperpigmentation Alopecia, stomatitis			
HEME	Infrequent bone marrow toxicity			↓ WBCs, platelets, and Hgb
CNS	Rare disorientation Aggressive behavior			

Key Reference: Waid-Jones MI, Coursin DB: Perioperative considerations for patients treated with bleomycin. Chest 1991; 99:993–999.

PERIOPERATIVE IMPLICATIONS

Preoperative Preparation

- Dyspnea, tachypnea, or dry cough should be evaluated prior to surgery
- Rales may indicate early toxicity
- Changes on physical exam may occur earlier than changes on CXR
- PFTs not predictive in subclinical disease

Preinduction/Induction

- Avoid marked vasodilation and fluid replacement

- Regional anesthesia may be preferred to avoid administering hyperoxic inspired gases; vigorous fluid administration should be avoided

Monitoring

- ABGs may be necessary to guide inspired oxygen concentration
- After induction of anesthesia, maintain FIO_2 at lowest level that allows for adequate oxygenation
- Restrict fluid administration in fashion appropriate to condition of patient and extent of surgery (hypotension might be treated with vasopressors rather than vigorous fluid replacement)

Extubation

- Verify adequate oxygenation on near normoxic inspired gas
- Auscultation for rales

Postoperative Period

- Monitor O_2 saturation closely for sustained period (12 h) if GA used

ANTICIPATED PROBLEMS/CONCERNS

- Animal and some human data suggest that hyperoxia may potentiate bleomycin-induced pulm damage, leading to postoperative pulm complications; this is controversial
- Fluid overload may be major contributing factor to postop pulm distress

BLINDNESS

Stanley W. Stead, M.D.

RISK

- Eye injuries represent 3% of claims analyzed in the ASA Closed Claims Project.
- Most common injury with GA is corneal abrasion, which is rarely associated with blindness.
- Blindness can result from injury to the eye, its surrounding structures (eyelid and conjunctiva), blood supply, and optic nerve.
- Injuries that may indirectly lead to blindness may involve the extraocular muscles and occipital lobe of the brain.

PERIOPERATIVE RISKS

- Procedures associated with blindness:
  - Cardiopulmonary bypass
  - Neurosurgical procedures
  - Plastic surgery of the face
- Intraocular procedures, procedures around the eye, prone position with padding around the face and eyes, exophthalmos or ophthalmic nerve blocks, and TURP with glycine irrigating solution

WORRY ABOUT

- Pressure or contact with eye by foreign objects or solutions
- Positioning of patient, especially prone
- Operations in physical proximity to the eyes
- During ophthalmic surgery:
  - movement of patient under either MAC or GA during intraocular surgery
  - coughing or substantial Valsalva maneuvers by patient following intraocular surgery
- During ophthalmic nerve block:
  - perforation of globe
  - trauma to the optic nerve, retinal artery, and vein

OVERVIEW

- Unless associated with glycine irrigating solution, blindness is an irreversible complication following anesthesia and surgery
- Blindness is most often associated with injury to the eye, its surrounding structures (eyelid and conjunctive), blood supply nad optic nerve.

ICD-9-CM Codes: 369.00 (acquired); 950.9 (due to nerve injury); 368.12 (transient)

ETIOLOGY

- Conditions that can result in blindness following anesthesia include
  - corneal abrasion, vitreous loss, hemorrhage, movement of patient while operating upon or in the eye, chemical injury to the cornea or conjunctiva from cleaning materials on the anesthetic mask, spillage of prep solution into the eye, and direct trauma to the eye due to OR table padding, needle used in retrobulbar block, anesthetic mask pressure upon the globe or foreign body falling into eye. Additionally, prone position, hypoxemia following cardiac arrest, prolonged hypotension resulting in central retinal artery occlusion, increased intraocular pressure, and embolization, occlusion, thrombosis, or spasm of the retinal artery
- Following absorption of glycine irrigating solution during TURP. Glycine distribution similar to that of γ-aminobutyric acid, an inhibitory neurotransmitter. Levels of glycine >143 mg/L associated with transient blindness.

USUAL TREATMENT

- In the case of glycine, supportive treatment is indicated until plasma glycine levels <143 mg/L. When actual blindness occurs from other causes, there is no treatment.

ASSESSMENT POINTS

SYSTEM	EFFECT	ASSESSMENT BY HX	PE	TEST
OVERALL	Retinal artery occlusion	Migraines Coagulopathies Hemoglobinopathies Oral contraceptives ↑ IOP		
HEENT	Ischemic retinopathy	Hypotension Hypoxemia Shock	Funduscopic: A normal retina but optic nerve head is swollen and ischemic	
	Orbital pressure		Funduscopic: An edematous retina with dilated arterioles and engorged veins	
GU	Transient blindness during or after TURP	TURP with glycine irrigating solution		Plasma glycine level (nml 13–17 mg/L)

Key Reference: Gild WM, Posner KL, Caplan RA, Cheney FW: Eye injuries associated with anesthesia. Anesthesiology 1992; 76:204–208.

INTRAOPERATIVE MANAGEMENT

Monitoring

- Proper positioning essential
- If prone, adequate padding so no pressure transmitted to either globe or nasal bridge.
- When face completely draped, consider use of a metallic Fox shield to protect eye from inadvertent pressure.
- In ophthalmic nerve blocks, needle does not enter globe or retinal artery, vein, or nerve. Avoid excessive volume of local anesthetic, which increases IOP and may compromise vascular supply of globe.

Airway

- Anesthetic masks may injure eye, either through inadequate drying and application of cleaning solution to eye or through direct pressure.

Surgical Stages

- Hypotension and hypoxemia implicated in cases of retinal artery occlusion.

Closure/Postoperative Considerations

- Protection of unoperated eye with the Fox shield is useful.
- When recovered in prone position, ensure that there is no pressure upon orbit or globe.

BOTULISM

Russell C. Raphaely, M.D.
Maureen M. O'Rourke, M.D.

RISK

• Infant botulism
  – Infants within USA: >1,000 confirmed cases since first recognized as distinct clinical entity in 1976
    – Regional preponderance: California, Pennsylvania, Utah, and Hawaii
    – Gender predilection: none
    – Average age at onset of Sx: 3–4 mo

PERIOPERATIVE RISKS

• Autonomic dysfunction may cause hemodynamic instability
• Muscle weakness results in vulnerability to aspiration, pulmonary infection, and respiratory failure

WORRY ABOUT

• Autonomic dysfunction
• Gastroparesis
• Respiratory gas exchange

OVERVIEW

• Three forms: foodborne, wound, and infant.
• Foodborne botulism intoxication results when improperly preserved food allows germination and toxin production by contaminating spores of *Clostridium botulinum;* consumption of food with preformed toxin results in absorption of potent neurotoxin; with education and control of food precessing industries, foodborne botulism has been uncommon in US in last 50 years
• Wound botulism, a rare entity, results when *C. botulinum* organisms contaminating traumatized tissue cause local infection and produce toxin that is absorbed
• Infant botulism is much more common; concepts described for infant botulism are referable to foodborne and wound forms
• Botulinum toxin binds irreversibly to synaptic membrane of cholinergic nerves and subsequently prevents release of acetylcholine

ICD-9-CM Code: 005.1

ETIOLOGY

• Infant: Ingestion of *C. botulinum* spores into intestinal tract that is transiently permissive to germination, subsequent colonization, elaboration of toxin, absorption into circulation, and delivery to acetylcholine receptors
• Foodborne: Consumption of preformed toxin with food
• Wound: Local infection with produced toxin causing symptoms after absorption

USUAL TREATMENT

• Nutritional support
• Insertion of artificial airway
• Mechanical ventilation
• Polyvalent antitoxin (may be helpful in patients with early identification of toxin in serum)

ASSESSMENT POINTS

SYSTEM	EFFECT	ASSESSMENT BY HX	PE	TEST
RESP	Pharyngeal constrictor and genioglossal hypotonia, paralysis of respiratory musculature	Drooling Poor feeding Decreased respiratory effort	Poor head control Absent gag	Negative inspiratory force; crying vital capacity
	Infection	Increased secretions	Fever Rhonchi Rales	WBC CXR
	Atelectasis	Poor color	Cyanosis Tracheal secretions	SpO_2 CXR
GI	Constipation	No bowel movement Irritability	Palpable stool Abdominal distention	
RENAL	UTI	Foul-smelling urine		Urine culture
CNS	SIADH		Diminished urine flow	Serum/urine Na Serum/urine osmolality
	Seizures	Twitching Altered consciousness	Seizure activity	EEG
	Cranial neuropathies	Ptosis Expressionless face Feeble cry	Fixed and dilated pupils Facial palsy Poor cough and gag	
PNS	Spinal neuropathies	Limp limbs	Hypotonia	EMG

Key Reference: Wohl DL, Tucker JA: Infant botulism: Considerations for airway management. Laryngoscope 1992; 102:1251–1254.

PERIOPERATIVE IMPLICATIONS

Preoperative Preparation

• Insert NG tube and apply vacuum to reduce retained gastric secretion volume
• Chest PT
• Treat infection

Monitoring

• Routine

Airway

• Select appropriately sized tracheal tube
• Monitor leak pressures (reduce risk for subglottic injury)

Induction

• Expect fluctuations in HR and BP
• Anticipate alveolar hypoventilation

Maintenance

• Recognize sensitivity to neuromuscular blockers and give (if needed) as gauged by evoked motor response
• Differentiate between blood loss, anesthetic effect, and autonomic dysfunction as causes for hemodynamic abnormalities

Extubation

• Examine for genioglossal tone
• Gag and cough reflex
• Observe and test for sufficient respiratory muscle strength

ANTICIPATED PROBLEMS/CONCERNS

• Respiratory failure from airway obstruction, bellows muscle weakness, chemical or infectious pneumonia, and fluid overload, added neuromuscular dysfunction associated with aminoyhcosides

BRAIN DEATH

Gwendolyn L. Boyd, M.D.

RISK

- People within USA: 29,000
- Potential organ donors: 10,000 to 12,000/y
- Actual organ donors: 4850 (1995 data)
- Race with highest prevalence debatable; Caucasians highest number or organ donors

PERIOPERATIVE RISKS

- Hemodynamically unstable
- Hypothermia
- Coagulopathy
- Diabetes insipidus
- Electrolyte imbalance

WORRY ABOUT

- Maintaining optimal organ function until procurement

OVERVIEW

- Irreversible cessation of all functions of entire brain: including brainstem
- There must be no evidence of hypothermia or depressant drugs as known cause of death.
- One factor in the failure of organ procurement is inadequate knowledge of the pathophysiology of brain death.
- Donor management should be considered the beginning of organ preservation.
- While the quality of organs from diseased donors should conform to that of the living, the pathophysiologic changes associated with brain death intervene.
- Diagnosed by cerebral unresponsiveness, absence of motor activity and brainstem reflexes, absent cough after deep tracheal suctioning, no HR response to atropine (2 mg), no respiratory response on apnea testing (P_{CO_2} >60 mmHg), and electrical silence without hypothermia, metabolic encephalopathy, or depressant drugs.

ICD-9-CM Code: 348.8

ETIOLOGY

- Massive intracranial trauma or primary CNS tumor
- Occurs when ICP exceeds systolic BP within 12–24 h of injury

USUAL TREATMENT

- Supportive until organ procurement

ASSESSMENT POINTS

SYSTEM	EFFECT	ASSESSMENT BY HX	PE	TEST
RESP	Neurogenic pulmonary edema Hypoxemia Infections DVT and pulmonary embolism		Rales	ABG, CXR
CV	CNS ischemia response Hypovolemia Ventricular dysfunction Depletion of myocardial substrates Unstable vasomotor center Brain herniation Nonfunctional sympathetic system Lack of ADH	} Need for inotrope support		BP Cardiac filling pressures Atropine resistance (2 mg) TEE for heart donors
HEME	Coagulopathy Anemia			Coagulation studies Hct
GU	Diabetes insipidus			UO >3 ml/kg/h Lytes SG <1.0005 Serum osmolality >310 mOsm
CNS	Lack of cerebral and brainstem function	Hx of drug ingestion, metabolic encephalopathy, and/or hypothermia excluded		Nonreaction of pupils to light Loss of corneal reflexes Oculocephalic or doll's eyes Oculovestibular Gag or cough absent Apnea to P_{CO_2} >60

PERIOPERATIVE IMPLICATIONS

Monitoring

- T
- A-line
- CVP or PA catheter
- UO
- ABGs for lung donors

Airway

- ETT already in place

Maintenance

- Rule of 100s:
  - Pa_{O_2} >100 mmHg
  - UO >100 ml/h
  - Systolic BP >100 mmHg
- Keep warm
- Hemodynamic states:
  - keep dopamine <10 µg/kg/min
- Good blood volume
- Muscle relaxant to racilitate surgery
- Drugs per procurement team, e.g., heparin, chlorpromazine

Extubation

- Not done
- Ventilation discontinued when cross clamp:
  - ascending aorta for heart-lung donors
  - descending aorta for liver-kidney donors above SMA and celiac

Adjuvants

- None

ANTICIPATED PROBLEMS/CONCERNS

- Expect an increase in BP and HR with incision—does not obviate criteria for brain death
- Knowledge of sequelae of brain death

BREAST CANCER

Vincent S. Cowell, M.D.

RISK

- Occurs predominantly in women: female > male, ~100:1
- 1 in 8 women develop breast cancer, most common cancer in USA for women
- Age and cigarette usage strongest risk factors
- Racial predilection: Caucasians > African-Americans
- 80% diagnosed in women with no family Hx
- BRCA-1 gene on chromosome 17 predicts familial carrier state
- High-fat diet and non-use of aspirin ↑ odds ratio for development

PERIOPERATIVE RISKS

- Mortality very rare
- Lymphedema of arm following axillary node dissection
- Ipsilateral brachial plexus injury from extensive abduction of the arm
- Injury to long thoracic and/or thoracodorsal n. during surgical dissection of axilla
- Rare incidence of unrecognized pneumothorax

WORRY ABOUT

- Systemic or regional impact of metastasis to lung, brain, or bone

- The use of muscle relaxants with axillary dissection interferes with response to stimulation for identification of major nerves
- Access to an upper extremity (e.g., venous access, monitoring) may be restricted or limited
- Potential adverse effects produced by cancer chemotherapeutic drugs, chest radiation therapy

OVERVIEW

- Abnormal growth of adenomatous tissue that results in systemic symptoms and metastasizes to liver, bone, lung and brain
- Early detection of breast cancer increases time of survival
- Women >50 y (?40 y) benefit from screening mammography
- Physical examination and mammography are complementary
- Incisional or excisional breast biopsy provides histologic Dx; needle core biopsy
- Presurgical needle localization may be necessary for nonpalpable lesions
- Most breast biopsies yield benign diagnosis

ICD-9-CM Code: 174.9

ETIOLOGY

- Unknown
- Possibilities under investigation include: breast cancer susceptibility genes, radiation exposure, and other environmental contributors
- ↑ Incidence if familial and mutant BRCA-1 on chromosome 17, cigarette usage, high-fat diet, and lack of aspirin use

USUAL TREATMENT

- Noninvasive breast cancer: mastectomy or local excision with follow-up and possible adjuvant treatment (radiation) when indicated
- Invasive breast cancer: modified radical mastectomy, total mastectomy or simple mastectomy, lumpectomy or segmental (partial) mastectomy with breast irradiation, chemotherapy
- Radical mastectomy rarely performed
- Reconstructive surgery integral part of management

PROGNOSIS

- 2nd major cause of cancer death among women, after lung cancer
- 5 y survival rate: 93% for nonmetastatic disease, 72% for regional metastasis, 18% for systemic metastic disease

ASSESSMENT POINTS

SYSTEM	EFFECT	ASSESSMENT BY HX	PE	TEST
CHEST	Lung lesions	Nipple discharge Chest pain or discomfort	Breast asymmetry Nipple discharge, erythema, crusting, or erosion Nipple retraction Skin dimpling	Physical exam Mammography Fine-needle aspiration biopsy CXR
GI	Liver metastasis	Fatigue, abdominal pain	Enlarged or nodular liver	Liver ultrasound or CT scan
HEME	Bone metastasis	Lethargy, SOB	Anemia, pancytopenia	CBC
CNS	Brain metastasis	Change in mental status, seizures	Neurologic exam	Head CT
MS	Bone metastasis Pathological fractures	Severe pain Immobility Arm swelling	Deformities Pain on palpation Axillary adenopathy	Bone scan X-rays Physical exam

Key Reference: 1994 Breast Cancer Facts. Atlanta, American Cancer Society, 1994.

INTRAOPERATIVE MANAGEMENT

Monitoring

- Routine noninvasive monitoring with attention to placement of ECG leads in reference to surgical field
- IV site and BP cuff on contralateral arm

Airway

- Proximity of surgical field to head and table arrangements by some surgeons warrant a secure airway

SURGICAL STAGES

Induction

- No special considerations for GA

- Thoracic epidural and intercostal nerve blocks have successfully been administered as adjuvants to general anesthesia, but have not replaced general anesthesia

Incision

- Over operative breast; can include axilla

Dissection

- Can include breast areolar tissue, muscle dissection down to chest wall, extension into axilla
- Identification of thoracodorsal and long thoracic nerves often requires stimulation that contraindicates presence of NM blocking agents
- Surgical field will be in view and allow for monitoring of active blood loss
- Surgical team leaning on chest can affect ventilatory performance

CLOSURE/POSTOPERATIVE CONSIDERATIONS

- BL varies from minimal for breast biopsy to 500–1000 ml for radical procedure
- Pain score: 2–6
- Pain adequately managed with PCA
- Communicate with PACU that no venous "sticks" or BP measurements should be performed on arm of operative side when axillary lymph node dissection is involved

ANTICIPATED PROBLEMS/CONCERNS

- Anxiety associated with the fear of breast cancer and altered body image can be quite significant

BRONCHIECTASIS

H. Michael Marsh, M.B., B.S.

RISK

- People within USA: <1/10,000 hospital admissions
- Gender prevalence: none
- Socioeconomic or ethnic prevalence: inbreeding and primitive health care, particularly lack of immunization and poor treatment of childhood bronchitides, increase the prevalence. Ciliary deformities have been shown in a Polynesian population

PERIOPERATIVE RISKS

- Spillage of infected secretions from bronchiectatic regions to normal lung → pneumonitis, retention of secretions
- Risk from bacteremia, after manipulation
- Risk of secondary acute respiratory failure

WORRY ABOUT

- Exacerbation of asthma
- Amount of sputum produced and its nature
- Fever, hemoptysis: acute pulmonary infection
- Right heart function
- Check frequency of cough and daily sputum volume; culture and smear for composition; check body T and WBC count for acute infection
- Exercise tolerance will indicate associated impairment or disability. Right heart function may need assessment

OVERVIEW

- Abnormal widening or dilatation of one or more branches of the bronchial tree. Widened segments commonly filled with purulent secretions; mucosa is swollen and inflamed and may be ulcerated with granulation tissue exposed. Extensive collateral flow occurs in these chronically inflamed bronchi (3–12% of CO)

ICD-9-CM Codes: 494; 748.61 (Congenital); 011.5 (Tuberculous)

ETIOLOGY/PATHOGENESIS

- Exact etiology for acquired form remains unclear but often involves necrotizing infection in tracheobronchial wall. Five mechanisms may predispose: (1) bacterial, viral, or fungal bronchopulmonary infections, including TB, pertussis, and measles; (2) bronchial obstruction; (3) immunodeficiency states, including IgG, IgA deficiency, and leukocyte dysfunction; (4) hereditary defects in ciliary-mucosal clearance, including Kartagener's syndrome, α_1-antitrypsin deficiency, and cystic fibrosis; and (5) miscellaneous disorders, including recurrent aspiration, inhaled irritants, Young's syndrome, and bronchiolitis obliterans following heart-lung transplantation

USUAL TREATMENT

- Medical therapy—postural drainage, deep breathing and assisted coughing, antibiotics, bronchodilators, and fluids/humidity. Drainage of sinuses
- Surgical therapy—resection indicated for uncontrolled hemoptysis; or lobar closely confined disease, age >20 y. Bronchopulmonary lavage under GA with divided airway

ASSESSMENT POINTS

SYSTEM	EFFECT	ASSESSMENT BY HX	PE	TEST
HEENT	Sinusitis	Postnasal drip Stuffiness, headache	Translucency	X-ray
CV	Clubbing, cyanosis	Exercise tolerance		ABGs
	CHF (cor pulmonale)	Pulm HTN, edema		Loud P_2 Right heart studies
	Kartagener's syndrome		Situs inversus	
RESP	Bronchiectasis	Cough, sputum	Rhonchi	Smear, culture, high-resolution CT, bronchogram
		Hemoptysis Wheezing		Bronchoscopy PFT
HEME	Immunodeficiency Infection			IgG, IgA, WBC
CNS	Brain abscess			CT/MRI

Key Reference: Marsh HM, Guffin AV: Preparation of the patient with chronic pulmonary disease. *In* Kaplan JA (ed): Thoracic Anesthesia, 2nd ed. New York, Churchill Livingstone, 1991.

PERIOPERATIVE IMPLICATIONS

Monitoring
- Routine: consider PA catheter for cor pulmonale or CHF

Airway
- Careful frequent suctioning and humidification of inspired gases

Induction
- Avoid asthma exacerbation
- Consider regional anesthesia when possible

Maintenance
- Routine

Extubation
- Depend upon degree of pulmonary and cardiac dysfunction

Adjuvants
- Routine

Postoperative Period
- Use stir-up regimen; monitor for retained secretions and respiratory failure
- Check for platypnea—orthodeoxia if right atrial pressures become elevated

ANTICIPATED PROBLEMS/CONCERNS
- Retained secretions, secondary respiratory failure
- Right heart decompensation if hypoxemia persists
- Bacteremia from airway manipulations

BRONCHIOLITIS OBLITERANS (BO)

William A. Lell, M.D.

RISK

- People within USA: 1/40,000
- Racial predilection: none

PERIOPERATIVE RISKS

- Hypoxemia
- Pulmonary infection

WORRY ABOUT

- Pulmonary dysfunction
- Pulmonary infection
- Steroid coverage
- Other effects of etiologic agents

OVERVIEW

- A nonspecific pulmonary inflammatory response affecting bronchiolar epithelium of small conducting airways and adjacent alveoli, sparing the interstitium.
- Two histopathologic types: (1) the more common proliferative form—organized connective tissue proliferating into the respiratory bronchioles and alveoli resulting in a reversible, restrictive ventilation defect; (2) the rarer constrictive type—extensive scarring and fibrosis of the more proximal conductive bronchioles resulting in a permanent obstructive abnormality. It may result from longer exposure to a more intense etiologic agent.

ICD-9-CM Code: 491.8

ETIOLOGY

- Diverse agents can trigger the BO response, including:
  - Inhalation: Toxic dusts, grains, gases (smoke inhalation, nitrogen dioxide from inhaled nitric oxide therapy)
  - Post Infections: Viral (most common cause in children), mycoplasmal, bacterial
  - Connective Tissue Diseases: Virtually all, but rheumatoid arthritis in particular
  - Drugs: amiodarone, cephalosporin, gold, free-base cocaine, many others
  - Post Organ Transplant: especially lung, heart-lung, bone marrow; possible liver, pancreas
  - Idiopathic: BO with cryptogenic organizing pneumonia (BOOP)

USUAL TREATMENT

- Varies with etiology and histopathology
- Mainly supportive with oxygen, chest physiotherapy
- Steroids controversial (usually effective with BOOP and toxic fume inhalation)
- Bronchodilators usually ineffective
- Specific antibiotics for active infection

ASSESSMENT POINTS

Use classification above to determine possible cause of BO. Then look for other manifestations of underlying disease (e.g., impaired joint mobility in patient with BO due to rheumatoid arthritis). (See other Diseases.)

SYSTEM	EFFECT	ASSESSMENT BY HX	PE	TEST
GENERAL	Active infection	Fever	$\uparrow$ T, tachycardia	WBC
RESP	*Proliferative Type* Restrictive defect (common) *Constrictive Type* Obstructive defect (rare)	Progressive, dry cough with dyspnea	Dry, inspiratory rales Wheezes (more common with constrictive type)	CXR ABG Spirometry V/Q scan bronchoalveolar lavage Lung biopsy (for diagnosis)

Key Reference: Ezri T, Kunichezky S, Eliraz A, et al: Bronchiolitis obliterans—current concepts. Q J Med 1994; 87:1–10.

PERIOPERATIVE IMPLICATIONS

Preoperative Preparation

- Treat active infections
- Consider prophylactic antibiotics, supplemental O_2
- Premedication useful but avoid excessive resp depression
- Steroid coverage if indicated

Monitoring

- Routine
- Consider arterial catheter if oximetry inadequate

Airway

- Prevent additional mechanical obstruction.
- Increase FIO_2.
- Use aseptic tracheal suction technique.

Induction

- Use short-acting agents to avoid prolonged CNS, resp depression

Maintenance

- Avoid fluid overload.

Extubation

- Delay until adequate ventilation assured

Adjuvants

- Consider regional technique for anesthesia/perioperative analgesia

Postoperative Period

- Monitor for and aggressively treat resp depression and infection.
- Continue steroids if indicated.

ANTICIPATED PROBLEMS/CONCERNS

- Many patients with resting hypoxia come to OR for diagnostic lung biopsy. A thoracoscopic technique may be impossible owing to adhesions post heart/lung transplant or inability to tolerate one-lung anesthesia.
- Anticipate further perioperative resp decompensation after open-lung biopsy and treat aggressively.

BRONCHITIS, CHRONIC

C. William Hanson III, M.D.

RISK

- People within USA: 8 million
- Race with highest prevalence: Caucasian
- Male:female ratio 2:1
- Smoking, occupational exposure to pulmonary toxic substances (radon, coal, asbestos)

PERIOPERATIVE RISKS

- Bronchospasm

WORRY ABOUT

- Airway stimulation at light levels of anesthesia
- Laryngospasm (due to secretions and hyperreactivity)
- Hypoxia
- Hypercarbia

OVERVIEW

- Chronic productive cough with periodic exacerbations
- Enlargement of the mucus-secreting glands in the airways with excessive sputum production
- Expiratory airways obstruction
- Derangement in V/Q relationships
- Chronic hypoxia with right heart failure

ICD-9-CM Code: 491.9

ETIOLOGY

- Acquired, and virtually always 2° to smoking

USUAL TREATMENT

- Cessation of smoking (preferably >8–10 wk prior to elective surgery)
- Antibiotics for acute exacerbations; inefficacious for prophylactic treatment
- Glucocorticoids of uncertain benefit; trial appropriate in acute exacerbations
- Bronchodilators, when response can be demonstrated by changes in either PFT or Sx

ASSESSMENT POINTS

SYSTEM	EFFECT	ASSESSMENT BY HX	PE	TEST
HEENT			Short, fat neck	
CV	Right heart failure	Exercise tolerance	RV heave Dependent edema	ECG ECHO
	Pulmonary HTN			PA catheter
RESP	Airways obstruction	Smoking Hx Exercise tolerance Sputum production	Cyanosis	PFT, DLCO, ABG
MS			Clubbing of fingers	

Key Reference: Clausen JL: The diagnosis of emphysema, chronic bronchitis, and asthma. Clin Chest Med 1990; 11(3):405–416.

PERIOPERATIVE IMPLICATIONS

Preoperative Preparation

- Smoking cessation
- Antibiotics to decrease sputum production
- Respiratory conditioning

Monitoring

- Consider arterial line to monitor blood gases
- Consider pulmonary artery catheter for large fluid shift operations

Airway

- Often, truncal obesity (especially with corticosteroids); may have redundant soft tissue in airway or short, fat neck

Preinduction/Induction

- Avoid stimulating the airway while in light levels of anesthesia; may precipitate bronchospasm (although less likely than with asthma)
- Regional anesthesia may be preferable

Maintenance

- Frequent suctioning of endotracheal tube
- Limit narcotic administration (danger of perioperative CO_2 retention)
- Adjuvant regional anesthesia for procedures that affect respiratory mechanics (e.g., intercostal nerve blocks, epidural analgesia)

Extubation

- Administer intratracheal bronchodilator in responsive patients prior to extubation

ANTICIPATED PROBLEMS/CONCERNS

- Postop respiratory complications (secretions, mucous plugging, atelectasis, pneumonia, prolonged requirement for mechanical ventilation)

BRONCHOPULMONARY DYSPLASIA (BPD) Mary A. Keyes, M.D.

RISK

- Severe resp distress at birth requiring prolonged mechanical ventilation and supplemental O_2
- Hyaline membrane disease (HMD) incidence inversely proportional to gestational age and weight (60–80% <28 wk; 15–30% between 32–36 wk, and rarely in term infants).
- Diabetic mothers, multiple gestations, C-section delivery, pulmonary infection with *Ureaplasma urealyticum,* asphyxia, and prior affected siblings.

PERIOPERATIVE RISKS

- Cardiopulmonary abnormalities in the first years include ↑ airway reactivity, ↑ airway resistance, ↑ FRC; ↑ arterial P_{CO_2}, ↓ arterial P_{O_2}, right or left ventricular hypertrophy, and pulmonary and systemic HTN. Tracheomalacia and bronchomalacia may be present.
- Pulmonary function generally improves with age.

WORRY ABOUT

- Adequate oxygenation and ventilation during intraoperative period and transport (hand ventilation to assess changes in compliance)
- Endotracheal tube dislodgement
- Retinopathy of prematurity (ROP).
- Increased airway reactivity exacerbated by endotracheal tube.
- Association between SIDS and BPD

OVERVIEW

- Chronic lung disease in premature infants treated for resp distress with mechanical ventilation.
- Have characteristic CXR—almost complete opacification with air bronchograms or of small, lucent areas alternating with areas of irregular density.
- Severe maldistribution of ventilation
- Prolonged mechanical ventilation, pulmonary HTN, cor pulmonale, and prolonged oxygen dependence are poor prognostic indicators.
- Most common chronic lung disease in infants in USA.

ICD-9-CM Code: 770.7

ETIOLOGY

- Multifactorial: pulmonary oxygen toxicity and barotrauma from positive pressure ventilation important

USUAL TREATMENT

- Bronchodilators, including aerosolized β_2-adrenergic agents and theophylline.
- Diuretics and fluid restriction as needed.
- Steroids improve ability to wean from mechanical ventilation but increase risk of HTN and infection.

ASSESSMENT POINTS

SYSTEM	EFFECTS	ASSESSMENT BY HX	PE	TEST
CV	Cor pulmonale LV failure	Inability to wean from ventilator Poor feeding and weight gain Dyspnea in extubated infant	Tachypnea Sternal retractions Nasal flaring Hepatomegaly Cardiomegaly Pulmonary rales	CXR ±ECHO
RESP	↑ Airway reactivity ↑ FRC ↑ Pa_{CO_2} ↓ Pa_{O_2}	Inability to wean from supplemental O_2 or ventilator Poor feeding and weight gain Frequent URI associated with bronchospasm	Tachypnea Sternal retractions Nasal flaring Wheezing Rhonchi	CXR ABG

Key Reference: Behrman R (ed): Nelson Textbook of Pediatrics, 14th ed. Philadelphia, WB Saunders, 1992, pp 463–469.

PERIOPERATIVE IMPLICATIONS

Preoperative Preparation

- Optimal management of pulmonary and cardiac systems.
- If URI, postpone all but life-death emergency surgery.

Monitoring

- Routine
- ABG monitoring indicated if tenuous cardiac or pulmonary status or major surgery

Airway

- Routine

Preinduction/Induction

- Ensure adequate anesthetic depth (once the cycle of bronchospasm and desaturation has been initiated, it is difficult to recover.)

Maintenance

- Routine

Extubation

- Awake with good respiratory pattern
- Postoperative apnea monitoring

Adjuvants

- Spinal anesthesia acceptable alternative in suitable procedures (avoiding endotracheal intubation may improve outcome)

ANTICIPATED PROBLEMS/CONCERNS

- Tenuous pulmonary status that is challenged during anesthesia and surgery
- Older child with Hx of BPD at risk for ↑ airway reactivity.

BUERGER'S DISEASE: THROMBOANGIITIS OBLITERANS (TAO)

Richard F. Davis, M.D.

RISK

- People within USA: 8–10/100,000 Caucasian males aged <45 y but up to 90–100/100,000 in 1950s Mayo Clinic data of entire age range
- Peak age 25–40 y, before appearance of occlusive atherosclerotic disease
- Male:female 10–100:1.
- Racial predisposition: Most common among males of Eastern European, Jewish, Indian, and Asian heritage
- Ten-year survival rate from Dx is approximately 2/3 that for the general population

PERIOPERATIVE RISKS

- No clinical data describing perioperative risks

WORRY ABOUT

- Enhanced temperature-related vasoconstrictor responsiveness
- Concurrent pulmonary disease due to tobacco abuse
- Coexistent thrombophlebitis

OVERVIEW

- Clinical common denominator is distal extremity ischemia, including gangrenous changes
- Dx established only by histopathology showing active vascular inflammatory lesion
- Vascular lesions most common in peripheral arteries of upper and lower extremities
- Lesions may occur in mesenteric, coronary, and cerebral vasculature
- Pathologic lesion includes a highly cellular organizing luminal thrombus with a panangiitis including venous involvement
- Significant association with tobacco abuse
- Significant temperature sensitivity

ICD-9-CM Code: 443.1

ETIOLOGY

- Entirely unknown, although a dramatic association with tobacco abuse exists together with marked temperature-related vasoconstriction.

USUAL TREATMENT

- Treatment is palliative
- Pentoxifylline 400 mg tid or calcium channel blocker
- Steroids often offered to diminish an acute inflammatory exacerbation
- Debridement and/or amputation frequently necessary owing to gangrene

ASSESSMENT POINTS

SYSTEM	EFFECT	ASSESSMENT BY HX	PE	TEST
CV	Coronary lesions and resultant myocardial ischemia	Angina, MI, CHF		ECG; more advanced testing guided by Hx
RESP	Concomitant cold	Cough, dyspnea, sputum production	Distant BS, coarse rhonchi, expiratory flow rate (match test)	Obstructive pattern on PFT
GI	Mesenteric ischemia	"Intestinal" angina	Abdominal bruit	
HEME	Carbon monoxide producing carboxyhemoglobin	Smoking		Blood gases with co-oximetry
CNS	Extra- or intracranial vascular disease leading to CNS ischemia	TIA, reversible ischemic neurodefecit, syncope	Carotid bruit	Carotid US to assess severity if extracranial disease suspected
EXTREMITIES	Digital ischemia; gangrene	Pain; cold intolerance	Poor capillary refill; hair loss; poor pulses; skin tropic changes	Doppler, plethysmography, arteriography

Key Reference: Juergens JL: Thromboangiitis obliterans (Buerger's disease, TAO). *In* Juergens JL, Spittell JA, Fairbairn JF (eds): Peripheral Vascular Disease. Philadelphia, WB Saunders, 1980, pp 468–491.

PERIOPERATIVE IMPLICATIONS

Monitoring
- T control
- Positioning with pressure point padding

Airway
- Routine

Maintenance
- Maintain normothermia
- Maintain normal to high cardiac output
- Be wary of myocardial ischemia issues
- Regional anesthesia acceptable choice

Recovery
- Avoid vasoconstrictor stimuli (hypothermia, hypovolemia)

Adjuvants
- None of specific importance

ANTICIPATED PROBLEMS/CONCERNS

- Thrombophlebitis, gangrene, ulcerations
- Impaired pulmonary function

BULIMIA

Robert J. Rose, M.D.

RISK

• Affects 5–18% of adolescent girls and young women
• Bulimic symptoms can be part of anorexia nervosa syndrome

PERIOPERATIVE RISKS

• Increased risks (which have not been quantified) of hypotension, cardiac arrhythmias, hypothermia, and aspiration of gastric contents, and their consequences.

WORRY ABOUT

• Reduced cardiac muscle mass with ↓ chamber size, impaired myocardial contractility with ↓ cardiac output, and relative hypotension
• Mitral valve prolapse and its arrhythmogenic effects
• Starvation, dehydration, hyponatremia, and hypokalemia

• Alterations (hypofunction) in autonomic nervous system function and a hypervagal state
• Abnormal T regulation
• ↓ Gastric emptying, gastric dilatation, aspiration of gastric contents, and gastric rupture
• Suicide

OVERVIEW

• Eating disorder characterized by binge-eating episodes followed by self-induced vomiting, fasting, and use of diuretics or laxatives
• Greatest perioperative risks are associated with low cardiac output and cardiac arrhythmias
• Hx is characterized by denial and is often unreliable

ICD-9-CM Codes: 783.6; 307.51
See also under Anorexia nervosa

ETIOLOGY

• Unknown; thought to be largely emotional

USUAL TREATMENT

• Tricyclic antidepressants and fluoxetine (Prozac) have been found effective in some patients (10–40 mg/d)

ASSESSMENT POINTS

SYSTEM	EFFECT	ASSESSMENT BY HX	PE	TEST
CV	Cardiomyopathy, mitral valve prolapse, arrhythmia, ipecac cardiomyopathy	Exercise intolerance, syncope	Heart sounds, BP, pulse	ECG, ECHO
GI	Gastric dilatation, diarrhea Hepatic dysfunction Inanition	Usually unreliable		Lytes Hepatic enzymes Serum glucose
ENDO	Amenorrhea, "euthyroid sick," ↓ norepinephrine, ↓ vasopressin secretion, abn T regulation	Cold intolerance		
HEME	Pancytopenia			CBC, Plt
RENAL	↓ GFR on basis of dehydration			BUN/Cr
CNS	Depression, ↓ CSF norepinephrine			
MS	Muscle mass	Marked weight fluctuation	Thin	

Key Reference: Arnold AE, Rose RJ, Stoddard P: Intraoperative cardiac dysrhythmias in a patient with bulimic anorexia nervosa. Anesthesiology 1987; 67:1003–1005.

PERIOPERATIVE IMPLICATIONS

Perioperative Preparation
• Assess cardiac, lyte, volume status

Monitoring
• Routine
• Arrhythmia, volume status, myocardial function
• T monitoring important

Airway
• May have ↑ risk of aspiration of gastric contents

Induction
• Hypovolemia, myocardial dysfunction, ANS dysfunction may make for CV instability

Maintenance
• CV instability, volume and lyte status, T should dictate anesthetic regimen.

Extubation
• Awake due to GI motility dysfunction
• Autonomic hypofunction may lead to sudden postop collapse

Adjuvants
• Vary if lyte, renal, or hepatic dysfunction exists

ANTICIPATED PROBLEMS/CONCERNS

• Gastric volume changes may increase risk of aspiration.
• Volume status, lyte, CV, and ANS changes increase risk of hypotension, arrhythmia, and sudden postoperative collapse.
• Habitus and metabolic changes may predispose to hypothermia.

BURN INJURY — CHEMICAL

Noel Lee Chun, M.D.

RISK

- >25,000 different chemicals can cause burns
- Compose ~10% of total burn population
- 85% of chemical burns are industrial and 75% occur in men 20–45 y from factories or labs
- US Poison Control Centers report 15,000 caustic ingestions/y; 80% involve children, mostly <5 y
- Majority of adult caustic ingestions are suicidal gestures and more severe burns; majority of caustic ingestions in children are accidental and less severe burns

PERIOPERATIVE RISKS

- If involve ≤30% BSA, less problematic; if >40% BSA, hypotensive shock, lyte abn, sepsis, arrhythmias, myoglobinemia, ATN, and compartment syndromes can occur
- Serious ingestion burns can cause injury to entire aerodigestive tract, including oropharyngeal injury, esophageal/gastric perforation, aspiration, and ARDS
- 40% BSA burns have 40% mortality in 60–75 y (90% survival in <45 y)

WORRY ABOUT

- Significant number of patients do not present until many hours after injury
- Chemical burns often look deceptively benign, often having a smooth, suntanned appearance
- Extent cannot be assessed for 2–3 d. Immediate treatment is irrigation with large amounts of sterile saline to dilute and wash away the agent

OVERVIEW

- The reaction of an acid or base with tissue liberates heat, damaging tissue
- Other agents injure by liquefaction necrosis (alkalis), delipidation (petroleum products), and vesicle formation (vesicant gases)
  - Mortality rare in <40% BSA burns and related to the extent of injury
  - Morbidity includes disfiguration and loss of function of tissue damaged, infection, loss of joint mobility due to scarring, and, particular to caustic ingestion, esophageal and gastric stricture/perforation

ICD-9-CM Codes: 949.0; 941 (Burn face)

ETIOLOGY

- Majority fall into two categories: accidental skin burns at work usually involving the extremities; caustic ingestions, accidentally by children or as suicidal gesture by adults

USUAL TREATMENT

- Immediate care usually focuses on the burn (occasional large BSA burns treated like large thermal burns, i.e., fluid resuscitation 3–4 ml/kg/%BSA over 24 h). Irrigate with sterile saline for at least 30 min to dilute agent, and cleanse wound
- Treat lyte abn, arrhythmias, ATN, ARDS
- Strict asepsis in dressing wounds, usually early debridement and tangential excision with flap reconstructions or skin grafting

ASSESSMENT POINTS

SYSTEM	EFFECT	ASSESSMENT BY HX	PE	TEST
HEENT	Chemical may burn eyes, oropharynx, trachea, esophagus, stomach	Consistent Hx, visual disturbances, dysarthria, dysphagia, chest/abdominal pain	Inspection for evidence of same, ocular analgesics, dye, slit-lamp exam	Early endoscopic exam Contrast x-ray
CV	Hypotensive shock, arrhythmias, myocardial depression	Hx dyspnea/orthopnea, palpitations or chest pain	Chest exam	CXR ECG Electrolytes
RESP	Aspirated chemical, ARDS	Hx dyspnea/SOB, chest pain, mental status changes	Chest exam	CXR ABGs
GI	Gastric, esophageal burns/perforation	Hx ingestion with chest or abdominal pain Hematemesis	Pharyngeal, chest, and abdominal exam	Endoscopic exam, contrast x-rays
RENAL	ATN from myoglobin, hypotension	Hx massive tissue injury, prolonged hypotension	Oliguria–anuria	BUN/Cr; Cr clearance Serum/urine myoglobin
EXTREMITIES	Compartment syndrome	Hx circumferential extremity burns	Weak pulses, neurologic deficits	Transduce compartment pressures

Key Reference: Singer A, et al: Chemical burns: Our 10-year experience. Burns 1992; 18:250–252.

PERIOPERATIVE IMPLICATIONS

Preoperative Preparation

- Stabilize first
- Most common operative procedures are panendoscopy, escharotomies/faciotomies emergently, and debridements with tangential excisions of eschar, flap reconstructions, and skin grafting procedures days and weeks later

Monitoring

- Attempt to minimize invasive lines to avoid sepsis; however, use whatever monitors necessary to manage patient's medical status; staple ECG leads on; staple pulse oximeter on

Airway

- If aerodigestive tract involvement, anticipate airway management problems and ARDS

Induction

- In more severely injured, considerations similar to those for thermal burns: In acute phase, anticipate homeostatic problems; electrolyte abn; hypovolemia. Chronic phase: scarring causing loss of function and positioning problems, infection, hyperkalemic response to succinylcholine, poor nutritional status, NMB resistance

Maintenance

- Cardiorespiratory stability is important to avoid renal and other organ dysfunction
- Significant blood loss can occur with debridements
- Avoid hypothermia (warm room and all fluids—warm air heating)

Extubation

- Assess resp status carefully; if in doubt, monitor patient and reassess later

Adjuvants

- NMB: consider avoiding succinylcholine; resistant to NM blockers
- Inhalation: patient may be esp. sensitive to depressant/arrhythmogenic effects of halothane

Postoperative Period

- Monitor cardiorespiratory status
- Heat loss in transfer to/from OR

ANTICIPATED PROBLEMS/CONCERNS

- Level of concern related to degree of injury
- Easy to underestimate extent of injury, esp. early on, and undertreat these patients

BURN INJURY — ELECTRICAL

J.A. Jeevendra Martyn, M.D.

RISK

• About 1% of the 100,000 accidental deaths or approximately 3% of the 150,000 burns in USA are caused by electrical or natural lightning injury.
• Low-voltage (<1000 V) injury usually occurs in the household; high-voltage (>1000 V) typically occurs in industry or in contact with high-tension wires.

PERIOPERATIVE RISKS

• Immediate sequelae are momentary or prolonged unconsciousness, temporary paralysis, and autonomic disturbances (arterial spasm and pupillary abnormalities).
• Possible destruction of muscle or visceral tissues, pancreatitis, diabetes, gastric stress ulceration, coagulation abnormalities.
• Possible fractures because of either intense muscle contraction or fall from height.

WORRY ABOUT

• Injury to CNS, fractures, visceral injuries, pneumothorax, renal shutdown.

OVERVIEW

• Injuries caused by either the current or its arc (flash burn). Burns can occur directly because of the flame or hot gases that are heated by the arc. Since electrical current chooses the shortest pathway between the contact points, any vital organs in its passage will be damaged during its path. Characteristic entry and exit wounds usually signal destruction of deeper tissues, severity of which cannot be predicted.
• Loss of vascular volume into damaged and undamaged tissue occurs.
• Injury to underlying tissues may necessitate amputation, excision of large amounts of muscle, and release of deep fascial compartments.

ICD-9-CM Code: 948

ETIOLOGY

• Heat produced is directly proportional to the resistance and the square of the current. Poor conductors of electricity develop heat when transmitting electrical energy. Thus, tissues such as the bone, which are poor conductors, damage the surrounding muscle owing to the heat developed.
• Skin and subcutaneous tissues, being better conductors, are damaged less severely, and such injury may not reflect organ/muscle damage.

ASSESSMENT POINTS

SYSTEM	EFFECT	ASSESSMENT BY HX	PE	TEST
DERMATOLOGIC	Burn injury. Loss of intravascular volume, edema.	↓ Urine, ↓ BP	↑ Heart rate	CVP Tilt test
CV	VFib, tachycardia, or cardiac arrest initially. Arrhythmias and conduction abnormalities, nonspecific ECG changes, myocardial rupture	Hemodynamic instability		↑ CPK-myocardial bands >4%. Increases in CPK-MB do not necessarily correlate with severity of cardiac damage
	Arterial or venous thrombosis, aneurysms, hemolysis	Will vary depending on site		Angiography
RESP	Pleural effusion, tracheobronchitis, bronchopleural fistula			X-rays, scans
NEURO	Unconsciousness, coma, paralysis, cerebral hemorrhage, spinal paralysis, transverse myelitis, neuropathies	Will vary depending on type of injury		X-rays, CT, or MRI C-spine injury
RENAL	Oliguria, albuminuria, myoglobinuria, acute renal failure			Urine volume, urine myoglobin
GI	Nausea, vomiting, paralytic ileus, Curling's ulcer, perforated bowel, pancreatitis	Peritonitis		Blood sugar, exploratory laparotomy
INFECTIONS	Local and systemic, anaerobic and aerobic			
MS	Release of myoglobin and CPK from muscle, fractures, or dislocation of bones			See above

Key Reference: Martyn JAJ (ed): Acute Management of the Burned Patient. Philadelphia, WB Saunders, 1990.

PERIOPERATIVE IMPLICATIONS

• Complications can occur acutely, during intermediate and late periods.
• Scans or x-rays needed to exclude CNS or bone damage.
• Measure UO because of high incidence of renal shutdown due to myoglobinuria.
• Monitor sensorium for any deterioration in consciousness.
• Continuous vigilance for evidence of perforation or visceral damage.

• Therapy for Curling's ulcer.
• Watch for direct injury to chest wall, pleural damage with hydrothorax, aspiration or pneumonia or frank bronchial perforation and mediastinal compression.
• Vascular damage to arteries and veins and evidence of thrombosis should be assessed.

MANAGEMENT OF ELECTRICAL INJURIES

• Basic or advanced life support for cardiac or respiratory arrest

• IV fluids to maintain urine ≥1 ml/kg/h.
• Furosemide and mannitol with alkalinization of urine may be indicated to maintain UO and prevent renal shutdown.
• Therapy for cardiac and neurologic dysfunction may be necessary.
• Monitor BUN, Hgb, blood gases.
• Administer anticlostridrial prophylaxis, including penicillin.
• Post-traumatic stress disorder of electrical injury has also been reported.

BURN INJURY — FLAME

Wendy Howard, M.D.
Enrico Camporesi, M.D.

RISK

- >2.5 million y in USA seek medical care for flame burn injury
- >100,000 require hospitalization
- Burn injuries are the second cause of accidental death, behind motor vehicle accidents.
- High-risk groups include the young and the old

PERIOPERATIVE RISKS

- Mean burn size with 50% mortality ranges from 65 to 75% BSA
- Inhalation injury significantly increases mortality by 30–40%
- Burn eschar readily supports infection, leading to high mortality due to systemic sepsis.

WORRY ABOUT

- Inadequate fluid resuscitation will leave significant hypovolemia

- Underlying medical condition (e.g., epilepsy, CVA), drug or alcohol overdose may have caused the burn
- Possibility of associated injuries, e.g., bone fractures, closed head injuries, spinal injuries, or blunt internal injuries

OVERVIEW

- Cause loss of microvascular integrity with consequent ↑ capillary permeability, fluid accumulation, ↓ perfusion
- Generalized edema results; maximal losses occur in the first 8 to 12 h
- Deep burns can constrict an extremity or chest wall causing circulatory or ventilatory insufficiency
- Inhalation injury may be associated with massive pulmonary edema

ICD-9-CM Codes: 940–949 (948—burn classified by % body affected)
See also under Carbon Monoxide Poisoning, Cyanide Toxicity

ETIOLOGY

- Hot liquid scalds, residential fires, ignition of clothing and cigarettes

USUAL TREATMENT

- Initially as a multiple trauma patient with a thorough systematic evaluation, first priority given to airway, ventilation, and then circulation
- Large-bore IV access ideally avoiding burnt skin
- Rule of nines for rapid assessment of BSA burnt
- IV fluid calculated with Parkland formula: 4 ml/kg/%burn in the first 24 h, half in first 8 h from time of injury (50% burn to 70 kg person—14L/24h)
- Maintain warm environment and body T
- Incremental narcotics for pain relief, continuous verbal reassurance

ASSESSMENT POINTS

SYSTEM	EFFECT	ASSESSMENT BY HX	PE	TEST
HEENT	Airway damage	Enclosed space Toxic fumes Dysphagia Lengthy exposure	Soot or burn to nose or mouth Stridor or cough	ABG CXR Carboxyhemoglobin level
CV	Hypovolemic shock Ischemia	Burn extent Associated injuries May be asymptomatic	Hypotension	CVP PVR ECG
RESP	Lung injury	Inhalation injury	See HEENT	See HEENT
RENAL	↓ Renal perfusion	Hypovolemic shock Massive tissue injury	Decreased UO	Creatinine Myoglobinuria
CNS	Hypoxia	Inhalation injury	Altered LOC	ABG Carboxyhemoglobin level
MS	Massive tissue injury	Burn extent	Myoglobinemia	

Key Reference: Griglak MJ: Thermal injury. Emerg Med Clin North Am 1992; 10(2):369–383.

PERIOPERATIVE IMPLICATIONS

Preoperative Preparation

- Elevate room T
- Consider use of warming devices: blankets, fluid, ventilator
- Secure adequate venous access

Monitoring

- Routine monitors
- If anticipating large blood losses, consider CVP, arterial line (for repeated lab work), and UO measurement
- Consider PA catheter or TEE if underlying CV disease or hemodynamically unstable (sepsis or shock)
- Consider suturing or stapling ECG leads and oximeter probe to attachment sites

Airway

- Anticipate difficulty due to generalized body edema

Preinduction/Induction

- Hypermetabolic state with high cardiac output, high O_2 demand, ↑ CO_2 output, and low PVR
- May be hypovolemic or have unrecognized sepsis
- Low serum albumin and protein binding

Maintenance

- Replace fluid losses rapidly (both evaporation and blood losses)
- Liberally transfuse blood and consider albumin or other oncotic agents (e.g., Hespan)
- Avoid hypothermia

Extubation

- Consider postop intubation if large fluid losses or suspected airway edema
- High risk of pulmonary edema and respiratory distress

Adjuvants

- Often rapidly metabolize drugs or increase binding sites for nondepolarizing muscle relaxants
- High narcotic demands
- Avoid succinylcholine owing to possibility of ↑ K^+

ANTICIPATED PROBLEMS/CONCERNS

- Avoid succinylcholine. Massive tissue damage associated with excessive K^+ release and CV collapse. Significant for unknown time, possibly for 6 mo.
- Airway difficulty due to burn or to inhalation injury. At risk of pulmonary edema
- Hypovolemia 2° to fluid loss from burn and generalized edema due to vascular permeability

CANCER — BRONCHIAL

John P. McCarren, M.D.

RISK

- 160,000 cases/y in USA
- Race with highest prevalence: ?
- Tobacco consumption is the major risk factor; males > females but this difference is decreasing as gender ratio of smokers of long duration is equalizing.

PERIOPERATIVE RISKS

- Respiratory insufficiency from severe COPD or from lung resection

WORRY ABOUT

- Endobronchial obstruction: obstructive pneumonitis, consolidation, atelectasis, or localized air trapping
- Metastasis: brain, bone, adrenal glands, pericardium, pleural
- Paraneoplastic syndromes: Cushing's, SIADH, hypercalcemia, neuromuscular (Eaton-Lambert, neuropathy, myelopathy, polymyositis), hematologic (migratory thrombophlebitis, marantic endocarditis, DIC)

OVERVIEW

- Malignancy of squamous cell, adenocarcinoma, large cell, and small cell types.
- Leading cause of cancer deaths in USA for both men and women with an overall 1/y survival of 20% and a 5-y survival of 8%.
- Cigarette smoking major risk factor for both lung cancer and COPD; hence, high incidence of COPD in patients with lung cancer.
- Severe COPD affects perioperative management and may limit lung resection.
- Paraneoplastic syndromes are rarely manifested.

ICD-9-CM Code: 162.9

ETIOLOGY

- 85% related to cigarette smoking; asbestos, radiation, heavy metal exposure, genetics contributing factors

USUAL TREATMENT

- Surgical resection of localized disease for non–small cell carcinoma
- Chemotherapy, radiation therapy for small cell carcinoma
- Unresectable endobronchial or endotracheal tumors treated with external beam radiation and/or bronchoscopic laser resection

ASSESSMENT POINTS

SYSTEM	EFFECT	ASSESSMENT BY HX	PE	TEST
HEENT	Possible tracheal fixation or obstruction by tumor	Dyspnea, cough, rhonchi	Poor air flow SOB	PFT CXR
CV	Pericardial effusion SVC syndrome	Dyspnea, cough	Dilated neck veins and facial swelling	ECHO CXR
RESP	Lung mass, airway consolidation and atelectasis, pleural effusion	Dyspnea, cough, feverish	Rhonchi Fever Dullness to percussion	CXR ABG
GI	Rarely pancreatitis from hypercalcemia	Anorexia, nausea, vomiting, constipation		Serum Ca^{2+}
CNS	Brain metastasis Paraneoplastic syndrome (optic neuritis, subacute cerebellar degeneration, peripheral neuropathy)	Headache, visual changes, unsteady gait, sensory or motor symptoms	Funduscopic or neurologic findings	
MS	Bone metastasis Eaton-Lambert syndrome Polymyositis with activity	Bone pain Fatigue and weakness Muscle soreness	Bone tenderness Decreased DTRs Improved strength	

Key Reference: Carr DT, Holoye PY, Hong WK: Bronchogenic carcinoma. *In* Murray J, Nadel J (eds): Textbook of Respiratory Medicine. Philadelphia, WB Saunders, 1994, pp 1528–1596.

PERIOPERATIVE IMPLICATIONS

Preoperative Preparation

- Adequate hydration, correction of electrolyte abnormalities, bronchodilators for bronchospasm, antimicrobials if infected, steroid coverage for adrenal insufficiency, if present
- Instruction in incentive spirometry

Monitoring

- Consider arterial line for lung resections

Airway

- Determine need for left- or right-sided double-lumen ETT

Preinduction/Induction

- Bronchodilators when appropriate
- Judicious use of neuromuscular blockers if Eaton-Lambert syndrome

Maintenance

- No one agent or technique is superior
  - Halogenated agents decrease bronchomotor tone and permit high FIO_2 but minimally decrease HPV
- CPAP and PEEP as needed

Extubation

- Change to single-lumen ETT if will remain intubated

Adjuvants

- Consider bronchodilators

Postoperative Period

- Consider epidural catheter for pain management

ANTICIPATED PROBLEMS/CONCERNS

- Potentially life-threatening postop problems include bronchial disruptions, cardiac herniation, tension pneuothorax, cardiac dysrhythmias.
- Adequate analgesia beneficial if severe COPD.

CANCER — LUNG PARENCHYMA

Roger A. Moore, M.D.

RISK

- 160,000 new cases/y
  - 75 deaths/100,000 males/y
  - 30 deaths/100,000 females/y
  - Asbestos exposure increases risk 5-fold.
  - Smoking increases risk 10-fold.

PERIOPERATIVE RISKS

- Associated coronary artery disease
- Pulmonary insufficiency following lung tissue resection

WORRY ABOUT

- Optimization of preop pulmonary status
- Myasthenic syndrome (Eaton-Lambert) with oat cell carcinoma
- Massive hemoptysis with cancer invasion of bronchial arteries
- Active pneumonia in pulmonary parenchyma distal to obstructed bronchioles

OVERVIEW

- Four primary types of lung cancers: (1) epidermoid or bronchogenic; (2) adenocarcinoma; (3) alveolar cell carcinoma; (4) undifferentiated carcinoma (large cell, small cell [oat cell])
- Oat cell metastasizes early
- 70% with COPD need extra postop pulmonary care
- Patients often nutritionally depleted
- Many have alcohol abuse history.
- Preop pulmonary state may limit option of lobectomy.
- Hormonal imbalances common
  - 3% of patients are cushingoid.
  - 70% of bronchogenic carcinomas have increased ACTH or pro-ACTH.
  - Up to 60% with lung cancer have inappropriate ADH.
- Myasthenic syndrome occurs owing to decreased release of nerve-ending acetylcholine →increased sensitivity to *all* muscle relaxants

ICD-9-CM Code: 162.9

ETIOLOGY

- Environmental factor important (i.e., smoking, asbestos exposure)
- Higher incidence in areas located near oil refineries

USUAL TREATMENT

- Oat cell cancer frequently treated with radiation and chemotherapy (need good renal function)
- Lobectomy or pneumonectomy common approaches in other types of lung cancers; DLCO of <60% predicts 75% mortality; >100% predicts 100% survival.

ASSESSMENT POINTS

SYSTEM	EFFECT	ASSESSMENT BY HX	PE	TEST
CV	Myocardial ischemia	Angina SOB	S$_3$ gallop	
	Arrhythmia	Palpitations	Irregular pulse	Exercise stress test ECG
	Cor pulmonale	SOB	Distended neck veins	Catheterization ECHO
RESP	Pneumonia	Productive cough	Rhonchi–rales	CXR
	Bronchospasm	Wheezing	Wheezes	PFTs: MBC; MMEFR; DLCO
	COPD	SOB, dyspnea	Decreased BS	ABG
ENDO	IADH	Lethargy, ↑ weight, ↓ urine Thin skin; poor wound healing	Hypometabolic	Electrolytes Elevated urine sodium (rarely needed)
	↑ ACTH	Weight gain; striae	Cushingoid; ↑ BP	Cortisone level (rarely needed)
NEURO-MUSCULAR	Eaton-Lambert (myasthenic)	Muscle weakness	Muscle strength with exercise	EMG (rarely needed)
NUTRITION	Wasting	Weight loss	Cachexia; BMI change	Liver function tests (esp albumin)
	DTs	Alcohol abuse	↑ Liver size	

Key Reference: Ferguson MK, Little L, Rizzo L, et al: Diffusing capacity predicts morbidity and mortality after pulmonary resection. J Thorac Cardiovasc Surg 1988; 96:894–900.

PERIOPERATIVE IMPLICATIONS

Preoperative Preparation

- Respiratory optimization with bronchodilatation, antibiotics, pulmonary hygiene, and smoking cessation
- Correction of lyte imbalances

Monitoring

- Routine monitors
- Capnography and pulse oximetry, esp during one-lung anesthesia
- Intra-arterial line and possible pulmonary catheter
- Neuromuscular blockade monitor

Airway

- Double-lumen tube needed—usually left-sided
- Fiberoptic bronchoscope available

Induction

- Anesthetic choice dependent on associated medical problems
- Light premedication to decrease CO$_2$ retention

- When right-sided double-lumen tube used, ensure right upper lobe ventilation (easiest with fiberoptic bronchoscope)

Maintenance

- Nerve damage with lateral position
  - use axillary roll
  - brachial plexus injury with arm hyperextension
  - pad all pressure points
- Substantiate pulse oximetric and capnographic readings with ABGs
- If oxygen saturation falls during one lung ventilation, PEEP on dependent lung may help. If not, CPAP on nondependent lung may help.

Extubation

- At end of procedure, double-lumen tube should be switched to single-lumen tube.
- Extubation should be determined by adequacy of respiratory variables.

Adjuvants

- Bronchodilators for intraoperative use, inotropes for myocardial depression, antiarrhythmics for post–lobectomy-pneumonectomy arrhythmias (some advocate prophylactic digoxin —but conflicting reported results)

Postoperative Period

- Adequate pain management usual for recovery of pulmonary function
  - PCA effective
  - thoracic epidural most efficacious
- Be watchful for DTs, inappropriate ADH, and ↓ neuromuscular strength.

ANTICIPATED PROBLEMS/CONCERNS

- Intensive pulmonary toilet postoperatively
- Careful suctioning of bronchial stump because of possibility of rupture
- Bronchopleural fistula or tension pneumothorax should be anticipated.

CANDIDIASIS

James M. Sonner, M.D.
Jeffrey A. Katz, M.D.

RISK

- Current or recent broad-spectrum antibiotic treatment
- Immunosuppression (e.g., AIDS, neutropenia, drugs)
- Breach of epithelial barriers (e.g., by surgery, indwelling catheters, burns)
- Lengthy critical illness
- IV hyperalimentation

PERIOPERATIVE RISKS

- Increased mortality (>50%) with candidemia
- Sequelae of sepsis

WORRY ABOUT

- Metastatic disease to brain, heart, lung, liver, kidney, bone may be involved with corresponding organ dysfunction
- Side effects of amphotericin treatment: hypotension, fever, azotemia, hypokalemia, emesis, thrombophlebitis
- Septic shock

OVERVIEW

- Clinical spectrum ranges from mild mucosal overgrowth of organisms to life-threatening disseminated infection. The former is easier to diagnose and treat; the latter, much more difficult
- Any organ can be affected. Mucosal surfaces are usually overgrown but may be invaded with microabscess formation and fungemia. *Candida* in solid organs reflects abscesses from disseminated disease

ICD-9-CM Code: 112.5 (Systemic)

ETIOLOGY

- Fungal infection due to *Candida* species. Disease occurs when normally commensal yeasts overgrow tissues that they colonize, e.g., thrush, or when *Candida* invades tissues (e.g., abscess).

- Infection facilitated by disruption of mucocutaneous barriers, immunosuppression, and following antibiotic treatment (kills bacterial flora that normally check *Candida* growth)

USUAL TREATMENT

- PO nystatin, clotrimazole, or ketoconazole for oral or esophageal candidiasis
- Topical antifungals for vaginal or cutaneous candidiasis
- IV amphotericin B for systemic candidiasis; IV flucytosine added for persistent or metastatic fungemia or septic shock
- IV and arterial catheters removed or replaced for candidemia
- Surgical excision for infected prostheses, endocarditis, thrombophlebitis
- Fluconazole in selected cases

ASSESSMENT POINTS

SYSTEM	EFFECT	ASSESSMENT BY HX	PE	TEST
HEENT	Endophthalmitis Thrush	↓ Visual acuity Dysphagia	Cottonball lesions on funduscopy White plaque in oropharynx	
CV	Endocarditis Myocardial invasion Shock		Murmur, hypotension Fever	ECHO ECG CVP, PCWP, CO
RESP	Pneumonia ARDS	Dyspnea, cough Cyanosis	Signs of consolidation not uniformly present	CXR
GI	Esophagitis Enteritis Peritonitis Intra-abdominal abscess	Dysphagia Abdominal pain	Hepatomegaly Splenomegaly Peritoneal signs Ileus	Endoscopy LFTs CT or MRI
RENAL	Bladder infection Kidney abscess	Urinary frequency Dysuria	Costovertebral tenderness	Urinalysis BUN/Cr, CT
CNS	Meningitis Brain abscess	Altered mental status	Altered mental status Meningeal signs	Lumbar puncture CT or MRI
MS	Osteomyelitis	Pain over bone	Tender over bone	X-ray, bone scan

Key Reference: Solomkin JS: Candida infection. *In* Scientific American Medicine: Care of the Surgical Patient, Vol 2, Section IX, Chap 10, 1993.

PERIOPERATIVE IMPLICATIONS

Preoperative Preparation

- Continue antifungal therapy
- Assess for presence of septic shock, impaired gas exchange, neurologic or cardiac involvement
- Check K, Cr if on amphotericin therapy
- Determine age of IV lines for possible changing in OR

Monitoring

- If septic shock is present, close monitoring of cardiac filling pressures, arterial pressure, ABGs, UO is required.

Airway

- None

Preinduction/Induction

- If sepsis is present ↑ risk of hypotension 2° to hypovolemia and myocardial depression
- With pulmonary involvement, rapid oxygen desaturation may occur

Maintenance

- Hypotension may be present because of sepsis and may be worsened by superimposing negative inotropic or vasodilating agents

Extubation

- Respiratory function can be compromised by pulmonary candidiasis or ARDS; may require postop ventilatory support

Adjuvants

- Depends on organ damage from disease or its treatment; often ↓ renal function and modification of anesthetic and neuromuscular blockers due to this organ impairment.

ANTICIPATED PROBLEMS/CONCERNS

- Fever and hypotension are associated with candidemia and its treatment; mortality is high
- Septic shock or multiple organ involvement may be present

CARBON MONOXIDE (CO) POISONING

Peter H. Breen, M.D., F.R.C.P.C.
Richard E. Moon, M.D.
Bryant W. Stolp, M.D., Ph.D.

RISK

- Most frequent toxic gas in smoke
- Major cause of death
- CO produced by all internal combustion engines, incomplete oxidative combustion (e.g., house fires, charcoal and gas grills, malfunctioning butane/propane stoves) and endogenous sources (e.g., by liver from exogenous exposure to paint stripper)
- During GA, use semi-closed circuits, esp when machine has not been used for 2–3 days
- No odor, taste, or color; nonirritating
- Toxicity potentiated by low inspired O_2 concentration (e.g., smoke inhalation)
- In carbon dioxide absorbers of anesthesia machines (esp. on Monday mornings)

PERIOPERATIVE RISKS

- Main target organs: heart and brain
- Heart: can resemble ischemia; potentiated by CAD
- Brain: acute loss of consciousness; after initial improvement, up to 30% risk of secondary syndrome: chronic psychiatric dysfunction and cerebral and cerebellar syndromes

WORRY ABOUT

- Seek other smoke inhalation injury
- Consider concomitant cyanide poisoning that potentiates CO toxicity

OVERVIEW

- CO, a colorless non-irritating and odorless gas, is a natural byproduct of combustion
- CO binds avidly to Hb ($> 200 \times > O_2$) to form carboxyhemoglobin (COHb), which carries no O_2 and causes left shift in oxyhemoglobin dissociation curve ($\downarrow O_2$ off-loading to tissues)
- CO binds to intracellular hemoproteins such as myoglobin and cytochrome aa_3 (especially cardiac) to inhibit O_2 uptake and metabolism
- "Classic" cherry-red complexion rarely observed
- COHb level correlates poorly with clinical condition.
- Treatment should be guided by symptoms and signs, not by blood COHb concentration

ICD-9-CM Code: 986

ETIOLOGY

- CO produced by incomplete oxidative combustion (e.g., house fires, malfunctioning butane/propane stoves, home heaters, and all internal combustion engines)
- Suicide attempts

USUAL TREATMENT

- Normobaric oxygen: $T_{1/2}$ of COHb decreases from 3.5 h (air-breathing) to 0.75 h (O_2-breathing)
- General supportive care, especially for other aspects of smoke inhalation injury
- Hyperbaric O_2 (2.5 atm) $\downarrow$ COHb $T_{1/2}$ to 20 min and has been shown to $\downarrow$ probability of development of delayed neurologic complication; for patients with neurologic Sx (including impaired consciousness), evidence of myocardial ischemia, fetal distress (if pregnant), or other Sx of significant exposure (e.g., COHb >25%), hyperbaric O_2 is recommended if feasible, within 6–8 h of exposure

ASSESSMENT POINTS

SYSTEM	EFFECT	ASSESSMENT BY HX	PE	TEST
HEENT	Thermal/toxic upper airway injury	Fire exposure/ smoke inhalation	Perioral burns Airway edema	Laryngoscopy/ bronchoscopy
RESP	CO diffuses rapidly into blood → COHb Thermal/toxic airway and parenchymal injury	Dyspnea, tachypnea	Bronchoconstriction and pulm edema	Co-oximetric COHb: Po_2 usually normal CXR Bronchoscopy
CV	$\downarrow$ Blood O_2 content and $\downarrow$ tissue O_2 unloading	Possibly angina or evidence of heart failure; tachycardia	Cardiac failure	ECG: ischemic ST-T changes; CXR
METABOL	Tissue hypoxia → acidosis			Lactic acidosis
CNS	Coma, cerebral edema	Temporal headache, N/V, restlessness	Muscle weakness, altered mental status	Abnormal neuropsychometric testing
	Neuropsychiatric syndrome	Cerebral, cerebellar		Can occur after initial recovery

Key Reference: Breen PH, et al: Combined carbon monoxide and cyanide poisoning: A place for treatment? Anesth Analg 1995; 80:681–687.

PERIOPERATIVE IMPLICATIONS

Preoperative Preparation

- Continuous 100% O_2
- Document CNS status
- Consider hyperbaric O_2 if mental status altered or patient has myocardial ischemia or is pregnant

Monitoring

- Routine monitors
- Pulse oximetry (Spo_2) unreliable in presence of COHb (Spo_2 overestimates oxyhemoglobin)
- Arterial cannula for frequent blood sampling
- Venous and arterial COHb levels are almost identical.

Airway

- Airway injury and edema often occur during smoke inhalation → may require emergent airway management

Induction

- Avoid cardiac depressant agents

Maintenance

- 100% O_2 (no N_2O)
- Assess muscle weakness to guide muscle relaxant dosage

Extubation

- Ensure CNS status permits natural airway maintenance and protection

Adjuvants

- Consider treatment for concomitant cyanide poisoning (see under Cyanide Poisoning)

Postoperative Period

- Maintain 100% O_2
- Consider hyperbaric O_2

ANTICIPATED PROBLEMS/CONCERNS

- Heart and brain affected most
- Follow CNS function carefully
- Seek concomitant smoke inhalation injury and cyanide toxicity
- CO toxic in trace quantities (breathing 0.1% inspired CO for 1 h results in significant toxicity, with COHb ~30%); CO not detectable with conventional gas analysis instruments (e.g., capnographs, mass spectrometers)
- Pulse oximeters do not specifically measure COHb, and O_2 sat readings only minimally affected, even by severe CO poisoning

CARCINOID SYNDROME

Stanley H. Rosenbaum, M.D.

RISK

- Most common GI endocrine tumor
- 15 cases/1 million population per year

PERIOPERATIVE RISKS

- Associated with patient's ability to tolerate abrupt hemodynamic change and/or bronchospasm

WORRY ABOUT

- Abrupt hypertension or hypotension with stress
- Right-sided valvular heart disease
- Bronchospasm

OVERVIEW

- Endocrinologically active tumor from GI mucosa
- May release histamine-like substances leading to hypotension and bronchospasm, or may release serotonin leading to hypertensive reactions (and hypovolemia)
- Commonly in ileum (especially appendix) or rectum, less so in pancreas and lung
- Systemically active when metastatic to liver, or when released substances avoid metabolism by liver (carcinoid syndrome)

ICD-9-CM Codes: 199.1 (Tumor); 259.2 (Syndrome)

ETIOLOGY

- Acquired disease
- May be associated with other ectopic humoral tumors, such as MEN-I syndrome

USUAL TREATMENT

- Surgery or arterial embolization to reduce tumor burden
- Histaminic effects blocked only partially by H_1 and H_2 blockers
- Serotonin synthesis blocked by parachlorophylalamine and effects blocked by ketanserin
- Octreotide blocks humoral release
- No specific medical Rx for established valvular heart lesions
- Catecholamines may ↑ humoral release and worsen symptoms

ASSESSMENT POINTS

SYSTEM	EFFECT	ASSESSMENT BY HX	PE	TEST
HEENT	Cutaneous flushing, lacrimation Pellagra-like skin lesions	Episodic flushing induced by stress, eating, alcohol consumption	Hyperkeratosis, hyperpigmentation	
CV	Histamine-induced hypotension Serotonin-induced HTN Endomyocardial fibrosis, especially in right heart	Sx of right-sided CHF	Murmurs of pulmonic stenosis, tricuspid regurgitation Ascites, edema	Echocardiogram Cardiac catheterization
RESP	Bronchospasm Endobronchial tumor with obstruction	Episodic asthma poorly responsive to medication Focal wheeze at site of obstructing tumor	Wheezing associated with episodes of flushing	
GI	Diarrhea Obstructing tumor	Episodic watery diarrhea		Bowel films Hepatic CT, ultrasound, angiograms
ENDO	Serotonin secretion			Urinary 5–HIAA levels elevated in most patients Occasionally need to measure plasma histamine
RENAL	Dehydration from chronic vasospasm or diarrhea			BUN/Cr, electrolytes
CNS	Hemodynamic instability, vasodilation	Hypertensive headache Syncope with flushing		
MS	Cutaneous flushing, lacrimation Pellagra-like skin lesions	Episodic flushing, induced by stress, eating, alcohol consumption	Hyperkeratosis, hyperpigmentation	

Key Reference: Buckley FP: *In* Barash, Cullen, Stoelting (eds): Clinical Anesthesia, 2nd ed. Philadelphia, JB Lippincott, 1992, pp 1180–1181.

PERIOPERATIVE IMPLICATIONS

Preoperative Preparation

- Assess adequacy of fluid balance
- Assess right-sided valvular status
- Somatostatin analogue (octreotide) available; its use has dramatically decreased hazards of anesthesia for patients with carcinoid syndrome

Monitoring

- Expect rapid fluctuation of BP
- Central venous pressures may not correlate well with fluid volumes

Airway

- Risk of stress-induced wheezing (Rx: somatostatin analogue)

Induction

- Chronic vasoconstriction and diarrhea may cause hemodynamic instability

Maintenance

- Volume assessments complicated by changing vascular tone
- Cardiac function limited by right-sided valvular lesions

Extubation

- Possible stress-induced hemodynamic instability (Rx: somatostatin analogue)

Adjuvants

- Caution! Catecholamines may increase humoral release and worsen symptoms
- Somatostatin analogue for hypo- or hypertension or bronchospasm has dramatically ↓ anesthesia risk for pts with carcinoid syndrome

Postoperative Period

- Humoral effects of hemodynamically active metastatic carcinoid usually not eliminated by surgery

CARDIOMYOPATHY, ALCOHOLIC

Gregory H. Botz, M.D.
Jonathan B. Mark, M.D.

RISK

- People within USA: 15 to 20 million chronic heavy ethanol users
- As much as 50% of dilated cardiomyopathy may be ethanol related.
- Population at risk: Unclear; likely includes chronic ethanol users with at least 5 oz daily ETOH for at least 5 y.
- Gender: male predominance

PERIOPERATIVE RISKS

- Alcohol withdrawal
- CHF
- Dysrhythmias common: AFib, PAC, PVC

WORRY ABOUT

- Myocardial ischemia: supply < demand (CAD rare)
- Abnormal systolic and diastolic function
- Chronic alcohol use alters myocardial response to inotropes
- Alcohol withdrawal symptoms

OVERVIEW

- Insidious onset; Sx uncommon unless severely stressed until late in course
- Dilated cardiomyopathy: ventricular hypertrophy early, chamber dilation later
- Low-output cardiac failure (as compared with high-output failure in cirrhosis and beriberi)
- Malnutrition often coexists.

ICD-9-CM Code: 425.5

ETIOLOGY

- Direct myocardial damage by ethanol and its metabolites
- Progressive chamber dilation and ventricular hypertrophy; microscopic fibrinoid deposition
- Possible intracellular calcium dysregulation
- Possible muscle excitation-contraction impairment

USUAL TREATMENT

- Abstinence—ventricular function improves markedly after abstinence.
- Pharmacologic management — digitalis, diuretics, vasodilators
- Address nutritional deficits — thiamine, folate, multivitamin

ASSESSMENT POINTS

SYSTEM	EFFECT	ASSESSMENT BY HX	PE	TEST
HEENT	Plethora, reflux, esophageal varices, friable mucosa	Reflux Sx Hematemesis	Spider angiomata	Endoscopy
CV	LV dysfunction CHF Myocardial ischemia Dysrhythmia	Fatigue, orthopnea PND Rare angina Palpitations	Narrow pulse pressure Cardiomegaly S_3, S_4, murmur JVD, peripheral edema	ECG ECHO Stress testing
RESP	Pulmonary edema	Dyspnea Cough	Rales	CXR
GI	Hepatic congestion	Poor appetite, distention	Hepatomegaly	PT, albumin, LFTs
HEME	Coagulopathy Anemia	Abnormal bleeding	Pallor Ecchymosis	CBC PT/PTT, plt
RENAL	↓ Renal perfusion	Oliguria		Cr, FENa
CNS	Poor perfusion	Confusion	Abn mental status	
MS	Proximal muscle weakness		Proximal limb weakness and muscle atrophy	

Key Reference: Piano MR, Schwertz DW. Alcoholic heart disease: A review. Heart Lung 1994; 23:3–17.

PERIOPERATIVE IMPLICATIONS

Preoperative Preparation

- Pharmacologic management of CHF

Monitoring

- ECG with ST segment analysis
- Consider arterial pressure catheter, pulmonary artery catheter, TEE depending on surgery and ventricular function

Airway

- None

Preinduction/Induction

- May have intravascular volume depletion

Maintenance

- Avoid tachycardia, increased sympathetic activity
- Avoid depression of myocardial contractility

Extubation

- Routine

Postoperative Period

- Consider monitoring in critical care unit.
- Observe for ethanol withdrawal.

Adjuvants

- Multivitamins, thiamine, B_{12}, folate, continued.
- Consider benzodiazepines, α_2 agonists for prophylaxis against withdrawal symptoms.
- Volume of distribution may be increased; consider adjusting drug dosages.

ANTICIPATED PROBLEMS/CONCERNS

- Postop ventricular dysfunction and CHF can occur
- Alcohol withdrawal symptoms can develop

CARDIOMYOPATHY, HYPERTROPHIC (HCM)
Edward Lowenstein, M.D.
J. Michael Haering, M.D.

RISK

- Incidence: rare; reported incidence between 0.025–1%
- Inherited as autosomal dominant with high degree of penetrance

PERIOPERATIVE RISKS

- Presence of dynamic outflow tract obstruction (either provoked or baseline) seen in 25% of patients with HCM
- ↑ Risk for myocardial ischemia due to profound LVH, high intraventricular pressures, and abnormal intramyocardial coronary arteries
- Little data to support worse perioperative outcome

WORRY ABOUT

- Worsening dynamic outflow tract obstruction with resultant hypotension due to:
  - ↓ in preload and afterload, esp with sudden volume loss or induction of anesthesia
  - ↑ in LV contractility
- Myocardial ischemia
- Diastolic dysfunction
- Supraventricular and ventricular dysrhythmias; loss of atrial contribution to LV diastolic filling

OVERVIEW

- Definition: presence of hypertrophied, nondilated LV in absence of other cardiac or systemic causes
- Histologically abnormal myocardium
- Septum usually disproportionately affected
- Hypertrophied myocardium may physically obstruct left ventricular outflow tract (LVOT) during systole, resulting in dynamic outflow tract gradient
- Anterior leaflet of mitral valve may contribute to dynamic obstruction as it is "drawn" into LVOT during systole
- May present as sudden death
- Other symptoms include dyspnea, syncope, and angina
- Diagnosis made echocardiographically or by demonstration of LVOT gradient at cardiac catheterization

ICD-9-CM Code: 425.1 (Obstructive cardiomyopathy)

ETIOLOGY

- Probable genetic abnormality of cardiac β myosin heavy chain

TREATMENT

- Medical: reduce LV contractility (e.g. β-blocker), improve LV diastolic function (e.g., calcium-channel antagonism), maintain preload and afterload, avoid provocative events (e.g., Valsalva)
- Surgical: septal myectomy, septal myotomy, mitral valve replacement, anterior mitral leaflet plication

ASSESSMENT POINTS

SYSTEM	EFFECT	ASSESSMENT BY HX	PE	TEST
CV	Myocardial ischemia	Angina, anginal equivalents, dyspnea		ECG, exercise tests
	LVOT obstruction	Angina, dyspnea, syncope	Systolic murmur accentuated by Valsalva	ECG, ECHO, cardiac catheterization
	Dysrhythmia	Syncope, sudden death	Pulse	ECG, Holter
	Diastolic dysfunction	See RESP section		ECHO, catheterization
RESP	Pulmonary congestion	Dyspnea	S_3, rales, wheezing	CXR
CNS	Syncope	Syncope, presyncope		

Key Reference: Maron BJ, et al: Hypertrophic cardiomyopathy. Interrelations of clinical manifestations, pathophysiology and therapy. N Engl J Med 1987; 316:780–789, 844–851.

PERIOPERATIVE IMPLICATIONS

Preoperative Preparation

- Replace any preoperative fluid deficit, ensure adequate ventricular volumes
- Consider preoperative β-blocker or calcium-channel blockade
- Sedate adequately to prevent anxiety-induced sympathetic stimulation

Monitoring

- Consider invasive arterial pressure monitoring
- Consider pulmonary artery catheter with atrial pacing capabilities given reduced LV compliance and dependence on sinus mechanism
- Transesophageal ECHO when blood loss or volume shifts anticipated

Airway

- None

Preinduction/Induction

- Phenylephrine infusion prepared, as worsening dynamic outflow tract gradient may be anticipated with any ↓ in SVR
- Avoid ketamine as induction agent
- Avoid prolonged laryngoscopy with attendant sympathetic stimulation
- Insertion of CVP/PAC may induce atrial or ventricular dysrhythmias

Maintenance

- Volatile agents that ↓ LV contractility without dramatic vasodilation desirable; halothane is the classic example
- Consider β-blocker or calcium-channel blockade for worsening LVOT obstruction
- Avoid agents that ↓ preload and afterload (e.g., nitroglycerin, nitroprusside), or any agent with significant histamine release
- Avoid agents that directly or indirectly ↑ HR and contractility (e.g., pancuronium, atropine, epinephrine, ephedrine)
- hypotension treated with:
  - volume expansion
  - pure α-adrenergic agonist (e.g., phenylephrine)
- Blood loss to be replaced promptly
- Spinal and epidural anesthesia may be associated with hypotension due to sympatholysis
- Risk of subendocardial ischemia
- Consider early electrical therapy for dysrhythmias

Extubation

- Avoid sympathetic stimulation
- Anticipate subendocardial ischemia

Postoperative Period

- Aggressive postop pain management

ANTICIPATED PROBLEMS/CONCERNS

- Myocardial ischemia
- Profound hypotension in setting of hypovolemia, ↓ preload/afterload, or ↑ contractility
- Dysrhythmias
- Diastolic dysfunction

CARDIOMYOPATHY, ISCHEMIC

Jonathan B. Mark, M.D.
Gregory H. Botz, M.D.

RISK

- Approximately 1:1000 incidence per annum
- Men > women (2:1)

PERIOPERATIVE RISKS

- Most important perioperative risk factor for cardiac morbidity and mortality
- Risk of CHF, hypotension, pulmonary edema, myocardial ischemia and infarction, renal insufficiency, arrhythmias

WORRY ABOUT

- CHF exacerbation, pulmonary edema, hypotension, myocardial ischemia and infarction, renal insufficiency, inability to tolerate fluid shifts associated with major surgery, arrhythmias

OVERVIEW

- Severe impairment of LVF leading to CHF; that arising from myocardial ischemia and infarction has extremely poor prognosis, with 30–50% 2 y mortality
- Patients may benefit from intensive medical therapy for underlying ischemia (nitrates, β-blockers, calcium antagonists, aspirin), CHF (ACE inhibitors, hydralazine, digoxin, diuretics), and prevention of cardiac thrombus (warfarin)
- Associated mitral regurgitation, left ventricular aneurysm, and ventricular arrhythmias may have specific perioperative considerations

ICD-9-CM Code: 414.8

ETIOLOGY

- Acquired disease with genetic predisposition
- Risk factors include associated hypertension, diabetes, hyperlipidemia, cigarette smoking, advanced age, peripheral vascular disease

USUAL TREATMENT

- Medical therapy (as indicated in Overview)
- Myocardial revascularization (angioplasty, atherectomy, coronary laser, stent, coronary bypass surgery)
- Cardiomyoplasty (generally experimental)
- Cardiac transplantation
- Associated cardiac surgery (mitral valve replacement/repair, left ventricular aneurysmectomy, implantation of AICD [automatic implantable cardioverter defibrillator])

ASSESSMENT POINTS

SYSTEM	EFFECT	ASSESSMENT BY HX	PE	TEST
CV	Myocardial ischemia Arrhythmias CHF	Angina Dyspnea, PND Palpitations	S_3, S_4, loud P_2 Narrow pulse pressure Displaced point maximal impulse	ECG Stress testing Echocardiogram Cardiac catheterization
RESP	Pulm congestion/ edema	Dyspnea on exertion Orthopnea Cough	Rales Wheezes	CXR
GI	Ascites	Abdominal distention	Shifting dullness Fluid wave Hepatomegaly	Liver function tests PT Albumin
CNS	Embolic stroke due to cardiac thrombosis	Weakness Vision problems Confusion	Altered mental status Focal deficits	CT or MRI
MS	Peripheral edema	Swollen ankles Weakness	Pitting edema	
RENAL	Insufficiency (prerenal)	Oliguria		Cr, BUN Excreted fraction of filtered sodium

Key Reference: Vlay SC: Innovations in the management of ischemic cardiomyopathy. Am Heart J 1994; 127:235–242.

PERIOPERATIVE IMPLICATIONS

Preoperative Preparation

- Pharmacologic control of myocardial ischemia and CHF

Monitoring

- ECG (V_5 or multilead) with ST-segment analysis
- Arterial catheter (close BP monitoring, ABG).
- Consider PA catheter or TEE for major operations and/or poor medical condition

Airway

- None

Preinduction/Induction

- Avoid tachycardia and increased afterload to prevent ischemia and reduced cardiac output
- Hypovolemia may result from diuretic therapy

Maintenance

- Limited ability to increase cardiac output in response to stress
- Attention to fluid balance (PCWP) to avoid pulmonary edema or low cardiac output
- High doses of inhaled anesthetics may be poorly tolerated because of myocardial depression superimposed on cardiomyopathy

Extubation

- May be time of greatest stress for developing myocardial ischemia or LV dysfunction
- Consider postoperative mechanical ventilation if a large fluid resuscitation was required intraoperatively

Adjuvants

- Extensive preoperative medical therapy may have circulatory consequences
- Preoperative anticoagulation may preclude regional anesthesia

Postoperative Period

- Epidural pain management techniques may limit stress if operation was major (beware of Coumadin therapy)
- Intensive care and hemodynamic monitoring may prevent complications if operation was major

ANTICIPATED PROBLEMS/CONCERNS

- Perioperative myocardial ischemia and CHF remain paramount concerns

CARNITINE DEFICIENCY

Raafat S. Hannallah, M.D.

RISK

• Rare

PERIOPERATIVE RISKS

• Hypoglycemia
• Massive rhabdomyolysis and cardiac arrest described following GA and succinylcholine. The response may be confused with malignant hyperthermia.

WORRY ABOUT

• Perioperative hypoglycemia: avoid prolonged fast; IV glucose should be administered.
• Neurologic and cardiopulmonary status: determine if a cardiomyopathy is present.

OVERVIEW

• Carnitine is essential cofactor in enzymatic transport of long-chain fatty acids into mitochondria in which they are oxidized.
• When carnitine deficient, peripheral tissues cannot use fatty acids for energy production and the liver cannot adequately make ketone bodies as an alternative substrate.
• The tissues become glucose dependent, and their metabolism exceeds liver's capacity for glucose production.
• This glucose dependency can lead to severe liver failure (↑ hepatic enzymes, lactic acidosis, hepatic encephalopathy) and hypoglycemia.

Common ICD-9-CM Code: 791.3

ETIOLOGY

• Rare inherited condition associated with lipid storage disorders ascribed to defect in hepatic biosynthesis of carnitine (systemic form) or reduced carnitine transport into muscle cells (myopathic form).

USUAL TREATMENT

• Dietary supplementation with L-carnitine and high-carbohydrate diet to prevent hypoglycemia.

ASSESSMENT POINTS

SYSTEM	EFFECT	ASSESSMENT BY HX	TEST
CV	Cardiomyopathy		ECHO
HEPATIC	Hypoglycemia	Lethargy	Blood glucose
HEME	Coagulopathy	Bleeding	Hypoprothrombinemia
CNS	Encephalopathy	Vomiting, diarrhea	Hyperammonemia

Key Reference: Rowe RW, Helander E: Anesthetic management of a patient with systemic carnitine deficiency. Anesth Analg 1990;71:295–297.

PERIOPERATIVE IMPLICATIONS

Preoperative Preparation

• Continue daily carnitine therapy
• Glucose infusion preoperatively
• For emergency surgery while in metabolic crisis, rehydrate; correct glucose, acid-base, and electrolyte imbalances, use IV carnitine if necessary, treat hypoprothrombinemia with FFP.

Monitoring

• Blood glucose

Airway

• Best to avoid succinylcholine for intubation

Maintenance

• IV glucose infusion, frequent monitoring of serum glucose level

Extubation

• No unusual concerns

Adjuvants

• Consider antiemetic prophylaxis to speed resumption of oral intake

ANTICIPATED PROBLEMS/CONCERNS

• Perioperative hypoglycemia

CAROTID SINUS SYNDROME (CSS)

Randall M. Schell, M.D.
Floyd S. Brauer, M.D.

RISK

- Carotid sinus hypersensitivity (CSH) may occur in ≈10% of adults
- True incidence is controversial
- >50 years of age and male
- Underdiagnosed cause of dizziness, falls, syncope
- Often associated with CAD, HTN
- Known complication of carotid endarterectomy

PERIOPERATIVE RISKS

- Potential for syncope, dizziness, falls
- CV causes of syncope carry ≈30% mortality and in cases of unexplained syncope ≈6% per annum; probably similar to standardized mortality for this age group

WORRY ABOUT

- High incidence of associated vascular disease (coronary, cerebrovascular) and aortic valvular disease
- Perioperative bradycardia, cardiac dysrhythmias, hypotension
- Associated with extravascular triggers (coughing, sneezing, micturition, acute biliary tract disease), classic triggers (neck hyperextension, forced head turning), and pathologic changes adjacent to carotid sinus (thyroid tumors, carotid body tumors)

OVERVIEW

- Cardinal symptom is syncope or near-syncope
- Diagnosed when CSH, defined as asystole >3 sec or, in the absence of asystole, a decrease in systolic BP >50 mmHg occurs with carotid sinus massage, in a patient with spontaneously occurring bradycardic or hypotensive symptoms
  - type I *cardioinhibitory:* asystole >3 sec with CSM
  - type II *vasodepressor:* ↓ systolic BP >50 mmHg independent of heart rate slowing
  - type III *mixed:* characteristics of both types I and II
- Cardioinhibitory type most common
- Only ≈5–20% with CSH demonstrate spontaneous Sx

ICD-9-CM Code: 337.0

ETIOLOGY

- Exaggeration of normal activity of baroreceptors in response to mechanical stimulation
- Symptoms (syncope, dizziness) result from baroreflex-mediated cerebral hypoperfusion due to bradycardia/asystole (cardioinhibitory), hypotension (vasodepressor), or both (mixed)
- Transmitted via branches of glossopharyngeal nerve to medulla; cardioinhibitory reflex is mediated by the vagus nerve, leading to asystole/bradycardia; the vasodepressor component is mediated by inhibition of sympathetic nervous system vasomotor tone, leading to ↓ SVR and ↓ BP

USUAL TREATMENT

- Controversial—surgical (carotid sinus denervation, pacemaker implantation, glossopharyngeal nerve transection), carotid sinus irradiation, and medical (vasopressors, anticholinergics, avoidance of cervical pressure, mineralocorticoid)
- Asymptomatic CSH→No treatment
- CSS
  - single episode→ ?no treatment
  - recurrent episodes→treatment
- Cardioinhibitory—VVI or DDD cardiac pacemaker
- Vasodepressor—cardiac pacemaker or if refractory to cardiac pacing, surgical ablation of carotid sinus
- Glossopharyngeal nerve block is alternative treatment in patients with CSS refractory to drug or pacemaker therapy
- Intraoperative
  - cardiac pacemaker: external vs internal
  - drugs: atropine, isoproterenol, epinephrine
  - other: infiltration of local anesthetic around carotid sinus, glossopharyngeal nerve block

ASSESSMENT POINTS

SYSTEM	EFFECT	ASSESSMENT BY HX	PE	TEST
HEENT	Bradycardia Hypotension	Syncope/near-syncope Falls with mechanical stimulation of neck	CSM	CSM (monitored) Electrophysiologic study
CV	See HEENT			
CNS	Syncope Stroke	See HEENT	Carotid bruit	Imaging studies of carotid artery
MS	Soft tissue injury Fx bone	Hx of falls		

Key Reference: Strasberg B, Sagie A, Erdman S, et al: Carotid sinus hypersensitivity and the carotid sinus syndrome. Prog Cardiovasc Dis 1989; 31:379–391.

PERIOPERATIVE IMPLICATIONS

Preoperative Preparation

- Evaluate for coexisting CAD and aortic valvular disease
- Evaluate cardiac pacemaker if in place to assure normal functioning (see under Pacemakers)

Monitoring

- Consider invasive BP monitoring

Positioning

- Avoid neck hyperextension, forced head turning, and pressure over carotid sinus (surgical preparation)

Airway

- Avoid neck hyperextension with intubation

Maintenance

- CSS may present as bradycardia/asystole, hypotension, or both
  - Esophageal pacing of the atria not expected to be of benefit

Adjuvants

- Digitalis, α-methyldopa, clonidine, and propranolol can enhance response to CSM
- Have epinephrine, atropine, and isoproterenol immediately available
- ?External pacemaker in OR
- Pancuronium may offer some advantages if muscle relaxant required

- Local anesthetic (lidocaine) available for infiltration around carotid sinus during carotid endarterectomy

ANTICIPATED PROBLEMS/CONCERNS

- Associated coronary, valvular, and/or cerebrovascular disease

CENTRAL NEUROGENIC HYPERVENTILATION

Cheri A. Sulek, M.D.
Roy F. Cucchiara, M.D.

INCIDENCE

• True central neurogenic hyperventilation (CNH) exceedingly rare; exact incidence unknown
• In patients with neurologic injury, not rare and most often associated with pulmonary dysfunction or shunting (aspiration, pneumonia, pulmonary edema, baseline disease)
• No association with age or gender

OVERVIEW

• A diagnosis of exclusion in neurologic disorders and hyperventilation
• Associated primarily with brainstem tumors with inconsistent involvement of midbrain, pons, and/or medulla

• CNS lymphomas and astrocytomas most common tumor types
• Gliomas, lymphomatoid granulomatosis, medulloblastoma, metastatic tumors also reported
• Effects of GA unknown

ETIOLOGY

• Exact etiology and level of brainstem dysfunction not known
• Probable etiology:
  – Loss of descending inhibitory control of ventilation by cerebral cortex with brainstem lesion
  – Postulated to be due to mesencephalic or pontine injury

– Ultimate control of respiration may lie in medulla (dorsal and ventral respiratory groups) with fine control from the pneumotaxic center of the pons with input from cerebral cortex, hypothalamus, chemo- and mechanoreceptors, and vagal nerve
– Stimulation of most areas of cerebral cortex except motor/premotor areas, which inhibit respiration
• Unlikely etiology:
  – Tumor pH: in vivo is alkalotic; does not appear to contribute to respiratory control
  – Mid- to caudal pontine lesions produce apneustic breathing, not CNH
  – Destructive lesions of midbrain or pons do not produce CNH, but animal models may not simulate the human brain

ASSESSMENT POINTS

SYSTEM	EFFECT	ASSESSMENT BY HX	PE	TEST
RESP	Tachypnea	Tachypnea that persists during sleep and is unpleasant to conscious patient	Resp rate	ABGs: • P_{CO_2} (low) • pH (alkalotic) • Pa_{O_2} (increased for age) • Decreased bicarbonate (all must be present to diagnose) • Alveolar-to-arterial gradient not larger than normal • Normal inspiratory and expiratory excursion
CNS		Patient cannot volitionally inhibit hyperventilation	Focal or nonfocal CNS findings	CSF pH may be normal CT/MRI

Key Reference: Jaeckle KA, Digre KB, Jones CR, et al: Central neurogenic hyperventilation: Pharmacologic intervention with morphine sulfate and correlative analysis of respiratory, sleep and ocular motor dysfunction. Neurology 1990; 40:1715–1720.

DIFFERENTIAL DIAGNOSIS FOR HYPERVENTILATION

• Anxiety
• Psychogenic
• Drug toxicity (salicylates, theophylline, cyanide)
• Pulmonary pathology with hypoxemia (pneumonia, pulmonary embolus, pulmonary edema, restrictive or obstructive lung disease)
• Cardiac (CHF, valvular disease)
• High altitudes
• Sepsis
• Hepatic dysfunction/encephalopathy
• Hyperthyroidism
• Pregnancy
• Metabolic acidosis
• Must exclude other etiologies for respiratory alkalosis with appropriate lab/Dx testing

ADVERSE EFFECTS

• Respiratory alkalosis shifts oxyhemoglobin curve to left
• Hypocapnia is a potent cerebral vasoconstrictor, subsequently decreasing cerebral blood flow and volume
• Hypocapnia in injured brains may result in ischemic insults
• Effect of severe hypocapnia in normal brains is less clear and may produce ischemia when combined with Bohr effect

TREATMENT

• No completely effective or consistent treatment
• Narcotics may attenuate respiratory rate and improve blood gases but will not correct rate or alkalosis
• Increasing dead space ventilation, administration of supplemental oxygen and benzodiazepines are not effective
• Treatment of tumor with steroids, chemotherapy, or radiation therapy; however, not always effective
• Mechanical ventilation with neuromuscular blockade and sedation during treatment of tumor has been attempted

OUTCOME

• Death from progressive neurologic deterioration or other complications (aspiration, pneumonia) likely
• Improvement with treatment of tumor or long-term narcotics

CEPHALOPELVIC DISPROPORTION (CPD) Ezzat I. Abouleish, M.D.

RISK

• 3% of pregnant population

PERIPARTUM RISKS

• Increased maternal and fetal mortality and morbidity
  – protracted labor
  – arrested labor
  – ruptured uterus
  – higher rate of C-section
  – higher rate of forceps delivery

WORRY ABOUT

• Increased need for operative delivery (including abdominal surgery)
• Increased incidence of fetal distress and need for emergency (stat) C-section

OVERVIEW

• Leads to abnormal labor pattern with subsequent high incidence of operative delivery
• Operative delivery associated with higher incidence of mortality and morbidity to mother and fetus
• Anesthesia: complete system exam, esp airway (for possible GA for "stat" section or failure of regional anesthesia), and landmarks at back (for regional anesthesia for labor and operative delivery)

ICD-9-CM Code: 660.1 (Obstructing labor)

ETIOLOGY

• Maternal causes: abnormality of mother's pelvis, e.g., android pelvis, scoliosis, old poliomyelitis, previous pelvis fracture
• Fetal causes: macrosomia

USUAL TREATMENT

• Obstetric: proper evaluation before and during labor
• Anesthesia: usually regional, for pain relief during labor and operative delivery, if required

ASSESSMENT POINTS

CPD can be diagnosed by clinical evaluation, radiographic cephalopelvimetry (rarely by x-ray, mostly by sonography), and failure of adequate response to oxytocin augmentation

Key Reference: Creasy RK, Resnik R: Maternal–Fetal Medicine, 3rd ed., Philadelphia, WB Saunders, 1994, pp 526–557.

PERIOPERATIVE IMPLICATIONS

• *Labor* usually more prolonged and painful than in absence of CPD
• Regional anesthesia adequate without interfering with course of labor

Anesthetic Technique

• Epidural analgesia: low concentration of bupivacaine supplemented with an opioid
• Combined spinal and epidural analgesia. *In early labor:* 10 µg sufentanil intrathecally (provides analgesia for 1–3 h) followed by epidural analgesia except reducing initial dose of fentanyl to 50 µg. *In late labor:* 10 µg sufentanil + 2.5 mg bupivacaine often sufficient for remainder of first stage + second stage. In delay of labor or if C-section required, epidural catheter can be used to administer epidural analgesia or anesthesia.

• *C-section:* In all cases: Anesthesia machine checked. Left uterine displacement, apply all monitors, e.g., BP, ECG, pulse oximeter, and capnograph with GA
• *Elective C-section:* Spinal anesthesia, prehydration 15 ml/kg within 20 min; bupivacaine injected at L2–L3. Supine with left uterine displacement. BP maintained >90% or original level with ephedrine drip.
• *Emergency C-section:* Following labor without fetal distress (failure to progress):
If patient already has reliable epidural block, epidural anesthesia is extended using 3% chloroprocaine + 75 µg fentanyl epidurally. If patient has not had epidural block during labor, spinal anesthesia can be used.
• *Following labor with fetal distress:* If patient has epidural, use as above. If no epidural and airway is acceptable, perform GA.

ANTICIPATED PROBLEMS/CONCERNS

• If airway expected to be difficult and no epidural catheter in place, use spinal anesthesia or perform awake intubation. Fiberoptic and laryngeal mask airway (LMA) available.

CEREBRAL ARTERIOVENOUS MALFORMATIONS (AVMs)

Barbara A. Dodson, M.D.

RISK

- Prevalence estimated at 0.2–0.5% of general population
- Account for ~1% of acute subarachnoid hemorrhages (SAHs)

PERIOPERATIVE RISKS

- ↑ ICP, seizures, neurologic deficits
- 4–10% perioperative mortality
- 4–10% incidence of associated aneurysms

WORRY ABOUT

- ↑ Risks for new neurologic deficits, severe intraoperative bleeding, and postop cerebral edema and hemorrhage (i.e., hyperemic complications)

OVERVIEW

- Neurovascular lesions with SAH as most common (80%) initial presentation. Morbidity and mortality from initial hemorrhage are 23–80% and 10–29%, respectively, and ↑ with each rebleed.
- May produce seizures and severe headaches. High-flow low-resistance shunt associated with AVMs can be severe enough to produce neurologic deficits (from ischemia in brain adjacent to AVM) or systemic effects (CHF is most common presentation for vein of Galen malformations in neonates)

ICD-9-CM Code: 747.81

ETIOLOGY

- Usually congenital, arising during primitive vasculature development
- Symptoms usually first occur between 2nd and 4th decades of life. Exceptions are great vein of Galen malformations.

USUAL TREATMENT

- Surgical removal, often with embolization, is treatment of choice.
- Inoperable (because of size or location) AVMs may be treated with radiation therapy or endovascular embolization

ASSESSMENT POINTS

SYSTEM	EFFECT	ASSESSMENT BY HX	PE	TEST
HEENT	Loss of airway protection	Aspiration	Gag reflex	Testing of lower cranial nerve function
CV	ECG changes, cardiac arrhythmias, CHF (in infants)	Sx CHF	Heart rate, S_3, rales	ECG, ECHO CXR
RESP	Hypoxia		Resp rate	ABGs
ENDO	Diabetes insipidus Syndrome of inappropriate antidiuretic hormone secretion		Volume status, BP	Serum and urine lytes and osmolality
CNS	Mass effect, CBF steal, neurologic deficits	Headaches, ataxia, seizures, LOC	Neurologic exam	CT, MRI, cerebral angiogram

Key Reference: Dodson BA: Interventional neuroradiology and the anesthetic management of patients with arteriovenous malformation. *In* Cotrell JE, Smith DS (eds): Anesthesia and Neurosurgery, 3rd ed. St. Louis, Mosby-Year Book, 1994, pp 407–424.

PERIOPERATIVE IMPLICATIONS

Preoperative Preparation

- Determine baseline neurologic status and evaluate for signs of mass effect
- Review results of preop endovascular procedures (embolization)

Monitoring

- Invasive arterial pressure monitoring
- Continuous end-tidal CO_2 and N_2 to detect venous air embolism, as applicable to surgical position
- Consider CVP

Airway

- May require early intubation if patient is hypoxic, with ↓ airway reflexes or ↑ ICP

Maintenance

- Tight BP control to prevent ↑ CPP (↑ mass effect or aneurysmal rupture) or ↓ CPP (ischemia in hypoperfused areas)
- Anesthetic technique dependent on medical and neurologic status, need for intraoperative neurologic testing, desire for early neurologic evaluation
- Deliberate hypotension or high-dose barbiturates should be considered

Extubation

- Need for tight BP control to prevent rebleeding

Adjuvants

- Nitroprusside, nitroglycerine, and/or β-blockers to prevent ↑ BP
- Consider hypothermia, barbiturates, propofol, etomidate, for brain protection

Postoperative Period

- Changes in CBF following AVM shunt removal can result in cerebral edema and hemorrhage due to (1) rebleeding from incomplete hemostasis or resection; (2) venous thrombosis or obstruction; (3) inability of previously hypoperfused areas to autoregulate at normal CPP (i.e., normal perfusion pressure breakthrough)

ANTICIPATED PROBLEMS/CONCERNS

- New neurologic deficits
- Severe intraoperative blood loss
- Hyperemic complications

CEREBROVASCULAR TRANSIENT ISCHEMIC ATTACK (TIA)

Renata Rusa, M.D.

RISK

- Incidence in USA: 1/100,000 for age <45 y, 293/100,000 for age ≥75 y
- Gender and race factors: extracranial disease more prevalent in whites; intracranial disease in blacks and Asians
- People at increased risk: white males
- Male > female 3/1 at age 75 y in 1990; female risk not decreasing as fast as male (thought because of increased cigarette usage in females)

PERIOPERATIVE RISKS

- Increased risk of CVA during CABG in patients with symptomatic carotid artery disease
- Increased risk for perioperative CVA in noncardiac noncarotid artery surgery: asymptomatic patients 0.0–3.0% vs. patient with TIAs: 0.0–17%
- Risk of coexisting heart disease

WORRY ABOUT

- Crescendo TIAs
- Critical carotid stenosis
- Impending basilar artery occlusion

OVERVIEW

- An episode of focal, nonconvulsive, neurologic deficit due to inadequate perfusion that is completely reversible in 24 h
- Disease of the carotid or vertebrobasilar system most often responsible
- Incidences of a stroke: 10%/y for first 3 y after TIA
- 50% survival time after first TIA is 7–8 y
- Heart disease the leading long-term cause of death
- Patients with TIA/CVA have 40% frequency of significant CAD
- Recommended by some that elective surgery be postponed for 6 wk after TIA

- Most perioperative CVAs in general surgery occur postop. Predictors: HTN, PVO, cerebrovascular and heart disease

ICD-9-CM Code: 435.9
See also Carotid Artery Surgery—Carotid Endarterectomy under Procedures

ETIOLOGY

- Atherosclerosis—risk factors: HTN, DM, heart disease, smoking, hyperlipidemia
- Cardioembolic—e.g., recent MI, AFib valvular heart disease
- Other—traumatic, mechanical compression, steal syndromes, nonatherosclerotic
- Carotid endarterectomy

USUAL TREATMENT

- Surgery in all but unstable patients; transluminal angioplasty still experimental
- Antithrombotics or anticoagulants in unstable patients if not a bleeding diathesis. Then surgery

ASSESSMENT POINTS

SYSTEM	EFFECT	ASSESSMENT BY HX	PE	TEST
HEENT		Trauma to neck	See CV	
CV	Cerebrovascular disease Other major artery disease	TIA Sx previous CVA	Funduscopic exam; carotid pulse, bruit; BP in both arms	Carotid duplex transcranial Doppler MRI: carotid, vertebrobasilar aortic arch
	CAD	History of MI, arrhythmias Exercise tolerance Cigarette smoking; HTN Atherosclerotic risk factors	Heart murmur, irregular heart beat S_3	ECG Stress test
GI		Nausea, vomiting can accompany other signs of brainstem ischemia		
CNS	Amaurosis fugax	Transient monocular blindness	Ischemic retina Presence of microemboli	See CV
	Transient focal neurologic deficit	Speech, language difficulties, visual disturbance, weakness, paresthesia, ataxia, vertigo, diplopia in combination with some other Sx	Neuro exam usually nml between attacks; disturbance of consciousness rare with TIAs	CT or MR brain scan

Key Reference: Fine-Edelstein VS, Wolf PA, O'Leary PH, et al: Precursors of extracranial carotid atherosclerosis in the Framingham study. Neurology 1994; 44:1040.

PERIOPERATIVE IMPLICATIONS

Preoperative Preparation

- Determine range of BP tolerated from both neuro and cardiac standpoint
- Avoid excessive sedation
- Need for preop work-up depends on risk assessment of perioperative CVA, cardiac morbidity, urgency of current procedure

Monitoring

- ECG, ST-segment analysis
- Consider invasive monitors for major procedures if significant atherosclerosis of major arteries or organs
- Use of intraoperative EEG has been limited, probably not practical in general surgery setting
- No data on sensitivity or specificity of transcranial Doppler

Airway

- Avoid extreme rotation and extension of neck during intubation, as such can impair flow through the vertebrobasilar system

Preinduction/Induction

- Maintain normal hemodynamics and adequate cerebral perfusion pressure
- Realize that cerebral autoregulation curve is shifted to the right if hypertensive

Maintenance

- Maintain glucose <250 mg/dl; avoid glucose in IV solutions
- Maintain slight hypocarbia to normocarbia for patient
- Theoretical advantage of isoflurane: allows lowest CBF before evidence of ischemia develops on EEG and is the least potent cerebral vasodilator.

Extubation

- Extubate deep to avoid HTN and tachycardia, or awake to ensure that patient can follow commands, protect airway, and is free of major neurologic deficit that could later result in significant cerebral edema

Postoperative Period

- Period of greatest risk for CVA in general surgery
- Resume antiplatelet and anticoagulation therapy ASAP

Adjuvants

- Barbiturates not clinically useful in prevention of perioperative stroke

ANTICIPATED PROBLEMS/CONCERNS

- TIA is marker for both cerebrovascular and cardiac disease

CERVICAL DISK DISEASE (CERVICAL SPINE DISEASE)

Andrew D. Rosenberg, M.D.

RISK

- 12,000 deaths in US/y; 70 million in US with cervical disk disease, spondylosis, or trauma
- Disk disease—normal consequence of aging (3rd–5th decades)
- Present in rheumatoid arthritis (RA), ankylosing spondylitis, other rheumatic disorders
- Trauma, esp motor vehicle accidents
- male > female (3:2)

PERIOPERATIVE RISKS

- Mortality (acute) 1–5% (depending on associated injuries)
- Spinal cord damage with C-spine movement
- Difficulty intubating or reintubating post extubation
- After neck surgery, swelling or hematoma can cause obstruction of airway
- Steroid-induced complications

WORRY ABOUT

- Airway management; C-spine movement during or after intubation
- Exacerbating or causing spinal cord damage with neck motion
- Osteoarthritis with osteophytes impinging on nerve roots

OVERVIEW

- Neck pain present in 30% of adults in USA
- Can cause radiculopathy, which can be aggravated by neck extension
- Root
  – C3—Unusual; C4—numbness rare, pain at root of neck; C5—numb over shoulder to lateral aspect of upper arm ("epaulet" area); C6—second most common radiculopathy: pain across top of neck, along biceps muscle into tips of thumb and index finger as well as biceps muscle weakness; C7—most common herniation: pain across back of shoulder triceps, and into middle finger as well as loss of triceps reflex; C8—numb small finger, interossei weak

ICD-9-CM Codes: 952.0 (cervical spine injury); 756.19 (cervical spondylosis)

ETIOLOGY

- Disk disease—natural process of aging
- Inflammatory arthropathy or trauma: In trauma, can have fractures, dislocations, or ligamentous damage causing spinal cord paralysis; can get swelling of soft tissues of neck

USUAL TREATMENT

- Neck should be stabilized, not forced into position: any movement can cause damage
- In patients with atlantoaxial subluxation, avoid flexion. Can have superior migration of odontoid as well as subaxial subluxation
- Stabilization and time to heal, repair
- Shoulder and strap muscle strengthening exercises
- Epidural steroids for recent disk disease
- Steroids for acute spinal cord injury

ASSESSMENT POINTS

SYSTEM	EFFECT	ASSESSMENT BY HX	PE	TEST
HEENT	Numbness and pain In RA: superior migration of odontoid, atlantoaxial subluxation, atlas-dens interval (ADI) increased (>4 mm unstable), subaxial subluxation Cricoarytenoid arthritis Airway abnormalities Trauma Swelling	Hoarseness, snoring	In RA: TMJ problems, hypoplastic mandible	In RA: Neck x-ray flexion and extension (measure ADI) Evaluate bones, ligament alignment, soft tissue swelling, motion
CV	Trauma: possible cardiac contusion/injury, spinal shock		Heart sounds distant Unstable BP	ECG, ECHO
RESP	Rheumatologic disorders: fibrosis, honeycombing Ankylosing spondylitis: restrictive pattern Trauma: diaphragm function (C3–C5), pneumothorax, hemothorax, contusion, aspiration, rib fractures	SOB	In trauma: Dyspnea, paradoxical ventilation, flail chest, breath sounds absent with pneumothorax	CXR, ABG
GI	Ulcers 2° to aspirin for RA			
HEME	RA: anemia 2° to medications		Trauma: look for signs of bleeding	Hgb
CNS	Vertebral artery compression: dizziness, vertigo, nausea, blurred vision			

Key Reference: Bracen MB, Shepard MJ, Collins WF, et al: A randomized controlled trial of methylprednisolone or naloxone in the treatment of acute spinal injury. Results of the Second National Acute Spinal Cord Injury Study. N Engl J Med 1990; 322:1405–1411.

PERIOPERATIVE IMPLICATIONS

- Assess neck in disk disease, rheumatic diseases, trauma
- Consider intubation with neck stabilized by assistant to avoid flexion or extension or awake fiberoptic intubation
- Avoid premedication (e.g., midazolam) that might interfere with spinal cord monitoring

Monitoring

- Acute spinal cord shock may require arterial and PA catheters or TEE to facilitate monitoring and treating hemodynamic disturbances

Induction

- Consider not initiating irreversible steps (e.g., muscle relaxants) until airway is secured

Extubation

- Consider not extubating until patient able to maintain airway without threat of swelling or airway obstruction

Adjuvants

- Steroids reduce injury in acute traumatic spinal cord injury

Postoperative Period

- Observe for neck swelling, hoarseness, airway obstruction
- Assess neurologic status

ANTICIPATED PROBLEMS/CONCERNS

- Anticipate difficulty intubating patients due to abnormal anatomy or limitation of motion. Prepare patient for fiberoptic intubation.
- Associated traumatic injuries—cardiac, brain, lung, abdomen, bladder, long bones—and their consequences
- ARDS from aspiration in preop traumatic event

CHAGAS' DISEASE

Charles W. Hogue, Jr., M.D.

- 16–18 million infected worldwide
- Rare in Southern US; chronic disease more likely in emigrants from endemic regions

PERIOPERATIVE RISKS

- Not defined
- Related to CV dysfunction

WORRY ABOUT

- LV dysfunction and CHF
- Conduction abnormalities (complete AV block)
- Ventricular arrhythmias
- Megaesophagus, achalasia, risk of pulmonary aspiration

OVERVIEW

- Acute infection, asymptomatic in ⅔ of patients, followed by chronic disease after latency of >2 decades
- In endemic areas, mild forms of disease common with benign course
- Pathogenesis to chronic, progressive end-organ disease poorly understood; autoimmunity, microvascular dysfunction, autonomic neuropathy implicated
- Cardiac involvement most serious end-organ manifestation; colon and esophagus also affected
- In USA, Dx usually not considered; presentation as CAD or dilated cardiomyopathy, or with AV heart block, CHF, ECG conduction abnormalities, sustained VTach
- Serologic test for Dx

ICD-9-CM Code: 086.0

ETIOLOGY

- *Trypanosoma cruzi*
- Transmission to humans by reduviid bug
- Transmission by blood transfusion possible
- Central and South America endemic areas

USUAL TREATMENT

- Nifurtimox (limited efficacy): for acute disease; usefulness for indeterminate phase or chronic disease not established
- Benznidazole (similar efficacy as nifurtimox) second agent

ASSESSMENT POINTS

SYSTEM	EFFECT	ASSESSMENT BY HX	PE	TEST
CV	Conduction abnormalities LV dysfunction and aneurysm	Syncope, DOE, orthopnea, fatigue	JVD, edema, rales, cardiomegaly	ECG ECHO MUGA Cardiac catheter
	Ventricular arrhythmias	Syncope, palpitations		Holter Electrophysiologic study
GI	Megaesophagus, megacolon	Dysphagia, GE reflux, constipation	Abdominal distention	Barium studies CXR Endoscopy

Key Reference: Hagar JM, Rahimtoola SH: Chagas' heart disease in the United States. N Engl J Med 1991; 325:763–768.

PERIOPERATIVE IMPLICATIONS

Preoperative Preparation

- LV function optimization with diuretics, ACE inhibitors
- Prophylaxis against pulmonary aspiration
- Assessment of conduction abnormalities, arrhythmias

Monitoring

Dictated by degree of LV dysfunction and proposed procedure; consider PA catheter or TEE
- ECG during entire perioperative period

Preinduction/Induction

- Consider temporary pacing if symptomatic AV block
- Caution with negative inotropic drugs
- Awake or rapid-sequence intubation

Maintenance

- Technique dictated by preferences, procedure, degree of cardiac involvement

Postoperative Period

- Continued monitoring depends on pre-existing LV dysfunction and operative procedure
- ECG monitoring for ventricular arrhythmias and AV conduction block

CHERUBISM

Daniel Siker, M.D.

RISK

- >200 cases in world literature
- Cherubs have a 40% chance of a cherub offspring

PERIOPERATIVE RISKS

- Swelling of lower face causing airway obstruction
- Displacement of ocular orbit and lower eye lid causing visual changes
- Excessive blood loss from curettage of vascular lesions
- Association with Noonan syndrome

WORRY ABOUT

- Pulmonary valve stenosis (Noonan syndrome)
- Undiagnosed hyperparathyroidism
- Convex, V-shaped hypertrophied hard palate
- Small mouth opening and mild trismus

OVERVIEW

- Progressive symmetric fullness of cheeks and jaw, with retraction of lower eyelids exposing an inferior rim of sclera.
- Onset age 2–12 y
- These round-faced, upwardly gazing infants look like Renaissance art "cherubs" (Jones)
- Diagnostic biopsy of mandible shows multinucleated giant cells
- Associated problems with speaking, breathing, swallowing, chewing
- Pathognomonic x-ray of jaw demonstrates radiolucent lesions

ICD-9-CM Code: 526.89

ETIOLOGY

- Familial—autosomal dominant
- Penetrance—100% for boys, 50% for girls
- Unknown but named alternatively familial fibrous dysplasia, bilateral giant cell tumors, familial multilocular cystic disease
- Multlocular cystic malformation of mandible and maxilla with painless submandibular lymphadenopathy

USUAL TREATMENT

- Operative curettage, removal of displaced teeth, cortical reshaping of mandible
- Selective embolization with operative excision of vascular lesions
- Bone grafts

ASSESSMENT POINTS

SYSTEM	EFFECT	ASSESSMENT BY HX	PE	TEST
HEENT	Orbits shifted Enlargement	Loss of binocular vision Photo review by age	Upward gaze Painless jaw swelling Lymphadenopathy	Jaw series
	Poor opening	Moderate trismus	Soft tissue swelling Concave palate	
	Malocclusion	Absence of third molar	Loose teeth	X-ray
CV	If associated with Noonan syndrome	Pulmonic valve disease	Pulmonary valve stenosis	ECHO
RESP	Generally unaffected	Obstructive airway		Sleep study
ENDO	Rule out hyperparathyroidism	Onset at older age		Normal Ca^{2+}, phosphorus
CNS	Midparental intelligence	No developmental delay, except with Noonan syndrome		
MS	Long bone lesions		Humerus, anterior ribs, femoral neck	

Key Reference: Maydew RP, Berry FA: Cherubism with difficult laryngoscopy and tracheal intubation. Anesthesiology 1985; 26:810–812.

PERIOPERATIVE IMPLICATIONS

Preoperative Preparation

- Rule out parathyroid disease
- Available blood for curettage replacement

Monitoring

- Routine

Airway

- Difficult airway protocol

Preinduction/Induction

- Spontaneous ventilation
- Laryngeal mask airway

Maintenance

- Consider hypotensive technique for minimizing blood loss

Extubation

- May require ICU admission for prolonged intubation

Adjuvants

- Routine

Postoperative Period

- Extubation awake with confirmation of no bleeding

ANTICIPATED PROBLEMS/CONCERNS

- Nasal intubation for oral procedures may be problematic, similar to Pierre Robin, Goldenhar's, and Treacher Collins syndromes. As mandibular rami approach midline, no space for visualization of airway

CHOLELITHIASIS

Fumito Ichinose, M.D.
Lydia A. Conlay, M.D., M.B.A.

RISK

- 15–20 million adults in USA have gallstones
- Present in 10% of males and 20% of females 55–65 YO

PERIOPERATIVE RISKS

- Differential diagnosis of severe epigastric pain and transient liver function abnormalities, including myocardial infarction and acute hepatitis
- Association with hiatus hernia and possible gastric reflux
- Possible coexisting liver dysfunction
- Risks of obesity (see under Morbid Obesity in Diseases section)

WORRY ABOUT

- Hypovolemia and full stomach if vomiting prominent
- Free abdominal air or peritonitis suggests perforation, necessitating emergency laparotomy
- Opioid-inducing choledochoduodenal sphincter spasm is rare (<3%)

OVERVIEW

- Acute cholecystitis is a severe, life-threatening condition
- Chronic cholelithiasis, with or without cholecystitis, more common
- Surgical/medical elimination of gallstones relieves symptoms and prevents cholecystitis, cholangitis, obstructive jaundice, pancreatitis
- Removal of asymptomatic gallstones is controversial

ICD-9-CM Code: 574.2

ETIOLOGY

- Abnormalities in physicochemical components of bile
- 90% of stones are composed primarily of cholesterol; remainder of calcium bilirubinate

USUAL TREATMENT

- Open or laparoscopic cholecystectomy
- Extracorporeal shock-wave lithotripsy and/or litholytic therapy in selected patients

ASSESSMENT POINTS

SYSTEM	EFFECT	ASSESSMENT BY HX	PE	TEST
CV	Hypovolemia if active vomiting *Beware MI*	Presence of vomiting Hx/Risk factors	Orthostatic hypotension	 ECG
GI	Ileus causing full stomach Perforated gallbladder may cause peritonitis	Nausea, vomiting Abdominal wall rigidity	Bowel sounds	Abdominal x-rays
LIVER	Mild dysfunction may coexist	Fatigue, weight loss, intermittent chills and fever	Jaundice	Liver function tests

Key Reference: Stoelting RK, Dierdorf SF: Anesthesia and Co-Existing Disease, 3rd ed. New York, Churchill Livingstone, 1993, pp 271–273.

PERIOPERATIVE IMPLICATIONS

Preoperative Preparation

- Consider H_2 blocker or metoclopramide if significant risk of aspiration (full stomach, gastric reflux, anticipated difficult airway)
- Avoid premedication with morphine and other opiates, which may constrict the sphincter of Oddi and precipitate abdominal pain. Fentanyl is less likely to cause sphincter constriction.
- Consider volume and electrolyte replacement before emergency surgery for acute cholecystitis or common bile duct obstruction associated with vomiting.

Monitoring

- End tidal CO_2 during laparoscopic cholecystectomy, to detect gas embolus or increased CO_2
- Routine for patient's illness

Induction

- Rapid-sequence induction with cricoid pressure for emergencies, and for reflux

Maintenance

- Paralysis and mechanical ventilation ensures adequate ventilation, attenuating systemic absorption of CO_2
- Opioids OK; since spasm rare (<3% in open cholecystectomy) and can be treated by naloxone or glucagon
- Minor alterations in volume status can be exacerbated by reverse Trendelenburg position and increased intra-abdominal pressure

Extubation

- Extubate when fully awake

Adjuvants

- Biliary tract obstruction may reduce clearance of muscle relaxants (e.g., vecuronium, pancuronium)

Postoperative Period

- Incision from open cholecystectomy ↓ pulmonary functions owing to depressed diaphragmatic function
- Patient-controlled analgesia or neuraxial opioids for intense postop pain
- Laparoscopic cholecystectomy may facilitate same day or next day.
- Potential complications of laparoscopic cholecystectomy: hemorrhage (half of all complications), venous gas embolism, pneumothorax, pneumomediastinum, mesenteric ischemia

CIGARETTE SMOKING

Kevin K. Tremper, Ph.D., M.D.

RISK

- People within US: 50 million
- No racial predilection
- Males > females (3/2). Young females fastest growing group

PERIOPERATIVE RISKS

- Increased risk of CAD × 2.0 of nonsmokers of same age
- Postop pulmonary complications × 6 of nonsmoker.
- Carboxyhemoglobin (COHb) ↑ (up to 15%)
- Hyperreactive airway

WORRY ABOUT

- CAD, COPD, PVD, productive cough, reactive airway
- Increases physiologic age by 8 y (30 pack years) relative to nonsmoker

OVERVIEW

- Addictive habit. Cigarette smoke contains >3000 identifiable constituents, many of which have toxic or tumorigenic effects. Acute effects relate to CO and nicotine.
- Nicotine stimulates the sympathetic ganglia, causing release of catecholamines from the adrenal medulla and sympathetic nerve endings, increasing BP, HR, and SVR, that persists for 30 min after one cigarette.
- Associated with ↓ MAO and ↑ dopamine levels in brain
- Inhaled CO produces up to 15% COHb. Combined effects of nicotine and COHb put diseased myocardium at risk.
- An irritant to pulmonary system, increasing mucus production while decreasing ciliary activity and mucus flow, markedly impairing tracheobronchial secretion clearance.
- Chronic use associated with CAD, HTN, COPD, peripheral vascular disease, numerous cancers.
- Cessation of smoking the night before surgery will reduce the COHb and nicotine levels to that of nonsmokers.

- Cessation of smoking for ≤ 8 wk has controversial additional benefits; cessation of >8 wk has demonstrated decreased incidence of postop pulmonary complications. Cessation for 2 y reduces risks of myocardial infarction to that of the nonsmoking population.
- Considered to be the cause of 1 of every 6 deaths in the US and is the leading cause of preventable mortality (400,000 preventable deaths/y).

ICD-9-CM Code: 305.1 (tobacco abuse)

ETIOLOGY

- Habituation

USUAL TREATMENT

- Nicotine patch and clonidine, Smokers Anonymous, or self-withdrawal.
- Cessation for a minimum of 12–24 h. Decrease in COHb and nicotine.
- Cessation for ≥ 8 wk or more will reduce postop pulmonary complications.
- Cessation for ≥ 2 y decreases risk of myocardial infarction.

ASSESSMENT POINTS

SYSTEM	EFFECT	ASSESSMENT BY HX	PE	TEST
HEENT	Oral, pharyngeal, head and neck cancers		Lesions on exam or intubation	Usually not needed
CV	↑ Heart rate, SVR, coronary vascular resistance → myocardial ischemia. ↑ PVR ↑ Blood viscosity	Exercise tolerance, angina (see CAD)	Two-flight walk	ECG
RESP	↑ COHb, COPD, ↓ FEV$_1$/FCV ↑ Secretion ↓ Clearance ↑ Airway reactivity	Exercise tolerance, chronic productive cough, character of sputum	Auscultation	CXR if symptomatic Hct, sputum (see COPD)

Key Reference: Egan TD, Wong KC: Perioperative smoking cessation in anesthesia: A review. J Clin Anesth 1992; pp. 4:63–72.

PERIOPERATIVE IMPLICATIONS

Preoperative Preparation

- Cessation overnight will ↓ COHb and nicotine.
- Cessation for 8 wk will ↓ postop pulmonary complications.
- If chronic productive cough, consider preop antibiotic treatment.

Monitoring

- Routine
- SpO$_2$ monitoring, may read higher SpO$_2$ than actual if COHb present (SpO$_2$ = % HbO$_2$ + % COHb).
- Consider invasive monitoring if symptomatic pulmonary or cardiac disease

Airway

- None

Premedication/Induction

- Consider deep induction if history of reactive airway disease

Maintenance

- Routine unless symptomatic cardiac or pulmonary disease

Extubation

- Consider deep extubation if severe reactive airway disease but is easy to intubate and ventilate, with no aspiration risk

Adjuvants

- Routine; smoking ↑ metabolism of theophylline, ↓ half-life from 265 to 180 min.

Postoperative Period

- Epidural analgesia may be beneficial in decreasing complications of hypercoagulability, CAD, or COPD.

ANTICIPATED PROBLEMS/CONCERNS

- Long-standing hx of smoking with symptomatic pulmonary disease leads to high risk of developing postop pulmonary complications (pneumonia) due to ↑ mucus production and ↓ ciliary function. Cessation for 8 wks is recommended.
- Airway reactivity significantly increased in smokers; abstinence for 24 h does not change this reactivity. Reactivity starts reducing after 24–48 h and reduces to near level of nonsmokers after 10 d of cessation.
- Risk of myocardial infarction decreases to that of nonsmokers after several years of cessation.

CIGARETTE SMOKING CESSATION

Talmage D. Egan, M.D., Ph.D.
K.C. Wong, M.D., Ph.D.

RISK

- Adults within USA: ¼–⅓ smoke cigarettes
- Higher prevalence of smoking among lower socioeconomic classes
- Prevalence among teens and women increasing

PERIOPERATIVE RISKS

- Risk not well defined through controlled studies; 25 pack-year Hx increases physiologic age 8 y of those 40–65 y
- ↑ Perioperative morbidity and mortality related to smoking-associated diseases
- ↑ Risk of postop lung complications

WORRY ABOUT

- Undiagnosed or poorly treated smoking-related disease that may require modification of the anesthetic plan (e.g., CAD, COPD)
- Propensity for bronchospasm and mucous plugging
- ↓ O_2 content 2° to high carboxyhemoglobin levels
- ↑ Autonomic activity (↑ heart rate and BP) 2° to nicotine in patients who have smoked just prior to anesthesia

OVERVIEW

- Smoking results in acute changes in cardiopulmonary function even in otherwise asymptomatic patients. With long-term use, smoking causes chronic changes in cardiopulmonary function that eventually culminate in irreversible cardiopulmonary disease.
- Acute changes include carbon monoxide–mediated decreases in O_2 content and nicotine-induced increases in heart rate and BP. Nicotine-mediated effects are relatively short-lived, whereas carboxyhemoglobin persists for many hours.
- Chronic changes include a gradual decline in lung function consisting of ↓ FEV_1, ↓ mucociliary activity, ↓ gas exchange surface, and ↓ pulmonary macrophage activity.
- Associated diseases include CAD, COPD and numerous cancers (e.g., lung, laryngeal, oral).

ICD-9-CM Code: 305.1 (Tobacco dependence)

ETIOLOGY

- Acquired behavior that is generally viewed as addiction
- Highest risk factors are low education level, low socioeconomic status

USUAL TREATMENT

- Counseling
- Group therapy (e.g., "12-step" program)
- Pharmacologic adjuncts such as nicotine patches/gum

ASSESSMENT POINTS

SYSTEM	EFFECT	ASSESSMENT BY HX	PE	TEST
HEENT	Oral/laryngeal cancer	Hoarseness	Oral exam (and inspection during direct laryngoscopy)	
CV	CAD (± altered LV function)	Exertional chest pain, dyspnea, poor exercise tolerance, orthopnea, paroxysmal nocturnal dyspnea	S_3 gallop, dysrhythmia	ECG, stress test, ECHO, angiography
RESP	COPD	Dyspnea, poor exercise tolerance	Tachypnea, rales, wheezing, pursed lip breathing	CXR, ABGs
OTHER	↑ Carboxyhemoglobin (with recent smoking)	Dyspnea	Tachycardia, tachypnea	ABGs with co-oximetry

Key Reference: Egan TD, Wong KC: Perioperative smoking cessation and anesthesia — a review. J Clin Anesth 1992; 4:63–72.

PERIOPERATIVE IMPLICATIONS

Preoperative Preparation

- Advise smoking cessation for at least 12 h before operation (so that carboxyhemoglobin levels fall to near-normal)
- Advise that a much longer period of cessation (i.e., ≈2 mo) is necessary to achieve a decrease in postop pulmonary morbidity; may rarely be worthwhile in true pulmonary cripples undergoing major procedures and very worthwhile for long-term motivation
- Suggest that this is an excellent time to quit smoking (and reduce future aging–related wrinkles and physiologic aging changes)

Monitoring

- Routine
- Current pulse oximeters cannot discriminate between carboxyhemoglobin and oxyhemoglobin. Significant levels of carboxyhemoglobin may exist without ↓ in pulse oximeter SpO_2 reading.

Airway

- Smokers vulnerable to bronchospasm or mucous plugging obstruction anytime

Induction

- Avoid instrumentation of airway until deep level of anesthesia
- Provide complete preoxygenation since less tolerance of apnea

Maintenance

- Routine; ensure adequate depth of anesthesia to avoid bronchospasm

Extubation

- Consider deep extubation if other considerations permit in order to avoid bronchospasm (e.g., empty stomach, easy laryngoscopy)

Postoperative Period

- Monitor for respiratory complications (e.g., pneumonia, bronchospasm)
- Encourage permanent smoking cessation

ANTICIPATED PROBLEMS/CONCERNS

- Propensity for bronchospasm
- ↓ O_2 content secondary to high carboxyhemoglobin levels

CLEFT PALATE

Andrei Cernea, M.D.

RISK

- ~1/800 live births
- Racial predominance: Caucasian
- Frequently associated with cleft lip
- Gender predominance: cleft lip/palate more common in males (2:1); isolated cleft palate more common in females (3:1)

PERIOPERATIVE RISKS

- Morbidity and mortality extremely low; only 5 life-threatening cases of postoperative airway obstruction described in literature

WORRY ABOUT

- Difficult airway when associated with syndromes such as Mohr, Shprintzen, 4-P, or Pierre Robin

- Intrainduction laryngospasm and airway obstruction due to chronic URIs, chronic otitis media, and/or tongue becoming wedged in cleft
- Difficult intraoperative oxygenation due to chronic aspiration syndrome
- ↑ Risk for transfusion if anemic due to poor ability to feed
- Intraoperative airway obstruction and extubation by Dingman gag
- Intraoperative dysrhythmias caused by surgical infiltration of epinephrine in presence of halothane
- Postoperative airway obstruction by forgotten pharyngeal packs and severe lingual edema
- Undiagnosed associated congenital heart and renal diseases

OVERVIEW

- Congenital condition occurs by 7th–12th wk of intrauterine life (associated with benzodiazepine usage)
- Cleft palate repaired at 12–18 mo
- Usually not associated with severe blood loss
- Postoperative airway obstruction may occur more frequently in prolonged procedures

ICD-9-CM Code: 749.00

USUAL TREATMENT

- If child is in otherwise good health, a palatoplasty is performed electively; all children with cleft palate should have repair by 18 mo to ensure:
  - normal speech development
  - appropriate social integration
  - normal growth of maxilla

ASSESSMENT POINTS

SYSTEM	EFFECT	ASSESSMENT BY HX	PE	TEST
HEENT	Otitis media Clear rhinorrhea	Ear pain	TM exam	
	Difficult airway	Snore, grunt	Airway exam (micrognathia)	
CV	Associated congenital heart disease	SOB, cyanosis, poor growth	CV exam, club feet	ECG, ECHO
RESP	URI	Cough, fever Congestion	Chest exam	
	Aspiration	SOB, cyanosis	Chest exam	CXR
GI	Impaired deglutition Malnutrition	Nasal regurgitation Poor growth		Observe feeding
HEME	Anemia	Malnutrition	Pallor	Hgb/Hct
RENAL	Associated congenital defects	UTI	Club feet	UA, BUN/Cr

Key Reference: Stehling L: Common Problems in Pediatric Anesthesia, 2nd ed. St Louis, Mosby–Year Book, 1992, pp 183–187.

PERIOPERATIVE IMPLICATIONS

Preoperative Preparation

- Recognize possibility of multiple future procedures and attempt to minimize stress during induction: consider oral premedication

Anesthetic Technique

- GA usually induced via mask using ↑ concentrations of volatile agent in oxygen
- Oral airway or gauze packing of cleft may help manual ventilation by preventing tongue from lodging in cleft
- Intubation, often with RAE endotracheal tube secured to mandible, as access to airway may be severely limited

Monitoring

- Precordial stethoscope
- Maintain normocapnia if epinephrine injection and halothane inhalation

Postoperative Considerations

- Significant risk for airway obstruction due to edema
- Often obligate mouth breathers
- Transfusion usually not required for cleft palate repair
- Rectal Tylenol frequently sufficient

ANTICIPATED PROBLEMS/CONCERNS

- Airway difficulty during induction and intubation, especially when associated with other facial anomalies
- Postoperative airway obstruction due to forgotten pharyngeal pack, severe lingual edema, or obligate mouth breathing

COAGULOPATHY — FACTOR IX DEFICIENCY

Thomas M. McLoughlin, Jr., M.D.

RISK

- People within US: 3000-4000 (15% of all hemophiliacs). Incidence = 1:25,000–50,000 males
- Race with highest prevalence: equal
- Gender with highest prevalence: overwhelmingly male

PERIOPERATIVE RISKS

- Increased risk of hemorrhagic complications from any and all operations

WORRY ABOUT

- Excessive and/or uncontrollable hemorrhage
- Tendency for recurrent hemorrhage after initial control
- Expansive deep and soft tissue hematomas
- Increased risk if hepatic or immune dysfunction present from prior plasma product transfusions

OVERVIEW

- Also called hemophilia B or Christmas disease
- Clinically indistinguishable from hemophilia A (classic hemophilia)
- Hemarthroses account for 75% of bleeding episodes; chronic debilitating arthritis is a common development
- Soft tissue hematomas and hematuria also common
- Intracranial hemorrhage is common fatal complication, accounting for death in 25%
- Severity of disease proportional to circulating factor IX activity (<1% normal activity = severe disease, >5% = generally mild disease)

ICD-9-CM Code: 286.1

ETIOLOGY

- Sex-linked recessive disorder

USUAL TREATMENT

- Restoration of circulating factor IX activity
- Solvent/detergent-treated pooled factor IX concentrates (AlphaNine SD, Alpha Therapeutic, Los Angeles, CA)
- Prothrombin complex concentrates and FFP are alternatives for life-threatening hemorrhage if concentrates unavailable

ASSESSMENT POINTS

SYSTEM	EFFECT	ASSESSMENT BY HX	PE	TEST
GI				LFTs if hepatitis Hx
HEME	Coagulopathy	Dental extractions, menses, lacerations, epistaxis	Ecchymoses, hematomas	Prolonged PTT; PT, TT, plt count usually normal
RENAL	Hematuria; eventual clot formation can obstruct collecting system	Discolored urine		BUN/Cr, urine dipstick or microscopic exam
CNS	Intracranial hemorrhage	Headache	Neurologic exam	
PNS	Discrete peripheral neuropathies	Hx of compressive hematoma	Sensory and motor exam	
MS	Hemarthroses, chronic arthritis	Painful, warm joints	↓ ROM	X-rays usually not necessary

Key Reference: Sampson J, Hamstra R, Aldrete J: Management of hemophilic patients undergoing surgical procedures. Anesth Analg 1979; 58:133–135.

PERIOPERATIVE IMPLICATIONS

Preoperative Preparation

- Collaboration with consulting hematologist
- Schedule surgery early in wk to allow optimal laboratory support of postop assessment of hemostasis; if multiple procedures are contemplated in near future, schedule simultaneously
- Assess preop factor IX activity; determine goal as guided by magnitude of hemostatic challenge (15–30% factor IX activity for minor lacerations/hematomas; 30–50% for hemarthroses or major hemorrhage, 50–75% for perioperative coverage or life-threatening bleeding)
- Units factor IX needed = (2)(wt in kg)(plasma volume in ml/kg)(fractional increase in factor IX activity desired); once-daily dosing is sufficient for maintenance

Monitoring

- *Confirm* expected increase in factor IX activity after preop dose but before incision

Airway

- Laryngoscopy to avoid tissue trauma, consider mask ventilation
- Nasotracheal route best avoided

Maintenance

- Consider tourniquets and local cooling to minimize blood loss

Extubation

- Avoid coughing on endotracheal tube
- Cautious oropharyngeal suction, best done under direct vision

Adjuvants

- Regional anesthesia not absolutely contraindicated but consider with caution; successful brachial plexus blockade at the axilla has been described
- Postop factor IX activity requirement: 15–40%

ANTICIPATED PROBLEMS/CONCERNS

- Excessive perioperative blood loss, hematoma formation
- Potential for delayed or recurrent bleeding after initial control
- Increased likelihood of infectious bloodborne disease (HIV, hepatitis)

COAGULOPATHY — INTRINSIC PATHWAY

Joel Bennett, M.D.

RISK

• Factor VIII hemophilia A: 1/10,000 male infants
• Factor IX hemophilia B: 1/60,000 male infants
• Von Willebrand disease types 1 and 2: 1/800–1000 individuals
• Von Willebrand disease type 3: 1/1 million individuals
• Factor XI: rare

PERIOPERATIVE RISKS

• Bleeding from operative sites
• Risk of hematomas from regional anesthetics
• Risk of airway bleeding

WORRY ABOUT

• Continued bleeding from surgical sites, drains (initial coagulation due to Plt plug but delayed bleeding in PACU)
• Hematoma formation, delayed wound healing
• Removal of epidural catheter

OVERVIEW

• Components of intrinsic pathway are factor XII (Hageman factor), factor XI (plasma thromboplastin antecedent), factor IX (Christmas factor), factor VIII (antihemophilic factor), Prekallikrein (PK), High molecular weight kininogen (HMWK)
• Quantitative deficiencies can occur in all factors
• All but factor XII deficiency result in excessive clinical bleeding
• Qualitative deficiencies can occur in factor VIII (von Willebrand disease)

ICD-9-CM Code: 286.9 (Coagulation defect)

ETIOLOGY

• Hereditary: hemophilia A and B (HA, HB)—x-linked; von Willebrand disease (vW), factor XI—autosomal recessive; factor XII
• Acquired: heparin administration, massive transfusion, liver failure, DIC (consumptive coagulopathy)

USUAL TREATMENT

• Deficiencies of HMWK, PK, factor XII are without clinical sequelae
• Factor XI deficiency replaced with FFP
• Factor VIII deficiency replaced with FFP, cryoprecipitate or factor VIII concentrate
• Factor IX deficiency replaced with FFP or factor IX concentrate
• Von Willebrand disease types 1 & 2 treated with cryoprecipitate
• Heparin reversed with protamine

ASSESSMENT POINTS

SYSTEM	EFFECT	ASSESSMENT BY HX	PE	TEST
HEENT		Epistaxis, bleeding after dental extractions (vW)		PTT (hemophilia A/B, vW) Bleeding time (vW) Ristocetin aggregation (vW)
GI		GI bleeding (HA, HB)		Hematest
CNS		CNS bleeds (CVA) (HA/HB)	Neuro exam	CT scan
MS		Bleeds into large joint spaces (HA, HB)	Joint deformity	

Key Reference: Horrow JC: Management of coagulation and bleeding disorders. *In* Kaplan JA: Cardiac Anesthesia. Philadelphia, WB Saunders, 1993, pp 951–994.

COARCTATION OF THE AORTA

Michael Nugent, M.D.

RISK

- 1 in 12,000 children
- Males > females: 2–5:1

PERIOPERATIVE RISKS

- Neonate: 10% mortality (preoperative CHF and associated cardiac anomalies)
- Children: 0.4% mortality

WORRY ABOUT

- Closure of ductus arteriosus causing severe CHF and hypoperfusion to body below coarctation
- Severe upper body hypertension in older children

- Risk of paraplegia: 0.5%
- Post-coarctectomy syndrome or mesenteric arteritis marked by abdominal pain, abdominal distention, N/V, and hypertension (postoperative day 1–3) treated with gastric decompression, IV fluids, and control of systemic hypertension

OVERVIEW

- Congenital constriction of aorta opposite insertion of ductus arteriosus
- Associated with bicuspid aortic valves, complex congenital anomalies, and aneurysms of circle of Willis (8–10%)

ICD-9-CM Code: 747.10

ETIOLOGY

- Aortic ampulla of ductus constricts obstructing aortic flow

USUAL TREATMENT

- Early surgical repair when diagnosed to minimize residual postoperative hypertension
- Subclavian flap used in coarctation repair of neonate
- Some prefer elective repair of asymptomatic children at age of 4–6 y to ↓ rate of re-coarctation

ASSESSMENT POINTS

SYSTEM	EFFECT	ASSESSMENT BY HX	PE	TEST
HEENT	Upper body hypertension	Older children may complain of headache and epistaxis		
CV			Decreased lower extremity pulses	2-D ECHO usually diagnostic
Neonates	Severe CHF	Poor feeding, irritability	Tachycardia, hepatomegaly	ABG: metabolic acidosis from hypoperfusion
Children >5 y	Collateral vessel formation	Older children asymptomatic	Visible or palpable collateral vessels	Rib notching on CXR
RESP	CHF (neonate)		Tachypnea Grunting Retractions	CXR of CHF: Cardiomegaly Pulmonary edema Pleural effusion "Figure 3" configuration of aorta
GI	Poor feeding in neonate			
RENAL	Renal failure 2° to CHF and poor distal aortic perfusion in neonate			Urinary catheter Electrolytes Creatinine
MS	Lower body hypoperfusion	Children may complain of lower extremity fatigue		

Key Reference: Davis BJ, Cook DR: *In* Kaplan J (ed): Vascular Anesthesia. New York, Churchill Livingstone, 1991, pp 491–498.

PERIOPERATIVE IMPLICATIONS

Preoperative Preparation

- Stabilize CHF in neonate using prostaglandin E_1 to reopen ductus arteriosus; severe CHF requires positive pressure ventilation, inotropic support, diuresis, and bicarbonate infusion

Monitoring

- Consider right radial arterial catheter and lower extremity BP cuff (arterial catheter if poor collateral circulation below coarctation)
- Temperature: incidental hyperthermia in neonate may predispose to paraplegia; moderate hypothermia to 34°C advocated in older children
- Consider evoked potentials, particularly if high gradient and poorly developed collateral circulation

Airway (Left Thoracotomy)

- Consider double lumen endotracheal in older patients

Induction

- Consider IV narcotic/relaxant-based anesthetic or slow induction with halothane and 50% nitrous oxide (<1% halothane) with severe CHF

Maintenance

- Nitroprusside often used to control hypertension during aortic cross-clamping (minimizes doses with labetalol)
- Hand ventilation when left lung retracted for exposure
- Prior to cross-clamp release, consider discontinuing inhalation agent and nitroprusside and administering volume
- Consider ABGs after cross-clamp release and bicarbonate as needed

Extubation

- Older children can be extubated at end of procedure
- Neonates in CHF generally remain intubated and ventilated; wean when CHF improves

ANTICIPATED PROBLEMS/CONCERNS

- Paroxysmal hypertension postoperatively
- Post-coarctectomy syndrome
- Paraplegia (0.5%)

COMPLEMENT DEFICIENCY

Christine Rinder, M.D.

RISK

- Incidence: <0.1% of general population
- Male-female ratio: 1:6
- Higher (6%) in patients with autoimmune disease (see Immune Disorders in Diseases section)
- Patients with Hx of *Neisseria* meningitis have incidence of 15%

PERIOPERATIVE RISKS

- ↑ Risk of postoperative infection, particularly if the deficiency affects the early complement components, C1–C3
- Risk for inflammatory complications, e.g., glomerulonephritis, vasculitis, etc.

WORRY ABOUT

- ↑ Infectious risk

OVERVIEW

- May affect any component of classical pathway, alternate pathway, or terminal common pathway
- Virtually all deficiencies show some ↑ risk of infection and/or autoimmune disease
- Deficiencies in early complement components, namely C1, C2, and C3 in particular, associated with immunocompromise, resulting in recurrent life-threatening infections due to variety of organisms
- ↑ Risk of autoimmune diseases
- Deficiency in any of the terminal components C5–C8 show selective risk of recurrent neisserial infections, usually not life-threatening

ICD-9-CM Code: 279.8

ETIOLOGY

- All complement proteins inherited in autosomal fashion, with possible exception of properdin, which appears to be X-linked

USUAL TREATMENT

- No specific therapy indicated
- Antibiotic treatment dictated by specific infection

ASSESSMENT POINTS

SYSTEM	EFFECT	TEST
IMMUNE	Infectious risk for all systems	CH50 screening test for complement-mediated lysis of sheep erythrocytes; tests for specific complement components available at reference laboratories Assess other specific organs as indicated by autoimmune disease (renal for SLE, etc.)

Key Reference: Ross SC, Densen P: Complement deficiency states and infection: Epidemiology, pathogenesis and consequences of neisserial and other infections in an immune deficiency. Medicine 1984; 63:243–273.

PERIOPERATIVE IMPLICATIONS

Preoperative Preparation

- Sterile technique strictly observed

Monitoring

- Routine
- Coagulation profile
- Minimize invasive lines

Airway

- Routine

Induction

- Routine

Maintenance

- Routine

Extubation

- Extubate and remove all lines at earliest opportunity

Postoperative Period

- Maintain sterile techniques

ANTICIPATED PROBLEMS/CONCERNS

- Meticulous sterile technique to minimize risk of infection

CONGENITAL METHEMOGLOBINEMIA

Bronwyn R. Rae, MB, BS(Syd), FANZCA

RISK

- Navajo Indians, Alaskan Indians, people of Puerto Rican and Cuban ancestry
- Normal life span (except for recessive congenital methemoglobinemia [RCM] type II)

PERIOPERATIVE RISKS

- No data available
- Pregnancies not compromised

WORRY ABOUT

- Measurement of SpO_2
- Oxidant drugs, e.g., prilocaine, benzocaine, nitroglycerin, sulfonamides, contraindicated

OVERVIEW

- Due to deficient reducing capacity of oxidized heme:
  - RCM types I and II: Deficient reducing capacity due to NADH cytochrome b5 reductase (diaphorase) deficiency. Shift of O_2 dissociation curve to left leads to mild erythrocytosis. Normal RBC life span.
  - RCM type I defect restricted to red cell soluble cytochrome b5 reductase only. Cyanosis is sole clinical symptom.
  - RCM type II: Defect in all tissues; involves both soluble and microsomal forms of cytochrome b5 reductase. Mental retardation, spasticity, opisthotonos, microcephaly, growth retardation. Death by 2–3 y.
- Due to structural abnormality in globin moiety:
  - HbM variations: Amino acid substitutions create abnormal environment for heme residues, displacing the equilibrium toward ferric state. Alpha chain variants affected from birth, beta chain variants by 3–6 mo of age. Mild hemolytic anemia.

ICD-9-CM Code: 289.7

ETIOLOGY

- RCM types I and II—autosomal recessive inheritance. Heterozygotes have increased susceptibility to metHb formation after exposure to oxidant drugs and chemicals.
- HbM variants—autosomal dominant inheritance

USUAL TREATMENT

- RCM types I and II: Reducing agents, e.g., riboflavin 20–60mg orally, methylene blue 1mg/kg IV. Effect lasts 10–14 d.
- HbM variants: Treatment not possible or indicated.

ASSESSMENT POINTS

SYSTEM	PE	TEST
RESP	Look cyanosed but more "blue" than "sick"	15–30% MetHb
HEME		RCM type I and II: mild erythrocytosis HbM variants: mild hemolytic anemia

Key Reference: Lukens JN: Methemoglobinemia and other disease accompanied by cyanosis. *In* Lee GR, Bithell TC, Foerster J, et al (eds): Wintrobe's Clinical Hematology, 9th ed. Philadelphia, Lea & Febiger, 1992, pp1262–1271.

PERIOPERATIVE IMPLICATIONS

Preoperative Preparation

- Can give reducing agents to patients with RCM type I but no data on whether treatment is indicated prior to anesthesia

Monitoring

- Pulse oximeter overestimates at low SpO_2, and underestimates at high SpO_2. In practice reads between 80–85% regardless of true saturation
- May need to measure ABGs, and estimate SpO_2 from ABG.

Airway

- None

Preinduction/Induction

- None

Maintenance

- Prilocaine, benzocaine, Emla cream contraindicated
- Lidocaine, bupivicaine, nitrous oxide, volatile agents OK

Adjuvants

- None

Postoperative Period

- Avoid acetanilids for pain relief; narcotics OK

ANTICIPATED PROBLEMS/CONCERNS

- Avoid oxidant drugs in both homozygotes and heterozygotes
- Pulse oximetry is inaccurate; use ABGs.

CONGESTIVE HEART FAILURE

Nicola D'Attellis, M.D.
Jean-Francois Baron, M.D.

RISK

• Complication and/or evolution of most cardiac diseases.
• 4.7 million in US; 400,000 new cases annually in US; 250,000 Americans die of CHF annually.

PERIOPERATIVE RISKS

• CHF is a major determinant of perioperative risk
• EF <40% associated with increased operative risk
• Single greatest risk factor for cardiac surgery: Use congestive heart failure score (CASS): Hx of CHF = 1; Rx digitalis = 1; Rales = 1; If overt symptoms after treatment = 1; Total 0–4: If score = 4, operative risk is 8× greater.

WORRY ABOUT

• Ventricular dysfunction preop; associated with increased operative mortality
• Diastolic dysfunction leads to increased left atrial pressures with pulmonary congestion
• Dysrhythmias due to cardiac ischemia
• Associated acute or chronic mitral insufficiency
• Volume status

OVERVIEW

• Different types of failure (left vs right; acute vs chronic; systolic vs diastolic; low output vs high output)
• Heart unable to pump blood to meet metabolic demands.
• Acute ischemia can lead to global diastolic dysfunction and CHF.
• Papillary muscle ischemia may lead to severe mitral regurgitation and pulmonary congestion.
• New York Heart Association classification: I: no limitation; II: slight limitation; III: marked limitation; IV: inability to carry out any physical activity. Overall 1-y mortality for classes III and IV 34–58%.

ICD-9-CM Code: 428.0

ETIOLOGY

• *Acquired, Acute or Chronic:* CHD, MI; cardiomyopathy (idiopathic, hypertrophic, hypertophic obstructive, congestive, alcoholic). Valvular heart disease: Arrhythmias, Severe HTN
• *Congenital:* Congenital heart disease, L→R shunts; intracardiac (ASD, VSD, atrioventricular canal), extracardiac (PDA, anomalous pulmonary venous connection). Obstructive (coarctation of the aorta, aortic stenosis). Complex (Ebstein's anomaly).
• *Multiple precipitating causes:* Noncompliance with medications (digitalis, diuretics), excessive Na+; excessive IV fluids; drugs (β-blockers, doxorubicin, corticosteroids, disopyramide, nortriptyline, NSAIDs, androgens and estrogens). Pulmonary embolism: High-output states (pregnancy, fever, hyperthyroidism, sepsis, AV fistula, anemia)

USUAL TREATMENT

Chronic

• Restriction of physical activity
• Restriction of sodium intake
• Improvement of pump performance (digitalis)
• Diuretics, vasodilators (ACE inhibitors)

Acute

• Optimize pre- and afterload before starting inotropes and vasodilators
• Inotropes (dobutamine, milrinone, amrinone)
• Vasodilators (IV nitroprusside)

Special Measures

• Surgical correction (CABG, CHD, valvular surgery, cardiac transplantation)
• Assist devices: (IABP, LV assist, artificial heart)

ASSESSMENT POINTS

SYSTEM	EFFECT	ASSESSMENT BY HX	PE	TEST
CV	Inadequate cardiac output, congestion	Tachycardia, arrhythmias	Peripheral edema Facial edema (infants/young children) Cardiomegaly, pulsus alternans, distended neck veins, Kussmaul's sign, abdominojugular reflex	Exercise testing ECG, CXR Circulation time
RESP	Pulmonary congestion, decreased lung compliance, VC, TLC, pulmonary diffusion capacity	Breathlessness (exertional dyspnea, orthopnea, paroxysmal nocturnal dyspnea) Frequent respiratory infections	Rales and wheezes Pleural effusions Expectoration: frothy blood-tinged sputum	PFT ABG CXR
GI	Hepatic and intestinal congestion	Nausea, bloating, fullness	Congestive hepatomegaly, ascites, icterus, cachexia	Liver enzymes
RENAL	Decreased GFR, activation angiotensin-renin-aldosterone system	Nocturia, oliguria	Ankle edema	BUN/Cr, K+, Na+ Proteinuria Specific gravity
CNS	Hypoperfusion	Confusion, impairment of memory	Mental status exam	
PNS	Increased sympathetic tone	Cool extremities	Peripheral vasoconstriction, pallor, diaphoresis, tachycardia, clubbing	

Key Reference: Braunwald E (ed): Heart Disease: A Textbook of Cardiovascular Medicine, 4th ed. Philadelphia, WB Saunders, 1992, pp 1348–1352.

PERIOPERATIVE IMPLICATIONS

Preoperative Preparation

• Stabilize patient by treating CHF before surgery
• Continue inotropic support, digitalis
• ACE inhibitors (may cause hypotension on induction)

Monitoring

• 5-lead ECG
  – Consider arterial line
  – Consider CVP, PA catheter, or TEE

Airway

• Frothy secretions may lead to difficult visualization

Induction

• Preop therapeutic regimen (diuretics) causes hypovolemia, hypokalemia, and hyponatremia, which are potential problems before surgery.
• Judicious volume replacement (avoid dehydration and overhydration)
• Avoid myocardial contractility depressants (e.g., barbiturates, inhalation agents)

Maintenance

• Maintain myocardial contractility, reduce afterload, and normalize PVR.

Extubation

• May be delayed owing to CV and pulmonary insufficiencies

Adjuvants

• Rx inotropes; digitalis, diuretics
• Regional anesthesia debated and not recommended by some (sympathectomy, volume status) or preferred (reduce preload) by others

Postoperative Period

• Inotropic support and mechanical assistance may be needed
• Pulmonary edema develops in 2–16% of patients.

ANTICIPATED PROBLEMS/CONCERNS

• Pulmonary edema may necessitate prolonged ventilation with high FIO_2.
• RV and/or LV failure in the postop period

CONN'S SYNDROME (HYPERALDOSTERONISM, PRIMARY)

Stephen P. Fischer, M.D.

RISK

- People within US: 0.5–1% of HTN patients without known etiology
- Female:male 2:1
- Age onset usually 30–50 y

PERIOPERATIVE RISKS

- Increased risk of CHF 2° to hypervolemia
- Increased risk of ischemic heart disease
- ↑ Diastolic HTN with LVH

WORRY ABOUT

- Volume/electrolyte imbalance, especially hypokalemia
- Nephropathy may impair renal function
- Pathologic fractures with positioning 2° to osteoporosis

OVERVIEW

- Primary aldosteronism; mineralocorticoid excess
- K^+ depletion, Na^+ conservation with ↑ extracellular volume
- Dx by ↑ urinary aldosterone and K^+ with ↓ plasma renin
- Proper treatment results in normal life expectancy

ICD-9-CM Code: 255.1

ETIOLOGY

- Unilateral adrenal functional adenoma (66%)
- Bilateral adrenocortical hyperplasia (33%)
- Adrenal carcinoma (<1%)
- Excess secretion of aldosterone

USUAL TREATMENT

- Initial treatment: K^+ supplement and competitive aldosterone antagonist (e.g., spironolactone 25–100mg bid)
- Surgical excision of adrenal gland(s)

ASSESSMENT POINTS

SYSTEM	EFFECT	ASSESSMENT BY HX	PE	TEST
HEENT		Visual disturbances		
CV	Cardiomegaly, diastolic HTN Arrhythmias 2° to ↓ K^+ ↑ Preload 2° to hypervolemia		BP ↑ JVD	CXR, ECG K^+
RESP	Hypoventilation Resp muscle weakness	Truncal obesity possible ↓ Exercise tolerance		
RENAL	Hypokalemic metabolic alkalosis Polyuria, polydipsia, nocturia Nephropathy, renal HTN			K^+, ABG Glucose BUN/Cr
GI	Hyperacidity	Reflux Hx		
SKIN	Atrophic	Easy bruising		
ENDO	Hyperglycemia (50% of patients) Hypernatremia, hypokalemia			Glucose, K^+, Na^+
HEME	Hypercoagulability with thromboembolism ↑ Infection susceptibility			
CNS		Headache		
PNS	Paresthesias			K^+
MS	Muscle weakness, fatigue, tetany Osteoporosis	 Pathologic fractures		K^+

Key Reference: Lampe GH, Roizen MF: Anesthesia for patients with abnormal function of the adrenal cortex. Anesthesiol Clin North Am 1987; 5: 245.

PERIOPERATIVE IMPLICATIONS

Preoperative Preparation

- Correct hypervolemia, hypokalemia, hypernatremia, hyperglycemia
- Treat hyperacidity: cimetidine/bicitrate

Monitoring

- Consider arterial or pulm artery catheter if suspect CV impairment, ↑ CO, or major surgery

Airway

- Tracheal intubation may be difficult with obesity

Induction

- No specific anesthesia technique for adrenalectomy

Maintenance

- Monitor intraoperative glucose, acid-base status, fluid balance
- Avoid hyperventilation: ↑ metabolic alkalosis and ↓ K^+

Extubation

- Prolonged emergence possible

Adjuvants

- Hypokalemia may potentiate response to muscle relaxants
- Use of enflurane questionable if hypokalemic nephropathy and polyuria

Postoperative Period

- CXR for pneumothorax; up to 20% postop if adrenalectomy

ANTICIPATED PROBLEMS/CONCERNS

- ↑ Pancreatitis with left adrenalectomy

CONSTIPATION

Takashi Asai, M.D.
Michael Rosen, F.R.C.A., C.B.E.

RISK

- Incidence in US: 2–25%
- Higher prevalence in elderly and in females

PERIOPERATIVE RISKS

- Increased risk of nausea, vomiting, abdominal pain, headache

WORRY ABOUT

- A possibility of increased risk of pulmonary aspiration of gastric contents
- Pseudo-obstruction of the intestine
- High airway pressure, decreased vital capacity, and decreased FRC due to elevated diaphragm

OVERVIEW

- Can cause nausea, vomiting, and abdominal pain
- By itself does not affect life expectancy

ICD-9-CM Code: 564.0

ETIOLOGY

- Idiopathic in most cases
- In some cases associated with congenital (e.g., Hirschsprung's disease) or acquired (whether genetic or not) diseases (diabetes mellitus, multiple sclerosis)

USUAL TREATMENT

- Ingestion of dietary fiber
- Laxatives and enemas
- Colectomy and ileorectostomy

ASSESSMENT POINTS

SYSTEM	EFFECT	ASSESSMENT BY HX	TEST
RESP	Elevated diaphragm Increased airway pressure	Abdominal distention	CXR
GI	Intestinal obstruction Nausea and vomiting Gastroparesis	Abdominal distention	Abdominal x-ray
CNS	Headache		

Key Reference: Stewart RB, Moore MT, Marks RG, Hale WE: Correlates of constipation in an ambulatory elderly population. Am J Gastroenterol 1992; 87:859–864.

PERIOPERATIVE IMPLICATIONS

Monitoring

- Airway pressure

Airway

- Decreased FRC

Induction

- Awake or rapid-sequence induction if there is an obstruction of the intestine

Maintenance

- Avoid using nitrous oxide if there is an obstruction of the intestine

Extubation

- Extubate after the airway reflexes have recovered

Adjuvants

- Opioids or atropine, but not NSAIDs, which delay gastrointestinal transit

ANTICIPATED PROBLEMS/CONCERNS

- Gaseous distention of gut and elevated diaphragm may be present. Avoid using nitrous oxide in such patients.
- Gastrointestinal transit may be delayed. Consider Rx enemas.

CONVERSION DISORDER

Michael Ho, M.D.

RISK

- Reported prevalence varies widely (11–300/100,000); may account for as much as 1–3% of outpatient psychiatric referrals
- Reported to be more common in rural populations, developing areas, lower socioeconomic groups, those less medically sophisticated

PERIOPERATIVE RISKS

- No definite association with increased perioperative morbidity or mortality, as long as patient's symptoms are due only to conversion disorder

WORRY ABOUT

- Presence of undiagnosed neurologic or general medical illnesses, which could take years to become evident
- Appearance of conversion symptoms mimicking medical disturbances, drug effects, or anesthetic or surgically related complications
- Malingering, factitious disorder, drug abuse, confabulation

OVERVIEW

- DSM-IV: Conversion disorder is one of 7 somatoform disorders (disorders whose physical symptoms suggest the presence of, but are not fully explained by, a general medical illness)
- Diagnosis based on involuntary appearance of one or more symptoms affecting voluntary motor or sensory function that suggest (but are not explained by) a neurologic or general medical condition ("pseudoneurologic" symptoms)
- Symptoms cannot be intentional or feigned, attributable to culturally sanctioned or religious experiences, limited to pain or sexual dysfunction, or better explained by another mental disorder, and must cause clinically significant distress or impairment in functioning
- Although individual symptoms are of short duration (<2 wk), recurrence is common (20% within 1 y)
- Patients may undergo numerous examinations, diagnostic procedures, and hospitalizations, potentially causing morbidity; diagnosis is usually tentative and provisional

ICD-9-CM Code: 300.11

ETIOLOGY

- Hypothesis that somatic symptoms represent symbolic resolution of an unconscious psychologic conflict by reducing anxiety and removing the conflict from awareness
- Although validity of hypothesis not essential, associated psychologic factors must be present
- Symptoms more frequently found among relatives of conversion disorder patients; risk is greater in monozygotic than dizygotic twins
- 1/4 to 1/2 of patients initially diagnosed actually have general medical conditions

USUAL TREATMENT

- First line: reassurance and relaxation
- Second line: amobarbital interview, hypnosis, behavior therapy, psychotherapy or psychoanalysis
- Anecdotal use of phenothiazines, lithium, ECT
- Direct confrontation not recommended

ASSESSMENT POINTS

SYSTEM	EFFECT	ASSESSMENT BY HX	PE	TEST
CNS	Four subtypes: 1. Motor: impaired coordination or balance, paralysis or localized weakness, aphonia, difficulty swallowing or sensation of lump in the throat, urinary retention 2. Sensory: loss of touch or pain sensation, double vision, blindness, deafness, hallucinations 3. Seizures or convulsions 4. Mixed presentation	Differential diagnosis includes almost any medical condition (e.g., myasthenia gravis, multiple sclerosis, porphyria, diabetic neuropathy, hyperparathyroidism, tumors, idiopathic or substance-abuse dystonias)	Findings do not conform to known anatomic pathways or physiologic mechanisms, symptoms inconsistent, e.g., unacknowledged strength in antagonistic muscles; normal muscle tone, intact reflexes; equal difficulty swallowing solids and liquids "Paralyzed" extremity moves on own with dressing: arm held over patient's head by examiner and dropped will not fall on head; stocking-glove anesthesia without proximal to distal gradient; equal loss of touch, temperature, and pain at sharply demarcated anatomic landmarks rather than dermatomes	Absence of expected findings (including EEG, EMG, lumbar puncture, CT, MRI, SPECT scan, nerve conduction velocity, drug screen) suggest and confirm diagnosis
GENDER		Gender tendencies: Men—antisocial personality, work-related or military injury Women—more common, especially on left side of body. Children <10 y: seizures, gait disturbances.		

Key Reference: Diagnostic and Statistical Manual of Mental Disorders. Washington, DC, American Psychiatric Association, 1994, pp 452–457.

PERIOPERATIVE IMPLICATIONS

Perioperative Preparation

- Careful history and PE, carefully documenting any pre-existing neurologic deficits
- Informed consent
- Confer with previous physicians (e.g., internist, neurologist, psychiatrist) when necessary
- Verify that tests are negative to rule out misdiagnosis
- Consider possibility that reason for surgery in patient with multiple procedures may involve conversion symptom

Monitoring

- Routine

Airway

- None

Premedication/Induction/Maintenance

- No specific technique clearly superior
- Regional anesthesia not contraindicated

Extubation

- None

Adjuvants

- Sedatives as appropriate

Postoperative Period

- Watch for reappearance of conversion symptoms

- Conversion symptoms may represent previously undiagnosed medical disease, unmasked by stresses of anesthesia and surgery

ANTICIPATED PROBLEMS/CONCERNS

- Previously undiagnosed medical disease is probably common among patients with psychiatric disease. The anesthesiologist may be the first to suggest the presence of both psychiatric disease and related medical conditions. In order to properly treat patients with somatic complaints, a preoperative screening clinic should be employed whenever possible and appropriate consultation sought whenever necessary

COR PULMONALE

Paul Zanaboni, M.D., Ph.D.

RISK

- Third most common cardiac Dx after age 50 y
- 10–20% of all CHF admissions have some aspect of right heart failure
- Gender predominance: male > female

PERIOPERATIVE RISKS

- ↑ Risk for respiratory failure, right heart failure, (≥ 10% if cor pulmonale Dx made preoperatively)
- Risk of prolonged postoperative ventilatory support

WORRY ABOUT

- ↑ Pulmonary vascular resistance (PVR) may cause systemic hypotension
- Hypoxia, hypoxemia, hypercarbia, and acidosis intraoperatively or in early postoperative period, which ↑ PVR
- Underlying CAD, LV dysfunction

OVERVIEW

- Alteration in RV structure (hypertrophy) and function
- Most common cause: COPD (↑ PVR 2° to chronic hypoxia and structural changes)
- Any disease that ↑ PVR chronically can induce RV changes, including idiopathic pulmonary hypertension and toxin-induced pulmonary hypertension, pulmonary fibrosis
- Prognosis: favorable for those who can maintain a near-normal PaO$_2$; unfavorable for those with structural changes

ICD-9-CM Code: 416.9

ETIOLOGY

- COPD: smoking or severe asthma
- Primary pulmonary hypertension: Pulmonary fibrosis; either drug-induced or idiopathic; chronic pulmonary embolism

USUAL TREATMENT

- ↓ PVR toward normal levels by ↑ PaO$_2$ to 60 mmHg (beware of depression of hypoxic drive to breathe; may have desensitized hypercarbic drive to breathe 2° to chronic ↑ PaCO$_2$); by giving diuretics, digoxin to relieve symptoms of CHF (caution: diuretics may increase Hct by hemoconcentration; if Hct already ↑ 2° to ↓ PaO$_2$, this may further ↑ viscosity of blood, increasing risk for sludging and microemboli); by administering vasodilators, only $\frac{1}{3}$ of patients improve (best would be selective pulmonary vasodilator: inhaled nitric oxide; other vasodilators, such as calcium channel blockers, have been tried; use caution because may ↓ SVR in face of fixed ↑ PVR, causing severe systemic hypotension [unable to increase CO]); and by giving antibiotics for prompt treatment of infection

ASSESSMENT POINTS

SYSTEM	EFFECT	ASSESSMENT BY HX	PE	TEST
CV	RV failure ↑ PVR Tricuspid regurgitation	DOE Effort-related syncope Chest pain	Accentuated pulmonary S$_2$ Diastolic or systolic murmur Dependent edema	CXR ECHO Right heart catheterization
RESP	COPD	DOE Chronic cough, sputum	Hyperinflated lungs Wheezing, rhonchi	CXR PFT
GI	Passive congestion of liver, spleen		Hepatosplenomegaly	LFT Albumin PT
RENAL	Impaired ability to excrete Na$^+$, H$_2$O	Edema	Edema	Urinary Osm Urine specific gravity
CNS	Stimulation of sympathetic nervous system 2° to hypoxia		Tachycardia	

Key Reference: MacNee W: Pathophysiology of cor pulmonale in chronic obstructive pulmonary disease: Parts I and II. Am J Respir and Crit Care Med 1994; 150:833–852, 1158–1168.

PERIOPERATIVE IMPLICATIONS

Preoperative Preparation

- Treat underlying infections
- Maximize treatment of reversible airway disease
- Maximize pulmonary toilet to expand airways and ↓ secretions
- Avoid preoperative medications that will depress ventilation

Monitoring

- Consider arterial line for ABG
- Consider pulmonary arterial catheter to monitor PA pressures, CVP monitoring for evaluation of RV function for large fluid shift reoperations

Airway

- Potential for bronchospasm

Induction

- Try to ↑ SVR in face of fixed ↑ PVR
- Deep anesthesia for intubation may ↓ incidence of bronchospasm and sympathetic stimulation, which ↑ PVR

Maintenance

- Potent inhalational agents for bronchodilation
- Consider avoiding nitrous oxide (which may ↑ PVR) and large doses of narcotics (which may cause postoperative hypoventilation)
- Although positive pressure ventilation may ↑ PVR 2° to alveolar expansion, it can ↓ PVR 2° to better oxygenation
- Aggresively prevent hypothermia, which may cause ↑ in PVR

Extubation

- Bronchospasm may occur during emergence

Adjuvants

- Regional anesthesia an option, but high level may cause ↓ SVR in face of fixed ↑ PVR
- Nitric oxide increasing in use

Postoperative Period

- Postoperative pain management with either low-dose epidural local anesthetics with low-dose opioids or low-dose intrathecal opioids can minimize respiratory depression

ANTICIPATED PROBLEMS/CONCERNS

- ↑ PVR and RV dysfunction from hypoxia/hypercarbia or hypothermia

CORONARY ARTERY DISEASE
(LEFT MAIN AND NON–LEFT MAIN DISEASE)

J. G. Reves, M.D.

RISK

- Incidence: 11 million in USA
- 1.5 million patients per year with CAD will have an acute MI; ⅓ of these will die
- CAD responsible for 51% of deaths in men and 49% in women (largest single disease cause in both)
- Male predominance <55 y, M = F >55 y
- Risk factors: HTN, diabetes, smoking, familial incidence, hyperlipidemia, and high cholesterol

PERIOPERATIVE RISKS

- Presence of disease by coronary anatomy is good predictor of survival with CAD
- Presence of left main disease with high degree of stenosis is life-threatening
- Recent MI ↑ risk, but revascularization interventions protect patient
- Impaired ventricular function, unstable anginal pattern, major surgery, and emergency surgery ↑ risk
- ↑ Risk if reoperation for bypass surgery

WORRY ABOUT

- Myocardial ischemia can lead to MI
- Postop MI carries very high mortality (>50%) in noncardiac surgical patients
- Atherosclerosis in other vascular beds (CNS, renal, mesentery)

OVERVIEW

- Atherosclerosis of vessels supplying blood to heart results in ↓ blood flow by either limitation of flow due to anatomy or due to vasoactive dysfunction (spasm, etc.)
- Single greatest cause of death in US population (500,000 deaths/y)
- Most prevalent form of cardiovascular disease: > 11 million of US population has CAD
- Leading cause of death in major noncardiac surgery

ICD-9-CM Code: 414.0
See also Angina, Chronic Stable in Diseases section

ETIOLOGY

- Atherosclerosis and obstructive deposits in coronary artery
- Interaction of genetics, diet, and environment: hypertension, cigarette smoking, and diabetes are three common predisposing factors
- Myocardial oxygen delivery does not meet myocardial oxygen demands: causes myocardial ischemia
- Myocardial oxygen supply does not reach myocardium after thrombosis of coronary artery: causes MI

USUAL TREATMENT

- Medical: nitroglycerin, ß rb's, calcium-channel blockers (low dose and in vasospastic component), diet, antihyperlipidemia drugs, aspirin, exercise, weight loss, antioxidants
- Catheter-based interventional cardiology (indicated in ≤ 2-vessel CAD: PTCA (has 30% 3-month closure rate), intracoronary stent (has good angiographic result and lower closure rate, but event-free survival is little different from PTCA), atherectomy
- Coronary artery bypass graft (CABG) surgery (indicated in ≥ 2-vessel CAD)

ASSESSMENT POINTS

CONCERN	EFFECT	ASSESSMENT BY HX	PE	TEST
Noncardiac Surgery				
Ischemia	Causes ventricular dysfunction Can herald and/or cause MI	Angina		Holter monitor, ECG exercise radionuclide, treadmill stress ECHO
Infarction	Indicates severe CAD Causes death			ECG, CK-MB and troponin enzyme release
Impaired function	Heart failure, shock	Activity history Stair climbing	Orthopnea gallop Neck veins	Ejection fraction (cath, ECHO radionuclide)
Cardiac Surgery				
Cardiac function	Best predictor of outcome			Ventricular angiogram (EF > 50% = good risk)
Coronary anatomy	Extent of disease and overall long-term survival			Coronary angiography
Renal function	↑ Risk if impaired			Cr ≥ 2.0 denotes ↑ risk
CNS	↑ Risk of stroke	Hx of TIA, symptomatic bruits		Carotid Doppler study

Key Reference: Mark DB, et al: Continuing evolution of therapy for coronary artery disease: Initial results from the era of coronary angioplasty. Circulation 1994; 89:2015–2025.

PERIOPERATIVE IMPLICATIONS

Preoperative Preparation

- Supportive preoperative interview to ↓ stress and anxiety
- Consider analgesic (opioid) if pain or likelihood of pain prior to anesthesia
- Give morning cardiac medications, especially the ß rb's
- Nitroglycerin at bedside

Monitoring

- Consider systemic arterial BP (invasive and continuous in unstable patients or in cases where BP swings are anticipated)
- Consider CVP and/or PA catheters; in cardiac surgical patients, EF ≤ 30% should trigger consideration of catheter

- Consider TEE if severe wall motion abnormalities and in major vascular cases

Anesthesia

- Principle is to maintain O_2 supply and to minimize myocardial O_2 consumption
  - maintain O_2 sat and Hgb concentration (O_2 carrying capacity)
  - maintain diastolic BP (perfusion pressure)
  - ↓ HR, contractility, and wall tension (O_2 consumption)
- No outcome difference demonstrated among general anesthetics
- Regional and conduction anesthesia with postoperative analgesia may be beneficial
- Transient periods of hypertension are well tolerated; prolonged periods of hypotension, tachycardia, and anemia are not well tolerated

Adjuvants

- Nitroglycerin, sublingual or (preferably) by continuous infusion (0.5–2.0 µg/kg/min), can treat myocardial ischemia
- ß rb's by bolus or infusion ↓ HR and myocardial contractility and can prevent and treat ischemia
- RBCs to maintain Hct ≥28%

Postoperative Period

- 2nd and 3rd postop days are most common time for MI in noncardiac surgical patients; ischemia intraoperatively, designate as "high risk" in postoperative period
- Maintain good analgesia to ↓ stress response
- Maintain cardiac medications (esp ß rb's)
- Consider use of aspirin or other medications to ↓ coronary thrombosis in high-risk noncardiac surgical patients

CORONARY ARTERY SPASM (CAS)

Robert G. Merin, M.D.

RISK

• Incidence of pure disease is very low, but CAS may complicate atherosclerotic CAD.
• Difficult to differentiate from transient microthrombotic episodes
• More common in females, diabetics, and hypertensives

PERIOPERATIVE RISKS

• Low (classical): Dx based on ST segment or wall motion evidence for myocardial ischemia without concurrent changes in determinates of myocardial oxygen balance (non–hemodynamically related [NHR]) may occur after CABG
• High (new view of cause of thrombosis in CAD): Not related to structural tight stenoses, but to humoral/endocardial factors that can also precipitate thrombosis

WORRY ABOUT

• Consequences of ischemia such as arrhythmia, ventricular failure, MI

OVERVIEW

• Classical: Diagnosed by normal coronary angiogram during chest pain and ST segment depression and exaggerated coronary vasoconstriction to ergonovine

Two Distinct Syndromes:

• Prinzmetal's (variant) angina (syndrome A): Demonstrable coronary vasospasm in epicardial vessels on coronary angiogram; regional, usually occurring at site of small nonobstructing atheroma; can be demonstrated in patients with hypercholesterolemia without coronary atherosclerosis; often occurs at rest; no gender predominance; without concurrent CAD, prognosis is excellent. With concurrent CAD can lead to infarction.
• Syndrome X (microvascular angina): No demonstrable coronary vasospasm on coronary angiogram; rarely associated with CAD; limited coronary vascular reserve (increased coronary blood flow with dipyridamole or papaverine); sometimes chest pain at rest, but accentuated by exercise; predominantly female (70:30); prognosis usually excellent.

ICD-9-CM Code: 413.1 (Prinzmetal)
See also Coronary Artery Disease

ETIOLOGY

• Vascular endothelial dysfunction with decreased release of nitric oxide (or increased degradation by oxygen free radicals)
• Same risk factors as for CAD but cigarette smoking even more prevalent
• Predominantly vascular smooth muscle dysfunction; present in peripheral vessels as well; diabetes and HTN special risk factors.

USUAL TREATMENT

• Medical therapy: Calcium channel blocking drugs (Ca^{2+} rb's) and nitroglycerin are Rx for both syndromes; also potassium channel agonists
• Angioplasty for discrete single proximal lesions in syndrome A.

ASSESSMENT POINTS

SYSTEM	EFFECT	ASSESSMENT BY HX	PE	TEST
CV	Chest pain Myocardial ischemia HTN	Chest pain at rest NHR ischemia relieved by Ca^{2+} rb's		ECG Coronary angio with ergonovine testing
RESP	Chest pain	May be caused by hyperventilation		
MS	Syndrome X ischemia	Claudication	Decreased or absent peripheral pulses	Angiography or Doppler

Key Reference: Maseri A, Davies G, Hackett D, Kaski JC: Coronary artery spasm and vasoconstriction: The case for distinction. Circulation 1990; 81:1983–1991.

PERIOPERATIVE IMPLICATIONS

Preoperative Preparation

• Continue Ca^{2+} rb's and nitrates. Consider IV nitroglycerin and nicardipine

Monitoring

• ST segment analysis
• Consider intra-arterial BP
• Consider TEE if available

Airway

• None

Preinduction/Induction

• Control HR and BP

Maintenance

• Careful HR, BP, and T control
• Consider thoracic epidural anesthesia

Extubation

• May be increased risk for vasospasm

Postoperative Period

• Adequate pain treatment
• Consider continuous epidural

Adjuvants

• Ca^{2+} rb's, nitroglycerin

ANTICIPATED PROBLEMS/CONCERNS

• Differentiate coronary vasospasm from microemboli because treatment is different; untreated, either may lead to arrhythmias, CHF, MI.

CRI DU CHAT SYNDROME (5p– SYNDROME)
Barbara W. Palmisano, M.D.

RISK
• 1/50,000 births

PERIOPERATIVE RISKS
• Difficult airway management due to micrognathia
• Congenital heart disease

WORRY ABOUT
• Difficult mask ventilation
• Inability to visualize larynx
• Behavioral problems due to profound retardation

OVERVIEW
• Chromosomal abnormality
• Microcephaly with profound mental retardation and somatic growth failure
• Characteristic facies including micrognathia and facial asymmetry
• Characteristic high shrill cry in infancy that is central in origin, although laryngeal malformations occasionally reported
• Congenital heart disease common (30–50%)
• Occasional malformations of CNS, GI tract, kidneys, MS system

ICD-9-CM Code: 758.3

ETIOLOGY
• Partial deletion of short arm of chromosome 5 occurring sporadically (85%) or as an unbalanced translocation inherited from a carrier parent (15%)

USUAL TREATMENT
• None for primary chromosomal abnormality

ASSESSMENT POINTS

SYSTEM	EFFECT	ASSESSMENT BY HX	PE	TEST
HEENT	Micrognathia Malocclusion High, vaulted palate Cleft lip/palate Asymmetric face	Feeding and swallowing difficulty	Receding mandible; reduced thyromental distance	
CV	Various congenital heart defects	Shortness of breath Night sweats	Murmur/gallop Dyspnea Tachycardia	ECHO ECG
RESP	Chronic aspiration Frequent URI with otitis media		Dyspnea Rales/rhonchi Wheezing	CXR
CNS	Retardation Seizures		Hypotonia in infancy Spasticity later	
MS	Scoliosis Various limb anomalies			

Key Reference: Gorlin RJ, Cohen MM, Levin LS: Syndromes of the Head and Neck. New York, Oxford University Press, 1990, pp 48–49.

PERIOPERATIVE IMPLICATIONS

Preoperative Preparation
• Develop strategies for difficult airway management

Monitoring
• Routine

Airway
• Laryngeal mask airway or fiberoptic bronchoscopy to facilitate endotracheal intubation

Preinduction/Induction
• Careful preop sedation in monitored setting for uncooperative patient

Maintenance
• Keep ectomorphic patients warm

Extubation
• Awake extubation for patients with difficult airway management

Adjuvants
• No specific concerns

ANTICIPATED PROBLEMS/CONCERNS
• Airway management may be difficult
• Associated malformations, especially congenital heart disease

CROHN'S DISEASE

Kelvin Yee, M.D.

RISK

- Incidence of 2 cases per 100,000/y: prevalence of 20 to 40 per 100,000
- Race: Caucasians > African-Americans
- Increased incidence 3- to 6-fold in Jews compared with non-Jews
- Peak occurrence: between ages 15 and 35 y

PERIOPERATIVE RISKS

- Risk of exacerbation of underlying liver disease

WORRY ABOUT

- Intravascular fluid volume and electrolyte status
- Nutritional status and adverse effects associated with hyperalimentation
- Colonic and extracolonic complications (anemia, liver disease, arthritis)
- Corticosteroids supplementation if chronically receiving steroids to maintain fluid and electrolyte balance, and vascular reactivity

OVERVIEW

- Anemia may be due to chronic disease, iron deficiency, chronic hemorrhage, or folate or vitamin B_{12} deficiency
- Decreased intravascular fluid volume due to malnutrition and hypoalbuminemia
- Electrolyte abnormalities, especially hypokalemia due to diarrhea
- Potential for malignancy and intestinal obstruction/perforation/toxic megacolon
- Rectocutaneous fistulas, rectal fissures, or perirectal abscesses with Crohn's disease

ICD-9-CM Code: 555.9

ETIOLOGY

- Unknown
- Features of the disease have suggested a relationship with familial or genetic, infectious, immunologic, and psychologic factors

USUAL TREATMENT

- Pharmacologic: anti-inflammatory agents, sulfasalazine, corticosteroids, antibiotics, and immunosuppressive therapy (azathioprine and cyclosporine)
- Surgical: surgery for symptomatic obstruction, fistula, abscesses, or perforation

ASSESSMENT POINTS

SYSTEM	EFFECT	ASSESSMENT BY HX	PE	TEST
CV	Dehydration, anemia	Bloody diarrhea, loss of weight	Postural hypotension, tachycardia	Hct, BUN/Cr, K^+, Mg^{2+}
GI	Fatty liver infiltration Pericholangitis Cirrhosis Toxic megacolon Intestinal perforation Proctitis/rectal abscess Malabsorption	Jaundice Fever Abdominal pain Bleeding/tenesmus	Hepatomegaly Rebound tenderness Cachexia, weight loss	Alkaline phosphatase LFTs Abdominal series WBC Albumin, B_{12}, folate
RENAL	Secondary amyloidosis Renal stones	Flank pain		Proteinuria
MS	Ankylosing arthritis	Joint mobility	↓ Joint ROM	

Key Reference: Hanauer SB: Inflammatory bowel disease. *In* Wyngaarden JB, Smith LH Jr, Bennett JC (eds): Cecil Textbook of Medicine, 19th ed. Philadelphia: WB Saunders, 1992, pp 699–708.

PERIOPERATIVE IMPLICATIONS

Preoperative Preparation

- Assess volume status and ensure normality
- Hyperalimentation: if given preoperatively, need to maintain intraoperatively; assess glucose, PO_4^{2-}
- Assess concurrent steroid use and need for supplementation

Monitoring

- Routine

Airway

- None

Preinduction and Induction

- Rapid-sequence induction in patients with gastric outlet or duodenal obstruction

Maintenance

- Consider avoiding nitrous oxide if bowel distention/obstruction
- Potential adverse effects of hyperalimentation must be noted, with serum glucose checked regularly

Extubation

- Awake extubation for "full stomach"

Postoperative Period

- Monitor volume status, as third space losses and fluid mobilization will ensue

Adjuvants

- With underlying liver disease consider avoiding halothane, and for muscle relaxants dependent on hepatic elimination, reduced plasma clearance necessitates smaller than normal maintenance doses

- Hypoalbuminemia results in diminished protein binding, higher free drug levels, and increased volume of distribution, thus enhancing effects and clearance of highly protein bound drugs while reducing effects of other drugs

ANTICIPATED PROBLEMS/CONCERNS

- Nutritional deficiency, often severe, particularly with small bowel involvement or with short bowel syndrome from extensive resection; may require supplementation of electrolytes, minerals, and vitamins
- Often marked hypovolemia and anemia exacerbated by third space losses; may need aggressive fluid hydration

CROUP (LARYNGOTRACHEOBRONCHITIS)

Maurice S. Zwass, M.D.

RISK

• Children between 6 mo and 6 y are at risk, (6 mo to 3 y at greatest risk)
• Children with underlying airway abnormalities (e.g., subglottic stenosis) or difficult intubations (e.g., micrognathia) and symptoms are at increased risk and require particular planning

PERIOPERATIVE RISKS

• Difficulty with intubation because of very narrowed subglottic region
• Obstruction of the small tracheal tube because of airway secretions

WORRY ABOUT

• Risk of rebound tracheal edema several hours after racemic epinephrine treatment
• Cardiorespiratory crisis if progressive or severe Sx, agitation, younger patients, or if exhibiting difficulties with oxygenation or ventilation, failure to oxygenate
• Bacterial superinfection of airway

OVERVIEW

• Common childhood ailment with prodromal illness accompanied by a characteristic cough (often sounds like seal barking)
• Sx and respiratory compromise from progressive swelling of subglottic region tracheal mucosa
• Frequently present when inspiratory stridor and respiratory distress develop
• Radiographs of neck often demonstrate gradual progressive tracheal narrowing, most narrow just below level of vocal cords (referred to as "steeple sign"); upper glottis on lateral neck radiograph is normal
• When obtained, evaluation of CBC is consistent with viral illness

ICD-9-CM Codes: 464.4 (Croup); 464.2 (Laryngotracheitis)

ETIOLOGY

• Viral agents are usual etiologies and include parainfluenza viruses (most common); adenoviruses, influenza virus, respiratory syncytial virus (RSV), and measles virus also associated

USUAL TREATMENT

• Cool mist often greatly improves Sx; supplemental O_2
• If symptoms more severe, aerosolized racemic epinephrine can dramatically reduce airway swelling (rebound tracheal edema risk several hours after administration necessitates observation in hospital)
• Steroid administration controversial; may ↓ severity of disease and reduce need for tracheal intubation or hasten improvement in first 24 h of illness
• Small percentage with this disease need tracheal intubation

ASSESSMENT POINTS

Differential points between croup (laryngotracheobronchitis) and epiglottitis

	CROUP	EPIGLOTTITIS
AGE	3 mo–3 y	1–7 y
ONSET	Gradual	More rapid (usually <24 h)
FEVER	Low grade	High
COUGH	Characteristic barking	None
SORE THROAT	Occasional	Frequently severe
POSTURE	Any	Frequently sitting forward, mouth open, drooling
AIRWAY SOUND	Inspiratory stridor	Inspiratory stridor
VOICE	Normal	Muffled
APPEARANCE	Nontoxic	Toxic
SEASONALITY	Peak winter, epidemic	Year round

Key Reference: McEniery J, Gillis J, Kilham H, Benjamin B. Review of intubation in severe laryngotracheobronchitis. Pediatrics 1991; 87:847–853.

PERIOPERATIVE IMPLICATIONS

Airway

• Airway support with good mask fit and positive pressure ventilation can generally overcome obstruction from swelling of airway
• Identification of larynx generally routine, but tracheal tube 0.5–1.0 mm diameter smaller than usual may necessitate having available extra-long or microlaryngeal tracheal tubes
• Tracheotomy rarely needed as therapy for these patients with current management and reserved only for unusual cases

Induction

• Induction common with IV access already obtained

ANTICIPATED PROBLEMS/CONCERNS

• Symptomatic patients who require intubation of trachea need tube 0.5–1.0 mm smaller in diameter than equivalent in children without croup.
• Patient who requires tracheal intubation usually requires sedative management to tolerate ventilation; often followed for development of leak around tracheal tube as a sign of improvement of edema; most patients improve within 2–4 days; when leak is present at 20–25 cm H_2O of pressure, extubation can be considered; complicated cases and patients with prolonged courses may benefit from examination of airway in operating room at time of extubation.
• Although viral illness, some patients may acquire bacterial superinfection of airway and require antibiotic therapy

CRYPTOCOCCUS INFECTION

David H. Wong, Pharm.D., M.D.

RISK

- 0.15% incidence in general population
- 7% incidence in AIDS patients
- 80–90% of infections occur in patients with AIDS as risk factor

PERIOPERATIVE RISKS

- Possible respiratory insufficiency

WORRY ABOUT

- Underlying disease

OVERVIEW

- Encapsulated yeast that reproduces by budding and causes cryptococcal meningitis. Dx usually made by CSF stain and culture
- Polysaccharide capsule prevents phagocytosis by PMNs
- Infection usually associated with defect in cell-mediated immunity
- Serum tests for Dx are unreliable.
- Pulmonary cryptococcosis diagnosed by bronchoscopy or biopsy
- With pulmonary cryptococcosis, look for disseminated cryptococcosis (do blood, urine, CSF, bone marrow cultures)
- Cryptococcal meningitis and pneumonitis can lead to disseminated disease
- Mortality rate as high as 50%
- Relapses are common, particularly in AIDS patients
- Not contagious from human to human

ICD-9-CM Code: 117.5

ETIOLOGY

- Organism present in soil, and particularly in pigeon feces
- Usually enters body via inhalation, then spreads hematogenously
- Associated with chemotherapy, corticosteroid therapy, immunosuppressive therapy (i.e., organ transplant recipients), hematopoietic cancer, AIDS

USUAL TREATMENT

- IV Amphotericin B
- IV 5-Fluorocytosine
- Cryptococcal meningitis may require intrathecal amphotericin treatment; may be less effective in AIDS patients
- Surgical drainage of abcesses as indicated
- If infection associated with corticosteroid therapy, discontinue or decrease corticosteroids

ASSESSMENT POINTS

SYSTEM	EFFECT	ASSESSMENT BY HX	PE	TEST
RESP	Pulm infection	Cough, sputum production, dyspnea	Wheezes or signs of infection	CXR, sputum culture, bronchoscopy if necessary
RENAL				Azotemia or decreased renal function
CNS	Meningitis	Headache, nausea, vomiting, seizures	Mental status	CSF culture, India ink stain, gram stain

Key Reference: Mandell G, Douglas R, Bennett J (eds): Principles and Practice of Infectious Diseases, 4th ed. New York, Churchill Livingstone, 1995, pp 2231–2240.

PERIOPERATIVE IMPLICATIONS

Preoperative Preparation

- Consider respiratory isolation circuit for anesthesia machine (for possible concomitant respiratory infections)
- Preop mental status may be depressed; may affect choice of anesthetic and need for airway protection

Monitoring

- Routine
- Pay particular attention to respiratory variables

Airway

- None

Preinduction/Induction

- None

Maintenance

- Administration of amphotericin B: if an anaphylactoid reaction occurs, may complicate interpretation of changes in vital signs or other physical signs

Extubation

- Consider if can adequately protect airway

Adjuvants

- None

Postoperative Period

- Pay particular attention to respiratory variables

ANTICIPATED PROBLEMS/CONCERNS

- Amphotericin B therapy associated with anaphylactoid reactions, hypotension, fever, chills, bronchospasm, nausea and vomiting. Chronic treatment can result in hypokalemia, hypomagnesemia, anemia, azotemia, renal tubular necrosis, and hepatic toxicity
- 5-Fluorocytosine therapy associated with thrombocytopenia, pancytopenia, and hepatitis

CUSHING'S SYNDROME

George H. Lampe, M.D.

RISK

- 10 million/y in USA treated with glucocorticoids
- Those treated for >21 d are at risk for Cushing's syndrome
- 7500 cases/y due to increased endogenous production

PERIOPERATIVE RISKS

- Acute adrenal insufficiency (addisonian crisis) if replacement is not provided
- Hyperglycemia, gastric ulceration, increased risk of infection with replacement

WORRY ABOUT

- Adequate gluco/mineralocorticoid replacement

OVERVIEW

- A constellation of physical signs caused by glucocorticoid excess (Cushing's disease specifically refers to pituitary excess resulting in Cushing's syndrome)
- Exogenous administration of glucocorticoids for more than 3 wk may suppress adrenal function for up to 1 y
- Epidural depot corticosteroid administration can cause adrenal suppression
- Acute adrenal insufficiency is rare but life threatening, prompting the guideline "When in doubt, treat"

ICD-9-CM Code: 255.0
Includes all causes except for congenital adrenal hyperplasia (255.2)

ETIOLOGY

- Exogenous administration prescribed by physicians—very common
- Pituitary ACTH overproduction (Cushing's disease)—rare
- Adrenal overproduction—rare

USUAL TREATMENT

- Rx must include gluco/mineralocorticoid activity (hydrocortisone is the gold standard)
- Physiologic (low-dose) replacement 25 mg of hydrocortisone IV q8h
- Supraphysiologic (extreme stress) doses 100 mg of hydrocortisone q8h

ASSESSMENT POINTS

SYSTEM	EFFECT	ASSESSMENT BY HX	PE	TEST
HEENT	Breathing difficult owing to fat or enlargement	Snoring	Uvula visible Neck and mandible ROM	
CV	HTN	Continue antihypertensives	BP CV exam for CHF S_3 gallop CHF with basilar rales	ECG CXR (if indicated)
GI	Gastric ulceration	Epigastric pain or black stools		Hgb Stool Hemoccult (if indicated)
METABOLIC-ENDO	Adrenal suppression Hyperglycemia with Rx Electrolyte abnormalities with metabolic alkalosis Overweight	Extended steroid exposure during last year	Centripetal fat, moon facies, cushingoid	ACTH stimulation test (rarely indicated) Glucose Na^+ and K^+ and electrolytes
CNS	Personality changes	Euphoria	Affect	
MS	Osteoporosis Delicate skin Muscle wasting	Pain Easy bruisability	Ecchymoses Thin extremities	X-rays (if indicated)

Key Reference: Roizen MF, Stevens A, Lampe GH: Perioperative management of patients with endocrine disease. *In* Nunn JF, Utting JE, Brown BR (eds): General Anaesthesia, 5th ed. London, Butterworths, 1989, pp 726–740.

PERIOPERATIVE IMPLICATIONS

Preoperative Preparation

- Steroid Rx in physiologic doses (25 mg q8h) for minor surgery; consider high dose (100 mg q8h) of hydrocortisone hemisuccinate for major surgery.

Airway

- Assume difficult airway due to moon facies and delicate mucosa that is easily traumatized

Induction

- Etomidate may further suppress adrenal function—might avoid in patients at risk
- Careful positioning to prevent stress fractures and skin trauma

Extubation

- Use great care when removing tape to avoid skin avulsion and bruising

Postoperative Care

- Monitor lytes and glucose
- Monitor hemodynamics
- Monitor for occult GI blood loss
- Taper steroids daily over 3 d

ANTICIPATED PROBLEMS/CONCERNS

- Hypotensive without supplementation
- Need for ulcer prophylaxis and attention to infection immune compromise and potential for CHF supplementation given

CYANIDE POISONING

Peter H. Breen, M.D., F.R.C.P.C.

RISK

- Potent and rapid-onset toxin, especially inhalation of hydrogen cyanide (CN)
- CN ingestion →slower onset
- Diffuses rapidly through body with high intracellular fixation to cytochrome aa_3 in cellular mitochondria to paralyze aerobic metabolism

PERIOPERATIVE RISKS

- Main target organs: CNS and heart
- Animal experiments: apnea precedes cardiac collapse

WORRY ABOUT

- If CN toxicity resulted from fire or smoke exposure, consider also carbon monoxide (CO) and other toxins
- ⅓ of patients from domestic fires with CO toxicity also have ↑ CN

OVERVIEW

- Major route of CN detoxification: conversion to thiocyanate, which requires sulfane sulfur donor (e.g., thiosulfate) and enzyme (e.g., rhodanase); without renal excretion, ↑ thiocyanate can cause CNS abnormalities
- Minor route: hydroxocobalamin (one form of vitamin B_{12}) chelates CN to form cyanocobalamin
- Methemoglobin (MetHb) ferric ion has high affinity for CN

ICD-9-CM Code: 989.0

ETIOLOGY

- Combustion product of natural and synthetic polymers
- Industrial chemistry (e.g., metals and plastics preparation)
- Plants: may contain cyanogenic glycosides
- Na nitroprusside: overtreatment (> 0.5 mg/kg/hr within 24 h)
- Abuse (e.g., suicide, Chicago CN–laced Tylenol murders [1982])

USUAL TREATMENT

- Intubation and ventilation with 100% O_2 (hyperbaric O_2, effective experimentally, is not practical)
- Na thiosulfate (25%) 150 mg/kg IV (minimal side effects but thiocyanate requires renal excretion or hemodialysis)
- Gastric decontamination (if necessary)
- Hydroxocobalamin, 4 g IV, safe and rapid but not yet available in US
- Methemoglobinemia induction (metHb, 30%) with 10% sodium nitrite (5–10 mg/kg IV) slow and unpredictable; can be hazardous in presence of carboxyhemoglobin (from CO toxicity) because neither metHb nor COHb carry O_2; can be fatal in G6PD deficiency
- Dicobalt EDTA (ethylenediaminetetraacetate), 300–600 mg IV, followed by glucose infusion; potent and rapid but unsafe (esp: arrhythmias, hypotension, and allergic reactions)

ASSESSMENT POINTS

SYSTEM	EFFECT	ASSESSMENT BY HX	PE	TEST
HEENT	↓ CNS → ↓ airway maintenance/protection	Concomitant smoke inhalation injury	Perioral burns Airway edema	Laryngoscopy/bronchoscopy
CV	Stimulation at low CN concn. Depression at high CN concn.	Hypertension, tachycardia Hypotension, bradycardia	↑ Cardiac output ↓ Cardiac output Arrhythmias	ECG: arrhythmias, esp ↓ conduction, VTach, VFib
RESP	Aerobic cellular respiration paralyzed Thermal/toxic airway and parenchymal injury	Concomitant smoke inhalation injury	Bronchoconstriction and pulm edema	↑ Blood PvO_2 and ↑ SvO_2 ↓ $\dot{V}O_2$ ↓ $\dot{V}CO_2$ ↓ $P_{ET}CO_2$ Chest x-ray Bronchoscopy
METAB	Cellular aerobic metabolism disabled	Combination of ↑ SvO_2 and lactic acidosis suggests CN		Lactic metabolic acidosis Whole blood CN levels (Not available in all labs)
CNS	Stimulation at low CN concn.	↑ Inhalatory CN intake Anxiety, dyspnea, headache Auditory/visual disturbances	↑ Resp rate Confusion	
	Depression at high CN concn.		Apnea, convulsions, coma	Funduscopy: red retinal veins (↑ SvO_2)

Key Reference: Breen PH, et al: Combined carbon monoxide and cyanide poisoning: A place for treatment? Anesth Analg 1995; 80:671–677.

PERIOPERATIVE IMPLICATIONS

Preoperative Preparation

- Continuous 100% O_2

Monitoring

- SpO_2 unreliable in presence of MetHb
- Mixed venous continuous SO_2 or blood PO_2 (SvO_2, PvO_2)
- $P_{ET}CO_2$
- Measure of $\dot{V}O_2$ or $\dot{V}CO_2$ helpful

Airway

- Protect and maintain airway

Induction

- Avoid CV depressant agents

Maintenance

- 100% O_2 (no N_2O)

Extubation

- Ensure CNS status permits natural airway maintenance and protection

Adjuvants

- Consider treatment for concomitant CO poisoning (see Carbon Monoxide)

Postoperative Period

- Maintain 100% O_2 breathing

ANTICIPATED PROBLEMS/CONCERNS

- Heart and brain are target organs
- Prompt CPR (ventilation with O_2) determines outcome
- Follow CNS function
- Seek concomitant smoke inhalation injury and CO toxicity

CYSTIC FIBROSIS

Theodore W. Striker, M.D.

RISK

- Prevalence 1:2500 births
- Incidence 20,000/y
- Race with highest prevalence: Caucasian

PERIOPERATIVE RISKS

- Increased risk of pulmonary problems:
  – pneumothorax
  – V/Q abnormalities
  – hypoxemia
  – obstructive pattern of ventilation

WORRY ABOUT

- Hypoxemia
- Pneumothorax
- Copious secretions with inspissation
- Cor pulmonale

OVERVIEW

- Multisystem disease of exocrine secretory glands involving salivary, sweat, digestive, and pulmonary secretions
- Frequent associated bronchiectasis, hemoptysis
- Recurrent pulmonary infection—frequently antibiotic resistant

ICD-9-CM Code: 277.00

ETIOLOGY

- Recessive inherited disorder—both parents must carry gene to inherit
- Mucus-secreting glands secrete abnormally—precipitation in ducts of secretory glands

USUAL TREATMENT

- Pulmonary therapy—antibiotics for infection, humidity, bronchodilators, chest physiotherapy
- Sweat electrolyte changes—adequate electrolyte intake. Diet: nutrition and enzyme replacement
- Gene therapy still experimental

ASSESSMENT POINTS

SYSTEM	EFFECT	ASSESSMENT BY HX	PE	TEST
HEENT	Frequent nasal polyps	Nasal obstruction Difficulty sleeping	Polyps of nose	
	Sinusitis	Fever, headaches	Sinus drainage	Sinus x-ray, culture
CV	Cor pulmonale	Dyspnea Cough Orthopnea Cyanosis	Tachypnea Rales, rhonchi, wheezing Clubbing of fingers Cyanosis	ECG (if indicated) CXR (if indicated)
RESP	Bronchiectasis Atelectasis Pneumonitis Bronchspasm	Dyspnea Poor exercise tolerance Orthopnea	Hyperinflation of chest Poor ventilation Cyanosis Clubbing Rales and rhonchi Cough, wheezing	CXR PFTs A:a gradient (if indicated)
GI	Cholelithiasis	Abdominal pain—may be asymptomatic	Jaundice	US (if indicated) Cholangiography (if indicated) Glucose
	Pancreatic insufficiency	Poor fat absorption Glucose intolerance		
	Hepatic fibrosis			LFTs
	Intestinal obstruction	Abdominal pain	Abdominal rigidity	GI x-rays (if indicated)
MS	Poor muscle development	Hx of poor nutrition Muscle weakness	Cachexia	

Key Reference: Boat TF, Boucher RC: Cystic fibrosis. *In* Murray JF, Nadel JA (eds): Textbook of Respiratory Medicine, 2nd ed. Philadelphia, WB Saunders, 1994, pp 1418–1450.

PERIOPERATIVE IMPLICATIONS

Preoperative Preparation

- Pulmonary function studies close to time of anesthesia
- CXR
- Blood gases, serum electrolytes, blood glucose
- Bronchodilators, antibiotics, cardiotonic drugs
- Chest physiotherapy

Monitoring

- Routine
- CVP if procedure and CV condition warrant
- Blood glucose—at frequent intervals

Airway

- Early oropharyngeal airway especially with nasal polyps
- Chest or esophageal stethoscope valuable if thorax not badly distorted

Induction

- Parenteral induction faster and more reliable than inhalation induction
- Avoid substances irritating to upper and lower respiratory tract

Maintenance

- High FIO_2
- Ventilatory assistance for severe obstructive airway and reactive airway disease
- Humidification of gases
- Regional techniques helpful for postanesthetic pain management. No evidence that better served by regional instead of general anesthesia

Extubation

- Should be delayed until adequacy of ventilation has reached preanesthetic levels
- May be accompanied by chest physiotherapy, endotracheal suction, and reinflation

Adjuvants

- Bronchodilators
- Digitalis and diuretics in presence of cor pulmonale

Postoperative Period

- Pain management (may include narcotics) to encourage coughing and deep breathing
- Chest physiotherapy
- Early activity

ANTICIPATED PROBLEMS/CONCERNS

- Pneumothorax
- Respiratory insufficiency
- Cor pulmonale
- Electroyte disturbance (Na^+, Cl^-)

CYTOMEGALOVIRUS (CMV) INFECTION

Andrew D. Badley, M.D.
Carlos V. Paya, M.D., Ph.D.

RISK

- Seroprevalence in US: <10 y—25%; 10–25 y—35%; 25–50 y—50%; >50 y—50+%
- Disease from CMV rare in immunocompetent individuals; can cause mononucleosis-like disease
- Disease from CMV in transplant recipients 10–40%
- Disease from CMV in HIV-positive patients 20–30% (increased risk with low CD4 count)
- Gender/race with highest prevalence: ?

PERIOPERATIVE RISKS

- Related to degree of CMV-induced organ dysfunction—pulmonary CNS, hepatic, GI, cardiac, bone marrow, adrenal
- Risk of acquiring CMV from tissue or blood products of CMV-seropositive donor

WORRY ABOUT

- Giving CMV-seropositive blood products to a CMV-seronegative immunocompromised host
- Abnormal hepatic metabolism if CMV hepatitis
- Elevated ICP if CMV encephalitis/meningitis
- Abnormal oxygenation if CMV pneumonitis

- Myocardial dysfunction or arrhythmias if CMV myocarditis
- Perforated viscus 2° to colonic/gastric CMV
- Abnormal bleeding from thrombocytopenia
- Adrenal insufficiency due to CMV adrenalitis

OVERVIEW

- Double-stranded DNA virus; member of herpes family of viruses. Vast majority of North American adults have had prior exposures and are CMV seropositive.
- CMV disease occurs in the following settings:
  – Perinatal infection
  – Intrauterine infection leading to congenital CMV disease
  – Infection of normal host is asymptomatic; rarely may cause a heterophile antibody negative mononucleosis-like syndrome.
  – Infection in immunosuppressed individuals leading to symptomatic or asymptomatic viremia with or without organ involvement: retinitis, encephalitis, meningitis, myelitis, polyneuropathy, pneumonitis, esophagitis, gastritis, colitis, hepatitis, cholangitis, myocarditis, adrenalitis, vasculitis, bone marrow suppression

ICD-9-CM Code: 078.5

ETIOLOGY

- Double-stranded DNA virus
- Transmission through blood/blood products, sexually, perinatally, other contact (daycare, ?medical facilities)

USUAL TREATMENT

- Medical treatment—ganciclovir (IV or oral maintenance), foscarnet (IV), occasionally IV immune globulin. Reduced immunosuppression
- Surgical treatment—none

ASSESSMENT POINTS

SYSTEM	EFFECT	ASSESSMENT BY HX	PE	TEST
RETINA	Destruction of retina	Decreased visual acuity, blind spots	Funduscopy; white and red lesion	Ophthalmology evaluation
CV	Myocarditis; LV dysfunction	CHF symptoms, palpitations	Irregular rhythm, displaced PMI S3	ECG, ECHO, heart biopsy
RESP	Pneumonitis; impaired gas exchange	Dyspnea, nonproductive cough	Wheezes, crackles	CXR, ABG, bronchoscopy ± biopsy
GI	Viral infection of organ	Hepatitis/cholangitis: – Right upper quadrant pain – Jaundice, itching, acholic stools – Esophagitis: dysphagia, odynophagia – Colitis: diarrhea, abdominal pain – Gastritis: pyrosis, anorexia	Signs of hepatic failure, fetor hepaticus, asterixis, jaundice, bruising, painful liver, nonspecific abdominal pain	Liver function tests, ERCP, US, viral blood cultures ± biopsy
HEME	Bone marrow suppression	Rash, fatigue	Petechiae, pallor, tachycardia	CBC
CNS	Encephalitis	Motor or sensory abnormalities, altered mental status	Motor weakness, sensory abnormality, cerebellar ataxia, abnormal tests of cortical function	CT MRI Lumbar puncture

Key Reference: Shepherd FA, Fanning MM, Dupeval R, et al: A guide to the investigation and treatment of patients with AIDS and AIDS-related disorders. Can Med Assn J 1986; 134:999.

PERIOPERATIVE IMPLICATIONS

Perioperative Preparation

- Evaluate for signs of cardiac/hepatic/CNS/bone marrow or adrenal dysfunction

Monitoring

- Routine

Airway

- May require high FIO_2 and PEEP

Preinduction/Induction

- Avoid tachycardia/hypotension

Maintenance

- Follow CO, PCWP, Sao_2, BP

Extubation

- None

Postoperative Period

- Monitor for clinical signs of disease progression

Adjuvants

- None

DEEP VEIN THROMBOSIS

Todd Dorman, M.D.

RISK

- 170,000 diagnosed new cases/y of deep vein thrombosis (DVT) in USA
- 90,000 recurrent cases/y
- True incidence (underdiagnosis) closer to 0.5 million cases/y
- Race with highest prevalence: ?
- Asthma ↑ with smoking, obesity, being bedridden, ↓ LVEF are predisposing factors
- Risk factors include age, previous DVT, paraplegia, spinal cord trauma, major orthopedic surgery, malignancy, hypercoagulable states
- Decreased risk with regional anesthesia vs general

PERIOPERATIVE RISKS

- Without prophylaxis, DVT develops in close to 30% of general surgery cases
- Incidence of fatal pulmonary emboli: 0.1% (general)–5% (total knee replacement)

WORRY ABOUT

- Pulmonary embolism
- Cardiac arrest, electromechanical dissociation
- Hypoxemia and increased dead space potentially leading to respiratory acidosis in patient with controlled ventilation

OVERVIEW

- Clinical findings (e.g., Homans' sign) helpful less than 50% of the time
- Ascending phlebography (venography) is standard for comparison, but has 2–3% incidence of inducing peripheral thrombosis
- Impedance plethysmography (IP), which detects proximal veins, reasonable in symptomatic patients, but lacks sensitivity and specificity in asymptomatic patients
- Compression ultrasonography with Doppler flow imaging better than IP (proximal veins), yet sensitivity falls off in asymptomatic patients. If IP or Doppler-supplemented ultrasonography negative, patient needs serial exams to detect potential progression of distal disease
- CT and MRI are reliable, yet are cumbersome, costly, and routinely not available

ICD-9-CM Code: 453.9 (Thrombosis, vein unspecified)

ETIOLOGY

- Stasis
- Activation of coagulation cascade by tissue trauma
- Hypercoagulability related to congenital or acquired antithrombin III, protein C, or protein S deficiency
- Hypercoagulability related to malignancy, smoking, sedentary lifestyle, ↑ physiologic age, ↓ LVEF
- Hyperviscosity states such as polycythemia vera

USUAL TREATMENT

- Heparin administration prior to warfarin to avoid acute decreases in endogenous anticoagulant protein C
- Thrombolytics

ASSESSMENT POINTS

SYSTEM	EFFECT	ASSESSMENT BY HX	PE	TEST
CV			SVT RV strain	ECG
RESP	Pulmonary embolism	Chest pain Hemoptysis	Tachypnea Wheezing possible	ABG End tidal CO_2
HEME				PT, aPTT Plt count Hgb
MS			Calf pain	Venography

Key Reference: Weinmann EE, Salzman EW: Medical progress: Deep-vein thrombosis. N Engl J Med 1994; 331:1630–1641.

PERIOPERATIVE IMPLICATIONS

Preoperative Preparation

- Sequential compression devices may decrease incidence by activating fibrinolytic system
- Anticoagulation needed for 6 mo after diagnosis and up to the time of procedure
- Consider preoperative placement of an IVC filter in high-risk patients

Monitoring

- Bleeding from residual anticoagulation or drug-induced thrombocytopenia

Airway

- None

Preinduction/Induction

- Regional anesthesia may reduce risk in some orthopedic and genitourinary procedures

Adjuvants

- Depends on etiology—examine specific etiology (e.g., Dilated Cardiomyopathy) in Diseases section
- Heparin, warfarin tissue plasminogen activator, streptokinase/urokinase, anisoylated plasminogen-streptokinase activator complex all increase perioperative bleeding diathesis. Some effect of these agents on other drugs (verify specific drug effects in Drugs section)

Postoperative Period

- In high-risk patients consider full anticoagulation postoperatively as prophylaxis
- Continue sequential use of elastic stockings until patient ambulatory, but do not start in patients suspected of having DVT.

ANTICIPATED PROBLEMS/CONCERNS

- Pulmonary embolism represents life-threatening complication of DVT

DEGENERATIVE DISK DISEASE

John E. Tetzlaff, M.D.

RISK

- Risk factors determined by spinal level
- Cervical spine—C3 and C4 most common, 10% of degenerative disk disease
- Thoracic—uncommon, can be related to trauma, tumor, 0.2–1.8% of disk disease
- Lumbar—very common, 85–90% of disk disease, third most common cause of chronic pain in US

PERIOPERATIVE RISKS

- Difficult airway
- Spinal cord injury from airway manipulation or positioning
- Positioning injury from prone position

WORRY ABOUT

- Cervical spine instability or chronic subluxation
- Difficulty with intubation
- Injury to the spinal cord
- Pressure injuries or ventilatory difficulty with the prone position

OVERVIEW

- Pain from degeneration and herniation of an intervertebral disk is the third most common chronic disease in the US and the most common indication for elective spine surgery
- Incidence varies among spinal segments, being absent in the sacral area, most common in the lumbar area, next with cervical and uncommon in the thoracic region

ICD-9-CM Codes: 722.0 (Cervical); 722.11 (Thoracic); 722.10 (Lumbar)

ETIOLOGY

- Osteoarthritis
- Trauma
- Connective tissue diseases such as rheumatoid arthritis—ankylosing spondylitis

USUAL TREATMENT

- Conservative measures, such as rest, exercises, physical therapy, heat and traction
- Symptoms are treated with analgesics and nonsteroidal anti-inflammatory drugs
- In acute phase, disk herniation can be treated with epidural steroid injection
- Surgery is performed to relieve compression on the spinal cord or specific nerve roots, and to expand the space for nerve root exit from the spinal column

ASSESSMENT POINTS

SYSTEM	EFFECT	ASSESSMENT BY HX	PE	TEST
HEENT	Difficult airway	Neck pain	Decreased ROM	Flexion/extension x-ray
RESP	Lung tumor can mimic symptoms of thoracic disk disease	Chest pain	Abnormal pulmonary auscultation	CXR
GI	GI malignancy can mimic symptoms of thoracic or lumbar disk disease	Truncal pain, abdominal pain	Abdominal mass	CT, MRI
RENAL	Pyelonephritis, cancer of prostate can mimic symptoms of lumbar disk disease	Lumbar pain, muscle spasm, fever/chills	Costovertebral angle tenderness to percussion	Urinalysis, prostate-specific antigen, lumbar spine x-ray
CNS	Myelopathy, anterior spinal cord syndrome	Radiating pain, incontinence, sexual dysfunction, paraplegia	Long tract signs, abnormal reflexes, pathologic, Babinski reflex	X-ray, MRI
PNS	Radiculopathy, absent deep tendon reflexes, peripheral nerve deficits	Sciatica Numbness Weakness of the extremities	Sciatic pain with ROM Motor deficits Patches of decreased sensation	EMG
MS	Pain, decreased ROM, calcification	Pain, night pain, disability from work	Decreased ROM spine	Spine x-ray, MRI

Key Reference: Rothman RA, Simeone FA: The Spine. Philadelphia, WB Saunders, 1989, Chapters 19–23.

PERIOPERATIVE IMPLICATIONS

Preoperative Assessment

- Evaluate coagulation if heavy NSAID use or symptoms of bleeding
- Airway assessment. If signs of cervical instability, flexion-extension x-ray of cervical spine.
- Antisialagogue if awake intubation

Monitoring

- Potential for air embolism, greater with sitting position for posterior approach to cervical spine.
- Consider multilumen right atrial catheter, precordial Doppler

Airway

- If cervical spine not involved, then routine
- If abnormal, choices include awake intubation, inhalation induction, and intubation with induction drugs and muscle relaxants with the head maintained in a neutral position, possibly with traction

Induction

- If airway secured, induction dictated by other aspects of patient's health
- If regional anesthesia, technical difficulty with placment due to anatomic abnormality of the spine
- Consider paramedian dural puncture. Higher levels for dural puncture may result in a better block with spinal stenosis.

Maintenance

- Movement while prone with spinal cord exposed is dangerous. Avoid muscle relaxants after induction if spinal stimulation is used.
- If regional anesthesia, be prepared to re-inject block if duration of surgery exceeds duration of action of local anesthetic injected

Extubation

- Awake and supine are ideal

Adjuvants

- Injury in the prone position to eyes, lips, teeth, tongue, chin, brachial plexus, ulnar nerves, genitalia, peroneal nerves, skin of the patella, and ankles.
- Identify full neurologic function prior to extubation, since re-exploration for compressive hematoma could be indicated for major deficit

Postoperative Period

- Neurologic checks to identify deficits, pain control
- H_2-blocker therapy to prevent GI hemorrhage if steroid Rx chosen for nerve root swelling.

ANTICIPATED PROBLEMS/CONCERNS

- Difficult airway if cervical involvement
- Air embolism—withdraw N_2O if any symptoms
- Transport bed availability and knowledge of how to remove frame, in case sudden transfer to supine position is necessary

DELIRIUM (POSTANESTHETIC)

David J. Cullen, M.D., M.S.

RISK

- Older patients (>70 y) and young patients
- Risk was 5.3% in 1961, although decreasing with newer drugs
- Premedication with barbiturates and/or scopolamine without opioids; phenothiazines; diphenhydramine
- Use of ketamine, Lomotil (atropine), meperidine
- Patients on high-dose steroids
- Withdrawal states—alcohol, barbiturates, meprobamate, or alprazolam
- Metabolic causes—hypoxia, hypercarbia, hyponatremia, hypochloremia, hyperosmolar states
- Incisional pain
- Gastric or urinary bladder distention, urethral irritation resulting from indwelling bladder catheter
- After major surgery (abdominal aortic and noncardiac thoracic surgery)

PERIOPERATIVE RISKS

- Attributing postanesthetic agitation, anxiety, or mental disturbances to drug effect when hypoxia and hypercarbia are the problem
- Patients can harm themselves and others

WORRY ABOUT

- Focusing on drug therapy while forgetting hypoxia and hypercarbia
- Damage to surgical site
- Violent behavior
- Residual hallucinations and nightmares (ketamine)
- Hyperthermia
- Augmenting resp depression from treatment with haloperidol or midazolam

OVERVIEW

- Rapid onset during early recovery from general anesthesia
- Specific cause that is usually reversible and diminishes with time
- Mental dysfunction: cognitive function impaired, emotional lability, inappropriate moods, agitation, belligerence, hallucinations, delusions, illusions, fluctuating state of consciousness

ICD-9-CM Code: 292.81 (drug induced)

ETIOLOGY

- Most important treatment principle: Establish a proper diagnosis. Hypoxia and hypercarbia must be ruled out. Treatment of delirium in presence of hypoxia and hypercarbia not only likely to fail but may accelerate resp depression and worsen hypoxia
- Consider other metabolic disorders such as hypoglycemia, hyponatremia, hepatic encephalopathy, hyperpyrexia
- Anticholinergics (atropine and scopolamine)—parenteral or in eye drops. Delirium associated with high serum levels of anticholinergics, though great variation in these levels in patients taking identical doses
- Drugs with nonspecific CNS effects—phenothiazines, tricyclic antidepressants, sedatives, tranquilizers (diazepam, benzodiazepines, butyrophenones), barbiturates, meperidine, high-dose steroids
- Drug withdrawal from alcohol, barbiturates, benzodiazepines, opioids, or meprobamate
- Unrelieved pain, urinary retention, and gastric distention

USUAL TREATMENT

- Temporary physical restraint
- Nonspecific: opioids, tranquilizers, esp. haloperidol in small IV doses
- Specific treatment: for anticholinergic-induced delirium, physostigmine, 0.5–2 mg IV

ASSESSMENT POINTS

SYSTEM	EFFECT	ASSESSMENT BY HX	PE	TEST
CNS	Postanesthetic delirium	Preop mental status, chronic drug therapy: Intraoperative anesthetic drugs, reversal drugs Oxygen status, ventilation, metabolic status, pain state	Anxiety, agitation, violent behavior, impaired cognition, emotional lability, agitation, hallucinations, fluctuating states of consciousness	O$_2$ saturation, ensurance of normal glucose and lyte status Response to physostigmine

Key Reference: Cassem EH, Lake CR, Boyer WF: Psychopharmacology in the ICU. *In* Chernow B (ed): The Pharmacologic Approach to the Critically Ill Patient, 3rd ed. Baltimore, Williams & Wilkins, 1994.

PERIOPERATIVE IMPLICATIONS

Preoperative Preparation

- Relieve anxiety by discussing anesthetic process with patient, answering all questions, providing assurances

Monitoring

- Routine

Airway

- Ensure clear airway, increase inspired oxygen concentration

Preinduction/Induction

- Avoid scopolamine without accompanying opioid

Maintenance

- Initiate analgesia coverage before ending anesthetic when appropriate

Extubation

- Evaluate for hypoxia and resp depression

Adjuvants

- Specific therapy: physostigmine 0.5–2 mg IV for anticholinergic-induced delirium
- Nonspecific drug–induced delirium:
  - Physostigmine 0.5–2 mg IV
  - Haloperidol 1–5 mg IV; wait 15–30 min to evaluate its effect and repeat or increase dose as needed
  - Midazolam 0.5–1 mg IV
- Assure a clear airway, monitor oxygen saturation, and increase inspired oxygen concentration

ANTICIPATED PROBLEMS/CONCERNS

- Use low-dose physostigmine 0.5–2 mg to avoid excess salivation and vomiting
- Prevention with physostigmine not as effective as treatment with physostigmine
- Opioid coverage during emergence helps limit incidence of delirium but may prolong awakening and promote resp depression
- Always rule out hypoxia/hypercarbia before treating delirium with drugs or restraints

DEMENTIA

David Eric Lees, M.D.

RISK

- People within USA: 4 million +
- Race with highest prevalence: ?
- Affects 20% of those over age 80 y; 50% of those over 50 y; women > men

PERIOPERATIVE RISKS

- Concomitant diseases in elderly patients include osteoarthritis, ASCVD, hypertension, renal disease, rheumatoid arthritis, and diabetes mellitus
- Risk increases with age and concomitant conditions

WORRY ABOUT

- Activities of other neurotransmitters (besides ACh) may be reduced: norepinephrine, serotonin, glutamate, and dopamine

OVERVIEW

- Dementia is a clinical diagnosis of progressive global intellectual impairment with 90% correlation at autopsy
- Alzheimer's disease is most common cause of dementia; more than 50% of all cases in US
- Another 10% due to alcohol abuse and 10% due to vascular disorders (multi-infarct syndrome); multiple metabolic and other causes for the few secondary (reversible) dementias
- Time from onset of symptoms until death, 2–15 y (average, 8 y)
- Dementia in young people may be due to HIV (more than 30% of all HIV cases)

ICD-9-CM Codes: 290.10 (Alzheimer's type); 290.40 (multi-infarct dementia)

ETIOLOGY

- Histopathology shows senile neuritic plaques and neurofibrillary tangles containing cholinergic neurons suggesting impaired cholinergic nerve transmission
- Extensive atrophy of cortical convolutions, especially in hippocampus and temporal lobes
- Changes normally seen in elderly brains, but markedly increased in Alzheimer's disease

USUAL TREATMENT

- Symptomatic treatment has been attempted with agents that affect cholinergic system, such as physostigmine, a centrally acting cholinesterase inhibitor; problems of short effect and high toxicity
- Tacrine has been of some benefit in early Alzheimer's disease, but almost 50% of patients suffer serious side effects

ASSESSMENT POINTS

SYSTEM	EFFECT	PE	TEST
CV	~10% of those with dementia have CVD and generalized ASCVD	Hypertension	ECG
GI	Hepatic injury possible with alcohol abuse etiology		Liver enzymes
ENDO	Hypothyroidism can mimic or exacerbate dementia		T_3, T_4
CNS	Subdural hematoma and hydrocephalus possible causes		EEG, MRI, CT
PNS	Poor motor skills	Neurologic exam	
MS	Generalized stiffness and slowness	Neurologic exam	

Key Reference: Beal MF, Richardson EP, Marin JB: Cecil's Textbook of Medicine, 18th ed. Philadelphia, WB Saunders, 1988, pp 2060–2065.

PERIOPERATIVE IMPLICATIONS

Preoperative Preparation

- Patient most likely cannot give consent or a history; determine if guardian or surrogate identified
- Centrally acting anticholinergics (atropine, scopolamine) and sedatives best avoided; glycopyrrolate is acceptable

Monitoring

- Routine

Airway

- Cervical ROM may be limited by arthritis

Preinduction/Induction

- Propofol may offer most rapid recovery

Maintenance

- No one technique or agent best
- Avoid sedatives and narcotics with long half-lives

Extubation

- Extubate when awake; orientation postoperatively may be further impaired by drugs

Adjuvants

- Can see prolonged effect with sedatives, hypnotics, and narcotics

ANTICIPATED PROBLEMS/CONCERNS

- Poor candidates for regional anesthesia or for PCA in postop period
- Disorientation and delirium postoperatively common—provide familiar person and radio, written orientation material

DEPRESSION — UNIPOLAR

Barbara A. Dodson, M.D.

RISK

- People within USA: 5–10 million
- Race/gender with highest prevalence: ?
- 4% of psychiatric admissions are for electroconvulsive therapy (ECT)

PERIOPERATIVE RISKS

- Risk of adverse drug interactions between antidepressants and anesthetic adjuncts resulting in cardiac arrhythmias and hypertensive crisis
- Cardiac arrythmias, hypertension ↑ cardiac output, and cerebral effects (↑ CMRO$_2$, ↑ CBF, ↑ ICP) 2° to ECT

WORRY ABOUT

- Cardiac arrhythmias, hypotension, hypertension
- ↑ Cardiac output, ↑ BP, bradycardia, tachycardia, myocardial ischemia, and ↑ ICP from ECT
- Neuroleptic malignant syndrome

OVERVIEW

- Most common psychiatric disorder, distinguished from reactive grief and sadness by the severity and duration of the disturbances and presence of fatigue, anorexia, and insomnia
- Most problems are the result of interactions between antidepressants and anesthetic agents:
  – Tricyclics have anticholinergic effects and can interfere with AV conduction
  – MAO ↑ norephinephrine stores, resulting in exaggerated responses to vasoactive agents
- ECT results in marked parasympathetic and sympathetic stimulation

ICD-9-CM Codes: 311; 296.2 (Single episode); 296.2 (Multiple episodes)
See also MAO Inhibitors, Tricyclic Antidepressants, ECT in Drugs and Procedures sections

ETIOLOGY

- Etiology is unknown
- ↓ Serotonin and norepinephrine levels in the CNS have been implicated
- Mechanisms underlying therapeutic effect of ECT remains unknown

USUAL TREATMENT

- Medical therapy—antidepressant drugs such as tricyclic and tetracyclic antidepressants, serotonin reuptake inhibitors, and MAO inhibitors (MAOIs)
- ECT used in cases that failed medical therapy or for whom antidepressants are contraindicated

ASSESSMENT POINTS

SYSTEM	EFFECT	ASSESSMENT BY HX	PE	TEST
HEENT	Dry mouth, blurred vision	Glaucoma, retinal detachment	↓ Visual acuity	Funduscopic exam
CV	AV conduction delays, bradycardia, tachyarrhythmias, hypertensive crisis	Angina, CHF symptoms, cardiac pacemaker, thrombophlebitis	Volume status, BP, S$_3$	ECG (±stress test) Echocardiography
RESP		CHF, severe pulmonary disease	S$_3$, rales, wheezing	CXR
GI	Delayed gastric emptying	Reflux		
ENDO		Symptoms suggestive of pheochromocytoma	Unexplained severe hypertension	Vanillylmandelic acid levels
RENAL	Urinary retention	Difficulty urinating		
CNS	Neuroleptic malignant syndrome	Recent CVA, intracranial surgery, intracranial mass lesion	Neurologic deficits, symptoms of ↑ ICP	CT, MRI, neurologic exam
MS		Severe osteoporosis or major fractures	Fractures, limited joint mobility	Skeletal x-rays, MRI

Key Reference: Psychiatric illness and substance abuse. *In* Stoelting RK, Dierdorf SF: Anesthesia and Co-Existing Disease, 3rd ed. New York, Churchill Livingstone, 1993, pp 517–538.

PERIOPERATIVE IMPLICATIONS

Preoperative Preparation
- Discontinuing MAOI 2 weeks prior to surgery may not be necessary

Monitoring
- Consider arterial pressure monitoring

Airway
- Risk of gastric reflux
- Maintain cricoid pressure during induction

Maintenance
- Combination of pancuronium, halothane, and exogenous epinephrine can result in malignant tachyarrhythmias

- Meperidine is absolutely contraindicated in patients on MAOI. Other opioids should be used with care
- Indirected vasopressors should be avoided
- ECT results in marked parasympathetic, followed by sympathetic, stimulation

Extubation
- Risk of aspiration following extubation

Postoperative Period
- Potential problems with seizures or agitation
- May exhibit respiratory depression and delayed emergence from anesthesia

Adjuvants
- Esmolol and phentolamine for hypertensive crises. Atropine for bradycardia
- ECT usually performed using a short-acting IV anesthetic (e.g., propofol or methohexital) and a short-acting muscle relaxant

ANTICIPATED PROBLEMS/CONCERNS

- Tricyclic antidepressants have anticholinergic effects and can interfere with AV conduction
- MAOI ↑ norepinephrine stores, which can result in exaggerated responses to vasoactive substances
- Patients should be monitored for signs of neuroleptic malignant syndrome, such as hyperthermia, autonomic dysfunction, and muscle rigidity

DIABETES INSIPIDUS

George J. Graf, M.D.

RISK

- Frequently occurs in childhood–early adulthood; males > females, males usually by sexlinked recessive transmission
- Nephrogenic diabetes insipidus (DI) rarely congenital; familial
- Racial predominance: none

PERIOPERATIVE RISKS

- Dehydration, hypernatremia, death
- Altered sensorium
- Hemodynamic instability
- Distended bladder, hydroureter

WORRY ABOUT

- Fluid and electrolyte imbalance during anesthesia
- New onset of central DI following serious head trauma
- Variable onset of central DI following pituitary surgery (1–6 days postop)
- Drug-induced renal tubular unresponsiveness to vasopressin (nephrogenic DI) (fluoride-related [or associated] toxicity, lithium, osmotic diuretics, etc)

OVERVIEW

- Endocrinopathy associated with serum electrolyte and volume abnormalities
- Polyuria, excessive thirst, and polydipsia regularly present
- Dehydration unusual in awake patient
- Inadequate fluid replacement of excreted urine leads to hypernatremia and dehydration causing weakness, fever, altered sensorium, hemodynamic instability, and death
- Monitor urine output, serum osmolality, and electrolyte concentrations during perioperative period
- Ensure adequate fluid replacement

ICD-9-CM Code: 253.5

ETIOLOGY

- Inadequate production or release of vasopressin (ADH) from posterior pituitary
- Most frequently caused by neoplastic or infiltrative lesions of pituitary, pituitary surgery, severe head injury following cardiac resuscitation; may be idiopathic
- Renal tubular unresponsiveness to endogenous or exogenous vasopressin (ADH) usually acquired
  - acute tubular necrosis
  - renal transplantation
  - drug-induced: lithium, amphotericin, osmotic diuretics, fluoride toxicity
  - hypokalemia, chronic hypercalcemia
  - systemic disorders: multiple myeloma, sickle cell disease

USUAL TREATMENT

- Hormone replacement: aqueous vasopressin, desmopressin
- Nonhormonal ADH stimulation: chlorpropamide
- Nephrogenic diabetes insipidus: hydrochlorothiazide, salt restriction

ASSESSMENT POINTS

SYSTEM	EFFECT	ASSESSMENT BY HX	PE	TEST
CV	Hypotension Tachycardia Myocardial ischemia	Orthostasis Reduced exercise tolerance	Orthostatic BP, HR	ECG
ENDO	Anterior pituitary dysfunction	Pituitary neoplasm or surgery	Multisystem effects 2° multiple hormone deficiencies	Levels assess anterior pituitary function
RENAL	Polyuria 1° or 2° nephropathy	Frequent dilute urine	Urine volume	24-h urine; simultaneous measurement of plasma and urine osmolality
CNS	Visual disturbance Altered sensorism	Excessive thirst Polydipsia	Neurologic function	CT scan

Key Reference: Braunwald E (ed): Harrison's Principles of Internal Medicine, 13th ed. New York, McGraw-Hill, 1994, pp 1923–1928.

PERIOPERATIVE IMPLICATIONS

Preoperative Preparation

- Dx and appropriate Rx
- Assess electrolytes, serum osmolality, and volume status
- Rule out additional hormone deficiencies
- Discontinue provocative medications: lithium, mannitol

Monitoring

- Urine output with Foley catheter
- Serum electrolytes
- Intravascular volume

Airway

- Generally not affected

Induction

- Patient may be hypovolemic with BP and HR fluctuation, electrolyte abnormalities, and arrhythmias

Maintenance

- CV instability
- Fluid and electrolyte replacement dependent on multiple factors

Extubation

- Altered sensorium; unable to protect airway

Adjuvants

- Fluoride toxicity from prolonged enflurane or sevoflurane extremely rare as cause of renal tubular dysfunction

- Variable neuromuscular relaxant activity in presence of hypokalemia or hypercalcemia
- Chlorpropamide treatment for DI may cause hypoglycemia

ANTICIPATED PROBLEMS/CONCERNS

- Vasopressin therapy causes vasoconstriction, and acute treatment could precipitate myocardial ischemia in unstable patient with CAD
- Plasma osmolality affected by increases in BUN or glucose; urine osmolality below that of serum in severe cases of DI; urine osmolality will not increase following ADH therapy of nephrogenic origin

DIABETES, TYPE I (INSULIN REQUIRING) Michael F. Roizen, M.D.

RISK

- People within USA: 1 million
- Race with highest prevalence: ↑ in Hispanics and Native Americans

PERIOPERATIVE RISKS

- Increase risk of CABG 5–10× if end-stage renal, CHF, or autonomic neuropathy; without renal, CHF, or autonomic dysfunction, risk is 1–1.5× of normal

WORRY ABOUT

- Autonomic neuropathy and gastroparesis and sudden postop death
- Painless myocardial ischemia
- Atlanto-occipital joint immobility
- Tight glucose control might be indicated if pregnant, difficult weaning from bypass (ECC), or predictable global or focal CNS ischemia

OVERVIEW

- Endocrinopathy associated with end-stage renal, myocardial, and neuropathic disease
- Blood sugar control per se not associated with increased perioperative risk in absence of
  - hypoglycemia
  - hyperosmolar coma
  - ketoacidosis
  - CNS ischemia
  - pregnancy
  - extracorporeal circulation
- Causes deranged autoregulation to CNS (blood sugar, 250 mg/dl), renal (blood sugar, 225 mg/dl), and cardiac (blood sugar, 100 mg/dl) vessels
- Thus need to control BP or blood sugar to decrease damage to these vessels and organs
- Check patient glucose log for degree of control
- Variable control may predict perioperative hypoglycemic episodes

ICD-9-CM Code: 850.09

See also Insulin; Diabetic ketoacidosis

ETIOLOGY

- Genetic predisposition to autoimmune destruction of glucose transporter on islet cells → increased blood glucose—affects proteins via nonenzymatic glycosylations?
- Swells cells (sorbitol is oncotically active)
- Increased viscous proteins (macroglobins), which impede blood flow
- Increased substrate for anaerobic metabolism
- Deranges autoregulation of blood flow

USUAL TREATMENT

- Insulin injections, diet, and exercise
- Pancreas transplant is rare option

ASSESSMENT POINTS

SYSTEM	EFFECT	ASSESSMENT BY HX	PE	TEST
HEENT	Possible atlanto-occipital dislocation prayer sign of opposing palms correlate with, 2° to abnormal collagen glycosylation	Pain	Neck ROM Prayer sign	Usually not needed Neck x-rays in extension
CV	Angiopathy LV dysfunction (4–10× with hypertension) Ischemic periph vascular disease	Exercise tolerance Angina CHF symptoms	2-flight walk Chest exam for signs of CHF BP lying and standing	ECG CXR
RESP	↓ Lung elastance ↓ FEV; ↓ FVC	Exercise tolerance		Generally not needed
GI	Gastroparesis	Early satiety		
RENAL	Nephropathy, especially if hypertensive	N/V; impotence; orthostatic Sx Non-protein foods		BUN/Cr
ENDO	↓ Insulin from islets			FBS, electrolytes
CNS	Autonomic dysfunction 2° to neuropathy	Early satiety; impotence; N/V; orthostatic symptoms		RR interval variation on ECG BP change on standing
PNS	Stocking-glove neuropathy → infections		PNS exam, especially regional planned	
MS	Impaired joint mobility 2° to non-enzymatic glycosylation of collagen	Joint mobility	↓ ROM of joints	

Key Reference: Roizen MF: Miller Anesthesia, ed 4. New York, Churchill Livingstone, 1994, pp 905–911.

PERIOPERATIVE IMPLICATIONS

Preoperative Preparation

- Metoclopramide (10 mg/70 kg) in patients with gastroparesis
- Assess myocardial and volume status

Monitoring

- Painless myocardial ischemia. Can have CHF if vol overload and LV dysfunction present
- Blood sugar

Airway

- Atlanto-occipital dislocation possible—see HEENT—do prayer sign test; may have gastroparesis

Induction

- Osmotic diuresis can make hypovolemic; ANS and CV dysfunction make BP and HR fluctuate

Maintenance

- CV instability; volume status key to avoid renal and myocardial dysfunction with operation

Extubation

- CV and pulm drive insufficiencies common with neuropathies

Adjuvants

- See Insulin in Drugs section
- Rx for tight control
- Muscle relaxants: no key point

- Regional: Diabetic nerves may be more prone to edema especially if epinephrine used. Reduce dose (e.g., lidocaine from 2.0% to 1.5%) for same effect

Postoperative Period

- Sliding scale of insulin Rx based on q 1–3 h blood glucose determinations

ANTICIPATED PROBLEMS/CONCERNS

- Gastroparesis with presence of solid food 24 hours after last meal if ANS dysfunction present. Consider Rx with metoclopramide 10 mg IM 1½ hours prior to induction
- ANS dysfunction associated with sudden death postop; can keep in ICU/PACU overnight; vested adult who can measure blood glucose and call 911 if sent home postop

DIABETES, TYPE II

Michael F. Roizen, M.D.
Stanley H. Rosenbaum, M.D.

RISK

- People within USA: 13–14 million
- Highest prevalence: Hispanics and Native Americans
- Gender predominance: none

PERIOPERATIVE RISKS

- Increased risk 5–10× if end-stage renal, CV, CHF, or autonomic neuropathy; without renal, CV, or autonomic dysfunction, risk is 1–1.5× normal
- Metabolic abnormalities increased with perioperative insulin Rx
- Unclear if same risks as for type I diabetes

WORRY ABOUT

- Autonomic neuropathy, gastroparesis, and sudden postop death
- Painless myocardial ischemia; CV instability
- Tight glucose control controversial in type II as opposed to type I diabetes, but might be indicated in pregnancy (see under Diabetes, Type III), difficult weaning from bypass (ECC), predictable global or focal CNS ischemia

- Disordered autoregulation makes hypertensive BP fluctuations more dangerous
- Fluid and electrolyte imbalance

OVERVIEW

- Endocrinopathy that can cause same organ dysfunction as in diabetes, type I: end-stage renal, myocardial, and neuropathic disease
- Associated with deranged blood flow autoregulation to CNS (at blood sugar 250 mg/dl), renal (at blood sugar 200 mg/dl), and cardiac (at blood sugar 100 mg/dl) vessels
- Ketosis is rare, since there is some endogenous insulin production
- Primarily controlled by diet and/or oral agents, although insulin sometimes required
- Usually has high insulin levels for glucose level, but peripheral resistance to insulin effect. Can develop hyperosmolar nonketotic coma
- Blood sugar control per se not associated with increased perioperative morbidity in absence of:
  - hypoglycemia
  - hyperosmolar coma
  - CNS ischemia
  - pregnancy
  - extracorporeal circulation
- Check patient glucose log for degree of control

ICD-9-CM Codes: 250.00; 250.02 (uncontrolled)
See also Diabetes, Type I

ETIOLOGY

- Familial predisposition with very high concordance in identical twins
- Autosomal dominant with variable expression accentuated by conditions that increase peripheral insulin resistance (obesity, inactivity, certain changes, hormones), increase glucose production or metabolic demands (glucocorticoids, pregnancy) or decrease insulin secretion (certain ß-adrenergic drugs)
- Increases non-enzymatic glycosylations
- Causes cell swelling
- Deranges autoregulation
- Increases viscous protein production
- Increases substrate for anaerobic metabolism

USUAL TREATMENT

- Hypoglycemic agents, diet, exercise, insulin

ASSESSMENT POINTS

SYSTEM	EFFECT	ASSESSMENT BY HX	PE	TEST
HEENT	Possible atlanto-occipital dislocation	Pain	Neck ROM, prayer sign	
CV	Premature CAD Hypertension Peripheral vascular disease	Angina Claudication Symptoms of CHF	Peripheral pulses	ECG CAD-related tests as indicated
RESP	↓ Pulm elastance	Exercise tolerance		
GI	Gastroparesis	Early satiety		
ENDO	Hyperglycemia Osmotic diuretic–caused hypokalemia	Polyuria		Blood glucose, K+
HEME	Infection from ↓ WBC phagocytic function		Site of infections	
RENAL	Nephropathy	Asymptomatic although often associated with neuropathy		BUN/Cr, UA for protein
CNS	Cerebrovascular disease Medication-induced hypoglycemia	TIAs, CVAs Long-acting oral hypoglycemic agents	CNS exam	
PNS	Distal neuropathy Postural hypotension	Impotence Foot infections	PNS exam, esp prior to regional anesthetic	
MS	Impaired joint mobility		ROM of joints	

Key Reference: Roizen MF: Miller's Anesthesia, 4th ed. New York, Churchill Livingstone, 1994, pp 905–911.

PERIOPERATIVE IMPLICATIONS

Preoperative Preparation

- Metoclopramide (10 mg/70 kg) if gastroparesis
- Assess myocardial and autonomic function and volume status, half-life of hypoglycemic agent(s) taken chronically

Monitoring

- Blood sugar (but ? tight control in type II diabetes and metabolic abnormalities)
- Painless myocardial ischemia can cause CHF if volume overload and LV dysfunction
- Peripheral vasculature and nerves vulnerable to pressure ischemia

Airway

- Atlantic-occipital dislocation possible—see HEENT, do prayer sign test

Induction

- Osmotic diuresis, autonomic nervous system and CV dysfunction can make BP/HR fluctuate

Maintenance

- CV instability: volume status and avoidance of hypertension key to avoiding renal and myocardial dysfunction perioperatively

Extubation

- CV and pulmonary drive insufficiencies common with neuropathies

Adjuvants

- See Oral hypoglycemics in Drugs section
- Regional: diabetic nerves may be more prone to edema, especially if epinephrine used. Reduce dose (e.g., lidocaine from 2.0% to 1.5%) for same effect

Postoperative Period

- Debate as to whether control to tighter than 60–250 ml/dl is of value in absence of hypertension

ANTICIPATED PROBLEMS/CONCERNS

- Autonomic nervous system dysfunction associated with sudden death postop; can need monitoring for respiratory function in ICU/PACU overnight; presence of adult at home who can measure blood glucose and call 911
- Infections and end-organ risk substantially increased with blood sugar >250 mg/dl. Hypoglycemic symptoms hidden by autonomic nervous system dysfunction, effects of regional, sedative-narcotic, and ß-adrenergic receptor blocking agents
- Avoid excess dextrose infusion as part of volume resuscitation

DIABETES, TYPE III (GESTATIONAL DIABETES MELLITUS)   Richard Clark, M.D.

RISK

- Incidence of gestational diabetes (GDM) is 10 × higher than that of overt diabetes
- Increased in African-American and Hispanic women
- Risk factors are:
  - Maternal age >25 y
  - Previous delivery of macrosomic infant
  - Previous unexplained fetal demise
  - Previous pregnancy with GDM
  - Strong immediate family history of NIDDM or GDM
  - Obesity (>90 kg)
  - Fasting glucose >140 mg/dl or random glucose >100 mg/dl

PERIOPERATIVE RISKS

- Unlikely renal, ocular, cardiac, neurologic, or orthopedic complications in GDM
- Hypoglycemia if insulin is used
- Fetal risk [if not controlled: polyhydramnios or macrosomia (6× normal)]
- RDS (2–3×normal); preeclampsia, neonatal hypoglycemia, prematurity

WORRY ABOUT

- Hyperglycemia and hypoglycemia

OVERVIEW

- Gestational diabetes is defined as a carbohydrate intolerance that occurs (or is first recognized) during pregnancy.
- A glucose tolerance test is used to identify GDM. For details of the test, see the Key Reference
- Maternal complications with GDM are few, but the fetus is at risk.
- Complications, such as fetal polyhydramnios, macrosomia (6×), prematurity, birth trauma, RDS (2–3× normal rate), neonatal hypoglycemia, or morbidity, are as common with type III diabetes (GDM) as with type I diabetes (insulin-requiring)

ICD-9-CM Code: 648.8
See under Pregnancy, Physiologic Changes and Diabetes, Type I and Type II

ETIOLOGY

- GDM occurs in genetically susceptible individuals
- Pregnancy through secretion of substances from uterus exerts diabetogenic effects

USUAL TREATMENT

- Use of insulin in GDM remains controversial. Diet has been used in management.
- Many clinicians obtain a single HbA_{1c} level at 6–12 wk gestation. In patients with mildly elevated plasma glucose levels and normal concentration of HbA_{1c}, dietary modification alone and a modest increase in exercise are often sufficient to normalize plasma glucose levels.
- If the fasting blood sugar exceeds 120 mg/dl, insulin may be required. Both regular and NPH insulin are used.

ASSESSMENT POINTS

SYSTEM	EFFECT	ASSESSMENT BY HX	PE	TEST
HEENT	Possible facial/pharyngeal edema	Snoring	Neck ROM Malampatti exam	
CV	CV changes of pregnancy—possible worse hypovolemia from osmotic diuresis		BP/HR with orthostatic maneuvers	
RESP	Resp changes of pregnancy, ↓ FRC, etc.			
GI	Gastroparesis of pregnancy	Early satiety		
ENDO	Neonatal hypoglycemia if maternal hyperglycemia Obesity			Blood sugar; glucose levels Acid-base status of fetus; HbA_{1c} in mother
HEME	Not present unless type I diabetes			
RENAL	↓ Renal function			BUN/Cr
CNS	ANS dysfunction	Gastroparesis, early satiety	Orthostatic BP	Tilt-table test
PNS	Neuropathy not present unless Type I diabetes			

Key Reference: Moore TR: Diabetes in pregnancy. *In* Creasy RK, Resnik R (eds): Maternal•Fetal Medicine. Philadelphia, WB Saunders, 1994, pp 934–978.

PERIOPERATIVE IMPLICATIONS

Preoperative Preparation
- Full stomach precautions: nonparticulate antacid administration usual

Monitoring
- Blood sugar in maternal and umbilical vein blood

Airway
- Examine for edema

Induction
- Regional anesthesia preferred to general anesthetic due to risks of aspiration and failed airway attainment if cesarean section is performed
- Osmotic diuresis can cause hypovolemia and increase BP and HR fluctuations

Maintenance
- CV instability: volume status is key to maintenance of uterine and other organ perfusion

Extubation
- Awake

Adjuvants
- Regional: Diabetic nerves may be more prone to edema especially if epinephrine used. Reduced dose (e.g., lidocaine from 1.5% to 1%) for same effect.

Postoperative Period
- Usually GDM cured by delivery

ANTICIPATED PROBLEMS/CONCERNS

- Fetal dysfunction, especially hypoglycemia and acidosis, if maternal hypoglycemia present
- Rapid changes in maternal blood glucose can accompany the pain/exertion of vaginal delivery of fetus and accompany the endocrine changes of uterine delivery

DIABETIC KETOACIDOSIS (DKA)

John R. Ammon, M.D.

John R. Ammon, M.D.

RISK

- Patients with type I diabetes mellitus; rare in type II (see Diabetes, Type I in Diseases section)
- Diabetic with local or systemic septic process requiring surgery (e.g., appendicitis, perinephric abscess)

PERIOPERATIVE RISKS

- Cardiovascular collapse 2° to severe dehydration (diuresis, fluid deprivation, fever) and myocardial depression (severe acidosis)
- CNS injury 2° to cerebral edema with rapid correction of DKA
- Worsening of pre-existing end-organ dysfunction (e.g., nephropathy → ATN, CAD → perioperative MI)

WORRY ABOUT

- Fluid deficit of 3–8 L in established DKA
- Cardiac arrest or severe shock with onset of GA or regional anesthesia
- Severe electrolyte derangements, esp total body potassium deficiency of several hundred milliequivalents
- Necessity of surgical therapy to treat etiology of DKA (abscess, gangrene)

OVERVIEW

- DKA is a metabolic emergency sometimes caused by a septic process requiring acute surgical care
- Absolute or relative deficiency of insulin and excess of glucagon causing severe hyperglycemia (300–800 mg/dl) with accompanying acidosis, dehydration, and organ dysfunction
- Perioperative approach as much hemodynamic as metabolic for favorable outcome

ICD-9-CM Code: 250.1

ETIOLOGY

- Type I diabetes with insulin deficiency caused by cessation of insulin therapy coupled with significant physical (infection, surgery) or emotional stress
- Glucagon, epinephrine, and cortisol operative in driving catabolic and ketogenic state
- Osmotic diuresis 2° to sustained hyperglycemia leads to volume depletion
- Metabolic acidosis a product of unrestrained free fatty acid release from adipose tissue and subsequent hepatic oxidation to ketone bodies from insulin lack and glucagon excess

USUAL TREATMENT

- Treat initiating cause
- Insulin, aggressive rehydration, correction of electrolyte derangements, hemodynamic support

ASSESSMENT POINTS

SYSTEM	EFFECT	ASSESSMENT BY HX	PE	TEST
CV	Hypovolemia	Duration of initiating event, postural symptoms	Tilt test, BP HR, skin turgor Mucous membranes	CVP ABG
RESP	Hyperventilation (Kussmaul respiration)		Ventilatory rate and depth	ABG
GI	Anorexia, N/V	Appetite, N/V		
RENAL	Diuresis	Urinary frequency, thirst		BUN/Cr
ENDO	Insulin deficiency, glucagon excess during severe catabolic stress	Type I diabetes		Blood glucose ABG Potassium
CNS	Depression from lethargy to coma; late cerebral edema in children		Assess LOC Signs of ↑ ICP	

Key Reference: Foster DW: Diabetes mellitus. *In* Harrison's Principles of Internal Medicine, 12th ed. New York, McGraw-Hill, 1991, pp 1752–1753.

PERIOPERATIVE IMPLICATIONS

Perioperative Preparation

- Vigorous isotonic saline infusion to restore hemodynamic stability (use 0.5 N saline if serum osmolality is >310 mOsm/L); CVP measurement appropriate in perioperative setting
- Insulin Rx usually begins with 0.1 U of reg insulin/kg IV with infusion of 0.1 U of reg insulin/kg/h

Monitoring

- Sequential glucose, pH, K⁺, anion gap, urine output determinations during perioperative period; CVP catheter, possibly PA catheter if pre-existing myocardial dysfunction known; high incidence of occult CAD

Airway

- Potential stiff joint syndrome with difficult intubation; full stomach status

Induction

- Hemodynamic instability likely if intravascular volume depletion not corrected; pre-existing autonomic neuropathy and CV dysfunction

Maintenance

- Protection of end-organs often compromised by diabetes mellitus, esp heart, CNS, renal

Extubation

- Awake

Adjuvants

- (See under Diabetes in Diseases section)

Postoperative Period

- Potential for hypoglycemic injury from rapid increase in insulin sensitivity when surgical cause of DKA corrected
- Medical management continued by physician with expertise in diabetes

ANTICIPATED PROBLEMS/CONCERNS

- Hemodynamic instability from combined volume deficiency, acidosis, and pre-existing CV disease
- CNS dysfunction from metabolic abnormalities, both early and late

DIAPHRAGMATIC HERNIA (CONGENITAL) Joan M. Niehoff, M.D.

RISK

- Occurs in ~1/5,000 births; 12–25% have associated anomalies.

PERIOPERATIVE RISKS

- 30–60% mortality in live births
- Pulmonary hypoplasia and associated CNS and CV malformations affect mortality
- Timing of diagnosis associated with the prognosis (high-risk newborn presents with respiratory failure within first 6 h of life)

WORRY ABOUT

- Hypoxemia and acidosis
- Shock
- Tension pneumothorax

OVERVIEW

- Classified by site of herniation.
- Posterolateral defects (Bochdalek) (90%), and left-sided defects occuring most frequently (80–90%); Morgagni hernias rare (5%), parasternal, less symptomatic; therefore, diagnosed at later age
- Degree of lung hypolasia determined by time of defect during fetal development and amount of abdominal contents in chest, result in decreased numbers and function of alveoli; hypoplastic lung has high vascular resistance
- Ipsilateral lung most affected; both lungs abnormal.
- Surgical treatment delayed for medical stabilization

ICD-9-CM Code: 756.6

INDICATIONS/USUAL TREATMENT

- Posterolateral defects require repair (does not resolve the pulmonary dysfunction)
- Small defects closed primarily; larger defects use artificial diaphragm, which contributes to postoperative respiratory failure
- ECMO indicated if severe pulmonary hypertension and/or hypercarbia despite maximal conventional management
- Fetal surgery still experimental

ASSESSMENT POINTS

SYSTEM	EFFECT	ASSESSMENT BY HX	PE	TEST
CV	Mediastinal shift Associated ASD, VSD, coarctation, tetralogy of Fallot (23%)	Displaced cardiac impulse	CV exam	ECHO
RESP	Respiratory distress, pulmonary hypertension	↓ Breath sounds on affected side Prominent ipsilateral chest	Pulmonary exam	CXR ABG
GI	Malrotation, atresia (20%)	Scaphoid abdomen	Abd exam	
GU	Hypospadias		Inspection	
CNS	Spinal bifida, hydrocephalus, anencephaly (28%)		Inspection and neurologic exam	Ultrasound, CT scan
METAB	Acidosis, hypoxemia, hypercarbia			ABG

Key Reference: Morin, et al: Prenatal diagnosis and management of fetal thoracic lesions. Semin Perinatol 1994; 18:228.

PERIOPERATIVE IMPLICATIONS

Perioperative Management

- ECMO provides temporary support until perinatal circulation matures and less sensitive to vasoconstrictive stimuli (1–2 wk)

Preoperative Preparation

- Avoid triggers for pulmonary vasoconstriction
- Goals include a $PaO_2 > 80$, $PaCO_2$ 25–30, normal or elevated pH, and normothermia
- Monitor pre- and postductal oxygenation
- NG tube
- Endotracheal intubation (unless small defect without respiratory distress)
- Sedation/analgesia/paralysis
- Watch for pneumothorax; consider prophylactic contralateral chest tube
- "Honeymoon" phase of adequate oxygenation after birth implies adequate alveolar surface

Anesthetic Technique

- Opioids well tolerated; inhaled halogenated anesthetics are not; avoid N_2O.

Monitoring

- Routine and (preductal) arterial line

Surgical Stages

- Left subcostal incision usual; occasionally, thoracic approach used
- Reduction of herniated viscera by gentle traction, followed by excision of hernia sac
- Suture repair of defect; large defects may require flap or prosthetic material
- Small peritoneal cavity may limit closure (staged closure may be required)
- Ipsilateral chest tube usual before diaphragmatic closure and placed on water seal; prophylactic con-tralateral chest tube often used

POSTOPERATIVE CONSIDERATIONS

- If A-aDO_2 gradient >400 mm Hg or if cardiopulmonary deterioration, continue respiratory assistance
- Persistent hypoxemia while on high FIO_2 suggests persistent pulmonary hypertension
- Minimize endotracheal suctioning, correct metabolic acidosis
- Deliver adequate nutrition
- Outlook dependent on pulmonary hypoplasia and bronchopulmonary dysplasia
- High degree of neurologic problems, whether or not infants placed on ECMO; seizures, developmental delay, and hearing loss in 20–30 %

DIARRHEA, ACUTE AND CHRONIC

Michelle Braunfeld, M.D.

RISK

- Acute: 20% of population at sometime during year
- Chronic: 5% of population; increasing with age
- Acute: male = female
- Chronic: female > male

PERIOPERATIVE RISKS

- Hypovolemia with hemodynamic instability
- Electrolyte abnormalities, especially hypokalemia
- Acid/base abnormalities: may be non–anion gap acidosis or alkalosis, depending on underlying cause

WORRY ABOUT

Chronic

- Underlying disease, especially iatrogenic (e.g., infection with antibiotic-induced diarrhea, end-stage liver disease with lactulose-induced diarrhea, or disaccharide [usually lactose] intolerance)
- Hormone-producing tumors (e.g., carcinoid, VIPomas, gastrinomas)
- Stress steroid therapy in inflammatory bowel disease
- Psychological symptoms in up to 50% of patients with irritable bowel syndrome; often alternates with constipation
- Postsurgical losses that may drain via ileostomy or fistula, or may be due to inadequate bowel absorption 2° to resection (short bowel syndrome)

Acute

- Viral, bacterial, or protozoan disease

OVERVIEW

- Acute: abrupt onset of loose stools in healthy individual: viral—self-limited, 1–3 days causing changes in small intestinal cells → shortened transit time; bacterial—tends to occur in groups of individuals (if within 12 h of a meal, usually due to preformed toxin); protozoan—prolonged watery diarrhea from contaminated water supply in endemic area.
- Chronic: Too frequent passage of stools that are too loose for too long; >200 g/day of stool for >1 mo
- Multifactorial medical problem that requires supportive therapy and attention to the underlying etiology
- Only one in a spectrum of medical problems associated with an underlying disease or with treatment of disease. Supportive therapy includes fluid and electrolyte repletion, and attention to acid/base balance.

ICD-9-CM Code: 558.9

ETIOLOGY

Chronic

- Osmotic—laxatives, indigestible carbohydrates.
- Secretory—hormone-producing tumors.
- Exudative—inflammatory bowel disease, pseudomembranous colitis.
- Decreased mucosal contact/mixing—short bowel syndrome.

Acute

- Viral or bacterial (with or without toxin) or protozoan (see Overview)

USUAL TREATMENT

- Volume and electrolyte replacement.
- Although acid/base correction often follows above, may occasionally need replacement.
- Seek and treat underlying cause.

ASSESSMENT POINTS

SYSTEM	EFFECT	ASSESSMENT BY HX	PE	TEST
CV	Hypovolemia	Postural symptoms, quantitation of bowel movements	Orthostatic changes Narrow pulse pressure Tachycardia Dry mucous membranes	
	Dysrhythmia 2° to electrolyte abnormalities			ECG
RESP	Compensatory hyperventilation			ABG
HEME	Derangement dependent on underlying cause			Lab values include ECG, Ca^{2+}, Mg^{2+}
RENAL	Pre-renal azotemia			BUN/Cr
CNS	Profound electrolyte abnormality		Range from drowsiness to obtundation	

PERIOPERATIVE IMPLICATIONS

Preoperative Preparation

- Assess volume status
- Repletion

Monitoring

- Consider arterial and central venous catheter (or some other fluid status monitor such as TEE) if significant hypovolemia and CV compromise present

Airway

- May require full-stomach precautions

Induction

- Hemodynamic instability and ↓ drug dosage if not repleted
- Sympatholytic drugs and sympathectomy with regional anesthesia can shorten transit time and increase diarrhea

Maintenance

- Tailor IV fluids to electrolyte and acid/base status (e.g., avoid normal saline if patient already has hyperchloremic acidosis).
- Continue electrolyte repletion if necessary.

Extubation

- Routine, dependent on underlying condition

Adjustments

- Acid/base status and electrolytes may affect muscle relaxant duration and ability of antagonists to reverse block.

ANTICIPATED PROBLEMS/CONCERNS

- Most operations do not affect underlying condition, but narcotics can make diarrhea less problematic or more problematic, and generally worsen constipation
- Regional anesthesia that causes sympathectomy leaves parasympathetic system unopposed, which can cause shortened transit time and increase diarrhea

DILATED CARDIOMYOPATHIES (DCMs)

Paul J. Dauchot, M.D.

RISK

- Prevalence varies from 8.3 to 36.5/100,000
- Higher mortality in elderly
- Racial predominance: African-American
- Gender predominance: male-to-female, 3:1
- 10,000 deaths from DCM reported annually in USA

PERIOPERATIVE RISKS

- Arrhythmias, systolic dysfunction, CHF, autonomic instability, intracardiac thrombi, diabetes, and ischemic heart disease
- Smoking history, diabetes mellitus, and high diastolic blood pressure are reportedly predictors of mortality from idiopathic DCM (IDCM)

WORRY ABOUT

- Malignant arrhythmias, sudden death
- Worsening systolic and diastolic function
- Fluid overload/CHF, "emboli," amiodarone- and implantable cardiac defibrillator (ICD)-related problems

OVERVIEW

- Disease characterized by dilatation of right, left, or both ventricles; increased EDV, ESV, and wall stress
- Systolic function is impaired; ejection fraction is below 0.4 or is 2 SD below normal values; SV may be normal
- Often CHF and tachyarrhythmias
- Intracardiac mural thrombi may be present
- High risk of sudden death

ICD-9-CM Code: 425.4 (Cardiomyopathy, idiopathic)

ETIOLOGY

- Acquired with genetic predispositions
- Majority: idiopathic
- Causes or associations include infectious (e.g., HIV) and noninfectious inflammatory (autoimmune) processes (myocarditis); ischemic heart disease; pregnancy; toxic (alcohol, anthracycline, cocaine); metabolic (thyroid, diabetes); and neuromuscular disorders (muscular dystrophy [myotonic, Duchenne]); asthma

USUAL TREATMENT

- Medical treatment is primarily based on diuretics, digitalis, and vasodilators (ACE). Further, ß-adrenergic receptor block agents, immunosuppressives, anticoagulants, and antiarrhythmics (e.g., amiodarone, sotalol) or an implantable cardioverter-defibrillator (ICD) may be needed
- Surgical treatment: cardiomyoplasty and cardiac transplant

ASSESSMENT POINTS

SYSTEM	EFFECT	ASSESSMENT BY HX	PE	TEST
CV	LV systolic dysfunction Myocardial ischemia CHF Intracardiac thrombi	Angina Dyspnea	Displaced posterior MI S_3 gallop JVD Pedal edema	CXR ECHO Ventriculography/angiography Electrophysiologic testing
RESP	CHF	Dyspnea Orthopnea	S_3 gallop Rales Wheezing	CXR ABG
GI		Anginal equivalent LUQ pain		see CV
HEME	Prolonged coagulation times	Bruising emboli		PT/PTT
RENAL	Hypoperfusion	Nocturia		Cr ↑ BUN:Cr ratio increased in prerenal azotemia, thought ideal for volume status of DCM patient for daily living
CNS	Cerebral infarcts	Stroke	Neurologic evaluation	CT scan
MS	Associated musculoskeletal disorders		Weakness	

Key Reference: Manolio TA, Baughman KL, Rodeheffer R, et al: Prevalence and etiology of idiopathic dilated cardiomyopathy (summary of a National Heart, Lung and Blood Institute workshop). Am J Cardiol 1992; 69:1458–1466.

PERIOPERATIVE IMPLICATIONS

Preoperative Preparation

- Optimization of cardiac condition for anesthesia (no volume depletion as is optimization for daily life)
- Checking of digoxin levels and coagulation condition

Monitoring

- Consider ST segment analysis
- Arterial line
- PA catheter if anticipation of large fluid shifts or PA introducer only, with or without central line
- TEE may be useful

Airway

- None

Preinduction/Induction

- Anesthetic principles based on afterload reduction, preload conservation, and prevention of myocardial depression
- Regional anesthesia techniques are not contraindicated provided hypotension is prevented
- ICD management precautions should be taken if applicable (see under Implantable Cardioverter-Defibrillators (ICDs) in Diseases and Procedures sections)

Maintenance

- Potent inhalation agents often poorly tolerated; a narcotic-based anesthesia technique may be preferable, and N_2O should be used with caution
- Fluid management should be conservative to prevent fluid overload and acute CHF

- Inotropic support and FFP may be necessary

Extubation

- Beware of hypertension, arrhythmias, hypothermia

Adjuvants

- DCM predisposes to decreased blood flow to liver and kidney, which prolongs action of many agents; DCM also predisposes to increased volume of distribution of many drugs, thus often requiring increased initial dose and smaller and rarer subsequent doses (as with neuromuscular blocking agents, lidocaine, etc.)

ANTICIPATED PROBLEMS/CONCERNS

- Tachyarrhythmias, CHF, sudden death, emboli, hemodynamic anesthesia, amiodarone interactions

DIPHTHERIA

Brian K. Bevacqua, M.D.

RISK

- People within USA: 5 cases/y (respiratory infections); 100 cases/y (cutaneous infections)
- Racial prevalence: none
- Age: children (age 15 y and younger) account for 25% of cases

PERIOPERATIVE RISKS

- Early (days after exposure): respiratory compromise; respiratory arrest; airway obstruction and hemorrhage; shock, coma, and death
- Late (2–6 wk after exposure): myocarditis; neuritis

WORRY ABOUT

- Early: progressive respiratory compromise caused by cervical and submandibular adenopathy, edema, and the characteristic "membrane" from the nasal pharynx to the bronchiolar level; systemic effects of exotoxin absorption (shock, coma, death)
- Late: myocarditis (10–25% of patients) characterized by tachycardia, S_3 gallop, dysrhythmias (atrial fibrillation, premature ventricular beats) and ECG changes (ST segment changes, T-wave inversions, bundle branch block), that can lead to complete heart block, CHF, cardiogenic shock, and myocardial fibrosis. Neuritis (10%) involving both cranial (III, VI, VII, IX, and X) and peripheral nerves (motor > sensory); can resemble infectious polyneuritis

OVERVIEW

- Infections and major complications are prevented by adequate levels of circulating antitoxic antibodies
- Requires complete primary immunization and periodic booster injections (every 10 y)
- Diagnosis of respiratory infections relies on recognition of the characteristic membrane
- Membrane begins as soft exudate patches that merge into a thin membrane, become thicker, and fuse to the underlying tissues
- Extent of membrane spread and exotoxin production determines degree of systemic involvement
- Myocarditis, the principal cause of death from diphtheria infections, begins as ST-segment and T-wave changes in the 2nd wk of illness

- Neuritis occurring 2–6 wk into the illness may involve cranial and peripheral nerves (motor > sensory) with compromise of speech, swallowing, and respiration

ICD-9-CM Codes: 032.0–032.9

ETIOLOGY

- Caused by *Corynebacterium diphtheriae*, a gram-positive rod with swellings at each end
- Encountered in patients who have never received complete primary immunization nor timely booster injections
- Can be spread from patients with respiratory or cutaneous infections (much more common than the respiratory form) or from chronic carriers

TREATMENT

- Early administration (within 48 h of onset) of equine antiserum essential
- Immunize inadequately immunized individuals after exposure
- Isolation, bedrest, careful observation (for respiratory compromise)
- Symptomatic treatment (e.g., intubation or tracheostomy for respiratory distress)
- Pacemaker insertion for arrhythmia control

ASSESSMENT POINTS

SYSTEM	EFFECT	ASSESMENT BY HX	PE	TEST
HEENT	"Membrane" spread and hemorrhage can cause airway obstruction	Altered speech, respiratory distress, croupy cough, hoarseness, chills, sore throat	Pharyngitis, fever, cervical and submandibular adenopathy and edema ("bullneck"); characteristic "membrane"	Gram stain and culture of "membrane," indirect laryngoscopy
CV	Conduction abnormalities, CHF, cardiogenic shock	Dyspnea with minimal exertion, symptoms of CHF, palpitations	Tachycardia, ectopic beats; atrial fibrillation, signs of CHF	ECG CXR
RESP	See HEENT	Tachypnea, dyspnea, presence of membrane	Progressive respiratory compromise	Indirect laryngoscopy
HEME/ IMMUNE	Systems compromised dependent on amount of exotoxin			CBC; blood culture
GU	Proteinuria			UA
CNS	Interference with phonation, swallowing, respiration, resembles Guillain-Barré syndrome	Symptoms depend on involved nerves	Cranial nerves (most often III, VI, VII, X), peripheral nerves (motor>sensory)	

Key Reference: Simon HB, Swartz MN: Infections due to gram-positive bacilli. *In* Rubenstein E (ed): Scientific American Medicine. New York, Scientific American, Inc., 1994.

PERIOPERATIVE IMPLICATIONS

Preoperative Preparation

- Assessment of respiratory distress/airway compromise (with observation, indirect laryngoscopy, etc.)
- Assessment of immunization status and early intervention (within 48 h of symptoms) with antiserum
- Assessment of the immunization status of health care workers exposed to diphtheria and aggressive use of purified diphtheria toxoid as needed
- Assessment (late) of cardiac and neurologic involvement

Monitoring

- Consider pulmonary artery catheter or transesophageal echocardiography to assess degree of myocardial involvement

Airway

- Careful manipulation, as membrane will bleed if manipulated
- Aggressive use of endotracheal intubation/ tracheotomy

Induction

- Compensate for problems of exotoxin shock (early) and possible CHF, cardiac arrhythmia (late)

Extubation

- Early: may need prolonged ventilation
- Late: cardiogenic shock/extensive polyneuritis may necessitate prolonged ventilating support

Adjuvants

- Cardiac pacemaker for arrhythmia control/ complete heart block
- Avoid digitalis preparations, as complete heart block is common

- Minimize use of sedatives, hypnotics, as development of respiratory difficulties may be obscured

Postoperative Period

- Careful observation for respiratory (early), cardiac (late), and neurologic (late) compromise

ANTICIPATED PROBLEMS/CONCERNS

- Airway obstruction requiring tracheostomy/ intubation
- Myocardial conduction problems that may necessitate pacemaker insertion
- Cardiogenic shock/CHF
- Neuritis that can present as a Guillain-Barré–like syndrome

DISSEMINATED INTRAVASCULAR COAGULATION (DIC)

Athos J. Rassias, M.D.
D. David Glass, M.D.

RISK

- Individuals at risk in USA: patients with sepsis, liver disease, shock, brain injury, tissue necrosis, leukemia, burns, fat embolism, retained placenta, amniotic fluid embolism, eclampsia, localized endothelial injury, disseminated malignancy, or intravascular hemolysis
- Gender/race predominance: None
- Mortality >50% in systemic DIC

PERIOPERATIVE RISKS

- Bleeding, poor coagulation
- Ischemic end-organ damage
- Concomitant problems (shock, hemolysis, obstetrical problems, etc.)

WORRY ABOUT

- Uncontrolled bleeding, from even minor sites of tissue trauma
- Usually occurs with other catastrophic problems, such as sepsis and major tissue damage
- End-organ damage from microthrombosis causing ischemic changes

OVERVIEW

- Syndrome consisting of activation of clotting cascade and fibrinolytic system
- Widespread formation of fibrin thrombi in microcirculation and resultant consumption of certain clotting factors and platelets
- Consumption of clotting factors responsible for bleeding
- Differential diagnosis: liver disease, massive transfusion, fibrinolysis, TTP, heparin overdose, dysfibrinogenemia/afibrinogenemia
- Diagnosis confirmed by fibrin degradation products (FDP); thrombin time (TT) is useful with suspected heparin overdose; D-dimer, if positive, excludes primary fibrinogenolysis as cause for positive FDP

ICD-9-CM Code: 286.6

ETIOLOGY

- Coagulation initiated and maintained by:
  - intrinsic processes that enzymatically activate procoagulant and protein
  - release of inherent tissue factor by external factor, such as tissue trauma
- Risk of developing DIC increases with associated diseases and processes

USUAL TREATMENT

- Correction of underlying problem is most important goal, including aggressive general supportive measures, such as correcting hypoxemia, acidosis, and hypovolemia
- DIC warrants treatment only if significant bleeding, organ dysfunction, significant thrombosis, or treatment of underlying disease (e.g., acute promyelocytic leukemia) will worsen DIC
- Blood products:
  - PRBC if significant hemorrhage is problem
  - cryoprecipitate for fibrinogen <50, aim to maintain at >100
  - platelets, to maintain >20,000, and some recommend >50,000; FDPs impair platelet function; need liver function to clear FDPs
- FFP can be used if clotting factor deficiency
- Pharmacologic agents (controversial):
  - heparin: used to turn off coagulation, allow coagulation factors to accumulate, and impede thrombus formation; amount given should not increase PTT
  - ε-aminocaproic acid, antifibrinolytic agent: can precipitate catastrophic thrombosis when used alone as single agent; thus, must be used with heparin; guideline is to load with 3–4 g and maintain at 1 g/h

ASSESSMENT POINTS

SYSTEM	EFFECT	ASSESSMENT BY HX	PE	TEST
HEENT	↑ Tendency for bleeding		Evidence of bleeding Engorged and friable mucous membranes	
CV	May have associated sepsis Microthrombi		Hypotension Signs of poor systemic perfusion	Invasive hemodynamic monitoring ECG ECHO
RESP	Bleeding Microthrombi	Dyspnea	Tachypnea	CXR ABG
GI	Bleeding Microthrombi of liver			Nasogastric suctioning Stool heme testing LFTs
ENDO	Pituitary and adrenal microthrombi			ACTH-stimulation test
GU	Microthrombi			BUN/Cr
CNS	Bleeding Microthrombi			
MS	Petechiae			

Key Reference: Bick RL: Disseminated intravascular coagulation. Med Clin North Am 1994; 78:511–543.

PERIOPERATIVE IMPLICATIONS

Preoperative Preparation

- Underlying disease process should be corrected as much as feasible
- Blood products should be transfused as indicated (see above)
- Type and cross for PRBCs
- Regional anesthesia relatively contraindicated if significant coagulopathy present

Monitoring

- Routine
- Consider invasive monitors as indicated by condition
- Monitor of coagulation

Airway

- Avoid tissue trauma

Induction

- Consider full stomach
- Septic patients likely hypovolemic and may have some degree of myocardial depression

Maintenance

- Coagulation monitoring frequently
- Transfusion of blood components according to clinical situation and coagulation status

Extubation

- Cardiovascular and pulmonary insufficiency may be present if acute DIC
- Consider postoperative mechanical ventilation

Adjuvants

- Muscle relaxants: may have concomitant hepatic and renal impairment, which alter metabolism of certain nondepolarizing muscle relaxants

ANTICIPATED PROBLEMS/CONCERNS

- Uncontrolled hemorrhage: patients may bleed from areas of even minor tissue trauma
- End-organ damage from microthrombosis
- Concomitant medical problems may present life-threatening situations

DIVERTICULOSIS

Stanley Deutsch, Ph.D., M.D.

RISK

• Age-dependent, ranging from 5% of the population by 40 y of age to 50% of the population after 80 y of age
• Common in the UK, North America, Northern Europe, Australia, and New Zealand, but uncommon in Black Africa, the Middle East, the Far East, and the Pacific Islands

PERIOPERATIVE RISKS

• Because age-related, greater incidence of atherosclerotic heart disease, systemic atherosclerosis, and CHF, as well as reduced pulmonary and renal reserve

WORRY ABOUT

• Possibility of pelvic abscess, peritonitis, or bleeding

OVERVIEW

• A chronic condition, often asymptomatic, but in some patients, chronic pain with inflammation and flare-ups

ICD-9-CM Code: 562.1 (Colon)

ETIOLOGY

• A degenerative acquired disease related to low-residue diet with long transit time, as opposed to diets with high-fiber content with shorter transit time; an incidence of 96% in the sigmoid colon, with an incidence of 16% of disease in the entire colon
• With long transit times intraluminal pressure ↑, colon becomes distended, followed by acute and then chronic inflammation of outpouches or diverticula

USUAL TREATMENT

• Anticholinergic antispasmodics, increased bulk by consuming a diet high in roughage (bran, fruit, and vegetables) to increase transit time
• With severe abdominal pain, fever, and clinical signs of peritonitis, or pelvic abscess, exploratory laparotomy and antibiotics are indicated

ASSESSMENT POINTS

SYSTEM	EFFECT	ASSESSMENT BY HX	PE	TEST
CV	Hypotension Tachycardia Fever CAD	Angina	BP, HR Auscultation for rales, S_3	Pulmonary artery catheter Arterial line, ECG Urine output
RESP		Dyspnea with CHF	Rales with CHF	ECG CXR
GI	Abdominal pain, rigidity, pelvic mass on rectal exam, ileus			Free air under diaphragm if perforation Mass on CT scan
HEME	Anemia, leukocytosis, DIC with sepsis			Hgb, WBC, differential PT/PTT, FSP, plt count, fibrinogen
RENAL		May pass air with urine if perforation into urinary bladder		Urinalysis Urine output
CNS	Disorientation with sepsis			

Key Reference: Boucher ID, Allan RN, Hodgson HJF, et al (eds): Gastroenterology: Clinical Science and Practice, 2nd ed. Philadelphia, WB Saunders, 1993.

PERIOPERATIVE IMPLICATIONS

Monitoring

• Routine, including urine output
• With sepsis, monitor arterial pressure; pulmonary artery occlusion pressure might be considered

Maintenance

• Optimize intravascular volume, high oxygen content, and treat CHF

Postoperative Period

• Maintain intravascular volume, continued monitoring of CV variables, and urine volume

Adjuvants

• Antibiotics and potential interactions of antibiotics in prolonging muscle relaxation; interaction more bothersome if antibiotics have "washed" an inflamed peritoneum
• Volume expanders
• Component therapy if DIC develops
• Vasopressor support if required; no interactions

ANTICIPATED PROBLEMS/CONCERNS

• Pelvic abscess or peritonitis
• Cardiac or cerebral ischemia with infarction

DO NOT RESUSCITATE (DNR) ORDERS

David E. Lees, M.D.

RISK

• More than ⅙ of all patients in tertiary care hospitals in USA now have DNR orders in force

PERIOPERATIVE RISKS

• Approximately 15% of patients with a DNR order come to surgery

WORRY ABOUT

• Most commonly performed resuscitative procedures: vascular access, feeding gastrostomies, tracheostomies

OVERVIEW

• The DNR order is a limited expression of an advance directive, which is a legal instrument to ensure that a patient's wishes are carried out in the event of incapacitation
• Resuscitation is the usual response to sudden death; there is a presumed consent to resuscitation
• DNR orders arose because effectiveness of CPR is no longer categorically presumed nor can the burden of a less than successful resuscitation be denied

ORIGIN

• In common law, unless contravened by statute or case law, the choices of a competent adult shall prevail
• US Supreme Court decision in the case of Nancy Cruzan affirmed that patients have the right to refuse treatment and that surrogates may act where patients have clearly and unequivocally made their views known
• Patient Self-Determination Act of 1991 and the JCAHO require that hospitals have written policies and procedures for dealing with advance directives under applicable state laws

TYPES/GOALS

• Several types of advance directives exist, including
  – DNR orders
  – Living wills
  – Health care proxies
• Advance directives have 3 specific goals
  – Give patient time to plan ahead
  – Provide someone to make surrogate decisions
  – Allow health care professionals and family members to make treatment plans in accord with patient's expressed wishes in event of incapacitation

Key Reference: Ethical Guideline for the Anesthesia Care of Patients with Do Not Resuscitate Orders or Other Directives That Limit Care. Park Ridge, IL, American Society of Anesthesiologists, 1993.

PERIOPERATIVE IMPLICATIONS

• Remember, existence of a DNR order does not preclude surgery
• A DNR order should be reassessed whenever surgery is planned and should be either reaffirmed or suspended
• A thorough explanation of care to be provided to patient must be given by the anesthesiologist; excluded procedures and temporal limits on any DNR suspension need to be established
• If personal views are in conflict with a patient's decision, all efforts should be made to find another anesthesiologist of comparable competence; an anesthesiologist does not have to surrender his/her own moral agency
• Anesthesiologists should be familiar with federal and state laws as well as local hospital policies
• When a patient with a DNR order is accepted for surgery, it must be remembered that a DNR order is not an excuse for suboptimal care
• These directives and policies should frequently be reviewed to determine the appropriateness of surgical and anesthetic care in these patients

• What is meant by *resuscitation*? Is treatment of hypotension on induction or correction of supraventricular dysrhythmia restricted in a DNR patient or is that part of total anesthetic care? Can only be answered by in-depth discussions with the patient
• Did DNR status arise from unilateral consent? Was the DNR order instituted by a physician, claiming a resuscitation would be medically futile? Was this communicated to patient? Does patient agree?

ANTICIPATED PROBLEMS/CONCERNS

Anesthesiologists' Objections to DNR in OR

• Consent for anesthesia automatically presumes consent for resuscitation
• Fear of administrative harassment that may follow an intraoperative death
• Perceived responsibility for a patient's intraoperative death regardless of cause
• Fear of being sought out by terminal patients as "angel of death"

DOUBLE AORTIC ARCH

Carol L. Lake, M.D.

RISK

- Most common form of vascular ring; a very rare lesion, accounting for < 1% of congenital heart disease.
- Race/gender predilection: none

PERIOPERATIVE RISKS

- Tracheal compression progressing to complete airway obstruction on induction and after neuromuscular blocking drugs

WORRY ABOUT

- Respiratory distress, wheezing, cyanosis
- Failure to thrive, poor growth, esophageal compression
- Associated cardiac disease such as transposition of the great arteries, tetralogy of Fallot, or VSD

OVERVIEW

- Double aortic arch produces a vascular ring around the trachea and esophagus, causing respiratory and esophageal obstruction of varying degrees.
- Symptoms occur at birth or within the first 3 mo of life in most patients
- Surgical division of the extra arch breaks the compressing ring, but coexistent tracheomalacia may necessitate prolonged postop ventilation.

ICD-9-CM Code: 747.21

ETIOLOGY

- Results from persistence of both arches during embryologic development instead of only the left arch. Ascending aorta divides into two arches passing on either side of the trachea and esophagus to join posteriorly to form the descending aorta. The left carotid and subclavian arteries arise from the smaller anterior arch, while the right carotid and subclavian arise from the dominant posterior arch.

USUAL TREATMENT

- Medical therapy: None.
- Surgery: Via a left posterolateral thoracotomy, the smaller (anterior) arch is divided at its distal end just proximal to the junction with the larger posterior arch. The persistence of the carotid, temporal, and descending aortic pulses should be verified during temporary occlusion of the arch to be resected. Trachea and esophagus are freed above and below the point of obstruction, avoiding injury to the recurrent laryngeal nerve.

ASSESSMENT POINTS

SYSTEM	EFFECT	ASSESSMENT BY HX	PE	TEST
HEENT	Airway obstruction Esophageal obstruction	Dyspnea, apnea, intermittent cyanosis, dysphagia	Intercostal retractions, head hyperextended	CXR Barium esophagogram
CV	Depends on presence of associated heart disease; none if *only* double aortic arch present			
RESP	Recurrent respiratory infection	Coughing, wheezing		CXR (hyperinflated lung fields)

Key Reference: Lake CL: Pediatric Cardiac Anesthesia, 2nd ed. Norwalk CT, Appleton and Lange, 1993, pp 368–370.

PERIOPERATIVE IMPLICATIONS

Preoperative Preparation

- Oxygen therapy if decreased arterial oxygen saturation present
- Antibiotics for bronchopneumonia

Monitoring

- Intra-arterial or central venous catheters with complex defects
- Doppler for persistent pulse presence

Airway

- Dynamic and static airway obstruction likely

Preinduction/Induction

- Inhalation induction without neuromuscular blockade until airway maintenance is documented by mask or tracheal tube is placed.
- Secure IV access essential, as bleeding may occur during resection of anomalous arteries

Maintenance

- Depends on procedure
- Usually: GA with combination of narcotic and volatile agent

Extubation

- Extubation at end of case if tracheomalacia and stenosis absent

Postoperative Period

- Epidural analgesia delivered via caudal route provides good postop analgesia to minimize respiratory complications if early extubation possible

Adjuvants

- Anesthetic choices may be modified by coexistence of other cardiac lesions

ANTICIPATED PROBLEMS/CONCERNS

- Patients with double aortic arch may have mild to life-threatening respiratory obstruction and apnea.

DOWN SYNDROME

James A. Greenberg, M.D.

RISK

- >300,000 individuals in the USA
- 80% of children with this condition survive beyond 1 y
- Number >50 y will ↑ by 200% by the year 2010
- Males > females 3:2
- No racial preponderance

PERIOPERATIVE RISKS

- Related to specific abnormalities in individual

WORRY ABOUT

- Congenital heart disease: 50% born with congenital heart disease (CHD), 8% with cyanotic CHD (usually tetralogy of Fallot)
  – may become profoundly hypoxic with R→L shunting; accidentally injected air bubbles may exit into systemic circulation (coronary and cerebral air emboli)
  – adults less likely to have CAD
- Upper airway obstruction:
  – Soft tissue obstruction of upper airway common immediately on induction of GA due to large tongue, small mandible, short neck
  – subglottic stenosis is present in 20–25% and of particular concern in children
- Obstructive and central sleep apnea
- Cervical extension during intubation can cause neurologic symptoms (neck pain, arm pain, upper extremity weakness, torticollis)
- Generalized joint laxity; TMJ may sublux with jaw thrust
- Endocrine: Hypothyroidism (4–6% in children; 15–20% in adults), hypothermia, obesity (difficult IV access)
- Mental retardation:
  – May have overwhelming fears of unknown
  – Can become physically resistant to entering OR
  – Alzheimer's disease and other forms of mental illness (depression, psychosis) may coexist

OVERVIEW

- Not a disease
- Incidence ↓ by prenatal screening and elective termination of pregnancy
- Wide variation in abilities and disabilities; neurologic development enhanced by external stimulation
- Institutionalized individuals have high incidence of seropositivity for hepatitis B
- More people living in group homes in community and becoming more self-sufficient in ADL

ICD-9-CM Code: 758.00

ETIOLOGY

- Genetic: trisomy 21
- Risk of parenting a Down syndrome fetus greatest in older (>35 y) parents (well characterized in mothers)

USUAL TREATMENT

- Depends on pathophysiology

ASSESSMENT POINTS

SYSTEM	EFFECT	ASSESSMENT BY HX	PE	TEST
HEENT	Large tongue Subglottic stenosis Hearing deficit in 66%	Hx of snoring Sleep apnea Intubation Hx		Audiology
CV	Tetralogy of Fallot in 4%	Sx of CHF "tet" spells	Cyanosis Murmur	ECHO
ENDO	Hypothyroidism Obesity	Hypothermia	Obesity	
MS	Subluxation of C1/C2 Joint laxity			Cervical spine radiographs (controversy over whether these should be routine)

Key Reference: Pueschel SM, Pueschel JK: Biomedical concerns in persons with Down syndrome. Baltimore, Brookes Publishing, 1992, pp 1–301.

PERIOPERATIVE IMPLICATIONS

Monitoring

- Temperature (hypothermia)
- ECG (arrhythmias, ischemia); treat bradycardia from halothane

Airway

- Have variety of alternative airway management devices available (e.g., oral and nasal airways, laryngeal mask, Bullard laryngoscope)
- Avoid neck extension during laryngoscopy if possible
- Smaller endotracheal tube may be necessary for narrowed subglottic space

Vascular Access

- Allow more time for IV placement
- Meticulously avoid injected air

Patient Management

- Soft, warm, kind, patient approach along with caregiver known to patient to help with initial management; warm, quiet OR

ANTICIPATED PROBLEMS/CONCERNS

- Hypoxia if R →L shunting develops
- Resistance to separation from caregiver
- Life-threatening upper airway obstruction with difficult vascular access
- Spinal cord ischemia with neurologic damage

DRUG ABUSE — LYSERGIC ACID DIETHYLAMIDE (LSD)

John M. Huffman, M.D.
Herbert D. Weintraub, M.D.

RISK

- Medical/surgical intervention usually necessary 2° to trauma related to hallucinations
- Highest prevalence: teens, 20s.

PERIOPERATIVE RISKS

- Potentiation of analgesic effects of narcotics
- Potentiation of neuromuscular blockade with succinylcholine, 2° to anticholinesterase activity
- Potentiation of ester local anesthetic toxicity 2° to anticholinesterase activity
- Inhibition of MAO activity, augmenting effects of sympathomimetic amines resulting in hypertension, tachycardia, and hyperpyrexia
- ↑ Levels of endogenous serotonin and histamine 2° to inhibition of MAO metabolism resulting in hypotension and bronchospasm

WORRY ABOUT

- Associated traumatic injuries (cervical spine fracture, pneumothorax)
- Concomitant drug or alcohol use
- Potential aspiration risk

OVERVIEW

- LSD is an illicit drug that is tasteless, odorless, and rapidly absorbed from the GI tract and nasal mucosa.
- Primary effect is intense visual and to a lesser extent auditory hallucinations.
- $T_{1/2}$ of 3 h. Effects may last up to 12 h.
- Depending on drug dose, insight usually remains intact; patients understand that they are experiencing drug-induced hallucinations.

ICD-9-CM Code: 305.3

ETIOLOGY

- Modulation of central serotonin receptors

USUAL TREATMENT

- Supportive reassurance
- Minimize external sensory stimulation
- Intravenous benzodiazepines or IM haloperidol for severe agitation

ASSESSMENT POINTS

SYSTEM	EFFECT	ASSESSMENT BY HX	PE
HEENT			Dilated, reactive pupils
CV	Sympathetic nervous system stimulation	Palpitations Sweating	Hypertension Tachycardia
RESP	No consistent changes		
ENDO			Mild hyperthermia
CNS	Euphoria, hallucinations Anxiety Tremors	Altered MS associated with illicit drug ingestion	

Key Reference: Micromedex—Drug Information Systems, Denver, CO, C.C.I.S. Expiration: May 1996.

PERIOPERATIVE IMPLICATIONS

Preoperative Preparation

- Rule out associated traumatic injury
- Aspiration prophylaxis
- Sedation if agitation is severe

Monitoring

- Temperature
- Neuromuscular blockade

Airway

- None

Preinduction/Induction

- Exaggerated response to endogenous and exogenous catecholamines
- May develop bronchospasm with histamine release

Maintenance

- Reduced anesthetic requirements
- Maintain normothermia

Extubation

- At risk for aspiration
- Continue supportive reassurance

Adjuvants

- May have exaggerated response to sympathomimetic agents due to MAO inhibition
- Potential of ester local anesthetic toxicity 2° to anticholinesterase activity
- Potentiation of succinylcholine neuromuscular blockade 2° to anticholinesterase activity

ANTICIPATED PROBLEMS/CONCERNS

- Avoid injuries associated with agitation
- Possible concomitant drug/alcohol use by patient

DRUG OVERDOSE — PROPYLENE GLYCOL
Winnie Y. Ruo, M.D.

OVERVIEW

• A commonly used solvent for parenteral, oral, and topical water-insoluble drugs
• Associated with many adverse side effects, many of which are attributable to high osmolality of propylene glycol–containing solutions
• Side effects esp. common in low birth weight infants

COMMONLY USED AGENTS DISSOLVED IN PROPYLENE GLYCOL

AGENT	PROPYLENE GLYCOL CONCENTRATION
Lorazepam	83%
Diazepam	45%
Etomidate	35%
Nitroglycerin (50 mg/vial)	33%
Nitroglycerin (100 mg/vial)	50%
Phenytoin	40%

Key Reference: Doenicke A, et al: Osmolalities of propylene glycol-containing drug formulations for parenteral use. Should propylene glycol be used as a solvent? Anesth Analg 1992; 75:431–435

PHARMACOKINETICS/METABOLISM

• Elimination half-life: 4 h
• Total body clearance: 0.1 L/kg/h
• Volume of distribution: 0.5 L/kg
• Renal excretion: 2.4–14.2%
• Propylene glycol is metabolized to lactaldehyde and then lactate, via hepatic alcohol and aldehyde dehydrogenases, with methylglyoxal providing an alternative pathway

TOXICITY/SIDE EFFECTS

• Cardiac—CV collapse, decreased contractility, peripheral vascular vasodilation, arrhythmias, asystole
• Pulmonary—resp depression, pulm HTN
• CNS—depression, coma, seizures
• Renal—diuresis, hemoglobinuria, microscopic damage
• Hepatic—microscopic damage
• Hematologic—intravascular hemolysis
• Acid-base—lactic acidosis, increased anion gap
• Others—pain on injection, thrombophlebitis, hyperosmolality, histamine release

DRUG OVERDOSE — RAT POISON (WARFARIN TOXICITY)   Michelle Braunfeld, M.D.

RISK

- Major risk is hemorrhage, esp. CNS or GI
- Incidence: Risk of hemorrhage is 2.4–8.1% of patients chronically anticoagulated. Risk is dose-related and proportional to PT prolongation. Thus patients with a higher therapeutic INR (e.g., those with prosthetic valves) have higher risk.
- Rx for: DVT, cerebral vessel atherosclerosis, prosthetic heart valves, mitral stenosis, paroxysmal atrial fibrillation

PERIOPERATIVE RISKS

- Bleeding
- Drugs that potentiate anticoagulant effects: antibiotics (esp. metronidazole, sulfonamides, cephalosporins), NSAIDs, phenytoin, cimetidine, barbiturates, alcohol

WORRY ABOUT

- Bleeding complications of invasive procedures
- Drug interactions
- Transient protein C deficiency preceding effect on procoagulant levels at initiation of warfarin therapy leading to thrombotic complications

OVERVIEW/PHARMACOLOGY

- Vit K antagonist
- Cleared by hepatic and renal transformation and excretion. $T_{1/2}$ is ≈ 40 h. Duration of action is 2–5 d.
- Onset of effect is delayed by 8–12 h because of time required to clear already synthesized clotting factors.

ICD-9-CM Code: 286.9 (Coagulation defect)

DRUG CLASS/MECH OF ACTION/USUAL DOSE

- Blocks vit K–mediated carboxylation of factors II, VII, IX, X (procoagulants); protein C, protein S (anticoagulants)
- Chronically taken for systemic anticoagulation for DVT, CVA, prosthetic valves, and atrial fibrillation either paroxysmal or associated with mitral stenosis
- Usual doses: Loading regimen varies, but maintenance dose is 2.5–10 mg/d.
- Alternatives: dicumarol, anisindione—while available, essentially never used. Neither shown to be superior to warfarin and both may have increased side effects.
- Heparin is drug of choice for acute anticoagulation, but must be given parenterally, usually as loading dose with an infusion.

DRUG EFFECTS

SYSTEM	EFFECT	ASSESSMENT BY HX	PE	TEST
HEME	Levels of factor II, IV, IX, X, and protein C, protein S	Easy bruising, prolonged bleeding time	Ecchymoses	PT

Key Reference: Stoelting RK: Pharmacology & Physiology in Anesthetic Practice. 2nd ed. JB Lippincott, Philadelphia, 1991, pp 472–474.

POSSIBLE DRUG INTERACTIONS

Preoperative

Increased effect	Decreased effect
Antibiotics, NSAIDs	Methylxanthines
Oral hypoglycemics	Rifampin
Diazepam	Antihistamines
Cimetidine	Corticosteroids
Diuretics	Barbiturates
Phenytoin	

Adjuvants/Regional Anesthesia/Reversal

- Regional block—relatively contraindicated without reversal of anticoagulation
- Peripheral block—relatively contraindicated without reversal of anticoagulation

SPECIAL CONSIDERATIONS/CONCERNS

- Relatively minor surgical procedures may be performed without reversal of warfarin anticoagulation.
- Major surgical procedures warrant discontinuation of drug 1–3 d preoperatively with a target PT within 20% of nml range. Alternatively, patient may be admitted 1–2 d prior to surgery. Warfarin is discontinued and heparin therapy instituted. Heparin is discontinued 6 h prior to surgery.
- In emergency surgery, patient may be given 10–20 ml/kg of FFP and 5–10 mg vit K, with additional amounts of both given as needed.

DUCHENNE MUSCULAR DYSTROPHY
(PSEUDOHYPERTROPHIC MUSCULAR DYSTROPHY)

Richard I. Cook, M.D.

RISK

- Males, (30/100,000 males); a few cases known in females
- Often undiagnosed until age 3–5 y
- Deterioration through puberty to death before age 25 y

PERIOPERATIVE RISKS

- Respiratory failure, prolonged mechanical ventilation
- Muscle weakness

WORRY ABOUT

- Poor cardiac function, cardiac arrhythmias, MVP (antibiotic prophylaxis)
- Poor respiratory function, pulmonary HTN from chronic sleep apnea, scoliosis
- Aspiration risk (delayed emptying)
- Hyperkalemic arrest with succinylcholine
- Association with malignant hyperthermia
- Consider supplemental steroids (if previous Rx with steroids)
- Poor long-term prognosis

OVERVIEW

- Most boys die from pneumonia but CHF is also seen in the later stages
- Gradual onset of the muscle wasting may go unnoticed for years after hyperkalemic response to depolarizing NM blockers develops. The infant may appear entirely normal. With age the body habitus may be normal or even athletic, but the muscle mass is gradually replaced by fat.
- ↑ Sensitivity to nondepolarizing neuromuscular blockers
- Use of Ca^{2+}-channel blocker (e.g., verapamil) may prolong or even cause neuromuscular blockade
- Up to 1/4 of patients may have mitral valve prolapse
- Resting tachycardia common; cardiac involvement in 70% of cases, cardiac debilitation usually late
- ECG abnormal (increased RS in V_1, deep Q in precordial leads)

ICD-9-CM Code: 359.1

ETIOLOGY

- X-linked recessive disease; the muscles (including myocardium) are gradually replaced with fat and connective tissue. The defect is in the muscle cell membrane protein *dystrophin*.

USUAL TREATMENT

- At least 25 drugs have been tried without success; early trials of steroids have shown some promise.
- Spinal rodding and fusion, often with AP approach, for the scoliosis that begins at 10–12 y can prolong comfort and ease of wheelchair use. Pulmonary deterioration continues, and life may be only minimally prolonged.
- Tendon releases for contractures
- Exploratory laparotomy for ileus

ASSESSMENT POINTS

SYSTEM	EFFECT	ASSESSMENT BY HX	PE	TEST
CV	Conduction	Tachycardia	Opening snap (MVP)	ECG, 24 h ambulatory ECG
	Contractile force	Difficult (Hx CHF Sx: orthopnea, DOE, PND)	CHF signs	ECHO, MUGA
RESP	↓ Volume and flows	Difficult	Unreliable	PFTs
	Sleep apnea/pulmonary HTN	Snoring, apneic spells	Unreliable	SaO_2?, sleep lab? ECHO?
GI	Dysmotility, gastric dilatation, paralytic ileus			
GU	Bladder paralysis, impotence			
CNS	↓ IQ		Mental status exam	
MS	Scoliosis, kyphosis Contractures			Spine films
	Muscle destruction	Progressive weakness		Abnormal myogram Elevated CK levels
	Macroglossia Poor IV access			

Key Reference: Emery AEH: Duchenne Muscular Dystrophy, 2nd ed. New York, Oxford University Press, 1993.

PERIOPERATIVE IMPLICATIONS

Preoperative Preparation
- Avoid or limit sedation

Monitoring
- Consider PA catheter/TEE based on EF and surgical procedure
- Nerve stimulator

Induction
- Succinylcholine contraindicated because of hyperkalemia
- Avoid MH triggering agents

- Consider avoiding depressants of cardiac contractility
- Consider long gastric emptying times, possible full stomach

Maintenance
- Variable response to neuromuscular blockers; titrate to effect
- Recommended to allow spontaneous recovery, as response to reversal agents varies

Emergence
- Potential for prolonged ventilator dependence when vital capacity <30% of predicted

- Late respiratory depression reported (cause unclear); may make outpatient surgery inadvisable

ANTICIPATED PROBLEMS/CONCERNS

- Respiratory failure
- Congestive failure
- Supraventricular tachydysrhythmias

WARNING

- The hyperkalemic response to succinylcholine (cardiac arrest) has been described in boys 4 mo old without clinical signs of Duchenne's muscular dystrophy.

ECHINOCOCCOSIS

Anis S. Baraka, M.D.
Zuhayr A. Tabbarah, M.D.

RISK

- Common to endemic in sheep-raising countries worldwide (e.g., Mediterranean basin, Australia, Argentina, Far East) and in dog-eating populations
- Rare in USA except among immigrants from sheep-raising countries and residents of sheep-raising areas
- Racial predilection: none

PERIOPERATIVE RISKS

- Organ dysfunction, depending on site of hydatid cyst
- Sepsis
- Communication of cyst with biliary tree bronchopleural communications

WORRY ABOUT

- Spillage of hydatid fluid:
  – anaphylactic reactions
  – dissemination of infestation
- Complications from scolicidal agents:
  – Methemoglobinemia with (cetrimide); hypernatremia and sclerosing cholangitis (hypertonic saline, 15–20%); air embolism (hydrogen peroxide); ethanol intoxication (75–95%)

OVERVIEW

- Zoonosis caused by larval stage of *Echinococcus granulosus,* which produces unilocular cystic lesions; larvae burrow through mucosa of small intestine, enter portal circulation, and travel to liver
- Liver involved in >50% of cases, followed by lungs
- Cysts can involve any organ system including muscles, spleen, brain, spinal cord, kidneys, bones, and omentum; hydatid cysts grow slowly
- Sx related to mechanical pressure of cyst on surrounding structures.
- Cyst may be infected and behave like abscess and/or acute cholangitis
- Spontaneous rupture/leak can occur causing anaphylactic reactions and dissemination of infestation
- *Echinococcus* should be suspected when cystic mass is discovered in liver, lung, or other organs by ultrasound, CT scan, or CXR, with Hx of past exposure
- Dx can be confirmed by serologic studies (indirect hemagglutininemia, ELISA, others)

ICD-9-CM Code: 122.9

ETIOLOGY

- Caused by *E. granulosus;* adult worm lives in jejunum of canines (mainly dogs) for 5–20 mo; in addition to scolex and neck, it has 3 proglottides (1 immature, 1 mature, and 1 gravid); gravid segment splits before or after passage of stools and releases eggs that contaminate environment; intermediate hosts (sheep and occasionally man) ingest food contaminated by *E. granulosus* eggs and develop cysts in liver, lungs, or other organs; life cycle of *E. granulosus* is complete when dogs consume infected viscera of sheep or other animals

USUAL TREATMENT

- Surgery, when feasible, principal definitive treatment; surgery may be conservative with use of scolicidal agent and evacuation of cyst or radical with pericystectomy or hepatic resection
- Puncture–aspiration–injection–reaspiration (PAIR) technique being used successfully in some countries
- Chemotherapy with albendazole is playing ↑ role as adjuct Rx to ↓ risk of dissemination and in nonoperable cases; usual dose, 10 mg/kg, to be started 1 mo–1 wk prior to surgery and for 1–6 mo postsurgery

ASSESSMENT POINTS

SYSTEM	EFFECT	ASSESSMENT BY HX	PE	TEST
CV	Hydatid cyst of heart Conduction defect Pericarditis	Chest pain		ECG ECHO Serology
RESP	Hydatid cyst of lung Rupture into bronchial tree	Cough, chest pain Hemoptysis		CXR Serology
GI	Hydatid cyst of liver, spleen, omentum	N/V Intermittent colic	Palpable mass Jaundice, fever	Ultrasound, CT scan Serology
RENAL	Hydatid cyst of kidney		Palpable mass	Ultrasound, CT scan, serology
CNS	Hydatid cyst of brain Space-occupying lesion ICP rupture into subarachnoid space	Headache	Signs of ICP Localizing signs	CT scan Serology
MS	Hydatid cyst mass of bones, muscles Pathologic fracture	Painless, localized swelling	Dull muscle ache on exertion	Ultrasound, CT scan, serology X-ray
SPINE	Mass effect	Weakness	Radicular distribution or paresis	X-ray CT scan

Key Reference: Craig PS: Current research in echinococcosis. Parasitology Today 1994; 10:209–211.

PERIOPERATIVE IMPLICATIONS

Preoperative Preparation

- Albendazole 10 mg/kg/day for 1 wk preoperatively
- LFTs, pulmonary function tests, depending on site of cyst
- Antihistamines part of premedication

Monitoring

- Routine monitors
- Other monitors depend on site of cyst

Airway

- Double-lumen tube for thoracotomy whenever hydatid cysts of lungs diagnosed

Induction

- Depends on site and function of organ involved

Maintenance

- 100% O_2 during one-lung ventilation for thoracotomy; cardiopulmonary bypass for cardiac hydatid
- Avoidance of spillage of hydatid fluid
- Irrigation with scolicidal agents, such as cetrimide or hypertonic saline

Extubation

- Routine extubation, except in cardiac, pulmonary, or brain hydatid cysts, when extubation is tailored according to situation

Postoperative Period

- Routine except:
  – complications such as anaphylactic reactions, methemoglobinemia, or excessive bleeding
  – specialized cases undergoing cardiopulmonary bypass, craniotomy, or thoracotomy complicated by bronchopleural fistula and/or excessive air leak

ANTICIPATED PROBLEMS/CONCERNS

- Anaphylactic reaction (2° to spillage); epinephrine first line of management
- Methemoglobinemia 2° to excessive cetrimide; methylene blue, 1–2 mg/kg, therapeutic

ECLAMPSIA

Therese K. Abboud, M.D.

RISK

- Pre-eclampsia: 6–8% of pregnant women
- Eclampsia: 0.2 to 0.67/1000 births
- Most often young primigravidas

PERIOPERATIVE RISKS

- Accounts for 20–40% of maternal mortality
- Severe hypertension, eclampsia, abruptio placentae, fetal distress, pulmonary edema
- Affects every organ system

WORRY ABOUT

- Hemodynamic variables and fluid changes
- Difficult airway
- Coagulopathy

OVERVIEW

- Pre-eclampsia Dx made if 2 or more of these criteria present: systolic BP >140 mmHg; diastolic BP >90 mmHg; proteinuria >2 g/24 h; and pedal edema
- Eclampsia implies seizures and may occur before, during, or after delivery; this worsens both maternal and fetal prognosis
- May manifest in virtually every organ system
- Disease process usually terminates 48 h after birth

ICD-9-CM Code: 624.4

ETIOLOGY

- Cause still speculative: genetic, immunologic, or simply ↓ in uterine blood flow
- Imbalance of thromboxane (↑) and prostacyclin (↓) with resultant ↑ vasoconstriction, platelet aggregation, uterine activity, and ↓ uteroplacental blood flow
- ↓ Placental perfusion releases fibronectin, which causes damage to tissues
- Seizures related to cerebral vasospasm, ischemia, edema, hemorrhage

USUAL TREATMENT

- Goal for eclampsia is stop convulsion, establish clear airway.
- Definitive: delivery of fetus/placenta
- Magnesium: ↓ irritability of CNS and direct vasodilation (Rx range, 4–6 mEq/L)
- Antihypertensives: hydralazine, trimethaphan, labetalol, nitroglycerin, nitroprusside (caution, cyanide toxicity)
- Chronic aspirin Rx ↓ incidence

ASSESSMENT POINTS

SYSTEM	EFFECT	ASSESSMENT BY HX	PE	TEST
CV	Hypertension, CHF	Palpitations, fatigue, edema	High BP, edema, rales	ECG, ECHO
RESP	Pharyngolaryngeal edema, pulmonary edema	Cough, stridor, breathlessness, chest tightness	Tachypnea, dyspnea, rales, wheezing	CXR ABG
HEME	Hypercoagulability, thrombocytopenia, platelet dysfunction, DIC, HELLP syndrome		Petechial oozing around IV puncture sites	Coagulation studies: platelet count PT, fibrin/fibrinogen
RENAL	Glomerulopathy, proteinuria, oliguria, ↑ Cr and BUN	↓ Urine output, edema	Rapid weight gain, edema	Urinalysis, 24-h urine protein, BUN/Cr
HEPATIC	↓ Hepatic blood flow, ↓ cholinesterase, periportal hepatic necrosis, subcapsular hemorrhage, abnormal LFT	Epigastric and subcostal pain	Tenderness over liver area, hepatomegaly	Liver enzyme assay, ultrasound

Key Reference: Patterson KW, O'Toole DP: HELLP syndrome: A case report with guidelines for diagnosis and management. Br J Anaesth 1991; 66:513–515.

PERIOPERATIVE IMPLICATIONS

Preoperative Preparation

- BP control
- Anticipate difficult airway
- Aspiration prophylaxis

Monitoring

- Routine
- Consider arterial catheter for severe cases
- PA catheter as indicated by: oliguria, pulmonary edema, refractory hypertension, and persistent arterial desaturation

Airway

- Anticipate difficult intubation due to tissue swelling and airway bleeding

Labor/Delivery

- Epidural if no coagulation problems
- Avoid high-level block, prehydrate with caution

Cesarean Section

- Epidural if no coagulation defect
- General if bleeding abnormalities or in emergency
- Control BP with rapid-onset, short-acting antihypertensives
- MgSO$_4$ may potentiate muscle relaxant
- Avoid narcotics, sedatives, and high concentration of inhalation agents prior to delivery of fetus
- Extubate fully awake

Postpartum

- Eclamptic: observe in highly monitored situation

- Continue MgSO$_4$, hemodynamic control, and fluid balance concerns
- Adequate pain management: pain score, 2–5
- Observe for coagulopathy

Adjuvants

- Mannitol (cerebral edema), furosemide (pulmonary edema)
- Digitalis (CHF)
- Barbiturates, benzodiazepine to control seizures

ANTICIPATED PROBLEMS/CONCERNS

- Eclamptic seizures
- Pulmonary edema
- Hypertensive encephalopathy
- DIC

ECTOPIC PREGNANCY

Joseph Rosa III, M.D.

RISK

- Implantation of fetus or blastocyst outside uterus
- Incidence, overall, 1/90. More common in non-whites and in 35–44 y age range than in 15–24 y

PERIOPERATIVE RISKS

- Second leading cause of maternal mortality (leading cause in 1st trimester), accounting for 14.7% of all maternal deaths; nearly 2 times greater in non-whites.
- 85% of deaths due to hemorrhage, 5% due to infection, 2% due to anesthetic complications
- Highest mortality associated with intra-abdominal and interstitial tubal pregnancies 2° to larger size at time of diagnosis and therefore ↑ blood supply

WORRY ABOUT

- Hemorrhagic shock, ↓ intravascular volume
- Blood availability—may need type-specific or O neg blood
- Full stomach/aspiration risk
- Consider physiologic changes of pregnancy if diagnosis made late in gestation, esp with intra-abdominal location (see under Intra-abdominal Pregnancy)
- If laparoscopic approach, consider effects of CO_2 insufflation, ventilation, and steep Trendelenburg position (see under Laparoscopy in Procedures section)

OVERVIEW

- Primary concerns with ruptured ectopic are intravascular volume, airway management
- Differential Dx of abd pain: appendicitis, any intra-abdominal infection or process. Dx made by Hx and physical—95% have pelvic pain, 75% amenorrhea, 60–80% uterine bleeding.
- ß-HCG—elevated in 100% of ectopics, US to rule out intrauterine pregnancy. Laparoscopy useful in Dx of acute pelvic pain and to rule out ectopic.

ICD-9-CM Code: 633

ETIOLOGY

- Mechanical factors: salpingitis, peritubal adhesions, previous ectopic, prior tubal surgery, multiple prior abortions
- Functional factors: external ovum migration, menstrual reflux, altered tubal motility

USUAL TREATMENT

- Surgical
  – 70% of ectopics diagnosed before rupture; an acutely ruptured ectopic is a surgical emergency.
  – Salpingo-oophorectomy—advocated by some if other adnexa appear normal and future pregnancy desired
    – Salpingectomy—most common treatment
    – Salpingostomy used to salvage unruptured tube
  – Laparoscopy—diagnostic and can be used to remove small ectopic; associated with decreased morbidity and hospital stay
- Medical
  – Methotrexate used for unruptured small ectopics. Surgery avoided and possibly increased potential for future fertility.
- Combined surgical/medical management—direct injection of methotrexate in fallopian tube
- Expectant management—primarily used for small ectopics following ß-hCG
- Prognosis: 40% of patients will never conceive again. Of the 60% who do conceive, 12% will have repeat ectopics and 15–20% will spontaneously abort.

ASSESSMENT POINTS

SYSTEM	EFFECT	ASSESSMENT BY HX	PE	TEST
HEENT		Snoring/difficult airway	Airway exam	
CV	Hypovolemia 2° to hemorrhage	Orthostatic dizziness	Vitals, neck veins, orthostatic vital signs Weak, thready pulse Cold legs and arms of vasoconstriction	
HEME	Blood loss 2° to rupture Hemoperitoneum/vaginal bleeding	Vaginal bleeding Orthostatic dizziness	Orthostatic vital signs	Hct
CNS	Hypoperfusion causing mental status changes and decreased urine production	CNS Hx	CNS exam	BUN/Cr UA

Key Reference: Chestnut DH: Obstetric Anesthesia Principles and Practice. St. Louis, Mosby–Year Book, 1994, pp 259–262.

PERIOPERATIVE MANAGEMENT

Preoperative Preparation

- Assessment of volume status; 2 large-bore IVs
- Blood availability—at least O neg; type-specific preferable
- Consideration of full stomach

Anesthetic Technique

- GA: preferable in unstable patient with ruptured ectopic, if laparoscopy to be used or contraindication to regional
- Regional anesthesia: spinal or epidural T2–T4 level needed; consider in hemodynamically stable patients

Monitoring

- Routine; once ectopic bleeding stopped, fluid resuscitation for replacement only; too zealous replacement can lead to pulm edema.

Airway

- If difficult airway, awake fiberoptic; otherwise rapid-sequence.

Induction/Maintenance

- If unstable, consider etomidate or ketamine, maintenance with O_2, inhalational, and narcotic with muscle relaxants
  – Choice of drugs less important than anesthetic management

SURGICAL STAGES

Induction

- Possible CV instabililty 2° to uncorrected hypovolemia, as well as full stomach/aspiration potential.
- Skin incision
  – If laparotomy for rupture, hemoperitoneum and hypotension and uncontrolled bleeding. Upon opening abdomen, a release of tamponade may result in ↓ BP.
    – Incision—Pfannenstiel or low midline
    – Laparoscopy—infraumbilical and 1–4 suprapubic incisions. Peritoneal insufflation: monitor end-tidal CO_2 and intraperitoneal pressures—should be <18 mmHg. Potential for CO_2 embolus or intra-abdominal injury during introduction of the Veress needle
- Dissection: minimal to extensive depending on location of ectopic and degree of bleeding

Definitive Surgery

- Salpingectomy, ipsilateral oophorectomy—used for ruptured ectopic hysterectomy; may be necessary if interstitial implantation
- Salpingotomy
  – Technique of fallopian tube conservation
  – Can be performed via laparoscope; used to remove small ectopic <2 cm; preferred technique for unruptured ectopic

- Approximate duration: 1–2 h
- Fluid shifts can be large with ruptured ectopic
- Closure: minimal if laparoscopy; low midline/or Pfannenstiel 15–20 min.

Extubation

- Awake

Postoperative Period

- EBL may be extensive; check Hct
- Pain score: 4–6 laparoscopy, 5–8 laparotomy
- PCA or neuraxial narcotics; local anesthetics if regional ± neuraxial narcotics

ANTICIPATED PROBLEMS/CONCERNS

- CV: instability from massive hemorrhage from ruptured ectopic
- Potential for pulm edema, fluid overload in postop period due to massive crystalloid infusion and subsequent mobilization of third-space fluid
- Postop shoulder and chest pain from unabsorbed gas and peritoneal irritation—30%
- Gastric dilation 3%, thrombophlebitis 3%, pulmonary embolism 2%, ureteral injury/stenosis 1% with laparotomy
- Postop infection, abscess

EISENMENGER'S SYNDROME

RISK

- 3% of all congenital heart disease patients with atrial, ventricular, or aortopulmonary shunt
- VSD is most common lesion

PERIOPERATIVE RISKS

- Mortality rate of patients with ES carrying pregnancy to viability is 27–30%
- Fetal risks: ↑ risk of preterm labor, intrauterine growth retardation; fetal demise of 75%
- Cesarean section carries higher mortality: 70% vs. 30% for vaginal delivery
- Death most often occurs at delivery or post partum

WORRY ABOUT

- R→L shunt, pulmonary hypertension, right and left ventricular failure, hypoxemia, arrhythmias, paradoxical emboli, thromboembolic phenomena, hemoptysis
- ↓ Systemic vascular resistance of pregnancy worsens R→L shunt
- Inability to meet ↑ demand for O₂ with gestation and labor
- Thromboembolic disease (hypercoagulation of pregnancy, venous stasis, polycythemia with chronic hypoxia)

- Delivery produces autotransfusion with RV failure
- Excessive bleeding with previous heparinization
- Acute blood loss produces systemic hypotension, ↓ pulmonary blood flow and hypoxia
- Postpartum increase in PVR

OVERVIEW

- Consists of pulmonary vascular occlusive disease with pulmonary hypertension with R→L shunt and right ventricular dysfunction
- Has poor prognosis; mean age at death, 25 y
- Hx of syncope, ↑ right-sided filling pressures, and systemic arterial desaturation below 85% indicate poor prognosis
- 50% of pregnant patients die in association with pregnancy; outcome is worst for patients with VSD (hemodynamic demands of pregnancy, labor, and delivery place excessive burdens)
- Some pulmonary vascular reactivity may exist in the pulmonary vasculature of pregnant women; may be due to systemic hormonal factors of pregnancy

ETIOLOGY

- Individuals with intracardiac shunts develop uncorrected L (systemic) →R (pulmonary) shunts
- Shunt occurs through ASD, VSD, patent ductus arteriosus, or aortopulmonary window

- L→R shunt overloads pulmonary vascular bed and RV
- Pulmonary vasculature becomes remodelled with relative fixed PVR
- ES follows with pulmonary hypertension, R→L or bidirectional shunt with peripheral cyanosis
- Pulmonary hypertension is fixed and not reversible by repair of intracardiac lesion

USUAL TREATMENT

- With expected high maternal mortality, pregnant patients with ES should initially be counseled to terminate pregnancy
- For the patient who wishes to continue with pregnancy:
  - hospital admission early in 3rd trimester
  - anticoagulation with heparin: SC heparin 5,000–10,000 U bid
  - patients with O₂ sat <80% on room air should be fully anticoagulated
  - O₂ Rx
  - Monitor for preterm labor
  - Medical Rx: diuretics, antiarrhythmics, inotropes
- Long-term and postpartum: Surgical treatment has been described: either heart and lung transplantation or lung transplantation with primary repair of congenital cardiac defects

ASSESSMENT POINTS

SYSTEM	EFFECT	ASSESSMENT BY HX	PE	TEST
CV	Right and left ventricular enlargement/failure	DOE, edema, orthopnea, anginal chest pain, syncope, fatigue	Elevated jugular venous pressure, increased intensity of S_2, split S_2 and S_3, rales Right ventricular heave	ECG CXR ECHO, angio
RESP	Pulmonary hypertension	Dyspnea, hemoptysis	Palpable pulmonary artery Cyanosis, clubbing	Pulse oximetry ABG, Hct (polycythemia)

Key Reference: Smedstad KG, et al: Pulmonary hypertension and pregnancy: A series of eight cases. Can J Anaesth 1994; 41:502–512.

PERIOPERATIVE IMPLICATIONS

Preoperative Preparation

- Discontinuation of heparin; consider reversal with protamine
- Avoid aortocaval compression at all times
- Antibiotic coverage for subacute bacterial endocarditis

Monitoring

- Pulse oximetry
- With uncorrected patent ductus arteriosus, use simultaneous right hand (preductal) and foot (postductal) pulse oximetry to estimate changes in shunt fraction
- CVP line
- PA catheter use is controversial, may be relatively contraindicated, potential complications may outweigh benefits:
  - difficult to position in PA
  - high risk of arrhythmias, thrombi, paradoxical emboli, PA hemorrhage
  - misleading data: unreliable PCWP and measurement CO with shunt

Airway

- Preoperative administration of Bicitra, metoclopramide, and ranitidine
- NPO for 8 h (if possible)

Preinduction/Induction

- For labor:
  - provision of effective analgesia prevents ↑ release of catecholamines, which ↑ PVR
  - coaxial technique: initial intrathecal dose of narcotic
- For cesarean section:
  - regional: slow induction of epidural anesthesia; counteract sympathectomy with vasopressor and maintenance of preload
  - general anesthesia: avoid rapid-sequence with risk of precipitating ↑ in PVR or inducing myocardial depression; maintain cricoid pressure through induction; avoid ↑ in PVR, ↓ in SVR, hypoxia, hypercarbia, and myocardial depressants

Maintenance

- For labor:
  - epidural infusion with low-dose local anesthetic/narcotic solution
  - avoid Valsalva maneuver, pushing; delivery with vacuum or forceps
- For cesarean:
  - high-dose narcotic technique
  - amnesia with benzodiazepine
  - avoid halogenated agents: myocardial depression, ↓ SVR
  - avoid nitrous oxide: ↑ PVR, higher FIO₂

Extubation

- High-dose narcotic technique neccessitates postop ventilation

Adjuvants

- Avoid N₂O
- Maintain SVR with dilute solution of phenylephrine
- Inotrope, vasodilator for treatment of failure
- Cautious use of oxytocin (systemic vasodilation)
- Avoid prostaglandin F (↑ in PVR)
- Resume anticoagulation in postpartum period

Postoperative Period

- Pain management is critical
- Death most often occurs at delivery or postpartum
- Possible hemodynamic changes:
  - excessive blood loss; replace volume
  - autotransfusion; treat with vasodilator, inotrope, judicious use of diuretic
  - arrhythmias: sinus bradycardia, AV block, EMD
  - pulmonary emboli
  - postpartum increase in PVR; reason unknown

ANTICIPATED PROBLEMS/CONCERNS

- Unresponsive, ↑ PVR or ↓ SVR with loss of oxygenation
- CHF

EMPHYSEMA

William Furman, M.D.

RISK

- Prevalence, incidence, mortality ↑ with age
- Higher in males than females
- Higher in whites than nonwhites

PERIOPERATIVE RISKS

- Intraoperative bronchospasm
- N_2O expansion of bullae
- Postop respiratory failure
- Postop pulmonary infection

WORRY ABOUT

- Worsening of baseline pulmonary function, caused by:
  – Bronchospasm
  – Acute bronchitis or pneumonia
  – Pulm embolism

OVERVIEW

- Anatomic: destruction of interalveolar septa and loss of pulmonary elastic recoil; leads to formation of bullae and development of irreversible expiratory airflow obstruction
- The prototypical "pink puffer" has dyspnea, hyperinflation, distant breath sounds, low diffusing capacity (↑ DLCO <60%)
- Patients often have elements of chronic bronchitis and asthma
- Hypoxia, hypercarbia, cor pulmonale are late developments
- Mucociliary clearance is often worsened after inhalational anesthetics
- Diaphragmatic mechanics are impaired by anesthetics, sedatives, NM blockers, conduction blocks, supine positioning

ICD-9-CM Code: 492.8 (Resection of bullae)

ETIOLOGY

- Acquired disease related to smoking tobacco products in most cases. Specific occupational exposures, such as coal mining, have also been implicated
- Genetic disease found in the presence of α_1-antitrypsin deficiency (accounts for very small fraction of cases)

USUAL TREATMENT

- Smoking cessation
- Relief of symptoms by treatment of bronchospasm and infection
- In advanced cases, if hypoxia and cor pulmonale have developed: oxygen
- Lung reduction surgery in cases of diaphragmatic dysfunction and disabling disease (experimental)

ASSESSMENT POINTS

SYSTEM	EFFECT	ASSESSMENT BY HX	PE	TEST
HEENT	Tumors 2° to smoking	Voice change	Hoarseness, stridor, inspiratory obstruction	
CV	Cor pulmonale (late)	Edema, severe dyspnea	Signs of pulm HTN, Hepatosplenomegaly, Pedal edema, cyanosis, pleural effusions, usually without pulmonary edema	CXR, ABG
	Pulmonary emboli	Episodic SOB, Arrhythmias and MS, Hard to differentiate from course of underlying illness	May reveal DVT in legs	CXR, V/Q scan, Pulmonary angiogram
RESP	Bronchospasm	Recent ↑ in dyspnea or ↓ in exercise tolerance	↑ Resp rate, ↑ Expiratory time, ↑ Accessory muscle use	Spirometry pre- and post bronchodilators
	Pneumonia	Fever, dyspnea, ↑ sputum	Signs of pulmonary consolidation	CXR

Key Reference: Pietak S, et al: Anesthetic effects on ventilation in patients with chronic obstructive pulmonary disease. Anesthesiology 1975; 42:160–166.

PERIOPERATIVE IMPLICATIONS

Preoperative Preparation

- Optimize bronchodilation
- Eradicate any underlying bacterial infection
- Encourage smoking cessation

Monitoring

- Be cognizant of potential for increased gradient between $PETCO_2$ and $PaCO_2$

Airway

- None, unless tumor present in airway

Preinduction/Induction

- If patient has airway reactivity, consider issues related to asthma
- Usually best to avoid N_2O when expansion of bullae is a risk

Maintenance

- Recumbent positions impair chest wall muscle function, and abdominal muscle function usually needed for spontaneous ventilation
- Ventilator settings: long expiratory times may be required; try to avoid high positive pressures, especially if bullae are present

Extubation

- Residual anesthetics may compromise the ventilatory response to CO_2, increasing the risk of postop respiratory failure
- Patients may be semiconscious and combative owing to hypoxia and hypercarbia on emergence
- Evaluate whether postop ventilation may be the safest approach until the residual anesthetic effects have dissipated

Adjuvants

- ß-adrenergic agonists, atropinic agents for airway reactivity

Postoperative Period

- Residual anesthetic effects may persist well into recovery period and predispose to postop respiratory failure
- Analgesics may depress ventilatory function; however, unrelieved incisional pain, especially after abdominal or thoracic surgery, will impair breathing

ANTICIPATED PROBLEMS/CONCERNS

- Postop respiratory failure
- Tension pneumothorax from ventilator-induced barotrauma
- Airway plugging from secretions

ENCEPHALITIS

Mary J. Njoku, M.D.
M. Jane Matjasko, M.D.

RISK

- Increased by exposure in endemic areas
- Increased during seasonal variation and epidemic outbreaks
- Associated with immunosuppression (HIV, transplant, oncology, chemotherapy)

PERIOPERATIVE RISKS

- Associated with mental status alteration, seizures, ↑ ICP, SIADH
- Associated with increased sensitivity to sedative and amnestic effects of anesthetics and adjunct drugs
- Unrecognized, unexpected deterioration in mental status may occur perioperatively

WORRY ABOUT

- Delayed awakening
- Hyperkalemic response to succinylcholine
- Postop delirium
- Electrolyte abn 2° to SIADH

OVERVIEW

- Inflammation of parenchymal brain tissue
- May be primary manifestation of disease process or a component of another CNS or systemic illness
- Organisms enter CNS via blood stream, peripheral nerves, olfactory nerves
- Sx include fever, headache, broad range of neurologic manifestations: altered mental status, lethargy, confusion, coma, personality disorders, memory loss, seizures, focal neurologic abn
- Dx is established by symptoms, epidemiologic Hx (exposure, season, geographic location), CSF culture, CSF bacterial and viral antigens, brain biopsy, CT scan, MRI, ^{99m}Tc scan, EEG

ICD-9-CM Code: 064

ETIOLOGY

- Infectious
  - Viral
  - Nonviral—bacteria, protozoa, nematodes, fungi
- Noninfectious
  - Toxic, vascular, SLE, Behçet's disease

USUAL TREATMENT

- Acyclovir effective for herpes simplex encephalitis
- Other antimicrobial therapy should be given according to culture and sensitivity
- Supportive care:
  - Intubate, ventilate, if dictated by mental status, airway reflexes
  - Hemodynamic support
  - Nutrition
  - DVT prophylaxis
  - GI prophylaxis
  - Physical therapy
  - Diagnosis and treatment of extracranial infections
- Management of complications: seizure, ↑ ICP, SIADH, ventilatory failure

ASSESSMENT POINTS

SYSTEM	EFFECT	ASSESSMENT BY HX	PE	TEST
HEENT	Colonization of nasopharynx	Preceding URI		Nasopharyngeal culture
CV	Autonomic dysfunction		Labile BP, HR	
HEME	↑ or normal WBC			CBC and differential
RENAL	SIADH	Water intoxication Anorexia N/V Personality disorders Neurologic abn	No evidence of volume depletion Normal skin turgor Normal BP Mental status changes from lethargy to coma	Serum Na⁺ and osmolarity Urine Na⁺ and osmolarity BUN, Cr
CNS	Focal, global neurologic disturbances	Fever Headache Seizure Personality change Memory loss Confusion Weakness	Focal neurologic deficits Altered mentation Papilledema	CSF culture Cell count, Gram stain, antigens CT MRI ^{99m}Tc scanning EEG Biopsy

Key Reference: Irani DN, Hanley DF, Johnson RT: Acute viral encephalitis: Diagnosis and clinical management. *In* Tyler KL, Martin JB (eds): Infectious Diseases of the Central Nervous System. Philadelphia, F.A. Davis, 1993.

COMPLICATIONS

Preoperative Preparation

- Document neurologic exam
- Elicit Hx of ↑ ICP or seizure
- If SIADH present, correct electrolyte and free water abn
  - Sodium administration or fluid restriction depending upon severity of hyponatremia
  - Beware of central pontine myelinolysis with rapid correction of hyponatremia

Monitoring

- Electrolytes
- Fluid I/O
- Consider ICP monitoring, EEG monitoring

Airway

- None

Induction

- Potential for hyperkalemic response to succinylcholine indicates preferred use of nondepolarizing NM blockers
- Autonomic instability

Maintenance

- If receiving seizure prophylaxis, be aware of potentiation of sedative effects and alteration of hepatic metabolism of anesthetics

Extubation

- Delayed awakening
- Seizures on emergence

Postoperative Period

- Delirium
- Possible progressive deterioration

Adjuvants

- See interactions under Induction and Maintenance

ANTICIPATED PROBLEMS/CONCERNS

- Delayed awakening
- SIADH
- Hyperkalemic response to succinylcholine

ENCEPHALOPATHY, HYPERTENSIVE

Jeffrey Katz, M.D.

RISK

- 1% of 60 million hypertensives
- Race with highest prevalence: African-American

PERIOPERATIVE RISKS

- ↑ Risk of MI
- CVA and renal failure, but not well documented

WORRY ABOUT

- Myocardial ischemia, failure
- Hemorrhagic CVA
- Neurologic deterioration postoperatively
- Aortic dissection
- Acute renal failure
- Microangiopathic hemolytic anemia

OVERVIEW

- Occurs with hypertension, renal failure, eclampsia
- On decline owing to better Dx and treatment; rare
- Follows rapid course leading to severe damage or death in hours if not treated
- Chronic hypertensives able to tolerate higher acute elevation in BP than others with recent onset of hypertension (e.g., eclampsia, renal failure)

ICD-9-CM Code: 437.2

ETIOLOGY

- Abrupt ↑ BP in chronic hypertensives
- Renovascular hypertension, parenchymal renal disease
- Drug ingestion (e.g., cocaine, amphetamines)
- Withdrawal from antihypertensive therapy, especially α-agonists (e.g., clonidine)
- Pre-eclampsia, eclampsia
- Pheochromocytoma
- Renin-secreting tumor
- Autonomic hyperactivity (cord lesions)
- Ingestion of tyramine with use of MAO inhibitor
- Head injury
- Thought to be precipitated by abrupt ↑ in SVR as a result of circulating levels of vasoconstrictors such as norepinephrine, angiotension II, or ADH

USUAL TREATMENT

- Antihypertensives
  - vasodilators: nitroprusside, nitroglycerin
  - ganglion blockers: trimethaphan
  - carbonic anhydrase inhibitors: diazoxide
  if not invasively monitored

ASSESSMENT POINTS

SYSTEM	EFFECT	ASSESSMENT BY HX	PE	TEST
CV	Hypertension (diastolic >140 mmHg) CHF Myocardial ischemia	Past hypertension Angina Sx of CHF ↓ Exercise tolerance	S_3 S_4 gallop Rales	CXR ECG
RESP	↓ Lung elastance ↓ FEV, FVC	Exercise intolerance Cough Orthopnea	Rales	CXR O_2 Sat
GI	Aortic dissection Encephalopathy	Abdominal pain Back pain N/V	Abdominal mass	Ultrasound or arteriogram (if indicated)
RENAL	Renal failure	Anuria		UO, UA BUN/Cr
CNS	Severe headache Visual disturbances Paralysis Convulsions Stupor, coma	Mental status examination	Retinal leak Arteriolar spasm	Retinoscopy

Key Reference: Calhoun DA, Oparil S: Treatment of hypertensive crisis: Review article. N Engl J Med 1990; 323:17, 1117–1183.

PERIOPERATIVE IMPLICATIONS

Preoperative Preparation

- Control BP: nitroprusside, nitroglycerin, trimethaphan
- Treat CV failure, renal failure

Monitoring

- Invasive BP monitoring
- Invasive blood volume monitoring (CVP or pulmonary artery cath) or TEE

Airway

- Control BP during intubation

Induction

- Avoid ↑ in BP
- Control volume preinduction

Maintenance

- CV instability; volume status key to avoid fluctuations
- Control BP aggressively

Extubation

- Under BP control

Adjuvants

- Continued aggressive BP control

ANTICIPATED PROBLEMS/CONCERNS

- Labile BP
- Myocardial ischemia/failure
- CNS symptoms
- End-organ ischemia owing to angiopathic changes

ENCEPHALOPATHY, METABOLIC

Charles Weissman, M.D.

RISK

- 3.4–11% of medical ICU admissions

PERIOPERATIVE RISKS

- With predisposing conditions, e.g., hepatic insufficiency, risk of developing or exacerbating metabolic encephalopathy
- Increasing severity of pre-existing encephalopathy

WORRY ABOUT

- Worsening hepatic insufficiency causing hepatic encephalopathy
- Diabetics becoming hypoglycemic
- Postop hyponatremia
- Deteriorating renal insufficiency leading to uremic encephalopathy
- Pre-existing encephalopathy may be exacerbated by anesthetics, e.g., benzodiazepines, in hepatic encephalopathy

OVERVIEW

- Altered sensorium, stupor, or coma without any other explanation in the setting of a metabolic disturbance
- Process affects global cortical function by altering brain biochemistry
- Distinguished from structural lesions by a nonfocal neurologic exam
- EEG shows diffuse background slowing, triphasic waves in hepatic encephalopathy
- Increased spontaneous motor activity—restlessness, asterixis, myoclonus, tremors, rigidity

ICD-9-CM Code: 348.3 (Unspecified encephalopathy)

ETIOLOGY

- Hypoglycemic encephalopathy—most commonly due to accidental or deliberate overdosing with insulin or oral hypoglycemic agents or prolonged ethanol intoxication
- Hepatic encephalopathy—acute or chronic hepatic insufficiency, Reye's syndrome
- Uremic encephalopathy—renal failure. After dialysis "disequilibrium syndrome" caused by acute fluid and electrolyte shifts
- Encephalopathy due to fluid and electrolyte abnormalities—hyperosmolar state, hyponatremia (acute decrease to <120 mEq/L), hypernatremia
- Pulmonary encephalopathy—combination of hypoxia and hypercarbia

USUAL TREATMENT

- Uremic encephalopathy—dialysis
- Hepatic encephalopathy—lactulose (oral or rectal), neomycin
- Hypoglycemic encephalopathy—intravenous glucose
- Septic encephalopathy—treatment of underlying infection
- Hyperosmolar/hyposmolar state—slow and careful restoration of electrolyte balance
- Pulmonary encephalopathy—quickly improve ventilation and oxygenation, mechanical ventilation

ASSESSMENT POINTS

SYSTEM	EFFECT	ASSESSMENT BY HX	PE	TEST
RESP	Sudden elevated $PaCO_2$ (>65 mmHg)	COPD, drug overdose	Hypoventilation, papilledema	Pulse oximetry and end-tidal capnography, or ABG
GI	Hepatic insufficiency	Liver disease, cirrhosis, alcoholism, portasystemic shunt	Asterixis, jaundice, ascites	AST, ALT, bilirubin, ammonia PT
ENDO	Diabetes	Use of insulin or oral hypoglycemic agents		Blood glucose
RENAL	Uremia Prerenal azotemia	Renal disease, ingestion of nephrotoxins, e.g., drugs	Asterixis	BUN/Cr, serum lytes Toxicology screen
CNS	Altered sensorium, stupor, coma, seizures		Nonfocal neurologic exam, altered mental status	EEG, CT Lumbar puncture
MS	Multifocal myoclonus, rigidity		Myoclonus	

Key Reference: Ravin PD, Walsh FX: Metabolic encephalopathy. *In* Rippe JM, Irwin RS, Alpert JS, Fink MP (eds): Intensive Care Medicine, 2nd ed. Boston, Little, Brown, 1991, pp 1553–1560.

PERIOPERATIVE IMPLICATIONS

Preoperative Preparation

- Assess and document preop mental status and neurologic function
- Uremic encephalopathy—preop dialysis, if possible

Monitoring

- Routine
- In hyperosmolar states, uremia and liver failure with ascites may need central monitoring

Preinduction/Induction

- Benzodiazepines should be avoided in hepatic encephalopathy.
- Increased potential for aspiration; consider rapid-sequence

Maintenance

- Carefully titrate anesthetics to avoid overdosing
- Careful attention should be paid to intravascular volume status, blood glucose, and lytes
- During TURP, sodium concentrations and volume status should be monitored
- In renal and hepatic failure, appropriate drugs and doses should be used. Long-acting drugs should be avoided

Extubation

- Extubate only if patient is able to protect airway and maintain adequate ventilation

ANTICIPATED PROBLEMS/CONCERNS

- Poor mental status at the conclusion of surgery may require continued intubation
- Hyponatremia is a cause of postop metabolic encephalopathy

ENCEPHALOPATHY, POSTANOXIC

Charles Weissman, M.D.

RISK

• After successful prehospital cardiac resuscitation: 59–65% of patients remain comatose
• 0–5% of successful resuscitations result in chronic vegetative state

PERIOPERATIVE RISKS

• Worsening of neurologic status; blindness most common residuum
• Postpone surgery in all but emergency situations
• Do what is necessary to treat precipitating cause and ↓ sequelae (e.g., ↓ ICP or edema by ↑ ventilation and slight ↑ in BP)

WORRY ABOUT

• Repeat of events that initially caused encepalopathy (e.g., arrhythmias leading to cardiac arrest)

OVERVIEW

• Definition: Brain injury resulting from "prolonged" period of insufficient cerebral oxygenation
• Clinical picture ranges from mild confusion to brain death
• Chances for acceptable neurologic recovery ~1% with continued coma after 24 h and lack of two of the following reflexes: pupillary, corneal, and oculovestibular
• Seizures occur in 25% of patients
• Anoxic damage may have been sustained by other organs (e.g., MI, shock liver, acute renal failure, stress ulcers, ARDS)
• Diabetes insipidus poor prognostic sign

ICD-9-CM Code: 348.1

ETIOLOGY

• Caused by inadequate O_2 delivery to CNS due to inadequate cardiac output, respiratory dysfunction, severe anemia, and/or ↑ICP
• Most often 2° to 1° cardiac (MI or arrhythmia) or pulmonary (asthma, pulmonary embolism) event
• May also be result of carbon monoxide poisoning, suffocation, and cyanide poisoning

USUAL TREATMENT

• Prevent recurrence of inciting event
• Ventilatory and hemodynamic support, as needed
• Stress ulcer prophylaxis
• Treatment of seizures (with anticonvulsants, e.g., phenytoin) and myoclonus

ASSESSMENT POINTS

SYSTEM	EFFECT	ASSESSMENT BY HX	PE	TEST
CV	MI	Assess if cardiac disease was cause of arrest		ECG, other cardiac assessment CPK, AST, LDH
RESP	ARDS	Assess if respiratory disease was cause of arrest Respiratory failure	Wheezing, stigmata of COPD	Pre-arrest PFTs ABG
GI	Shock liver		Jaundice	AST, ALT, bilirubin, alkaline phosphatase
	Stress ulceration	Hx of GI bleeding		Hct NG output
RENAL	Renal failure	Assess if electrolyte abnormalities or acidosis caused initial event	Urine output	BUN/Cr
CNS	Altered mental status, diffuse and focal neurologic abnormalities	Changes in neurologic signs since hypoxic event	Neurologic and mental status exams, apnea test	CT scan EEG
MS	Myoclonus, posturing	Hx of abnormal movements, posturing	Decerebrate or decorticate postures	
	Contractures	Prolonged immobility	Contractures	

Key Reference: Lippa CP: Generalized anoxia/ischemia of the nervous system. In Rippe JM, et al (eds): Intensive Care Medicine, 2nd ed. Boston, Little, Brown, 1991, pp 1561–1564.

PERIOPERATIVE IMPLICATIONS

Preoperative Preparation

• Assess and document neurologic function and mental status
• Review cause of anoxic event
• Assess damage to other organs

Monitoring

• If arrest was due to cardiac arrhythmias or MI/ischemia or if patient is hemodynamically unstable, may need specialized monitoring

Airway

• Assess potential for aspiration: gag reflex, ability to cough and clear secretions

Induction

• Avoid succinylcholine

Maintenance

• Must consider that patients may have pain perception and will require analgesia
• Do what is appropriate to ↓ sequelae (e.g., prevent cerebral edema, ↓ ICP with mild hyperventilation and slight ↑ in BP)

Extubation

• If unable to maintain patent airway or sustain adequate minute ventilation, should remain intubated

Adjuvants

• Avoid long-acting anesthetics so that neurologic status can be assessed soon after surgery
• Avoid drugs that ↓ seizure threshold

ANTICIPATED PROBLEMS/CONCERNS

• Repeat of events (e.g., arrhythmias) that initially led to anoxic encephalopathy
• Worsening of neurologic condition during perioperative period
• Postpone all but emergency surgery if fluctuating neurologic deficits or acute encephalopathic condition exists

ENDOCARDIAL CUSHION DEFECT

Carol L. Lake, M.D.

RISK

- 0.3% of newborns affected
- Male:female ratio 1.3:1

PERIOPERATIVE RISKS

- Paradoxical embolism, esp with shunt reversal caused by anesthetic drugs, airway stimulation during light anesthesia, airway obstruction
- Subacute bacterial endocarditis prophylaxis
- Pulm hypertensive crisis in patients with reactive pulm vasculature
- AV valve regurgitation, arrhythmias after surgical repair of lesion

WORRY ABOUT

- Reversal of shunt and development of pulm vascular obstructive disease
- Development of supraventricular arrhythmias, particularly AFib

OVERVIEW

- Endocardial cushion defects result from failure to grow and fuse to create portions of the interatrial and interventricular septa and clefts in anterior mitral and septal tricuspid valve leaflets.
- Causes shunting at atrial or ventricular (or both) sites with or without associated AV valvular regurgitation
- Dx established by ECHO and cardiac catheterization
- Endocardial cushion defects place patients at risk for development of shunt reversal leading to Eisenmenger's syndrome and pulm vascular obstructive disease.

ICD-9-CM Code: 745.69

ETIOLOGY

- Result when the endocardial cushions in the 6 mm embryo fail to fuse with each other and with interatrial septum primum.

USUAL TREATMENT

- Medical: Symptomatic therapy with digitalis and diuretics for heart failure.
- Surgical: Definitive therapy requires closure of the septal defects and repair of the clefts in the AV valves

ASSESSMENT POINTS

SYSTEM	EFFECT	ASSESSMENT BY HX	PE	TEST
HEENT	Feeding difficulties	Failure to thrive	< Normal wt/ht for age	
CV	CHF	Dyspnea, diaphoresis, coughing	Wheezing, rales	Cardiac catheterization, ECG
RESP	Pulm HTN			CXR
RENAL	Renal dysfunction due to heart failure			BUN, Cr
MS	Decreased exercise compared with peers			

Key Reference: Lake CL: Pediatric Cardiac Anesthesia, 2nd ed. Norwalk, CT: Appleton and Lange, 1993, pp 233–241.

PERIOPERATIVE IMPLICATIONS

Preoperative Preparation

- Prophylactic antibiotics for subacute bacterial endocarditis
- Premedication to minimize anxiety and possible shunt reversal
- Diuretic if prone to CHF

Monitoring

- Intra-arterial catheter and central venous catheter if required by surgical procedure
- TEE if available and appropriate to anesthetic and surgical procedure

Airway

- May be difficult if associated congenital anomalies such as Down syndrome

Preinduction/Induction

- Meticulous air removal to avoid paradoxical embolism
- IV or inhalation induction depending on patient preference/cooperation. Choice of intravenous induction agent, depends on severity of CHF and pulm HTN

Maintenance

- Volatile agents that decrease systemic vascular resistance may worsen R → L shunting. Combinations of narcotic with low concentrations of volatile agents may be appropriate in patients with moderate disease.

Extubation

- At end of operation in patients without CHF or pulm HTN. If reactive pulm vasculature, may develop pulm hypertensive crisis requiring hyperventilation, $\uparrow FIO_2$, and sedation, which is more easily accomplished during mechanical ventilation.

Adjuvants

- Nitric oxide, nitroglycerin, prostaglandin to control pulm vascular tone. Inotropes for heart failure

Postoperative Period

- Observe left and right atrial pressures, as LAP more than 6 mm >RAP suggests mitral valve incompetence/stenosis
- Residual shunting at atrial or ventricular level should be excluded by echocardiography.
- Heart block or other conduction defects may result from surgical repair.
- Effective analgesia to minimize pulmonary hypertensive crisis

ANTICIPATED PROBLEMS/CONCERNS

- Patients with partial or complete AV canal defects 2° to endocardial cushion defects who have CHF are likely to have moderate to severe AV valvular incompetence or pulm HTN.
- Significantly increased pulm blood flow 2° to L → R cardiac shunting increases the risk of developing pulm vascular obstructive disease and shunt reversal.

EPIDERMOLYSIS BULLOSA

Nancy B. Kenepp, M.D.

RISK

- 1/50,000, equal racial distribution
- 1/300,000 for dystrophic form

PERIOPERATIVE RISKS

- Iatrogenic blister formation, secondary acute airway obstruction, hemorrhage, septicemia, scarring, stricture

WORRY ABOUT

- Difficult intubation (23%) 2° to microstomia
- Establishing monitoring, IV access
- Dehydration, malnutrition
- Anemia, hypoalbuminemia, electrolyte imbalance, thrombocytosis
- Septicemia
- Renal and adrenal dysfunction

OVERVIEW

- Characterized by epithelial blistering as a result of minor trauma by lateral shearing forces, not pressure
- 4 types: simplex (SEB), junctional (JEB), dystrophic, acquired
- Associated conditions: porphyria, amyloidosis, pyloric stenosis, multiple myeloma, diabetes mellitus, hypercoagulable states, mitral valve prolapse
- SEB: Blisters form at the keratocyte level, generally mild. In Dowling-Meara form, blisters are herpetiform
- JEB: Blisters form within basement membrane at the lamina lucida. Most die by age 2 y. Scarring absent, but blistering more extensive and involves resp, GI, GU mucosa. Sepsis, malnutrition, esophageal and laryngeal strictures result.
- Dystrophic: Blisters form in lamina densa with scarring (either atrophic or hypertrophic) and involve mucosa, mouth, esophagus, GI tract. Syndactyly, milia, nail dystrophy, dental lesions, microstomia, esophageal stricture result
- Acquired: Blisters occur on skin and in mouth in 50% of cases; may be extensive, with resulting fluid and protein loss

ICD-9-CM Code: 757.39

ETIOLOGY

- SEB: Inherited autosomal dominant mutation on chromosome 1, 12, or 17, producing abnormal type I keratin K 5 and 14
- JEB: Inherited autosomal recessive defect in hemidesmosomes that lack BM600 and epiligrin
- Dystrophic: 2 inherited types: recessive (RDEB) and dominant (DDEB). DDEB (Cockayne-Touraine) is less severe and linked with the type VIII collagen gene on short arm of chromosome 3. RDEB is a heterogeneous group with mutant type VIII collagen affecting the anchoring fibrils, and increased collagenase and matrix metalloproteins, e.g., stromolysin-degrading collagen.
- Acquired: development of antibodies to epiligrin and type VIII collagen

USUAL TREATMENT

- Acquired: cyclosporine, steroids
- Inherited: no definitive Rx, usual wound care, steroids, vitamin E
- Aggressive nutritional support, gastrostomy, balloon dilatation of esophagus, hydration, laxatives, fiber
- Phenytoin inhibits collagenase and has been used for RDEB, but effectiveness unpredictable, probably related to collagenase activity

ASSESSMENT POINTS

SYSTEM	EFFECT	ASSESSMENT BY HX	PE	TEST
HEENT	Enamel hypoplasia (JEB)	Delayed eruption, impaction of teeth	Poor oral hygiene, malocclusion	None
	Blisters, microstomia, ankyloglossia (RDEB)	Pain: lesions of hard palate, tongue, buccal mucosa, lips, gingiva	Obliteration of vestibular sulci, atrophy of tongue, viscous saliva	Airway assessment
	Supraglottic ulceration, cysts, or narrowing; rare subglottic stenosis	Hoarseness, resp obstruction	Vocal cord bullae, webs, or stenosis (JEB)	Endoscopy
	Mucosal bullae	Painful swallowing, spasm, food impaction, obstruction, onset age 4 y	Cervical stricture (70%), diverticula, web, "double-barrel"	Endoscopy
GI	Bullae (JEB) Perianal blisters, poor absorption, diarrhea	Anal pain, tenesmus, constipation, onset age 3 y	Anal fissure or stricture	Barium enema, endoscopy
GU (JEB)	Blisters	Urinary diversion	Obstruction, sepsis	Renal function
MS (dystrophic)	Scarring	Growth retardation	Flexural contractions, pseudosyndactyly of hands and feet, dystrophy of nails	
SKIN	Blisters	Age at onset, Hx of remissions, infections	Scars, milia, nail dystrophy, cancer	Skin biopsy

Key Reference: Griffin RP, Mayou BJ: The anesthetic management of patients with dystrophic epidermolysis bullosa. A review of 44 patients over a 10 year period. Anesthesia 1993; 48:810–815.

PERIOPERATIVE IMPLICATIONS

Preoperative Preparation

- Difficult intubation, incidence 23%
- Assess for infection, nutritional status, fluid and lyte balance
- Plan positioning and padding on operating table; have patient move to avoid skin traction

Monitoring

- Pad BP cuff; use sparingly, or use arterial line.
- No esophageal stethoscope
- Monitoring without adhesive

Induction

- Regional anesthesia may be used
- Agent: no anesthetic or muscle relaxant specifically contraindicated; consider ketamine or propofol infusion.

Airway

- All techniques reported successful; use least traumatic. Consider fiberoptic intubation; mask with port for endoscopy; LMA or endotracheal tube for SEB without mucosal involvement. Avoid endotracheal tube with JEB to prevent laryngeal lesions. If larynx involved, tracheostomy indicated as tracheal mucosa is more resistant to scarring than glottic mucosa.
- Lubricate masks, tubes; and laryngoscopes everywhere. Use small endotracheal tube, soft lubricated gauze to prevent movement in the mouth, no lateral force on mouth corners from tube. Avoid nasal or oral airways.

Emergence

- Aim for a quiet emergence
- No suction on intraoral mucosa

ANTICIPATED PROBLEMS/CONCERNS

- Blisters of ears, head (1%), eyes (1%), pharynx (0.5%) from positioning and managing airway. Treat hemorrhage with epinephrine-soaked sponge
- IV and arterial lines sutured rather than taped, pour prep, no rubbing
- Consider stress dose steroids
- Perioperative regurgitation incidence 1.5%
- Avoid sweating, warming blanket, high ambient temp; exacerbates bullae
- Extremity tourniquets and IM injections can be used
- Common procedures: repair syndactyly, dilatation of esophageal stricture, colonic interposition, gastrostomy tube, dental extractions, excision of skin tumor, anal fissure, urinary diversion, endoscopy, airway surgery

EPIGLOTTITIS

Maurice S. Zwass, M.D.

RISK

- Children 1–7 y, although epiglottitis (sometimes called supraglottitis) does occur in adults. (Decreasing incidence in children >3 y, ? related to recent vaccine against *H. influenzae* type B.)

PERIOPERATIVE RISKS

- Acute deterioration of airway patency resulting in complete obstruction
- Difficulty in tracheal intubation because of airway obstruction, and severe edema of epiglottis and arytenoids

WORRY ABOUT

- Airway compromise in children who appear "toxic," with increasing distress, drooling, hypoxemia. The acute risks of airway compromise (of principal concern in small children with epiglottitis) appear to be less critical in adult patients, most likely because of their larger airway size.
- Loss of airway control and aspiration during induction of anesthesia

OVERVIEW

- An acute, potentially life-threatening cause of upper airway obstruction (etiologic agents may include bacteria other than *H. influenzae* type B)
- Produces inflammatory edema of epiglottis and other supraglottic structures
- Onset usually rapid; progression to severe obstruction can occur in several hours
- High fever, sore throat, and dysphagia frequently so severe that swallowing is inhibited and drooling results.

ICD-9-CM Codes: 464.30; 464.31 (with obstruction)

ETIOLOGY

- *H. influenzae* type B is most often associated pathogen, though can be caused by β-hemolytic streptococci

USUAL TREATMENT

- Antibiotic therapy against bacterium (usually *H. influenzae*) and airway support, which generally requires tracheal intubation
- Because of high incidence of ampicillin-resistant strains, ampicillin plus a β-lactamase inhibitor (such as sulbactam) and/or chloramphenicol, cefuroxime, ceftazidime, or another penicillinase-resistant antibiotic as indicated by blood and epiglottis culture results.
- Tracheal intubation classically performed in OR in a controlled fashion with surgical support for possible tracheotomy or cricothyrotomy present and gowned

ASSESSMENT POINTS

Differentiation between epiglottitis and croup (laryngotracheobronchitis):

	CROUP	EPIGLOTTITIS
Age	3 mo–3 y	1–7 y
Onset	Gradual	More rapid (usually <24 h)
Fever	Low grade	High
Cough	Characteristic barking	None
Sore throat	Occasional	Frequently severe
Posture	Any	Frequently sitting forward, mouth open, drooling
Airway sound	Inspiratory stridor	Inspiratory stridor
Voice	Normal	Muffled
Appearance	Nontoxic	Toxic
Seasonality	Peak winter, epidemic	Year round

Radiographic studies may be helpful, because AP view of trachea appears normal but lateral neck view usually shows a markedly swollen, edematous epiglottis ("thumbprinting").

Key Reference: Emmerson SG, Richman B, Spahn T: Changing patterns of epiglottitis in children. Otolaryngol Head Neck Surg 1991; 104:287–292.

PERIOPERATIVE IMPLICATIONS

Preoperative Preparation

- With suspected epiglottitis, other personnel on patient care team can set up care (e.g., OR or ICU). Radiographs can be obtained, *but a team member capable of monitoring the patient and securing the airway if urgently needed should be present.*
- Allow to remain in a position of comfort (often sitting with parent). Direct exam of oropharynx generally avoided, as are attempts to secure vascular access, because these may cause agitation leading to acute tracheal obstruction.
- Humidified oxygen should be delivered as tolerated.

- Aerosol therapy with racemic epinephrine may provide slight improvement of Sx, but not definitive. If Dx is confirmed, patient is taken to the location for intubation (most commonly OR)

Airway Management

- Anesthesia with halothane and O$_2$, maintaining spontaneous ventilation
- IV catheter placed after induction of anesthesia, followed by direct laryngoscopy.
- Large, swollen epiglottis can make viewing and identification of airway structures difficult, but once the epiglottis is identified, arytenoids and larynx are immediately below and tracheal tube can be inserted.
- Because of upper airway swelling, a tracheal tube 0.5–1.0 mm smaller in diameter may be needed (tracheal tube of adequate length can be made available).

- Rarely is emergency tracheotomy necessary, but surgical consultants are "gloved" until airway secured and stable.
- Frequently orotracheal tube is changed to a nasotracheal tube for ease of securing and patient comfort.

Post Airway Management Plans

- Once airway secured, cultures of blood and epiglottis are obtained, antibiotic therapy is initiated, and sedation plans are instituted.

ANTICIPATED PROBLEMS/CONCERNS

- Resp support often for 24–72 h until swollen epiglottis returns to normal.
- Usually require sedative management to facilitate tolerating mechanical ventilation
- Many patients (approx. 25%) have associated pneumonia that requires treatment

ESOPHAGEAL CANCER

Dawn P. Desiderio, M.D.
Anne C. Kolker, M.D.

RISK

- People within USA: 6 in 100,000 men, 1.6 in 100,000 women
- African-Americans three times greater incidence than Caucasians
- Increase in patients with tobacco abuse, excessive alcoholic intake

PERIOPERATIVE RISKS

- Reflux as a risk for aspiration
- Malnutrition with dehydration due to swallowing dysfunction
- 30% 300-day serious morbidity and 1–3+% 30-day operative mortality

WORRY ABOUT

- Pulmonary compromise due to either chronic aspiration or extensive tobacco history
- Hydration status
- Airway protection at time of anesthesia induction and postop
- Alcohol withdrawal syndromes

OVERVIEW

- Primarily either squamous cell from esophageal squamous epithelium or adenocarcinomas of gastric origin
- Usually 55 to 65 y, with a long-standing Hx of tobacco and alcohol intake
- Dysphagia and weight loss are initial symptoms, often present for 3–4 mo
- Characterized by extensive local growth and lymphatic involvement before becoming widely disseminated

ICD-9-CM Code: 150.9

ETIOLOGY

- Achalasia of 25 y or longer, tobacco use, excessive alcohol intake, lack of aspirin use are associated with an increased incidence of squamous cell cancer
- Reflux esophagitis (Barrett's esophagus) is associated with adenocarcinoma
- Nutritional factors and ingestion of hot liquids have been implicated

USUAL TREATMENT

- Treatment depends on extent of disease and patient's medical status
- Surgery with or without chemotherapy the only possibly curative option
- Patients who are unacceptable surgical risks or with advanced disease may benefit from radiation
- Palliative placement of an internal esophageal stent allows for swallowing of liquids and secretions

ASSESSMENT POINTS

SYSTEM	EFFECT	ASSESSMENT BY HX	PE	TEST
HEENT	Airway assessment for intubation—rapid-sequence or awake fiberoptic	Prior difficult intubation	Neck ROM Visualize uvula, mandibular space	
CV	Alcohol abuse–induced cardiomyopathy	DOE Exercise tolerance		ECG ECHO
RESP	Tobacco abuse Chronic aspiration Radiation/chemotherapy	Pneumonias; RV HTN Cough, dyspnea Sputum	Wheezing RV heave	CXR PFT, diffusion capacity ABG
GI	Obstruction Reflux Malnutrition	Difficulty swallowing Unable to sleep flat Weight loss	Debilitated	UGI Endoscopy
CNS	Alcohol abuse Delirium tremens	Last alcohol ingestion and amount		
MS	Weakness	Poor nutrition	Muscle wasting	Serum albumin
RENAL	Dehydration	Limited intake		Lytes, Cr, BUN

Key Reference: Baue AE (ed): Glenn's Thoracic and Cardiovascular Surgery. Norwalk, CT, Appleton & Lange, 1991, pp 767–827.

PERIPERATIVE IMPLICATIONS

Preoperative Preparation

- Premedication not to obtund a patient at risk for aspiration
- Antisialogogue (atropine 0.4 mg or glycopyrrolate 0.2 mg)
- Premedication with H_2 blocker for acid aspiration prophylaxis plus Reglan to promote gastric emptying
- Steroids given if recently used

Monitoring

- Central venous or PA catheter placement for volume assessment and replacement, and for volume loading prior to surgical compression of the mediastinal structures
- Arterial line for BP monitoring and ABGs

Airway

- Rapid-sequence induction or awake fiberoptic intubation
- The surgical need for one-lung ventilation requires a double-lumen endotracheal tube, a bronchial blocker, or a Univent tube and proper positioning

Induction

- Hypovolemia often results in BP fluctuation
- Aspiration risk during intubation

Maintenance

- No one agent or technique shown superior
- Volume requirements due to mediastinal compression, blood loss, and initial dehydration status
- Oxygenation concerns during one-lung ventilation, the use of 100% O_2 and chemotherapy Hx (bleomycin, mitomycin), prior pulmonary compromise due to tobacco history
- Hypothermia of concern in long procedures
- Placement of nasogastric tube with surgical guidance

Extubation

- Continuing risk of aspiration
- Extubation after postop ventilation to allow for prior resp problems to be resolved and adequate pain control
- Patients with double-lumen endotracheal tubes in place should be reintubated or bronchial blockers pulled back (Univent) or removed.
- Reintubation difficult because of edema and fluid shifts. With solid paralysis and pharyngeal suctioning, double-lumen tube withdrawn under direct vision and replaced with a styletted single-lumen tube
- In difficult patients, a tube exchanger (Cook Airway Exchanger Catheter 5mm) can be inserted in the tracheal lumen, the double-lumen tube withdrawn, and a single-lumen threaded.

Adjuvants

- Patients who have received chemotherapy (mitomycin or bleomycin) might be administered an O_2 concentration of 28% or as low as possible (see Bleomycin in Drugs section)

Postoperative Period

- Epidural analgesia may be beneficial

ANTICIPATED PROBLEMS/CONCERNS

- Airway management: aspiration risk, reintubation problems, extubation criteria
- Volume status in a dehydrated patient undergoing a lengthy surgical procedure with mediastinal compression

FAMILIAL DYSAUTONOMIA
(RILEY-DAY SYNDROME)

Thomas J. Ebert, M.D., Ph.D.
William Hope, M.D., Ph.D.

RISK

- 1:10,000–20,000 in Jews originating from Eastern Europe (Ashkenazi)

PERIOPERATIVE RISKS

- Hemodynamic instability 2° to an erratic autonomic nervous system
- Pulmonary insufficiency 2° to a relative insensitivity to hypoxemia and hypercarbia

WORRY ABOUT

- Precipitation of a dysautonomic crisis characterized by intractable vomiting, HTN, tachycardia, and diaphoresis

OVERVIEW

- Rare, inherited disease of nervous system involving mainly peripheral sensory and sympathetic nerves
- Primarily a disease of children because mortality is high, particularly in early years; usually due to repeated aspiration pneumonias

ICD-9-CM Code: 742.8

ETIOLOGY

- Inheritance is autosomal recessive
- Symptoms due to diffuse sensory defect and an autonomic insufficiency with superimposed supersensitivity to acetylcholine and catecholamines

USUAL TREATMENT

- Symptoms are managed by conventional therapies

ASSESSMENT POINTS

SYSTEM	EFFECT	ASSESSMENT BY HX	PE	TEST
CV	Orthostatic hypotension	Dizziness, syncope	Supine and standing BP, HR	Autonomic function
RESP	Pneumonia Bronchiectasis	Pleuritic chest pain Secretions	Minimal	CXR
GI	Poor swallowing Aspiration pneumonia	Drooling Vomiting, Hx of "attacks"		Swallow study
GU	Dehydration	Emesis	Dry mucosa	Serum Cr
CNS	Seizure	Seizure		EEG

Key Reference: Axelrod, FB, Donenfeld RF, Danziger F, Turndorf H: Anesthesia in familial dysautonomia. Anesthesiology 1988; 68:631–635.

PERIOPERATIVE IMPLICATIONS

Preoperative Preparation

- Difficulty swallowing: abundant secretions plus diminished laryngeal reflexes. Treat with antisialogogues
- Avoid medications interacting with autonomic nervous system
- Vomiting crises: intractable vomiting associated with tachycardia, HTN, apprehension can be prevented by preop sedation with benzodiazepines
- H_2 blockers can decrease gastric volume and acidity
- Phenothiazines are associated with erratic hemodynamics at induction
- Treat chronic dehydration 2° to dysphagia and emesis
- Insensitivity to hypoxia, hypercarbia: minimize narcotics as premedication
- Insensitivity to superficial pain: lines placed without discomfort

Monitoring

- Routine
- Consider arterial line

Induction

- Consider rapid-sequence induction with etomidate because of poor airway reflexes and BP instability
- Use of nondepolarizing agents must be balanced against the risk of postop hypotonia and unpredictable effect of reversal agents on autonomic nervous system
- Lubricate eyes to avoid corneal abrasions

Maintenance

- Dysfunctional temp regulation can require exogenous treatment
- Aggressively treat blood loss, as hemodynamic instability exacerbated by ↓ intravascular volume
- Very sensitive to effects of exogenous catecholamines. If vasopressors required, use direct-acting agents
- Control ventilation

Postoperative Care

- Although peripheral pain sensation is diminished, visceral pain sensation is usually intact, and present as anxiety, HTN, tachycardia or can precipitate dysautonomic crisis. Treat complaints of pain with narcotics and anxiety with benzodiazepines

ANTICIPATED PROBLEMS/CONCERNS

- Respiratory function often compromised by aspiration, hypotonic musculature, and scoliosis, and abnormal response to hypoxemia and hypercarbia; some authors advocate endotracheal intubation until pain Rx no longer needed

FAMILIAL PERIODIC PARALYSIS (HYPERKALEMIC)

W. John Russell, M.D.

RISK

- Rare, probably about 1/400,000
- Race appears to be exclusively Caucasian

PERIOPERATIVE RISKS

- No reported increase in mortality with any procedure, but severe myotonia could create respiratory difficulty
- Use of succinylcholine may not result in relaxation, and therefore a difficult intubation may result
- Risk of precipitating hyperkalemia and cardiac arrhythmia after succinylcholine

WORRY ABOUT

- Patient getting cold, triggering an attack
- Hypoglycemia triggering an attack. Should be only minimal fasting

OVERVIEW

- Intrinsic defect in muscle membrane allows depolarization of the muscle, but Na^+ channel does not close. Membrane thus remains inexcitable and a variable K^+ efflux continues.
- Patient may experience profound global stiffness and weakness, after succinylcholine, exposure to cold, or spontaneously.
- Dx by family Hx.

ICD-9-CM Code: 359.3

ETIOLOGY

- Na^+ channel in skeletal muscle membrane has a defective α subunit
- Defect associated with chromosome 17 is substitution of a single base pair, usually methionine replacing threonine in fifth transmembrane segment of second domain
- An autosomal dominant condition; allows a persistent Na^+ influx with activation threshold ~10mV more negative than normal
- Persistence of a Na^+ influx is associated with K^+ leak from cell
- Episodes of weakness associated with elevated serum K^+ levels

USUAL TREATMENT

- Avoid succinylcholine, cooling during anesthesia, hypoglycemia.
- Do not give K^+-containing solutions.
- Preop treatment with furosemide has been used.
- Severe postop weakness may alleviated with Ca^{2+}.

ASSESSMENT POINTS

SYSTEM	EFFECT	ASSESSMENT BY HX	PE	TEST
MS	Weakness	Exercise, fatigue	Limb tone	Electromyography (discharges) K^+ load

Key Reference: Ashwood EM, Russell WJ, Burrows DD: Hyperkalaemic periodic paralysis and anesthesia. Anaesthesia 1992; 47:579–584.

PERIOPERATIVE IMPLICATIONS

Preoperative Preparation

- 24 h furosemide for K^+ depletion

Monitoring

- Temperature (esophageal) (keep warm)
- ECG (detection of hyperkalemia)
- Neuromuscular (minimize relaxant dose)

Induction

- Avoid ketamine and succinylcholine
- Relaxation with nondepolarizing agents as indicated

Maintenance

- Keep warm
- Warm all IV fluid, use glucose 5% as maintenance

Extubation

- Normal reversal as indicated clinically
- Evidence of muscle weakness should be treated with IV calcium gluconate or chloride 10% 10 ml slowly over 5 min

Adjuvants

- Some experimental evidence suggests that postop weakness may be helped by phenytoin.
- Anticipate normal analgesic requirements for age and surgery.
- Regional techniques are appropriate.

FAMILIAL PERIODIC PARALYSIS (HYPOKALEMIC)

W. John Russell, M.D.

RISK

- Rare, probably ~1000 people affected in USA
- Appears to occur in most races
- Presents in childhood or adolescence

PERIOPERATIVE RISKS

- Associated with supraventricular or conduction defect–type cardiac arrhythmias
- Treatment with lidocaine is contraindicated.
- Weakness may be enhanced or percipitated by β rb drugs. General muscle weakness including resp muscles may occur postoperatively.

WORRY ABOUT

- Attacks after cold exposure, glucose intake, insulin administration
- Cold triggers attacks
- Serum K+ levels should be maintained above 4.0 mEq/L.
- Cardiac dysrhythmias, especially bradycardias, during an attack

OVERVIEW

- Any severe hypokalemia may induce paralysis in susceptible persons even if no familial disease. Limb weakness and paralysis have been reported after thyrotoxicosis, starvation, autoimmune and renal disease.
- An autosomal dominant condition. Usually patient will be aware of onset of weakness. Prompt treatment with K+ will usually abort an attack, although as much as 40 mEq of K+ may be required hourly. Attacks most likely with increased muscle activity, precipitated by exercise and cold, presumably because of shivering.
- Symptoms controlled by regular K+ supplements and acetazolamide.

ICD-9-CM Code: 359.3

ETIOLOGY

- Intrinsic defect in muscle membrane appears to be associated with gene localized to 1q31-1q32 region near dihydropyridine receptor gene.
- Unrelated to familial hyperkalemic disease
- Gene defect impairs voltage-sensitive Ca^{2+} channel, which may cause compensatory increase in the $Na^+/K^+/Cl^-$ cotransport and a reduced overall efflux in K^+.

USUAL TREATMENT

- Avoid succinylcholine, cooling during anesthesia, hyperglycemia.
- Give K+-containing solutions.
- Acetazolamide preoperatively
- Severe postop weakness may be aggravated by Ca^{2+}.
- Ventilation during anasthesia should be normocarbic to avoid K^+ shifts.
- Maintenance by IPPV if evidence of weakness in postop phase.

ASSESSMENT POINTS

SYSTEM	EFFECT	ASSESSMENT BY HX	PE	TEST
RESP	Inadequate	Noticeable SOB	Resp rate high	ABG
MS	Weakness	Exercise, fatigue	Limb tone	Serum K+ elevation < normal (N = 0.8 ± 0.2 mEq/L) Glucose/insulin infusion, ACTH infusion induce paralysis attack Plasma biochemistry after attack: elevated myoglobin, creatine kinase Muscle fiber conduction velocity may be slower than normal

Key Reference: Lema G, Urzua J, Moran S, Canessa R: Successful anesthetic management of a patient with hypokalemic familial periodic paralysis undergoing cardiac surgery. Anesthesiology 1991; 74:373–375.

PERIOPERATIVE IMPLICATIONS

Preoperative Preparation

- 24-h acetazolamide if not already given. Only glucose-free solutions IV. If Hx of frequent instability, set up K+ infusion

Anesthetic Technique

- Regional techniques are appropriate.

Monitoring

- Temperature
- ECG (detection of hypokalemia may not be seen until late)
- Neuromuscular (minimize relaxant dose)

Induction

- Successful relaxation with succinylcholine and with atracurium has been reported.

Maintenance

- Warm all IV fluid, use glucose-free solutions as maintenance

Extubation

- Normal reversal as indicated clinically
- Evidence of muscle weakness should be treated with IV potassium chloride up to 40 mEq/h.

Adjuvants

- Calcium channel blockers do not appear to be contraindicated in patients with concomitant CV disease
- Anticipate usual analgesic requirements for age and surgery.

FAT EMBOLISM

Brian J. McGrath, M.D.

RISK

- With long bone fractures, pelvic fractures, multiple fractures: 80–100% fat embolism; 0.5–11% fat embolism syndrome (FES)
- With total hip or total knee replacement: 27–100% fat embolism; ?incidence of FES
- Rare: Lymphangiography; liposuction; bone marrow transplantation; pancreatitis; corticosteroid use; closed cardiac massage; burns

PERIOPERATIVE RISKS

- FES carries 10–20% mortality
- Pre-existing FES: respiratory failure/ARDS; RV dysfunction; coagulopathy; neurologic dysfunction
- Intraoperative fat embolism: shock; hypoxemia (severe)

WORRY ABOUT

- Pre-existing FES: hypoxemia; poor pulmonary compliance; HTN; RV failure; abnormal CNS response to anesthetics; coagulopathy
- Intraoperative embolism: myocardial failure (right heart), hypoxemia (severe)

OVERVIEW

- Fat particles (globules of marrow fat) traveling into blood and lung
- Must distinguish fat embolism, which is common, from fat embolism syndrome, a much less common consequence of fat embolism
- FES can produce mild pulmonary dysfunction to severe ARDS
- Pulmonary HTN and acute right ventricular failure may occur in severe cases of FES
- Typically, there is delay in onset of signs and symptoms of up to 72 h following injury
- Occurs commonly during femoral reaming and cementing in hip arthroplasty and with tourniquet release in knee arthroplasty

ICD-9-CM Codes: 958.1; 673.8 (Obstetric)

ETIOLOGY

- Usually occurs following orthopedic or obstetric trauma with release of marrow fat into venous circulation
- Pathology produced by intravascular fat passage into the arterial circulation or by production of endogenous inflammatory mediators

USUAL TREATMENT

- Early fracture fixation to ↓ embolization
- Use of noncemented prosthesis or venting of femoral shaft may reduce risk during hip arthroplasty
- O_2 therapy to maintain SaO_2 >90%
- Positive pressure ventilation with PEEP for ARDS
- Aggressive hemodynamic support with fluid and/or inotropes with shock
- Factor replacement for coagulopathy with bleeding
- Corticosteroids, heparin, ethanol, dextran: unproven benefit

ASSESSMENT POINTS

SYSTEM	EFFECT	ASSESSMENT BY HX	PE	TEST
CV	Intravascular fat	Fever		?Fat staining of blood ?Bronchoalveolar lavage, macrophage staining PA catheter
	Hypoperfusion Pulm HTN RV failure	Syncope Obtundation	Hypotension Tachycardia Oliguria Vasoconstriction	
RESP	ARDS Hypoxemia	Dyspnea	Tachypnea Cyanosis, rales	CXR, ABG
HEME	Thrombocytopenia DIC Anemia		Bleeding (rare)	CBC Platelets PT, PTT D-dimer Fibrinogen
SKIN	Capillary fat embolism		Petechiae (60%) • Axilla, chest • Base of neck • Conjunctiva • Uvula	
CNS	Neurologic injury Cerebral edema	Agitation	Delirium Confusion Focal deficits (rare) Seizure (rare) Coma (rare)	

Key Reference: Fleischer E, LeBel LA: Fat embolism syndrome. Nurse Anesth 1993; 4:18–27.

PERIOPERATIVE IMPLICATIONS

Preoperative Preparation

- Avoid sedatives/narcotics if hypoxemic and not mechanically ventilated

Monitoring

- Arterial catheter; PA catheter may be helpful in severe cases

Airway

- May already be intubated and ventilated in severe cases
- Decreased FRC and oxygen "reserve" with ARDS

Induction

- Minimize myocardial depression

Maintenance

- CV: Patients with RV dysfunction may require inotropic treatment
- Resp: Patients with ARDS may require high FIO_2 and PEEP
- Watch for embolism during femoral reaming, prosthesis cementing, and tourniquet deflation

Extubation

- Maintain intubation and mechanical ventilation in hemodynamically unstable patients and those requiring high FIO_2, high PEEP, or high minute ventilation
- Patients with CNS involvement may have a prolonged or exaggerated response to anesthetics and narcotics

ANTICIPATED PROBLEMS/CONCERNS

- Embolism during femoral reaming, prosthesis cementing, tourniquet deflation
- Patients with ARDS may be difficult to ventilate and oxygenate

FOREIGN BODY ASPIRATION

Frederic Berry, M.D.

RISK

• Foreign body aspiration into the airway or esophagus is one of the most frequent and frightening pediatric surgical emergencies.

PERIOPERATIVE RISKS

• Risk of aspiration is present but is very small. The danger period for vomiting or regurgitation with aspiration is primarily during the induction and recovery from anesthesia.
• Unless foreign body is immediate threat to survival, further consultation should be sought and, if necessary, transfer of the patient to a specialized facility.

OVERVIEW

• Acute presentation, with parent or caretaker observing the child swallowing or aspirating a foreign body and immediately developing respiratory distress or dysphagia; or chronic presentation after 1–2 wk of unexplained coughing, wheezing, or dysphagia; often with secondary infection behind the foreign body.

ICD-9-CM Code: 934.0 (Trachea through orifice)

USUAL TREATMENT

• Bronchoscopy

ASSESSMENT POINTS

SYSTEM	EFFECT	PE	TEST
CV	Dehydration	Skin turgor	UO
RESP	Main stem bronchus may have ball-value effect	Involved lung cannot fully expire Reactive airway with secretions	Chest exam CXR

Key Reference: Woods AM: Pediatric endoscopy. *In* Berry FA (ed): Anesthetic Management of Difficult and Routine Pediatric Patients, 2nd ed. New York, Churchill Livingstone, 1990, pp 199–242.

PERIOPERATIVE MANAGEMENT

• Divided into three time periods: preoperative, intraoperative, and postoperative.

Preoperative Concerns

• Unclear whether or not to allow an NPO period—the stomach will not empty
• IV fluids assessment, anticholinergic and sedative premedication. Premedication should be reserved for the uncooperative child.

Induction

• Done in OR without presence of parents
• A technique of spontaneous ventilation usually with inhalation anesthetic
• If IV present, small doses (1mg/kg) of IV Pentothal or propofol to gently sedate and make inhalation induction smoother

Intraoperative Management

• If child is struggling to breathe or cyanotic, induction is with halothane and O_2.
• If only mild airway distress, nitrous oxide used for initial inhalation induction to facilitate administration of halothane (very insoluble volatile anesthetics, e.g., sevoflurane, have disadvantage that if ventilation is interrupted for short periods the level may decrease so rapidly that the child awakens). After initial inhalation induction, nitrous oxide is discontinued, halothane increased, and ventilation gently assisted.
• Small amounts of PEEP (3–5 cm water) useful for any degree of obstruction.

• Topical anesthesia of larynx and cords with 4% or 10% solution of lidocaine, 5–6 mg/kg (4% lidocaine contains 40 mg lidocaine/ml) prior to laryngoscopy so no response to introduction of ventilating bronchoscope. This often requires an inspired concentration of halothane (3–4%).

Monitoring

• End-tidal CO_2 (also the wave form) may be elevated into the 80s or 90s. As long as saturation remains in 85–95 range, the CO_2 is usually not a problem.
• Ventilating bronchoscope with a sidearm attachment for anesthesia circuit. Bronchoscope advanced through larynx into trachea and often into main stem bronchus. Desaturation may result from inadequate ventilation of contralateral lung. If this occurs consider administering PEEP until saturation can be returned to reasonable range.
• With pneumonia, saturations may not be able to be raised higher than the low 90s. Saturation of 85–90 is acceptable as long as it is stable. If rapidly falling oxygen saturation, bronchoscope must be withdrawn into trachea and ventilation assisted with PEEP.
• The surgeon grasps foreign body and starts to extract it from airway. If child starts to move or cough, management includes (1) releasing foreign body and reanesthetizing; or (2) administering either muscle relaxant such as succinylcholine 1 mg/kg or ketamine, propofol, lidocaine, or Pentothal 1–2 mg/kg to deepen anesthesia.

Postoperative Management

• After trachea and bronchus rechecked with ventilating bronchoscope, trachea is intubated and awake extubation performed. If patient coughing but not sufficiently awake, lidocaine 1.5 mg/kg can be administered.

ANTICIPATED PROBLEMS/CONCERNS

• If PVCs develop because of elevated CO_2, can administer lidocaine 1.5 mg/kg, which can be repeated 2 times in 5 minutes, or switch anesthetic to isoflurane.

FRIEDREICH'S ATAXIA

Mark Helfaer, M.D.

RISK
- Prevalence 2/100,000; 80–90% have cardiac involvement

WORRY ABOUT
- Cardiac involvement does not correlate with neurologic involvement

OVERVIEW
- Progressive degeneration of posterior columns and corticospinal and posterior spinocerebellar tracts
- Usual onset in childhood
- Proprioceptive sensory loss, areflexia, ataxia of limbs, Babinski's sign
- Pes cavus and scoliosis
- Cardiomyopathy

ICD-9-CM Code: 334.0

ETIOLOGY
- Inherited—usually autosomal recessive, but occasionally dominant

USUAL TREATMENT
- Usually untreatable and progressive
- Can be mistaken for metabolic disorders (hexosaminidase A deficiency, adrenomyeloneuropathy, vitamin E deficiency)

ASSESSMENT POINTS

SYSTEM	EFFECT	ASSESSMENT BY HX	TEST
CV	LV hypokinesia Concentric and asymmetric hypertrophy Cardiomyopathy		ECG ECHO
RESP	Severe scoliosis Neuromuscular impairment	Noncardiac dyspnea	Lung functions
MS	Pes cavus Scoliosis		

Key Reference: Campbell AM, Finley GA: Anaesthesia for a patient with Friedreich's ataxia and cardiomyopathy. Can J Anaesth 1989; 36:89–93.

PERIOPERATIVE IMPLICATIONS

Preoperative Preparation
- Usual premedication

Monitoring
- Train of four to monitor effects of neuromuscular blocking agent with unpredictable response due to NM disease

Airway
- None

Preinduction/Induction
- Case report of sensitivity to curare (0.06 mg/kg caused 90 min apnea)
- Possibility of hyperkalemia and cardiac arrhythmias after succinylcholine

Maintenance
- Case reports of successful spinal and epidural anesthesia
- Case reports of successful GA with cautious use of nondepolarizing agents
- Case report of successful use of hypotensive anesthesia with isoflurane
- Case report of marked decrease in cardiac output and supraventricular tachycardia with nitroprusside for hypotensive anesthesia
- Case report of successful use of epidural narcotic

Extubation
- If adequate strength from neuromuscular blocker and adequate pulmonary function, extubation is appropriate

Adjuvants
- See under Maintenance

Postoperative Period
- ECG monitoring for dysrhythmias

GASTRINOMA

Jane Eyrich, M.D.

RISK

- Annual incidence: 2–4/million
- More common in men than women: 3:2
- Predominantly diagnosed in patients 40–60 y
- 60% of gastrinomas are malignant

PERIOPERATIVE RISKS

- Risks associated with peptic ulcer disease
- Associated tumors (MEN type 1)
- Risks associated with metastatic lesions (liver, bone, lungs)

WORRY ABOUT

- Likelihood of large gastric fluid volume
- Esophageal reflux (common)
- Electrolyte imbalance 2° to watery diarrhea
- Malnutrition 2° to chronic diarrhea and peptic ulcer disease
- 20–25% with other functioning endocrine adenomas (parathyroid, pituitary, thyroid, adrenal cortex)

OVERVIEW

- Gastroenteropancreatic neuroendocrine tumor arising from gastrin-secreting cells, occurring in pancreatic and extrapancreatic sites
- Secrete gastrin autonomously, leading to severe ulcer diathesis, abdominal pain, and diarrhea
- May occur sporadically or as part of the MEN-1 syndrome (benign or malignant cellular proliferation of at least two endocrine glands, mainly pancreatic islets, and parathyroid, pituitary, and adrenal glands)
- Constitutes part of the Zollinger-Ellison syndrome: gastric acid hypersecretion, intractable ulcer diathesis, and non–beta islet cell tumor of the pancreas

ICD-9-CM Code: 235.2
See also under Multiple Endocrine Neoplasia Type 1

ETIOLOGY

- Often familial—may be inherited as autosomal dominant trait with a high but variable degree of penetrance

USUAL TREATMENT

- Correct gastric acid hypersecretion with H_2 blockers and proton pump inhibitors (omeprazole)
- Surgical exploration and resection

ASSESSMENT POINTS

SYSTEM	EFFECT	ASSESSMENT BY HX	PE	TEST
CV	Hypovolemia	Weakness, dizziness	Orthostatic BP	ECG
RESP[1]	Hypoxia	Dyspnea, decreased exercise tolerance	Breath sounds	CXR
GI	Gastric hyperacidity	Abdominal pain, esophageal reflux, diarrhea	Abdominal exam	Secretin stimulation test
ENDO[2]	Hyperparathyroidism	Multiple systems involved		Serum parathyroid hormone
RENAL[2]	Nephrolithiasis	Flank pain, hematuria	Costovertebral angle tenderness	Urinalysis
CNS[2]	Pituitary adenoma	Headaches, visual changes	Visual fields	MRI of sella turcica; prolactin levels
PNS[2]	Hypercalcemia	Somnolence, psychosis	Hyperreflexia	Ca^{2+} levels
MS[2]	Weakness, arthralgias	Proximal muscle weakness	Motor strength	Serum, urinary Ca^{2+}

[1] In the presence of pulmonary metastases.
[2] If gastrinoma presents as components of MEN-1.
Key Reference: Gagel RF: Multiple endocrine neoplasia. Endocrinol Metab Clin North Am 1994; 23:1.

PERIOPERATIVE IMPLICATIONS

Preoperative Preparation

- Assess electrolyte and volume status
- Control of gastric hypersecretion

Monitoring

- Intravascular volume status. Can have significant volume shifts due to gastroduodenal pancreatic manipulations and resections. May need arterial line and central venous pressure monitoring. Measure urinary output with bladder catheter.

Airway

- Increased risk for aspiration and pneumonitis

Induction

- Rapid-sequence induction with cricoid pressure (awake intubation if extremely difficult airway by Hx or physical exam.)
- May be hypovolemic from chronic diarrhea, abdominal pain

Extubation

- Careful assessment of pulm function and airway reflexes prior to extubation

Adjuvants

- Epidural catheter for postop pain control

Postoperative Period

- Possibility of continued acid hypersecretion
- Worry about pulmonary complications, e.g., decreased vital capacity and FRC—exacerbated by pain, ileus

ANTICIPATED PROBLEMS/CONCERNS

- 60% of gastrinomas are malignant and may metastasize to lymph nodes, liver, or lung, resulting in ↓ survival rate
- Lower cure rates after resection for patients with multiple gastrinomas

GLAUCOMA — CLOSED ANGLE

John V. Donlon, Jr., M.D.

RISK

- One tenth as common as open-angle glaucoma
- 200,000/prevalence in US, for angle-closure glaucoma
- More common in white Northern Europeans
- No clear hereditary pattern

PERIOPERATIVE RISKS

- Acute angle-closure glaucoma (ACG) attack, optic nerve damage, visual loss

WORRY ABOUT

- Mydriasis precipitating acute attack of ACG
- Intraocular pressure (IOP) > 30 mmHg
- Prolonged, stationary mid-dilation of the pupil at 3–6 mm

OVERVIEW

- Development of primary ACG a multifactorial phenomenon
- Usually associated with small eyes with flat anterior chambers but normal trabecular meshwork
- Attacks can be sudden and severe, with IOP reaching 60–70 mmHg within 1 h

ICD-9-CM Code: 365.20

ETIOLOGY

- Angle closure occurs when peripheral iris comes to rest against trabecular meshwork and covers it, preventing outflow of aqueous humor.
- Relative pupillary block a common factor in most ACG episodes. Resistance of aqueous flow from posterior chamber increased owing to iris-lens apposition or synechia

USUAL TREATMENT

- Acute episodes: promptly, pilocarpine 2% eye drops, a sympathomimetic used to cause miosis. Also consider topical β rb drops and acetazolamide 500 mg PO or IV. If IOP does not resolve to ≤30 mmHg, a peripheral or laser iridectomy can be performed.
- Chronic ACG: surgical iridotomy

ASSESSMENT POINTS

SYSTEM	EFFECT	ASSESSMENT BY HX	PE	TEST
EYE	Increased IOP	Visual blurring	Red eye	IOP > 30 mmHg
		Eye pain	Corneal edema	
		Nausea	Dilated pupil, fixed	Gonioscopy
		Vomiting	Narrow angle	
		Visual halos	Optic nerve edema	
			Shallow anterior chamber	

Key Reference: Campbell DG: Primary angle-closure glaucoma. *In* Albert DM, Jakobiec FA (eds): Principles and Practice of Ophthalmology, Vol 3. Philadelphia, WB Saunders, 1994, pp 1365–1388.

PERIOPERATIVE IMPLICATIONS

Preoperative Preparation

- Avoid mydriasis
- Continue glaucoma medication regimes
- Check lytes of patients on chronic acetazolamide treatment
- Systemic premedication with antisialogogue such as glycopyrrolate or atropine has no significant effect on IOP.

Induction

- Anesthetic agents do not increase IOP
- Laryngoscopy and intubation may cause temporary, mild, clinically insignificant increase in IOP placement, and removal of laryngeal mask airway disturbs IOP less than endotracheal intubation.

Extubation

- Avoid coughing and bucking
- Combinations of systemic neostigmine and atropine used to reverse the effects of nondepolarizing muscle relaxants will not cause mydriasis.

Postoperative Period

- Observe patient for signs of acute ACG attack

ANTICIPATED PROBLEMS/CONCERNS

- β rb eye drops such as timolol may have systemic effects: bradycardia, asthma. Selective β rb eye drops such as betaxolol are less likely to produce pulmonary effects.

GLAUCOMA — OPEN ANGLE

John V. Donlon, Jr., M.D.

RISK

- People within USA: 2 million
- African-Americans: Primary cause of blindness, 5× incidence of glaucoma among Caucasians
- Age: 10.5% prevalence in 70–79 y group

PERIOPERATIVE RISKS

- Optic nerve ischemia

WORRY ABOUT

- Mydriasis
- Sudden, significant increase in IOP
- Eye pain: dull, periorbital ache with a dry, pale, firm eye

OVERVIEW

- Primary open angle glaucoma (POAG) is most common form
- Gradual, asymptomatic onset in midlife
- Bilateral disease with significant hereditary predisposition
- Untreated, leads to progressive optic nerve damage and blindness (4% of glaucoma patients in US become blind)
- Chronic, incurable disease that requires lifetime control of IOP by medication or surgery

ICD-9-CM Code: 365.10

ETIOLOGY

- Pathogenesis unclear. Increased resistance to outflow of aqueous humor at videocorneal angle, probably in the cribriform layer of trabecular meshwork near canal of Schlemm.
- Multifactorial hereditary predisposition. Within families with Hx of POAG there is 6-fold prevalence for glaucoma.
- Risk factors for developing optic nerve damage include family Hx, age, African-American race, diabetes, and CV disease.

USUAL TREATMENT

- Early detection, control IOP
- Topical eye drops: β rb such as timolol or, less often, ecothiophate, a long-acting anticholinesterase agent
- Laser trabeculoplasty
- Surgical intervention: iridectomy, Molteno valve, trabeculotomy, cyclodialysis, filtering procedures

ASSESSMENT POINTS

SYSTEM	EFFECT	ASSESSMENT BY HX	PE	TEST
EYE	Increased IOP	Myopia	Asymmetric optic cups	IOP > 23 mmHg
	Optic nerve damage	Family Hx of POAG	Firm, pale eyeball	Gonioscopy
		Dull eye pain		Slit lamp
		Visual changes		Visual fields

Key Reference: Thomas JV: Primary open angle glaucoma. *In* Albert DM, Jakobiec FA (eds): Principles and Practice of Ophthalmology, Vol 3. Philadelphia, WB Saunders, 1994, pp 1342–1345.

PERIOPERATIVE IMPLICATIONS

Preoperative Preparation

- Do not interrupt routine glaucoma medication regime (except ecothiophate)
- Discontinue ecothiophate 2 to 3 wk before surgery
- Chronic acetazolamide therapy can cause modest Na^+ and bicarbonate diuresis and metabolic acidosis. Evaluate lytes.
- Topical eye drops such as the β rb timolol may have systemic effects causing bradycardia or exacerbation of asthma.
- Avoid mydriasis.
- Premedication with systemic antisialogogue such as glycopyrrolate or atropine has no significant effect on IOP.

Induction

- Anesthetic agents tend to decrease IOP.
- Succinylcholine may be used. (See Anticipated Problems/Concerns)
- Laryngoscopy and intubation may cause a temporary, mild, clinically insignificant increase in IOP. Placement and removal of laryngeal mask airway disturb IOP less than endotracheal intubation.

Extubation

- Minimize cough and bucking.
- Combinations of systemic neostigmine and atropine used to reverse effects of nondepolarizing muscle relaxants will not cause mydriasis or increase IOP.

Postoperative Period

- Acute glaucoma attack presents as dull, periorbital headache. Eye will appear pale, dry, and firm. Treatment includes acetazolamide IV 5–7 mg/kg.

ANTICIPATED PROBLEMS/CONCERNS

- Ecothiophate eye drops rarely used today for treatment of glaucoma. Patients on ecothiophate therapy have decreased plasma cholinesterase activity. Succinylcholine may be safely used in these patients if titrated IV in small (5 mg) increments to a monitored train-of-four effect.

GLOMUS JUGULARE TUMORS

Ghaleb A. Ghani, M.D.

RISK

- 0.6% of head and neck tumors
- Slow-growing
- Can coexist with other paragangliomas
- Histologically benign but can be malignant with metastases

PERIOPERATIVE RISKS

- Hypothermia
- Massive blood loss
- Venous air embolism
- HTN
- Hypotension, bronchospasm
- Tumor part emboli

WORRY ABOUT

- Multiple locations, persistence of symptoms after resection of the tumor

OVERVIEW

- Tumors of neural crest at base of skull in jugular bulb area
- May extend into posterior fossa
- May damage lower cranial nerves (IX–XII)
- May secrete catecholamines
- May secrete serotonin, histamine
- May grow into lumen of jugular vein as far as the right atrium

ICD-9-CM Codes: 194.6 (Malignant); 227.6 (benign)

ETIOLOGY

- Congenital (usually benign) hypertrophied arteriovenous anastomosis.
- Epithelial cells with abundant capillary network common

USUAL TREATMENT

- Radiation
- Embolization, alone or preop
- Resection

ASSESSMENT POINTS

SYSTEM	EFFECT	ASSESSMENT BY HX	PE	TEST
HEENT	Cranial nerve injury	Hoarseness Dysphagia Tinnitus	Soft palate motion Gag reflex ↓ Hearing	Indirect laryngoscopy
CV	HTN Intravascular growth	Headaches	BP	Catecholamine level (if indicated) MRI/CT scans, Angio (if indicated)
RESP	Aspiration	Cough Fever SOB	Rhonchi, wheezing	CXR
GI	Delayed gastric emptying	Heartburn Regurgitation		
GU		No different from normal		
CNS	Intracranial extension	Hearing loss Headaches Dizziness		CT scan (if indicated) MRI (if indicated) Paragangliomas in other locations

Key Reference: Jensen NF: Glomus tumors of the head and neck: Anesthetic considerations. Anesth Analg 1994; 78:112–119.

PERIOPERATIVE IMPLICATIONS

Preoperative Preparation

- Control HTN (in cathecholamine-secreting tumors). Preparation is similar to pheochromocytoma (see under Pheochromocytoma)
- Treat pneumonia
- Metoclopramide for delayed gastric emptying
- Adequate venous access for rapid fluid infusion

Monitoring

- Consider A-line, CVP
- Monitor for venous air embolism (end-tidal CO_2, N_2; precordial Doppler)

Maintenance

- Watch out for
  – Massive blood loss
  – HTN
  – Hypotension
  – Bronchospasm
  – Venous air embolism
  – Tumor part emboli
  – Provide controlled hypotension if needed
  – Measure to ↓ the ICP for intracranial extension:
    – Mannitol
    – Hyperventilation
    – Optimize venous return from brain

Extubation

- Evaluate for cranial nerve (IX–XII) injury

Adjuvants

- Controlled ventilation
- Muscle relaxants to prevent spontaneous ventilation intraoperatively
- Controlled hypotension

ANTICIPATED PROBLEMS/CONCERNS

- Loss of upper airway reflexes
- Airway obstruction
- Aspiration
- Delayed gastric emptying
- Ileus
- CNS insult

GLOSSOPHARYNGEAL NEURALGIA

Evelina Worwag, M.D.

RISK

- Patients with multiple sclerosis
- Age ≥40 y
- Increased in patients with carotid artery occlusive diseases, arachnoiditis, and extracranial tumors of larynx, pharynx, and tonsils
- Male to female prevalence 2:3

PERIOPERATIVE RISKS

- Manipulation in throat can trigger pain and arrhythmia
- Profound bradycardia or even asystole can accompany attack of pain

WORRY ABOUT

- Cardiac arrhythmias, sudden death
- Chronic opioid use
- Signs of major depression and anxiety

OVERVIEW

- Involves episodic bursts of pain in distribution of cranial nerves IX and X
- Attacks can be precipitated by chewing, yawning, or swallowing
- Pain usually located in pharynx, tonsil, or ear (unilaterally)
- Bradycardia, tachycardia, syncope, hypotension, or seizures may accompany painful episodes
- Easily confused with sick sinus syndrome, carotid sinus syndrome, or atypical trigeminal neuralgia
- Pain and cardiac arrhythmia can be relieved by topical anesthesia to oropharynx
- Sick sinus syndrome can be ruled out by the absence of ECG changes (see under Sick Sinus Syndrome)
- Glossopharyngeal nerve block rules out trigeminal neuralgia

ICD-9-CM Code: 352.1

ETIOLOGY

- Usually idiopathic
- Can be caused by vascular compression in region of cerebellopontine angle, the entry zone of vagus and glossopharyngeal nerves especially by cross-compression of the nerve
- Seen with vertebral and carotid artery occlusive disease, arachnoiditis, and extracranial tumors arising in area of pharynx, larynx, and tonsils

USUAL TREATMENT

- Anticonvulsants—Tegretol
- Surgical exploration in posterior fossa (microvascular compression of cranial nerve)
- Rhizotomy
- Local anesthetic block at jugular foramen or topical anesthesia of pharynx

ASSESSMENT POINTS

SYSTEM	EFFECT	ASSESSMENT BY HX	PE	TEST
CV	Bradycardia, tachycardia, syncope, hypotension	Syncope, palpitation, orthostatic symptoms	BP HR	ECG when pain triggered
CNS	Cranial nerves IX and X; seizures	Pain in cranial nerves IX and X distribution precipitated by chewing, yawning, or swallowing	Triggering of pain and pain relief	CT scan with infusion for microvessel localization and to rule out tumors

Key Reference: Rao NL, Drupin BR: Glossopharyngeal neuralgia with syncope—anesthetic considerations. Anesthesiology 1981; 54:426–428.

PERIOPERATIVE IMPLICATIONS

Preoperative Evaluation

- Adequate assessment of intravascular fluid volume and cardiac status with emphasis on ruling out treatable causes of syncope and bradycardia

Monitoring

- Consider arterial line and central venous line when need for pacemaker is possible

Airway

- Topical anesthesia to oropharynx before laryngoscopy
- Drying agent before induction
- Consider glossopharyngeal nerve block as premedication and prophylaxis

Maintenance

- Constant preparedness to treat cardiac arrhythmias, HTN

Extubation

- Worry about vocal cord paralysis

GONORRHEA

Jerry M. Calkins, Ph.D., M.D.

RISK

- Decreasing; ~700,000/y in USA
- Incidences highest in young adults (men 20–24 y; women 18–24 y)
- Highest among the unmarried, urban poor, minority ethnic, prostitutes, homosexual males

WORRY ABOUT

- Universal blood and body fluid precautions

OVERVIEW

- Sexually transmitted disease
- Pathogenesis—initial attachment and mucosal colonization

Clinical Features

- Mucosal infections: Urethritis in men, urogenital tract disease in women, anorectal infections, pharyngeal infections, conjunctivitis in neonates and adults
- Invasive gonococcal disease: Pelvic inflammatory disease (PID), perihepatitis (Fitz-Hugh–Curtis syndrome), disseminated gonococcal infection, septic arthritis, gonococcal endocarditis and meningitis

ICD-9-CM Code: 098

ETIOLOGY

- *Neisseria gonorrhoeae*
- Gram-negative intracellular diplococcus

USUAL TREATMENT

- Penicillin, ampicillin, tetracycline
- Antibiotic-resistant—spectinomycin, third-generation cephalosporins (ceftriaxone, cefotaxime)
- Untreated gonococcal urethritis often spontaneously resolves after several wk
- In some, asymptomatic carriage develops
- Resolution of symptoms after treatment suggests cure—follow-up cultures are recommended

ASSESSMENT POINTS

SYSTEM	EFFECT	ASSESSMENT BY HX	PE	TEST
Mucosal HEENT	Conjunctivitis, ophthalmia neonatorum, adult gonococcal conjunctivitis Pharyngeal infection			
GI	Anorectal infections Proctitis	Purulent discharge, bloody diarrhea		
GU	*Women* Urogenital tract disease *Men* Acute epididymitis Prostatitis	Abnormal vaginal discharge, dysuria, urinary frequency, lower abdominal pain, labial pain, abnormal menstruation	Mucopurulent cervicitis	Cultures from urethra and vagina
Invasive CV	Gonococcal endocarditis			
GI	Perihepatitis (Fitz-Hugh–Curtis syndrome)	RUQ tenderness		Liver enzyme elevation
GU	*Women* PID *Men* Urethritis	Lower abdominal pain, vaginal discharge, fever, palpable adnexal mass		Endocervix cultures
CNS	Gonococcal meningitis			
MS	Septic arthritis	Most common cause of septic arthritis in young adults Tends to involve single joints		

Key Reference: Stephens DS, Del Rio C: Gonococcal infections. *In* Kelley WN (ed): Textbook of Internal Medicine. Philadelphia, JB Lippincott, 1991, pp 1382–1387.

PERIOPERATIVE IMPLICATIONS

Monitoring
- Awareness—Foley catheter placement; temperature

Airway
- Awareness if pharyngitis exists

Maintenance
- Awareness of extent of disease

Adjuvants
- Vary with hepatic involvement

ANTICIPATED PROBLEMS/CONCERNS

Measures to Control
- Follow-up cultures
- Effective antibiotics
- Testing isolates for antibiotic susceptibility
- Routine culturing of high-risk populations
- Diligent contact tracing and prompt referral; treatment of sexual partners
- Education targeted at high-risk groups
- Use of condoms and other barriers

GUILLAIN-BARRÉ SYNDROME

Jay B. Brodsky, M.D.

RISK

- Prevalence: both sexes, all races, all ages but mostly afflicts young and middle-aged adults
- Worldwide illness, occurs all times of year
- Mortality rate 5–20%. Most patients eventually fully recover, 15% have significant residual weakness

PERIOPERATIVE RISKS

- Resp failure 2° to polyneuropathy
- Autonomic dysfunction with profound CV instability

WORRY ABOUT

- Rapidity of symptoms—resp paralysis may occur within 24 h of onset
- Pulmonary complications

OVERVIEW

- Polyneuropathy most often encountered in critical care practice
  - Patients present initially with lower limb weakness that spreads
- Widespread, patchy, inflammatory demyelination of peripheral and autonomic nervous systems
- Dysautonomia from chromatolysis of anteromediolateral cell column and autonomic ganglia: fluctuating BP, HTN, hypotension, postural hypotension, tachycardia, arrhythmias
- CSF protein usually nml during first few days of illness, steadily rises and remains elevated for several months, even after recovery

ICD-9-CM Code: 357.0

ETIOLOGY

- Believed to be hypersensitivity reaction
- Cause unknown—slow virus, metabolic or autoimmune etiology speculated
- Antecedent illness within 4 wk of onset (resp or GI infection in 60–70% of cases)
- Other predisposing factors include surgery, pregnancy, malignancy, acute seroconversion to HIV
- Epidural anesthesia may be antecedent event or cause recurrence

USUAL TREATMENT

- Basis of treatment is symptomatic care
- Daily bedside evaluation of vital capacity and resp muscle strength; patients with ↓ resp reserve should be moved to ICU
- Elective tracheal intubation and mechanical ventilatory support when signs of resp distress are present *even before* $PaCO_2$ rises or vital capacity falls
- Guidelines for ventilatory support:
  - Alveolar-arterial tension difference >300 mmHg with FIO_2=1.0
  - $PaCO_2$ >50 mmHg
  - Maximum static inspiratory pressure <30 cm H_2O
  - Vital capacity <14 ml/kg
- Steroid therapy, immunosuppressants
- Plasmapheresis reduces hospital stay and time spent on ventilator if given to patients who do not improve or who worsen within first 7 d of onset of symptoms

ASSESSMENT POINTS

SYSTEM	EFFECT	ASSESSMENT BY HX	PE	TEST
HEENT	Inability to close eyes	Dry eyes	Dry eyes	
CV	Fluctuating hypo- and hypertension, postural hypotension, sinus tachycardia, arrhythmias	Orthostatic Sx Palpitations	BP/pulse	ECG
RESP	Respiratory failure 2° to weakness	Stamina— for breathing	↓ Strength on repeated ventilation	Macrophage-inhibiting factor
GI	Bowel obstruction	Inability to move bowels	Abdominal exam	Abdominal x-ray
CNS	Autonomic dysfunction	Early satiety Orthostatic hypotension Lack of sweating	BP lying and standing	ECG with RR interval on deep breathing
MS	Weakness, joint fixation	Lack of stamina		

Key Reference: Perel A, Reches A, Davidson JT: Anaesthesia in the Guillain-Barré syndrome. Anaesthesia 1977; 32:257–260.

PERIOPERATIVE IMPLICATIONS

Preoperative Preparation

- Avoid rapid turning of patient—autonomic instability and postural hypotension may result
- Avoid head-up (reverse Trendelenburg) position—inability of patient to maintain CV stability with tilt
- Increased gastric acidity—treat with antacid and metoclopramide, 10 mg/70 kg
- Maintain appropriate environmental temperature

Monitoring

- Arterial line for continuous pressure monitoring started prior to anesthetic induction
- CVP or PA line to monitor for potential fluid shifts that result from positional changes and cardiac dysrhythmias
- Temperature—patients may become poikilothermic
- Neuromuscular monitoring

Airway

- Most patients have early tracheostomy; airway access should not be a problem; previous patients may have tracheal stenosis
- Fusion of TMJ—may make orotracheal intubation difficult

Induction

- Avoid barbiturates and phenothiazines, which may produce profound CV depression

Maintenance

- Local anesthesia preferred
- GA: nonsympatholytic technique such as nitrous oxide–oxygen supplemented by opioids or ketamine
- Sensitive to positive pressure ventilation and tracheal suction—may result in autonomic instability

Extubation

- Continue to ventilate postop if patient required ventilatory support preop
- Residual weakness from anesthetic agents and muscle relaxants may necessitate postop ventilation in patients not ventilated preop
- In ICU—wean from mechanical ventilation when vital capacity > 10 mL/kg

Adjuvants

- Muscle relaxants
  - Avoid succinylcholine; can cause hyperkalemia with cardiac arrest
  - Patients have increased sensitivity to nondepolarizing muscle relaxants
  - May have residual muscle weakness after apparent full recovery from GA
- Volume
  - Maintain blood volume
  - Use colloid to maintain CVP >5 cm H_2O

ANTICIPATED PROBLEMS/CONCERNS

- Autonomic instability
- Respiratory failure

Special Problems

- Parturient: during third trimester, risk of exacerbation; for labor a regional anesthetic indicated to avoid exaggerated hemodynamic response to pain from autonomic dysfunction. For C-section a regional anesthetic contraindicated even for patient with mild resp involvement
- Fecal impaction
- Stress ulcers

HASHIMOTO'S THYROIDITIS

M. Lawrence Berman, M.D.

RISK

• People within USA: 100,000–400,000 new cases/y
• Most common cause of primary hypothyroidism in adults (10% over age 65)
• Race with highest prevalence: none known
• Gender predominance: F>M (8:1; age 30–50 y)

PERIOPERATIVE RISKS

• ↑ Risk of thyroid storm even if euthyroid preop
• Some risk of resp insufficiency and ↑ bleeding perioperatively

WORRY ABOUT

• Hyperthyroidism in perioperative period with thyroid storm (see under Hyperthyroidism in Diseases section)
• Chronic hyperthyroidism with its concomitants
• Coexisting autoimmune disease with adrenal failure

OVERVIEW

• Chronic inflammation of thyroid (painful or painless) with lymphocytic infiltration due to autoimmune factors
• Acute inflammation results in ↑ release of preformed hormone with hyperthyroidism
• Chronic inflammation results in ↓ thyroid gland function with resistant hypothyroidism

ICD-9-CM Code: 423.9

ETIOLOGY

• Autoimmune disease associated with other autoimmune disease: Sjögren's syndrome; SLE, RA, pernicious anemia, autoimmune endocrinopathies, Addison's disease, hypoparathyroidism, diabetes mellitus, gonadal failure
• ↑ Incidence in patients with a family Hx and with chromosomal disorders — Turner's, Down, and Klinefelter's syndromes

USUAL TREATMENT

• Thyroid hormone replacement chronically in hypothyroidism
• NSAIDs in acute thyroiditis (painful) and propranolol to control symptoms of hyperthyroidism

ASSESSMENT POINTS

SYSTEM	EFFECT	ASSESSMENT BY HX	PE	TEST
HEENT	Swollen tender neck Enlarged tongue Tracheal compression	Neck pain, hoarseness	Examine airway and neck	Lateral neck x-rays or CT of neck
CV	Dehydration, tachy- or bradydysrhythmias	Orthostatic symptoms		Tilt test ECG
RESP	↓ Resp muscle strength	SOB, DOE	Standard	
GI	Ileus Constipation			
ENDO	Acutely hyperthyroid Chronically hypothyroid	Shaking, anxiety, emotional lability	Reflex speed, HR Tremor, nervousness Mental status	Free T_4 estimate
	Other autoimmune dysfunction	Weakness	Ability to arise from chair without using hands	Serum K^+/Na^+
HEME				
CNS	Cold intolerance Slow or fast movement, depending on stage	Cold intolerance	Reflexes, mental status exam	
MS		Arthralgias and myalgias		

Key Reference: Murkin JM: Anesthesia and hypothyroidism: A review of thyroxine physiology, pharmacology, and anesthetic implications. Anesth Analg 1982; 61:371–383.

PERIOPERATIVE IMPLICATIONS

Preoperative Preparation
• Ensure that euthyroid (to avoid thyroid storm)
• Assess fluid status
• Assess for co-morbidities (autoimmune/adrenal/pancreatic dysfunction)

Monitoring
• Temperature (consider placing cooling blanket on OR table as Rx for thyroid storm)
• Consider invasive monitoring if CV or resp compromise

Airway
• If normal preop, routine
• If displaced or distorted, consider awake fiberoptic and armored tube

Induction/Maintenance
• No data indicate one technique better than any other

Extubation
• Consider extubation in optimal situation for reintubation

Postoperative Concerns
• Routine + treatment of co-morbidities if coexisting autoimmune disease

Adjuvants
• Esmolol for acute hyperthyroidism
• Steroids sometimes needed for adrenal dysfunction
• Oral hypoglycemics (if chronic Rx) can cause hypoglycemia for longer duration and of greater severity in perioperative patient

ANTICIPATED PROBLEMS/CONCERNS

• Thyroid storm—clinical diagnosis of life-threatening illness if hyperthyroidism severely exacerbated by illness or operation—manifested by hyperpyrexia, tachycardia, alterations in consciousness
• Resp failure

HEADACHE — MIGRAINE

P. D. Randolph, M.D.
S. I. Dagher, M.D.
G. B. Racz, M.D.

RISK

- People within USA: 20 million
- More frequent in women, declines after age 40 y
- Familial aggregation

PERIOPERATIVE RISKS

- ↑ Incidence of HTN, stroke, CAD
- Gastric stasis
- Drug toxicity and side effects

WORRY ABOUT

- Toxic and side effects of antimigrainous preparations, adverse interaction with anesthetic drugs
- Associated intracranial disorders
- ↑ Aggregation of plt with ↑ risk of stroke and CAD

OVERVIEW

- Periodic unilateral headache, often preceded by aura; associated with systemic symptoms.
- Diagnosis history dependent
- Migrainous infarction with permanent neurologic damage is rare

ICD-9-CM Codes: 346.0 (classic migraine); 346.1 (common migraine. 5th digit sub-classification: 0 without mention of intractable migraine, 1 with intractable migraine, so stated.)

ETIOLOGY

- Central or peripheral mechanisms incited by internal or external stimuli

- Precipitated by trigger factors
- Cerebral and extracerebral arteries are most likely sources of pain
- Pain results from exaggerated pulsations in association with sensitization of nociceptors around blood vessels

USUAL TREATMENT

- No permanent cure
- Elimination of trigger factors, chronobiologic regulation
- Abortive therapy: sumatriptan; ergotamine, sphenopalatine ganglion block, nonopioid and opioid analgesics
- Prophylactic therapy: β-blocking agents, Ca²⁺ channel blockers, TCAs, and MAO inhibitors

ASSESSMENT POINTS

Mainly side effects and toxicity of antimigrainous therapy.

SYSTEM	EFFECT	ASSESSMENT BY HX	PE	TEST
CV	Ergotamine, sumatriptan – Worsening of HTN, ischemic heart disease, and peripheral vascular disease	Symptoms of angina and peripheral vascular insufficiency		ECG Stress ECG
	Beta adrenergic receptor blocking agents and Ca channel blockers – Excessive depression of myocardial function	Symptoms of CHF	S_3 Rales	CXR
	Methysergide – Pericardial fibrosis		↓ Heart sounds	CXR
	TCAs and Ca channel blockers – Cardiac conduction abnormalities	Syncope		ECG
RESP	β rb – Worsening of COPD	Dyspnea	Expiratory wheezing	CXR ABG
	Methysergide – Pleuropulmonary fibrosis	Dyspnea	Rapid shallow breathing	PFTs
GI	Gastroparesis	Early satiety		
CNS	Intracranial disorders TCAs, MAO inhibitors – Anticholinergic and CNS stimulation	Tachycardia, dry mouth, blurred vision, urinary retention, delayed gastric emptying	Focal deficit	Neuroimaging

Key Reference: Dalessio DJ, Silberstein SD: Wolff's Headache and Other Head Pain, 6th ed. New York, Oxford University Press, 1993, pp 96–170.

PERIOPERATIVE IMPLICATIONS

Preoperative Preparation

- Detailed pharmacotherapy Hx
- Discontinue MAO inhibitors 14–21 d in advance, if possible (see in Drug section)
- Gastroparesis: Metoclopramide (10mg/70kg patient)

Monitoring

- Routine, unless signs of ischemic heart disease

Airway

- None

Preinduction/Induction

- Patients receiving β rb's and Ca channel blockers may develop reduced CO and hypotension

Maintenance

- Exaggerated response to indirect-acting vasopressors may occur with patients on ergotamine, sumatriptan, TCAs, and MAO inhibitors

Extubation

- Increased risk of CNS stimulation with sumatriptan, ergotamine, TCAs, and MAO inhibitors

Postoperative Period

- Pain management may be critical
- Avoid withdrawal syndromes

ANTICIPATED PROBLEMS/CONCERNS

- Possible adverse interactions of anesthetic drugs and antimigrainous preparations
- No unique hazards of anesthesia administered to patients with migraine

HELLP SYNDROME

David J. Birnbach, M.D.

RISK

- If severe preeclampsia, 20% may exhibit HELLP syndrome.
- Preeclampsia occurs in 5–10% of pregnancies.

PERIOPERATIVE RISKS

- High maternal and fetal morbidity and mortality
- Increased C-section rate (up to 94%)
- Immediate delivery after diagnosis to prevent maternal and fetal death

WORRY ABOUT

- Confused with hepatitis, thrombotic thrombocytopenic purpura, gallbladder disease, and acute fatty liver of pregnancy
- Thrombocytopenia and coagulopathy increase risk of hematoma after regional anesthetic
- Upper airway and laryngeal edema leading to airway obstruction and difficult or failed intubation. Fluid management difficult; pulmonary edema may ensue

OVERVIEW

- HELLP is an acronym for the findings that suggest hepatic involvement in preeclampsia patient: Hemolysis, Elevated Liver enzymes, Low Platelets
- Diagnostic criteria include: hemolysis, defined by abnormal peripheral smear and ↑ bilirubin levels, elevated liver enzymes (AST >70 μ/L, LDH >600 μ/L), and thrombocytopenia (<100,000 / mm^3)
- Failure to treat may lead to eclampsia or death due to hepatic hematoma or rupture
- Not always associated with HTN

ICD-9-CM Code: 642.5 (Severe pre-eclampsia)

ETIOLOGY

- Poorly understood
- May be severe form of preeclampsia resulting from abnormal prostaglandin control, intravascular plt activation, and microvascular endothelial damage. Microangiopathic hemolytic anemia usual

USUAL TREATMENT

- Definitive treatment is delivery as quickly as possible.
- After delivery, many experience uneventful recovery with plt counts returning to normal within 1 wk.
- In the presence of immaturity, two doses of glucocorticoids may accelerate fetal lung maturity.
Plts, FFP, and cryoprecipitate administered as needed.
- Magnesium sulfate for CNS irritability and antihypertensives for HTN

ASSESSMENT POINTS

SYSTEM	EFFECT	ASSESSMENT BY HX	PE	TEST
HEENT	Upper airway edema	Dyspnea, voice change	Poor visualization on airway exam	Mallampati assessment
CV	LV failure	Dyspnea, desaturation	Adventitious sounds	CVP and/or PA pressures
RESP	Resp depression	Magnesium administration	↓ Reflexes	$MgSO_4$ level
GI	Liver swelling Subcapsular hematoma	Epigastric pain Nausea, vomiting		Elevated AST, ALT
HEME	Thrombocytopenia Hemolytic anemia	Bruising Pallor, jaundice	Bleeding	Plt count LDH, bilirubin Peripheral smear
RENAL	Acute renal failure	Oliguria		Elevated uric acid, BUN, serum Cr
CNS	Eclampsia, cerebral edema	Seizures		

Key Reference: Crosby ET: Obstetrical anaesthesia for patients with the syndrome of haemolysis, elevated liver enzymes and low platelets. Can J Anaesth 1991; 38:227–233.

PERIOPERATIVE IMPLICATIONS

Preoperative Testing

- Obtain CBC, PT, PTT, fibrinogen, ALT, AST, LDH, BUN, Cr

Monitoring

- Consider arterial line if unstable
- Consider CVP or PA catheter if decreased UO or CHF.

Airway

- Assess airway early and repeat airway exam periodically
- Laryngeal edema may preclude normal tracheal intubation in the event of emergency C-section
- Difficult intubation equipment should be readily available
- Consider preemptive epidural anesthetic

Induction

- Slow, controlled epidural with incremental dosing, if not contraindicated

Adjuvants

- If significant HTN, antihypertensive therapy prior to laryngeal intubation
- If receiving magnesium sulfate and needs GA, small doses of neuromuscular blocking agents with close monitoring

HEMOPHILIA

Vincent S. Cowell, M.D.

RISK

- Incidence: 20/100,000 male births
- Estimated that <20,000 persons in US are diagnosed with hemophilia
- Hemophilia A, factor VIII (FVIII) deficiency, affects 80–85% of hemophiliacs; remainder have hemophilia B (Christmas disease) due to factor IX (FIX) deficiency
- Mode of inheritance and clinical features of hemophilias A and B are similar
- Females may be asymptomatic carriers of the hemophilia gene and may have partial deficiency of factor VIII or IX
- Hemophilia is without ethnic or geographic predilection

PERIOPERATIVE RISKS

- Prolonged and potentially fatal hemorrhage both during and after surgery
- Closed-space bleeding can lead to nerve injury or vascular or airway obstruction
- Surgery should not proceed without adequate supply of factor concentrate to support the procedure and postop course

WORRY ABOUT

- Spontaneous bleeding
- Postop hemorrhage despite optimal replacement therapy of deficient plasma coagulation factor

- Approximately 5–15% develop inhibitors, antibodies, to factor VIII or factor IX (VIII much more often than IX)
- Factor replacement therapy risks exposure to viruses, including hepatitis and HIV

OVERVIEW

- Hemophiliacs can have severe deficiency (no detectable factor), moderate deficiency (1–4% of nml levels), or mild deficiency (5–25% of nml levels)
- Congenital disorder, inherited as an x-linked recessive trait, affecting males almost exclusively
- Acute and chronic complications often due to recurrent spontaneous bleeding, e.g., cycle of joint hemorrhage, inflammation, synovial proliferation, and erosion of cartilage causing pain and disability
- Treatment follows bleeding episodes; high cost of products inhibits prophylactic therapy
- PTT is often elevated and used as a screening test for hemophilia; PTT and factor assays are used to monitor factors VIII and IX levels (PT and plt count are nml)

ICD-9-CM Code: 286.0

ETIOLOGY

- Hereditary disorder, x-linked recessive
- Dx made by abn plasma concentrations of factor VIII or IX

USUAL TREATMENT

- Plasma concentrations of deficient factors maintained at minimum of 40–70% throughout the perioperative period (2–7 d postop) for adequate hemostasis
- Preparations for hemophilia A include purified factor VIII concentrates, recombinant factor VIII, and desmopressin (DDAVP; leads to release of von Willebrand factor and concomitant increase in FVIII; may be used for persons with mild hemophilia A)
- Factor IX deficiency treated with purified factor IX concentrates
- 1 U of factor VIII is amount of factor VIII activity contained in 1 ml of nml plasma
- Dose of factor VIII is 50 U/kg to attain 100% factor VIII levels; 70 kg patient = 70 × 50 U/kg = 3500 U of factor VIII concentrate ($T_{1/2}$ of factor VIII is 10–12 h); treat every 12 h
- Dose of factor IX is twice that of factor VIII to attain 100% factor IX levels; 70 kg patient = 70 × 100 U/kg = 7000 U of factor IX concentrate ($T_{1/2}$ of factor IX is 20–24 h) treat every 24 h
- FFP no longer used in routine treatment of hemophilia A or B, but consider in urgent situations if factor concentrates are not available
- Cryoprecipitate is concentrated source of factor VIII but is not often used because of availability of purified factor VIII concentrates
- Gene insertion therapy under investigation

ASSESSMENT POINTS

SYSTEM	EFFECT	ASSESSMENT BY HX	PE	TEST
HEENT	Pharyngeal bleeding	Often seen in children	Tongue and mouth lacerations	Examination
GI	GI bleeding not common	When it occurs, bleeding can be excessive	Stool exam, endoscopy	Hemoccult, Angio
HEME	Anemia, hematoma formation, bruising	Lethargy, SOB, skin discoloration	Hematomas	PT/PTT Factor VIII and factor IX assay, gene analysis
GU	Hematuria	Blood in urine		Urinalysis, cysto, IVP
CNS	Intracranial hemorrhage	Head trauma, headache, change in mental status	Any sign or symptom of head injury or trauma	Head CT
MS	Joint hemorrhage Joint deformities Muscle hemorrhage Compartment syndrome Chronic pain	Painful distention of the joint Bruising Restricted movement Narcotic dependence	Hemarthroses Limited ROM Tenderness	Physical exam X-ray

Key Reference: Furie B, Limentani SA, Rosenfield CG: A practical guide to the evaluation and treatment of hemophilia. Blood 1994; 84:3–9.

PERIOPERATIVE IMPLICATIONS

Preoperative Preparation

- Therapeutic levels (40–70%) of plasma factor VIII or factor IX before proceeding with surgery
- Avoid unnecessary IM injections

Monitoring

- Consider avoiding invasive monitoring unless absolutely essential

Airway

- Extra care to avoid trauma from instrumentation of airway

Induction

- No special considerations

Maintenance

- Risk of bleeding may outweigh the benefits of regional anesthetics

Extubation

- Be sensitive to extubating patients who have potential for bleeding in neck or pharynx that could compromise airway

Adjuvants

- When selecting anesthetic drugs, consider presence of coexisting liver disease due to hepatitis from previous transfusion

ANTICIPATED PROBLEMS/CONCERNS

- Transmission of blood-borne viruses (HIV, hepatitis viruses, and recently reported parvovirus) by clotting factor concentrates
- Universal precautions should be observed
- 5–15% of persons with hemophilia A develop inhibitors to factor VIII; treatment becomes individualized and complex
- May want to avoid drugs that interfere with nml plt function such as aspirin and NSAIDs
- Chronic pain due to bleeding in joints or muscle tissue may lead to narcotic addiction

HEPATIC ENCEPHALOPATHY

Jeffrey M. Baden, M.D.

RISK

• People in the USA: Approximately 2000/y from fulminant liver failure and many more from chronic liver disease
• Race/gender with highest prevalence: Unknown

PERIOPERATIVE RISKS

• Increased risk of CV depression, arrhythmias, sudden cardiac arrest
• Coagulopathy
• Cerebral edema, resp arrest, sepsis, renal failure, hypoglycemia, sodium abnormalities.

WORRY ABOUT

• Deteriorating liver function
• Deteriorating renal function requiring hemodialysis
• Deteriorating CV and resp function

OVERVIEW

• Complex mental state associated with liver disease
• Key symptom is changed mental state ranging from confusion to coma
• Nature, extent, and complications of liver disease are main determinants of long-term survival.

ICD-9-CM Code: 572.2

ETIOLOGY

• In ⅔ of cases, failure of liver to remove ammonia and possibly other comogenic substances before they enter systemic circulation.
• Non-nitrogenous encephalopathy occurs in ⅓ of cases and is often precipitated by drugs that depress consciousness

USUAL TREATMENT

• Most important measures:
  – Decrease dietary protein intake
  – Suppress ammoniagenic intestinal flora with oral neomycin
  – Stimulate ammonia fixation and removal with oral lactulose

ASSESSMENT POINTS

SYSTEM	EFFECT	ASSESSMENT BY HX	PE	TEST
CV	CV depression Arrhythymias Sudden cardiac arrest		Low BP Abnormal pulse	ECG ECHO
RESP	Increased AV shunts Hypocapnia Lower O_2 consumption	Dyspnea	Cyanosis Hyperventilation	Pulse oximetry and capnography (if indicated) Blood gases
GI	Liver disease	Numerous causes, e.g., alcohol and viral hepatitis	Stigmata of liver disease Liver biopsy	Blood chemistry Viral hepatitis screens
HEME	Coagulation defects	Bleeds easily	Petechiae	CBC, prothrombin time
RENAL	Hepatorenal syndrome			Blood chemistries
CNS	Cerebral edema	Worsening mental state		EEG
METAB	Hypoglycemia Hypernatremia Hyponatremia			Blood chemistries

Key Reference: Brown, BR Jr: Liver failure and hepatic encephalopathy. *In* Brown BR Jr (ed): Anesthesia in Hepatic and Biliary Tract Disease. Philadelphia, FA Davis, 1988, pp 243–249.

PERIOPERATIVE IMPLICATIONS

Preoperative Preparation

• Avoid opiates and sedatives

Monitoring

• Routine monitors
• ECG—sudden arrhythmias
• Consider intra-arterial and CVP monitoring—remember coagulopathy
• Frequent blood glucose and lyte analysis

Airway

• Bleeding of instrumented upper airway

Preinduction/Induction

• Avoid "fixed agents" when possible

Maintenance

• Volatile anesthetic of low arrhythmogenicity may be good choice

Extubation

• Remember hypoxia from disease itself

Adjuvants

• Use muscle relaxants sparingly and titrate carefully to effect
• Atracurium may be a good choice

ANTICIPATED PROBLEMS/CONCERNS

• Bleeding
• Prolongation of drug effects
• Cardiovascular depression and arrhythmias
• Tendency to hypoxia
• Sepsis
• Renal dysfunction
• Hypoglycemia

HEPATITIS, ALCOHOLIC

Johnathan L. Pregler, M.D.

RISK

- People within USA: 10% of men and 3–5% of women develop alcoholism, 10–15% of alcoholics will develop alcoholic hepatitis and cirrhosis.

PERIOPERATIVE RISKS

- Mortality rate of 60–100% of patients undergoing surgery during active alcoholic hepatitis. (Some reports of lower mortality rate if alcohol intake stopped, and hepatitis is chemical without jaundice.)
- Elective surgery should be postponed.
- >10% develop DTs without prophylaxis.

WORRY ABOUT

- Bleeding disorders and anemia
- Pulmonary shunting
- Altered mental status/encephalopathy/alcohol withdrawal with DTs
- Insulin resistance

OVERVIEW

- Acute inflammatory lesion of liver. As mild as nausea and vomiting or as severe as fulminant hepatic failure.
- In-hospital mortality 50% if elevated bilirubin, Cr, PT, ascites, and/or encephalopathy.
- An intermediate stage between fatty liver and alcoholic cirrhosis
- May be preceded by period of heavy alcohol consumption

ICD-9-CM Code: 571.1

ETIOLOGY

- Daily consumption of a pint or more of alcohol or equivalent in wine/or beer for 10 or more y.
- Amount and duration of consumption more important than type of alcohol or pattern of consumption
- Women at risk with lower consumption levels.
- Inflammatory lesion with leukocytic infiltration. Progresses to hepatocellular necrosis and deposition of alcoholic hyaline.
- Repeated episodes precursor to cirrhosis after healing and scar tissue formation

USUAL TREATMENT

- Abstinence
- Recovery varies from several weeks to months.
- Supportive care includes diet adjustment, multivitamin supplementation, lactulose, and neomycin if needed.

ASSESSMENT POINTS

SYSTEM	EFFECT	ASSESSMENT BY HX	PE	TEST
CV	High CO Low SVR Low CO (in advanced disease)	Exercise tolerance	Hyperdynamic cardiac exam	ECG ECHO
RESP	Pulmonary shunts Restrictive disease Pulmonary effusions Central hyperventilation	Orthodeoxia Ascites	Effusions on chest exam. Ascites on abdominal exams	Respiratory alkalosis on ABG
GI/LIVER	Disrupted synthetic and metabolic function	Anorexia, N/V, malaise, wt loss, fever	Jaundice, ascites, tender hepatomegaly, splenomegaly	Elevated transaminases (AST/ALT>2), PT, Alk phos, bilirubin Decreased albumin
RENAL	Mg^{2+} and PO_4 wasting Free water retention		Ascites	Serum Mg^{2+} and PO_4 Hyponatremia
ENDO	Insulin resistance			Glucose
HEME	Anemia and thrombocytopenia GI blood loss Hypersplenism	Bruising/bleeding	Splenomegaly	Hgb/Hct, platelets
CNS	Decreased clearance of amines	Altered mental status	Neurologic exam	NH_3 levels

Key Reference: Gholson CF, Provenza JM: Hepatologic considerations in patients with parenchymal liver disease undergoing surgery. Am Gastroenterol 1990; 85:487–496.

PERIOPERATIVE IMPLICATIONS

Preoperative Preparation

- Elective procedures should be postponed.
- Extreme sensitivity to sedative medications
- Ascites may be treated by diuretics (spironolactone) or percutaneous drainage.
- Hypokalemia and hyponatremia should be corrected slowly (over 24–36 h).
- Assess/correct coagulopathy by vit K administration and FFP, platelets if needed.

Monitoring

- Glucose levels
- Large fluid shifts during abdominal procedures due to drainage of ascites may necessitate CVP or PA catheter.

Airway

- At risk for aspiration if ascites and increased abdominal pressure.

Induction

- Hypoalbuminemia may decrease V_d (Pentothal)
- H_2O-soluble drugs may have increased V_d owing to ascites
- Regional anesthesia well tolerated (if coagulation status permits)

Maintenance

- Maintain normocarbia.
- Decreased clearance of hepatically metabolized drugs (meperidine, fentanyl, barbiturates)
- Conjugative metabolic pathways better preserved (morphine)
- Maintain hepatic blood flow (isoflurane is best inhalation agent). (No contraindication to N_2O)

Extubation

- Extubate when patient fully awake

Adjuvants

- MVI and vit K 10mg SQ or IM.

Postoperative Period

- Pain control ideally via regional to avoid sedative effects of system drug; however, must assess coagulation system.
- Morphine metabolism is better preserved than other narcotics.
- Monitor or treat for alcohol withdrawal.

ANTICIPATED PROBLEMS/CONCERNS

- Poor regulation of glucose levels
- Need for prolonged airway protection because of altered mental status and pulmonary dysfunction
- Acute withdrawal from alcohol
- Multiple coagulation abnormalities due to synthetic dysfunction and hypersplenism.

HEPATITIS B

Arnold J. Berry, M.D.

RISK

- General population of USA: 3–5% have had the disease and 0.3–1.0% are carriers of hepatitis B virus (HBV)
- High-risk groups include immigrants from endemic areas, IV drug users, homosexual men, household contacts of HBV carriers, patients on hemodialysis, clients in mental institutions
- About 20% of susceptible anesthesiologists have serologic evidence of prior HBV infection

PERIOPERATIVE RISKS

- Depends on activity and stage of infection
- Worsening liver function, hepatic encephalopathy, coagulopathy

WORRY ABOUT

- With acute hepatic failure or end-stage liver disease: coagulation abnormalities, decreased hepatic metabolism of drugs, decreased levels of plasma cholinesterase, hypoxemia from pulmonary shunting, ascites and Na+ overload, hepatic encephalopathy, impaired glucose metabolism, portal HTN and GI bleeding, hepatorenal syndrome
- Maintenance of liver blood flow and O_2 delivery
- Use of universal precautions by anesthesia personnel

OVERVIEW

- Hepatotropic viral infection: 90% have self-limiting acute hepatitis; 1% develop fulminant hepatitis; 10% become chronic HBV carriers with about half progressing to chronic active hepatitis, cirrhosis, or hepatocellular carcinoma
- 50% with acute infection asymptomatic whereas others have jaundice, malaise, nausea, abdominal pain
- HBV carriers are diagnosed by persistent positive serology for hepatitis B surface antigen (HBsAg)
- Hepatitis B surface antibody (anti-HBs) confers immunity (after resolution of infection or with immunization)

ICD-9-CM Codes: 070.30 (Acute); 070.32 (Chronic)

ETIOLOGY

- HBV (42 nm DNA virus) carried in and spread by blood and body fluid contact
- Transmitted to health care workers via parenteral or mucocutaneous exposure to HBV-infected blood or body fluids. One in four to one in five exposures causes disease in previously uninfected contact.

USUAL TREATMENT

- Prevention with hepatitis B vaccine
- Hepatitis B immune globulin for passive immunization after susceptible individual is exposed
- No specific Rx, bed rest for acute hepatitis B
- Orthotopic liver transplantation for liver failure

ASSESSMENT POINTS

(The following are for patients with fulminant hepatitis or cirrhosis from chronic hepatitis.)

SYSTEM	EFFECT	ASSESSMENT BY HX	PE	TEST
CV	Hyperdynamic circulation		Tachycardia Skin spiders	Measure CO, SVR
RESP	Hypoxemia		Tachypnea	SpO_2
GI	Bleeding Ascites Jaundice Hypoalbuminenia Hepatitis	Hx of bleeding Increasing abdominal girth Dark urine	Ascites, pedal edema Abdominal pain	Hct, endoscopy Bilirubin Serum albumin ALT, AST
ENDO	Hypoglycemia	Altered consciousness		Blood sugar
HEME	Anemia Thrombocytopenia Immunosuppression Coagulopathy	Easy bruisability Infections Abn bleeding	Bruises	Hct Plt count PT (low factors V, VII, IX, X, fibrinogen)
RENAL	Hepatorenal syndrome Hyponatremia Hypokalemia	Altered consciousness, seizures Taking diuretics	Oliguria	Urinary Na+ Serum Na+ Serum K+
CNS	Encephalopathy	Mental status exam	Level of consciousness Asterixis	

Key Reference: Koff RS: Viral hepatitis. In Schiff L, Schiff ER (eds): Diseases of the Liver, 7th ed. Philadelphia, JB Lippincott, 1993; pp 492–577.

PERIOPERATIVE IMPLICATIONS
(for patients with end-stage liver disease from hepatitis B) — emergency surgery only with acute infection

Preoperative Preparation

- Correction of clotting abnormalities with FFP, Plt, cryoprecipitate as needed
- Paracentesis if resp compromise from massive ascites

Monitoring

- Arterial line for ABG and BP
- Consider need for central venous or pulmonary artery catheter

Airway

- Consider rapid-sequence induction if pt has ascites or upper GI bleeding

Preinduction/Induction

- Ketamine or etomidate in hypovolemic patients
- Duration of action of succinylcholine may be prolonged
- Increased bioavailability of IV drugs with low serum albumin
- Limit sedative drugs

Maintenance

- Inhalation agent with high FIO_2 useful for maintaining hepatic blood flow; should probably avoid halothane
- Choose muscle relaxants not dependent on liver metabolism
- Increased blood loss with coagulopathy

Extubation

- May need postop ventilation to ensure time for adequate metabolism of depressant drugs

Adjuvants

- Hypocalcemia may occur with citrate administration

ANTICIPATED PROBLEMS/CONCERNS

- Worsening of hepatic or renal function
- Fluid overload
- Delayed awakening from prolonged drug metabolism or encephalopathy
- Need to protect airway with reduced consciousness, esp with upper GI bleeding
- Hypoglycemia

HEPATITIS C

Arnold J. Berry, M.D.

RISK

- Majority of cases of sporadic and post-transfusion non-A, non-B hepatitis are caused by hepatitis C virus (HCV)
- High-risk groups include IV drug users, sexual or household contacts of HCV carriers; transfusions account for 6% of new cases (90% of post-transfusion hepatitis is caused by HCV); increased prevalence in patients on hemodialysis
- About 2–3% of cases occur in health care workers

PERIOPERATIVE RISKS

- Worsening liver function, hepatic encephalopathy, coagulopathy
- Risk of transmission of HCV from carrier to anesthesia personnel is 3–4% after percutaneous exposure

WORRY ABOUT

- With end-stage liver disease: coagulation abn, ↓ hepatic metabolism of drugs, ↓ levels of plasma cholinesterase, hypoxemia from pulm shunting, ascites and Na+ overload, hepatic encephalopathy, glucose metabolism, portal HTN and GI bleeding, hepatorenal syndrome
- Maintenance of liver blood flow and O₂ delivery
- Use of universal precautions by anesthesia personnel

OVERVIEW

- Hepatotropic insidious viral infection; fulminant acute hepatitis C rare
- After HCV infection, 50% remain carriers and progress to chronic active hepatitis; 10–20% develop cirrhosis

- Anti-HCV found in 60–85% after HCV infection, but this antibody does not correlate with resolution or confer immunity.

ICD-9-CM Codes: 070.51 (acute); 070.54 (chronic)

ETIOLOGY

- HCV (30-60 nm RNA virus) carried in and transmitted by blood and body fluid contact

USUAL TREATMENT

- Interferon α-2b for chronic HCV infection but high relapse rate after discontinuation
- Orthotopic liver transplantation for liver failure

ASSESSMENT POINTS

(The following are for patients with end stage liver disease from cirrhosis or chronic hepatitis.)

SYSTEM	EFFECT	ASSESSMENT BY HX	PE	TEST
CV	Hyperdynamic circulation		Tachycardia Skin spiders	Measure CO, SVR
RESP	Hypoxemia		Tachypnea	ABG
GI	Bleeding Ascites Jaundice Hypoalbuminenia Hepatitis	Hx of bleeding Increasing abdominal girth Dark urine	Hemoccult+ material Fluid wave on abdominal exam Icteric sclera Ascites, pedal edema Abdominal pain	Hct, endoscopy Bilirubin Serum albumin ALT, AST
ENDO	Hypoglycemia	Altered consciousness		Blood sugar
HEME	Anemia Thrombocytopenia Immunosuppression Coagulopathy	Easy bruisability Infections Abn bleeding	Bruises	Hct Plt count PT (low factors V, VII, IX, X, fibrinogen)
RENAL	Hepatorenal syndrome Hyponatremia Hypokalemia	Altered consciousness, seizures Taking diuretics	Oliguria	Urinary Na+ low Serum Na+ Serum K+
CNS	Encephalopathy	Mental status exam	Level of consciousness Asterixis	

Key Reference: Koff RS: Viral hepatitis. *In* Schiff L, Schiff ER (eds): Diseases of the Liver, 7th ed. Philadelphia, JB Lippincott, 1993, pp492–577.

PERIOPERATIVE IMPLICATIONS (for patients with end-stage liver disease from hepatitis C)

Preoperative Preparation

- Correction of clotting abnormalities with FFP, Plt, cryoprecipitate as needed
- Paracentesis if resp compromise from massive ascites

Monitoring

- Arterial line for ABG and BP
- Consider central venous or pulm artery catheter

Airway

- Consider rapid-sequence induction with ascites or upper GI bleeding

Preinduction/Induction

- Ketamine or etomidate in hypovolemic patients
- Duration of action of succinylcholine may be prolonged
- Increased bioavailability of IV drugs with low serum albumin
- Limit sedative drugs

Maintenance

- Inhalation agent with high FIO_2 useful for maintaining hepatic blood flow; should probably avoid halothane
- Choose muscle relaxants not dependent on liver metabolism
- Increased blood loss with coagulopathy

Extubation

- May need postop ventilation to ensure time for adequate metabolism of depressant drugs

Adjuvants

- Hypocalcemia may occur with citrate administration

ANTICIPATED PROBLEMS/CONCERNS

- Worsening of hepatic or renal function
- Fluid overload
- Delayed awakening from prolonged drug metabolism or encephalopathy
- Need to protect airway with reduced consciousness, especially with upper GI bleeding
- Hypoglycemia

HEPATITIS — HALOTHANE

Aisling Conran, M.D.

RISK

• Greater if repeated exposures, obese, taking P450 inducing agent, middle age (>40 y, esp. 50–60 y) female, genetic susceptibility
• Rare in infants and children: 1/10,000 to 1/40,000 halothane anesthetics

PREOPERATIVE RISKS

Pre-existing liver disease; site, duration, or degree of surgery has NOT been shown to contribute to development

WORRY ABOUT

• Enzyme induction of hepatic cytochrome P450 system by other pharmacologic agents may predispose (esp INH).

OVERVIEW/PHARMACOLOGY

• Liver damage within 28 d of halothane exposure when other causes of liver dysfunction have been excluded
• Viral hepatitis, pre-existing liver disease, blood transfusion, sepsis, drug reactions, and intraop and postop hypoxia and hypotension must be excluded as causes of liver dysfunction.
• In past, undiagnosed viral hepatitis, especially non-A, non-B hepatitis, confused clinical picture.

• Clinical features include nausea, jaundice, fever, eosinophilia, rash and arthralgias, ↑ liver function test results, presence of autoantibodies

ICD-9-CM Code: 997.4 (Postoperative acute)

ETIOLOGY

• Hepatic hypoxia has been postulated as mechanism for development. While halothane, enflurane, and isoflurane decrease portal blood flow, both isoflurane and enflurane maintain hepatic blood flow better than halothane by increasing hepatic arterial flow. While persistent global hypoxia occurs rarely, local liver hypoxia may occur and contribute to the development of halothane hepatitis.
• Two forms: more common, mild form is associated with reductive metabolites of halothane metabolism. Fulminant form, occurring in approx 1:35,000 halothane anesthetics, is associated with a high mortality and is likely immune-mediated. This hypersensitivity hypothesis is supported by prevalence of eosinophilia, fever, Hx of previous or repeated exposures to halothane, Hx of drug allergy or atopy, and presence of IgG autoantibodies. IgG autoantibodies are found in 70%. The autoantibodies react with trifluro-acetyl halide (TFA), a reactive metabolite that can bind to cellular components, changing "self" to "non-self." This new hapten provokes an immune hypersensitivity reaction in genetically susceptible individuals.
• Increased Ca^{2+} levels in cell may be final common pathway to cell destruction in liver. Halothane can inactivate endoplasmic reticulum's Ca^{2+} transport mechanism, resulting in an intracellular release of Ca^{2+}.

DRUG CLASS/METABOLISM

• Halothane is a nonflammable, halogenated alkene which is a potent volatile anesthetic agent. Undergoes biotransformation by the liver via two pathways, an oxidative and a reductive pathway. Oxidative pathway is favored in the presence of high oxygen tensions and the reductive pathway is more prevalent under both hypoxic conditions and in the presence of enzyme induction. Approximately 20% metabolism, a much higher rate than either enflurane (2.4%) or isoflurane (0.2%). Trifluoroacetic acid and bromide ion are the metabolites of the oxidative pathway and 2-chloro-1,1,1-trifluoroethane, 2-chloro-1,1-difluoroethylene, and fluoride ion are produced via the reductive pathway. None of the metabolites shown to be directly hepatotoxic. Binding of metabolites to hepatic cells is more likely under hypoxic conditions and therefore more likely to occur with the reductive pathway.

ASSESSMENT POINTS

SYSTEM	ASSESSMENT BY HX	PE	TEST
GI	Nausea	Jaundice (5th–6th d after exposure)	Eosinophilia Elevated LFTs Serum transaminases markedly increased Alkaline phosphatase may double Liver biopsy: centrilobular necrosis Antibody tests (still experimental but available)

Key Reference: Ray DC, Drummond GB: Halothane hepatitis. Br J Anaesth 1991; 67:84–99.

PREOPERATIVE IMPLICATIONS

• Assess patient for risk factors; review anesthetic records for possible prior halothane exposures.

ANTICIPATED PROBLEMS/CONCERNS

• When evaluating a patient with postop liver dysfunction, many causes of postop jaundice need to be excluded, anesthesia records need to be reviewed, LFTs obtained and followed serially.
• Hx of any contact with person with jaundice elicited, drug Hx and transfusion Hx obtained, serologies for viral hepatitis, antibody testing for volatile anesthetics, and liver biopsy obtained prior to making Dx.

HEREDITARY HEMORRHAGIC TELANGIECTASIA (Osler-Weber-Rendu Disease)

Kamla K. Prasad, M.D.

RISK

- Annual incidence in USA: 1/50,000
- Caucasians > other races
- No gender preponderance

PERIOPERATIVE RISKS

- Paradoxical air, bland, or septic embolism to brain (due to pulmonary AVMs in 20% of patients)

WORRY ABOUT

- Anemia 2° to hemorrhage, especially recurrent epistaxis
- High incidence of HIV, hepatitis B and C due to frequent transfusions (may exceed 100 units over a lifetime)

OVERVIEW

- A fibrovascular dysplasia
- Triad of telangiectases, AVMs, aneurysms distributed throughout body
- Great variability in severity of vascular lesions and organ dysfunction
- May present as frequent epistaxis, mucosal or GI bleeding, hypoxemia, central neurologic deficit, brain abscess, high-output CHF or hepatic encephalopathy

ICD-9-CM Code: 448.0

ETIOLOGY

- Autosomal dominant disease with variable penetrance

USUAL TREATMENT

- High-dose estrogen therapy (may increase risk of thromboembolism)
- Multiple transfusions

ASSESSMENT POINTS

SYSTEM	EFFECT	ASSESSMENT BY HX	PE	TEST
HEENT	Nasopharyngeal AVMs	Frequent epistaxis		
CV	High-output CHF Thromboembolism		Rales Neurologic deficit	CXR
RESP	AVMs/hypoxemia (R→L shunting)	Fatigue Exertional dyspnea Hemoptysis	Cyanosis Clubbing	ABG CXR (rounded homogeneous masses of consistent density, rib notching)
HEPATIC	Hepatic failure (L→R shunting)	Bleeding Jaundice		PT, PTT LFTs
HEME	Anemia Coagulopathy	Recurrent epistaxis	Pallor	CBC Bleeding time ($\downarrow$ plt aggregation) PT, PTT (Factor XI deficiency, hepatic failure)
CNS	Paradoxical embolism	CVA Bacterial encephalitis Brain abscess	Neurologic deficits Fever	Brain CT Diagnostic lumbar puncture

Key Reference: Radu C, Reich DL, Tamman R: Anesthetic considerations in a cardiac surgical patient with Osler-Weber-Rendu disease. J Cardiothorac Vasc Anesth 1992; pp 461–464.

PERIOPERATIVE IMPLICATIONS

Preoperative Preparation

- Debubble IV lines to prevent paradoxical air embolism
- Meticulous aseptic line techniques to avoid septic embolism to brain

Monitoring

- Presence of esophageal varices or AVMs increase risk of esophageal stethoscope placement and gastric suctioning

Airway

- Risk of airway hemorrhage if oropharyngeal telangiectases
- Nasal intubation contraindicated if nasal telangiectases

Maintenance

- Risk of hepatic failure and high-output CHF modify anesthetic management

Postoperative Period

- Immobilization may predispose to CNS embolism

Adjuvants

- Precipitation of incompatible drugs in IV line or peripheral vein may send particulate matter to brain; avoid by careful technique or filter
- Prophylactic antibiotics to decrease risk of aerobic and anaerobic CNS infections
- NSAIDs, including ketorolac, may precipitate GI or mucosal bleeding
- Regional: AVMs may be present in epidural space

ANTICIPATED PROBLEMS/CONCERNS

- Anemia due to recurrent bleeding
- Transfusion is complicated: low hematocrit may increase the risk of high-output CHF by increasing extent of arteriovenous shunting ($\downarrow$ viscosity effect), but a high hematocrit may increase risk of thromboembolism.
- Coagulopathy: Multiple hemostatic defects, including low-grade DIC, reduced plt aggregation, and Factor XI deficiency, may aggravate bleeding caused by local vessel wall pathology.
- Paradoxical embolism: Owing to pulmonary AVMs, peripheral microemboli (air, bland, or septic) bypass normal pulmonary capillary filtering and embolize, causing transient or permanent neurologic defects or brain abscess.

HERNIATED NUCLEUS PULPOSUS

Garfield B. Russell, M.D.

RISK

- Incidence: 1% of low back pain; cervical 1/1 million individuals.
- Can be lumbar (most common), cervical, or thoracic (least common).
- 70% of adults experience low back pain; 40% experience sciatica.
- 4–6% of the population experience clinically significant sciatica.
- 20% of sciatica is caused by lumbar herniation.
- Lumbar disks most prevalent ages 25–40 y
- Race with highest prevalence: equal

PERIOPERATIVE RISKS

- Mortality rare: 0–0.5%
- Related to underlying conditions

WORRY ABOUT

- Associated psychologic problems if pain has been chronic; possible medications—narcotics, muscle relaxants, tranquilizers, antidepressants
- Potential litigious issues if injury is job- or accident-related

OVERVIEW

- Occurs in relatively healthy patients without increased risk for significant end-organ disease
- Injury risks of patient positioning:
  – Patients may be supine with arms tucked (cervical disks), prone on bolsters, prone on a Wilson frame, prone on an Andrew's table, in the Georgia-prone position (lumbar disks), in the lateral decubitus position (lumbar or anterior approaches to thoracic disks)
  – If supine, these include: peripheral nerve injury (particularly ulnar) from poorly padded arm tucking, hyperextension injuries of the cervical spine, corneal abrasions
  – If prone, these include:
    - eyes—corneal abrasions, retinal artery or vein thrombosis from pressure, scleral edema
    - nose—pressure necrosis
    - mouth/pharynx—glossal edema, laryngeal edema, endotracheal tube kinking, pressure necrosis from poorly positioned oral airways.
  - CV—↓ venous return and associated hypotension, particularly if in Georgia-prone position; venous air embolism—the free abdomen may generate pressure gradient in relation to the surgical incision, allowing air to be entrained; the incidence is unknown.
  - Resp—Respiratory compromise if abdomen and diaphragm are not free and dependent. The endotracheal tube is at risk if not well secured.
  - GI—Patients prone to reflux may experience passive regurgitation.

ICD-9-CM Code: 722

ETIOLOGY

- Trauma
- Degenerative changes
- Risk factors include: frequent lifting of objects >25 lb, exposure to whole body vibration, cigarette smoking, narrow lumbar vertebral canals.

USUAL TREATMENT

- Medical therapy with short period of rest, physiotherapy, analgesics, muscle relaxants, and behavioral modification with a continued exercise program are usually successful.
- Chemonucleolysis—much less frequently practiced because of anaphylactic reactions to chymopapain.
- Traction
- Manipulation
- Surgical diskectomy

ASSESSMENT POINTS

SYSTEM	EFFECT	ASSESSMENT BY HX	PE	TEST
HEENT	↓ ROM, pain, difficult airway	Pain and limited ROM	Neck ROM	Cervical spine x-rays usually available for C-spine cases
CV	None primary	Predispositions: rheumatoid arthritis, obesity, family Hx	Murmurs Weight	None usually needed
CNS	None usual	Personality changes with pain or analgesic dependency	None	None usual
PNS	Pain ↓ Strength ↓ Sensation	New pain, paresthesias Impotence Bowel and urinary incontinence	Strength and sensory evaluation	None usual, possible EMG
MS	Muscle wasting Muscle spasm Limited motion Pain with activity	Strength changes Mobility	Spine ROM	None usual

Key Reference: Shapiro HM, Drummond JC: Miller's Anesthesia, 4th ed. New York, Churchill Livingstone, 1994, pp 1777–1779.

PERIOPERATIVE IMPLICATIONS

Preoperative Preparation

- Continued analgesia if necessary

Monitoring

- Routine
- Dermatomal somatosensory evoked potentials (dSSEP) have questionable clinical and practical applicability.
- If spinal instrumentation with pedicle screw fixation used, free-run and triggered EMG monitor for bone cortex disruption and possible nerve root injury.

Airway

- Associated with poor neck mobility and possible worsening with "sniffing" position
- Reinforced endotracheal tube
- Consider nasal endotracheal tubes for anterior cervical disks.

Induction

- Routine

Maintenance

- Simple diskectomies can be done with regional anesthesia (spinal preferable to epidural).

Extubation

- Prone positioning predisposes to significant upper airway edema.
- Cervical disk patients may have a soft or hard neck collar in place.

Adjuvants

- Some prefer no or limited NM blockade.
- If neurophysiologic monitoring used: NMB can alter EMG and many anesthetics, particularly volatile agents, interfere with dSSEP recording.
- For anterior cervical diskectomies, esophageal stethoscope affords reliable landmark for the esophagus.

Postoperative Period

- Analgesia requirements depend on surgical approach.

ANTICIPATED PROBLEMS/CONCERNS

- Resolution of airway/facial/scleral edema for those positioned prone, particularly for longer cases.
- Atelectasis after thoracic surgery
- Interference with swallowing by edema and discomfort from cervical surgery, particularly the anterior approach
- Possible postop stridor due to hematoma development after anterior cervical surgery

HERPES — TYPE I

Eugene Y. Cheng, M.D.

RISK

- Rare in the immunocompetent host
- Frequency and severity markedly increased in patients with AIDS, hematologic and lymphoreticular malignancies, or recent organ transplantation

PERIOPERATIVE RISKS

- No evidence that surgery or anesthetics affect extent or duration of infection

WORRY ABOUT

- Transmitting infection to uninfected
- ↑ Risk of spreading HSV to other sites through examination or instrumentation
- Secondary infection of herpetic lesions with bacteria or fungi

OVERVIEW

- Transient viremia common; abnormal nonspecific and immune defenses unable to limit virus replication and spread, esp. in immunosuppressed patients
- Recurrent infection slow to resolve and more likely to spread by contiguous extension
- Disseminated viral skin infection is usually self-limiting and resolves in 7–14 d
- Dx: Gold standard—viral culture
  Rapid Dx—Tzanck smear; electron microscopy; polymerase chain reaction

ICD-9-CM Codes: 054.7 (Infection with specified complications); 054.8 (infection with unspecified complications)

ETIOLOGY

- Ubiquitous human virus; HSV-1 responsible for 90% of infections above waist. Approx. 80% of genital herpetic lesions caused by HSV-2 (genital herpes). In the family of Herpesviridae; other human herpesviruses are varicella-zoster (HHV-3), Epstein-Barr virus (HHV-4), cytomegalovirus (HHV-5), and human herpes virus 6 (HHV-6).
- Humans the only natural reservoir; no vectors are involved with transmission
- Intact immune system will not prevent infection, but differences in immune system produce variations in pattern of disease (e.g., asymptomatic or disseminated)

USUAL TREATMENT

- Acyclovir for acute or recurrent infections
- Foscarnet or vidarabine for acyclovir-resistant mutants

ASSESSMENT POINTS

SYSTEM	EFFECT	ASSESSMENT BY HX	PE	TEST
RESP	Pneumonitis	Aspiration of oral secretions; previous HSV esophagitis	Bilateral crackles	CXR—bilateral interstitial infiltrates
GI	Esophagitis	Odynophagia, dysphagia, substernal pain	Multiple shallow mucosal ulcers	
GU	Cystitis			
CNS	Encephalitis Meningitis	Headache, confusion, lethargy	Anosmia, memory loss, expressive aphasia, focal seizures	Brain biopsy
SKIN	Stevens-Johnson syndrome	Extensive painful skin lesions	Deep bullous-erosive lesions	

Key Reference: Moulin GC, Hedley-Whyte J: Hospital-associated viral infection and the anesthesiologist. Anesthesiology 1983; 39:51–65.

PERIOPERATIVE IMPLICATIONS

Preoperative Preparation

- Cover exposed herpetic lesions
- Strict adherence to univeral precautions

Monitoring

- Avoid inserting catheters through any herpetic infected areas

Regional Anesthesia

- Contraindicated if needle must be inserted through herpetic infected area

Postoperative Period

- Thorough disinfection of any surface area that might have been in contact with oral secretions or herpetic lesions

ANTICIPATED PROBLEMS/CONCERNS

- No effective pre- or postexposure prophylaxis
- Most effective therapy is high-dose intravenous acyclovir for at least 10–14 d

HERPES — TYPE II

Rosa M. Navarro, M.D.
Woo Chan Kim, M.D.

RISK

- People within USA: Estimated 40–60 million
- Highest prevalence in women, African-American, and lower socioeconomic groups
- Frequency and severity of infection increased in immunocompromised patients
- Incidence of neonatal HSV infection estimated at 1/2000–1/5000 deliveries

PERIOPERATIVE RISKS

- Vertical transmission from infected mother to fetus during vaginal birth
- Intrauterine fetal infection after rupture of membranes

WORRY ABOUT

- Transmission of infection to health care personnel resulting in herpetic whitlow via inoculation of virus into fingers
- Neonatal herpetic infection during vaginal births
- Viremia 2° to needle placement within infected area during regional anesthesia
- Extension of genital infection to adjacent areas during examination and instrumentation
- Secondary bacterial or fungal infection of herpetic lesions

OVERVIEW

- Causative primarily of infections below waist transmitted by sexual contact
- Maternal primary HSV-2 infection associated with spontaneous abortion
- Newborns infected with HSV-2 during vaginal delivery from the mother's genital infection (high neonatal mortality)
- Primary genital HSV-2 infection with highest incidence of systemic symptoms (malaise, fever, headache, myalgias)
- Latent infection remains dormant in sensory ganglia innervating infected area until reactivation
- Recurrent infection involves vesicular, ulcerative lesions in genital tract, labia, vulva, perineum, cervix, urethra
- Neuraxial opioid anesthesia does not reactivate or increase risk of recurrent genital HSV-2 infection
- Chronic recurrent HSV-2 infection associated with development of cervical cancer
- Diagnosis by viral culture most sensitive and specific (rapid Dx by Tzanck smear)

ICD-9-CM Codes: 054.9 (infection); 771.2 (congenital)

ETIOLOGY

- Double-stranded DNA virus in family of Herpesviridae
- Acquired genital infection primarily by sexual transmission of HSV-2
- Immunosuppression and increased number of sexual partners are risk factors for acquisition
- Diagnosed by multinucleated giant epithelial cells with intranuclear inclusion bodies on Giemsa stain smears (Tzanck preparation) taken from vesicle or tissue biopsy

USUAL TREATMENT

- IV acyclovir for neonatal HSV-2 infection
- Oral acyclovir and topical cream shorten duration of lesions for recurrent infections
- Most recommend that full-term parturients with visible genital lesions (especially primary infection) undergo abdominal delivery to decrease incidence of neonatal HSV infection

ASSESSMENT POINTS (PRIMARY AND RECURRENT)

SYSTEM	EFFECT	ASSESSMENT BY HX	PE	TEST
HEENT	Pharyngitis (primary)		Cervical adenopathy Mucosal ulceration	
GU (mucous membranes)	Cystitis (primary) Genital ulcers (recurrent)	Dysuria	Vaginal or urethral discharge Ulcerated lesions of penis or labia or cervix	Viral culture Tzanck smear; direct immunofluorescent assay Biopsy; intranuclear inclusion bodies
LYMPHATICS		Lymphadenopathy	Tender inguinal nodes	
SKIN	Herpetic whitlow (recurrent)	Painful vesicular or papular lesion	Pain	Tzanck smear
CNS	Aseptic meningitis (primary)	Headache	Cauda equina syndrome	
RECTAL	Herpes proctitis (primary)	Constipation Tenesmus Discharge		Proctosigmoidoscopy

Key Reference: Roizman B, Whitley RJ, Lopez C (eds): The Human Herpesviruses. New York, Raven Press, 1993.

PERIOPERATIVE IMPLICATIONS

Preoperative Preparation

- Universal precautions

Monitoring

- Routine

Regional Anesthesia

- Needle placement in infected area contraindicated 2° to risk of viremia and local extension into deep tissues
- Preferred in pregnant women with recurrent infection, no systemic symptoms, and no infection in area of block placement

Postoperative Period

- Universal precautions

ANTICIPATED PROBLEMS/CONCERNS

- Difficulty identifying asymptomatic carriers of HSV-2 with viral shedding
- No effective prophylaxis for newborns

HIRSCHSPRUNG'S DISEASE

Donald C. Tyler, M.D.

RISK

• Incidence: 1:5000 live births

PERIOPERATIVE RISKS

• Intestinal obstruction with full stomach
• Electrolyte abnormalities and inadequate volume replacement

WORRY ABOUT

• Abdominal distention
• Intestinal obstruction
• Enterocolitis with shock
• Electrolyte abnormalities
• Anemia

OVERVIEW

• Presents as intestinal obstruction or chronic constipation
• Vomiting and diarrhea may result in electrolyte and fluid status abnormalities
• Enterocolitis may occur with dehydration and shock.

ICD-9-CM Code: 751.3

ETIOLOGY

• Intestinal obstruction results from absence of ganglion cells in bowel wall. The aganglionic segment, usually in rectosigmoid, causes functional intestinal obstruction.

USUAL TREATMENT

• Laparotomy and colostomy with multiple biopsies to determine extent of aganglionic segment. Later (age 6–12 mo) a "pull-through" operation is done to ensure ganglia in rectosigmoid area.

ASSESSMENT POINTS

SYSTEM	EFFECT	ASSESSMENT BY HX	PE	TEST
CV	Hypovolemia	UO, IV replacement Extent of vomiting	Mucous membranes Orthostatic vital signs	BUN and Cr BUN/Cr ratio
GI	Intestinal obstruction	No meconium Diarrhea Vomiting	Mass in abdomen No feces in rectum Protruding abdomen Wasting	Abdominal films Barium enema

Key Reference: Motoyama EK, Davis PJ: Smith's Anesthesia for Infants and Children. St. Louis, CV Mosby, 1990, pp 598–599.

PERIOPERATIVE IMPLICATIONS

Preoperative Implications

• Assess volume status
• Other congenital anomalies

Monitoring

• Routine

Airway

• No special problems except those of newborns

Induction

• May need rapid-sequence induction
• Be careful to monitor BP as anesthesia is deepened

Maintenance

• Prevent heat loss
• Need for muscle relaxation
• Concern about risk of retrolental fibroplasia if baby is premature

Extubation

• Awake

Adjuvants

• Concern about apnea after opioids in newborns

ANTICIPATED PROBLEMS/CONCERNS

• Aspiration pneumonitis

HISTIOCYTOSIS

Hugh L. Preas, II, M.D.

RISK

- Uncommon (1:2 million) worldwide
- Males > females

PERIOPERATIVE RISKS

- Depends on organ system involved and extent of dysfunction

WORRY ABOUT

- Specific organ dysfunction caused by infiltration with reactive histiocytes including hepatic, pulmonary, bone marrow, hypothalamic, and bone (lytic lesions, especially head and face, can include vertebrae and other bones)
- Treated with steroids and chemotherapy; may require perioperative steroid supplementation
- Diabetes insipidus due to infiltration of hypothalamus

OVERVIEW

- Clinical syndromes involving infiltration of organs with histiocytes or macrophages. Severity of clinical symptoms varies markedly. Can involve primarily skin and/or bone or liver, lung, or brain.
- Limited or progressive and fatal. More commonly progressive in patients under 2 y and those with multiple or severe organ involvement
- Clinical presentation in first decade of life

ICD-9-CM Codes: 277.8 (Acute); 202.3 (Malignant)

ETIOLOGY

- Unknown, some variants may have autosomal dominant or recessive inheritance
- Hypothesized to be related to viral infection or autoimmune disease

USUAL TREATMENT

- Chemotherapy (methotrexate, vincristine, etoposide, cyclophosphamide, others) and steroids
- Surgery required for biopsy and diagnosis, lytic bony lesions, and occasionally splenectomy

ASSESSMENT POINTS

SYSTEM	EFFECT	ASSESSMENT BY HX	PE	TEST
HEENT	Soft tissue distortion of airway, loose teeth		Airway and dental evaluation	
RESP	Pneumothorax, reactive airways, infiltrates	Wheezing, dyspnea		CXR, ABG
GI	Ulceration, obstruction Hepatic dysfunction		Jaundice Hepatomegaly	Bilirubin SGOT, SGPT PT
CNS	Diabetes insipidus, neuropathy, exophthalmos	Polyuria, polydipsia	Neuro exam	Urine and serum osm, electrolytes
HEME	Thrombocytopenia, anemia, leukopenia	Bruising or bleeding	Splenomegaly	CBC

Key Reference: Egeler RM, Nesbit ME: Langerhans cell histiocytosis and other disorders of monocyte-histiocyte. Crit Rev Oncol Hematol 1995; 18:9–35.

PERIOPERATIVE IMPLICATIONS

Preoperative Preparation

- Indicated by degree of organ dysfunction

Monitoring

- Routine

Airway

- Airway soft tissue or mandibular involvement may distort anatomy

Preinduction/Induction

- Usual precautions depending on severity of organ involvement

Maintenance

- Usual precautions depending on severity of organ involvement

Extubation

- If anatomy distorted and airway difficult, consider awake extubation

Adjuvants

- Vary depending on hepatic function

ANTICIPATED PROBLEMS/CONCERNS

- Organ dysfunction (hepatic, pulmonary, hematologic, hypothalamic, or bone)
- Diabetes insipidus
- Adrenal suppression due to chronic steroid therapy

HYDROCEPHALUS

Joseph R. Tobin, M.D.

RISK

- Newborns and children with anatomic CNS abnormalities (including myelomeningocele)
- Head trauma and intracranial hemorrhage patients
- CNS tumors
- Meningitis

PERIOPERATIVE RISKS

- Cerebral ischemia and neurologic sequelae
- Impaired airway reflexes, level of consciousness, gastric emptying
- Cardiorespiratory arrest

WORRY ABOUT

- Intracranial HTN
- Persistent nausea and vomiting
- Bradycardia
- Decreased level of consciousness

OVERVIEW

- Excess accumulation of CSF due to obstruction in normal CSF flow pattern from ventricular system to cortical surface (obstructive hydrocephalus); or from impaired reabsorption of CSF at arachnoid villi (communicating hydrocephalus)
- Slow progressive hydrocephalus well tolerated for weeks with slowly worsening symptoms (headache, nausea, papilledema)
- Acute hydrocephalus results in acute symptoms and may be life-threatening owing to herniation of brain with catastrophic ischemic injury; bradycardia, HTN, depressed level of consciousness, depressed airway reflexes and respiratory drive, and gastric atony.

ICD-9-CM Codes: 331.4 (Obstructive); 331.3 (Communicating)

ETIOLOGY

Congenital

- Anatomic abnormalities: aqueductal stenosis, Arnold-Chiari malformation, Dandy-Walker syndrome.

Posthemorrhagic/Post-traumatic

- Intraventricular hemorrhage (newborns or adults) with blood clot in ventricular system

Neoplastic

- Brain tumor obstructing normal CSF flow

Postinflammatory

- Meningitis, abscess, meningoencephalitis

USUAL TREATMENT

- Surgical correction of underlying cause or CSF diversion procedures (ventriculoperitoneal, ventriculoatrial, or lumboperitoneal shunts)
- Glucocorticoids are used acutely to diminish edema associated with neoplasm or abscess and may diminish associated intracranial HTN
- Acetazolamide to diminish CSF production

ASSESSMENT POINTS

SYSTEM	EFFECT	ASSESSMENT BY HX	PE	TEST
CV	Bradycardia, HTN		Pulse, BP	
RESP	Impaired respiratory drive and airway reflexes		Cranial nerve exam, stridor Swallowing abnormalities	Pulse oximetry
GI	Nausea, vomiting, aspiration Abnormal feeding	Hx of progression of nausea/vomiting		
CNS	Depressed level of consciousness Increased ICP	Timing of onset	Arousability and neurologic exam Tense fontanelle, inferior eye deviation	CT scan

Key Reference: Cheek WR (ed): Pediatric Neurosurgery: Surgery of the Developing Nervous System. Philadelphia: WB Saunders, 1994.

PERIOPERATIVE IMPLICATIONS

Preoperative Preparation

- Assessment of urgency of presentation. Catastrophic increased ICP requires emergent intubation and hyperventilation. In young infants, direct neurosurgical needle puncture of a proximal lateral ventricle or previously inserted shunt may diminish ICP sufficiently to avoid a catastrophe.
- Secure IV access if possible

Monitoring

- Level of consciousness
- Routine

Airway

- Head up 10–20° and midline may diminish ICP.
- Aspiration risk due to gastric atony

Preinduction/Induction

- Sedatives usually not indicated so that resp compromise or sedation does not increase ICP. Minimal sedation or use of Emla cream to secure IV access without causing increased ICP due to crying and struggling
- Rapid-sequence IV induction preferred (because of aspiration risk) unless in doubt of airway anatomy
- Debate over use of succinylcholine vs. rapid-onset nondepolarizing muscle relaxant (rocuronium); thiopental, propofol or etomidate IV agents preferred; avoid ketamine
- Mask induction may increase ICP by increasing cerebral blood volume
- Isoflurane associated with coughing and not recommended for induction
- Lidocaine 1–1.5 mg/kg IV may be useful adjunct to minimize increase in ICP due to laryngoscopy and endotracheal intubation.

Maintenance

- Volatile anesthetic (most commonly isoflurane) <1 MAC, N_2O 0–70% and opioid (i.e., fentanyl 2–5 µg/kg or equivalent)
- Maintain normothermia, cardiac output. Hyperventilation may be acutely helpful until shunt is placed.
- Isotonic crystalloid at restricted or maintenance rate. Glucose support for infants.

Extubation

- Ensure return of airway reflexes, level of consciousness, and respiratory drive.
- Failure of achieving above criteria may require CT scan and/or ICU monitoring

Postoperative Period

- Usually unremarkable; depressed level of consciousness is concern for perioperative ischemic insult or hemorrhage
- EBL: minimal

Adjuvants

- Lidocaine, mannitol, furosemide, spontaneous hyperventilation by patient

ANTICIPATED PROBLEMS/CONCERNS

- Immediate postop neurologic exam should demonstrate improvement. If not improved, urgent CT scan and secure airway must be maintained. Postop ICU admission not required unless impaired neurologic status continues.

HYPERALDOSTERONISM (SECONDARY)

R. Lee Wagner, M.D.

RISK

- Risk: 0.5 to 2.0% of patients with renal tubular dysfunction and cirrhosis, congestive heart failure, severe vomiting, and severe intravascular volume depletion (primary hyperaldosteronism [Conn's syndrome] occurs in 0.5 to 1% of patients with hypertension of unknown etiology)
- Mild hypokalemia, metabolic alkalosis make Dx more likely

PERIOPERATIVE RISKS

- Electrolyte disorders: K^+, Mg^{2+}, Na^+, HCO_3^-
- Fluid retention
- HTN
- ↑ Risk of ischemic cardiomyopathy

WORRY ABOUT

- Preop management of fluids, lytes, worsening CHF
- HTN

OVERVIEW

- Physiologic action of aldosterone is on collecting tubules of nephron: Na^+ reabsorption, K^+, H^+ secretion. Maintains BP by controlling intravascular volume. Hyperaldosteronism is pathologic accentuation of these actions: HTN, hypokalemia, metabolic alkalosis.
- Hyperaldosteronism in response to high renin activity is secondary hyperaldosteronism.
- May be unrecognized when patient presents to OR for unrelated operation

ICD-9-CM Code: 255.1

ETIOLOGY

- Secondary hyperaldosteronism involves dysfunctional kidney or decreased effective intravascular volume in kidney: cirrhosis, CHF, GI lyte loss, chronic renal disease

USUAL TREATMENT

- All etiologies: consider spironolactone
- Treat underlying disease

ASSESSMENT POINTS

SYSTEM	EFFECT	ASSESSMENT BY HX	PE	TEST
CV	HTN, fluid overload, possible overdiuresis	Presyncope	S_3, diastolic HTN, edema, jugulovenous distention	ECG, CXR CVP or PA measurements
RESP	CHF	Dyspnea, orthopnea	Rales, wheezing, tachypnea	CXR
GI	Hepatic cirrhosis causing intravascular volume depletion and ascites Laxative abuse, diuretic abuse, bulimia causing lyte disorders	Known cirrhosis? Psychological issues suggesting self-induced disorders	Ascites Spider angiomas Muscle wasting, edema Postural hypotension	Na^+, K^+, HCO_3^-, Mg^{2+}
RENAL	Intrinsic renal dysfunction	Known renal disease?	Edema	Na^+, K^+, HCO_3^-, in all pts. Probably ABG for acid-base status. Consider ionized Ca^{2+}, PO_4^-, Mg^{2+}, BUN/Cr, urine lytes in selected pt (renal or hepatic disease)

Key Reference: Gill JR Jr.: Hyperaldosteronism. *In* Becker KL (ed): Principles and Practice of Endocrinology and Metabolism, 2nd ed. Philadelphia, JB Lippincott, 1995, pp 716–729.

PERIOPERATIVE IMPLICATIONS

Preoperative Preparation

- Assess and normalize K^+, Mg^{2+}, Na^+, HCO_3^-
- Normalize intravascular volume. For diuresis, consider spironolactone, amiloride, triamterene to spare K^+.
- Control BP. Consider ACE inhibitors, Ca^{2+} channel blockers, K^+-sparing diuretics
- Diagnose etiology of hyperaldosteronism if unknown—appropriate endocrine work-up

Monitoring

- Consider CVP or PA line if volume status in question
- Consider arterial line if BP labile

Airway

- Routine, unless obesity present

Preinduction/Induction

- Consider problems presented by underlying disease (see under Congestive Heart Failure; Renal Failure, Chronic)

Maintenance

- Hypokalemia may accentuate neuromuscular blockade
- Hyperventilation may exacerbate hypokalemia
- If hyperaldosteronism caused by renal disease, consider avoiding enflurane, sevoflurane
- Consider monitoring intraoperative glucose, acid-base status

Extubation

- Hypokalemia may prolong and potentiate response to muscle relaxants

Postoperative Period

- Continue close attention to lytes, volume status

Adjuvants

- Hypokalemia may prolong and potentiate response to muscle relaxants
- Volume depletion (effective) may alter distribution and clearance of many drugs (e.g., lidocaine with ↑ volume of distribution and ↓ clearance)

ANTICIPATED PROBLEMS/CONCERNS

- Hypoperfusion from underlying disease(s) may be worsened by effects of anesthesia and surgery

HYPERCALCEMIA

Michelle Braunfeld, M.D.

RISK

- Most often due to hyperparathyroidism in ambulatory outpatient—risk increased age >50
- Most often due to malignancy in patient
- Female > male (2.5/1)
- 0.15%/y (1.5/1000 persons/y)

PERIOPERATIVE RISKS

- Hypovolemia and acid/base abnormalities
- Renal insufficiency
- Other electrolyte abnormalities, esp. phosphorus
- Full stomach and (in)ability to protect airway with altered mental status

WORRY ABOUT

- Volume status
- PUD associated with primary hyperparathyroidism

- Other manifestations of underlying disease, e.g., cardiopulmonary status in sarcoid, lytic bone lesions (esp. in spine) in patient with malignancy with pathologic fractures
- Fluid overload and sodium retention

OVERVIEW

- Multifactorial medical problem that requires both supportive therapy and attention to underlying problem
- One in spectrum of problems associated with underlying disease or may be due to treatment of that disease (e.g., milk-alkali syndrome in PUD).
- Therapy includes volume replacement and possible further fluid/Lasix administration to induce Ca^{2+} excretion in exchange for Na^+

ICD-9-CM Code: 275.4

ETIOLOGY

- Increased GI absorption, e.g., milk-alkali syndrome, sarcoid
- Increased bone resorption, e.g., hyperparathyroidism, malignancy (8% renal cell carcinoma; 20% of squamous carcinomas including lung, female genital tract, head and neck; 8% of breast, lymphoma), Paget's
- ↑ Renal reabsorption

USUAL TREATMENT

- <14 mg/dl in asymptomatic patient—no acute therapy more than hydration and diuresis aimed at lowering Ca^{2+} needed. Maintain good hydration and UO.
- >14 mg/dl or symptomatic patient <14 mg/dl—forced diuresis with saline (2–3 ml/kg/h) and Lasix (1–2 mg/kg/h). More potent agents (steroids, mithramycin, calcitonin, and bisphosphonates) needed if Ca^{2+} levels not reduced
- Seek and treat underlying cause

ASSESSMENT POINTS

SYSTEM	EFFECT	ASSESSMENT BY HX	PE	TEST
HEENT	Band keratopathy			
CV	Hypovolemia	Postural symptoms	Orthostatic VS changes Narrowed pulse pressure Tachycardia	
	Conduction abnormalities, esp. short QT_c^* interval			ECG Shortens QT_c^* interval—can follow in any one individual
GI		Nausea/vomiting		
ENDO	Excess PTH or production of PTH-related hormone			Radioimmunoassay of PTH or PTH-related peptides
CNS	Altered mental status	Confusion, obtundation, even coma		
MS		Bone pain		
RENAL	Calculi Renal insufficiency			Abd x-ray, IVP BUN/Cr

*$QT_c = QT/\sqrt{RR}$; RR = RR interval.

Key Reference: Federman DD: Scientific American Medicine 1992, Endocrinology Section VI, pp 1–15.

PERIOPERATIVE IMPLICATIONS

Preoperative Preparation

- Assess volume, renal function
- Assess need to reduce serum calcium if level >14 mg/L
- Consider H_2-receptor antagonist metoclopramide

Monitoring

- UO—important to keep well hydrated
- Consider central venous catheter or other monitor of fluid status (such as TEE) if aggressive fluid therapy required and cardiovascularly compromised

Airway

- Full stomach precautions
- Rule out lytic C-spine lesions

Induction

- Hypovolemia can lead to hemodynamic instability if usual dose of drugs given

Maintenance

- Hemodynamic instability if hypovolemic or myocardial contractility abnormalities
- Aggressive hydration—tailor IV fluids to lyte and acid/base status (avoid hypernatremia and acidosis from excessive N/S).
- Continue lyte replenishment if necessary (esp. K^+, Mg^{2+})

Extubation

- Related to preop condition and underlying disease

Adjuvants

- May alter NMB duration and ability of antagonists to reverse block
- Associated acid/base and lyte derangements or renal insufficiency may affect duration of NMBs and ability to reverse block

ANTICIPATED PROBLEMS/CONCERNS

- Fluid and lyte overload from too aggressive hydration
- Bone fractures (pathologic)
- Lethargy, stupor, coma from high levels of Ca^{2+}

HYPERCHOLESTEROLISM

Uday Jain, Ph.D., M.D.

RISK

- People in USA: About 50 million
- Low-density lipoprotein (LDL) similar in African-Americans and Caucasians; high-density lipoprotein (HDL) higher in African-Americans. Death rate higher in African-Americans
- Familial hypercholesterolemia (LDL >260 mg/dl)—0.2% population
- Severe polygenic hypercholesterolemia (LDL >220 mg/dl)—1% population
- Familial combined (multiple lipoprotein type) hyperlipidemia: elevated LDL and/or VLDL—1% population

PERIOPERATIVE RISKS

- Risk of myocardial ischemia and infarction
- Worsened CHF

WORRY ABOUT

- New-onset angina or increasing frequency or severity of angina
- Worsening or new-onset CHF
- TIAs of the CNS
- Peripheral atherosclerosis

OVERVIEW

- Normal total cholesterol <200 mg/dl, 200–239 mg/dl borderline high ≥240 mg/dl high
- HDL <35 mg/dl low; ≥60 mg/dl high
- CAD: Keep LDL (total LDL – triglyceride/5) ≤100 mg/dl
- Lp(a) resembles LDL, is risk factor for CAD
- Secondary to diabetes, nephrotic syndrome, chronic renal failure, and hypothyroidism

ICD-9-CM Code: 272.0,2
See also Coronary Artery Disease, Atherosclerosis, Lipidemias, Hypertriglyceridemia

ETIOLOGY

- Can be inherited or due to systemic illness

USUAL TREATMENT

- Diet and exercise
- Cholestyramine and colestipol inhibit bile acid absorption
- Neomycin inhibits cholesterol absorption
- HMG CoA reductase inhibitors (lovastatin, pravastatin, simvastatin) reduce cholesterol synthesis and are commonly used
- Thyroid hormone clears LDL
- Probucol reduces LDL but also HDL
- Nicotinic acid inhibits VLDL, LDL production
- Fibric acids clofibrate and gemfibrozil cause catabolism of triglyceride-rich lipoproteins
- Partial ileal bypass surgery

ASSESSMENT POINTS

SYSTEM	EFFECT	ASSESSMENT BY HX	PE	TEST
CV	Myocardial ischemia and infarction	Angina or its equivalents	Displaced PMI	ECG, CXR, stress testing,
	LV dysfunction	Dyspnea, edema, exercise intolerance	S_3	ECHO, coronary Angio
RESP	CHF	Dyspnea, orthopnea, cough	Rales and rhonchi	CXR
SKIN	Lipid deposits		Xanthelasma, xanthoma, arcus juvenilis	
RENAL	Impaired renal perfusion	Nighttime urinary frequency		Cr
CNS	Cerebrovascular atherosclerosis	TIAs	Carotid bruit	Carotid US and Angio

Key Reference: Stein JH: Internal Medicine. Boston, Little, Brown, 1987, pp 2035–2057.

PERIOPERATIVE IMPLICATIONS

Preoperative Preparation

- Assess for CAD and peripheral vascular disease
- β rb and nitrates perioperatively, as tolerated

Monitoring

- Consider PA catheter, TEE, in presence of large fluid shifts, ischemic Hx

Airway

- May be overweight and difficult to intubate

Induction

- Hypovolemia may lead to hypotension

Maintenance

- Maintain hemodynamic stability without hypothermia or anemia (ideal HCT may be 30%)
- No anesthetic agent or technique proven superior
- Monitor for ischemia and failure

Extubation

- For noncardiac surgery, this is the period of greatest risk for ischemia

Postoperative Period

- High incidence of tachycardia, ischemia, and MI for several days after noncardiac surgery
- Treat pain, hemodynamic and biochemical abnormalities aggressively

Adjuvants

- Depends on end-organ disease

ANTICIPATED PROBLEMS/CONCERNS

- Problems are related to atherosclerosis

HYPERGLYCEMIA

William L. Lanier, M.D.

RISK

- People within US: can occur in virtually any anesthetized or critically ill patient
- Race with the highest prevalence: Equal

PERIOPERATIVE RISKS

- Increased likelihood of neurologic injury following brain ischemia, and perhaps traumatic brain injury and spinal cord injury
- Dehydration resulting from osmotic diuresis

WORRY ABOUT

- Electrolyte abnormalities, particularly hypokalemia, while treating hyperglycemia
- Hypoglycemia following insulin, resulting in insult to the CV system and CNS
- Polyuria complicates assessment of fluid balance

OVERVIEW

- Is not a disease
- Typically produces adverse effects by two mechanisms: increases in plasma osmolality and increases in postischemic tissue lactic acidosis
- Dx made by measuring blood glucose concentrations
- In acute setting, blood glucose concentrations can be estimated using indicator impregnated strips; confirmation can be made by mechanized techniques

ICD-9-CM Code: 790.6
See also under Diabetes, Diabetic Ketoacidosis, Hyperosmolar Nonketotic Coma, Cushing's Syndrome, Acromegaly, Pheochromocytoma, Morbid Obesity, Steroids

ETIOLOGY

- Results from DM (both insulin-requiring and non–insulin-requiring), other endocrinopathies (Cushing's syndrome, acromegaly, obesity, pheochromocytoma), physiologic stress, drug administration (particularly corticosteroids), and glucose-containing fluid infusions

USUAL TREATMENT

- Insulin
- Isotonic intravenous crystalloid solutions to treat hypovolemia and dilute existing blood glucose
- If possible, treat underlying cause (e.g., discontinue infusion of glucose-containing solutions, discontinue corticosteroids, reduce physiologic stress to patient)

ASSESSMENT POINTS

SYSTEM	EFFECT	ASSESSMENT BY HX	PE	TEST
HEENT	Dehydration in extreme cases		Dry mucosa in extreme cases	
CV	Mild inotropic effect with mild hyperglycemia Dehydration		Tachycardia, orthostatic hypotension	
GI		Polydipsia in extreme cases		
RENAL	Osmotically induced diuresis	Polyuria, urinary frequency		Elevated urine glucose
ENDO		See under Etiology		Elevated blood glucose
HEME	Diminished WBC activity; changes in serum sodium concentrations			Serum sodium concentration decreases 1.6 mEq/L for each 100 mg/dl increase in glucose concentration
CNS			Altered consciousness; neurologic deficits	Plasma osmolality

Key Reference: Ewald GA, McKenzie CR: Manual of Medical Therapeutics. Boston, Little, Brown, 1995, pp 46, 437–463.

PERIOPERATIVE IMPLICATIONS

Preoperative Preparation

- Glucose reduction with insulin
- Hydration
- Normalization of lytes

Monitoring

- Blood glucose concentrations in all cases
- In severe cases, blood lytes, blood osmolality, urine output

Airway

- Abnormalities typically related to DM (↓ range of motion and abn atlanto-occipital contractions), acromegaly (distorted anatomy), or chronic corticosteroid use or Cushing's syndrome (cushingoid Sx, friable tissues)

Maintenance

- Maintain hydration
- Insulin therapy
- K+ replacement

Extubation

- No special considerations, other than those related to underlying disease

Adjuvants

- Limit attempted reduction of blood glucose concentration to ~75 mg/dl/h to avoid problems with osmotic injury to brain and lyte disturbances
- Monitor ECG during correction of profound hyperglycemia

Postoperative Period

- Variations in physiologic stress, fluid administration, and drug usage make postop blood glucose concentrations difficult to predict and control

ANTICIPATED PROBLEMS/CONCERNS

- Increases in blood glucose concentrations by a mere 40 mg/dl may worsen outcome following cerebral ischemic insult. In contrast, hypoglycemia resulting from excessive use of insulin may result in irreversible neurologic injury, independent of ischemic event.

HYPERKALEMIA

Irving Hirsch, M.D.

RISK

• Any patient with plasma K$^+$ concentration > 5.5 mEq/L

PERIOPERATIVE RISKS

• Cardiac conduction system abnormalities
• VFib
• Cardiac standstill in diastole

WORRY ABOUT

• Adverse effects are likely to accompany acute increases in K$^+$
• Depolarizing muscle relaxants, esp if given to patients with burns, spinal cord transection, or muscle trauma
• Digitalis toxicity
• Acidosis

OVERVIEW

• Condition that can be due to ↑ total body K$^+$ content or alterations in distribution between intracellular and extracellular sites

ICD-9-CM Code: 276.7

ETIOLOGY

• Diminished renal excretion
  – Acute oliguric renal failure
  – Chronic renal failure
  – Addison's disease
  – Hyporeninemic hypoaldosteronism
  – Potassium-sparing diuretics
  – Ingestion of potassium-rich foods by patient with renal insufficiency
• Transcellular shifts
  – Acidosis
  – Cell destruction—trauma, burns, rhabdomyolysis, hemolysis, tumor lysis
  – Hyperkalemic periodic paralysis
  – Diabetic hyperglycemia
  – Depolarizing muscle relaxant causing K$^+$ release esp in patients with burns, spinal cord transection, muscle trauma, or denervating muscle
• Factitious hyperkalemia
  – Tourniquet method of drawing blood
  – Hemolysis of drawn blood due to delay in chemical determination

USUAL TREATMENT

• Promote transfer of K$^+$ from ECF to ICF
  – Glucose and insulin—25 gm glucose with 10–15 U regular insulin/70 kg
  – Sodium bicarbonate—40–150 mEq/70 kg
  – Hyperventilation: With each pH change of 0.1, there is an inverse change in K$^+$ of 0.6 mEq/L
• Enhance K$^+$ elimination: diuretics, exchange resins (Kayexalate), dialysis
• Calcium gluconate: 10–30 ml of a 10% solution over 10–20 min/70 kg counteracts cardiac effects

ASSESSMENT POINTS

SYSTEM	EFFECT	ASSESSMENT BY HX	PE	TEST
CV	Tall peak T waves ↓ Amplitude R wave Widened QRS complex Decreased and eventual disappearance of P wave QRS blends into T wave—"sine wave of hyperkalemia"			ECG
	Ventricular arrhythmia	Possible hemodynamic instability		ECG
	Cardiac arrest	CV collapse		ECG
NM	Weakness Paralysis			
HORMONAL	↑ Aldosterone Insulin release ↑ Glucagon Epinephrine release	↑ BP, HR		K$^+$, renin, aldosterone, glucose

Key Reference: Kokko JP: Disorders of fluid volume, electrolyte, and acid-base balance. *In* Bennett JC, Plum F (eds): Cecil Textbook of Medicine, 20th ed. Philadelphia, WB Saunders, 1996, pp 525–551.

PERIOPERATIVE IMPLICATIONS

Preoperative Preparation

• Normal K$^+$ levels before elective surgery
• Avoid sedatives (↓ ventilation) prior to K$^+$ normalization

Monitoring

• ECG
• Plasma K$^+$ levels
• ABG concentration
• Peripheral nerve stimulator

Maintenance

• Adequate ventilation to avoid respiratory acidosis
• Avoid metabolic acidosis—arterial hypoxemia or excessive depths of anesthesia
• IV fluids—avoid lactated Ringer's or others containing K$^+$

Adjuvants

• Muscle relaxants—avoid depolarizing agents. Increase K$^+$ 0.3–0.5 mEq/L with succinylcholine
• Dose of nondepolarizing relaxants required is unclear—may need diminished dose

ANTICIPATED PROBLEMS/CONCERNS

• Acute increases in K$^+$ leading to acute ECG changes or adverse cardiac effects. Rx: see Usual Treatment
• Avoid use of depolarizing muscle relaxants in patients with burns, neuropathies, para- or quadriplegia, or muscle trauma

HYPERMAGNESEMIA

David R. Gambling, F.R.C.P.C.

RISK

- Patients with renal insufficiency, especially those receiving Mg^{2+}-containing cathartics or antacids
- Parturients on $MgSO_4$ therapy

PERIOPERATIVE RISKS

- Potentiates nondepolarizing neuromuscular blocking agents
- May increase risk of modest hypotension during administration of regional anesthesia
- Potentiates hypotension associated with use of volatile anesthetics, calcium channel blockers, and butyrophenones
- Can exacerbate local anesthetic toxicity

WORRY ABOUT

- Intraoperative hypotension
- Muscle weakness (esp. respiratory)
- Excessive sedation
- Myocardial depression and cardiorespiratory arrest with very high levels

OVERVIEW

- Defined as an elevated Mg^{2+} concentration in plasma, in excess of 1.1 mmol/L
- Magnesium elimination is dependent on glomerular filtration rate; with GFR <30 ml/min patients are at significant risk
- Sx vary with plasma concentration and become more serious as the plasma concentration increases >4 mmol/L
- CV, resp, MS systems are predominately affected.

ICD-9-CM Code: 275.2

ETIOLOGY

- Patients with chronic renal failure who are receiving Mg^{2+}-containing antacids or laxatives
- Often iatrogenic, e.g., excessive administration of $MgSO_4$ infusion to parturient with preterm labor or pregnancy-induced HTN
- Rarely Addison's disease, myxedema, or lithium therapy

USUAL TREATMENT

- Discontinue Mg^{2+} therapy and delay nonessential surgery
- Fluid load and diuretic therapy
- Adults — IV calcium gluconate 1g (temporary but effective). Neonates — IV calcium gluconate 100–200 mg/kg over 5 min and continuous infusion 100–300 mg/kg/d
- Peritoneal dialysis or hemodialysis for persistent or life-threatening hypermagnesemia
- Assist ventilation/protect airway if necessary

ASSESSMENT POINTS

The side effects of hypermagnesemia are more serious as the serum level of magnesium increases.

	SIGNS AND SYMPTOMS	SERUM Mg^{2+} CONCENTRATION
	Normal	0.7–1.1 mmol/L (normal range)
CV	Warmth, flushing, headache, nausea, dizziness	2–3 mmol/L (range during parenteral treatment)
	Decreased AV and intraventricular conduction	>2.5 mmol/L
	ECG—prolonged PQ and widening of QRS	
	Possible hypotension	
	Cardiac arrest in diastole	>12.5 mmol/L
CNS	Sedation	2–3 mmol/L
MS	Absent deep tendon reflexes	4–5 mmol/L
	Progressive muscle weakness and resp arrest	6–7.5 mmol/L

Patients with chronic renal failure frequently have Mg^{2+} levels up to 3 mmol/L but are seldom symptomatic.
Acidemia will decrease serum level at which side effects occur, e.g., in presence of acidemia cardiac arrest can occur at a serum level of 8–10 mmol/L.
Key Reference: Gambling DR, et al: Magnesium and the anesthetist. Can J Anaesth 1988; 35:644–654.

PERIOPERATIVE IMPLICATIONS

Preoperative Preparation

- Discontinue $MgSO_4$ unless being used to treat seizures or ventricular dysrhythmias
- Check serum level
- ECG, Cr, lytes

Monitoring

- Routine

Airway

- Use full dose of succinylcholine for intubation
- Reduce dose of nondepolarizing neuromuscular blocking drugs (NMBs) by 1/3–1/2

Preinduction/Induction

- Avoid sedative premedications
- Ensure full denitrogenation of lungs

- Avoid pre-curarization or priming dose of NMB

Maintenance

- May decrease requirement for anesthetics owing to decreased neurotransmitter release.

Extubation

- Ensure full return of train-of-four, ability to sustain head lift and vital capacity >10 ml/kg
- Ensure patient responsiveness

Adjuvants

- Hypemagnesemia may exacerbate hypotension associated with hypovolemia, calcium channel blockers, volatile inhalation anesthetics, butyrophenones, lumbar epidural or subarachnoid anesthesia
- Treat with IV calcium gluconate 1g and fluid load and diuretics

Postoperative Period

- Beware of excessive sedation, weakness, hypoventilation, cardiac arrest
- May cause or aggravate neonatal hypotonia and hypotension

ANTICIPATED PROBLEMS/CONCERNS

- Hypermagnesemia potentiates action of nondepolarizing NMBs by inhibiting release of acetylcholine from motor nerve terminal, decreasing sensitivity of postjunctional membrane, and reducing excitability of muscle fibers.
- Many common anesthestic drugs exacerbate weakness and sedation associated with hypermagnesemia.
- Potentiates local anesthetic toxicity
- Excessively high plasma Mg^{2+} concentrations can cause cardiorespiratory arrest.

HYPERNATREMIA

John K. Hayes, Ph.D.
K.C. Wong, M.D., Ph.D.

RISK

- People with chronic liver disease treated with certain drugs (lactulose, mannitol, fructose)
- Children with diarrhea
- Elderly and pediatric populations with decreased H_2O acquiring skills

PERIOPERATIVE RISKS

- Increased risk of CV hemorrhage
- Coma
- High incidence of mortality and morbidity

WORRY ABOUT

- Development of hypertonic encephalopathy
- High mortality rate associated with hypernatremia; of those recovering >40% may develop neurologic sequelae

OVERVIEW

- Serum sodium and intra- to extracellular ratio is important for maintaining cellular integrity and electronic activity of excitable cells. High serum sodium occurs most commonly in very young or very old patients with inadequate water-acquiring skills
- Can result from diseased osmoregulatory centers, CNS histiocytosis, pineal tumors, head trauma, craniopharyngioma, cranial surgery, and hypophysectomy

ICD-9-CM Code: 276.0

ETIOLOGY

- Elevated serum [Na+] with large UO of free water in excess of salt may potentiate cellular dehydration and shrinkage
- Impaired thirst — medicated H_2O acquisition
- Excessive water loss

— Renal: nephrogenic diabetes insipidus (DI) (tubular damage)
— Pituitary: Pituitary diabetes insipidus (PDI)
— Extrarenal: sweating, solute diuresis from glucose (diabetic ketoacidosis, nonketotic hyperosmolar coma) or mannitol or glycerol administration, kidney dialysis
- Brain tumors, head trauma, cranial surgery can cause DI states
- Children—diarrhea
- Elderly—reduced water intake, ingestion of sodium bicarbonate

USUAL TREATMENT

- Adequate water intake/administration
- Fluid volume supplement:
  — [Na+] < 160 mEq/L: for moderate acidosis give hypotonic saline slowly over 48 h
  — Circulatory collapse: give rapid plasma or blood substitutes to correct shock; then give normal saline (N/S)
- Acute hypernatremia without circulatory collapse: give 5% glucose at slow infusion rates
- Drug therapy (PDI)
  — Desmopressin (nasal spray, 5–10 μg)
  — Chlorpropamide (oral, 250–750 mg/d)

ASSESSMENT POINTS

SYSTEM	EFFECT	ASSESSMENT BY HX	PE	TEST
HEENT	Dry mouth Swollen tongue		Exam of mouth	
CV	Tachycardia Hypotension Possible circulatory collapse	BP on arising	HR BP	ECG
METABOL	Fever			Temp
CNS	Restlessness Weakness Maniacal behavior Delirium		CNS exam	
SKIN	Flushed		Skin exam	
RENAL	Polyuria Hyposthenuria	Urinary frequency and color		Na+, K+, and Osm both urine and serum

Key Reference: Reeves WB, Andreoli TE: The posterior pituitary and water metabolism. *In* Wilson JD, Foster DW (eds): Textbook of Endocrinology, 8th ed. Philadelphia, WB Saunders, 1992, pp 332–356.

PERIOPERATIVE IMPLICATIONS

Monitoring

- Blood lytes (esp. Na+ and K+), UO, temp

Airway

- None unless patient is unconscious

Maintenance

- Give adequate fluids (see under Usual Treatment)
- Sustain blood lytes and temp in physiologic ranges

Extubation

- Dependent on neurologic function

ANTICIPATED PROBLEMS/CONCERNS

- Development of neurologic dysfunction/coma
- Enhanced mortality and morbidity with higher incidence in children

HYPEROSMOLAR NONKETOTIC COMA

John R. Ammon, M.D.

(see also under DIABETES, TYPE II)

RISK

- Middle-aged or elderly type II diabetic who is ketoacidosis-resistant
- Occurrence of perioperative catabolic stress state in type II diabetic
- Elderly diabetic with stroke or gram-negative infection, esp. pneumonia

PERIOPERATIVE RISKS

- CV collapse due to extreme osmotic diuresis from elevated glucose
- End-organ injury from deranged volume status and hemodynamic instability (renal, myocardial, in situ thrombosis) and hyperosmolarity (CNS)

WORRY ABOUT

- Underlying cause of hyperosmolar crisis, e.g., infection, CVA, loss of metabolic control perioperatively
- Hypovolemia
- CNS hyperosmolar dysfunction and/or injury

OVERVIEW

- A grave metabolic emergency with mortality > 50%
- Characterized by extreme hyperglycemia, serum osmolality > 350 mOsm/L, profound fluid depletion
- Prevented perioperatively by appropriate metabolic monitoring and support

ICD-9-CM Code: 250.2

ETIOLOGY

- Type II diabetic in severe catabolic state resulting from infection, CVA, or uncontrolled perioperative metabolic stress
- Inadequate insulin present to prevent extreme hyperglycemia but enough to prevent or suppress diabetic ketoacidosis (DKA)

USUAL TREATMENT

- Urgent volume resuscitation for an average fluid deficit of 10 L; must reestablish circulation and urine flow (oliguria or anuria in late stage)
- 0.9% saline, then 0.45% saline; add 5% dextrose as blood sugar approaches normal
- Insulin usually required, although patients more sensitive than those in DKA
- Sodium bicarbonate only if significant lactic acidosis present from poor tissue perfusion

ASSESSMENT POINTS

SYSTEM	EFFECT	ASSESSMENT BY HX	PE	TEST
CV	Severe volume contraction, shock, and acidosis in extreme cases		Vital signs	ABG CVP ECG
RESP	Inadequate ventilation with brainstem hypoperfusion		Ventilatory rate and depth	ABG
ENDO	Inadequate insulin during severe catabolic stress	Type II diabetes Recent CVA, infection, or surgical procedure		Blood glucose
RENAL	Profound diuresis →oliguria, →anuria			UO BUN/Cr
CNS	Clouded sensorium to coma; seizure; delayed anesthesia emergence	Altered CNS status over hours to days	Loss of consciousness	Serum osmol, CSF culture

Key Reference: Foster DW: Diabetes mellitus. *In* Harrison's Principles of Internal Medicine, 12th ed. New York, McGraw Hill, 1991, pp 1752–1753.

PERIOPERATIVE IMPLICATIONS

Monitoring

- Sequential glucose determinations during surgical period in type II diabetic, esp. when catabolic stress severe, e.g., CABG, trauma, major vascular surgery

Airway

- Airway protection lost by depressed CNS function

Induction

- If surgical procedure necessary (unlikely), volume resuscitation key step before induction; usual concerns for diabetic end-organ dysfunction (see under Diabetes, Type II)

Maintenance

- Ongoing treatment of metabolism (blood glucose, insulin) and volume status; end-organ support

Extubation

- Intact CNS function crucial for airway and ventilatory adequacy

Postoperative Period

- Risk of hyperosmolar coma continues after surgery with ongoing catabolism and potential for inadequate insulin, extreme hyperglycemia

ANTICIPATED PROBLEMS/CONCERNS

- High mortality and severe morbidity (CNS and myocardial ischemia, shock, ATN, widespread thrombosis)

HYPERPARATHYROIDISM

Michael L. Nahrwold, M.D.
Srinivas Mantha, M.D.

RISK

- People within USA: 50,000 patients/y
- Race with highest prevalence: none
- Male/female: 1:2
- Prevalence: 50–100/100,000 (increases with age)

PERIOPERATIVE RISKS

- Hypovolemia and lyte abn
- ↑ Risk of cardiac dysrhythmias 2° to hypercalcemia
- Aspiration from full stomach

WORRY ABOUT

- Signs of hypercalcemia and other lyte irregularities
- Intravascular volume changes
- Fluid overload and Na⁺ retention in CV fragile patients
- Renal, cardiac, and CNS abnormalities

OVERVIEW

- Endocrinopathy associated with elevation in parathyroid hormone (PTH) levels
- Primary problem is hypercalcemia
- Dx supported by ↑ PTH level associated with hypercalcemia
- Most patients with primary hyperparathyroidism are hypercalcemic but asymptomatic
- Hypercalcemia in pregnant patient may lead to neonatal hypocalcemia and tetany

ICD-9-CM Code: 252.0
See also Parathyroid Adenoma Resection under Procedures, Hypercalcemia under Diseases

ETIOLOGY

- Primary hyperparathyroidism usually due to benign parathyroid adenoma (80–90%), hyperplasia (15%), or parathyroid carcinoma (uncommon)
- May be manifestation of MEN II, which includes pheochromocytoma, hyperparathyroidism, and medullary thyroid carcinoma

USUAL TREATMENT

- Surgically with parathyroidectomy
- Medically with saline hydration and furosemide
- Mithramycin (for more resistant Ca^{2+} elevators), calcitonin, and steroids (for hypercalcemia associated with hyperphosphatemia)
- IV phosphates, indomethacin

ASSESSMENT POINTS

SYSTEM	EFFECT	ASSESSMENT BY HX	PE	TEST
CV	HTN, dysrhythmias	Palpitation, headache	Abn pulse rate and/or rhythm, ↑ BP	ECG*, lytes, total and ionized Ca^{2+}
RESP	↓ Bronchial clearance of secretions	Cough	Adventitious sounds	
GI	Peptic ulcers, pancreatitis	Constipation, anorexia, nausea and vomiting, epigastric pain		
RENAL	Nephrocalcinosis, nephrolithiasis →renal dysfunction	Polyuria, hematuria		BUN, Cr
CNS	EEG abn, seizures	Depression, personality change, psychomotor retardation, memory impairment	Psychosis, disorientation, obtundation, coma	
MS	Hyporeflexia, osteopenia, osteitis fibrosa cystica	Weakness, bone pain	Muscular atrophy, arthritis, pathologic fractures	

$$* \; Q_A T_C = \frac{Q_A T}{\sqrt{RR}} \; ; RR = RR \text{ interval.}$$

Key Reference: Rogers MC, Tinker JH, Covino BG, Longnecker DE: Principles and Practice of Anesthesiology. St. Louis, Mosby-Year Book, 1993, pp 284–285.

PERIOPERATIVE IMPLICATIONS

Preoperative Preparation

- Assess total and ionized Ca^{2+} levels
- Reduce serum total calcium to <14 mg/dl
- No intervention for Ca^{2+} level ≤12 mg/dl
- For higher levels use saline hydration and furosemide (rapid action), mithramycin (acts in 6–12 h), calcitonin (acts in 1–2 h), or glucocorticoids (cover intraoperatively with stress dose); reduce Ca^{2+} to <14 mg/dl
- Consider H_2 receptor antagonists and metoclopramide

Monitoring

- Routine; pay attention to changes in QT_c interval (QT_c by itself poorly correlated with ionized Ca^{2+}, but changes correlate)

Airway

- Possibility of pathologic fractures requires careful positioning for laryngoscopy

Preinduction/Induction

- No preferred agents or techniques
- Hypovolemia can lead to hemodynamic instability if usual dose of drugs is given

Maintenance

- No preferred agents or techniques. Possibility of pathologic fractures requires careful positioning and padding of pressure points

Extubation

- Swelling of or bleeding into the neck or recurrent laryngeal nerve injury during surgery may cause airway compromise

Adjuvants

- Response to NM blockers may be unpredictable if Ca^{2+} level elevated

ANTICIPATED PROBLEMS/CONCERNS

- Cardiac arrhythmias due to hypercalcemia
- Postop airway compromise 2° to bleeding or recurrent laryngeal nerve injury
- Pneumothorax 2° to surgical procedure
- Fluid and lyte overload from too aggressive hydration

HYPERTENSION

Simon J. Howell, M.D.
Pierre Foëx, M.D.

RISK

• Prevalence in the US population: 4% aged 18–29 y; 75% aged ≥80 y
• Ideal pressure of 115/76 or less present in only 4% of adult US population

PERIOPERATIVE RISKS

• Not proven significant risk factor of serious cardiac complications or death perioperatively
• Associated with perioperative HTN, bradycardia, myocardial ischemia

WORRY ABOUT

• Stages 3 and 4 hypertension (>180/110 mmHg)
• Evidence of end-organ damage (see Assessment Points)

OVERVIEW

• Hypertension can be essential or secondary
• Increased risk of coronary heart disease, stroke, CHF, renal insufficiency

ICD-9-CM Code: 401

ETIOLOGY

• Essential hypertension not fully understood: many putative factors: genetic factors (linkage to angiotensin gene), race, age, lifestyle (exercise), obesity, sodium intake, alcohol intake, childhood influences (birth weight, blood pressure tracking), socioeconomic status
• Secondary hypertension uncommon; 5% of all HTN. Possible causes include renal artery stenosis, Cushing's syndrome, pheochromocytoma, Conn's syndrome

USUAL TREATMENT

• Nonpharmacologic treatment: weight loss, reduction of alcohol intake, salt restriction, exercise, behavior modification
• Pharmacologic treatment: diuretic, β blockers, calcium channel blocking drugs, ACE inhibitors, α blockers

ASSESSMENT POINTS

SYSTEM	EFFECT	ASSESSMENT BY HX	PE	TEST
CV	CAD	MI, angina		ECG Exercise ECG Radionuclide scintigraphy Coronary Angio
	LVH/LVF	Dyspnea, orthopnea	Displaced apex beat S₃, basal crepitations Rales	CXR ECHO Radionuclide Angio
	Peripheral vascular/aortic disease	Claudication	Peripheral pulses Brachial-ankle BP ratio	Doppler Angio
RENAL	Renal impairment			Cr
CNS	TIA/CVA	Hx of TIA/CVA	Neurologic signs Carotid bruit	CT scan Doppler Angio

Key Reference: Stone JG, Foex P, Sear JW, et al.: Risk of myocardial ischaemia during anaesthesia in treated and untreated hypertensive patients. Br J Anaesth 1988; 61:675–679.

PERIOPERATIVE IMPLICATIONS

Preoperative Preparation

• Continue usual antihypertensive medications through surgery
• No clear evidence that acute management of moderate HTN is indicated
• Severe hypertension should be controlled

Monitoring

• Routine
• Consider intra-arterial catheter for severe HTN
• Consider CVP if significant hypovolemia suspected

Airway

• None

Preinduction/Induction

• May develop hypotension at induction and HTN at intubation
• Consider preload
• Consider use of opiates or vasoactive drugs to control response to intubation

Maintenance

• No technique demonstrated to be superior
• Risk of CV liability

Extubation

• Risk of HTN

Adjuvants

• β-blockers, calcium channel blockers, nitroglycerin, hydralazine, phentolamine, labetalol

Postoperative Period

• Resume normal antihypertensive medication ASAP
• For certain procedures, e.g., vascular surgery and neurosurgery, parenteral treatment of BP may be required if patient unable to take drugs orally

ANTICIPATED PROBLEMS/CONCERNS

• Hypertensive patients with end-organ damage are at greatest risk of developing complications

HYPERTENSION, UNCONTROLLED, WITH CARDIOMYOPATHY

Edward D. Miller, Jr., M.D.

RISK

- People within USA: 1 million
- Race with highest prevalence: African-American
- Male=female

PERIOPERATIVE RISKS

- Increased risk of myocardial ischemia and/or infarction
- Increased risk of stroke
- Increased risk of renal failure

WORRY ABOUT

- Tachycardia
- Severe elevations or depressions in BP

OVERVIEW

- Severe volume depletion may be present
- Silent myocardial ischemia
- May be forerunner of renal failure and/or stroke
- CHF may be presenting sign
- May develop left ventricular hypertrophy (LVH) ± strain pattern on ECG
- May require >6 wk of treatment for regression of LVH

ICD-9-CM Code: 402

ETIOLOGY

- Genetic predisposition
- Secondary forms related to abnormalities of kidney or adrenal glands
- High peripheral resistance is accelerated with time

USUAL TREATMENT

- Variety of antihypertensive agents to decrease BP
- Surgical correction of secondary forms of HTN

ASSESSMENT POINTS

SYSTEM	EFFECT	ASSESSMENT BY HX	PE	TEST
CV	LV function LVH	Exercise tolerance	2-flight walk	ECG, CXR ECHO Stress thallium
RESP	Pulm edema	Orthopnea Dyspnea	Rales	CXR
CNS	Stroke	Blackouts	Carotid bruit	Carotid study
RENAL	Nephropathy		Edema	BUN/Cr

Key Reference: Roizen MF: Patients with comorbidities. *In* Miller RD (ed): Anesthesia, 4th ed. New York, Churchill Livingstone, 1994, pp 933–937.

PERIOPERATIVE IMPLICATIONS

Preoperative Preparation

- Continue and/or increase antihypertensive medicine
- Short-acting vasodilator prepared
- Assess myocardial and volume status

Monitoring

- Consider direct arterial monitoring
- Volume status monitoring depending on LV function (e.g., PA cath, CVP, or TEE)

Induction

- Preintubation narcotics to prevent exacerbation of HTN
- Generous induction dose of IV agent
- Volume repletion prior to induction
- Consider short-acting β rb to prevent tachycardia

Maintenance

- CV stability best maintained by careful volume control and anticipation of noxious stimuli

Extubation

- Adequate pain relief prior to termination of anesthesia
- Short-acting vasodilator and/or β rb to prevent HTN and tachycardia

Adjuvants

- Regional: may prevent severe increases in BP, since intubation not needed. Severe dehydration may be present, resulting in profound hypotension
- Continuous infusions of nitroglycerin, nitroprusside, or esmolol
- Severe hypotension may not respond to usual doses of vasoconstrictor due to prior drug treatment

Postoperative Period

- Restart antihypertensive medication ASAP in postop period
- Patch therapy for some drugs must start 12 h prior to anticipated need due to slow absorption from skin

ANTICIPATED PROBLEMS/CONCERNS

- Watch for Sx of CNS, renal, or myocardial dysfunction
- Preop period affords opportunity to educate patient about importance of complying with antihypertensive therapy

HYPERTHYROIDISM

Michael F. Roizen, M.D.

RISK

- People within USA: 400,000/y develop hyperthyroidism plus 5% of pregnant females (highest prevalence in 2nd trimester); 1/1000 females; 1/3000 males.
- Race with highest prevalence: Not known

PERIOPERATIVE RISKS

- Pre- and intraoperative goals of management of extrathyroidal surgery are no different from those of thyroid surgery
- Risk related to occurrence of thyroid storm; ↑ risk of thyroid storm, even if made euthyroid prior to surgery
- Some increased risk of respiratory insufficiency
- Progressive increased risk of hypothyroidism after surgery on thyroid, radioactive Rx of hyperthyroidism, and thyroiditis

WORRY ABOUT

- Assessing that patient is euthyroid
- Securing airway in patient with large goiter or displaced trachea
- Postop risks of nerve injury (immediate stridor requires immediate reintubation), surreptitious bleeding (examine wound—can drain externally—prior to PACU discharge), and thyroid storm (uncommon without another acute illness or after 3 d postop)

OVERVIEW

- Endocrinopathy with CV disease—tachycardia (commonly idiopathic if no prior Dx of hyperthyroidism has been made), CHF, dysrhythmias (AFib) as major manifestation.
- Other target systems are respiratory and CNS (decreases drive to breathe; worsens anxiety, psychoses) and metabolic (hypermetabolism and increased protein turnover resulting in weakened muscles and malnourishment)
- If euthyroid prior to operation, risk of thyroid storm and of perioperative CV problems diminished by >90%
- If not euthyroid, try to delay operation until euthyroid
- If emergency (life-threatening trauma, ruptured viscus), use ß rb agents and iodides to decrease perioperative effects of released thyroid hormones and decrease further synthesis and release of thyroid hormones; keep in ICU until risk of thyroid storm has passed.

ICD-9-CM Codes:
242.9 (Hyperthyroidism [thyrotoxicosis]); 242.0 (Graves' disease); 245 (Thyroiditis); 193 (Malignant thyroid disease); 198.89 (Metastatic malignant thyroid disease)

ETIOLOGY

- Multinodular diffuse enlargement (Graves' disease); almost never malignant, soft large gland, thought autoimmune as associated with thyroid-stimulating IgGs that bind to TSH receptors on thyroid associated with goiter and ophthalmopathy
- Pregnancy (ectopic TSH-like substance production)
- Thyroiditis (autoimmune)
- Thyroid adenoma—toxic multinodular goiter (firm gland) later in life and rarely (almost never) malignant; unilateral solitary nodule with autonomous function earlier in life, also almost always benign
- Choriocarcinoma
- TSH-secreting pituitary adenoma
- Surreptitious ingestion of T_4 or T_3

USUAL TREATMENT

- Antithyroid drugs for 2–6 mos; if recurs, re-treat; if recurs again, consider surgery or radioiodine Rx

ASSESSMENT POINTS

SYSTEM	EFFECT	ASSESSMENT BY HX	PE	TEST
HEENT	Weakened tracheal rings, distorted/displaced trachea Ophthalmopathy	Snoring, hoarseness, neck pain	Ask to vocalize "e"; examine airway and neck Look at eyes; test for diplopia	Check CXR (PA and lateral) lat neck films; CT scan of neck
CV	Dysrhythmias, AFib, sinus tachycardia, mitral valve prolapse CHF cardiomyopathies	Palpitations; ↑ HR during sleep DOE, orthostatic SOB	Standard exam	Rhythm strip or full ECG CV system is involved in either Hx or PE
GI	Weight loss, diarrhea, dehydration	Dizziness on arising; Hx of diarrhea, constipation	Skin turgor; other measures of volume status such as orthostatic vital signs	Increased serum alkaline phosphatase (common, no need to assess)
HEME	Mild anemia, thrombocytopenia Agranulocytosis 2° to propylthiouracil or methimazole		Skin/mucous membranes for infection/petechiae	CBC with plt count and differential
CNS		Shaking, anxiety, emotional lability	Reflex speed, tremor, nervousness, mental status	
METABOLIC	Need to assess if euthyroid Malnourished	Refer to all other systems, esp. reflex speed, tremor, heat intolerance; fatigue; weakness; weight loss; anorexia, increased appetite	Reflex speed; HR	Free T_4 estimate

Key Reference: Roizen MF: Anesthetic implications of concurrent diseases. *In* Miller RD (ed): Anesthesia, 4th ed. New York, Churchill Livingstone, 1994, pp 926–928.

PERIOPERATIVE IMPLICATIONS

(See also under Thyroidectomy, Subtotal)

Preoperative Preparation

- Assess if euthyroid
- Assess if associated autoimmune diseases are present and need Rx

Preinduction/Induction

- Prehydrate liberally if CV status will tolerate
- Check and protect eyes

Anesthetic Technique

- No one technique has proved superior
- Hyperthyroidism is associated risk factor for halothane hepatitis

Monitoring

- T (also place cooling blanket on OR table to treat thyroid storm if it occurs)
- Consider invasive monitoring if patient has dilated cardiomyopathy/thyroid storm/severe dysrhythmia
- If considerable head-up position is utilized, consider air embolus monitoring and therapy strategies

Airway

- Consider awake fiberoptic intubation if questions about adequacy of airway or distortion/involvement of trachea present
- Consider armored tube or equivalent if tracheal rings are affected

Induction/Maintenance

- Routine

Adjuvants

- Usually no requirement for muscle relaxants for thyroidectomy

ANTICIPATED PROBLEMS/CONCERNS

- Thyroid storm is life-threatening illness if hyperthyroidism has been severely exacerbated by illness or operation. Manifested by hyperpyrexia, tachycardia, striking alterations in consciousness. Early signs include delirium, confusion, mania, excitement. Differential Dx: malignant hyperthermia, pheochromocytoma crisis, NMS
- Rx includes: supportive care, propylthiouracil followed in 1 h by iodides and propranolol, decrease conversion of the less active T_3 to the more active T_4.
- Surreptitious bleeding behind neck bandages can suddenly compromise airway function
- Recurrent laryngeal nerve injuries post thyroidectomy usually result in damage to abductor fibers, which results in hoarseness (test by asking to vocalize the letter "e") and compensatory overadduction of normal side.
- Bullous glottic edema can require immediate reintubation
- Occasionally late tetany (usually 2–3 d post thyroidectomy) can occur from accidental removal of or damage to parathyroid glands: results in hypoparathyroidism

HYPERTRIGLYCERIDEMIA

Uday Jain, Ph.D., M.D.

RISK

- People within USA: Combined with hypercholesterolemia in up to 1/5th of population
- Racial predilection: None

PERIOPERATIVE RISKS

- Some causes such as dysbetalipoproteinemia can cause atherosclerosis
- Primary chylomicronemia not atherogenic
- Acute pancreatitis and its complications (fatal hemorrhagic pancreatitis, pseudocyst, pancreatic exocrine insufficiency and impaired insulinogenesis)

WORRY ABOUT

- Myocardial ischemia and infarction
- Acute pancreatitis when triglycerides >1000 mg/dl
- Serum electrolytes, hydrophilic species underestimated in laboratory
- Transient eruptive cutaneous xanthomas

OVERVIEW

- Not independent risk factor for CAD in absence of hypercholesterolemia
- Triglyceride is glycerol esterified by 3 fatty acid molecules of variable chain length and degree of saturation
- Chylomicrons and very low density lipoproteins (VLDLs) are lipoproteins primarily containing triglycerides
- Normal value of triglycerides <200 mg/dl; values >1000 mg/dl associated with ↑ risk of pancreatitis
- Spinal or epidural anesthesia and β rb agents reduce FFA levels
- Sympathetic stimulation, stress, insulin, increase FFA levels
- Heparin releases lipoprotein lipase inhibited by protamine and hepatic lipase resistant to protamine

ICD-9-CM Code: 272.1–3
See also Hypercholesterolemia, Lipidemias, Coronary artery disease, Atherosclerosis

ETIOLOGY

- Primary hypertriglyceridemia or chylomicronemia; primary hyperprebetalipoproteinemia and mixed lipemias caused by several genetic disorders; combined hyperlipidemia and multiple lipoprotein type hyperlipidemia (excess of VLDLs and/or LDLs); familial dysbetalipoproteinemia (broad β disease, type III hyperlipoproteinemia)
- Due to diabetes, nephrotic syndrome, renal failure, rare dysproteinemias, oral contraceptives, thiazide diuretics, and β blockers

USUAL TREATMENT

- Diet and exercise
- Nicotinic acid inhibits production of VLDLs and LDLs
- Fibric acids clofibrate and gemfibrozil may cause abdominal discomfort, cholesterol gallstones, or myalgias accompanied by high serum creatine phosphokinase

ASSESSMENT POINTS

SYSTEM	EFFECT	ASSESSMENT BY HX	PE	TEST
CV	Coronary and peripheral atherosclerosis (not without ↑ cholesterol) LV dysfunction	Hx of CAD—angina, CHF, MI Exercise tolerance	2-flight walk Displaced posterior MI S$_3$	ECG, CXR, ECHO, stress testing, Angio
RESP		Exercise tolerance		Generally not needed
GI	Acute pancreatitis	Epigastric pain, obesity		
ENDO	Caused by poorly controlled DM	Ketoacidosis Hyperosmolar coma		Blood glucose level
SKIN	Markedly elevated VLDLs may lead to transient eruptive xanthomas		Xanthomas occur on extensor surfaces such as elbows, knees, buttocks	
RENAL	Caused by nephrotic syndrome, renal insufficiency	Urinary problems		BUN, Cr
CNS	Lipemia retinalis when triglycerides >3000 mg/dl		Whitish cast of venous vascular bed of retina	

Key Reference: Stein JH: Internal Medicine. Boston, Little, Brown, 1987, pp 2035–2057.

PERIOPERATIVE IMPLICATIONS

Preoperative Preparation

- If serum triglycerides high, lytes may be underestimated. Cholesterol and glucose may be high while thyroid hormone may be low
- Assess CV system and abdomen

Monitoring

- Routine

Preinduction/Induction

- FFAs are competitive inhibitors of barbiturates and other acidic drugs binding to albumin
- FFAs increase the likelihood of ventricular arrhythmias

Maintenance

- No agent or technique superior
- Negative inotropic properties of anesthetics may be enhanced
- Blood-gas partition coefficient of inhalational anesthetics is increased in hyperlipemia, slowing their uptake

Extubation

- Period of greatest risk for developing myocardial ischemia
- Epigastric pain may be felt if acute pancreatitis

Adjuvants

- Depends on etiology and end-organ diseases
- Lipid stores of anesthetic agents may alter awakening and return of psychomotor normality

ANTICIPATED PROBLEMS/CONCERNS

- Complications of CAD
- Acute pancreatitis

HYPOKALEMIA

Irving A. Hirsch, M.D.

RISK

- Any patient with plasma K^+ <3.5 mEq/L
- Patients on diuretic therapy for HTN or other conditions
- HTN affects 60 million people
  - Higher prevalence in African-Americans than in Caucasians
  - Increased with age in all groups
  - Increased in men vs. women <50 y
  - Increased in women vs. men >50 y

PERIOPERATIVE RISKS

- Cardiac arrhythmias—atrial and ventricular premature beats
- Muscle weakness
- Autonomic insufficiency

WORRY ABOUT

- Recent evidence suggests that cardiac arrhythmogenicity is dependent on acuteness or chronicity of hypokalemia
- Acute alkalosis
- β_2 adrenergic agonists may shift K^+ intracellularly, worsening hypokalemia
- Potential for prolonged response to nondepolarizing muscle relaxants

OVERVIEW

- Serum K^+ and its extracellular to intracellular ratio important for electrical excitation of excitable cells, including heart, skeletal muscles, nerves
- Acute shifts, in face of chronic hypokalemia, are more likely to produce life-threatening complications
- Chronic condition less dangerous because ratio of intracellular to extracellular K^+ is maintained

ICD-9-CM Code: 276.8

ETIOLOGY

- Inadequate intake: diet; alcoholism; anorexia nervosa; geophagia
- Excess renal loss: mineralocorticoid excess; primary or secondary hyperaldosteronism; Cushing's syndrome; chronic licorice ingestion; Bartter's syndrome; diuretics: pre–late distal tubule locus of action (such as hydrochlorothiazide and furosemide [Lasix]), osmotic diuretics, carbonic anhydrase inhibitors (acetazolamide); chronic metabolic alkalosis; antibiotics: carbenicillin, genta-micin, amphotericin B; renal tubular acidosis; Liddle's syndrome; acute leukemia; ureterosigmoidostomy
- Gastrointestinal losses: vomiting; diarrhea; nasogastric suctioning; villous adenoma
- Etiology of acute hypercalemia
  - Acute alkalosis
  - Hypokalemic periodic paralysis
  - Barium ingestion
  - Insulin therapy
  - Vitamin B_{12} therapy
  - Thyrotoxicosis (rarely)

USUAL TREATMENT

- Plasma K^+ decrease from 4 to 3 mEq/L = 100–200 mEq deficit
- Plasma K^+ <3 mEq/L = 200–400 mEq deficit
- Replacement:
  - Oral—potassium gluconate or citrate
  - IV—potassium chloride 10–20 mEq/L/h, larger amounts only under adequate monitoring of cardiac electrophysiology

ASSESSMENT POINTS

SYSTEM	EFFECT	ASSESSMENT BY HX	PE	TEST
CV	Arrhythmias ECG changes	PACs, PVCs	Prolonged PR and QT intervals Flattened T waves, V waves ST segment depression	ECG
ENDO	↓ Aldosterone ↓ Insulin release			Aldosterone Glucose
NM	Weakness Areflexic paralysis Ileus, abdominal pain Autonomic insufficiency Rhabdomyolysis	Muscle pain	Respiratory insufficiency Absence of bowel sounds Orthostatic hypotension	ABG (rarely needed) BP CPK
RENAL	K^+ conservation Polyuria Polydipsia ↑ Renal ammonia Edema and sodium retention	Frequent urination Frequent drinking		Urine K^+ Urine ammonia Urine sodium

Key Reference: Hirsch IA, Tomlinson DL, Slogoff S, Keats AS: The overstated role of preoperative hypokalemia. Anesth Analg 1988; 67:131–136.

PERIOPERATIVE IMPLICATIONS

Preoperative Preparation

- K^+ levels (>2.7 and <5.8 mEq/L) before elective surgery
- Determine if hypokalemia is acute or chronic in onset

Monitoring

- ECG
- Plasma K^+ levels
- ABG
- Peripheral nerve stimulator

Maintenance

- Adequate ventilation to avoid respiratory alkalosis (avoid hyperventilation)
- Avoid hyperglycemia—IV fluids with glucose
- Avoid epinephrine or other β_2 agonist, which may shift K^+ intracellularly

ANTICIPATED PROBLEMS/CONCERNS

- Decision to proceed with elective surgery depends on level and acuteness or chronicity of hypokalemia
- Hypokalemia may lead to arrhythmias, esp. with catecholamines, digitalis, calcium, or hyperventilation
- Hypokalemia due to diuretics may cause or be associated with volume depletion
- Hypokalemic patients may be sensitive to vasodilators or cardiac-depressant effects of volatile anesthetics

HYPOMAGNESEMIA

James M. Feld, M.D.

RISK

• 60% of all patients admitted to either a surgical or medical ICU were hypomagnesemic

PERIOPERATIVE RISKS

• ↑Risk for arrhythmias (atrial and ventricular)
• ↑Risk for worsening ischemia/CHF
• ↑Susceptibility to seizures, bronchoconstriction, vasospasm
• ↑Mortality from endotoxin challenge

WORRY ABOUT

• Giving $MgSO_4$ too fast may cause burning at IV site, overall sense of warmth (has been used for postop shivering), mild transient hypotension
• As long as renal function is intact, excessive levels will be cleared over several hours
• Prolongation of neuromuscular blockade with all nondepolarizing drugs.

OVERVIEW

• Common deficiency from multiple causes that results in decreased stability of excitable cells, decreased contractility and ↑SVR
• Safe to give even if levels are high—may not truly reflect intracellular levels
• Must replete Mg^{2+} levels before correcting K^+ and Ca^{2+} deficiencies
• Primary concern is increasing susceptibility to worsening myocardial ischemia

ICD-9-CM Code: 275.2

ETIOLOGY

• Poor nutrition, diuretic therapy, aminoglycosides, digitalis, prolonged IV therapy, diabetes mellitus, large blood transfusions, increased alcoholic intake

USUAL TREATMENT

• Acute administration of 2 g $MgSO_4$ over 20–30 min
• 1 g $MgSO_4$ with every 20 mEq of KCl
• Give at beginning of case, as it may interfere with neuromuscular blockade reversal
• Keep in mind usual preeclamptic doses are 4–6 g bolus and 1–2 g/h; monitoring levels between 6–8 mg/dl

ASSESSMENT POINTS

SYSTEM	EFFECT	PE	TEST
CV	Myocardial ischemia HTN Arrhythmias		ECG BP
RESP	Bronchospasm	Wheezing Airway pressure	
NEURO	Seizures (more marked in presence of cocaine) Vasospasm		
UTERUS	HTN of preeclampsia, eclampsia	Seizures	
MS	Weakness	Difficulty weaning	

Key Reference: James M: Clinical use of magnesium infusions in anesthesia. Anesth Analg 1992; 74:129–136.

PERIOPERATIVE IMPLICATIONS

Preoperative Preparation

• In patients susceptible to hypomagnesemia, give 2–5 g $MgSO_4$ over the first 1–2 h of surgery
• Initial 2 g will alter the catecholamine response to intubation and may contribute some analgesic effect

Intraoperative Period

• Give more Mg^{2+} only if patient is to be kept intubated postop and if UO is adequate, as reversibility of neuromuscular blockade may not be complete
• Mg^{2+} will potentiate vasodilators and slowing effect of digitalis in supraventricular arrhythmias.

Postoperative Period

• Rarely measure blood levels in routine case unless patient with heart disease is going to ICU and is on vasoactive drugs or requiring large amounts IV fluids
• 1–2 g $MgSO_4$ slow push in PACU may attenuate postop shivering

ANTICIPATED PROBLEMS/CONCERNS

• Levels above 8–10 mg/dl cause diaphragmatic weakness and are rarely reached with above recommendations
• Other than potentiating neuromuscular weakness, Mg^{2+} administration is safe
• In suspected MIs it should be given as early as possible.

HYPONATREMIA

Kuang C. Wong, M.D., Ph.D.
John K. Hayes, Ph.D.

RISK

- Patients with adrenocortical insufficiency (Addison's disease) or syndrome of inappropriate secretion of antidiuretic hormone (SIADH)
- Up to 25% of elderly males subjected to transurethral resection of the prostate (TURP), from irrigating fluid absorption
- Females subjected to endoscopic gynecologic surgery with excessively absorbed irrigating fluid
(See Addison's disease and SIADH in Diseases section, and under Transurethral Resection of Prostate in Procedures section)

PERIOPERATIVE RISKS

- Adrenocortical insufficiency associated with ↑ risk of inability to cope with stress and of CV collapse
- Iatrogenic dilution associated with CNS, cardiopulmonary, and skeletal muscle abnormalities

WORRY ABOUT

- Intraoperative TURP syndrome with iatrogenic hyponatremia
  – Water intoxication (cerebral and/or pulmonary edema)
  – Cardiac dysrhythmias
  – Visual or motor disturbance from glycine irrigating fluid toxicity
  – Hypothermia

OVERVIEW

- Can occur in isotonic, hypertonic, and hypotonic forms—all require that excretion of renal water is impaired despite continued intake of dilute fluid(s)
- Serum sodium and intra- to extracellular ratio is important in maintaining cellular integrity and electrical activity of excitable cells. Low serum sodium from inadequate dietary intake, too vigorous diuresis, or absorption of sodium-free irrigating solutions.

- Dilutional hyponatremia is inevitable during TURP, so pre-existing conditions should be optimally stabilized before coming to the OR (e.g., lyte disturbance, cardiac ischemia, chronic pulmonary disease).

ICD-9-CM Code: 276.1

ETIOLOGY

- Dilutional hyponatremia results from absorption of sodium-free irrigating fluid.
- SIADH can be caused by CNS or pulmonary tumors or dysfunction

USUAL TREATMENT

- Restricting free water administration (rate of rise of Na^+ to be <1 mEq/L/h lest central pontine myelinolysis occur)
- Intravenous hypertonic saline
- IV diuretic
- Decrease symptomatic organ dysfunction (CHF Rx with diuresis, vasodilation)

ASSESSMENT POINTS

SYSTEM	EFFECT	ASSESSMENT BY HX	PE	TEST
CV	Dysrhythmias	Palpitations		ECG
	CHF	Orthopnea, DOE	S_3, rales	CXR
RESP	Pulm edema		S_3, rales	CXR
CNS	Confusion Restlessness Visual disturbances Seizure, coma			Usually serum Na^+ <123 mEq/L
MS	Hyporeflexia Cramps, weakness	Cramps, weakness	Weakness	Reflexes
RENAL				Serum Na^+ Serum and urine osmolality

Key Reference: Liu WS, Wong KC: Anesthesia for genitourinary surgery. *In* Barash PG, Cullen BF, Stoelting RK (eds): Clinical Anesthesia. Philadelphia, JB Lippincott, 1992, pp 1160–1164.

PERIOPERATIVE IMPLICATIONS

Monitoring
- Blood lytes and serum osmolality
- ECG
- Body temp
- EEG if patient is under GA

Airway
- None

Maintenance
- Ensure optimal general or regional anesthesia
- Prevent hypothermia by using warmed irrigating and IV fluid

Extubation
- Cardiopulmonary problems should be stabilized following hyponatremia and water intoxication

Postoperative Period
- Pain management
- Restore lyte balance
- Replace blood loss if necessary (hypovolemia, tachycardia, hypoxemia)

ANTICIPATED PROBLEMS/CONCERNS

- Dilutional hyponatremia is generally related to the skill of the resectionist and the duration of resection
- Patient with pre-existing cardiopulmonary problems should be optimally stabilized
- ASA class 1 and class 2 patients will tolerate hyponatremia and water load better than classes 3 and 4 patients; chronic hyponatremia tolerated better than acute hyponatremia
- Risk of central pontine myelinolysis if hypertonic saline is administered

HYPOPHOSPHATEMIA

Alan S. Tonnesen, M.D.

RISK

- 0.3–1.5% of "healthy" adults; 5–20% of hospitalized patients
- Alcoholism, ketoacidosis, osmotic diuresis, acidosis, catabolism, acute burn injury
- Depressed intake: starvation, malabsorption, familial hypophosphatemia, hemodialysis, binding within gut, vitamin D deficiency
- Increased urinary losses: hyperparathyroidism, osmotic diuresis, acute volume expansion, acetazolamide, diuretic phase ATN, renal transplantation, acidosis
- Redistribution: glucose-insulin infusion, β adrenergic agonists, resp alkalosis, recovery from malnutrition, alcohol withdrawal, theophylline overdose

PERIOPERATIVE RISKS

- Acute resp or cardiac failure of unclear etiology.

WORRY ABOUT

- Postop resp or cardiac failure
- Hypocalcemia and vascular calcification if PO_4 administered too rapidly

OVERVIEW (P_i mol wt = 31)

- Requirements: 10 mmol/1000 kCal; 1 mmol/kg/d
- 60–70% absorbed in duodenum and jejunum, stimulated by vitamin D, from dairy products, meat, eggs
- Excretion: Kidney: filtered, reabsorbed proximally (inhibited by PTH, cortisol, glucagon, calcitonin, osmotic diuresis, high dietary PO_4 intake); 10% absorbed distally
- Gut: secreted, then reabsorbed; may be trapped by Al antacids, Ca^{2+}, sucralfate: may be lost by diarrhea or drainage via ostomies or fistulas
- Distribution: Total body content about 15 g/kg; volume of distribution about 400 ml/kg. Bone contains 85% of total.
- Intracellular: (50–75 mmol/L), bound organic form, as high-energy phosphates, phosphorylated proteins, metabolic intermediates.
- Factors favoring intracellular movement include glucose, fructose, alkalosis (especially resp), insulin, β adrenergic stimulation, anabolism (rapid tumor growth, refeeding), osteoblastic metastases.
- Extracellular fluid volume (ECFV): 1 mmol/L: 10% protein bound, 5% chelated. Normal P_i is 3.5–5.0 mg/dl (1.1–1.6 mmol/L); falls by 30% after carbohydrate ingestion; higher in females, childhood, postmenopausal women; lower in am than pm; elevated after PO_4 ingestion; serum concentration is not closely related to body stores. Body stores assessed better by measuring excretion of PO_4, $FePO_4$, tubular reabsorption of PO_4/GFR.
- Functions:
  – Buffer: binds 1, 2, or 3 hydrogen ions/mole, depending on pH. Store and release energy. Structure of proteins, cell membrane lipids, and bone; enzyme phosphorylation for activation. Carbohydrate metabolism: phosphorylate glucose during cellular entry; glycerol-PO_4 serves as gluconeogenic precursor.

ICD-9-CM Code: 275.3

ETIOLOGY

- Depressed intake, increased loss, redistribution

USUAL TREATMENT

- Measure Ca^{2+}, Mg^{2+}, and K^+. Administer 10–15 mmol/1000 calories, 20–30 mmol/d in critically ill. Dietary supplement may be limited by diarrhea.
- For severe hypophosphatemia (<1 mg/dl): Na or K phosphate, intravenously or enterally: multiply volume of distribution by the desired change in $[P_i]$; rate of administration not >0.04 mmol/kg/h to avoid hypocalcemia and tissue precipitation.

ASSESSMENT POINTS

SYSTEM	EFFECT	RESULT
CV	Depressed ATP generation	Heart failure
	Impaired pressor response to norepinephrine and angiotensin	
HEME	Impaired phagocytosis,	
WBC	bacteriocidal and migration functions	
Platelets		Thrombocytopenia, defective aggregation, megakaryocytosis
		Impaired clot retraction
RBC	Reduced RBC 2,3-DPG level	Increased Hgb O_2 affinity
	Spherocytosis, splenic sequestration	Hemolytic anemia (<0.2 mg/dl)
CHO Metabolism	Insulin resistance, impaired insulin secretion	Hyperglycemia
RENAL	Reduced GFR	
	Hypercalciuria	
	Hypermagnesiuria	Hypomagnesemia
	Hypophosphaturia	
	↓ Proximal Na^+ reabsorption	
	↓ Tm for bicarbonate, reduced titratable acid excretion	
	↓ Tm for glucose	Bicarbonaturia, metabolic acidosis
CALCIUM	Inhibits PTH secretion	Hypercalcemia
CNS	Neurologic depression	Irritability, paresthesia, dysarthria
		Anisocoria, hyperreflexia
MS	Weakness	Proximal > distal
	Resp failure	Rhabdomyolysis
		CPK
		Myoglobinuria
		Aldolase
	Increased osteoclast activity	Bone pain
		Pseudofractures

Key Reference: Rubin MF, Narins RG: Hypophosphatemia: pathophysiological and practical aspects of its therapy. Semin Nephrol 1990; 10:536.

PERIOPERATIVE IMPLICATIONS

- Severe hypophosphatemia corrected slowly over hours to days to fully replete body stores and avoid hypocalcemia and vascular and interstitial calcium precipitation

HYPOPITUITARISM

Johnathan L. Pregler, M.D.

RISK

• Pituitary tumor most common cause, with incidence of 0.2–2.8/100,000/y; prevalence of 8.9/100,000 for total of ~22,500 people in US.
• 30% of pituitary macroadenomas (>10 mm) cause one or more hormone deficiencies.
• 50% of patients after pituitary radiation therapy by 4.2 y have hypopituitarism.

PERIOPERATIVE RISKS

• In patient with adequate hormone replacement, surgery presents no increased risk.
• If due to secreting tumor, then ↑ risk of Cushing's disease, acromegaly, SIADH, or hyperthyroidism.

WORRY ABOUT

• Hypoglycemia
• Airway abnormalities if due to GH-secreting adenoma
• Altered volume status due to ↑ urinary losses
• Adequacy of adrenal function

OVERVIEW

• Partial or complete disruption of pituitary gland secretion. Symptoms result from end-organ hypofunction or dysfunction. Organs affected include adrenals, thyroid, reproductive system, liver (glucose production), and kidneys
• May manifest cortisol deficiency, hypothyroidism, amenorrhea, infertility, insulin-induced hypoglycemia, diabetes insipidus
• Pituitary apoplexy is sudden loss of pituitary function with hypotension, eye pain, blindness, ophthalmoplegia

ICD-9-CM Codes: 253.2 or 253.7 (if due to radiotherapy, post ablative, post hypophysectomy, or secondary to hormone therapy)

ETIOLOGY

• Common causes include pituitary adenoma, pituitary surgery, pituitary radiation therapy, pituitary apoplexy from hemorrhage or infarction
• Other causes: empty sella syndrome, head trauma, infiltrative disease, and internal carotid artery aneurysms
• Mechanical compression of normal pituitary cells by mass effect, impaired blood flow, and interference with hypothalamic regulatory hormone delivery may all be causes of dysfunction.

USUAL TREATMENT

• Surgical resection of adenoma with appropriate hormonal replacement therapy includes: for ACTH: prednisone or cortisone PO; for TSH: thyroxine PO; for LH and FSH: women: estrogen and progesterone PO; men: testosterone esters IM; for ADH: desmopressin intranasal.

ASSESSMENT POINTS

SYSTEM	EFFECT	ASSESSMENT BY HX	PE	TEST
HEENT	Mandibular and oral soft tissue hyperplasia in acromegalics		Airway exam Check ring size	
CV	Hypovolemia Catecholamine resistance		Orthostatic hypotension	AM cortisol level Serum corticotropin Give cortisol and observe BP effect
GI	Hypoaldosteronism	Anorexia, N/V, weight loss, abdominal pain		Hyperkalemia, hyponatremia, hypovolemia
ENDO	Decreased LH, FSH	Decreased libido and sexual function Amenorrhea	Regression of secondary sexual characteristics	FSH, LH serum levels Serum estradiol and testosterone
	Decreased GH	Fatigue		Insulin-induced hypoglycemia Serum IGF-1
	Decreased TSH	Weight gain, cold intolerance, depression, constipation, hair loss	Myxedema, hyporeflexia	TSH, T_4
	Increased prolactin	Lactation, amenorrhea	Galactorrhea	Serum prolactin
MS	Increased GH in acromegalics		Large hands, feet, mandible, tongue	
RENAL	↑ Vasopressin ↓ Vasopressin	Excessive thirst Increased UO and thirst	Hypovolemia Hypotension	Hyponatremia Hypernatremia Dilute urine

Key Reference: Vance ML: Hypopituitarism. N Engl J Med 1994; 330:1651–1662.

PERIOPERATIVE IMPLICATIONS

Preoperative Preparation

• Ensure adequacy of hormone replacement therapy
• Check serum Na⁺ and K⁺ and correct if necessary
• Determine volume status and adequacy of fluid replacement
• In acromegalics: careful airway assessment
• Steroid supplementation considerations (hydrocortisone 100 mg/70 kg/d)

Monitoring

• Consider central venous pressures if indicated by coexisting CV abnormalities or inadequate preop correction of fluid status

• Frequent monitoring of electrolytes if hypo- or hypernatremia is not corrected preop
• Consider glucose monitoring

Airway

• Acromegalics with normal airway exam may be difficult to intubate. Have fiberoptic available.

Induction

• Little risk of ↑ ICP with pituitary adenomas
• No special technique if hormone replacement and volume status are adequate

Maintenance

• Maintain normocarbia for pituitary surgery

Extubation

• Routine (for nonpituitary surgery; for pituitary surgery—see under *Procedures*)

Adjuvants

• Intraoperative diabetes insipidus treated with vasopressin 5–10 IU SC or IM q 4–6 h.

Postoperative Period

• Polyuria and polydipsia with dilute urine may indicate development of diabetes insipidus
• Postop hypopituitarism may require steroid replacement therapy

ANTICIPATED PROBLEMS/CONCERNS

• Acromegalic should be treated as a difficult airway with possible awake fiberoptic intubation and extubation only when fully awake
• Patient with GH deficiency may manifest hypoglycemia

HYPOTHERMIA, MILD (Core temperature 34–36°C) — Daniel I. Sessler, M.D.

RISK

- Greater in infants and children
- Greater in longer, larger operations
- Similar in regional and GA

PERIOPERATIVE RISKS

- Myocardial ischemia
- Surgical wound infections
- Coagulopathy
- Altered drug kinetics
- Shivering and thermal discomfort

PERIOPERATIVE BENEFITS

- Resistance to cerebral ischemia
- Decreases triggering and severity of malignant hyperthermia

OVERVIEW

- Core temperature normally protected by responses including sweating, vasoconstriction, shivering
- Typical doses of general anesthetics ↑ the sweating threshold ≈1°C and ↓ vasoconstriction and shivering thresholds 2–4°C, thus increasing the range of temp *not* triggering protective responses from ≈0.2°C to ≈4°C
- Regional anesthesia inhibits thermoregulatory control by preventing peripheral responses (such as vasoconstriction) and centrally by altering afferent input

ICD-9-CM Code: 991.6 (accidental)

ETIOLOGY

- Initial 0.5–1.5°C decrease in core temp from core-to-peripheral *redistribution* of body heat
- Subsequently, slow, linear decrease in core temperature from *heat loss exceeding heat production*
- Finally, a core-temp plateau results when thermoregulatory *vasoconstriction decreases cutaneous heat loss and constrains metabolic heat* to core thermal compartment

USUAL TREATMENT

- Forced-air is most effective non-invasive warming method, typically increasing mean body temp 1.5°C/h
- Fluids administered can be warmed. One L of crystalloid at 20°C or 1 U of blood at 4°C decreases mean body temp ≈0.25°C in adults
- Passive insulation (eg, surgical drapes, cotton blankets) decreases heat loss only 30%
- Circulating-water mattresses less effective and may cause burns. Airway heating and humidification is less effective

ASSESSMENT POINTS

SYSTEM	EFFECT	DX	TREATMENT
CNS	Ischemia protection Thermal discomfort	None Visual analog scale	Maintain hypothermia Active cutaneous warming
CARDIAC	Myocardial ischemia (usually postop)	ST segment depression ECHO	Active cutaneous warming
VASCULAR	Precapillary dilation; reduced SVR Arteriovenous shunt constriction; little effect on SVR	Associated with sweating Fingers feel cold	Active or passive cooling Active cutaneous warming
MUSC (shivering)	2–3-fold ↑ metabolic rate Patient discomfort Interference with monitoring	Visual inspection Oxygen consumption	Prevent hypothermia Meperidine 25 mg IV Clonidine 75 µg IV Active cutaneous warming
IMMUNE	Incidence of infections increases 2–3-fold	Clinical infections	Prevent hypothermia
COAGULATION	10% ↑/°C in blood loss	Bleeding time PT/PTT *falsely* normal	Prevent hypothermia Defect probably *not* reversed by FFP and plt transfusions
METAB (increased drug action)	MAC decreases ≈5%/°C ↓ drug metabolism	Monitor drug action (rather than dose)	Titrate drug administration to desired endpoint Monitor twitch depression

Key Reference: Sessler DI: Temperature monitoring. *In* Miller RD (ed): Anesthesia, 4th ed. New York, Churchill Livingstone, 1994, pp 1363–1382.

PERIOPERATIVE IMPLICATIONS

Preoperative Preparation

- "Prewarming" with forced-air for 30–60 min usually minimizes hypothermia

Monitoring

- Four core temp sites are accurate: pulmonary artery, distal esophagus, tympanic membrane, nasopharynx
- Four additional sites suitable except during cardiopulmonary bypass: mouth, axilla, rectum, bladder
- Skin-surface temp is 2–4°C < core temp and not a substitute for coretemp

Intraoperative

- Maintain normothermia (core temp >36°C) unless otherwise indicated
- Sufficient passive or active reduction of heat loss will prevent hypothermia. Active warming often required
- Once triggered, thermoregulatory vasoconstriction effective in preventing further core hypothermia

Postoperative

- Hypothermic patients can be aggressively rewarmed
- Shivering and thermal discomfort can be specifically treated
- Postop warming not a routine substitute for maintaining intraoperative normothermia

ANTICIPATED PROBLEMS/CONCERNS

- Thermal discomfort is not life-threatening, but many patients consider it the *worst* part of surgery.

HYPOTHYROIDISM

RISK

• Subclinical hypothyroidism may be present in as many as 8–10% of adult women and 1–2% of adult men; overt hypothyroidism occurs in 0.5–1.5% of adult women and about 0.05–0.15% of adult men

PERIOPERATIVE RISKS

• Potential increased risk for hypothermia, hypotension, cardiac failure, and perioperative gastrointestinal dysfunction
• Perioperative mortality rate not increased unless overtly hypothyroid

WORRY ABOUT

• Predisposition to hypothermia
• Neuromuscular weakness may impair weaning from mechanical ventilation

OVERVIEW

• A common condition, particularly in adult women
• Dx established by decreased total and free thyroxine (T_4) (and usually triiodothyronine [T_3]) concentrations, and elevated thyrotropin (TSH) concentrations in blood

• Patients presenting with severe, untreated hypothyroidism or myxedema coma may also demonstrate hypothermia, hypoventilation, hyponatremia, hypotension, heart failure, bowel obstruction, and hypoglycemia

ICD-9-CM Code: 244.9

ETIOLOGY

• Hypothyroidism (decreased thyroid hormone secretion) may result from disease of thyroid or pituitary glands, or hypothalamus
• Most (95%) of cases result from primary disease of gland, most commonly autoimmune thyroiditis; previous ^{131}I treatment for hyperthyroidism and previous total thyroidectomy are also relatively common causes of hypothyroidism
• Patients with critical illness often have reduced total T_4 and reduced total and free T_3 with normal TSH concentrations ("euthyroid sick syndrome"), but usually do not require treatment
• Primary TSH deficiency may result from pituitary tumors and cysts or their treatment (either surgery or radiation), pituitary infiltration, necrosis, or infarction; secondary TSH deficiency may result from congenital deficiency of thyrotropin-releasing hormone (TRH), radiation therapy, infections, or tumors or cysts impinging on the hypothalamic–pituitary portal circulation.

USUAL TREATMENT

• Maintenance outpatient therapy for adults consists of oral thyroxine 0.1–0.2 mg (1–3 µg/kg) daily
• Long $T_{1/2}$ of T_4 (about a week) permits oral T_4 to be withheld safely for several NPO days
• Rifampin and phenytoin increase metabolism of T_4 and increase T_4 dosage requirements
• Patients with angina may not tolerate full (or any?) T_4 replacement doses
• Myxedema coma may require use of intravenous T_3 (liothyronine) 0.15–0.3 µg/kg every 6 h and IV hydrocortisone 0.5–1 mg/kg every 8 h to cover for possible hypothyroid-impaired adrenal response to stress
• Intravenous liothyronine may also be indicated in other circumstances when peripheral conversion of T_4 to T_3 is impaired (e.g., hypothermic cardiopulmonary bypass)

ASSESSMENT POINTS

SYSTEM	EFFECT	ASSESSMENT BY HX	PE	TEST
HEENT	Enlarged tongue	Snoring	Enlarged tongue	
CV	↓ Heart rate, ↓ BP, heart failure	Palpitations, myocardial ischemia, arrhythmias, peripheral edema	Bradycardia, tachycardia	TSH, T_4 concentrations, ECG
RESP	Hypoventilation			Arterial P_{CO_2}; or HCO_3^- / serum electrolytes
GI	Ileus		Bowel sounds	
RENAL	Decreased free water clearance	Fluid retention, edema	Edema	Serum Na^+ concentration
CNS	Obtundation, muscular weakness	Lethargy, weakness, mental slowness	Decreased deep tendon reflexes, impaired mental status examination	TSH, T_4 concentrations

Key Reference: Toft AD: Thyroxine therapy. N Engl J Med 1994; 331:174–180.

PERIOPERATIVE IMPLICATIONS

Preoperative Preparation
• Thyroid replacement to maintain clinically euthyroid state

Monitoring
• Temperature (particularly in those who have not received full T_4 replacement)
• Routine

Airway
• Usually no abnormalities, but may have large tongue

Maintenance
• No significant effect of hypothyroidism on MAC for inhaled anesthetics
• Keep the patient warm
• Possible increased risk of perioperative heart failure, hypotension, and GI dysfunction (controversial)

Extubation
• Keep the patient warm
• Weaning from mechanical ventilation may be impaired

Adjuvants
• None (except in cases of myxedema coma, in which IV liothyronine and hydrocortisone are indicated)

ANTICIPATED PROBLEMS/CONCERNS

• Only patients who have been inadequately treated with T_4 carry risks; those receiving an appropriate dose of T_4 probably have (at most) minimally increased risks compared with other patients.
• Inadequately treated hypothyroidism can lead to lethargy and fatigue, dementia, heart failure, resp weakness, fluid retention and edema, hyponatremia, clotting abnormalities, and generalized weakness.

DISEASES   **185**

HYPOXEMIA

Ted J. Sanford, Jr., M.D.

RISK

• All patients undergoing anesthesia and surgery (7–35% in large series have PaO_2 <60 mmHg in OR or PACU)
• Patients with preexisting pulmonary disease

PERIOPERATIVE RISKS

• Hypoxemia may lead to hypoxia and eventual severe neurologic/cardiac sequelae or death

WORRY ABOUT

• Inadequate delivery of O_2 to blood—greatest concern to the anesthesiologist is inadequate delivery of O_2 to patient
• Concern that inadequate delivery of O_2 to blood will lead to inadequate delivery of O_2 to tissues
• Misinterpretation of clinical manifestations of hypoxemia

OVERVIEW

• Hypoxemia—denotes low PO_2 in blood (vs. hypoxia, which denotes inadequate delivery of O_2 to tissues)
• Hypoxemia defined as (1) resting PO_2 >2 SD below normal for age and FIO_2, (2) SaO_2 <90%, (3) PaO_2 <60 mmHg on room air, (4) a fall in SaO_2 >5%
• Multiple clues in vital signs and patient symptoms that should be assumed to be due to hypoxemia

ICD-9-CM Code: 799.0 (Hypoxia)

ETIOLOGY

• Decreased FIO_2—failure to provide adequate inspired O_2 (e.g., O_2 supply failure, gas machine disconnect, airway disconnect, patients at higher altitude)
• Inadequate alveolar ventilation or alveolar hypoventilation: venous admixture accounts for majority of causes
  – V/Q mismatch—asthma, COPD, pulm embolism, pulm vascular disease, passive atelectasis due to pneumonia. Resorption atelectasis is most common when O_2 is taken up from an obstructed area of tracheobronchial tree; adhesive atelectasis seen with decreased surfactant; alveoli filled with blood, vomitus; FRC > closing capacity.
  – R→L cardiac shunts—ASD, VSD (*Note:* will not respond to increased FIO_2)
  – Diffusion problems—very rare cause

USUAL TREATMENT

• Determine cause of decreased O_2 delivery and treat
• Increase FIO_2—this will help in all situations of hypoxemia except those due to R→L shunts

ASSESSMENT POINTS

• Subjective signs
  – anxiety, confusion, altered mental status, diaphoresis, seizures, cyanosis (both central and peripheral)
• Objective signs
  – Tachypnea—increased ventilation due to stimulation of carotid body chemoreceptors, lactic acidosis. May not occur in patients with severe lung disease or history of bilateral carotid endarterectomies
  – Tachycardia—early signs due to sympathetic stimulation, not to be ignored as just light anesthesia or patient anxiety
  – Hypertension
  – Arrhythmia—due to myocardial ischemia
  – Hypotension
  – **BRADYCARDIA—LATE SIGN! ! !**
• Pulse oximeter—decreased or decreasing saturation. May be interpreted as artifacts or problems with machine. Be wary of pulse oximeter readings of 85% (equal saturated). May have many false positive results because of movements, cautery, or peripheral circulation problems.
• Arterial and venous blood gases—decreased PaO_2
  Alveolar-arterial oxygen difference—$P(A-a)O_2$ will be normal if hypoxemia is due to decreased PaO_2, increased if hypoxemia due to venous admixture problems
• CXR—look for areas of atelectasis, lung collapse, or evidence of aspiration

Key Reference: Gaba DM, Fish KJ, Howard SK: Crisis Management in Anesthesiology. New York, Churchill-Livingstone, 1994, pp 79–82.

PERIOPERATIVE IMPLICATIONS

Monitoring
• Routine
• ABG

Airway
• Must assure patency and intact circuit at all times

Maintenance
• Adequate FIO_2 and alveolar ventilation

ANTICIPATE PROBLEMS/CONCERNS

• Must have a high index of suspicion whenever SaO_2 decreases or any of the clinical subjective or objective signs and symptoms are present. Always assume the decreased SaO_2 does not reflect a problem with the pulse oximeter, but signifies a real problem.

186 DISEASES

IgA DEFICIENCY

David Bui, M.D.
Paul R. Knight III, M.D., Ph.D.

RISK

- The most common immunodeficiency disorder
- Incidence has been estimated to be 1 in 400 to 1 in 3000, depending on ethnic groups
- More prevalent among European descendants

PERIOPERATIVE RISKS

- Increased incidence of pulmonary complications, atopic disorders, and postoperative infections

WORRY ABOUT

- Recurrent sinopulmonary infections leading to decreased pulmonary reserve
- Associated autoimmune disorders
- Associated GI disorders leading to volume depletion
- Anaphylactic reactions from transfusion of blood products containing IgA

OVERVIEW

- An immunodeficiency syndrome with increased susceptibility to nosocomial infection
- Most patients are healthy
- Cell-mediated immunity is usually normal
- Co-existing diseases may include allergies, recurrent sinopulmonary infection, GI disease, and autoimmune disease
- Decreased synthesis or secretion of IgA

ICD-9-CM Code: 279.01

ETIOLOGY

- Specific cause has not been conclusively identified
- Increased prevalence of histocompatibility groups HLA-A1, -B8, and -Dw3 has been identified in patients with IgA deficiency and autoimmune diseases
- There have been several reported cases of acquired IgA deficiency
- Associated with decreased synthesis or secretion of IgA rather than absence of IgA-producing lymphocytes

USUAL TREATMENT

- Should not be treated with gamma globulin
- Aggressive use of antibiotics
- Therapy directed toward specific co-existing diseases

ASSESSMENT POINTS

SYSTEM	EFFECT	ASSESSMENT BY HX	PE	TEST
CV	Decreased reserve, hypovolemia	Dyspnea on exertion	Tachycardia, orthostatic hypotension	ECG, ECHO
RESP	Recurrent infection, hemosiderosis, asthma	↓ Exercise tolerance	Wheezing, rales	CXR, PFTs
GI	Chronic gastroenteritis, malnutrition, malabsorption	Chronic diarrhea	Cachexia	Electrolytes, BUN, serum albumin
HEME	Nonspecific	Depends on the extent of co-existing diseases		Serum IgA, anti-IgA antibody, Coombs test
RENAL	Nonspecific	Varies in severity depending on the extent of co-existing diseases		BUN, Cr
CNS	Degenerative, demyelinating	Mental retardation associated with ataxia-telangiectasia		MRI

Key Reference: Knight PR: *In* Lema MI (ed): Problems in Anesthesia. Philadelphia, JB Lippincott, 1993, pp 375–391.

PERIOPERATIVE IMPLICATIONS

Preoperative Preparation

- Continue or initiate antibiotic therapy
- Optimize any underlying organ dysfunction and volume status

Monitoring

- Consider invasive hemodynamic monitoring in debilitated patients

Airway

- Strict aseptic technique
- Universal precautions
- May encounter difficult intubation in patients with associated rheumatoid arthritis

Induction

- Hypotension secondary to hypovolemia and/or decreased cardiac reserve
- Wheezing due to allergic condition relatively resistant to conventional therapy

Maintenance

- May require high inspired O_2
- Regional anesthesia and careful titration of anesthetic agents due to potential underlying cardiovascular and pulmonary diseases

Extubation

- Careful assessment of neuromuscular function due to potential drug-drug interaction

Adjuvants

- Depend on organ dysfunction

Postoperative Period

- May require intensive pulmonary therapy
- Maintain strict antiseptic precaution

ANTICIPATED PROBLEMS/CONCERNS

- Anaphylactic reaction from transfusions of blood or blood products containing IgA to individual with IgA antibodies
- Asthmatic patient with IgA deficiency is relatively resistant to treatment
- Increased risk of nosocomial infection

IMMUNE SUPPRESSION

Paul R. Knight III, M.D., Ph.D.

RISK

- 0.25 to 1.5% of US population have HIV or other cause of immune suppression

PERIOPERATIVE RISKS

- 22.2% 30-day mortality in one study of AIDS patients undergoing intra-abdominal surgery
- Mortality greatest at the extremes of age
- Greatest source of morbidity and mortality is 2° to infection
- Pneumonia accounts for ~40% of all deaths
- Increased incidence of postoperative pneumonia, wound infection, postoperative sepsis, respiratory insufficiency, and hypotension due to cardiovascular instability
- Increased healing time

WORRY ABOUT

- Nosocomial transmission of infection
- Transmission of pathogenic drug-resistant strains of microbial agents to medical personnel (e.g., new strains of TB)
- ↓ Pulm reserve due to repeated infections
- Decreased myocardial reserve secondary to underlying disease and generalized poor health

OVERVIEW

- Immune suppression can arise from multiple causes
- Intraoperatively, surgical trauma, anesthetic agents, blood transfusion with/without severe hemorrhage decreases the immune response

ICD-9-CM Code: 279.3 (Immune deficiency)

ETIOLOGY

- Drugs, cancer, infections (HIV), massive burns, or trauma
- Primary immune deficiency
- Very young have immature immune systems
- The aged develop thymic involution and decreased T-cell mediated responses
- Smoking decreases respiratory defense mechanisms

USUAL TREATMENT

- Preoperative antibiotics
- Strict sterile procedures and universal precautions
- Immune-enhancing adjuvants
- Fastidious personal hygiene

ASSESSMENT POINTS

SYSTEM	EFFECT	ASSESSMENT BY HX	PE	TEST
BLOOD	Anemia, neutropenia, lymphocytopenia, hypoglobulinemia, recurrent bacteremia	Easy fatigue, recurrent fever, sweats, and chills	Pale, petechiae	Hct/Hgb, WBC, plasma proteins, special lymphocyte counts (e.g., CD4+ cells)
CV	SBE, decreased cardiovascular reserve, hypovolemia, drug-induced injury (e.g., arabinomycin), mycotic aneurysms	Decreased exercise tolerance	Murmurs: orthostatic hypotension, abnormal HR	ECG, ECHO
RESP	Recurrent pulm infections, pulm fibrosis	Decreased exercise tolerance		CXR, spirometry
GI	Chronic gastroenteritis, chronic malnutrition	Chronic diarrhea	Cachexia	Electrolytes, albumin
RENAL	Chronic pyelonephritis, bladder infections, chronic cystitis, drug-induced injury (e.g., cyclosporine)	Recurrent urinary tract infections, frequency		BUN, Cr, pyelogram
CNS	Mycotic infarcts	Minor strokes	Focal lesions	Brain scan
MS	Osteomyelitis	Deep pain located over involved area	Point tenderness	X-ray

Key Reference: Knight PR: *In* Lema MJ (ed): Problems in Anesthesia. JB Lippincott Co, 1993, pp 375–391.

PREOPERATIVE IMPLICATIONS

Preoperative Preparation

- Continue or initiate antibiotic therapy and immune therapy
- Optimize underlying organ system dysfunction.
- Assess volume status

Monitoring

- Consider arterial line, PA line, or other invasive hemodynamic monitors in severely debilitated patients

Airway

- Strict aseptic technique and universal precautions when handling the airway

Induction

- Chronic respiratory injury may cause increased tendency to desaturate
- Hypotension due to decreased myocardial reserve and/or relative hypovolemia

- Decreased drug requirements 2° to decreased plasma proteins

Maintenance

- Increased inspired O_2 may be required due to chronic lung infections
- Decreased myocardial reserve may require careful selection and titration of anesthetic agents or local or regional anesthesia for peripheral procedures
- Preemptive pain management may protect against additional immune suppression

Extubation

- Due to weakness and drug-drug interactions, return of strength should be carefully evaluated.

Adjuvants

- Transplantation and anti-cancer drug interactions need to be considered (e.g., cyclosporine and barbiturates, narcotics, and muscle relaxants); bleomycin and O_2 administration

Postoperative Period

- Resp adequacy should be carefully followed and may require intensive care monitoring
- Maintain careful antisepsis procedures for extended periods

ANTICIPATED PROBLEMS/CONCERNS

- The greatest intraoperative risk to these patients is infection; therefore, strict hygienic practices are required
- The general state of nutrition, recurrent infections, and the underlying cause of the immune suppression all tend to generally decrease respiratory reserve and cardiovascular stability
- Risk of transmission of drug-resistant pathogenic microbial agents to medical personnel via blood products

IMPLANTABLE CARDIOVERTER-DEFIBRILLATORS (ICDs) — MANAGEMENT

Paul D. Eckenbrecht, M.D.

RISK

- Persons within US: 300,000/y suffer sudden cardiac death (SCD); 10,000/y undergo ICD implantation, and more than 30,000 live with an ICD.
- 76% of ICD patients are male.

PERIOPERATIVE RISKS

- Presence of ICD is not a risk in itself
- Associated diseases: spontaneous dysrhythmias (VTach/VFib)—100%; CAD—65%; cardiomyopathy—19%; LV dysfunction with mean LVEF 35±10%; valvular disease—8%; mitral valve prolapse—4%; hypertrophic cardiomyopathy—1%.
- ↑ Risk of perioperative ventricular dysrhythmias, myocardial ischemia, and LV dysfunction with hypotension and CHF.

WORRY ABOUT

- Electromagnetic interference (EMI) can cause ICD malfunctions.
- Strong, continuous EMI can (1) inhibit therapy because system can no longer sense intrinsic rhythm; (2) activate or deactivate a CPI Ventak AICD depending on its present mode; (3) temporarily suspend both VT and VF detection and therapy capability of a Medtronic PCD or Ventritex Cadence.
- EMI may cause incorrect sensing and deliver inappropriate therapy.
- Transthoracic paddles should be positioned perpendicular to a line between the epicardial patches.

OVERVIEW

- All ICDs have two interrelated functions: dysrhythmia detection and dysrhythmia therapy.
- Dysrhythmia detection may be based on morphology (electrogram shape) or rate criteria.
- For dysrhythmia therapy, the CPI Ventak AICD treats both VT and VF with countershocks only.
- The Medtronic PCD and Ventritex Cadence have tiered therapy: VVI pacing for bradycardia, antitachycardia pacing (ATP) and low energy cardioversion for VT, and high-energy defibrillation for VF.
- Epicardial patch-patch leads are most frequently present in devices implanted before 1993.
- Newer, more recently implanted devices often have a left pectoral subcutaneous patch, and/or transvenous sense/pace and defibrillating leads.

ICD-9-CM Codes: VT, 427.1; VF, 427.41

ETIOLOGY

- SCD is a multifactorial problem: A structural cardiac abnormality interacts with an acute trigger and results in death via a final common pathway of VT/VF.
- Myocardial damage is the primary dysrhythmic substrate
- Low LVEF (≤35%) is a strong, independent predictor for SCD
- Acute triggers include myocardial ischemia, sympathetic stimulation, lyte abn (K+, Mg2+), prodysrhythmic drug effects

USUAL TREATMENT

- Survivors of cardiac arrest due to VT/VF not associated with acute MI and/or sustained VT who at EP study are noninducible, nonsuppressed by drug or surgical therapy, or intolerant of drugs: No randomized trial demonstrates that ICDs are superior to EP-directed, antidysrhythmic drug therapy for sustained VT.
- First-line therapy for poorly tolerated VT in association with impaired LV function, or VT in patients who are not inducible at EPS
- 80% with an ICD receive concomitant antidysrhythmic therapy to reduce required device interventions.

ASSESSMENT POINTS

SYSTEM	EFFECT	ASSESSMENT BY HX	PE	TEST
CV	Myocardial ischemia LV dysfunction	Angina symptoms Exercise tolerance DOE, anginal equivalent	S_3, rales	ECG, thallium exercise stress test ECHO, MUGA Ventriculography
RESP	Amiodarone toxicity CHF	Exercise tolerance, DOE PND, orthopnea	S_3, rales	PFTs, ABG CXR
NEURO	CV disease	Stroke, TIAs	Bruits	Carotid duplex
RENAL	Renal insufficiency		Edema	BUN, Cr
LYTES	Reversible VT/VF	Diuretic Rx		Serum K+ and Mg2+

Key Reference: Nacarelli GV, Veltri EP: Implantable Cardioverter-Defibrillators. Cambridge, MA, Blackwell, 1993.

PERIOPERATIVE IMPLICATIONS

Preoperative Preparation

- All ICD dysrhythmia detection and therapy functions should be turned off preoperatively.
- The Ventak AICD can be deactivated with an external magnet. When a magnet is applied to an active unit, R-wave synchronized tones will be heard, after which a continuous tone will indicate device deactivation. *Reactivate AICD postop* by applying a magnet until intermittent tones are heard again.
- Both Medtronic PCD and Ventritex Cadence should have their VT and VF detection and therapy programmed OFF. Such programming leaves their VVI pacing intact.
- An external magnet will temporarily suspend both VT and VF detection and therapy functions of a PCD or Cadence. Removing the magnet restores both functions (done under emergent conditions when a programmer is not available).
- Transthoracic countershock becomes necessary for VT/VF once ICD is turned off. Transthoracic paddles should be positioned perpendicular to a line between the epicardial patches.

Monitoring

- Routine
- When PACs are removed they may dislodge defibrillating leads positioned in SVC.
- Dislodgment of transvenous sense/pace and defibrillating leads placed in the RV apex is less likely, especially those >6 wk of age.
- TEE a reasonable alternative to a PAC if hardware dislodgment is serious concern.

Airway

- Tracheal intubation may cause sympathetic stimulation and myocardial ischemia, acute triggers of VT/VF in patients at risk for SCD.

Preinduction/Induction

- None

Maintenance

- Maintain normothermia and Hct ≥28 with CAD and LV dysfunction.
- ↑ Incidence of intraoperative conduction defects, atropine-resistant bradycardia, CHB, pacemaker and inotropic dependency, α blockade with low SVR and hepatic, thyroid, and pulmonary dysfunction in patients taking chronic, preop amiodarone.

Extubation

- Same concern as intubation

Postoperative Period

- Consider epidural for postop pain.
- Reactivate ICD postop after electrocautery no longer needed.

ANTICIPATED PROBLEMS/CONCERNS

- Transthoracic paddles should be positioned perpendicular to a line between the ICD epicardial patches (energy requirements for defibrillation increase with antidysrhythmics [class IA, B, C, including lidocaine, propranolol, amiodarone, verapamil]; halogenated hydrocarbons; hypothermia; myocardial ischemia; acidosis).
- Temporary pacing can cause a Ventak AICD to deliver needless countershocks. Use bipolar pacing electrodes, the lowest possible mA output for capture, and the maximum sensitivity.
- Skin potential produced by ICD discharge not harmful to caregivers in contact with patient.

INFRATENTORIAL TUMORS

Marie L. Young, M.D.

RISK

• ~⅔ of intracranial tumors in children are in the posterior fossa
• Primary intra-axial lesions are generally malignant; extra-axial lesions are generally benign

PERIOPERATIVE RISKS

• Signs, symptoms of brainstem compression

WORRY ABOUT

• ↑ ICP, hydrocephalus
• Impaired protective airway reflexes, aspiration
• Irregular respiration due to brainstem compression, swelling
• Impaired level of consciousness

OVERVIEW

• Prognosis is poor with glioblastoma, infiltrating brainstem glioma
• Pediatric cystic cerebellar astrocytoma is associated with 80% survival at 20 years
• Benign lesions such as meningioma, acoustic neuroma have low morbidity, mortality, but may recur if resection is incomplete
• Degree of head elevation influences incidence, severity of air embolism (sitting > prone > park bench/lateral position)

ICD-9-CM Codes: 191.6; 191.7; 225.1; 225.2

ETIOLOGY

• Astrocytoma, medulloblastoma, brainstem glioma are the most common posterior fossa tumors in children
• Acoustic neuroma, metastases, meningioma are the most common posterior fossa tumors in adults

USUAL TREATMENT

• Surgical removal or debulking
• Primary or adjuvant radiotherapy
• CSF diversion (ventriculostomy or shunt)
• Steroids to ↓ peritumor edema

ASSESSMENT POINTS

SYSTEM	EFFECT	ASSESSMENT BY HX	PE	TEST
HEENT	Tonsillar herniation Cranial nerve VII compression	Dysphagia, change in voice Tinnitus, ipsilateral hearing impairment	Gag dysfunction	Indirect laryngoscopy Hearing exam
CV	Progressive brainstem compression Ischemic cardiomyopathy		Bradycardia Hypertension S₃ gallop, CHF	ECG
RESP	Progressive tonsillar herniation		Hyperventilation Irregular respiration Apnea	CT exam MRI
GI	↑ ICP	Nausea Vomiting		CT scan MRI
CNS	↑ ICP	Listlessness, headache, nausea, drowsiness, diplopia	Papilledema	CT scan MRI
MS	Lesion in cerebellar midline Lesion in cerebellar hemisphere	Truncal ataxia	Nystagmus Hypotonia, limb ataxia Intention tremor	Extraocular movement abnormalities

Key Reference: Wen DY, Haines SJ, Young ML: In Cottrell, Smith (eds): Anesthesia and Neurosurgery, 3rd ed. St. Louis, Mosby–Year Book, 1994, pp 323–363.

PERIOPERATIVE IMPLICATIONS

Preoperative Preparation

• Individualize to physical status, presence of ↑ ICP, anxiety level
• Avoid narcotic premedication if risk of ↑ ICP
• Oral benzodiazepines effective in reducing anxiety

Monitoring

• Goals are maintenance of adequate CNS perfusion and cardiorespiratory stability, detection/treatment of air embolism, and surgical brainstem compression
• Capnography, precordial Doppler ultrasound, right atrial catheter for air embolism detection/retrieval (TEE if available)
• Brainstem auditory evoked responses and cranial nerve VII stimulation may reduce morbidity from surgical manipulation

Airway

• Verify appropriate endotracheal tube position after final positioning; avoid large bite blocks and oral airways to minimize tongue and soft tissue compression, postoperative airway swelling

Induction

• Hypotension on induction can be offset by preinduction IV hydration

Maintenance

• Preserve autonomic reflexes; avoid long-acting vasodilators
• Monitor for changes in electrolyte balance due to loop and osmotic diuretics
• Avoid severe hypothermia (<32°C), hyperglycemia
• Controlled positive pressure ventilation, adequate hydration decrease risk of air embolism

Extubation

• Patient should be awake, following commands, and showing return of protective airway reflexes

Adjuvants

• Short-acting vasopressors or vasodilators for maintenance of cardiovascular stability

Postoperative Period

• Suspect brainstem compression or hematoma if postoperative hypertension or profound bradycardia persists in previously normotensive patient
• Avoid potent narcotic analgesic drugs that may produce hypercarbia, decreased intracranial compliance

ANTICIPATED PROBLEMS/CONCERNS

• Patients with higher grade malignancy have greater likelihood of postoperative brain swelling

INSULINOMA

Jesse J. Muir, M.D.

RISK

- Rare tumors
- Clinically important hyperfunctional islet cell tumors have an incidence of <1:100,000

PERIOPERATIVE RISKS

- Hypoglycemia

WORRY ABOUT

- Intraoperative hypoglycemia
- Possibility of multiple endocrine neoplasia syndrome type I (MEN-I), i.e., pituitary tumors, parathyroid tumors, islet cell tumors (often multiple)
- Multiple insulinomas are possible, even in absence of MEN-I

OVERVIEW

- Hypoglycemia has many causes; extensive endocrine evaluation is needed to make diagnosis.
- Diagnosis strongly suggested by Whipple's triad: (1) symptoms of hypoglycemia provoked by fasting; (2) blood glucose levels < 50 mg/dl; and (3) relief of symptoms with glucose
- Diagnosis made by showing circulating insulin level is inappropriately high for existing blood glucose level; esp at time of hypoglycemia, two types of measurement can be made: during fasting (up to 72 h) and after provocative testing
- In normals, the ratio of plasma insulin (μU/ml) to blood glucose (mg/dl) is <0.4. A higher ratio suggests inappropriately high insulin levels for existing blood glucose.
- Tumor(s) localization vital if blind pancreatic resection is to be avoided

ICD-9-CM Code: 211.7 (Benign)

ETIOLOGY

- Unknown: most are solitary adenomas
- MEN-I syndrome present in 4% of patients with insulinomas

USUAL TREATMENT

- Surgery
- Diazoxide if surgery fails or if patient not a surgical candidate

ASSESSMENT POINTS

SYSTEM	EFFECT	ASSESSMENT BY HX	PE	TEST
RENAL	May have renal stone if MEN-I	Renal colic	Flank pain	Serum Ca^{2+}
ENDO	MEN-I, possible hyperparathyroid Pituitary tumors	Renal colic Vision changes	Flank pain Look for signs of pituitary dysfunction	Serum Ca^{2+} Skull x-rays Appropriate endocrine testing
	Insulinoma	Seizures or "spells"	Mental status evaluation	Fasting blood glucose and insulin levels
CNS	Seizures or abnormal behavior secondary to hypoglycemia	Hx of seizure or spells Frequent meals to avoid "spells"	Mental status evaluation	Blood glucose

Key Reference: Muir JJ, et al: Glucose management in patients undergoing operation for insulinoma removal. Anesthesiology 1983; 59:371–375.

PERIOPERATIVE IMPLICATIONS

Preoperative Preparation

- Monitor mental status for hypoglycemia
- Rule out MEN-I

Monitoring

- Measure plasma glucose every 10–15 min
- Intermittent sampling is safe as long as plasma glucose is kept above 60 mg/dL
- Consider arterial line or CVP to facilitate sampling ease

Airway

- None

Induction

- None

Maintenance

- Tend to be long procedures; careful attention to fluid status
- Have dextrose solutions available to Rx hypoglycemia

Extubation

- None

ANTICIPATED PROBLEMS/CONCERNS

- It has been proposed that glucose solutions be avoided intraoperatively so that hyperglycemic rebound can be used to confirm tumor removal; less than half of patients will have this "rebound" in first 30 min following tumor removal
- Hyperglycemic rebound cannot be used as proof of complete tumor removal; some patients who have hyperglycemia rebound continue to have hypoglycemic episodes
- Thorough pancreatic exploration combined with intraoperative sonography has been reported to be technique of choice to identify insulinoma intraoperatively
- Although patients may appear to have had successful tumor removal, they must be monitored for hypoglycemia in the postoperative period.

INTRACRANIAL HYPERTENSION (ICH)

Joseph Dooley, M.D.
Kevin J. Gingrich, M.D.

RISK

- People within US: >50% of patients presenting with head trauma or other intracranial pathology (>600,000/y).
- Gender predominance: depends on etiology

PERIOPERATIVE RISKS

- ↑ Risk of brain ischemia and herniation leading to brain infarction, disability, coma, and death
- ↑ Risk of permanent CNS dysfunction

WORRY ABOUT

- Controlling intracranial pressure and preventing brain ischemia/herniation
- CV and resp instability
- Coexisting injuries in trauma patients (occult cervical spine and intra-abdominal injuries)

OVERVIEW

- Intracranial compartment has fixed volume with three components (brain = 85%, CSF = 10%, cerebral blood volume [CBV] = 5%)
- Increased volume of one component (e.g., tumor, hydrocephalus, or hemorrhage) elevates ICP, causing intracranial HTN (ICH: ICP >20 mmHg)
- ICH reduces cerebral perfusion pressure (CPP = MAP – ICP), causing brain ischemia/infarction
- ICH causes intracranial pressure gradients that may extrude brain parenchyma through dural or bony passages, resulting in herniation
- Some anesthetic agents, HTN, hypercapnia, and hypoxemia increase cerebral blood flow (CBF), increasing CBV and ICP

ICD-9-CM Code: 348.2 (benign)

ETIOLOGY

- Usually a secondary process accompanying other pathology (e.g., head injuries, hemorrhage, hydrocephalus, abscess, primary and metastatic brain tumors, cerebral infarcts, hypertensive and metabolic encephalopathies, venous thrombosis, infection, burns, near-drowning, and status epilepticus) that increases brain, CSF, or cerebral blood volumes

USUAL TREATMENT

- Treatment of primary disease (e.g., removal of tumor, hematoma, or abscess)
- Avoid hypercapnia/hypoxemia and deliver moderate hyperventilation acutely
- Establish stable hemodynamics
- Head elevation (head above heart) and neutral neck position to promote cerebral venous return
- Osmotic therapy (mannitol) to decrease neuronal size
- Corticosteroids (neoplasm or abscess)
- CSF drainage
- Sedation and NMB in responsive patients

ASSESSMENT POINTS

SYSTEM	EFFECT	ASSESSMENT BY HX	PE	TEST
CV	Dysrhythmias, unstable vital signs Inferior wall myocardial ischemia		BP Pulse S_3 gallop	Tachycardia, bradycardia, prolonged QT interval, ECG, ECHO
RESP	Irregular breathing		Resp rate and pattern	
GI	Reduced gut motility	Vomiting		
RENAL	SIADH Central diabetes insipidus		Oliguria Polyuria	Urinalysis, serum electrolytes
CNS	Altered function	Headache, vomiting, unconsciousness	Neurologic deficits, papilledema	Head CT

Key Reference: Schweitzer JS, Bergsneider M, Becker DP: Intracranial pressure monitoring. *In* Cottrell JE, Smith DS (eds): Anesthesia and Neurosurgery, 3rd ed. St. Louis, Mosby-Year Book, 1994, pp 117–135.

PERIOPERATIVE IMPLICATIONS

Preoperative Preparation

- Judicious or no preop sedation because of risk of hypoventilation
- Assess volume status

Monitoring

- Consider arterial catheter for BP monitoring and for serial ABGs to properly manage mechanical ventilation
- Consider ICP monitor and CVP line
- Glucose

Airway

- Neutral cervical spine position for tracheal intubation if possible traumatic injury
- Possible aspiration risk (emergency procedure or severe ICH)

Preinduction/Induction

- Neutral neck position and head elevation
- If patient cooperative, establish voluntary hyperventilation; otherwise hyperventilate as soon as possible.
- Induction technique should maintain CV stability and not ↑ CBF (e.g., fentanyl, thiopental, nondepolarizing NM blocker; avoid succinylcholine unless airway concerns override)

Maintenance

- O_2, N_2O (controversial) or hypnotic (thiopental or propofol) infusion, and narcotic infusion with 0.25% isoflurane or equivalent sevoflurane. Up to 1.2% isoflurane without narcotic infusion. Avoid halothane and Ethrane.
- Moderate hyperventilation (Pa_{CO_2} to ~30 mmHg) and avoid PEEP.
- Maintain mean arterial pressure such that estimated CPP >60 mmHg

Extubation

- Maintain tracheal intubation if concerns about postop resp function; otherwise, prompt extubation for early neurologic evaluation

Adjuvants

- Benzodiazepines, β-blockers, antihypertensives

Postoperative Period

- If ICH persists, adequate ventilation/oxygenation, pain control, sedation essential

ANTICIPATED PROBLEMS/CONCERNS

- Use isotonic crystalloid or colloid IV solutions to minimize brain water and cerebral edema. Avoid dextrose since it may exacerbate effects of brain ischemia.
- Renal dysfunction and severe hypovolemia are possible from preop osmotic therapy.

INTRAOPERATIVE RECALL

Randall C. Cork, M.D., Ph.D.

RISK

- People within USA: 2.5 million
- Gender/race prevalence: None

PERIOPERATIVE RISK

- 0.2–2.0% of all GA
- Incidence of recall is increased in obstetrics (7–28%), major trauma (11–43%), cardiopulmonary bypass (up to 23%), and bronchoscopy (8%), all associated with a "light level" of anesthesia

WORRY ABOUT

- Post-traumatic stress syndrome (PTSS)
- 7% of closed claims from intraoperative recall
- Poor postop recovery

OVERVIEW

- Explicit recall is conscious, deliberate recollection of events
- Implicit recall is change in behavior attributable to intraoperative event
- Both can lead to PTSS
- Underdiagnosed because of inadequate questioning by anesthesiologist and denial by patient

ETIOLOGY

- 70% due to technique, e.g., accidental or purposefully light anesthesia
- 20% due to equipment, e.g., empty vaporizer or faulty ventilator/circuit
- 10% unknown

USUAL TREATMENT

- Discuss the memories/feelings with patient
- Consult with psychologist or psychiatrist for treatment of PTSS

ASSESSMENT POINTS

SYSTEM	EFFECT	TEST
CV	HTN	BP
	Tachycardia	ECG
RESP	Tachypnea	Resp rate
	Sighing	Ventilatory compliance
	Breath holding	Observation
	Bronchospasm	
	↑ Peak inspiratory pressure for same volume	
CNS	Increased autonomic activity	ECG
	HTN	BP
	Tachycardia	Observation
	Diaphoresis	
	Lacrimation	
MS	Spontaneous movement	Ventilatory compliance
	Increased tone	Observation

Key Reference: Hameroff SR, Polson JS, Watt RC: Monitoring anesthetic depth. *In* Blitt C, Hines R (eds): Monitoring in Anesthesia and Critical Care Medicine, 3rd ed. New York, Churchill Livingstone, 1995, pp 491–507.

PERIOPERATIVE IMPLICATIONS

Preoperative Preparation

- Inform patient about risk of explicit and implicit memory and assure that you will be there at all times
- Perhaps allow patient option of earplugs, music, or tape to listen to during anesthetic (certainly for patients with this problem after prior operations/anesthetics)
- Use an amnesiac agent as part of preop medication

Monitoring

- If using muscle relaxants, use twitch monitor to maintain at least one twitch.
- There is no monitor to indicate whether patient is alert or not.

Airway

- Delaying endotracheal intubation beyond the normal period after a short-acting induction agent may result in recall.

Induction

- Use excess induction agent if possible, and supplement if more time is required to control airway.
- Use an amnesiac agent.

Maintenance

- Use spontaneous ventilation, if possible.
- Supplement with volatile agent, and monitor end-tidal concentration.
- Monitor twitch, and maintain one visible.
- Apply earplugs or play audio tapes to patient.

Extubation

- Reverse muscle relaxation well before decreasing anesthetic.

Adjuvants (to decrease incidence)

- Amnesiac agents
- Volatile anesthetics

Postoperative Period

- Always ask
  - Last thing remembered before?
  - First thing remembered after?
  - Anything in between?
  - Dream?
- If evidence of recall, discuss memories/feelings with patient and consult a psychologist or psychiatrist to treat for PTSS

ANTICIPATED PROBLEMS/CONCERNS

- Post-traumatic stress syndrome
- Talkative OR personnel

JAUNDICE

William T. Merritt, M.D.

RISK

- Chronic liver disease consistently 9th most common cause of death in US.
- Male/Female 2/1
- African-American/Caucasian 2/1

PERIOPERATIVE RISKS

- Jaundice per se poses no special risks
- Risks associated with co-existing or underlying conditions

WORRY ABOUT

- Esophageal varices (incompetent lower esophageal sphincter)
- Ascites
- Low systemic vascular resistance
- Bleeding
- Inability to extubate at end of surgery

OVERVIEW

- Mostly unconjugated
  - Excess production
    - Hemolytic anemias (e.g., sickle cell anemia; β-thalassemia major)
  - Extravascular hemolysis (tissue infarction; hemorrhage into tissue, "postoperative jaundice")
  - Ineffective erythropoiesis
  - ↓ Hepatic uptake
    - Sepsis
  - Drugs (e.g., flavaspidic acid, novobiocin, some cholecystographic dyes)
  - Severe, prolonged fasting
  - ↓ Conjugation
  - Neonate: Physiologic jaundice of the newborn; "breast milk" jaundice; hypothyroidism; galactosemia
    - Sepsis
  - Acquired transferase deficiency: drug inhibition (e.g., pregnanediol, chloramphenicol); hepatocellular disease (cirrhosis, hepatitis)
    - Gilbert's disease — ↓ glucuronyl transferase
    - Crigler-Najjar 1 (absent) and II (partial decrease) in glucuronyl transferase
- Mostly conjugated
  - ↓ Hepatic excretion
  - Hereditary/familial: Dubin-Johnson, Rotor syndromes; recurrent intrahepatic cholestasis, benign; gestational cholestatic jaundice—(≈1/13,000 deliveries; 3rd trimester; preeclampsia, nulliparity; twin; ↓ plt)
  - Acquired: Sepsis; hepatocellular disease (drug- and viral-induced hepatitis); postoperative jaundice (pigment overload [transfusions, resorption of hematomas, hemolysis]; hepatocellular damage [drugs, including halothane, shock]; benign postoperative jaundice); drug-induced cholestasis (e.g., oral contraceptives, methyltestosterone)
  - Extrahepatic biliary obstruction (e.g., mechanical, from stones, stricture, tumor)
- Pseudojaundice
  - Dietary carotenoids (primarily infants; excessive intake of vegetables, such as carrots, tomatoes)
  - Poisoning (picric acid)

ICD-9-CM Code: 782.4 (Jaundice, unspecified, non-newborn)

USUAL TREATMENT

- No specific treatment outside of newborn period
- For neonates: fluids, phototherapy, exchange transfusion, albumin, tin mesoporphyrin and IV immunoglobulin Rx have been shown to decrease the level of unconjugated bilirubin below levels regarded to be toxic to the neonatal brain.
- The smaller and sicker the premature infant, the more aggressive the therapy needed.

ASSESSMENT POINTS

SYSTEM	EFFECT	ASSESSMENT BY HX	PE	TEST
HEENT		Duration	Yellow sclerae	
CV	Hyperdynamic Poss ↓ SVR	General Sx	↑ HR; ↓ BP	
RESP	Cirrhotics have 6× increase in pulm HTN	Severe dyspnea, hypoxia, clubbing	Clubbing Cyanosis	ECHO; right heart catheterization if indicated
GI	Severe dysfunction Prolonged effects of most anesthesia drugs	General Sx, reflux, ascites, varices, edema	Signs of chronic liver disease	LFTs Coagulation time HgB, plt
ENDO/ METAB	↓ Synthetic function ↑ Enzymes, ↓ albumin, ↓ hepatic coag factors; ↓ clearance of toxins	General malaise Sx Easy bruising/ bleeding	Jaundice Ecchymoses Hematoma Ascites	LFTs Coagulation time NH$_3$
HEME	↓ Plt	Easy bruising/bleeding	Ecchymoses, hematoma	
SKIN		Duration; evidence of bleeding	Yellow color	
RENAL	↓ Function		Edema	BUN, Cr; Cr may be spuriously lower with high bilirubin
CNS	Recurrent encephalopathy in cirrhosis Cerebral edema in fulminant hepatic failure Autonomic dysfunction	Mental status: Duration of illness Abnormal autonomic function	Normal to encephalopathy/ comatose Orthostatic BP changes	

Key Reference: LaMont JT, Isselbacher KJ: Postoperative jaundice. N Engl J Med 1973; 288:305–307.

PERIOPERATIVE IMPLICATIONS

- Drug— ↓ protein production leads to ↓ albumin binding and potentially more active drug
  - Cimetidine/ranitidine—clearance reduced, esp. in patients with ascites, hypoproteinemia, encephalopathy
  - Benzodiazepines—clearance of oxidative pathway benzodiazepines markedly ↓; glucuronidation path (e.g., lorazepam) not greatly altered. Excessive sedation may occur in severe liver disease.
  - Narcotics—morphine metabolism is fairly normal; meperidine clearance is severely affected; succinylcholine activity may be prolonged somewhat because of ↓ levels of pseudocholinesterase
  - Miscellaneous—β rb's and lidocaine have reduced clearance; diuretics may have reduced natriuretic efficacy
  - Halogenated agents—halothane should be avoided, although the relationships between halothane toxicity and patients with preexisting liver disease are unclear; association of enflurane with hepatic toxicity is less clear; isoflurane preferred agent in setting of liver disease and best preserves liver hemodynamics.

Preoperative Preparation

- Hydration should be adequate; if chronic liver failure, may be total body fluid ↑, but intravascularly ↓.

Monitoring

- NMB—dose muscle relaxants to effect and consider path of elimination
- As appropriate for overall hepatic and other system illness

Airway

- May have bleeding disorder

Induction

- Avoid benzodiazepines
- Consider cricoid pressure if varices present, or Hx of sclerotherapy

Maintenance

- Be mindful of metabolic clearance paths of drugs used
- When practical, use drugs cleared chiefly by nonhepatic paths

Extubation

- May have delay in awakening

ANTICIPATED PROBLEMS/CONCERNS

- Inability to extubate immediately postop due to prolonged action of NMB and sedative/hypnotic/narcotic medications

JEHOVAH'S WITNESS PATIENT

Meg A. Rosenblatt, M.D.

RISK

• Approximately 2 million members in US, 4.9 million worldwide
• Headquartered in Brooklyn, New York

PERIOPERATIVE RISKS

• Mortality 2° to massive hemorrhage

WORRY ABOUT

• Understanding the rights and desires of patient vs. rights of physician prior to need to administer blood or blood products
• Problems arise in emergencies when little time is available for discussion of transfusion issues
• Competent adults are those who know the nature and consequences of their actions; such adults have the right to refuse specific therapies
• *Parens patriae*, the power of the state, represents the duty and interest of the state to preserve the health of minors

OVERVIEW

• Began as Bible study group in early 1800s; became Jehovah's Witnesses in 1931
• Strict interpretation of Bible passages, which forbid eating of blood, interpreted as prohibition of acceptance of blood products to sustain life
• Witnesses believe acceptance of blood products precludes achievement of eternal salvation

USUAL TREATMENT

• Discuss and document preoperatively the potential for life-threatening hemorrhage and therapies and interventions that would be acceptable to the patient
• Seek evidence of advance directive, an affidavit that confirms the patient's refusal to accept a transfusion (which forces discussion and releases physicians/hospitals of responsibility for outcome of the patient's decision)
• Optimize hematocrit, with erythropoietin, prior to elective procedures in which risk for transfusion is high
• Consider contacting a Jehovah's Witness Hospital Liaison Committee, which consists of a group of individuals trained to work as intermediaries in avoiding conflict between patients and physicians
• Contact legal counsel if patient is a minor, is unconscious, or is an incompetent adult

ASSESSMENT POINTS

SYSTEM	ASSESSMENT BY HX	TEST
HEME	Evaluate for treatable forms of anemia	Iron, folate, B_{12} levels BUN/Cr

Key Reference: Mann MC, et al: Management of the severely anemic patient who refuses transfusion: Lessons learned during the care of a Jehovah's Witness. Ann Intern Med 1992; 117:1042–1048.

PERIOPERATIVE IMPLICATIONS

Preoperative Preparations

• Oral iron supplementation
• Consider erythropoietin, 75–100 U/kg SC or IV, 3 times/wk for 3 to 4 wk

Monitoring

• Minimize phlebotomies/pediatric sampling tubes
• Consider oximetric pulmonary artery catheter if high possibility of hemorrhage

Maintenance

• Hypervolemic hemodilution
• Hypotensive anesthetic techniques
• Hypothermia
• Colloid volume expanders: dextran, hydroxyethyl starch, gelatin
• Desmopressin and aprotinin may reduce blood loss in cardiac procedures

Extubation

• Consider postoperative ventilation with neuromuscular blocking agents, sedation, and hypothermia for severe anemia; supplement with IV hyperalimentation, erythropoietin, iron dextran (which may add ~ 100 mg of iron per liter of TPN)

Adjuvants

• May accept use of red blood cell scavenging devices or hypervolemic hemodilution when the equipment is arranged in circuit with patient's circulatory system
• May accept use of closed drainage systems that allow reinfusion of shed mediastinal or wound blood
• May accept use of "minor" blood fractions, such as albumin and clotting factors
• Progesterone decreases blood loss in menstruating patients

JEUNE SYNDROME (ASPHYXIATING THORACIC DYSTROPHY) Anne Marie Lynn, M.D.

RISK

- Rare: 106 reported cases in literature
- Some cases in offspring of consanguineous parents
- Seen in families of Norwegian, African-American, and Japanese descent

PERIOPERATIVE RISKS

- 75% mortality in newborn period from restrictive lung disease
- Respiratory failure from small thoracic cage and hypoplastic lungs
- Affected individuals surviving infancy are reported to have progressive renal disease with cystic lesions
- Liver involvement with fibrosis, cysts, and pancreatic cysts also sometimes seen

WORRY ABOUT

- Respiratory failure with hypoxia and hypercapnia

- Barotrauma with positive-pressure ventilation
- Renal failure may require careful fluid and electrolyte management and selection of non-renally cleared muscle relaxants

OVERVIEW

- Rare autosomal recessive form of dwarfism with a 75% mortality in the newborn period
- Respiratory failure from restrictive thorax and hypoplastic lungs
- If pulmonary involvement is milder, allowing survival, then changes in renal, hepatic, and pancreatic systems (often with cystic lesions and/or fibrosis) are reported
- Postaxial polydactyly is often seen, but nail dysplasia and facial changes are not, helping to separate this from Ellis–van Creveld syndrome
- Cardiac anomalies infrequent except for pulmonary hypertension

- Surgical enlargement of the thorax has been undertaken to increase pulmonary compliance; in some cases respiratory function improves with age, so long-term ventilatory support (months to years) has been attempted
- Larynx is reported to be small in affected children

ICD-9-CM Code: 756.4

ETIOLOGY

- Autosomal recessive inheritance
- Gene involved has not been identified as of yet

USUAL TREATMENT

- Surgical thoracic enlargement requires long-term ventilation, which can be difficult and has a high incidence of barotrauma
- Older children require surgery related to renal failure (dialysis catheters, renal transplantation)

ASSESSMENT POINTS

SYSTEM	EFFECT	ASSESSMENT BY HX	PE	TEST
HEENT	Small larynx			
CV	Pulmonary hypertension	Syncope	↑ 2nd heart sound	ECG (RVH) ECHO
RESP	Stiff, small rib cage Hypoplastic lungs	Assisted ventilation Asynchronous ventilation with agitation/crying	Small chest Horizontal ribs Cyanosis with crying	ABG CXR Oximetry
GI	Hepatic fibrosis/cysts Pancreatic fibrosis/cysts			Abdominal ultrasound
RENAL	Cysts Nephritis			BUN, Cr, abdominal ultrasound
CNS	Retinal degeneration			
MS	Short limbs Polydactyly of hands and feet			

Key Reference: Holtby HM, Relton JES: Orthopedic diseases. *In* Katz J, Steward DJ (eds): Anesthesia and Uncommon Pediatric Diseases, 2nd ed. Philadelphia, WB Saunders, 1993, pp 483–484.

PERIOPERATIVE IMPLICATIONS

Preoperative Preparation

- Assess ventilation
- Evaluate for possible pulmonary hypertension

Monitoring

- Consider arterial catheter

Airway

- Small larynx requires ↓ endotracheal tube size

Induction

- Agitation may make respiration asynchronous (chest/abdomen), causing hypoxemia

Maintenance

- Lung hypoplasia makes barotrauma high risk; consider with acute respiratory deterioration

Extubation

- Document adequate ventilation before extubation; postoperative ventilation may be needed for a prolonged period, especially after thoracoplasty

Adjuvants

- Renal function assessment guides selection of muscle relaxant and fluid management

ANTICIPATED PROBLEMS/CONCERNS

- Asynchronous ventilation during crying with hypoxia
- Barotrauma during assisted mechanical ventilation
- Renal failure
- Postoperative respiratory failure requiring ventilatory support

KARTAGENER'S SYNDROME

Russell C. Raphaely, M.D.
Maureen M. O'Rourke, M.D.

RISK

- In USA and Europe, prevalence of situs inversus varies from 1/6800 to 1/35,000
- ~20% of all persons with situs inversus have bronchiectasis and chronic paranasal sinusitis to complete syndrome described by Kartagener

PERIOPERATIVE RISKS

- Morbidity: Lung infection, pulm edema, atelectasis, sinusitis

WORRY ABOUT

- Airway obstruction due to ineffective clearance of mucus
- Bronchiectasis, which can lead to cor pulmonale and pulm edema

- Chemical injury from aspiration in left lung, which is the larger lung in patients with Kartagener's syndrome
- Unintended bronchial intubation with single-lumen tracheal tube resulting in nonventilation of right lung (in those with pulmonary inversion)
- Left-sided double-lumen tube may occlude orifice of left upper lobe
- Nasal catheters relatively contraindicated because of risk of paranasal sinusitis and ear infections

OVERVIEW

- Situs inversus (including dextrocardia)
- Primary ciliary dyskinesia resulting in chronic resp tract infections, bronchiectasis, sinusitis

ICD-9-CM Code: 759.3

ETIOLOGY

- Congenital defect in synthesis of the protein dynein; genetic—autosomal recessive
- 1/70 persons involved are heterozygous

USUAL TREATMENT

- Aerosol administration to reduce secretion viscosity
- Antimicrobial therapy for chronic resp tract infections, sinusitis
- Surgical intervention for pulm lobectomy as needed
- Chest physical therapy
- Chronic disease with variable onset

ASSESSMENT POINTS

SYSTEM	EFFECT	ASSESSMENT BY HX	PE	TEST
CV	Dextrocardia			CXR ECHO
RESP	Bronchiectasis Ciliary dyskinesia	Dyspnea Cough Halitosis	Decreased breath sounds Rhonchi	CXR Bronchoscopy Spirometry Bronchography
INFECTION	Chronic paranasal	Nasal drainage Morning sore throat	Frontal and maxillary tenderness	Sinus films (CT)
	Bronchitis	Cough Mucus production	Rhonchi	Sputum and tracheal aspirate for culture and Gram stain
	Pneumonia	Cough Fever	Rales Rhonchi	CXR SpO_2
	Otitis media	Earache	Erythematous tympanic membrane	Audiometry Tympanotomy

Key Reference: Ho AMH, Friedland MJ: Kartagener's syndrome: Anesthetic considerations. Anesthesiology 1992; 77:386–388.

PREOPERATIVE PREPARATION

- Consider omitting anticholinergics and cough suppressant from preanesthetic medication.

PERIOPERATIVE IMPLICATIONS

Monitoring

- In dextrocardia, position of ECG leads should be the mirror image of normal, as should be that of paddles of external defibrillation, cardioversion, and pacing.
- Since the great vessels and thoracic duct are likely to be reversed, consider cannulation of the internal jugular vein from the left.

Airway

- Emphasize aseptic technique
- Humidify inspired gases
- Inhalation injury usually occurs in left lung, which is also larger lung

- Bronchial intubation with a single-lumen tracheal tube usually involves left side
- Right bronchial suctioning will be more difficult to perform with nonangulated suction catheters
- Left-sided double-lumen tube may occlude orifice of left upper lobe
- When lung isolation is needed, consider tracheal intubation first with a bronchial blocker in the appropriate bronchus
- If double-lumen tube is required, consider inserting the left-sided tube with the bronchial tube on the right; the endobronchial stylet and the upper part of tube must be bent 180° from original orientation prior to insertion such that the normal curvature of the oropharynx is still followed. The same principles apply to use of a right-sided tube.

Anesthetic Technique

- Employ regional techniques when possible

Extubation

- As soon as possible

Postoperative Considerations

- Consider conduction and non-narcotic analgesia if possible

ANTICIPATED PROBLEMS/CONCERNS

- Lung infection common as result of ciliary dyskinesia
- Fluid overload can precipitate cor pulmonale and pulm edema.
- Avoid nasal catheters/airways to minimize chances of paranasal sinusitis

KEARNS-SAYRE SYNDROME

Jeremy M. Geiduschek, M.D.

RISK

- Less than 300 reported cases
- Same incidence in males and females
- Onset of symptoms before age 20 y

PERIOPERATIVE RISKS

- Cardiac conduction defects progress to complete heart block

WORRY ABOUT

- Cardiac rhythm
- Increasing demand for O_2 leading to lactic acidosis
- Decreased respiratory efficiency 2° to muscle weakness

OVERVIEW

- Triad of findings: chronic progressive external ophthalmoplegia, retinal pigmentary degeneration, and cardiac conduction block.
- Other findings may include: short stature, muscle weakness, developmental delay, dementia, cerebellar ataxia, epilepsy, hypoparathyroidism, diabetes, hypogonadism, nephropathy, hepatic dysfunction, asymmetric septal hypertrophy, cardiomyopathy, ↑ CSF protein, and ↑ serum lactate

ICD-9-CM Code: None listed; Use 759.89 (Congenital malformation affecting multiple systems not elsewhere classified)

ETIOLOGY

- Caused by rearrangement of mitochondrial DNA, KSS is part of spectrum of mitochondrial myopathies and encephalomyopathies
- Heterogeneous disorders that are still being defined
- Sporadic inheritance
- Diagnosis based on clinical findings and muscle biopsy that show abnormal accumulation of mitochondria ("ragged red fibers"); more sophisticated genetic analyses are able to demonstrate mitochondrial DNA deletions or insertions

USUAL TREATMENT

- Complete cardiac evaluation, including Holter monitor and echocardiogram; prophylactic pacemaker insertion for any evidence of AV block
- Treatment with steroids may precipitate hyperglycemia and severe metabolic acidosis
- Routine medical management of any associated findings

ASSESSMENT POINTS

SYSTEM	EFFECT	ASSESSMENT BY HX	PE	TEST
CV	Conduction defect Cardiomyopathy	↓ Exercise tolerance Sx CHF	Bradycardia	ECG, Holter ECHO Electrophysiology
RESP	CHF and muscle weakness may affect respiratory function	↓ Exercise tolerance		
RENAL	Nephropathy			BUN/Cr
ENDO	Hypoparathyroidism Diabetes		Tetany Chvostek's sign Weakness	Calcium FBS
CNS	Ophthalmoplegia Retinal pigment degeneration Hearing loss Cerebellar ataxia Elevated CSF protein	Visual disturbance ↓ Night vision ↓ Mobility	↓ ROM of ocular muscles ↓ Visual acuity "Salt and pepper" pigment changes of retina on funduscopy ↓ Hearing Dysdiadochokinesia Wide-based gait	MRI Lumbar puncture
PNS	Peripheral neuropathy	Weakness	↓ Strength	
MS	Variable muscle weakness	↓ Mobility	↓ Strength Impaired gait	Muscle biopsy

Key Reference: DeVivo DC: The expanding clinical spectrum of mitochondrial diseases. Brain Dev 1993; 15:1–22.

PERIOPERATIVE IMPLICATIONS

Preoperative Preparation

- Be prepared to provide cardiac pacing
- Have magnet if pacemaker already present
- Assess cardiac status

Monitoring

- Routine, assuming no cardiomyopathy or CHF present

Airway

- Routine

Induction

- Consider regional or local anesthesia if applicable
- Avoid administration of muscle relaxant; if needed, use reduced dose.

Maintenance

- No specific technique proven superior

Extubation

- Muscle weakness may delay extubation

Adjuvants

- Sedatives carefully titrated

Postoperative Period

- Watch for respiratory failure 2° to muscle weakness
- Continuous cardiac monitoring

ANTICIPATED PROBLEMS/CONCERNS

- Progression to complete heart block; consider pacemaker insertion with any degree of AV block; have ability to provide cardiac pacing (e.g. transcutaneous pacer)
- So far, mitochondrial myopathies have not been associated with malignant hyperthermia
- Not known if KSS or other mitochondrial myopathies create risk for severe hyperkalemia following succinylcholine administration

KLIPPEL-FEIL SYNDROME

Ronald S. Litman, D.O.

RISK

- Incidence estimated at 1:40,000 live births (probably underestimate, as milder cases go unrecognized)
- Gender/race predilection: none

PERIOPERATIVE RISKS

- Cervical spine instability and cardiopulmonary complications

WORRY ABOUT

- Exacerbation of cervical spine instability during airway maneuvers, endotracheal intubation, and subsequent positioning

OVERVIEW

- Not a disease
- Congenital abnormality consisting of the following triad of findings: (1) fusion of two or more cervical vertebrae; (2) low posterior hairline; (3) cervical immobility
- Severity ranges from mild (often not recognized until late in life) to severe (recognized at birth because of obvious deformity)
- Careful preoperative assessment of cervical spine anatomy and degree of instability
- Review of systems for other congenital abnormalities (many reported; see below)

ICD-9-CM Code: 756.16

ETIOLOGY

- Unknown

USUAL TREATMENT

- None

ASSESSMENT POINTS

SYSTEM	EFFECT	ASSESSMENT BY HX	PE	TEST
HEENT	Head and neck immobility		ROM of cervical spine, facial asymmetry, cleft palate, torticollis, vocal cord dysfunction	Flexion/extension radiographs of cervical spine Consider MRI of cervical spine
CV	Bradyarrhythmias and AV conduction pathway abnormalities (due to CNS malformations) Cardiac defects (most commonly VSD)	Syncope	Murmurs	ECG ECHO
RESP	Central alveolar hypoventilation Pulmonary agenesis or hypoplasia Restrictive lung disease (due to severe scoliosis)	Sleep apnea, snoring, difficulty breathing		ABG CXR (if symptomatic)
RENAL	Urinary tract abnormalities			BUN, Cr if indicated
CNS	Hindbrain abnormalities (e.g., syringomyelia, Arnold-Chiari malformation) Mental retardation	Peripheral neurologic dysfunction (e.g., weakness, paresthesias, paraplegia, quadriplegia)	Neurologic exam	
MS	Scoliosis, Sprengel's deformity (scapular elevation)		Exam of spine and shoulders	Radiographs if indicated

Key Reference: Hall JE, et al: Instability of the cervical spine and neurological involvement in Klippel-Feil syndrome. J Bone Joint Surg Am 1990; 72:460–462.

PERIOPERATIVE IMPLICATIONS

Preoperative Preparation

- Careful and complete evaluation of cervical spine anatomy and instability and of other major organ system abnormalities

Monitoring

- Depends on patient's physical condition

Airway

- If indicated, awake intubation using maneuvers to stabilize cervical spine; complete immobility with use of fiberoptic intubating bronchoscope ideal

Preinduction/Induction

- Depends on patient's physical condition

Maintenance

- Careful positioning of head and neck with maintenance in neutral position

Extubation

- Depends on extent of cervical spine pathology and respiratory compromise

Adjuvants

- No special considerations

ANTICIPATED PROBLEMS/CONCERNS

- Exacerbation of preexisting cervical spine instability leading to neurologic deterioration

LEIGH SYNDROME (SUBACUTE NECROTIZING ENCEPHALOPATHY)

Jeremy M. Geiduschek, M.D.

RISK

- Onset of symptoms usually in infancy
- Rare disorder

PERIOPERATIVE RISKS

- Depends on degree of involvement and presence of renal disease or cardiomyopathy

WORRY ABOUT

- Abnormal regulation of respiration may lead to respiratory failure following sedation for procedures
- Decreased respiratory efficiency 2° to muscle weakness

OVERVIEW

- Neuropathologic entity; diagnosis made at autopsy
- Also called "subacute necrotizing encephalomyelopathy"
- Lesions usually subcortical and symmetric, often in midbrain, pons, basal ganglia, thalamus, and optic nerves; may be present on CT or MRI (cysts, vascular proliferation, demyelination, and neuronal loss)
- Clinical features
  – Age <1 y: diarrhea, poor weight gain, hypotonia, motor regression
  – Age >1 y: progressive CNS dysfunction, ataxia, optic atrophy, ptosis, nystagmus, dystonia, tremor, peripheral neuropathy, abnormal breathing patterns
  – Terminal phase (age variable): muscle atrophy, dysphagia, dysarthria, progressive respiratory insufficiency
  – Renal disease and cardiomyopathy may occur

ICD-9-CM Code: 330.8

ETIOLOGY

- Defects in cytochrome-c oxidase and pyruvate dehydrogenase complex have been implicated as causes

USUAL TREATMENT

- Supportive measures only; use of thiamine has resulted in improved status in a small number of patients

ASSESSMENT POINTS

SYSTEM	EFFECT	ASSESSMENT BY HX	PE	TEST
HEENT	Swallowing difficulties		Sialorrhea	
CV	Cardiomyopathy	Sx CHF	Murmur, gallop holosystolic murmur, pulm edema	ECG CXR ECHO
RESP	CNS disease will affect resp regulation Muscle weakness will affect resp regulation	Response to sedatives History of pneumonia		
GI	Chronic diarrhea	Episodes of dehydration	Hydration status	Electrolytes
ENDO/METAB	Lactic acidosis			Lactate
GU	Nephropathy			BUN/Cr
CNS	Ophthalmoplegia Optic atrophy Ataxia Seizures	Developmental history Loss of milestones	↓ ROM of ocular muscles ↓ Visual acuity Abnormal reflexes Wide-based gait	Cranial CT MRI
PNS	Peripheral neuropathy	Weakness	↓ Strength	
MS	Progressive hypotonia and weakness	↓ Mobility	↓ Strength	

Key Reference: VanCoster R, et al. Cytochrome c oxidase-associated Leigh syndrome: Phenotypic features and pathogenetic speculations. J Neurol Sci 1991; 104:97–111.

PERIOPERATIVE IMPLICATIONS

Preoperative Preparation

- Determine extent of cardiac involvement
- Give preoperative anticholinergic if oral secretions are copious

Monitoring

- Routine, assuming no cardiomyopathy or CHF present

Airway

- Routine

Induction

- No specific technique has been proven superior
- Succinylcholine avoided if peripheral neuropathy present

Maintenance

- No specific technique proven superior

Extubation

- Muscle weakness may delay extubation

Adjuvants

- Sedatives carefully titrated due to ↓ consciousness and weakness

Postoperative Period

- Watch for respiratory failure

ANTICIPATED PROBLEMS/CONCERNS

- Not associated with malignant hyperthermia
- Not known if risk present for severe hyperkalemia following administration of succinylcholine (peripheral neuropathy would theoretically create risk)
- Fatal disorder, with death usually resulting from either progressive cardiac or pulmonary involvement

LESCH-NYHAN SYNDROME

Lawrence O. Larson, M.D.

RISK

- X-linked recessive disorder
- Incidence ~5.2 per million male births

PERIOPERATIVE RISKS

- Airway problems 2° to scarification from self-mutilation
- Impairment of renal function due to obstructive uropathy

WORRY ABOUT

- Aspiration pneumonia
- Drug metabolism and prolonged drug effects 2° to metabolic defect and impaired renal function

OVERVIEW

- Patients usually mentally subnormal
- Patients exhibit characteristic pattern of compulsive self-mutilation, spasticity, and choreoathetosis
- Primary biochemical defect is almost complete absence of hypoxanthine-guanine-phosphoribosyltransferase (HGPRT)
- Enzyme defect leads to excessive purine production and elevated uric acid concentrations

ICD-9-CM Code: 277.2

ETIOLOGY

- Genetic disease inherited as X-linked recessive trait

USUAL TREATMENT

- No specific treatment of enzyme deficiency
- Benzodiazepines frequently used to control self-mutilation and spasticity
- Gene therapy possibility

ASSESSMENT POINTS

SYSTEM	EFFECT	ASSESSMENT BY HX	PE	TEST
HEENT	Distortion of airway structures due to self-mutilation		Examine airway	
CV	Hypertension, CAD Adrenergic pressor response to stress is absent	Angina, angina equiv. symptoms PND	Displaced PMI S_3	ECG Pharmacologic stress testing Coronary angiography and ECHO
RESP	Aspiration pneumonia	SOB following vomiting episode	Rales Wheezing	CXR
GI	Vomiting Athetoid dysphagia	Dysphagia		
RENAL	Decreased renal function due to obstructive uropathy			BUN Cr IVP
CNS	Retardation Seizure disorders Decreased MAO activity		Mental status questioning	EEG Mental function tests
MS	Spasticity Contractures		ROM	

Key Reference: Wilson JR, et al: A molecular survey of hypoxanthine-guanine, phosphoribosyltransferase deficiency in man. J Clin Invest 1986; 77:188.

PERIOPERATIVE IMPLICATIONS

Preoperative Preparations

- Antacids
- H$_2$ blockers
- Metoclopramide
- IV access may be difficult

Monitoring

- Routine
- ST segment analysis if CAD present

Airway

- Rapid-sequence induction
- Avoid succinylcholine
- Awake fiberoptic intubation

Preinduction/Induction

- Restraints
- Avoid agents with renal metabolism

Maintenance

- Avoid agents with renal toxicity
- No one agent or technique shown superior
- Administer exogenous catecholamines with caution

Extubation

- Awake to avoid aspiration

Adjuvants/Postoperative Period

- Restraints
- Benzodiazepines for spasticity

ANTICIPATED PROBLEMS/CONCERNS

- History unavailable or inaccurate because of retardation

LEUKEMIA

Subhash Jain, M.D.
Nolan Tzou, M.D.

RISK

- Incidence in USA: 2.8% all new cancers, 5/100,000 (acute) (children and adult)
  - CLL: 2.5/100,000
  - CML: 1/100,000
- 15× greater incidence in patients with Down's syndrome

PERIOPERATIVE RISKS

- Immunosuppression creates risk of both minor and major infections; sepsis, interstitial pneumonitis, encephalopathy
- Hematoma/bleeding 2° to thrombocytopenia and splenic sequestration of platelets

WORRY ABOUT

- Bone marrow suppression with nitrous oxide; no evidence that nitrous oxide adversely affects bone marrow engraftment
- Clinical case reports of patients with ALL who developed malignant hyperthermia
- Neuropathy related to chemotherapy

OVERVIEW

- Hematologic malignancy with proliferation of cells may cause ↓ in amino acids causing fatigue and metabolic starvation
- Invasion possible in all organ systems
- Usually outpatient treatment, but may require several procedures including bone marrow aspiration, central venous access placement, lumbar puncture, bronchoscopy, pericardiocentesis

ICD-9-CM Codes: 208.0 (undifferentiated, acute, blastic); 204.0 (lymphoblastic)

ETIOLOGY

- Unknown
- Strong suspicion that leukemia and lymphoma are virus-induced

USUAL TREATMENT

- AML
  - Ara-C
  - Anthracyclines: daunorubicin, idarubicin
  - Vinca alkaloids: epipodophyllotoxin, vincristine/vinblastine
  - Bone marrow transplant
- CML
  - Busulfan
  - Hydroxyurea
  - α interferon
  - Bone marrow transplant
- CLL
  - Cyclophosphamide
  - Corticosteroid
  - Fludarabine
  - Cytarabine

ASSESSMENT POINTS

SYSTEM	EFFECT	ASSESSMENT BY HX	PE	TEST
HEENT	Ulceration, oral lesions	Dysphagia	Airway assessment	
CV	Rare: Pericardial effusion, conduction defects, murmurs, CHF	Dyspnea, fatigue	Narrow pulse pressure, pericardial friction, rub, cardiomegaly	CXR ECG ECHO
GI	Hepatosplenomegaly Nutritional support may be necessary to prevent hypoalbuminemia and loss of immunocompetence	Loss of appetite	Hepatosplenomegaly	Albumin
HEME	Anemia Leukostasis Thrombocytopenia	Weakness, fatigue	Pallor Ecchymoses Petechiae	CBC Bone marrow aspirate results
RENAL	Renal failure from tumor lysis syndrome (acute loss of tumor)	↓ Urine output	↓ Urine output	BUN/Cr ↑ Phosphate, ↑ or ↓ Ca^{2+} ↑ K$^+$
CNS	Cranial nerve infiltration (very rare) Meningeal leukemia (less common in adults) Vincristine neuropathy	Cranial nerve palsies, clouding of mental status Peripheral neuropathy	Weakness	EMG
MS	Infiltration of bony cortex and periosteum, synovial membranes	Bone pain	Bone swelling	X-ray CT scan

Key Reference: Dewhirst WE, Glass DD: Hematologic disease. *In* Katz J, et al (eds): Anesthesia and Uncommon Diseases, 3rd ed. Philadelphia, WB Saunders, 1990, pp 404–406.

PERIOPERATIVE IMPLICATIONS

Preoperative Preparation

- Assess volume status, evidence of N/V, diarrhea, oral mucositis

Monitoring

- Routine

Airway

- Signs of dysphagia, ulcerations from chemotherapy and candidiasis
- Oral leukemia lesions can occur prior to or during therapy

Induction

- Brief heparinization and thrombocytopenia before bone marrow aspiration may influence choice of spinal or epidural

Maintenance/Extubation

- Based on clinical status of patient

ANTICIPATED PROBLEMS/CONCERNS

- Risk of infection, aseptic technique with placement of all lines

LIPIDEMIAS

Uday Jain, Ph.D., M.D.

RISK

- People within the USA: 10% of children, 25% of adult population
- Race with highest prevalence: None

PERIOPERATIVE RISKS

- Myocardial ischemia, infarction, CHF
- Stroke and TIAs
- Pancreatitis with hypertriglyceridemia

WORRY ABOUT

- New-onset angina, increasing frequency or severity of angina
- Worsening or new-onset CHF
- Transient ischemic attacks of CNS
- Peripheral atherosclerosis

OVERVIEW

- Hypertriglyceridemia, hypercholesterolemia (see separate sections)
- Hypolipidemia: Autosomal recessive Tangier disease (severe deficiency of HDL); familial hypoalphalipoproteinemia (HDL deficiency); LDL deficiency (autosomal recessive abetalipoproteinemia, autosomal dominant familial hypobetalipoproteinemia); normotriglyceridemic abetalipoproteinemia (LDL absent); 2° to cancer, myeloproliferative disorders, liver failure
- Lipodystrophy: Familial generalized lipodystrophy (Berardinelli-Seip syndrome: autosomal recessive, leads to macrosomia); Köbberling-Dunnigan syndrome (familial lipodystrophy of limbs and trunk, autosomal dominant, may lead to macrosomia)

ICD-9-CM Codes: 272.0–9
See also Coronary Artery Disease, Atherosclerotic Disease, Hypercholesterolism, and Hypertriglyceridemia in Diseases section

ETIOLOGY

- Autosomal dominant or recessive inheritance
- Secondary to systemic illness

USUAL TREATMENT

- Diet and exercise
- Cholestyramine and colestipol inhibit absorption of bile acids derived from cholesterol
- Neomycin blocks cholesterol absorption
- HMG CoA reductase inhibitors (lovastatin, pravastatin, simvastatin) reduce cholesterol synthesis and are commonly used
- Thyroid hormone clears LDL
- Probucol reduces LDL but also HDL
- Nicotinic acid inhibits VLDL, LDL production
- Fibric acids clofibrate and gemfibrozil cause catabolism of triglyceride-rich lipoproteins

ASSESSMENT POINTS

SYSTEM	EFFECT	ASSESSMENT BY HX	PE	TEST
HEENT	Tangier disease		Lobulated, bright orange-yellow tonsils	
CV	Myocardial ischemia and infarction LV dysfunction	Angina or its equivalents Dyspnea, edema, exercise intolerance	Displaced posterior MI S_3	ECG, CXR, stress testing, ECHO, coronary angiography
RESP	CHF	Dyspnea, orthopnea, cough	Rales and rhonchi	CXR
RENAL	Impaired renal perfusion	Nighttime urinary frequency		Cr
CNS	Cerebrovascular atherosclerosis	TIAs	Carotid bruit	Carotid ultrasound and angiography

Key Reference: Stein JG: Internal Medicine. Boston, Little, Brown, 1987, pp 2035–2057.

PERIOPERATIVE IMPLICATIONS

Preoperative Preparation

- Assess for CAD and peripheral vascular disease
- ß rb agents and nitrates perioperatively, as tolerated

Monitoring

- Consider PA catheter, TEE in the presence of large fluid shifts, history of ischemia

Airway

- Patients may be overweight, have large head and neck, difficult to intubate

Maintenance

- Monitor for ischemia and cardiac failure
- Avoid hypothermia and anemia
- Heparin releases two triglyceride hydrolases: lipoprotein lipase inhibited by protamine and hepatic lipase resistant to protamine
- Insulin increases activity of lipoprotein lipase and releases free fatty acids (FFAs)
- Sympathetic stimulation, stress, and catecholamines release FFAs
- Spinal or epidural anesthesia and ß rb reduce FFA levels

Extubation

- For noncardiac surgery, this may be period of greatest risk for ischemia

Adjuvants

- Depends on end-organ disease and lipid-drug binding

Postoperative Period

- High incidence of tachycardia, ischemia, and MI for several days after noncardiac surgery
- Treat pain, hemodynamic and biochemical abnormalities

ANTICIPATED PROBLEMS/CONCERNS

- Problems are related to atherosclerosis

LYME DISEASE

Sophia Socaris, M.D.
Philip D. Lumb, M.B.

RISK

- Most common arthropod-borne infection in USA
- Coastal areas in the east (3.7/100,000), from Maryland (6.1/100,000 [mid-Atlantic]) to Massachusetts; the Midwest in Wisconsin and Minnesota (0.7/100,000); and the far west, in northern California (0.6/100,000), southern Oregon (0.9/100,000), and western Nevada (0.6/100,000)
- Gender predilection: none
- Children <15 y; adults 25–44 y

PERIOPERATIVE RISKS

- Increased risk of arrythmias and CHF in patients with cardiac involvement

WORRY ABOUT

- Fluid overload
- CHF
- AV block

OVERVIEW

- Stage 1 — Early localized infection: Erythema chronicum migrans (rash spreads centrifugally; lesion usually occurs at site of bite)
- Stage 2 — Early disseminated infection: Aseptic meningitis, cranial neuritis, and peripheral radiculoneuritis are neurologic manifestations
  - Carditis occurs in 4–8% of patients during this stage of disease
  - 2nd and 3rd degree AV block and myocarditis may be documented by ECG and heart failure; symptoms resolve in days to weeks
- Stage 3 — Late persistent infection: Intermittent episodes of asymmetric pain and swelling in a few large joints, especially the knees, over years; 62% of untreated patients develop frank arthritis, a mean of 6 mo after disease onset; 10% of untreated Americans with joint involvement develop chronic Lyme arthritis

ICD-9-CM Code: 088.81

ETIOLOGY

- Lyme disease is caused by the spirochete *Borrelia burgdorferi,* which is transmitted by the tick *Ixodes dammini*

USUAL TREATMENT

- Antibiotic therapy typically shortens stage 1 and generally aborts stages 2 and 3

ASSESSMENT POINTS

SYSTEM	EFFECT	ASSESSMENT BY HX	PE	TEST
CV	AV node block CHF	Palpitations Fatigue Dyspnea Dizziness with exercise	Bradycardia Tachycardia	ECG
RESP		SOB	Rales	CXR
SKIN	Erythema chronicum migrans	Erythematous annular lesions	Erythematous circular rash	
CNS	Meningitis Bell's palsy Radiculoneuritis	Headache Cognitive impairment Memory deficit	Cranial nerve facial palsy	Serology Lumbar puncture EMG
MS	Arthritis	Joint pain and swelling Musculoskeletal pain	Swelling of one or a few joints Erythema of joints	

Key Reference: Karsh R: Lyme disease. Rheum Dis Clin North Am 1993; 19:339–426.

PERIOPERATIVE IMPLICATIONS

Preoperative Concerns

- Ensure antibiotic Rx and cure of carditis prior to all but life-death emergency operations

Monitoring

- Routine

Airway

- Routine

Preinduction/Induction

- Avoid depolarizing muscle relaxants

Maintenance

- Routine

Extubation

- Routine

Adjuvants

- Avoid depolarizing muscle relaxants on induction, because of hyperkalemia

Postoperative Period

- Routine

ANTICIPATED PROBLEMS/CONCERNS

- Patients may develop arrhythmias

LYMPHOMAS

Alisa C. Thorne, M.D.

RISK

- Hodgkin's disease (HD) USA: 7/100,000 annually Dx
- Non-Hodgkin's lymphoma (NHL) USA: 13.7/100,000 annually Dx
- Race with highest prevalence of HD and NHL: Caucasian (90% of all cases)

PERIOPERATIVE RISKS

- Morbidity and mortality related to compression of organs and chemotherapy
- Mediastinal mass
- Superior vena cava syndrome; anthracycline cardiac toxic effects
- Bleomycin pulm toxic effects
- Pericardial effusion
- Radiation pneumonitis

WORRY ABOUT

- Tracheal or bronchial compression by large mediastinal mass
- Increased cardiac/pulm toxic effects with combination chemotherapy/radiation therapy (RT)

OVERVIEW

- Two major types of lymphoma: HD and NHL
- 7th most common cause of cancer-related death in USA
- Average age at diagnosis: 42 y
- Often curable
- Accurate Dx and staging critical in determining Rx and prognosis

ICD-9-CM Codes: 200–202.8

ETIOLOGY

- HD: Possibly associated with prior mononucleosis; woodworking; increased educational level; familial
- NHL: Increased risk with exposure to phenoxyherbicides or ionizing radiation; collagen vascular diseases; possible viral and hereditary etiologies

USUAL TREATMENT

- Radiation therapy (RT)
- Chemotherapy with multiple agents
- Combination RT and chemotherapy
- Chemotherapy commonly includes: bleomycin, doxorubicin, prednisone, nitrogen mustard, vincristine
- RT commonly includes: neck, chest
- Both chemotherapy and RT have cardiac and pulmonary toxic effects

ASSESSMENT POINTS

SYSTEM	EFFECT	ASSESSMENT BY HX	PE	TEST
HEENT	Bulky nodal disease Compression	SOB, DOE Tracheal deviation	Neck mass Wheeze, stridor	Indirect laryngoscopy CXR CT/MRI
CV	Mediastinal mass	SOB, DOE	Facial swelling, wheeze, may be asymptomatic	CXR, CT/MRI ECHO CT of airway
	SVC syndrome (SVC obstruction)	Cough, orthopnea Mental status change	Dilated veins upper half of body Edema of head, neck, and upper extremities, cyanosis	
RESP	Pericardial effusion CHF due to anthracyclines Bronchial compression Obstructive pneumonia Pneumonitis due to bleomycin and/or RT	Frequently asymptomatic SOB, DOE Cough Wheeze Sx worse in supine position Fever, cough	↑ HR, ↓ BP, neck vein distention Rales, pedal edema	CXR, ECHO CT/MRI Flow-volume loop ABG, PFTs, DLCO
GI	Abdominal mass Upper/lower GI bleed Perforated viscus	Abdominal pain, GI bleeding	Palpable mass	CT/MRI
HEME	Bone marrow involvement			Alk phos, CBC, Plts, bone marrow biopsy
CNS	Leptomeningeal disease or single or multiple mass lesions	Headache Cranial nerve abnormalities	Abnormal neuro exam	Spinal tap CT/MRI
RENAL	Ureteral compression			IVP, BUN/Cr

Key Reference: DeVita VT Jr, et al (eds): Cancer: Principles and Practice of Oncology, 4th ed. Philadelphia, JB Lippincott, 1993, Chs 51 and 52.

PERIOPERATIVE IMPLICATIONS

Preoperative Preparation

- Assess extant bulky nodal disease causing upper or lower airway and/or cardiac compression
- Assess LV function after anthracyclines
- Assess pulmonary function after bleomycin, RT
- If large mediastinal mass, use local anesthetic if possible

Monitoring

- Routine

Airway

- Routine, unless large anterior mediastinal mass calls for awake fiberoptic intubation
- Use armored ETT
- Rigid ventilating bronchoscope on hand

Induction

- If large mediastinal mass: consider awake fiberoptic intubation, maintaining spontaneous ventilation, and semi-Fowler's position

Maintenance

- Spontaneous ventilation as above; avoid muscle relaxants
- After bleomycin use lowest FIO_2 possible

Extubation

- If mediastinal mass, extubate patient awake and breathing spontaneously and have rigid ventilation bronchoscope on hand

Adjuvants

- If asymptomatic with mediastinal mass, airway obstruction and/or cardiac compression may develop on induction

Postoperative Period

- Airway obstruction if mediastinal mass: observe longer in intensive nursing setting
- Monitor fluid status if significant LV dysfunction

ANTICIPATED PROBLEMS/CONCERNS

- If bulky nodal disease in neck and chest, at risk for SVC syndrome, difficult airway, and tracheobronchial compression on loss of spontaneous ventilation
- May have significant cardiac/pulmonary impairment due to combination chemotherapy/RT

MALIGNANT HYPERTHERMIA (MH) AND OTHER ANESTHETIC-INDUCED MYODYSTROPHIES (AIMs)

Henry Rosenberg, M.D.
John G. Shutack, D.O.

RISK

- Incidence of MH: 1/15,000–20,000 anesthetics in children; 1/50,000–100,000 in adults depending on use of trigger agents, gene pool
- Male > female

PERIOPERATIVE RISKS

- Mortality with MH in North America <10%
- Mortality with other AIMs ~50%
- Masseter muscle rigidity (MMR)—10–20% of patients experiencing MMR develop clinical MH; generalized rigidity predicts clinical MH in >60%
- Central core myopathy—very high risk for MH
- Hyperkalemia and cardiac arrest with Duchenne, Becker's dystrophy when succinylcholine used and sometimes with volatile agents only
- Certain forms of myotonia lead to risk for MH and/or hyperkalemia with succinylcholine

WORRY ABOUT

- Potent volatile anesthetics and succinylcholine contraindicated in MH and patients with AIM
- Availability of dantrolene
- Purge machine with 100% O_2 15–20 min prior to case
- Recrudescence of MH (about 25% of cases)
- Counseling family regarding risk and muscle biopsy testing

OVERVIEW

Malignant Hyperthermia

- Autosomal dominant myopathy
- Hypermetabolic disorder manifested by ↑ CO_2 production/O_2 consumption, acidosis, hyperkalemia, myoglobinuria/emia, tachycardia, tachypnea, increased end tidal CO_2
- Untreated, mortality >80%
- Dantrolene only specific treatment
- Dx by halothane/caffeine contracture test of biopsied muscle

ICD-9-CM Code: 995.89 (MH)

Other AIMs

- Patients with muscular dystrophy/myotonia may develop hyperkalemic arrest with succinylcholine and occasionally with potent volatiles only.
- Signs of dystrophy subtle or not apparent in young children.
- Obtain muscle specimens for dystrophin analysis, genetic testing if cardiac arrest.
- Test for CK elevation in suspicious cases.

ETIOLOGY

MH

- Defect in calcium release/control leads to ↑ intracellular calcium

- Heterogenetic predisposition
  – ? Ryanodine receptor, ? sodium channel, ? fatty acid production, ? inositol triphosphate system defect(s)
- Chromosome 19, 17, 7, 3 linked in some cases

Other AIMs

- Muscular dystrophies: X-linked inheritance, several mutations
- Myotonia—genetic abnormality of sodium, chloride channels, or protein kinase, linked to chromosome 19, 17, ? others
- Central core disease—in some families, linked to ryanodine receptor

USUAL TREATMENT

MH

- Discontinue triggers
- Hyperventilate patient with 100% O_2
- Dantrolene 2.5 mg/kg IV; may use more to treat acute episode
- Treat metabolic acidosis; actively cool
- Increase fluids 1½ to 2 × maintenance
- No calcium channel blockers
- Maintain UO 1–2 ml/kg, diuretics if necessary
- Assess for hyperkalemia and treat appropriately
- Coagulation profile, DIC a problem

Other AIMs

- Treat for hyperkalemia

ASSESSMENT POINTS

SYSTEM	EFFECT	ASSESSMENT BY HX AND PE	TEST
HEENT	Masseter muscle rigidity	Difficult intubation	ABG/acidosis Hypercarbia Myoglobinuria
CV	MH: Tachycardia, arrhythmias AIM: Sudden bradycardia VFib, asystole	Hyper/hypotension	Mixed venous and ABG: ↑ End tidal CO_2, myoglobinuria Hyperkalemia
RESP	Tachypnea	Tachypnea	↑ End tidal CO_2
MS	Generalized rigidity	Developmental delay Muscle weakness	CK Muscle biopsy
RENAL	Renal failure	Low UO Dark urine	Myoglobinuria
SKIN	Vasoconstriction Heat	Mottled appearance (late) Hot skin Sweating	Core temperature

*The caffeine/halothane contracture test is used to assess MH susceptibility.

Key Reference: Rosenberg H, Seitman D: Pharmacogenetics. *In* Barash P, Cullen B, Stoelting K (eds): Clinical Anesthesia. Philadelphia, JB Lippincott, 1989. Revised edition (with J E Fletcher), 1996.

PERIOPERATIVE IMPLICATIONS

Perioperative Preparation for Known MH

- Avoid triggers (succinylcholine, all potent volatile agents)
- Use local anesthesia (amides and ester OK)
  – Regional anesthesia (epidural, spinal, regional block)
  – General: all following drugs are *not* triggers: pentothal (barbiturates), etomidate, ketamine, propofol, nitrous oxide, all nondepolarizing muscle relaxants, narcotics, benzodiazepines

- Anesthesia machine
  – Change circuit and bag
  – Remove and/or drain vaporizers
  – Oxygen flow at 10 L/min for 15–20 min prior to use
- Dantrolene prophylaxis not necessary
- Dantrolene and calcium channel blockers together produce hyperkalemia

Monitoring

- Routine including end tidal CO_2, core temperature

Perioperative Implications, Other AIMs

- Some, not all, patients with DMD and Becker's dystrophy will develop hyperkalemia with MH triggers.
- Avoid succinylcholine in patients with myotonia

ANTICIPATED PROBLEMS/CONCERNS

- Sudden cardiac arrest in PACU
- Myoglobinuria, renal failure
- Rhabdomyolysis—follow CKs
- Hyperkalemia

MALNUTRITION

Srinivas Mantha, M.D.

RISK

- People within US: Generally 28% in surgical patients on admission to hospital
- Race with highest prevalance: Unknown

PERIOPERATIVE RISKS

- 18-fold increase for same operations compared with nonmalnourished
- Related to poor wound healing, infection, sepsis
- Presence of hypoalbuminemic malnutrition associated with poor outcome compared with protein-calorie malnutrition (PCM).
- 16.6% incidence of wound infections

WORRY ABOUT

- CHF
- Impaired cellular immunity
- Respiratory muscle strength

OVERVIEW

- Results from inadequate intake of macronutrients (carbohydrate, protein, fat); referred to as PCM.
- There are two types of PCM:
  – Marasmic form (MF-PCM), which results in uniform loss of fat and muscle mass in all tissues and a concomitant loss of water in proportion to nonaqueous mass.
  – Stress-induced hypoalbuminemic form of protein-calorie malnutrition (HAF-PCM), which results from neurohumoral modulation leading to depletion of visceral protein (in excess of muscle mass) and fat and is associated with an expansion of extracellular fluid compartment. Stress may be surgery, infection, inflammation, trauma, neoplasia

ICD-9-CM Code: 261

ETIOLOGY

- Prolonged fasting and stress
- Surgical conditions associated with nausea and vomiting
- Malignant conditions involving GI tract. Tumors involving the neck. End-stage liver disease awaiting liver transplantation. Patients undergoing anterior and posterior spinal fusion.

USUAL TREATMENT

- If albumin level does not increase after 3–7 d of enteral or parenteral nutrition, mortality rate perioperatively exceedingly high

ASSESSMENT POINTS

SYSTEM	EFFECT	ASSESSMENT BY HX	TEST
CV	↓ Preload and stroke volume		ECHO
RESP	↓ FRC and diaphragmatic activity		CXR Expiratory spirogram
GI	↓ Gastric motility Gastric ulceration Gastric and intestinal atrophy	Anorexia, vomiting	Generally not needed
GENERAL	Malnutrition	Weight loss, edema, anorexia, vomiting, diarrhea, ↓ food intake, chronic illness	Anthropometric measurements (midarm circumference, pectoral skinfold thickness) Decreased serum albumin (<3.5 mg/dl) and serum transferrin
IMMUNO	Impaired cell-mediated immunity Surgical wound infection and sepsis		Delayed hypersensitivity to skin testing
RENAL	↓ Mass ↓ Cr clearance and impaired ability to concentrate urine	↓ UO	Serum Cr/BUN
LIVER	↓ Protein synthesis		↓ Serum albumin and transferrin
PNS	↓ Peripheral nerve conduction and sensory abnormailities	Tingling and numbness in extremities	Generally not needed

Key Reference: Askanazi J, et al: Influence of total parenteral nutrition on fuel utilization in injury and sepsis. Ann Surg 1989; 191:40.

PERIOPERATIVE CONSIDERATIONS

Preinduction

- Consider prophylaxis for aspiration of gastric contents

Monitoring

- Routine

Induction

- None

Maintenance

- Careful titration of volatile agents
- Hydration and UO

Extubation

- Resp muscle failure may preclude early extubation

Adjuvants

- Vecuronium metabolism impaired
- ↓ Binding (volume of distribution) of protein-bound drugs.

ANTICIPATED PROBLEMS/CONCERNS

- Since edema is prominent feature of HAF-PCM, interpretation of anthropometric measurements may be difficult.
- Perioperative nutritional support, if given for at least 10 d, reduces morbidity and mortality in patients with biochemical evidence of severe malnutrition, manifested as a low serum albumin (<3 mg/dl) and excessive weight loss.
- Patients with end-stage chronic obstructive lung disease usually have malnutrition, and sudden refeeding perioperatively may precipitate acute respiratory failure.

MARFAN'S SYNDROME

Scott R. Schulman, M.D.
William J. Greeley, M.D.

RISK

- Prevalence is 4–6 cases/100,000 population
- Inherited as autosomal dominant trait

PERIOPERATIVE RISKS

- Aortic arch dissection, mitral or aortic regurgitation, coronary artery abnormalities

WORRY ABOUT

- Symptoms referable to progressive dilatation or rupture of ascending thoracic aortic aneurysm (e.g., chest pain radiating to interscapular region)
- Sx of mitral (midsystolic click) or aortic valvular insufficiency
- Myocardial ischemia (angina) due to medial necrosis of coronary arterioles
- Arrhythmias and conduction disturbances (palpitations)
- Shortness of breath (dyspnea) due to restrictive lung disease

OVERVIEW

- Familial disorder of connective tissue with underlying defect of collagen synthesis resulting in decreased tensile strength and elasticity of connective tissue manifests as CV, musculoskeletal, ocular disturbances
- Most common causes of death are CV complications: aortic dilatation, dissection, or rupture; aortic or mitral valvular regurgitation; coronary artery insufficiency
- Skeletal features include increased length of long bones leading to tall stature; pectus excavatum/carinatum and scoliosis are common
- Ocular findings include lenticular subluxation or dislocation and cataracts

ICD-9-CM Code: 759.82

ETIOLOGY

- Abnormality in the genes coding for fibrillin and decorin, which are involved in the synthesis of microfibrils and the proteoglycan matrix of connective tissue

TREATMENT

- No specific treatment available, supportive care

ASSESSMENT POINTS

SYSTEM	EFFECT	ASSESSMENT BY HX	PE	TEST
HEENT	Lens dislocation	Myopia	Retinal detachment	Ophthalmoscopy
CV	Aortic dissection Myocardial ischemia	Chest pain Angina		MRI, ECHO ECG Exercise ECG Radionuclide studies Pharm stress testing Angio
	Arrhythmias	Palpitations	Pulse	Ambulatory ECG Electrophysiology
RESP	Restrictive lung disease	Dyspnea	Pectus Scoliosis	PFTs
MS	Tall stature Joint hypermobility Recurrent dislocation Hernias			Arm span > height

Key Reference: Pyeritz RE, McKusick VA: The Marfan syndrome. Diagnosis and management. N Engl J Med 1979; 300:772–777.

PERIOPERATIVE IMPLICATIONS

Preoperative Preparations

- If aortic aneurysm present, preop β receptor antagonist therapy to mitigate increases in myocardial contractility and aortic wall tension (decrease dP/dT)
- Antibiotics for subacute bacterial endocarditis prophylaxis if indicated

Monitoring

- ST segment analysis; consider TEE
- Invasive hemodynamic monitoring as appropriate for planned surgery

Airway

- Potential for TMJ dislocation with laryngoscopy

Preinduction/Induction

- No specific anesthetic technique, but avoid sudden increases in aortic wall tension
- Careful positioning to avoid dislocations

Maintenance

- Monitor for myocardial ischemia and airway pressures
- No one technique has demonstrated superiority

Extubation

- Avoid sudden increases in CO, as this may increase dP/dT
- High risk for developing ischemia

Postoperative Period

- Adequate pain management important
- Doses of local anesthetics for regional blockade may be increased by increased size

MASTOCYTOSIS

Ron Yaniv, M.D.
Azriel Perel, M.D.

RISK

- People within USA: very rare
- Race/gender with highest prevalence: equal

PERIOPERATIVE RISKS

- Increased risk of hypotension and bronchospasm as consequence of paroxysmal release of mast cell mediators
- Anesthetic drugs and procedure may induce mast cell degranulation
- Perioperative mortality rate—fatal cases reported

WORRY ABOUT

- Increased risk of hypotensive shock and bronchospasm
- Clotting factors may be disturbed as result of vitamin malabsorption, hepatic fibrosis, and massive heparin release from mast cells (uncommon).

OVERVIEW

- A spectrum of mast cell proliferative disorders (MPD) Common—indolent cutaneous MPD: Localized—solitary mastocytoma: Generalized—diffuse mastocytomas, urticaria pigmentosa (UP), telangiectasia macularis eruptiva perstans (TMEP)
- Initial manifestation is cutaneous eruption in many
- Episodic flushing, headaches, nausea, and vomiting
- Sometimes vascular collapse with syncope and palpitations, abdominal pain, wheezing
- Main concern—to avoid mast cell degranulators
- Rare—mast cell lymphoma/leukemia; rule out carcinoid syndrome as cause of symptoms (elevated urinary 5-HIAA)

ICD-9-CM Codes: 202.6 (Mastocytosis); 238.5 (Mastocytoma); 757.33 (Mastocytosis Syndrome)

ETIOLOGY

- Unknown
- Mast cell proliferative disorder
- Also hypersensitive degranulation response of neoplastic mast cell

USUAL TREATMENT

- H_1 blockers—e.g., chlorpheniramine maleate, hydroxyzine, terfenadine; H_2 blockers—e.g., cimetidine, ranitidine followed by aspirin to block PGD_2 synthesis
- Disodium cromoglycate PO for GI symptoms
- Ketotifen
- Shock—IV epinephrine 2–10 µg/min and volume repletion
- EpiPen and epinephrine inhalers
- PUVA (psoralen plus ultraviolet A) for cutaneous manifestation
- Steroids—topical and systemic
- Anticholinergic agents
- Chemotherapy
- Splenectomy
- Protamine sulphate *rarely* necessary when endogenous heparin prolongs prothrombin time.

ASSESSMENT POINTS

SYSTEM	EFFECT	ASSESSMENT BY HX	PE	TEST
HEENT	Rhinorrhea	Allergic rhinitis		
CV	Episodic vascular collapse			Episodic elevations of plasma histamine levels
RESP	Asthma	Wheezing		
GI	Malabsorption, GI bleeding Abdominal pain N/V; diarrhea		Hepatosplenomegealy	
HEME	Anemia, thrombocytopenia, leukopenia, mast-cell leukemia			CBC Clotting studies Bone marrow biopsy
SKIN	Mastocytoma Urticaria pigmentosa (UP) Telangiectasia macularis eruptiva perstans (TMEP)	Pruritus Urticaria	Skin biopsy	(+ Giemsa)
PNS	Polyneuropathy		CNS exam	
MS	Bone pain			X-ray, ^{99m}Tc bone scan

Key Reference: Parris WCV, Scott HW, Smith BE: Anesthetic management of systemic mastocytosis: experience with 42 cases. Anesth Analg 1986; 65:5117.

PERIOPERATIVE IMPLICATIONS

Preoperative Preparation

- Refrain from ethanol, aspirin, NSAIDs
- Premedication with histamine-releasing drugs might be avoided
- Diazepam premedication—reported to be safe
- Start prophylactic H_1 and H_2 blockers
- Prophylactic disodium cromoglycate—yet to be confirmed (100 mg q6h)
- Predictive prick tests for drugs such as muscle relaxants—controversial

Monitoring

- Routine monitors
- Intra-arterial catheter (sudden BP changes)

Airway

- Intubation may be dangerous in the presence of mucosal lesions, as pressure can cause degranulation and bronchospasm or hypotension

Preinduction/Induction

- Avoiding atropine, scopolamine, and sodium thiopental has been recommended. Preinduction with H_1 blocker such as 25–50 mg diphenhydramine
- Inhalational agents—safe (may even increase mast cell stability)

Maintenance

- Maintain normothermia
- Hypotension due to histamine release—IV epinephrine, 1–3 mg/kg
- Dopamine—not helpful
- Avoid dextran as colloidal solution

Extubation

- Should be smooth
- Keep patient warm

Adjuvants

- Blood transfusion—should be warmed and given only when essential

- Muscle relaxants: Vecuronium recommended. Avoid potential histamine-releasing muscle relaxants in large doses, such as ditubocurarine, atracurium, gallamine
- Regional: has been advocated but hypotension and bronchospasm reported to be even more common as well as urticaria and pruritus
- Antibiotics: Avoid polymyxin B sulfate. Used safely: amikacin, cefazolin, metronidazole (± vancomycin)
- Miscellaneous drugs: Avoid dipyridamole, papaverine, quinine, thiamine
- Radiologic contrast dyes can induce acute episode

Postoperative Period

- Continue with analgesics, H_1 and H_2 blockers

ANTICIPATED PROBLEMS/CONCERNS

- Hypotensive and bronchospastic crisis due to mast cell degranulation induced by anesthetic or surgical procedures

MEDIASTINAL MASSES

Jeffrey Rosenberg, Ph.D., M.D.

RISK

- Congenital lesion: 1/5000, M:F 1:1
- Thymoma, lymphoma, retrosternal goiter

PERIOPERATIVE RISKS

- Perioperative mortality rare
- Inability to ventilate or oxygenate
- Hypotension or tamponade

WORRY ABOUT

- Airway obstruction and inability to ventilate
- Vascular compression with hypoxia, hypotension, arrest
- Superior vena cava syndrome with airway edema and increased bleeding
- Recurrent laryngeal nerve injury
- Patients at risk with: cough and pain, dyspnea and dysphagia, superior vena cava syndrome, tracheal deviation, Horner's syndrome, cyanosis, mediastinal widening and hoarseness

OVERVIEW

- Severity of symptoms does not predict intraoperative course
- Airway obstruction or hemodynamic compromise has occurred with induction of GA, intubation, muscle relaxation, position change, and after extubation

ICD-9-CM Codes: 164.0 (Malignant thymoma); 201.9 (Hodgkin's lymphoma); 202.8 (Non-Hodgkin's lymphoma)

ETIOLOGY

- Adults: 97% malignant—80% metastatic bronchogenic carcinomas; 17% lymphomas (50% of lymphomas have mediastinal involvement); 20% thymomas (50% malignant; 35% association with myasthenia gravis).
- Pediatric: 87% malignant—16–36% of non-Hodgkin's lymphomas and 54–81% of Hodgkin's lymphomas, bronchial cysts, and teratomas

- Superior vena cava syndrome in 6–7% of lung cancer
- Others include parathyroid or thyroid tumors; lymphoid tumors; teratomas, aortic aneurysms, esophageal achalasia or diverticula, diaphragmatic hernia, bronchogenic or pericardial cysts, neurofibromas

USUAL TREATMENT

- For tissue diagnosis: biopsy under local
- If no tissue can be obtained or patient is uncooperative, approach is selective radiotherapy sparing some tumor for later diagnosis – if not diagnostic, then biopsy under GA
- Surgical resection for some tumors
- Cardiorespiratory complications during anesthesia are usually fewer after radiation

ASSESSMENT POINTS

SYSTEM	EFFECT	ASSESSMENT BY HX	PE	TEST
HEENT	Compression of trachea by mass	Cough Cyanosis Dyspnea Orthopnea	Wheezing Stridor	CXR Flow-volume loop CT scan
CV	Compression of PA or heart SVC syndrome	Fatigue, faintness Headache Dyspnea	Neck edema JVD Pulsus paradoxus $\downarrow$ BP	CXR ECHO supine and sitting
RESP	$\downarrow$ Lung volume	Cough, cyanosis dyspnea, orthopnea	$\downarrow$ Breath sounds Wheezing; stridor	CXR, CT scan, PFTs
CNS	Compression of recurrent laryngeal nerve, sympathetic chain, spinal cord	Stridor Sympathetic instability Focal neuro Sx	BP changes with postural changes Paresthesias Focal weakness	Flow-volume loops Tilt table testing SSEP EMG

Key Reference: Pullerits J, Holzman R: Anaesthesia for patients with mediastinal masses. Can J Anaesth 1989; 36:681–688.

PERIOPERATIVE IMPLICATIONS

Preoperative Preparation

- Consider (including pediatric patients) an IV prior to induction (lower extremity if SVC syndrome)
- Those with PA or heart compression may need cardiopulmonary bypass (check availability prior to induction with cannulation sites prepped and draped)
- Consider light or no premedication except for anticholinergic

Monitoring

- Consider light intra-arterial catheter, central venous, or pulm artery catheter
- If SVC syndrome, insert central venous access or PA catheter via femoral vein

Airway

- Tracheal or distal compression; may become obstructed with induction and muscle relaxation
- Maintain spontaneous ventilation throughout procedure unless ET tube is below obstruction
- Symptomatic patients in supine position are best maintained sitting or semi-sitting during

induction
- Awake fiberoptic intubation not necessary if asymptomatic in supine position and CXR and/or CT scan do not reveal airway obstruction or compression
- If in doubt consider awake fiberoptic bronchoscopy to rule out obstruction or compression
- If compression seen in thoracic trachea, then consider a single-lumen armored endotracheal tube with its tip distal to the compression
- If compression is at level of carina or distal, endobronchial intubation is recommended or a double-lumen endobronchial tube

Preinduction/Induction

- May develop airway obstruction with inability to ventilate
- May develop hypoxia from obstruction of pulm artery and blood flow to lungs

Maintenance

- Consider local anesthesia; otherwise keep patient breathing spontaneously
- If obstruction occurs consider altering patient's position, attempt rigid bronchoscopy, median sternotomy, or femorofemoral cardiopulmonary

bypass

Extubation

- Deep extubation during spontaneous breathing recommended; try to minimize straining, coughing, or bucking with an increase in intrathoracic pressure
- Observe several hours after extubation to detect and treat delayed airway obstruction.

ANTICIPATED PROBLEMS/CONCERNS

- Airway obstruction, hypotension, and hypoxia are major concerns
- Consider radiation and/or chemotherapy before GA
- If GA required, consider inspection of tracheobronchial tree with fiberoptic bronchoscopy
- If GA required, maintaining spontaneous ventilation preferable

MESOTHELIOMA

John R. Moyers, M.D.

RISK

- Diffuse mesothelioma: 15/1 million population
- Male:female 6–7:1
- 0.16% of all malignancies
- Localized mesothelioma extremely rare

PERIOPERATIVE RISKS

- Usually discovered in geriatric male undergoing lung biopsy
- Pleural effusion
- Previous needle biopsy of lung and thoracentesis make pneumothorax a concern
- General debilitation from malignancy

OVERVIEW

- Diffuse malignant mesothelioma is a sheet-like growth usually originating in lower part of chest cavity, invading diaphragm, and encasing lung and other mediastinal structures
- Peak incidence 20–40 y after asbestos exposure
- Usual onset of symptoms at age 55–70 y
- Median survival after onset of symptoms is 18 mo

ICD-9-CM Codes: 162.9 (Lung neoplasm); 199.1 (Mesothelioma, malignant site unspecified)

ETIOLOGY

- Diffuse mesothelioma related to asbestos exposure in 12–93% of cases
- Also associated with radiation therapy, erionite exposure, chronic inflammation and fibrosis, and other agents

USUAL TREATMENT

- Treatment has been controversial and largely ineffective
- Therapy has consisted of radiation to hemithorax, chemotherapy, and sometimes surgery (parietal pleurectomy and decortication or extrapleural pneumonectomy)

ASSESSMENT POINTS

SYSTEM	EFFECT	ASSESSMENT BY HX	PE	TEST
HEENT	Tracheal displacement			Lateral and AP CXR
CV				ECG
RESP	Pneumothorax	Cough, chest pain, increased SOB		ABGs, PFTs (rarely necessary) CXR (post biopsy; in expiration)
	Restrictive lung disease	Dyspnea, exercise	Percussion and auscultation of chest	
GI	Weight loss, debilitation, peritoneal tumors	Past body weights		CT scan of abdomen (not for perioperative care) Albumin (for degree of malnutrition) CBC (for malnutrition)
ENDO	Not associated with paraneoplastic syndromes			

Key Reference: Rusch VW: Diagnosis and treatment of pleural mesothelioma. Semin Surg Oncol 1990; 6:279–288.

PERIOPERATIVE IMPLICATIONS

Perioperative Preparation

- Usually come to surgery for lung biopsy via thoracoscopy
- Assess pulmonary status; size of effusion, no pneumothorax
- Have often had one or more recent needle biopsies of lung or thoracenteses
- Review CT scan for size and location of tumor

Monitoring

- Routine monitors
- Resp system via stethoscope, SpO_2 and $P_{ET}CO_2$
- Intra-arterial catheter for complex surgical procedures

Airway

- Look for tracheal and mediastinal displacement on CXR and CT scan

Induction

- Propensity for hypoxia, particularly from restrictive lung disease

Maintenance

- High FIO_2 may be necessary
- One-lung ventilation
- Lateral positioning

Extubation

- Ensure patient meets extubation criteria

Adjuvants

- Pain control after thoracoscopy or thoracotomy
- No special considerations for muscle relaxants, reversal agents, local anesthetics, or special drug interactions

Postoperative Period

- Monitor ventilation and oxygenation
- Pain relief; consider epidural or spinal analgesia after thoracotomies
- May have air leak postop

ANTICIPATED PROBLEMS/CONCERNS

- Anesthesia with one-lung ventilation for a geriatric patient with incurable malignancy
- Recent lung biopsy and thoracentesis prior to surgery and potential for complications from those procedures, including pneumothorax and dehydration
- Effective pain relief and monitoring of respiratory function postop
- Consider ICU stay for those undergoing complex procedures

METHEMOGLOBINEMIA

H. Michael Marsh, M.B.

RISK

- People within USA: rare
- Gender prevalence: none
- Socioeconomic/ethnic prevalence: none

PERIOPERATIVE RISKS

- Inadequate oxygen carriage and delivery to tissues

WORRY ABOUT

- % of methemoglobin or sulfhemoglobin. Acutely developing methemoglobinemia or sulfhemoglobinemia may become symptomatic at 1% with cyanosis; at 60% acute CV collapse, coma, or death may occur.

OVERVIEW

- Present when >1% of circulating hemoglobin is oxidized to ferric form.
- Two hereditary forms: (1) due to NADH-diaphorase (cytochrome b5 reductase) deficiency, inherited as an autosomal recessive trait; (2) due to abnormal globins, hemoglobin M, which are inherited as autosomal dominant traits
- Toxic methemoglobinemia occurs from exposure to agents that directly oxidize hemoglobin or facilitate its oxidation by molecular oxygen: nitrates ingested, nitroglycerin, isobutyl nitrite, and some local anesthetics

ICD-9-CM Code: 289.7

ETIOLOGY/PATHOGENESIS

- Fe^{2+} in hemoglobin is constantly oxidized in vivo, by NO and reactivity with O_2, to Fe^{3+}, methemoglobin. NADPH-diaphorase utilizes NADH generated by glyceraldehyde dehydrogenase, in the Embden-Meyerhof pathway, to reduce cytochrome b5, which in turn reduces Fe^{3+} in methemoglobin to Fe^{2+} in hemoglobin.

USUAL TREATMENT

- Medical therapy: ascorbic acid 300–600 mg/d in divided doses. Methylene blue 1 mg/kg IV, repeated once provided that patient is not G6PD-deficient, since hemolysis will occur in this case.
- Methylene blue may also be taken orally as 60 mg tid.

ASSESSMENT POINTS

SYSTEM	EFFECT	ASSESSMENT BY HX	PE	TEST
RESP	SOB DOE	Hx of cyanosis if hereditary form	RR	Co-oximetry
HEME	Cyanosis if 1% methemoglobin is present or sulfhemoglobin seen	Cyanosed	Cyanosis	Spectrometry at 630 nm

Key Reference: Beutler E: Erythrocyte disorders: Diseases with cyanosis. In Williams WJ, Beutler E, Erslev AJ, Lichtmann MA (eds): Hematology, 4th ed. New York, McGraw-Hill, 1990.

PERIOPERATIVE IMPLICATIONS

Preoperative Preparation

- Consider treatment if methemoglobin level is >1%. If sulfhemoglobin is present, may mean exchange transfusion.

Monitoring

- Use co-oximeter (IL282), since presence of methemoglobin will render pulse oximetry unreliable.

Airway

- Routine

Induction

- Routine

Maintenance

- Routine

Extubation

- Routine

Adjuvants

- Avoid nitrates and local anesthetics that act as oxidizing agents

Postoperative Period

- See Monitoring concerns

ANTICIPATED PROBLEMS/CONCERNS

- O_2 carriage is interfered with, proportional to concentration of altered hemoglobin present, and the interference with O_2 release and shift of tension-saturation curve from normal position.
- Pulse oximetry overestimates SaO_2 in presence of methemoglobin. Methylene blue will decrease the SaO_2 for about 30 min after injection

MITRAL REGURGITATION

Keith L. Stein, M.D.

RISK

- People within USA: 5–10% of population (if mitral valve prolapse included)
- Race with highest prevalence: unknown
- Female > male

PERIOPERATIVE RISKS

- Risk of atrial tachyarrhythmias, LV dysfunction, pulm edema, CHF, acute RV failure
- Bacterial endocarditis
- Acute mitral regurgitation (MR) associated with MI, CAD, and all associated risks (see under Angina in Diseases section)
- Low LV ejection fraction or severe symptoms associated with poor outcome

WORRY ABOUT

- Worsening symptoms of fatigue, DOE, nocturnal dyspnea, orthopnea, cachexia
- New-onset AFib

- Evidence of right heart failure: hepatic congestion and hepatopathy, peripheral edema, jugular venous distention

OVERVIEW

- Disease of abnormal flow in heart, allowing some of systolic outflow to go back into left atrium
- Offloads LV by allowing low-pressure retrograde ejection
- Resulting hyperdynamic LV allows long period before symptoms; eventually, LV dilatation and hypertrophy progress to cardiac failure; left atrial distention leads to pulmonary HTN, pulmonary edema, and possible RV failure
- The more precipitous the onset, the more significant the acute heart failure
- Diagnosis made by Doppler, ECHO, cardiac catheterization

ICD-9-CM Code: 424.0

ETIOLOGY

- Chronic: degenerative (mitral prolapse, ruptured chordae), rheumatic, endocarditis, CAD, papillary muscle dysfunction, dilated LV, hypertrophic cardiomyopathy, SLE, rarely congenital (see also under mitral valve prolapse)
- Acute: ruptured chordae, endocarditis, MI with papillary muscle dysfunction, left atrial myxoma, trauma, prosthetic valve dysfunction
- May be accelerated by systemic HTN, ↓ left atrial compliance

USUAL TREATMENT

- Medical therapy: cardiac glycosides, angiotensin inhibitors, hydralazine, antibiotic endocarditis prophylaxis, CHF regimen (diuretics, nitrates)
- Surgical therapy (with symptoms or cardiomegaly): mitral valvuloplasty or mitral valve replacement

ASSESSMENT POINTS

SYSTEM	EFFECT	ASSESSMENT BY HX	PE	TEST
CV	Mitral regurgitation	Fatigue, exertional or nocturnal dyspnea	Pansystolic and late systolic murmur, rales	Doppler, ECHO Cardiac catheterization
	RV failure	Peripheral swelling RUQ pain, tenderness	Ankle edema Hepatomegaly Hepatojugular reflux	
	Cardiomegaly Left atrial enlargement		Displaced posterior MI	CXR
	AFib	Palpitations	Irregular rhythm	ECG
RESP	CHF, pulm edema	Dyspnea, orthopnea	Gallop, rales	CXR
GI	Cachexia Congestive hepatopathy	Weight loss Bleeding with minor trauma	Muscle wasting Bruises	Weight PT, PTT, LFTs
RENAL	↓ Perfusion Diuretic-induced ↓ in K$^+$, Mg^{2+}	Oliguria Palpitations	Muscle weakness ↓ Reflexes	BUN, Cr Serum K$^+$, Mg^{2+} ECG
MS	Cachexia		Muscle wasting	

Key Reference: Waller BF, Howard J, Fess S: Pathology of mitral valve stenosis and pure mitral regurgitation. Clin Cardiol 1994; 17:330–336 (Pt I); 395–402(Pt II).

PERIOPERATIVE IMPLICATIONS

Preoperative Preparation

- Continue chronic medications for AFib rate control, CHF, afterload reduction
- Avoid hypoxemia, hypercarbia to limit increase in PVR and resultant risk of RV failure
- Consider antibiotic prophylaxis

Monitoring

- Consider PA catheter or TEE if LV dysfunction, aortic operations, or procedures with large fluid shifts or BP variations

Airway

- None

Preinduction/Induction

- Avoid bradycardia or acceleration of AFib ventricular response
- Maintain preload, reduce afterload
- Avoid myocardial depression

Maintenance

- Any technique that avoids ↑ afterload or myocardial depression, both of which manifest as cardiac failure
- Regional anesthetic technique may help ↓ afterload
- Maintain normovolemia, normocarbia, normotension, normal SaO$_2$
- Avoid excessive PEEP
- Follow CO, utilize IV vasodilators and vasodilating inotropes as needed

Extubation

- ↑ Risk of HTN inducing MR and CHF
- ↑ Risk of hypoventilation and hypoxemia inducing RV dysfunction

Adjuvants

- No known drug interaction problems unless CHF develops and ↓ liver or renal perfusion

Postoperative Period

- Maintain afterload reduction, digoxin levels, fluid balance
- Pain management may be critical to avoid HTN
- PCA, epidural analgesia potentially beneficial

ANTICIPATED PROBLEMS/CONCERNS

- Depressed LV ejection fraction, severe pulmonary HTN, and RV dysfunction may be best predictors of high perioperative risk.
- ↑ LV afterload (HTN) rapidly worsens MR and induces pulm edema and CHF

MITRAL STENOSIS

Albert T. Cheung, M.D.

RISK

- Bimodal age distribution: 20–39 y and 50–60 y patients
- Most common among USA immigrants from regions where rheumatic fever is prevalent (e.g., Middle East, Asia, Latin America)

PERIOPERATIVE RISKS

- ↑ Risk of perioperative cardiac complications that include infectious endocarditis, pulm edema, heart failure, new-onset AFib or atrial flutter, embolic stroke of cardiac origin

WORRY ABOUT

- Fluid status
- Paroxysmal AFib or flutter
- Limited ability to increase cardiac output in response to ↑ metabolic demands
- Cardiomyopathy, pulm HTN, RV failure, hepatic dysfunction, tricuspid regurgitation, and associated aortic valve disease

OVERVIEW

- Diastolic emptying of blood from the left atrium into the left ventricle is impaired
- Transmitral pressure gradient varies directly with cardiac output; acute increases in cardiac output and venous return to heart cause acute increases in pulm venous pressure. Pulm edema occurs when the pulm venous pressure > pulm capillary oncotic pressure
- Left atrial dilation, AFib, left atrial thrombosis, pulm HTN, RV failure, tricuspid regurgitation may develop
- Symptoms of mitral stenosis can be elicited by conditions (fluid overload, exercise, pregnancy, sepsis, operation) that demand an increase in cardiac output

ICD-9-CM Code: 394.0

ETIOLOGY

- Congenital heart disease (rare)
- Acquired mitral stenosis is sequela of rheumatic carditis developing after group A streptococcal pharyngitis
- Rheumatic carditis produces exudative and inflammatory lesions that lead to fibrosis, calcification, thickening, and fusion of the mitral valve leaflets

USUAL TREATMENT

- Anticoagulation to ↓ risk of thromboembolic events
- Digoxin to control ventricular rate in patients with AFib
- Diuretic therapy for symptomatic pulm edema
- Percutaneous balloon valvotomy or open valvotomy
- Mitral valve replacement or reconstruction

ASSESSMENT POINTS

SYSTEM	EFFECT	ASSESSMENT BY HX	PE	TEST
CV	Mitral stenosis	DOE Chest pain or tightness	Diastolic murmur	ECHO Cardiac cath
	AFib Pulm HTN	Palpitations DOE	Irregular pulse Sternal heave Prominent S_2	ECG
RESP	Pulm edema	DOE Orthopnea Paroxysmal nocturnal dyspnea Hemoptysis	Tachypnea Rales Wheezes	CXR
GI	CHF		Hepatomegaly	Liver function tests
RENAL	Fluid retention Diuretic therapy	Dependent edema	Pedal edema	Serum lytes
CNS	Embolic stroke	Neurologic deficits TIAs	Focal neurologic deficits	Head CT scan TEE

Key Reference: Savino JS, Cheung AT: Rheumatic mitral stenosis. *In* Oka Y, Konstadt S (eds): Transesophageal Echocardiography: A Problem Oriented Approach. Philadelphia, Lippincott-Raven, 1996.

PERIOPERATIVE IMPLICATIONS

Preoperative Preparation

- Optimize fluid status of patients in CHF
- Control ventricular rate in patients with AFib
- Replete K⁺ in patients with hypokalemia on digoxin therapy
- Antibiotic prophylaxis for infectious endocarditis
- Keep patient calm using reassurance, anxiolytics, and analgesics

Monitoring

- ECG to detect paroxysmal AFib or flutter
- Consider arterial catheter for continuous BP monitoring and ABG sampling
- Consider PA catheter or TEE to guide intravascular volume status when large fluid shifts are anticipated.

Preinduction/Induction

- Cautious administration of drugs that decrease myocardial contractility, or cause arterial dilation or tachycardia
- Vasoconstrictors may worsen pulm HTN
- Hypoventilation and hypoxia may worsen pulm HTN

Maintenance

- Control fluid administration

Extubation/Postoperative Period

- Provide adequate analgesia
- ↑ Risk of postop resp failure

Adjuvants

- Consider regional anesthesia or perioperative epidural anesthesia and analgesia

ANTICIPATED PROBLEMS/CONCERNS

- Patients have a limited ability to increase their cardiac output
- Acute pulm edema is precipitated by ↑ cardiac output, pregnancy, anxiety, fluid overload, exercise, and postop mobilization of sequestered (third space) interstitial and extracellular fluid

MITRAL VALVE PROLAPSE

Albert T. Cheung, M.D.

RISK

- Present in ~3.9% of men and 5.2% of women
- Severity increases with age (symptoms most common > age 50 y)

PERIOPERATIVE RISKS

- Infectious endocarditis
- Heart failure as a consequence of acute or chronic mitral regurgitation
- Embolic stroke
- Cardiac dysrhythmias

WORRY ABOUT

- Associated conditions: Marfan's syndrome, Ehlers-Danlos syndrome, pseudoxanthoma elasticum, sudden cardiac death, pectus excavatum, scoliosis, hyperadrenergic state

OVERVIEW

- Caused by structural weakness of valve apparatus
- Ventricular systole causes displacement or prolapse of valve leaflets into left atrial side of mitral valve annulus
- Progressive annular dilation, elongation of chordae tendineae, and stretching of valve leaflets leads to development of mitral regurgitation
- Rupture of weakened chordae produces acute mitral regurgitation
- Surface abnormalities on valve apparatus increase risk of infectious endocarditis and embolic stroke

ICD-9-CM Code: 424.0

ETIOLOGY

- Inherited connective tissue disorders
- Myxomatous degeneration (replacement of collagen and elastin by mucopolysaccharide)

USUAL TREATMENT

- Antihypertensive therapy (experimental)
- Mitral valve replacement or reconstruction in patients with severe mitral regurgitation

ASSESSMENT POINTS

SYSTEM	EFFECT	ASSESSMENT BY HX	PE	TEST
CV	Mitral valve prolapse	Atypical chest pain DOE	Mid- and late-apical nonejection systolic clicks	ECHO
	Mitral regurgitation	DOE	Mid- to late-apical systolic murmur	ECHO
	Dysrhythmias	Palpitations Syncope	Abn pulse	ECG Holter
CNS	Stroke	Neurologic deficits TIAs	Focal neurologic signs	Head CT scan
MS	Skeletal deformities		Pectus excavatum Scoliosis	CXR

Key Reference: Fontana ME, Sparks EA, Boudoulas H, Wooley CF: Mitral valve prolapse and mitral valve prolapse syndrome. Curr Probl Cardiol 1991; 16:309–375.

PERIOPERATIVE IMPLICATIONS

Preoperative Preparation

- Assess existence and severity of mitral regurgitation
- Antibiotic prophylaxis for infectious endocarditis in patients with mitral regurgitation detected by ECHO

Monitoring

- Routine

Preinduction/Induction/Maintenance

- Avoid HTN and acute increases in sympathetic tone

Adjuvants

- Medicines that decrease preload, increase contractility, or decrease or increase heart rate, or decrease sympathetic tone, may make CV sequelae and severity of MVP and mitral regurgitation worse, and increase the risk of chordal rupture

Extubation/Postoperative Period

- Avoid HTN and acute increases in sympathetic tone

ANTICIPATED PROBLEMS/CONCERNS

- HTN and positive inotropic stimulation may increase severity of MVP, the regurgitant LV ejection fraction when mitral regurgitation is present, and risk of acute rupture of chordae tendineae.
- Presence of severe mitral regurgitation or associated connective tissue disorders may alter routine management of patients with isolated MVP (see under Mitral Regurgitation and individual connective tissue disorders in Diseases section)

MOBITZ I (SECOND DEGREE ATRIOVENTRICULAR BLOCK)

James R. Zaidan, M.D.

RISK

• Occurs after inferior myocardial infarction, or occasionally in trained athletes or in normal, sleeping people

PERIOPERATIVE RISKS

• Without associated heart disease and without symptoms, should not present undue risk during anesthesia
• If occurs secondary to inferior myocardial infarction, the perioperative risk depends on extent of ischemic area

WORRY ABOUT

• Advancing to a higher degree block if ischemic zone extends to anterior wall
• Papillary muscle dysfunction may occur

OVERVIEW

• Found usually in presence of CAD
• Block generally occurs in AV node, resulting in normal QRS complexes
• ECG reveals progressive lengthening P-R intervals at decreasing increments and progressively shortening R-R intervals
• Bradycardia usually responds to atropine

ICD-9-CM Code: 426.13 (Mobitz I)

ETIOLOGY

• Acquired, usually with MI
• Increased resting parasympathetic tone relative to resting sympathetic tone (i.e., may be some parasympathetic and decreased sympathetic tone)

USUAL TREATMENT

• Specific therapy in absence of heart disease not necessary unless patient is symptomatic
• Treatment of an infarction-related Mobitz I block includes observation and medical therapy with atropine
• Temporary pacing is necessary only if medically unresponsive patient is symptomatic
• Permanent pacing seldom required and considered only if persistently blocked, symptomatic patients.

ASSESSMENT POINTS

SYSTEM	EFFECT	ASSESSMENT BY HX	PE	TEST
CV	Commonly no Sx Bradycardia on occasion	Exercise tolerance Angina SOB	Signs of CHF and ↓ perfusion	ECG CXR
RENAL	Likely normal			Renal function testing?
CNS	No effect or ↓ perfusion of CNS	No Sx or only mild Sx: fainting, dizziness	Normal Bruits	PE Carotid US

Key Reference: Rardon DP, Miles WM, Mitraini RD, et al: Electrocardiographic recognition. *In* Zipes DP, Jalife J (eds): Cardiac Electrophysiology: From Cell to Bedside, 2nd ed. Philadelphia, WB Saunders, 1995, pp 935–942.

PERIOPERATIVE IMPLICATIONS

Preoperative Preparation

• Consider availability of transcutaneous pacing

Monitoring

• Based upon coexisting disease
• Observe for and prepare to treat third degree block when positioning PA catheter in patient with Mobitz I block

Airway

• None

Induction/Maintenance

• Regional or general
• No contraindications to any standard anesthetic drugs
• Intraoperative processes and drugs that increase atrial rate could decrease ventricular rate.

Extubation

• None

Adjuvants

• Cautious use of drugs that slow AV conduction

ANTICIPATED PROBLEMS/CONCERNS

• Extension of infarcted area with higher degree block and CHF

MOBITZ II (SECOND DEGREE ATRIOVENTRICULAR BLOCK)

James R. Zaidan, M.D.

RISK

• Occurs after anterior infarction and can quickly proceed to a third degree heart block

PERIOPERATIVE RISKS

• Risk of developing third degree block

WORRY ABOUT

• Rapid development into a third degree block, which requires temporary transvenous pacing

OVERVIEW

• Block is located in bundle of His or bundle branches, resulting in lengthening QRS duration
• P-P and R-R intervals are constant, and PR intervals are constant prior to the dropped QRS complex

ICD-9-CM Code: Mobitz II: 426.12

ETIOLOGY

• Acquired, usually associated with MI

USUAL TREATMENT

• Temporary pacemaker insertion should be considered soon after onset of this block, because third degree block commonly occurs
• Pacing does not improve survival
• Atropine usually does not improve conduction

ASSESSMENT POINTS

SYSTEM	EFFECT	ASSESSMENT BY HX	PE	TEST
CV	Bradycardia	Exercise tolerance Angina SOB	Signs of CHF and ↓ perfusion	ECG CXR Other tests as indicated
GU	Likely normal			Renal function testing?
CNS	↓ Perfusion of CNS	Fainting, dizziness	Normal? Bruits	PE Carotid US

Key Reference: Rardon DP, Miles WM, Mitrani RD, et al: Electrocardiographic recognition. *In* Zipes DP, Jalife J (eds): Cardiac Electrophysiology: From Cell to Bedside, 2nd ed. Philadelphia, WB Saunders, 1995, pp 935–942.

PERIOPERATIVE IMPLICATIONS

Preoperative Preparation

• Evaluation of CAD important
• Likely a transvenous pacemaker will be in place
• Transcutaneous pacing should be available if temporary transvenous pacing was not established prior to induction of anesthesia

Monitoring

• Based on severity of heart disease and extent of infarcted area
• Prepare to treat third degree block when positioning a PA catheter

Airway

• None

Induction/Maintenance

• No contraindications to any standard anesthetic drugs
• Any intraoperative process or drug increasing atrial rate could worsen block and decrease ventricular rate

Adjuvants

• Cautiously use drugs that slow conduction through AV node unless they also slow SA nodal rate and allow 1:1 AV conduction and ↑ ventricular rate
• First degree AV block will persist if 1:1 conduction occurs

MORBID OBESITY

Susan L. Polk, M.D., M.S.Ed.

RISK

- About 5% of Americans

PERIOPERATIVE RISKS

- Morbidity or mortality twice normal, owing to associated CV and resp abnormalities, hypercoagulability

WORRY ABOUT

- Technically difficult procedures: intubation, establishing IV lines
- Restrictive ventilatory dysfunction and hypoxemia
- Associated sleep apnea (may be associated with problematic narcotic epidural analgesia)
- Systemic and pulm HTN
- LV and RV failure

- Hypercoagulability
- ↑ Gastric emptying time and hiatus hernia
- Liver disease
- Psychologic disorders

OVERVIEW

- Defined as twice ideal body weight [ideal body weight (kg) = height (cm) −100] or body mass index >35 [BMI = weight (kg)/height^2 (meters)]
- CV and resp dysfunction due to increased body mass to be perfused and oxygenated. Increased demand for O_2 and CO_2 excretion from metabolic demand of increased tissue mass. Increased work of breathing due to decreased chest wall compliance
- Obstructive and/or central sleep apnea due to increased upper airway soft tissue mass relaxing during sleep. Patients extremely sensitive to resp depressant effects of sedatives and hypnotics
- Psychologic dysfunction may interfere with

postop stir-up routine and contribute to pulm and thromboembolic phenomena

ICD-9-CM Code: 278.0

ETIOLOGY

- Unknown. Presumed genetic predisposition but an acquired disease

USUAL TREATMENT

- Dietary intervention with exercise and behavioral modification
- Surgical: Gastric stapling or bypass, or intestinal bypass

ASSESSMENT POINTS

SYSTEM	EFFECT	ASSESSMENT BY HX	PE	TEST
CV	HTN	Dyspnea, pounding	BP Cardiomegaly	ECG, CXR, BUN
	Pulm HTN	Dyspnea at rest and on exertion, orthopnea	Rales	CXR, ECG
	Ventricular dysfunction	Dyspnea Orthopnea, poor exercise tolerance	Venous engorgement Rales, S_3 and S_4 Cardiomegaly	CXR, ECG, ECHO
	CAD	Angina, poor exercise tolerance		Stress ECHO, ECG, Angio
RESP	Restrictive dysfunction	Dyspnea at rest or on exertion Orthopnea	Rapid resp rate Shallow breathing, ruddy color	ABGs, PFTs, Hct, CXR (pulm HTN) Pulse oximetry on room air while supine
	Sleep apnea	Snoring, frequent sleep interruptions Daytime somnolence	Upper airway tissue, ruddy color	ABGs, Hct, polysomnogram
GI, METAB	Hepatic dysfunction	Jaundice Bleeding disorders Ascites	Hepatomegaly, ascites, spider angiomas, jaundice	LFTs, PT, PTT BUN and Cr
	Full stomach NIDDM	Heartburn, hiatus hernia Polydipsia, polyuria		Fasting glucose Urinalysis, GTT
DIFFICULT AIRWAY		Snoring	Visualization of uvula and tonsillar pillars	Lateral neck x-ray may be helpful

Key Reference: Buckley FP: Anesthesia and obesity and gastrointestinal disorders. *In* Barash PG, Cullen BF, Stoelting RF (eds): Clinical Anesthesia, 2nd ed. Philadelphia, JB Lippincott, 1992, pp 1169–1184.

PERIOPERATIVE IMPLICATIONS

Preoperative Preparation

- Metoclopramide 10 mg, cimetidine 300 mg PO the night before and IV preoperatively
- Assess myocardial and volume status

Monitoring

- Routine monitors plus consider arterial line if BP cuff does not fit well or takes too long to inflate
- Frequent ABGs
- UO
- Possible CVP or PA catheter if volume status likely to be significantly altered

Airway

- Awake intubation may be indicated if difficulty anticipated on basis of examination
- Elevation of shoulders and head on a bolster facilitates insertion of laryngoscope

Induction

- Patient may need to remain semi-sitting if SaO_2 drops when supine
- Preoxygenation should be complete

Maintenance

- Volume status can change precipitously, esp with position change
- Oxygenation may deteriorate with upper abdominal surgery or increased intra-abdominal pressure
- All agents tapered at the end to minimize postop sedation

Extubation

- As soon as adequate to maintain normocapnia and patient is responsive to command

Adjuvants

- Initial dose of induction agent and narcotics calculated on a mg/kg basis and muscle relaxants calculated on estimated lean body mass

- Subsequent doses of sedatives, hypnotics, relaxants, narcotics calculated on estimated lean body mass. Regional anesthesia if physically poss and if patient can use accessory muscles to help with breathing

Postoperative Period

- Pain control necessary to facilitate early stir-up routine. PCA acceptable in sleep apnea, but not in continuous mode. Some think epidural narcotic infusions are contraindicated unless continuously monitored for resp depression

ANTICIPATED PROBLEMS/CONCERNS

- Resp insufficiency and pneumonia postop avoided by minimal sedation, appropriate pain control, early ambulation
- Postop thromboembolic phenomena also avoided by above
- Poor motivation, resulting in poor ambulation, avoided by intensive preop teaching and postop coaching

MUCOPOLYSACCHARIDOSES

James J. Fehr, M.D.

James J. Fehr, M.D.

RISK

- Only males affected in Hunter syndrome (X-linked)
- People within USA: Incidence estimated to be 1/30,000

PERIOPERATIVE RISKS

- Estimated perioperative mortality: 20%
- Difficult intubation (25%), failed intubation (8%)

WORRY ABOUT

- Difficult airway, cardiac lesions, poor IV access, resp failure

OVERVIEW

- Child may appear normal at birth; by age 1 y often shows signs of both growth and mental retardation. Dx made by characteristic physical findings and ↑ urinary mucopolysaccharides (MPs).
- Hurler syndrome, considered prototype, is characterized by involvement of heart, liver, and bones. Most severe form and also associated with corneal clouding, developmental delay, frequent respiratory infections, stiff joints, abnormal airway.
- Scheie syndrome is milder form of Hurler syndrome; patients have normal intelligence and life expectancy but may have stiff joints and aortic regurgitation.
- Hunter syndrome has diffuse joint limitations, short neck, short stature, ischemic cardiomyopathy.
- Morquio syndrome has severe kyphoscoliosis, possible cervical subluxation and aortic regurgitation.
- Maroteaux-Lamy syndrome has kyphoscoliosis, cardiac involvement, mild joint stiffness.
- Recurrent hernias often occur in mucopolysaccharidoses.

ICD-9-CM Code: 277.5

ETIOLOGY

- Hereditary, progressive disorders of lysosomal enzymes responsible for metabolism of mucopolysaccharides resulting in intracellular accumulation of incompletely metabolized MPSs in tissues throughout body. Leads to progressive alteration of cellular structure and function. Death often results from cardiac or pulmonary failure.
- All forms are autosomal recessive except for Hunter syndrome, which is X-linked recessive.

USUAL TREATMENT

- None at present; prenatal diagnosis is available

ASSESSMENT POINTS

SYSTEM	EFFECT	ASSESSMENT BY HX	PE	TEST
HEENT	Large tongue, small mouth, micrognathia Difficult airway anticipated Atlantoaxial subluxation possible		Neck ROM	X-ray
CV	Difficult IV access Frequent valvular lesions Compliance often reduced Possible ischemic disease (even at a young age)	Exercise tolerance Angina Hx		ECG CXR ECHO
RESP	Propensity to develop pneumonia Obstructive apnea Bronchospasm			
GI	Frequent hepatomegaly Hepatic function usually normal			
CNS	Mental retardation, deafness are frequent Cervical myelopathy in Morquio syndrome Hydrocephalus in Hurler and Hunter syndromes			
MS	Short neck, severe skeletal abnormalities Anticipate difficulty in positioning			

Key Reference: Walker et al: Anesthesia and mucopolysaccharidoses. Anaesthesia 1994; 49:1078–1084.

PERIOPERATIVE IMPLICATIONS

Preoperative Preparation

- May be resistant to sedative premedications
- Anticipate possible airway obstruction/cardiopulmonary difficulties
- Antisialagogue, e.g., glycopyrrolate
- Antibiotic prophylaxis for cardiac lesions

Monitoring

- Routine

Airway

- Abnormal airway and short neck predispose to complicated airway management, including difficulty in performing a tracheostomy.
- Consider fiberoptic bronchoscopy.
- LMA may be useful.

Preinduction/Induction

- IV placement before induction
- Padding and positioning

Maintenance

- Avoid myocardial ischemia

Extubation

- Conscious with intact airway reflexes prior to extubation

Adjuvants

- Utilize local anesthetics and regional techniques when appropriate

Postoperative Period

- Delayed emergence
- Respiratory complications including pneumonia, bronchospasm, and apnea

ANTICIPATED PROBLEMS/CONCERNS

- Airway is likely to be difficult to manage
- Cardiac and pulmonary systems frequently affected

MULTIPLE ENDOCRINE NEOPLASIA (MEN) TYPES I AND II

Burnell R. Brown, Jr., M.D., Ph.D.
Edward J. Frink, Jr., M.D.

RISK

• People within USA: 1:15,000 (?)
• Racial predominance: unknown

PERIOPERATIVE RISKS

(See specific syndrome)

OVERVIEW

• MEN I (Werner's syndrome) and II (Sipple's syndrome) are group of familial diseases involving hyperplasia and malignancies of several endocrine organs.

• MEN I: characterized by parathyroid, pancreas, and pituitary tumors. 90% have hyperparathyroidism (hyperplasia); 20–40% peptic ulcers (hypergastrinemia); 80% have islet cell tumors (Zollinger-Ellison syndrome); 25% have acromegaly.
• MEN II: characterized by medullary carcinoma of thyroid; pheochromocytoma (50%); hyperparathyroidism (25% incidence, primarily adenomas). Any combination of tumors is possible with these diseases.

ICD-9-CM Code: 258.0

ETIOLOGY

• Both are genetic diseases inherited in autosomal dominant fashion.

USUAL TREATMENT

• MEN I: Parathyroid disease treated by subtotal parathyroidectomy. Pancreatectomy (partial or total) may be required for control of hyperinsulinism (hypoglycemia). Diazoxide and streptozocin may be helpful for hypoglycemia. Therapy for gastrin-secreting tumors is total gastrectomy.
• MEN II: Excision of pheochromocytoma, if present, is lifesaving (usual site is adrenal glands). All those patients displaying either pheochromocytoma or hyperparathyroidism (hypercalcemia) should have total thyroidectomy.

ASSESSMENT POINTS

DISEASE	EFFECT	ASSESSMENT BY HX	PE	TEST
MEN I	Parathyroid hyperplasia	Family Hx essential	Acromegaly	Glucose Ca^{2+}
	Nephrolithiasis; nephrocalcinosis Pancreatic tumors, severe hypoglycemia Pituitary tumors, acromegaly			CT scan of sella; CT scan of abdomen; growth hormone level
MEN II	Pheochromocytoma	Family Hx Sweating; tachycardia	HTN (paroxysmal)	CT scan Urinary catecholamines
	Medullary cancer of thyroid Parathyroid adenoma	Metastatic disease Family Hx	Thyroid gland	Calcitonin levels Ca^{2+}
		Hx urinary stones		Cr BUN Pelvic x-rays

Key Reference: Thomas JL, Bernardino ME: Pheochromocytoma in multiple endocrine adenomatosis. JAMA 1981; 245:1467–1469.

PERIOPERATIVE IMPLICATIONS: MEN I

Monitoring

• Cardiac arrhythmias, prolonged QT interval (hypercalcemia)
• UO
• CNS monitoring for pituitary adenomas
• Blood glucose

Airway

• Acromegalics very difficult to intubate

Maintenance

• Monitor blood glucose
• Maintain renal function, NaCl infusion (high-output diuretics such as furosemide)
• Usual neurosurgical precautions for operations for adenomas of pituitary

PERIOPERATIVE IMPLICATIONS: MEN II

Monitoring

• Usual monitoring for pheochromocytoma removal (intra-arterial line, PA cath); ECG
• UO
• Venous pressure
• Thyroidectomy (possible air embolism)

Airway

• Usually no problem. Post thyroidectomy may precipitate problem (severed recurrent laryngeal nerve, tracheomalacia)

Maintenance

• Keep BP at acceptable levels (volatile anesthetics, nitroprusside, phentolamine)
• Carefully monitor volume status
• Be prepared to treat hypercalcemic cardiac arrhythmias

• For thyroidectomy, metabolic maintenance

Adjuvants

• Pretreatment with phenoxybenzamine for pheochromocytoma
• Calcium-lowering drugs (mithramycin) preop, if necessary

ANTICIPATED PROBLEMS/CONCERNS

• MEN I: Hypoglycemia; hypercalcemia; postparathyroidectomy hypocalcemia with tetany
• MEN II: Problems associated with pheochromocytoma (HTN, stroke, MI)

MULTIPLE MYELOMA

Kamla K. Prasad, M.D.

RISK

- Incidence in USA 3/100,000/y
- 1% of all malignant disease
- African-American 2× >Caucasians
- Median age at diagnosis: 61 y; only 2% < 40 y
- Median survival 3 y; nearly 100% fatality rate

PERIOPERATIVE RISKS

- ↑ Risk of acute renal failure and exacerbation of chronic renal failure
- ↑ Risk of neurologic sequelae

WORRY ABOUT

- ↑ Risk of infection from multifactorial causes
- Multifactorial coagulopathy

OVERVIEW

- Neoplastic proliferation of a single clone of plasma cells
  - Pathology by bone marrow invasion and excessive monoclonal Ig production
- Potentially severe adverse renal, neurologic, hemostatic, immunologic, pulmonary consequences perioperatively

ICD-9-CM Code: 203.0
See also under Waldenström's macroglobulinemia

ETIOLOGY

- Unknown, with possible genetic predisposition
- Massive production of monoclonal Ig's causes derangements in most organ systems and overwhelms host

USUAL TREATMENT

- Alkylating chemotherapeutic agents
- Glucocorticoids (high dose)
- Localized irradiation

ASSESSMENT POINTS

SYSTEM	EFFECT	ASSESSMENT BY HX	PE	TEST
HEENT	Instability of axial spine	Vertebral bone pain	Neurologic deficits	Neck radiographs
CV	Hyperviscosity syndrome (microvascular sludging)	Angina, fatigue, CHF	Venous thrombosis	Serum viscometry
RESP	Pneumonia Resp insufficiency	Recurrent infections Rib/thoracic spine pain	Pathologic rib fractures	CXR Thoracic spine x-ray
ENDO	Malnutrition	Cachexia		
HEME	Abnormal plt function Thrombocytopenia Factor I, II, XI inhibition Normochromic, normocytic anemia	Easy bruisability Prolonged bleeding		Bleeding time PT, PTT CBC
RENAL	Glomerular and tubular failure (due to precipitated Ig's, hypercalcemia, hyperuricemia)			Bence-Jones proteinuria BUN/Cr Serum Ca^{2+} Uric acid
CNS	Spinal cord compression	Radicular pain	Neurologic deficits	X-rays (vertebral collapse, lytic lesions)
PNS	Peripheral nerve compression	Carpal tunnel syndrome	Neurologic deficits	
METAB	Hypercalcemia ↑ Infection susceptibility	Lethargy; weakness Recurrent infections		ECG (QT, PR) WBC
MS	Pathologic fractures	Bone pain	Pathologic fractures	X-rays: fractures, punched-out bony lesions

Key Reference: Barlogie B: Plasma cell myeloma. *In* Beulter E, et al (eds): Williams Hematology, 5th ed. New York, McGraw-Hill, 1995, pp 1109–1126.

PERIOPERATIVE IMPLICATIONS

Preoperative Preparation

- Positioning to prevent pathologic fractures
- Prophylactic antibiotics

Monitoring

- UO: maintain to prevent hypercalcemia and renal failure
- Temp: maintain normothermia to prevent microvascular sludging

Airway

- Axial spine fractures/cord compression may be present
- Macroglossia if amyloidosis

Maintenance

- Adequate hydration to minimize renal failure, hypercalcemia, hyperviscosity

Extubation

- Pulm insufficiency due to rib and vertebral fractures and pneumonia

Adjuvants

- All protein-bound drugs: unpredictable pharmacokinetics due to alterations of relative proportions of globulins and albumin in plasma
- Regional: relatively contraindicated owing to multifactorial coagulopathy and pre-existing neurologic deficits

Postoperative Period

- ↑ Pulm complications: venous thrombosis (hyperviscosity) and pneumonia (presence of rib fractures)—adequate hydration/aggressive pulm toilet mandated
- Encourage early ambulation to prevent hypercalcemia and venous thrombosis
- ↑ Infection risk due to functional hypogammaglobulinemia/neutropenia

ANTICIPATED PROBLEMS/CONCERNS

- Transfusion to treat anemia may precipitate hyperviscosity syndrome; plasmapheresis may be indicated before transfusion.
- Treat hypercalcemia with hydration, furosemide—consider mithramycin, diphosphonates, calcitonin (see under Hypercalcemia)

MULTIPLE SCLEROSIS

Armin Schubert, M.D.

RISK

• Prevalence: 1/1000 in North America
• Occurs primarily in temperate climates
• Female predominance 8:1
• Onset usually in 3rd decade of life
• Racial predominance: Caucasian 6 × incidence of all other races

PERIOPERATIVE RISKS

• Exacerbation of Sx with hyperpyrexia, stress of surgery, infection, emotional trauma, postpartum state
• Muscle wasting with ↑ risk for positioning injury, neuromuscular blocking agent overdose, and hyperkalemia with succinylcholine
• Steroid therapy predisposes to adrenal suppression, gastric ulceration

WORRY ABOUT

• Fluctuating Sx and advisability of major conduction block

• Presence of transverse myelitis and other major motor neuron disease (risk of hyperkalemia with depolarizing NMB)
• Cranial nerve involvement with loss of airway integrity
• Major temp changes (hyperthermia may exacerbate Sx)
• Autonomic dysfunction

OVERVIEW

• Demyelinating disease of brain and spinal cord (peripheral nerves are not affected), with chronically remitting and relapsing or progressive course
• Associated conditions include seizures and uveitis; CNS components involved are cortex (cognitive dysfunction, memory loss, personality change, emotional lability)
• Chronic dysesthetic pain and spasticity contribute to disability
• Paroxysmal Sx may mimic cerebral ischemia, spinal cord compression, tic douloureux.

ICD-9-CM Code: 340

ETIOLOGY

• Cause unknown
• Autoimmune, genetic, environmental factors thought to combine to attack CNS myelin

USUAL TREATMENT

• No treatment curative
• Steroids ameliorate relapses
• Carbamazepine used for paroxysmal Sx (including pain), baclofen and, occasionally, surgery for spasticity (thalamotomy)
• Beta interferon now thought to shorten attacks, prolong time between attacks, delay onset of disability

ASSESSMENT POINTS

SYSTEM	EFFECT	ASSESSMENT BY HX	PE	TEST
HEENT	Pseudobulbar palsy	Hx of swallowing difficulty	Cranial nerves IX, X	
RESP	May have aspirated during seizure	Review with family	Auscultation	CXR, oximetry
GI	GI effects of steroids	HX of pain, bleeding		
CNS	Cognitive dysfunction, optic neuritis, seizures, dysesthesias, ophthalmoplegia, autonomic dysfunction Monoplegia, transverse myelitis, quadriplegia	Hx of memory loss, emotional lability, "dropping" things, visual problems Lhermitte's sign (electric shock to legs); check with family for description of seizures	Mental status exam Neurologic exam (esp motor and sensory) Orthostatic vital sign changes	CSF electrophoresis, MRI, evoked potentials, EEG

Key Reference: Kytta J, Rosenberg PH: Anaesthesia for patients with multiple sclerosis. Ann Chir Gynaecol 1984; 73:299–303.

PERIOPERATIVE IMPLICATIONS

Preoperative Preparation

• Consider steroid supplementation for stress coverage
• May need benzodiazepine premedication
• Carefully document preop neurologic status
• Adequate volume status

Monitoring

• Routine

Airway

• None

Preinduction/Induction

• Spinal anesthesia implicated in aggravating MS symptoms and considered contraindicated

• Epidural anesthesia not contraindicated but less popular because of coincident exacerbation of MS symptoms
• Peripheral nerve blocks OK
• Succinylcholine may precipitate hyperkalemia
• Avoid elevation of body temp

Maintenance

• Avoid large temp swings, esp. hyperthermia
• Continue steroid stress coverage
• Careful titration of nondepolarizing NMBs

Extubation

• Patients with brainstem involvement should be extubated awake
• Spasticity may diminish maximal inspiratory effort

Adjuvants

• Duration of most NMBs shortened by phenytoin and carbamazepine

Postoperative Period

• Be aware of exacerbation of MS symptoms
• Continue supplemental steroid coverage
• Unknown benefit/risk from beta interferon prophylaxis
• Treat hyperthermia
• Spasticity may interfere with pulmonary toilet

ANTICIPATED PROBLEMS/CONCERNS

• Unpredictable appearance of new neurologic deficits perioperatively
• Exacerbation of MS symptoms with hyperthermia
• Hyperkalemia with succinylcholine
• Emotional lability and need for sedative premedication

MULTISYSTEM ORGAN FAILURE, LUNG DYSFUNCTION IN

Bhaskar Deb, M.D.
Thomas W. Feeley, M.D.

RISK

- Lung dysfunction in multisystem organ failure (MSOF) occurs in 150,000 people/y in USA
- Multiple risk factors include systemic sepsis, pulmonary contusion, inhalation of toxic substances, near-drowning, long bone fractures, severe pancreatitis, diffuse pneumonia, DIC, multiple emergency blood transfusions
- Risk of developing lung dysfunction (adult respiratory distress syndrome—ARDS) in MSOF is additive based on number of risk factors involved.
- Age does not appear to be an important risk factor, although COPD increases risk of lung dysfunction in MSOF

PERIOPERATIVE RISKS

- Hypoxemia
- ↓ Venous return and preload 2° to PEEP and ↑ intrathoracic pressure
- Pulm HTN with RV dysfunction

- Mortality perioperatively 10–90% determined by ability to oxygenate and underlying cause of MSOF

WORRY ABOUT

- Barotrauma and oxygen toxicity
- Mechanical device malfunction
- Unsuspected auto-PEEP
- Death from primary cause of MSOF

OVERVIEW

- MSOF is the result of multiple disease processes often with a common pathologic pulmonary endpoint, ARDS. Pathogenesis of lung dysfunction involves uncontrolled inflammatory response to massive insult, leading to vascular endothelial damage and allowing pulm edema to occur.
- Physiologic changes: Lung dysfunction in MSOF consists of hypoxemia, ↓ FRC, ↓ compliance, ↑ intrapulmonary shunt and pulm interstitial infiltrates

- Long-term resp function good for survivors of MSOF

ICD-9-CM Code: 518.4 (Lung edema, not of cardiac etiology)

ETIOLOGY

- Pulm and systemic infections, especially gram-negative septic shock, have high association with lung dysfunction of MSOF with mortality as high as 90%.
- MSOF from DIC caused by systemic agent often associated with severe lung dysfunction

USUAL TREATMENT

- Treatment of underlying cause and supportive lung treatment
- Reversal of life-threatening hypoxemia of utmost importance
  – Administration of supplemental O_2
  – Intubation and mechanical ventilation employing PEEP (see under ARDS)

ASSESSMENT POINTS

SYSTEM	EFFECT	ASSESSMENT BY HX	PE	TEST
CV	Hypovolemia ↓ CO RV dysfunction	Hypotension	Gallops S_3 Dysrhythmias Edema	ECG PA catheterization
RESP	Hypoxemia Noncompliant lungs Pulm HTN Pulm edema	Tachypnea Dyspnea	Crackles ↑ P_2	Oximetry, ABG PA catheterization CXR Peak pressures
GI	Ileus Distention Hemorrhage	Abdominal discomfort Nausea/vomiting Hemorrhage	↓ Bowel sounds Guaiac + stool	KUB, endoscopy
HEME	Anemia (↓ Hct) Thrombocytopenia DIC		Pallor Bleeding	CBC with plt count PT/PTT Fibrinogen level, FSPs
RENAL	Renal failure	Oliguria	Edema	BUN/Cr
CNS	Cerebral hypoxia	Altered mental status		

Key Reference: Taylor RW, Norwood SH: The adult respiratory distress syndrome. *In* Civetta JM, Taylor RW, Kirby RR (eds): Critical Care, 2nd ed. Philadelphia, JB Lippincott, 1992, pp 1237–1247.

PERIOPERATIVE IMPLICATIONS

Preoperative Preparation

- Be able to maintain stable oxygenation with standard Ambu bag and PEEP valve. Check ventilator settings and verify lack of movement of ET tube during transport.
- Re-evaluate least PEEP required to maintain adequate arterial saturation

Monitoring

- Routine and consider PA catheter and airway pressure to follow changes in compliance and reduce barotrauma.
- Consider TEE or PA catheter and arterial catheter to follow blood gases and maintain cardiac filling volumes

Airway

- Ensure airway is secure; loss could lead to rapid cardiopulmonary decompensation and hypoxemia that may take many minutes or even hours to reverse

Preinduction/Induction

- Hypoxemia and hypercarbia may exacerbate pulm HTN leading to RV dysfunction.
- Reduced FRC impacts negatively on shunt fraction and V/Q imbalance.

Maintenance

- PEEP is mainstay in the supportive therapy of lung dysfunction in MSOF by restoring FRC, decreasing shunt, and improving V/Q mismatch.
- Administer fluids to maintain adequate pulm capillary wedge pressure and cardiac index.
- Administer blood and inotropes as needed to optimize O_2 delivery.
- Underlying cause (sepsis/bleeding/DIC) can be made much worse by surgical trespass.

Extubation

- Usually left intubated on ventilatory support until improvement in lung function
- Prevent ↑ in O_2 consumption, e.g., shivering

Adjuvants

- Unconventional modes of ventilation, artificial gas exchange, specific therapies targeted at pathogenic pathways, and more recently nitric oxide, prostacyclins, thrombolytics, and surfactant

Postoperative Period

- Close monitoring of volume status, PEEP requirements
- Reduce FIO_2 to nontoxic level ASAP

ANTICIPATED PROBLEMS/CONCERNS

- Significant complications of supportive therapy for lung dysfunction in ARDS are pulm infections and pulm barotrauma, including pneumothorax, pneumomediastinum, pneumopericardium, and venous or arterial air embolism.
- Maintaining adequate oxygenation on a nontoxic FIO_2 requires vigilant and creative attention to volume status and mechanical ventilation.

MYASTHENIA GRAVIS

Cecil O. Borel, M.D.

RISK

- Individuals within USA: 10,000–15,000
- Affects all races
- Females: males 2:1

PERIOPERATIVE RISKS

- Postop neuromuscular ventilatory failure
- Postop pneumonia due to poor cough and secretion clearance

WORRY ABOUT

- Preop optimization of muscle strength
- Anticholinesterase medications, steroids, plasmapheresis

OVERVIEW

- Characterized by weakness and fatigability of skeletal muscles:
  - Inspiratory muscle weakness from residual paralysis from nondepolarizing neuromuscular blocking agents
  - Exacerbation of underlying bulbar (airway) musculature
  - ↑ Sensitivity to hypoventilation with narcotic analgesics
- Muscle strength improves similarly in both myasthenia gravis and nondepolarizing blockade after administration of anticholinesterase drugs

ICD-9-CM Code: 358.0

ETIOLOGY

- Autoimmune disease of neuromuscular junction mediated by reduction in number of acetylcholine receptors at neuromuscular junction

USUAL TREATMENT

- Anticholinesterase medications (pyridostigmine, Mestinon)
- Immunosuppression: steroids, azathioprine, IV immunoglobulin
- Plasmapheresis
- Thymectomy

ASSESSMENT POINTS

SYSTEM	EFFECT	ASSESSMENT BY HX	PE	TEST
NEUROMUSCULAR	Peripheral muscle weakness	Easy fatigability	Arm adduction times <1 min	Repetitive nerve stimulation
RESP Airway	Bulbar weakness	Difficulty swallowing	Head lift <5 sec	Formal swallowing evaluation
Ventilation	Inspiratory muscle weakness	Orthopnea, breathlessness	Paradoxical inspiratory motio	NIF <30 cm H_2O FVC <1000 ml
Ventilatory drive	CO_2 retention headache	Morning		ABGs
Secretion clearance	Weak cough	Recurrent pneumonia	↓ Ventilation of bases	CXR

Key Reference: Borel CO, Hanley DF: Muscular paralysis—myasthenia gravis and polyneuritis. *In* Parrillo JE, Bone RC (eds): Critical Care Medicine: Principles of Diagnosis and Management. Philadelphia, Mosby–Year Book; pp 1994, 1193–1215.

PERIOPERATIVE IMPLICATIONS

Preoperative Preparation

- Anticholinesterase medications: Hold 2–4 h preop, then start IV neostigmine 1 h before emergence at 1/30–1/60 daily pyridostigmine dose, infuse over 24 h
- Steroid maintenance

Monitoring

- Routine
- Train-of-four twitch monitor if short-active nondepolarizers used

Induction/Intubation

- Consider breathe-down techniques
- Intubation without muscle relaxation in severe disease

Maintenance

- Minimize or avoid use of muscle relaxants

Extubation

- Check NIF (>30 cm H_2O), head lift, cough, gag, assure full return of twitch

Adjuvants

- Avoid or minimize use of nondepolarizing muscle relaxants
- Depolarizing relaxants may have ↑ or ↓ efficacy

ANTICIPATED PROBLEMS/CONCERNS

- Postop ventilatory failure, pneumonia, aspiration

MYCOPLASMA PNEUMONIAE INFECTION

Bobby Su-Pen Chang, M.D.
Scott C. Streckenbach, M.D.

RISK

- Infections in the USA population: 60/1000/y
  - Asymptomatic infections—12/1000/y
  - Tracheobronchitis, pharyngitis—46/1000/y
  - Pneumonia—2/1000/y (2 million cases annually)
- Ages 5–20 y common; all ages possible
- Virulent in neonates
- Closed populations such as military camps and schools
- Epidemic outbreaks during fall and early winter in temperate climates
- Patients with Down syndrome, sickle cell disease (functional asplenism), and immunocompromised hosts may manifest more severe disease

PERIOPERATIVE RISKS

- No perioperative risk data; ↑ hemagglutination and hemolysis with hypothermia during CPB

WORRY ABOUT

- Progression or unmasking of pulmonary and extrapulmonary disease

OVERVIEW

- Atypical pneumonia: differential Dx includes influenza, adenovirus, RSV, CMV, *Chlamydia,* and *Legionella*
- Clinical disease
  - Incubation period 2–3 wk
  - Insidious onset—fever (101–102°F), malaise, headache, scratchy throat, nonproductive cough.
  - 5–10% progress to pneumonia
- Diagnosis
  - Hx and clinical picture
  - CXR—bronchopneumonia, plate-like atelectasis, nodular infiltration, hilar adenopathy
  - Gram stain—polymorphonuclear leukocytosis only. Organism does not stain because of absence of cell wall
  - Culture—gold standard; organism may take 5–20 d to culture
  - Serologic
  - Cold agglutinins—IgM antibodies directed to I-antigen on RBC membranes (nonspecific). A titer >1:32 during acute stage is presumptive evidence of *M. pneumoniae*
  - Rapid diagnostic tests of *M. pneumoniae*-specific antigen, antibody, and nucleotide sequences

ICD-9-CM Code: 483.0

ETIOLOGY

- Transmitted by respiratory droplets

USUAL TREATMENT

- Antimicrobial therapy is not necessary for most cases of *Mycoplasma* upper respiratory infections
- Antibiotics (erythromycin, ciprofloxacin, tetracycline) will shorten course of pneumonia

ASSESSMENT POINTS

SYSTEM	EFFECT	ASSESSMENT BY HX	PE	TEST
HEENT	Pharyngitis, sinusitis, myringitis, conjunctivitis			
CV	Pericardial effuson Pericarditis Myocarditis	Reported incidence as high as 10%. ↑ Incidence with advanced age	Distant heart sounds S_3, JVD Pericardial rub	ECG ECHO Effusion tap
RESP	Tracheobronchitis Pneumonia Pleural effusion Bullous disease ARDS Hemoptysis	See above	Rhonchi, wheeze, ↓ breath sounds, egophony, substernal pain	CXR Sputum
HEME	Hemagglutination and hemolysis due to cold agglutinins Raynaud's phenomenon Anemia	Effect of cold agglutinins occur when surface or core temperature falls below critical temp	Physical signs rare at room temp except for peripheral cyanosis	Cold agglutinins Blood smear CBC Free Hgb UA Direct Coombs
SKIN	Stevens-Johnson syndrome	Most patients with rash have associated pneumonia	Erythematous maculopapular and vesicular exanthems	
CNS	Aseptic meningitis Meningoencephalitis Transverse myelitis Guillain-Barré dysfunction Peripheral neuropathy	0.1% of infections have CNS involvement 7% of patients with pneumonia have CNS involvement	Meningeal signs Focal or generalized neurologic deficits	CSF Blood culture MRI

Key Reference: Park JV, Weiss CI: Cardiopulmonary bypass and myocardial protection: Management problems in cardiac surgical patients with cold autoimmune disease. Anesth Analg 1988; 67:75–78.

PERIOPERATIVE IMPLICATIONS

Preoperative Evaluation

Hypothermic procedures—cardiopulmonary bypass:
- Routine 20°C crossmatch
- If crossmatch reveals presence of cold agglutinins (CA), determination of titer, thermal amplitude, critical temperature recommended. If CA, then agglutination test at 4°C as well.
- If significant low thermal amplitude CA, postpone elective procedures. CA may persist up to 2–3 mo.
- If emergent procedure: warm fluids, blood, room, and gases. Limit transfusions as donor RBCs lack protective C3d. Transfuse washed cells only.

Normothermic procedures:
- Limit transfusions as donor RBCs lack protective C3d. Transfuse washed cells only.

Monitoring

- Consider invasive monitoring if cardiac disease suspected

Airway

- Rapid desaturation 2° to reduced FRC
- Hyperreactive airway 2° to inflammation

Maintenance

- Warm all fluids and blood products, humidified inspired gases
- If hemolysis suspected, maintain UO with maintenance of intravascular volume, osmotic and/or loop diuretics, alkalinization of urine

Adjuvants

- Vary if hepatic or renal insufficiency exists

Extubation

- Clear sensorium and adequate analgesia to participate in postop mechanical toilet

ANTICIPATED PROBLEMS/CONCERNS

- Cold agglutinins
  - Normothermic procedures
  - Limit transfusions as donor RBCs lack protective C3d.
  - Transfuse washed cells only
  - Hypothermic procedures—cardiopulmonary bypass, hypothermic arrest

MYOCARDIAL CONTUSION
Andrew L. Rosenberg, M.D.

RISK (BLUNT CHEST TRAUMA)

- 2 million motor vehicle accidents/y with ≈ 40% involving closed chest injury
- 20–70% incidence by clinical criteria
- 16–20% incidence by autopsy
- Motor vehicle > falls > crush injuries
- Males > females (5/1)

PERIOPERATIVE RISKS

- Abnormal ECG
- Nonspecific ST-T wave changes (70%) in trauma patients
- Ventricular arrhythmias most common in contusion
- Q wave and ST elevation
- 7–17% false negative
- 60% false positive
- Other cardiac conditions: thrombosed, lacerated coronary arteries in spasm; ventricular hypofunction; pericardial effusion/tamponade; pericarditis; valvular insufficiency, left-sided > right-sided; ventricular wall rupture

- Possible ↑ risk of cardiac complications (arrhythmias, hypotension) with ↑ CK-MB and abnormal ECHO
- No evidence of ↑ mortality associated with GA

WORRY ABOUT

- Malignant ventricular arrhythmia
- Cardiac conduction blocks
- Volume status
- Acute hypotension
- Associated injuries: pulmonary contusion–hypoxemia, thoracic aorta injuries, flail chest

OVERVIEW

- Traumatic injury with hemorrhagic, well-circumscribed lesions of partial or full thickness from myocardial contusion
- Usually of RV but can be multichambered
- Frequently in severe blunt chest trauma and after CPR, precordial thumps, but difficult to definitively diagnose
- Incorporation of clinical suspicion, anginal chest pain unrelieved by nitrates, ECG—especially ventricular dysrhythmia, CK-MB levels, 2-D ECHO for Dx
- Amount of malignant arrhythmias may be proportional to severity of myocardial contusion

ICD-9-CM Code: 861.01
See also under Trauma

ETIOLOGY

- Mechanical contusion of myocardium from posterior sternum
- "Ram effect" from ↑ transdiaphragmatic pressure
- Automobile accident = 15%
- Falls ≈ 10%
- Crash, sports-related assaults ≈ 15%

USUAL TREATMENT

- Supportive
- Adequate volume replacement

ASSESSMENT POINTS

SYSTEM	EFFECT	ASSESSMENT BY HX	PE	TEST
CV	Ventricular contusion	Angina-like chest pain unrelieved by nitrates	Chest wall, sternal tenderness	ECG, serial
		Dyspnea	Hypotension with severe dysfunction	CK-MB
			S_3	ECHO
			Rales	SPECT
	Arrhythmia	Palpitations, dizziness, syncope	Pulse	ECG monitoring
	Valvular disruptions	Dyspnea	Auscultatory murmurs	ECG
	Coronary artery injury: thrombosis, laceration, spasm	Chest pain		Angio
	Effusion/tamponade			
		Chest pain	Pericardial friction	2-D cardiography
			Diminished heart sounds	PA catheter
			Distended neck veins	
RESP	CHF			
	Pulm contusion	Dyspnea	S_3	
		Orthopnea	Rales	
		Chest tightness	Wheezing	CXR
			Tachypnea	Oxygen saturation

Key Reference: Capan L, et al: Management of thorocoabdominal injuries. *In* Caplan LM, Miller SM, Turndorf H (eds): Trauma, Anesthesia and Intensive Care, Philadelphia, JB Lippincott, 1991, pp 492–495.

PERIOPERATIVE IMPLICATIONS

Preoperative Preparation

- 2-D ECHO—abnormalities predict perioperative hypotension
- Assess and ensure adequate volume replacement
- Assess and treat associated concurrent injuries
- No evidence for benefit of prophylactic antiarrhythmic agents

Monitoring

- Continuous ECG for arrhythmias
- PA catheter for large fluid shift operations or patients with signs of LV dysfunction
- ↑ Risk of perioperative arrhythmias without ↑ mortality

Airway

- Evaluation for associated airway injury

Preinduction/Induction

- Adequate volume replacement
- Hypotension more likely with large contusions
- Extra attention to avoid hypoxia, hypovolemia

Maintenance

- No one agent or technique shown superior
- Avoid known pulm vasoconstrictors: catecholamine, hypoxia, acidosis, histamine-releasing agents ($MgSO_4$, mivacurium)
- Consider high inspired oxygen if contusion
- Nitrous oxide can aggravate pulm HTN
- Elevations in PVR may unmask RV failure
- ↑ LV filling pressures and ↓ cardiac output often reflect hypovolemia or are 2° to RV failure, not LV failure

Extubation

- May leave intubated if concerns for resp failure and hypoxia present

Adjuvants

- Combination of appropriate intravascular volume replenishment and vasodilators (nitroglycerin) for pulmonary HTN

Postoperative Period

- Delayed hypoxia from pulmonary injury common and can cause pulmonary HTN leading to hypotension if RV severely contused

ANTICIPATED PROBLEMS/CONCERNS

- Variable diagnostic criteria, total CK-MB >50 U/L and ≥5% total CK.
- Possible higher risk of cardiac complications with ↑ CK-MB
- Almost any arrhythmia reported, especially conduction delays; more severe contusion associated with ↑ malignant ventricular arrhythmia
- Watch for RV failure leading to ↑ LV pressure but ↓ LV diastolic filling.

MYOCARDIAL ISCHEMIA (MIsch)

Dennis T. Mangano, M.D., Ph.D.
Michael F. Roizen, M.D.

RISK

• People within USA:
  – 1.5 million/y develop acute myocardial infarction (MI)
  – 8 million have ≥70% narrowing of 1 or more coronary arteries
• European and African-American heritage > Japanese, but environment of North America equalizes risks
• Highest in patients with known other atherosclerotic disease (including prior MI): smokers (3.5-fold ↑); hypertensives (3-fold ↑); diabetics (4-fold ↑); hypercoagulable diseases (3-fold ↑); stressed, divorced, or unstable marriage (2.5-fold ↑); with weight gain since age 20 y (1.5-fold (3-fold ↑ for each 5 kg ↑); ↑ LDL cholesterol in those who do not exercise (1.4–3.4-fold ↑); who do not drink or take vitamin E or folate or aspirin; whose parents died of CAD at < age 40 y.

PERIOPERATIVE RISKS

• Increases risk 9-fold of perioperative CV complication (MI, CHF, arrhythmia requiring Rx)
• 2 y survival: rate in high-risk patient with perioperative MIsch is 25% vs 85% for those without preop MIsch
• Inadequate coronary perfusion (3 to 6% reinfarction rate with general surgery; higher with vascular/thoracic/upper abdominal surgery); lower with cataract/prostate/peripheral surgery with 1-limb anesthesia only

• Can lead to ↓ LV or RV compliance and CHF and dysrhythmias
• Can lead to inadequate perfusion of other organs and their insufficient function (brain/kidney/liver/gut)

WORRY ABOUT

• Postop period if stressed by perturbations that increase demand (pain, sepsis, fever, hyper- and hypovolemia, and tachycardia), or limit supply (thrombosis, hyperviscosity states, diseases limiting pulm function and gas exchange [restrictive, obstructive, parenchymal], hematocrit <28%)

OVERVIEW

• Condition of inadequate supply of O_2 and nutrients to myocardial cells relative to need associated with the ↑ stress of perioperative period
• Treatment and prophylaxis of this and related disorders consumes 5–20% of total health expenditures. Perioperative CV complications increased one fold with MIsch, with 3-fold reduction in 2 y survival and survival and 3-fold increase in perioperative costs for major surgery
• Major focus of clinical and basic studies to decrease incidence of and risks from concern over benefit:risk ratio and cost-effectiveness, identifying high-risk patients prior to surgery

and segregating them for prior therapy (smoking cessation, control of HTN, hypercholesterol states, hypercoagulable states, PTCA, CABG) or increased perioperative vigilance and care (PA lines, TEE, ICU care, prophylactic pain therapy, stepped-care)

ICD-9-CM Code: 410.09

ETIOLOGY

• Known atherosclerotic risks (genetic predisposition, smoking, HTN, diabetes, divorced or unstable marriage, hypercoagulable states, ↑ LDL cholesterol, weight gain)
• Known conditions that increase perioperative demands on heart (tachycardia, 2-fold greater for HR >90; 11-fold greater for HR >110); or limit supply (vasospastic states; $PaCO_2$ <25: Hct <28%; hyperviscosity and hypercoagulable states; inadequate O_2 exchange)

USUAL TREATMENT

• Decrease atherogenic risk factors
• Decrease perioperative demands on heart
• Consider preop segregation for ß rb and nitrate therapies, antispasm and sympatholytic therapies, PTCA or CABG considerations, or stepped-up postop care of increased monitoring, intensive normalization of hemodynamics, greater prophylactic pain therapies

ASSESSMENT POINTS

SYSTEM	EFFECT	ASSESSMENT BY HX	PE	TEST
HEENT	Plaques in other areas	Risk factor search: smoking stain; hypercholesterolemic lesions	McArdle's earlobe	
CV	↓ LV or RV compliance ↓ Pump function arrhythmias Autonomic pain	SOB, DOE Angina ↓ Exercise tolerance Palpitations PND	HR/BP prior to and after 2-stair climb; S_3; rales; JVD; use character and rhythm	ECG, CXR, stress ECHO or dipyridamole thallium or ambulatory Holter
RESP		Nocturnal cough, orthopnea		
RENAL	Perfusion insufficiency	Nocturia		BUN/Cr
CNS	Autonomic pain syndromes Other atherosclerotic syndromes	Pain in neck or left arm Stroke/TIA Hx	CNS and cranial nerve exam	Carotid Doppler Autonomic NS testing

Key Reference: Browner WS, Li L, Mangano DT, SPI Research Group: In-hospital and long-term mortality in male veterans following noncardiac surgery. JAMA 1992; 268:228–232.

PERIOPERATIVE IMPLICATIONS

Preoperative Preparation

• Consider segregation procedures and prophylactic regimens (see under Usual Treatment)

Monitoring

• ST-T waves of area of myocardium identified as at risk (or II and V_5) (II esp. for CNS surgery); ST segment trend analysis
• Consider PA line or TEE and arterial line and approaches to intensively normalize hemodynamics

Airway

• Routine

Induction

• Without hemodynamic disturbance and especially with HR control

Maintenance

• Tachycardia or hypovolemia and Hct <28 can precipitate ischemia
• No one agent with demonstrated outcome superiority
• Intensively normalize hemodynamics and HR control

Extubation

• In nonstressful fashion for patient without compromising supply of O_2 to myocardium
• Aggressive stepped pain therapy recommended

Adjuvants

• CHF decreases liver blood flow and clearance of drugs requiring hepatic metabolism (such as lidocaine)
• Beta adrenergic receptor antagonists and nitrates can be associated with profound hemodynamic disturbances if drug interactions or sudden preload/afterload/or contractility perturbations (such as rapid onset of spinal anesthesia) occur

ANTICIPATED PROBLEMS/CONCERNS

• Pre- and postoperative periods at least as great a cause of morbidity as intraoperative period
• Consider compassionate anxiety-relieving yet aggressive preop consultation and intensive stepped pain prophylaxis consultations postop

MYOTONIA DYSTROPHICA (MYOTONIC DYSTROPHY, STEINERT'S DISEASE)

Arthur J. Klowden, M.D.

RISK

- 2.4–5.5/100,000 births

PERIOPERATIVE RISKS

- Operative/anesthetic and postop morbidity/mortality are increased.
- High incidence of cardiopulmonary complications

WORRY ABOUT

- Increasing frequency of symptoms
- Signs of resp or cardiac decompensation

OVERVIEW

- Degenerative disease of skeletal muscles. Triad of characteristic features described as frontal baldness, cataracts, and mental retardation
- Onset of symptoms in 2nd and 3rd decades of life. Death frequently in 5th or 6th decade of life, usually due to cardiopulmonary complications.
- Inability of skeletal muscle to relax is diagnostic. EMG is corroborative and pathognomonic showing continuous, low-voltage activity with high-voltage, fibrillation-like potential bursts.
- Abnormal calcium metabolism seems causative, with inadequate incomplete return of Ca^{2+} by cellular adenosine triphosphate system to sarcoplasmic reticulum. The unsequestered calcium is then available to produce sustained skeletal muscle contractions. Myotonia persists even after denervation or paralysis.

ICD-9-CM Code: 359.2

ETIOLOGY

- Inherited autosomal dominant trait

USUAL TREATMENT

- Quinine, procainamide, phenytoin, tocainide, mexiletine (depress Na^+ influx).

ASSESSMENT POINTS

SYSTEM	EFFECT	ASSESSMENT BY HX	PE	TEST
HEENT	Visual disturbance		Presenile cataract, ptosis, strabismus	Exam by ophthalmologist
	Speech/swallowing impaired		Generalized weakness of pharyngeal, mandibular (and thoracic) musculature Dysarthria, facial weakness Expressionless facies	
CV	Dysrhythmias Cardiomyopathy	CHF uncommon but may occur with pregnancy	Delayed intraventricular conduction Heart block Up to 20% with mitral valve prolapse	ECG ECHO, Holter Cardiology consult
RESP	Restrictive lung disease	Weak cough Dyspnea Hx of pneumonias	Wasting of sternocleidomastoid muscles; resp muscle weakness Lungs intrinsically normal; ↓ VC, ERV	PFTs ABG
GI	High aspiration potential Delayed esophageal and gastric emptying Gastric dilation/atony ↑ incidence of cholelithiasis	Weak swallowing ability		
ENDO	Gonadal atrophy Diabetes mellitus ↓ Thyroid function Adrenal insufficiency Frontal balding ?Malignant hyperthermia		Thyroid nodules	Blood/urine glucose tests Thyroid function tests
CNS	Mental retardation Associated with central sleep apnea and hypersomnolence Emotional abn		Myotonic handgrip (delayed, incomplete release), ↑ CPK in serum Myotonia can be initiated or worsened by exercise or cold temp	EMG CPK
GYN	Pregnant patient is a challenge. Resp function threatened by ↓ FRC and myotonic weakness, which may be exacerbated by pregnancy. Seems to be added risk for uterine hemorrhage at delivery due to uterine atony and retained placenta. C-section may be safer.			

Key Reference: Aldredge LM: Anaesthetic problems in myotonic dystrophy. A case report and review of the Aberdeen experience comprising 48 general anesthetics in a further 16 patients. Br J Anaesth 1985; 57:1119–1130.

PERIOPERATIVE IMPLICATIONS

Preoperative Preparation

- Ensuring NPO status
- No preop analgesics or sedatives
- Warm ambient room air in OR may ↓ incidence and severity of myotonia

Monitoring

- Routine

Airway

- Propensity for frequent jaw dislocation
- Potential inability to secure airway because of jaw muscle spasm

Preinduction/Induction

- Risk for aspiration of gastric contents
- Succinylcholine-induced skeletal muscle contraction may be so severe and prolonged (2–5 min) as to make adequate ventilation difficult.

Maintenance

- Halothane may cause more postop shivering and myotonia.
- Regional or local anesthesia acceptable, but will not block myotonic response.
- IV regional may be preferable when suitable.

Extubation

- Beware airway obstruction because of jaw muscle weakness.
- Delayed recovery from anesthetic common

Adjuvants

- ↑ Sensitivity to ventilatory depressant effects of all premedicants, sedatives, opioids.

- Reversal agents can theoretically precipitate skeletal muscle contraction by facilitating depolarization of NMJ, but adverse responses do not predictably occur

Postoperative Period

- ↑ Sensitivity to respiratory depressant effects of opioids or sedatives.
- Pulm complications due to poor cough possible.

ANTICIPATED PROBLEMS/CONCERNS

- If myotonia develops intraoperatively, neither general or regional anesthesia, nor NMBs will attenuate it. Local infiltration of involved muscles may help. Even asymptomatic patients may have some degree of cardiomyopathy. Beware premature extubation, consider postop ventilation

MYXOMA

Solomon Aronson, M.D.

RISK

- Although primary cardiac tumors are rare (< 0.01%) this is the most common (50%)
- 75% develop in left atrium
- Rarely develop in ventricle
- More common in females (70%)

PERIOPERATIVE RISKS

- May be friable and embolize
- Risk of LV or RV inflow obstruction
- May simulate pulm HTN and/or constrictive pericarditis

WORRY ABOUT

- Hypotension due to obstruction of ventricular inflow and/or incompetence of tricuspid (right) or mitral (left) valve
- Tumor "flips" on stalk across valves, causing stenotic or incompetent symptoms
- RV hypertrophy due to long-standing left inflow obstruction
- Rare pulm or systemic embolization

OVERVIEW

- Is a true neoplasm and distinct from a thrombus
- Usually polypoid with 1 to 2 cm stalk projecting into cavity, round shape with smooth margins
- Typically grows very slowly before symptomatic (10–20 y)

ICD-9-CM Code: 215.4 (Thorax myxoma)

ETIOLOGY

- Polyhedral cells with small nuclei are separated by an afibrillar, eosinophilic myxomatous stroma that is predominantly a mucopolysaccharide
- Rarely extends deeper than endocardium
- Although "benign," this tumor can undergo malignant degeneration

USUAL TREATMENT

- Surgical
- Cardiopulmonary bypass required
- Atriotomy with transseptal approach through fossa ovalis

ASSESSMENT POINTS

SYSTEM	EFFECT	ASSESSMENT BY HX	PE	TEST
CV	Mitral stenosis or insufficiency syndromes	Edema, CHF	Left atrial enlargement Systolic murmur (MI) Diastolic murmur (mitral stenosis)	ECHO ECG CXR
RESP	Pulm emboli (right)	DOE, cough	Rales, wheezing, $\uparrow P_2$	ECHO, CXR, ECG
GI		CHF	Hepatic enlargement	Hepatic enzymes (if Sx of CHF)
RENAL	Emboli (left)			Urinalysis Cr clearance
CNS	Stroke (left)	CNS dysfunction	CNS dysfunction	ECHO
GENERAL	Constitutional symptoms	Fever, malaise	Weight loss	

Key Reference: Larsson S, Lepore V, Kennergren C. Atrial myxomas: Results of 25 years experience and review of the literature. Surgery 1989; 105:695.

PERIOPERATIVE IMPLICATIONS

Preoperative Preparation

- Differential Dx includes mitral stenosis/insufficiency (left), tricuspid stenosis/insufficiency (right), constrictive pericarditis, pulm HTN, subacute bacterial endocarditis.
- Mitral stenosis: hemodynamic aim is to keep in normal sinus rhythm with adequate preload and high normal afterload (see under Mitral Stenosis).
- Mitral insufficiency (regurgitation): hemodynamic aim is to keep HR normal or fast and vasodilate.
- Hemodynamics can mimic any or all of above depending on load-dependent variables prevailing in the cardiac cycle at the time (e.g., preload, afterload, HR).

Monitoring

- Routine monitors otherwise needed for cardiopulmonary bypass (e.g., temp, ECG, coagulation, Foley)

- Intra-arterial catheters
- Beware of central line with right-sided atrial myxoma (may cause dislodgment of friable debris as pulm emboli)
- TEE most sensitive way to guide hemodynamic management and assess therapeutic approach

Airway

- Routine

Preinduction/Induction

- May develop hypotension if preload ↓ or HR ↑
- Avoid insertion of central venous or PA monitoring catheters or cannula with right-sided tumor

Maintenance

- May dislodge pieces during CPB venous cannulation; direct assessment of anatomy, physiology; and even placement of cannula can be guided by TEE

- If pedunculated, tumor may obstruct inflow track and hemodynamics may present as low BP, low CO; ↑ CVP (right) or ↑ PCWP (left)

Extubation

- Expect excellent recovery from primary myxomatous lesion and ventricular function
- Criteria should be based on myocardial protection techniques and post-CPB bleeding risk
- Early extubation consideration is reasonable

Postoperative Period

- Beware residual ASD (as tumors typically originate in atrial septum in region of fossa ovalis)
- Beware conduction, dysrhythmia disturbance (especially in pediatric population)
- Symptoms of pulm HTN usually regress quickly

ANTICIPATED PROBLEMS/CONCERNS

- Hypotension with inadequate preload when lesion obstructs inflow dynamics

NARCOLEPSY

RISK

- People within US: >200,000
- Race with highest prevalence: equal

PERIOPERATIVE RISKS

- Risks related to treatment medications

WORRY ABOUT

- Tricyclic drugs increase incidence of perioperative hypotension
- Tricyclic drugs blunt pressor response to indirect-acting sympathomimetic agents (e.g., ephedrine) and exaggerate pressor response to direct-acting sympathomimetic agents (e.g., phenylephrine).
- ↑ Incidence of postop apneic episodes
- Possible ↑ sensitivity to anesthetic agents

OVERVIEW

- Lifelong disease that usually develops in childhood/adolescence
- Initial symptom is excessive daytime sleepiness with irresistible sleep attacks
- Secondary symptoms of cataplexy, hypnagogic hallucinations, disrupted nocturnal sleep, and automatic behavior have variable incidence and occur later in the disease
- Sleep attacks appear as clinically normal sleep lasting from seconds to minutes. Can be easily awakened by auditory or tactile stimulation
- 80% incidence of cataplexy (sudden brief loss of voluntary muscle control). Usually precipitated by strong emotional response (e.g., laughter, anger, surprise). Patient remains conscious. Majority of patients develop a flat affect to suppress the emotional trigger
- Diagnostic work-up includes nocturnal polysomnogram (documents adequacy of sleep and rules out obstructive sleep apnea) followed by a Multiple Sleep Latency Test (MSLT) to document hypersomnolence and REM onset sleep. Patients with narcolepsy fall asleep quickly (usually < 5 min) and have early onset of sleep.
- Often confused with obstructive sleep apnea syndrome

ICD-9-CM Code: 347

ETIOLOGY

- Association with HLA DR2 antigen

USUAL TREATMENT

- Psychosocial support, therapeutic naps, medications
- Sleep attacks treated with CNS stimulants. Methylphenidate (Ritalin) is drug of choice
- Cataplexy and other secondary symptoms treated with tricyclic antidepressants (e.g., imipramine, protriptyline)

ASSESSMENT POINTS

SYSTEM	EFFECT	ASSESSMENT BY HX	TEST
HEENT		Obstructive symptoms (rare)	
CV	Conduction abnormalities due to tricyclics		ECG
CNS	Flat affect Fatigue	Daytime sleep attacks	

Key Reference: Chaudhary BA, Husain I: Narcolepsy. J Fam Pract 1993; 36:207–213.

PERIOPERATIVE IMPLICATIONS

Preoperative Preparation

- Avoid sedative premedication
- Continue medical therapy on day of surgery
- If antisialagogue needed use non–central acting agent

Monitoring

- May have conduction abnormalities on ECG

Induction

- May have exaggerated hypotension if taking tricyclics
- Prehydrate prior to induction

Maintenance

- ↑ Sensitivity to anesthetic agents
- Exaggerated pressor response to direct acting sympathomimetics (e.g., phenylephrine) if taking tricyclics. Use small doses if clinically indicated
- Blunted/unpredictable pressor response to indirect acting sympathomimetics if taking tricyclics. Probably best to avoid

Adjuvants

- Muscle relaxants: Life-threatening arrhythmias have been reported with the use of pancuronium in patients on tricyclics
- Anesthetic agents: Life-threatening arrhythmias have been reported with the use of halothane in patients on tricyclics

Postoperative Period

- May be prone to postoperative apneic episodes

ANTICIPATED PROBLEMS/CONCERNS

- Patients often on tricyclic therapy and CNS stimulant therapy. Will often be sensitive to anesthetic agents. If on tricyclics need to be concerned about exaggerated pressor responses with direct acting sympathomimetics. Indirect-acting sympathomimetics have a blunted pressor response and probably should be avoided. Postoperative apnea is of theoretical concern. Postoperative obstruction symptoms are extremely rare

NECROTIZING ENTEROCOLITIS

I. David Todres, M.D.

RISK

Most common acquired life-threatening intestinal disease in newborn
• Occurs predominantly in premature infant, 75% in infants <1500 g wt
• Incidence increases with decreasing weight and gestational age

PERIOPERATIVE RISKS

• Bowel ischemia, hypoxemia, acidosis, shock, drugs (e.g., indomethacin), patent ductus arteriosus, polycythemia

WORRY ABOUT

Persistent acidosis is an ominous sign

OVERVIEW

• Ileum most commonly involved followed by ascending colon. Bowel ischemia may lead to gangrene of bowel with perforation, followed by peritonitis, shock, and death.
• Part of syndrome of multisystem failure involving the resp, CV, renal, hepatic, and hematopoietic systems. ↑ Cytokine levels of TNF, IL-6, PAF are seen
• Infant, usually premature, may show generalized signs of sepsis such as temp instability, feeding intolerance, apnea, bradycardia, hypotension, metabolic acidosis.
• In severe cases, abdominal wall is erythematous, reflecting peritonitis or localized cellulitis 2° to bowel inflammation.

• Pneumatosis intestinalis (classic sign) is seen as linear collection of air in wall of dilated loop of bowel; may extend into portal venous circulation. Free intraperitoneal air reflecting perforation of bowel is not seen in all infants.

ICD-9-CM Code: 777.5

ETIOLOGY

• Unknown: appears to be multifactorial in origin in infant with immature GI tract and immature host defenses in whom enteral feeds, especially artificial feeds, in high concentration have been administered; this sets stage for pathogenic organisms to colonize gut, with serious consequences.

ASSESSMENT POINTS

SYSTEM	EFFECT	ASSESSMENT BY HX	PE	TEST
CV	PDA Shock		Murmur BP/HR	ABGs UO
RESP	Resp failure	Hyperpnea		ABGs
GI	Malabsorption: hypoglycemia, hypovolemia, acidosis Peritonitis, sepsis		Weight UO Local cellulitis of bowel wall	Glucose, BUN, Cr ABGs Abd x-ray Pneumatosis intestinalis Temp instability
RENAL	Prerenal failure			BUN, Cr
HEME	Coagulopathy Polycythemia	Bleeding		Plt count, Hct, Hgb Fibrinogen PTT

Key Reference: Höllworth ME: Necrotising enterocolitis symposium. Acta Paediatr 1994; 83:396 (S).

PERIOPERATIVE MANAGEMENT

Preoperative Preparation

• Many infants may be treated successfully medically, i.e., fluid resuscitation, antibiotics, IV hyperalimentation.
• Surgery indicated for pneumoperitoneum due to bowel wall perforation, intestinal gangrene (detected by abdominal paracentesis), and presence of portal vein gas. Relative indications include clinical deterioration, erythema of abdominal wall, and a fixed abdominal mass.
• Discontinue enteral feeds and insert orogastric tube connected to suction to decompress abdomen
• Goals of therapy include ensuring adequate oxygenation and ventilation, e.g., tracheal intubation, mechanical ventilation, adequate perfusion.
• Fluid resuscitation (the third-space loss due to peritonitis is profound) must be aggressive to achieve an adequate UO.
• Correct metabolic acidosis—achieved primarily through fluid resuscitation.
• Avoid sodium bicarbonate.

• Inotropic agents such as dopamine may be required to optimize cardiac output.
• Correct coagulopathy with FFP and plts to achieve a plt level >50,000/ml.
• Administer broad-spectrum antibiotics (ampicillin and gentamicin with clindamycin for anaerobe cover).

Monitoring

• Routine, plus glucose

Induction/Maintenance

• Potent anesthetic agents are poorly tolerated.
• A carefully titrated narcotic and muscle relaxant technique is satisfactory.
• Nitrous oxide is usually avoided because of its potential for causing bowel distention.
• Fluid resuscitation (lactated Ringer's, 5% albumin, and, in some cases, blood) is actively carried out during surgical procedure.

Postoperative Period

• Closely monitor in ICU for ongoing fluid requirements as third-space loss continues.
• Often require prolonged TPN.
• Stricture formation a complication in both medically and surgically treated infants.
• Short bowel syndrome can occur (most outgrow this problem).

ANTICIPATED PROBLEMS/CONCERNS

• Hypovolemia leading to bowel ischemia, acidosis, shock, and death
• PDA with hypoxia, hypothermia, and hypercarbia leading to R→L shunt

NECROTIZING FASCIITIS

RISK

- Rare: 5000 in USA
- No race or gender preference
- Risk factors include diabetes (20–50% of cases), atherosclerosis (20–30%), CV or renal disease, alcoholism, malnutrition

PERIOPERATIVE RISKS

- Highly lethal condition with 30–60% mortality depending on speed of Dx and spread of infection
- Death by septic shock and associated multiorgan system failure
- Need for surgery often emergent
- Associated chronic medical conditions complicate anesthetic care.

WORRY ABOUT

- Incomplete initial fluid and pressor resuscitation
- Associated CV, renal, liver disease
- Metabolic derangements: acidosis, hypocalcemia, DIC

OVERVIEW

- Progressive, usually polymicrobial, soft tissue infection involving subcutaneous tissue and spreading along fascial planes
- Can progress rapidly to severe systemic toxicity with septic shock, pulm and renal dysfunction, and extreme third-space sequestration of fluid
- Extensive surgical debridement usually performed. Hyperkalemic responses to succinylcholine usually not a concern, as necrotizing infection spares muscle
- Use of N_2O not a concern if gaseous pockets exist, as surrounding tissue is avascular and necrotic

ICD-9-CM Code: 729.4

ETIOLOGY

- Minor trauma, wounds, or decubiti in patients with diabetes, alcoholism, chronic CV and renal disease or poor nutrition. Subsequent bacterial seeding event
- Can also occur in young, otherwise healthy patients following surgery or cuts/abrasions
- Spread of necrotic infection along fascial planes with sparing of skin
- Onset of severe systemic toxicity, septic shock, end-organ dysfunction, death
- Malignant bacterial species

USUAL TREATMENT

- Antibiotics
- Wide, often repeated surgical debridement
- Hemodynamic, resp, nutritional support perioperatively

ASSESSMENT POINTS

SYSTEM	EFFECT	ASSESSMENT BY HX	PE	TEST
HEENT	Possible infection	Edema complicating intubation	Airway exam	
CV	↓ SVR ↑ CO	↓ Mentation	Orthostatic hypotension	Invasive monitoring
RESP	ARDS Pulm edema	SOB Dyspnea	Rales	ABG CXR
ENDO	Metabolic abn			ABG, electrolytes PT/PTT, Hct
RENAL	↓ Renal function	↓ UO		BUN/Cr
CNS	Disoriented 2° to sepsis		Neuro exam	

Key Reference: Conly J: Necrotizing fasciitis. *In* Hall, Schmidt, Wood (eds): Principles of Critical Care, 1st ed. New York, McGraw-Hill, 1992, pp 1329–1333.

PERIOPERATIVE IMPLICATIONS

Preoperative Preparation

- Surgery often emergent
- Verify adequacy of initial resuscitation including volume status
- Patient may not be on NPO status

Monitoring

- Often persistently hypotensive, tachycardic, with septic physiology
- Consider invasive monitoring including arterial line, CVP or PA catheter or transesophageal ECHO to manage intraoperative volume status

Airway

- Spread of fascial infection can be clinically silent
- Can cause airway edema if infectious spread to neck or face

Induction

- May be severely septic and hypotensive with massive fluid requirements
- Relative hypovolemia may accentuate hypotensive response to anesthetic induction.

Maintenance

- Hemodynamic instability. Monitor volume status and adequacy of cardiac output.

Extubation

- Often need repeat exploration within 24 h if sepsis and hemodynamic instability continue postop. Consider postop intubation and ICU management between debridements.

Adjuvants

- No contraindication to N_2O
- Efficacy of hyperbaric oxygen therapy for anaerobic infection unproven but felt worthwhile by some

Postoperative Period

- Consider ICU level care
- Will likely need repeat debridement within 24 h
- Prognosis worst with perineal/truncal infection, extensive spread, associated diabetes/CV disease

ANTICIPATED PROBLEMS/CONCERNS

- Need for emergent surgery in potentially unstable patient
- Massive fluid requirements 2° to edema formation and septic physiology
- Associated metabolic abnormalities

NEUROFIBROMATOSIS

Zeev N. Kain, M.D.

RISK

- Prevalence: 1:3000 people

PERIOPERATIVE RISKS

- Risk depends upon tumor and location

WORRY ABOUT

- Difficult intubation
- Intraoperative HTN and tachycardia

OVERVIEW

- Genetic disorder in which multiple organs, such as skin and nervous system, are site of tumors and hamartomas
- Hallmark is café-au-lait spots (more than 6 that are >1.5 cm in diameter) and multiple neurofibromas
- Laryngeal and tracheal compression may occur 2° to associated tumors
- Surgery may be indicated for patients with NF-1, esp. for removal of tumors (e.g., neurofibromas, pheochromocytoma), skeletal dysplasia (e.g., tibial pseudoarthrosis), scoliosis, and renovascular HTN

ICD-9-CM Codes: 237.7; 171.# (malignant)

ETIOLOGY

- Autosomal dominant, although about 50% of cases represent new mutations. The gene for NF-1 appears to reside on the long arm of chromosome 17.

USUAL TREATMENT

- Radiation and surgical treatment for various tumors involved

ASSESSMENT POINTS

SYSTEM	EFFECT	ASSESSMENT BY HX	PE	TEST
HEENT*	Pharyngeal compression Laryngeal compression Airway obstruction	Dyspnea, dysphonia	Evaluation of airway	X-ray CT of neck
CV	Renovascular HTN Pheochromocytoma	Headache, perspiration		BP/HR Urinary catecholamines
RESP*	Restrictive lung disease Cor pulmonale Interstitial lung disease Hypoxemia	Exercise tolerance	Cyanosis Clubbing	CXR ECG ABG PFTs (rare)
GU*	Obstruction and uremia			
CNS	Mental retardation Seizures Neurofibromas			
MS*	Kyphoscoliosis Macrocephaly Craniofacial/vertebral dysplasia			

*In severe cases

Key Reference: Listernick R, Charrow J: Neurofibromatosis type 1. J Pediatr 1990; 116:845–853.

PERIOPERATIVE IMPLICATIONS

Preoperative Preparation

- Evaluation of airway for possible laryngeal and pharyngeal tumors
- Asymptomatic intraspinal neurofibromas can make identification and entry into epidural and subarachnoid spaces very difficult. A careful examination of the back is indicated before any regional technique is considered.

Monitoring

- Routine
- Consider arterial line depending on resp status and presence of pheochromocytoma

Airway

- Consider awake fiberoptic intubation or tracheostomy if laryngeal and pharyngeal involvement

Preinduction/Induction

- No particular anesthetic drug or technique recommended
- Consider potential for spinal cord neurofibromas if regional considered
- Consider potential for increased ICP
- Consider potential of pheochromocytoma (see under Pheochromocytoma)

Maintenance

- CV instability if pheochromocytoma present
- Several reported cases of prolonged NMB in response to administration of succinylcholine, pancuronium, d-tubocurarine

Extubation

- Routine considerations

Postoperative Period

- Pain management may be critical

Adjuvants

- Prolonged response or resistance to NMBs

ANTICIPATED PROBLEMS/CONCERNS

- Presence of pheochromocytoma
- Potential for increased ICP if expanding intracranial tumor

OCCLUSIVE CEREBROVASCULAR DISEASE

Ian A. Herrick, M.D., F.R.C.P.C.

RISK

• People within USA: stroke incidence = 0.1%/y (all causes)
• Races with highest prevalence: Japanese/Eastern European (incidence 0.3%/y)

PERIOPERATIVE RISKS

• Stroke
  – Major general surgery at age >50 y = 0.4%; at age >80 y = 2.5%
  – Major peripheral vascular reconstruction = 1%
  – CABG = 1–5%, carotid endarterectomy (CEA) = 3% or less

WORRY ABOUT

• Cerebral ischemia
• Myocardial ischemia (CAD, leading cause of morbidity following CEA)
• Control of coexisting CAD, DM, HTN

OVERVIEW

• Two main clinical presentations
  – Patients with known occlusive CVD undergoing CEA. Risk factors include: CAD/CHF; stroke in evolution, frequent TIAs; severe HTN; carotid siphon stenosis; COPD; poor cerebral collateral flow; age >70 y; intraluminal thrombus.
  – Patients with known or possible CVD presenting for other surgery. Risk factors are poorly defined. Most perioperative strokes occur postop and do not correlate with presence of CVD. Highest risk with CABG.
• Asymptomatic carotid bruits are inconsistent predictors of CVD, but predict poor CVD survival.

ICD-9-CM Code: 434.9

ETIOLOGY

• Vasculopathy 2° to advanced atherosclerosis
• Risk factors include age, HTN, diabetes mellitus, smoking
• High incidence of concomitant CAD and peripheral vascular disease

USUAL TREATMENT

• Antiplatelet drugs (esp. ASA); CEA

ASSESSMENT POINTS

SYSTEM	EFFECT	ASSESSMENT BY HX	PE	TEST
HEENT	Possible positional cerebral ischemia	Sx of cerebral ischemia with head movements	Neck ROM	
CV	HTN Vasculopathy LV dysfunction, CHF	Exercise tolerance Angina, MI, CHF Claudication	Arterial BP S_3 Peripheral pulses	ECG, CXR ECHO Stress test
RESP	COPD due to smoking Irritable airway	Dyspnea Chronic cough Smoker	Wheezing Accessory muscles	CXR ?ABGs ?PFTs
ENDO	Possible diabetes			Glucose
RENAL	Possible nephropathy	Diabetes, HTN		Cr, urea
CNS	Cerebral ischemia	TIA, stroke	Neurologic deficits	Cerebral Angio prior to CEA

Key Reference: Herrick IA, Gelb AW: Occlusive cerebrovascular disease. *In* Cottrell/Smith Anesthesia and Neurosurgery, 3rd ed. St. Louis, CV Mosby, 1994, pp 481–494.

PERIOPERATIVE IMPLICATIONS

Preoperative Preparation

• Neurologic assessment
• Optimize control of coexisting HTN, CAD, diabetes, COPD
• Evaluate normal BP range

Monitoring

• Arterial catheter and inferior lead ECG (as well as V_5)
• Consider neurologic monitor: EEG often used for CEA, regional anesthetic with awake patient (if practical)

Induction/Maintenance

• Have surgeon block carotid sinus nerve if bradycardic
• Maintain hemodynamic stability based on preop BP range
• Maintain normocapnia based on preop pH and $PaCO_2$

Extubation

• Be prepared to manage hemodynamic instability following CEA
• Avoid straining on ET tube with fresh arteriotomy following CEA

Postoperative Period

• Hemodynamic instability due to baroreceptor dysfunction following CEA
• Adequate analgesia, supplemental O_2
• Awake patient allows early and frequent neurologic evaluation

ANTICIPATED PROBLEMS/CONCERNS

• Most patients with CVD also at high risk for CAD. Consistent approach to management of both problems includes hemodynamic stability, adequate oxygenation, normocapnia, adequate analgesia, normoglycemia.
• Caution regarding use of succinylcholine in patients with previous paretic CVA.

OPITZ-FRIAS SYNDROME (The G Syndrome)

Bruno Bissonnette, M.D.

RISK

- Overall incidence not reported
- Very rare congenital disorder

PREOPERATIVE RISKS

- Very high risk of recurrent pulmonary aspiration; hypoplasia of both pulmonary and vascular components of one lung
- High mortality rate in infancy

WORRY ABOUT

- Neuromuscular dysfunction of laryngo-esophageal apparatus
- Laryngotracheoesophageal cleft or fistula
- Difficult tracheal intubation due to craniofacial deformity
- Associated congenital anomalies

OVERVIEW

- Known also as the hypospadias-dysphagia syndrome
- Emergency presentations are for cardiopulmonary resuscitation, upper resp obstruction, severe resp stridor, regurgitation, aspiration
- Presence of one hypoplastic lung
- Laryngeal hypoplasia
- Laryngotracheoesophageal cleft or fistula
- Anticipate very difficult tracheal intubation
- Any male infant presenting for TEF with genital defect should be suspected

ICD-9-CM Code: 759.9 (Congenital anomaly, unspecified)

ETIOLOGY

- X-linked recessive inheritance
- Autosomal dominant inheritance or new mutation
- Partial male sex limitation
- Autosomal recessive inheritance, high parenteral consanguinity
- Females can be equally or nearly as severely affected as males

USUAL TREATMENT

- Prophylactic gastrostomy
- Feeding jejunostomy
- Cervical esophagostomy if unable to swallow
- Prophylactic antibodies (pulm infection)

ASSESSMENT POINTS

SYSTEM	EFFECT	ASSESSMENT BY HX	PE	TESTS (if indicated)
HEENT	Cleft lip–palate (35%) Ankyloglossia Micrognathia	Feeding difficulties Speech anomalies	Short lingual frenulum	
CNS	Dolichocephaly (20%) Large metopic sagittal suture and anterior fontanel	Mental dysfunction Prominent forehead	"Cone-head" Palpation	CT (if indicated)
FACIES	Hypertelorism/telecanthus(90%) Mongoloid palpebral fissures Strabismus	Mother-related disease	Large nasal bridge downslanting	Face x-ray
CV	Congenital heart defects (40%) (ASD, VSD, PDA, coarctation of aorta)	Failure to thrive	Auscultation	ECG TEE, ABG
RESP	Agenesis, hypoplasia of one lung Tracheoesophageal cleft, fissure Hypoplasia of vocal cord Tracheomalacia Short trachea, high carina	Polyhydramnios on delivery Coughing, choking, cyanosis Hoarse, weak cry Stridorous resp	Auscultation Tracheal stenosis	CXR Bronchogram Esophagogram
GI	Achalasia of the cardia (70%) Neuromuscular dysfunction of esophagus	Dysphagia		Esophagogram (if indicated) Cinefluoroscopy of swallowing (if indicated)
GU	Hypospadias with descended testis Ureteral stenosis or duplication		Perineal or penoscrotal	Nephrogram

Key Reference: Bershof JF, Guyyron B, Olsen MM: G syndrome: A review of the literature and a case report. J Craniomaxillofac Surg 1992; 20:24–27.

PERIOPERATIVE IMPLICATIONS

Preoperative Preparation

- Evacuation of the stomach with NG tube
- Feeding: clear water or apple juice
- Consider H_2-blocker
- No atropine IM or metoclopramide
- Give sodium citrate through NG tube
- IV access 24 h before surgery to reduce stomach content

Monitoring

- All standard monitors

Airway

- Tubes smaller than normal 2° to laryngeal hypoplasia

Preinduction

- Warm OR
- Decompress stomach with suction
- Atropine and succinylcholine backup

Induction

- Maintain spontaneous respiration
- Danger of regurgitation and aspiration requires careful inhalation induction
- Cricoid pressure should be applied
- Atropine 20 µg/kg before intubation may prevent bradycardia

Maintenence

- Hand ventilation (low PPV)
- Avoid hypothermia

Extubation

- Based on patient's lung condition

Adjuvants

- All medications can be used

ANTICIPATED PROBLEMS

- Regurgitation and pulm aspiration. Difficult tracheal intubation. ↑Incidence of pneumothorax. High mortality rate in infancy.

OSTEOARTHRITIS

Denise J. Wedel, M.D.

RISK

- Osteoarthritis (OA) most common cause of impairment in the elderly
  - 63–85% of Americans >65 y have radiographic signs
  - 35–50% have pain, stiffness, or limitation of movement
  - 9–12% are significantly disabled
  - 46 million MD visits and 68 million work days lost per annum
- Risk factors differ across joints: knee—obesity, injury; hand—repetitive use; hip—congenital or developmental abn, male preponderance

PERIOPERATIVE RISKS

- Often associated with obesity
- Common analgesics include NSAIDs and intra-articular steroid injections
- Rarely affects neck or jaw
- Reported association with diabetes, hypothyroidism, hyperparathyroidism, gout

WORRY ABOUT

- Anesthetic problems with associated obesity
- Positioning may be difficult owing to joint pain and stiffness
- Possible associated metabolic conditions
- Effect of medications on plt function and frequent steroid injections

OVERVIEW

- OA is age-related but not caused by aging
- Early radiographic findings include joint space narrowing, osteophytes, subchondral stenosis
- With progression, osteophytes, subchondral cysts, intra-articular osseous bodies seen
- Subchondral bony collapse is a late finding
- Knees most common joint affected (41%), followed by hands (30%), and hips (19%)
- Risk factors for symptoms are obesity (knees) and severe radiographic findings

ICD-9-CM Code: 715.0 (Generalized)

ETIOLOGY

- Cartilage shows ↑ water with softened cartilage and depletion of keratan sulfate
- Age-related decreases in blood supply, followed by changes in distribution of forces causing damage to cartilage nutrition
- Repetitive use or previous injury may cause subchondral microfractures over time with strain on overlying cartilage
- Autosomal dominant in some with co-segregation of OA with a mutation in type II procollagen gene

USUAL TREATMENT

- Conservative therapy: weight loss, physical therapy to maintain function and mobility, analgesics (aspirin, acetaminophen, NSAIDs), steroid injections, surgical replacement

ASSESSMENT POINTS

SYSTEM	EFFECT	ASSESSMENT BY HX	PE	TEST
HEENT	Rare C-spine involvement	Pain	Neck ROM	Usually not needed C-spine x-rays
CV	Age-related changes	Exercise tolerance may be limited by joint changes	HR and tolerance to 2-flight stair climb	ECG CXR
RESP	Nonspecific	Exercise tolerance		CXR
GI	Sensitivity to NSAIDs	Gastric upset		
ENDO	Associated diabetes			Fasting blood sugar
CNS	Age-related changes	TIAs or stroke		
MS	Multiple joint involvement	Joint pain	Joint ROM	
RENAL	Age-related changes			Cr

Key Reference: Felson DT: Osteoarthritis. Rheum Dis Clin North Am 1990; 16:499–512.

PERIOPERATIVE IMPLICATIONS

Preoperative Preparation

- Assess joint involvement and ROM
- Question patient regarding nonprescription analgesics
- Consider regional anesthetic techniques
- Evaluate for steroid need

Monitoring

- Routine

Airway

- Assess neck ROM

Induction

- Age-related considerations: elderly patients may have slow circulation times, CV disease, fluctuations in BP

Maintenance

- Position with consideration of other joint involvement

Extubation

- No special considerations

Adjuvants

- Elderly patients may be more sensitive to narcotics

Postoperative Period

- Consider continuous regional technique with local anesthetic and/or narcotic for pain management

ANTICIPATED PROBLEMS/CONCERNS

- Usually neck and airway normal
- Concomitant risk factors—esp. obesity
- Often several joints involved with pain and decreased ROM
- Regional anesthesia well suited

OSTEOPOROSIS

David B. Albert, M.D.

RISK

- All elderly patients of European descent considered at risk. Female > male 3/1
- Postmenopausal female, small frame, low wt
- Risk factors: Positive family history, nulliparity, long-term glucocorticoid fracture, long-term anticonvulsant fracture, thyrotoxicosis, hyperparathyroidism, smoking, heavy alcohol use

PERIOPERATIVE RISKS

- Concomitant medical conditions in elderly
- Pneumonia
- Coexisting metabolic or endocrine disorders
- Fractures

WORRY ABOUT

- Positioning because of ↑ risk of bone fractures
- Vertebral fractures
- Pulm function/restrictive disease, esp. if kyphosis present

OVERVIEW

- Imbalance between bone resorption and formation causes loss of bone substance, resulting in bone fractures.
- Most common fracture sites: vertebral body, neck of femur, distal radius, proximal humerus, pelvis
- Severe kyphosis common
- Type I (postmenopausal) osteoporosis: women 15–20 years after menopause; vertebral and Colles' fractures most common
- Type II (age-related) osteoporosis: men and women ≥70 y. Hip and vertebral fractures most common. Also pelvis, humerus, femur
- Biphasic pattern of bone loss
  – slow phase occurs in both sexes beginning at age 40 y; 0.5–1%/y, cortical and trabecular bone
  – accelerated phase in women after menopause: 2–3%/y cortical bone; 4-6%/y trabecular bone

ICD-9-CM Code: 733.00

ETIOLOGY

- Insufficient accumulation of bone mass during skeletal growth
- Age-related factors: Decreased bone formation at cellular level begins in 4th decade and becomes more severe with age. Age-related ↑ in parathyroid function with age-related ↓ in calcium absorption
- Menopause: Accelerated phase of bone loss is the result of estrogen deficiency.
- Sporadic factors: Twofold increased risk with cigarettes and high alcohol consumption

TREATMENT

- Calcium; estrogen (newer nonestrogen bone matrix–enhancing drugs); calcitonin; discontinuation of glucocorticoid if due to chronic use; sodium fluoride; surgical stabilization of fractures

ASSESSMENT POINTS

SYSTEM	EFFECT	ASSESSMENT BY HX	PE	TEST
HEENT	Osteoporosis of skull Vertebral fractures	Pain		Skull x-ray Neck x-ray
RESP	Kyphosis	Dyspnea	Dowager's hump	Flow-volume loop ABGs
ENDO	Parathyroid function ↓ in Type I ↑ in Type II Calcium absorption ↓ Metabolic disorders of vitamin D			Ca^{2+}
MS	Back pain Loss of height Spinal deformity Fractures	Acute back pain Remittance and recurrence until chronic	Dowager's hump ↓ Height Multiple fractures	X-ray Vertebral bone density

Key Reference: Riggs BL: Osteoporosis. *In* Wyngaarden JB, Smith LH (eds): Cecil Textbook of Medicine, 18th ed. Philadelphia, WB Saunders, 1988, pp 1510–1515.

PERIOPERATIVE IMPLICATIONS

Preoperative Preparation

- Move and position carefully owing to risk of bone fractures

Monitoring

- Routine
- Consider ABGs if pulm disease or pneumonia present

Airway

- Cervical fractures may require neck stabilization and fiberoptic intubation.
- Acromegaly may occur with osteoporosis.

Musculoskeletal

- Vertebral collapse may make spinal/epidural anesthesia more difficult.

ANTICIPATED PROBLEMS/CONCERNS

- Susceptible to fracture with routine positioning and moving

OTITIS MEDIA

Donald C. Tyler, M.D.

RISK

• 70% of infants have at least one episode

PERIOPERATIVE RISKS

• Laryngospasm from upper respiratory secretions
• Airway problem after surgery increases if anesthesia in patients with productive vs. nonproductive URI

WORRY ABOUT

• Risk of airway obstruction from hypertrophied adenoids and tonsils

OVERVIEW

• Common condition seen in most children. Results from obstruction of eustachian tube and interference with drainage of middle ear
• Usually treated with antibiotics. May come to surgery for ear tubes, which are placed to drain middle ear fluid. Procedure is short (10 min), and child should be able to leave day of surgery shortly after.

ICD-9-CM Codes: 381.0 (chronic); 382.0 (acute)

ETIOLOGY

• Obstruction of eustachian tube results in collection of fluid in middle ear.
• Infection with common respiratory bacteria including *S. pneumoniae* and *H. influenzae* occurs (less *H. influenzae* since vaccine).
• After treatment with antibiotics, fluid may remain in middle ear, which may produce hearing loss.

USUAL TREATMENT

• Antibiotics
• Myringotomy and tubes may be used to drain persistent effusions if hearing loss is a concern.

ASSESSMENT POINTS

SYSTEM	EFFECT	ASSESSMENT BY HX	PE	TEST
HEENT	Mucous secretions Adenoid and tonsil hypertrophy	Acute vs. chronic Snoring, sleep apnea	?Acute infection Adenoid facies	Pulse oximetry
RESP	Pneumonia	Degree of illness	Auscultation	Pulse oximetry, CXR
CNS	Systemic illness	Degree of illness		

Key Reference: Bluestone CD, Klein JO: Otitis media, atelectasis, and eustachian tube dysfunction. *In* Bluestone CD, Stool, SE (eds): Pediatric Otolaryngology, 2nd ed. Philadelphia, WB Saunders, 1990, pp 320–486.

PERIOPERATIVE IMPLICATIONS

Monitoring
• Routine

Airway
• Concern about upper airway obstruction due to adenotonsillar hypertrophy

Maintenance
• Brief, rapidly reversible anesthetic for 10 min procedure

Extubation
• Usually not intubated, except when specifically indicated

Adjuvants
• Usually none, may elect not to place intravenous catheter

Postoperative Concerns
• Prolonged respiratory status evaluation and parent education if productive URI

ANTICIPATED PROBLEMS/CONCERNS

• Prefer to have child ready to go home soon after surgery

PACEMAKERS

Mark F. Trankina, M.D.

RISK

- People within USA: 0.5 million
- >115,000 permanent pacemakers implanted/y

PERIOPERATIVE RISKS

- No proven increase in risk due to pacemaker itself
- Risk related to associated medical problems

WORRY ABOUT

- Perioperative loss of capture due to electromechanical interference (EMI)—underlying rhythm
- Magnet should be placed on generator only if (1) response to magnet is absolutely known in that patient or (2) patient has become hemodynamically unstable owing to pacemaker failure and failure of other measures.
- Newer designs (rate-adaptive) may alter rate by perioperative hemodynamic/respiratory manipulations and have very unpredictable responses to magnet placement.

OVERVIEW

- While pacemaker is indication of cardiac disease, it can be considered adjunct to successful anesthetic management and not a problem in itself
- Indications (permanent): symptomatic brady-dysrhythmias, asymptomatic Mobitz II or greater, sinus-node dysfunction, some types of SVT or VTach, orthotopic heart transplantation, hypertrophic and ?dilated cardiomyopathy, ?long Q-T syndrome
- Indications (temporary): following cardiac surgery, treatment of drug toxicity resulting in dysrhythmias, certain dysrhythmias complicating MI
- Codes: 1st letter refers to the chamber paced, 2nd to the chamber sensed, and 3rd to response to sensed event. Final 2 letters refer to programmability and antitachycardia (AICD) functions. In 1st position A refers to atrium, V to ventricle; D implies that both atrium and ventricle are paced. For 2nd position the same letters are utilized for chamber or chambers sensed. O indicates that no chamber is sensed. In 3rd position I refers to inhibition, T to triggering, D to double (atrium-triggered, ventricle-inhibited), O to none. A newer class of pacemakers, designated by R (rate-adaptive) in 4th position (i.e., DDDR), is designed to deliver more physiologic response by changing rate in response to exercise.

ICD-9-CM Code: v45.0 (Pacemaker status postsurgical)

ETIOLOGY

- Congenital
- Acquired: CAD, MI, HTN, post cardiac surgery, post evoked potential study, dilated and infiltrative cardiomyopathy, inflammatory, infectious, neoplastic, radiation, neuromuscular, idiopathic, neurally mediated

USUAL TREATMENT

- Possible electrophysiology study
- Permanent pacemaker placement followed by regular telephone evaluations

ASSESSMENT POINTS

SYSTEM	EFFECT	ASSESSMENT BY HX	PE	TEST
CV	Dysrhythmia Pacemaker 50% significant CAD 20% HTN	Pacemaker indication, syncope Review recent phone checks Exercise tolerance, angina, Sx CHF BP control	ECG/pulse 2-flight walk	ECG ?programming; CXR (leads)
ENDO	10% insulin-dependent diabetes			
CNS	Other causes of syncope	TIA, CVA	Bruits	
MS		PNS exam if regional planned		

Code	Indication	Function	Perioperative Management
VVI	Bradycardia without need for preserved AV conduction	Demand ventricular pacing	Magnet utilization may be helpful and converts to asynchronous pacing, usually at 72 bpm
VVIR	Bradycardia without need for preserved AV conduction, chronotropic incompetence	Allows somewhat physiologic response to exercise	Pacemaker may sense perioperative changes (e.g., temp and respiratory rate) as related to exercise, unpredictable response to magnet placement
DDD	Bradycardia when AV synchrony can be preserved	Provides more physiologic response, maintains AV concordance	Unpredictable response to magnet placement
DDDR	Patients requiring physiologic response of heart rate, i.e., chronotropic incompetence	Allows somewhat physiologic response to exercise, maintains AV concordance	Pacemaker may sense perioperative changes (e.g., temp and respiratory rate) as related to exercise, unpredictable response to magnet placement.

Key Reference: Atlee JL: Arrhythmias & Pacemakers: Practical Management for Anesthesia and Critical Care Medicine. Philadelphia, WB Saunders, 1996, pp 205–329.

PERIOPERATIVE IMPLICATIONS

Preoperative Preparation

- Magnet available
- Alternate pacing modality (e.g., esophageal, transcutaneous)
- IV chronotropes (isoproterenol, ephedrine)
- Discuss cautery precautions with surgeon
- Regional offers CNS perfusion monitoring
- ?Cardiology consult—probably not needed if patient asymptomatic and recent evaluations of generator OK. Generator programming check always advisable if feasible

Monitoring

- ECG/pulse relationship, especially during cautery (consider arterial catheter)

Induction

- Succinylcholine may cause pacemaker inhibition with myopotentials in older pacemakers

Maintenance

- Vigilant ECG/pulse monitoring
- Electrocautery, which emits radiofrequency energy, has potential to cause transient or permanent changes in pacemaker function. Most common problem is inhibition of pacemaker. In one study, 21% of patients exposed to electrocautery during surgery had pacemaker reprogram to the backup mode. Grounding plate away from operative site (circuit should not go through generator/leads), bipolar if possible, short bursts, lowest current. X-rays OK, MRI not advisable
- Magnet: should be applied only if effect known or if pacemaker dysfunction has caused hemodynamic compromise. Once placed, removed only with pacemaker programmer's presence

Extubation

- ECG/pulse, recheck generator status before proceeding

Adjuvants

- K+ rapid fluctuations could affect capture

Postoperative Period

- Programming recheck advisable, especially after cardioversion/defibrillation or if magnet has been placed

ANTICIPATED PROBLEMS/CONCERNS

- Intraoperative reprogramming, loss of pacing capture
- Postop generator failure, loss of pacing capture
- Risks related to associated medical problems

PANCREATITIS, ACUTE

Jeffrey J. Schwartz, M.D.

RISK

- Incidence of 100–200/1 million in larger cities
- No gender/racial predilection

PERIOPERATIVE RISKS

- Most mortality occurs with surgery for complications of acute pancreatitis: 10–40%
- Risk of nonpancreatic surgery probably dependent on severity of attack

WORRY ABOUT

- Severe hypovolemia 2° to sequestration of fluid in retroperitoneal space
- Electrolyte abn, including hypocalcemia, hyperglycemia, acidosis
- Systemic complications such as alcohol withdrawal, ARDS, acute renal failure, DIC, multisystem organ failure, sepsis (see the above topics in Diseases section)

OVERVIEW

- Intense inflammatory response caused by release of activated pancreatic enzymes with resultant tissue destruction, fluid and electrolyte loss
- Most commonly a mild self-limited disease diagnosed by abdominal pain radiating to the back, elevated serum amylase, CT imaging
- Occasionally severe with renal, pulm, coagulation, septic complications

ICD-9-CM Code: 577.0

ETIOLOGY

- Many diverse causes
- Most commonly alcohol, gallstones, trauma, CPB, medications, hypertriglyceridemia, infection
- 10% of cases idiopathic

USUAL TREATMENT

- In most cases, nonspecific and supportive only
- Adequate volume replacement and correction of electrolyte abn
- Intensive care of organ system failures
- Parenteral analgesia; meperidine preferred to morphine
- Rarely, judiciously timed surgery to drain abscesses or debride necrotic tissue

ASSESSMENT POINTS

SYSTEM	EFFECT	ASSESSMENT BY HX	PE	TEST
CV	Hypovolemia	Orthostatic dizziness Cold	Lying and sitting BP and HR Hypotension Oliguria	BUN/Cr
RESP	ARDS	Dyspnea Tachypnea	Chest exam may be nonspecific	ABG CXR
GI	Ileus GI bleed	Nausea, vomiting Hematemesis		
ENDO	Hyperglycemia			Serum glucose
HEME	DIC		Bleeding	PT/PTT, Plt FSP, fibrinogen Hct
RENAL	Acute renal failure Hypocalcemia		Tetany	BUN/Cr Serum Ca^{2+}
CNS	Psychosis Encephalopathy		Mental status	

Key Reference: Steinberg W, Tenner S: Medical progress: Acute pancreatitis. N Engl J Med 1994; 330:1198–1210.

PERIOPERATIVE IMPLICATIONS

Preoperative Preparation

- Assess and correct volume status, hypocalcemia, hyperglycemia, acidosis

Monitoring

- Consider arterial catheter if need for blood draws or hypovolemia
- Consider CVP or PA catheter for monitoring of volume status

Airway

- Routine

Induction

- Peritoneal irritation frequently leads to ileus and ↑ risk of aspiration
- Anticipate hypovolemia

Maintenance

- CV instability due to massive sequestration of fluid; depending on severity >10 L of isotonic fluid may be required over 24 h

Extubation

- Will likely require postop mechanical ventilation

Adjuvants

- Multiple interaction of protein-bound drugs, esp. if patient malnourished or undergoing alcohol withdrawal (see under Malnutrition; Alcohol Abuse)

ANTICIPATED PROBLEMS/CONCERNS

- Patients with pancreatitis presenting for abdominal surgery are typically critically ill and require postop intensive care to manage hypovolemia, ARDS, DIC, acute renal failure, sepsis.
- Hypoglycemia, hyperglycemia are life-threatening risks after pancreatectomy.
- Alcohol withdrawal can be life-threatening.

PANCREATITIS, CHRONIC

Jeffrey J. Schwartz, M.D.

RISK

- Unknown

PERIOPERATIVE RISKS

- Perioperative mortality directly related to chronic pancreatitis (rare)
- Associated malnutrition may lead to difficulty with wound healing and infection.
- Endocrine insufficiency leads to glucose intolerance but ketosis, coma, and chronic diabetic complications are rare.

WORRY ABOUT

- Management of pain and narcotics if patient is addicted owing to chronic administration

OVERVIEW

- A nonlethal condition characterized by fibrosis, inflammation, loss of exocrine pancreatic tissue
- Characterized by severe persistent or episodic abdominal pain
- Malabsorption and diabetes mellitus are consequences of loss of pancreatic tissue.
- Endocrine insufficiency occurs later than exocrine insufficiency.

ICD-9-CM Code: 577.1

ETIOLOGY

- Most commonly chronic alcohol use leads to proteinaceous plugs in the ducts and atrophy of acinar tissue with fibrosis.
- Other causes are pancreatic duct obstruction, cystic fibrosis, protein-calorie malnutrition.
- Acute pancreatitis does not lead to chronic pancreatitis.
- 30–40% of cases are idiopathic.

USUAL TREATMENT

- Strict avoidance of alcohol
- Pancreatic enzyme supplements for exocrine insufficiency
- Insulin for glucose intolerance
- Selected patients may occasionally receive pain relief with surgery

ASSESSMENT POINTS

SYSTEM	EFFECT	ASSESSMENT BY HX	PE	TEST
GI	Malabsorption	Diarrhea	Orthostatic hypotension	BUN/Cr
ENDO	Glucose intolerance	Polyuria, polydipsia		Serum glucose

Key Reference: Steer ML, Waxman I, Freedman S: Medical progress: Chronic pancreatitis. N Engl J Med 1995; 332(22):1482–1490.

PERIOPERATIVE IMPLICATIONS

Preoperative Preparation

- If patient is receiving chronic narcotics, the usual dose should be given on the day of surgery
- Glucose/insulin management

Monitoring

- Routine

Airway

- Routine

Induction

- Consider full stomach if abdominal pain

Maintenance

- Consideration of narcotic tolerance must be incorporated in plan

Extubation

- Routine

Adjuvants

- Multiple interventions and adjustments needed for protein-bound drugs if patient is malnourished (see under Malnutrition)

ANTICIPATED PROBLEMS/CONCERNS

- Difficulty managing pain and narcotics in patients on large doses of narcotics for chronic pain
- Pancreatic endocrine insufficiency may lead to impaired glucose intolerance without chronic sequelae of diabetes mellitus

PARKINSON'S DISEASE (PARALYSIS AGITANS)

Michael D. Sharpe, M.D.
William Zimmermann, M.D.

RISK

- People within USA: ~1% of population >50 y
- Gender with higher prevalence: males; 40–60 y (1.4:1)

PERIOPERATIVE RISKS

- Associated with ↑ incidence of arteriosclerosis and obstructive lung disease

WORRY ABOUT

- Increased sensitivity to anesthetic agents
- Laryngospasm/diaphragmatic spasms
- Visual and tactile hallucinations
- Reduced vital capacity leading to pulm complications
- Violent tremors
- Muscle tremors mimicking VFib
- Postop delirium/psychiatric disturbances
- Side effects of L-dopa therapy

OVERVIEW

- Degenerative disease of extrapyramidal system characterized by bradykinesia, rigidity, tremor
- Dementia in up to 50% of patients
- Symptoms may worsen on emergence from GA
- Classic signs: (1) poverty of movement (bradykinesia), (2) muscular rigidity, (3) resting tremor, (4) postural instability

ICD-9-CM Code: 332.0

ETIOLOGY

- Parkinsonism or Parkinson's disease
  – Unknown
  – Some clusters related to 1927 influenza epidemic

- Secondary Parkinsonism
  – Postencephalitis, CO poisoning, manganese poisoning, n-MPTP poisoning, chronic ingestion of dopamine-inhibiting antipsychotic drugs

USUAL TREATMENT

- Levodopa (L-dopa) in combination with α-methylhydrazine (carbidopa) (Sinemet)
- Bromocriptine and lergotrile: provide direct stimulation of dopaminergic receptors. Use in combination with Sinemet
- Amantadine: reduces symptoms via presumed anticholinergic and enhanced dopamine effect
- Anticholinergics (benztropine): cholinergic side effects limit use
- Stereotaxic surgery in rare cases
- Experimental treatment with fetal adrenal implantation

ASSESSMENT POINTS

SYSTEM	EFFECT	ASSESSMENT BY HX	PE	TEST
HEENT	Laryngospasm Cervical/facial muscle rigidity		Mouth opening Neck ROM	
CV	Orthostatic hypotension Hypovolemia	Fainting Sx		BP drop with postural change
RESP	Aspiration pneumonitis Obstructive lung disease	Exercise tolerance, chest tightness, cough	Rales, wheezing Fever Assess cough, ability to take deep breath	CXR O$_2$ sat PFTs
	↓ Vital capacity	Difficulty with coughing, deep breathing exercises, resp infection Sx		
GI	Gastroparesis, N/V	Early satiety		
CNS	Agitation, confusion, depression, dementia Visual/tactile hallucinations			
MS	Impaired joint mobility due to rigidity Violent skeletal muscle tremors	Joint mobility		ROM of joints Tremor severity
RENAL	Urinary retention	Frequency, incontinence, suprapubic pain	Bladder distention	Residual urine volume

Key Reference: Stoelting RK, Dierdorf SF, et al: Diseases of the Nervous System, Anesthesia and Co-existing Diseases, 2nd ed. New York, Churchill, Livingstone, 1988, pp 304–306.

PERIOPERATIVE IMPLICATIONS

Preoperative Preparation

- Administer anti-Parkinson's therapy up to time of surgery; benefits last 6–12 h
- Avoid phenothiazines, butyrophenones, and metoclopramide—exacerbate extrapyramidal Sx
- Assess intravascular volume status
- Preop instruction of deep breathing/incentive spirometry

Monitoring

- Close attention to ECG in presence of arrhythmogenic anti-Parkinson's agents (e.g., L-dopa)

Airway

- Muscle rigidity may impede airway manipulation and impair ventilation
- Increased risk of aspiration

Induction

- Intravascular volume depletion and inadequate response to hypotension (due to ↓ renin release and depletion of noradrenaline stores 2° to L-dopa therapy) make BP and HR fluctuate
- Ketamine may cause exaggerated sympathetic response
- Potential hyperkalemic response to succinylcholine

Maintenance

- Normal response to nondepolarizing muscle relaxants
- Use agents that have rapid recovery

Extubation

- Ensure full recovery of NMB
- Laryngospasm and impaired ventilation 2° to muscle rigidity
- Violent tremors/hallucinations on emergence

Adjuvants

- Avoid indirect-acting sympathomimetics if patient is on deprenyl
- Regional: preferred over GA owing to emergence problems
- N/V and ileus following GA may prevent reinstitution of oral anti-Parkinsonian therapy
- Muscle relaxants eliminate rigidity

Postoperative Period

- Close attention to respiratory status (e.g., physiotherapy, incentive spirometry)
- Close attention to CNS state—potential for delirium and other psychotic disturbances
- Begin anti-Parkinsonian therapy immediately postop

ANTICIPATED PROBLEMS/CONCERNS

- Skeletal muscle tremor may mimic VFib on ECG monitor

PAROXYSMAL ATRIAL TACHYCARDIA

Jeffrey R. Balser, M.D., Ph.D.
Michael J. Breslow, M.D.

RISK

- Common in surgical ICU patients
- Incidence in US population estimated at 1.9%
- No racial prevalence
- Commonly with mitral valve prolapse

PERIOPERATIVE RISKS

- Rapid heart rate impairs LV filling and may adversely affect LV function in patients with LV failure, LV hypertrophy, aortic stenosis, or mitral stenosis.

WORRY ABOUT

- Hypotension—esp. in patients with systolic or diastolic dysfunction
- Ischemia—patients with CAD
- VFib—in Wolff-Parkinson-White (WPW) patients who develop AFib

OVERVIEW

- Paroxysmal atrial tachycardia (PAT), aka paroxysmal supraventricular tachycardia (PSVT), describes supraventricular arrhythmias other than AFib and atrial flutter
- Usually seen postop in critically ill patients, most commonly after major vascular surgery, pneumonectomy, cardiac procedures; also in patients who develop postop infectious complications
- Causes poorly defined, probably multifactorial, and may include catecholamine excess and pericardial inflammation.
- Common types of PAT
  - Re-entrant rhythms: AV nodal re-entrant tachycardia; AV reciprocating tachycardia through accessory pathway
  - Unifocal or ectopic atrial tachycardia
  - Multifocal atrial tachycardia

ICD-9-CM Code: 427.0

ETIOLOGY

- Re-entrant rhythms
  - AV nodal re-entry: re-entrant pathway within AV node. Most common form of PAT; seldom associated with organic heart disease.
  - Accessory pathway mediated: re-entrant rhythm that involves an accessory pathway from atrium to ventricle. In sinus rhythm, the bypass tract may cause a pre-excitation pattern on ECG (WPW syndrome: short P-R interval and δ wave on ECG) or may not be apparent.
- Unifocal atrial tachycardia: arising from a single atrial muscle site other than SA node. Associated with catecholamine excess states (light anesthesia) or digitalis toxicity (triggered activity with 2:1 or 3:1 AV block).
- Multifocal atrial tachycardia: arising from multiple atrial sites, usually seen in patients with pulm disease or CHF

USUAL TREATMENT

- First-line therapy: vagal maneuvers or adenosine. Adenosine 6 mg/70 kg to be followed (if no hypotension) by 12 mg/70 kg is effective in 90% of re-entrant PAT. The effect lasts <20 sec. Carotid sinus massage may be dangerous if used with carotid artery disease.
- When PAT immediately recurs following adenosine, second-line therapy aims for reduced AV conduction to control ventricular rate.
  - Ca channel blockers: verapamil and diltiazem equally effective and both long-acting. Hypotension most likely with verapamil.
  - Digoxin: delayed onset of action even when given IV; not recommended for symptomatic PAT.
  - Beta blockers: often effective, but negative inotropic effects and bronchoconstriction possible
- WPW syndrome—procainamide blocks conduction through accessory pathway. Avoid digoxin and Ca channel blockers if patient at risk for AFib, since these drugs may accelerate antegrade conduction through accessory pathway, leading to VFib
- Multifocal and unifocal PAT: Correct underlying abn (hypoxia, lytes). Rx digoxin toxicity: lidocaine, phenytoin, or digoxin-specific Fab antibody fragments. Class IA agents (quinidine, procainamide) sometimes effective in re-entrant unifocal PAT.

ASSESSMENT POINTS

SYSTEM	EFFECT	ASSESSMENT BY HX	PE	TEST
CV	WPW AV nodal re-entry Symptomatic unifocal atrial tachycardia	Palpitations Diaphoresis	Prominent jugular venous pulsations	ECG Electrophysiologic studies

Key Reference: Ganz LI, Friedman PL: Medical progress: Supraventricular tachycardia. N Engl J Med 1995; 332:162–173.

PERIOPERATIVE IMPLICATIONS

Preoperative Preparation

- If possible, continue Ca channel blockers and β-blockers perioperatively to avoid withdrawal-associated arrhythmias

Monitoring

- Continuous intraoperative ECG monitoring and postop ECG monitoring in high-risk patients

Induction/Maintenance/Extubation

- Avoid tachycardia, light anesthesia, hypoxia, and lyte abn
- Aim for effective postop analgesia
- Consider β-blockers in hyperadrenergic postop patients with adequate cardiac output

Adjuvants

- Limit use of vagolytic agents such as pancuronium and atropine

ANTICIPATED PROBLEMS/CONCERNS

- Adenosine, digoxin, and verapamil shorten refractoriness in accessory pathways and may induce VFib in WPW patients with AFib.
- Hemodynamic collapse may occur when verapamil is used to treat patients with VTach, which is sometimes mistaken for SVT with aberrancy. Avoid by using adenosine.

PATENT DUCTUS ARTERIOSUS

George A. Gregory, M.D.

RISK

- People within USA: 20,000–30,000/y
- Highest in preterm infants
- No race prevalence

PERIOPERATIVE RISKS

- Hemorrhage: <2%
- Hypoxia with collapsing lung for surgery
- Hypotension due to hypovolemia and preop dehydration

WORRY ABOUT

- Hypovolemia
- Chronic lung disease
- CHF

OVERVIEW

- PDA primarily occurs in preterm infants
- Present in ~70% of birth wt <1250 g
- CHF in 10–20% of patients
- Onset 1–10 d of age as lung function improves
- ↑ Pulmonary blood flow—85% of cardiac output may flow through lungs

ICD-9-CM Code: 747.0

ETIOLOGY

- Prematurity
- Prostaglandin
- Inadequate innervation of ductus arteriosus

USUAL TREATMENT

- Restrict fluid intake to 120 ml/kg/d
- Indomethicin (0.1–0.25 mg/kg) IV q12 h × 3
- Mechanical ventilation
- Ligation of ductus arteriosus

ASSESSMENT POINTS

SYSTEM	EFFECT	ASSESSMENT BY HX	PE	TEST
CV	Pulmonary edema	↑ O_2 and myocardial ventilation requirement ↑ O_2 desaturation	Palmar pulses Hypotension Low diastolic pressure Bounding pulses and precordium	ECHO
RESP	CHF	↑ Myocardial ventilation requirement, worsening oxygenation	Rales; ↓ breath sounds	CXR
GI	Necrotizing enterocolitis	Abdominal distention Poor feeding Blood in stool Free air in peritoneum	Distended tense abdomen Edema of abdominal wall Tender abdomen	Abdominal x-ray
RENAL	Oliguria	↓ UO due to ↓ renal blood flow		Volume of urine
CNS	CNS hemorrhage	↑ Fontanel pressure ↓ Hct	↑ Fontanel size and tension	Head sonogram

Key Reference: Yu VY: Patent ductus arteriosus in the preterm infant. Early Hum Dev 1993; 35:1–14.

PERIOPERATIVE IMPLICATIONS

Preoperative Preparation

- Stabilize ventilation
- Replete intravascular volume
- Optimize vasopressors

Preinduction/Induction

- Mechanical ventilation
- Consider inducing anesthesia with fentanyl (10–50 µg/kg) or other opioid

Monitoring

- Intra-arterial pressure (continuous)
- SaO_2 right arm (preductal); end-tidal CO_2; CVP if available
- Airway pressure

Airway

- Routine

Maintenance

- Support arterial pressure with fluid (Ringer's lactate or 5% albumin) and vasopressors
- Ensure adequacy of blood gases; keep SaO_2 87–92% to reduce risk of retinopathy of prematurity
- Provide adequate anesthesia to prevent HTN

Extubation

- Continue mechanical ventilation postop
- Maintain normal blood gases

Adjuvants

- None

Postoperative Period

- Provide adequate pain relief
- Maintain normal blood gases and pH

ANTICIPATED PROBLEMS/CONCERNS

- Patients may develop necrotizing enterocolitis due to low gut blood flow
- Intracranial hemorrhage may occur if BP increases with ligation of PDA

PEMPHIGUS

James M. Sonner, M.D.
Jeffrey A. Katz, M.D.

RISK

• Incidence in US: 0.1–0.5/100,000/y for pemphigus vulgaris (the most common form of pemphigus)
• Age: Most common from age 30–60 y; can occur in children or elderly
• Most common in people of Mediterranean descent

PERIOPERATIVE RISKS

• Infection
• Electrolyte abn with extensive lesions

WORRY ABOUT

• Pharyngeal blisters, sloughing of mucosa, bleeding produced by airway manipulations
• Consequences of steroid treatment (e.g., HTN, hyperglycemia, gastric or duodenal ulceration, myopathy, infection, psychic disturbances, osteoporosis) or immunosuppressive therapy (bone marrow suppression)

OVERVIEW

• Autoimmune, intraepidermal blistering disease of skin and mucous membranes. Oral lesions most common. Blisters rupture easily, heal slowly, usually do not scar.
• Four types: vulgaris (most common and severe form), vegetans, foliaceus, erythematosus
• 5-y mortality 5–15% for treated pemphigus vulgaris. Most common cause of death is infection, usually with *Staphylococcus aureus*.
• Occasionally coexists with other autoimmune diseases, thymoma (with or without myasthenia gravis), or malignancies

ICD-9-CM Code: 694.4

ETIOLOGY

• Autoimmune disease in which autoantibodies are produced to antigens on epidermal cells. More common in patients with certain HLA haplotypes. Immune response leads to acantholysis and blistering.
• Uncommonly, pemphigus is drug-induced.
• Rarely, may occur in association with malignancy (paraneoplastic pemphigus)

USUAL TREATMENT

• Corticosteroids
• Adjuvant therapy
  – Immunosuppressive agents (such as azathioprine and methotrexate) commonly used
    – Oral gold or dapsone occasionally used
    – Plasmapheresis occasionally used for refractory disease

ASSESSMENT POINTS

SYSTEM	EFFECT	ASSESSMENT BY HX	PE	TEST
HEENT	Oral and pharyngeal erosions and blisters	Painful oral lesions ↑ Salivation Painful swallowing	Oral lesions	
CV	HTN (due to steroids)		BP	
RESP	At risk for pneumonia	Fever, cough, sputum	Diminished breath sounds, Dullness to percussion	CXR
GI	Gastric or duodenal ulcer (due to steroids)	Epigastric pain Dark stools		
MS	Myopathy (due to steroids)	Fatigability, weakness		
CUTANEOUS	Blisters Denuded areas Lyte abn	Blisters	Blisters Denuded or crusted areas of skin	Electrolytes

PERIOPERATIVE IMPLICATIONS

Preoperative Preparation

• Patients may require supplemental steroids
• Avoid tape on skin—it can generate new lesions
• Secure IV with loose cloth bandage or suture

Monitoring

• Consider monitors that do not adhere to skin. Consider removing adhesive from ECG pads and oximeter probes and securing with loose bandage. Place soft padding (e.g., Webril) under BP cuff.

Airway

• Patients may have oral erosions or blisters; new blisters may form from airway management. Risk is of airway obstruction or bleeding. Consider lubricating mask and laryngoscope blade to decrease friction, using small ET tube; minimal cuff inflation; and suture or hold tube in place. Avoid LMA owing to unquantified risk of pharyngeal trauma.

Preinduction/Induction

• Lubricate eyes—do not tape
• Allow patient to position self on well padded OR table, to decrease risk of blister formation with positioning. Ensure all pressure points are padded once patient is on table.

Maintenance

• Neither general nor regional anesthesia clearly superior
• Local infiltration probably contraindicated owing to risk of blister formation

Extubation

• Minimize coughing during extubation

Postoperative Period

• New lesions of skin or mucous membranes may appear.

Adjuvants

• Depends on agents and effects of agents used for chronic treatment
• Consider need for steroid supplementation

ANTICIPATED PROBLEMS/CONCERNS

• Minor frictional trauma to skin or mucosa may generate new lesions. Airway must be instrumented gently and tape avoided anywhere on the skin.
• Patients are at risk of infection and lyte abnormalities from pemphigus and of side effects of steroid and immunosuppressive therapy.

PERICARDIAL EFFUSION

Bruce D. Spiess, M.D.

RISK

- Occurs rarely
- Postop open heart or PTCA—blood/serous
- Infection: viral, bacterial, fungal
- Neoplastic—lymphoma, leukemia
- Post: acute MI (especially transmural)
- Gender predominance: Male > female

PERIOPERATIVE RISKS

- If unknown, tamponade causing CV collapse possible with low probability of determining cause ante mortem
- If known, risk of CV collapse, especially with induction and institution of positive pressure ventilation

WORRY ABOUT

- Hypovolemia
- Limited filling of cardiac chambers

OVERVIEW

- Found in sac surrounding heart; if severe can restrict filling of heart
- Ventricular filling is depressed in both RV and LV
- Fluid bolus and inotropes do little to improve cardiac output
- Must have surgical drainage for proper treatment

ICD-9-CM Code: 423.9

ETIOLOGY

- Postsurgical and catheterization procedures
- During or after viral, bacterial, or fungal infection
- Postinflammatory process: acute transmural, SLE, RA
- Neoplastic

USUAL TREATMENT

- Drainage either percutaneous or open

ASSESSMENT POINTS

SYSTEM	EFFECTS	ASSESSMENT BT HX	PE	TEST
CV	Tamponade limiting CO Hypotension		Neck veins HR BP	Equalization of all pressures in heart
	Arrhythmias			ECG
RESP	↓ CO on institution of IPPB (mechanical ventilation)	Change in BP on institution of mechanical ventilation		PA, RA, LA pressures
METAB	Metabolic acidosis			ABG

PERIOPERATIVE IMPLICATIONS

Preoperative Preparation

- Appropriate monitoring before induction
- Preoxygenation—not always effective
- Support hemodynamics-catecholamines, acid-base—keep "full and fast"
- Consider draining transthoracally if hemodynamic compromise severe
- Consider prep and drape prior to induction with surgeon ready
- Positive pressure ventilation may significantly worsen hypotension, resulting in shock and death
- Consider placing external defibrillator patches prior to anesthetic induction

Monitoring

- Arterial line indicated as BP may change suddenly; sampling of Hct for bleeding and acid-base status in low cardiac output state is useful
- Consider PA catheter—useful in making diagnosis and following surgical treatment. If pressures not relieved on surgical drainage, question original diagnosis
- TEE—useful but less so than PA monitoring

Induction/Maintenance

- Do not decrease preload
- Avoid moderate to full dose barbiturates or propofol
- Monitor hemodynamics and use anesthetic, if tolerated, or etomidate
- Ketamine and pancuronium have been advocated for new tamponade situations
- Initiation of positive pressure ventilation may cause severe CV compromise due to ↓ filling of RV and LV

Subject Approach

- Post open heart hemorrhage—reopening sternum to explore for sites of hemorrhage—usually relieved by first few sutures released
- Infections/neoplasia—subxyphoid pericardial window
- Small incision—open pericardium under direct vision—chest tube placed behind heart

Adjuvants

- Depends upon etiology

Extubation

- Consider awake extubation or postop mechanical ventilation, depending on etiology

ANTICIPATED PROBLEMS/CONCERNS

- Many different causes, all with different sequelae
- Hypotension on induction of anesthesia or positive pressure ventilation

PERICARDITIS, ACUTE

John P. Williams, M.D.
Michael Sopher, M.D.

RISK

• Most common pathologic process involving pericardium; exact incidence unknown (3.5–5% of all autopsies)
• Following MI, males > females, anterior > inferior

PERIOPERATIVE RISKS

• MI: Risk is for acute MI not pericarditis per se
• Associated with lower cardiac output, evidence of greater myocardial damage (akinetic and dyskinetic segments), higher incidence of pericardial effusions (possible tamponade)
• Infectious acute pericarditis of little risk unless evidence of severe myocarditis intervenes (displaced PMI, Sx of CHF)

WORRY ABOUT

• MI—Differentiating pain of pericarditis from extension of MI. Alterations in ST segments may make Dx of myocardial ischemia difficult

• Infectious—extension of pericarditis into myocarditis
• Tamponade physiology in patients with rapidly accumulating pericardial effusions
• Atrial and ventricular dysrhythmias

OVERVIEW

• Inflammatory pericardial process associated with MI, infection, collagen vascular disorders, trauma
• Inflammation results in typical ECG changes: widespread elevation of ST segments, followed days later by inversion of T-waves.
• Easily differentiated from MI where ST segments are depressed, Q-waves appear, and T-wave inversions occur within hours following onset of pain. Check for paradoxical pulse as cardinal sign of significant pericardial effusion.

ICD-9-CM Code: 420

ETIOLOGY

• Infectious—in young adults, viral or idiopathic, typically occurring after Hx of URI often associated with pleural effusions and pneumonitis
• MI—Post myocardial infarction, pericarditis associated with patients in their 5th and 6th decades

USUAL TREATMENT

• If no effusion, NSAIDs and treatment of primary disease, if identified
• Corticosteroids may be necessary for NSAID failures.
• If effusion present, serial ECG or ECHO may be necessary to follow effusion size.
• Drainage may be indicated if Sx of tamponade intervene.

ASSESSMENT POINTS

SYSTEM	EFFECT	ASSESSMENT BY HX	PE	TEST
CV	Pericarditis Myocarditis Pericardial effusion Tamponade	Chest pain: pleuritic anginal equivalents Dyspnea Tachycardia	Friction rub Tachycardia Hypotension Displaced PMI	ECG CXR ECHO ?Cardiac enzymes ?Pericardiocentesis
RESP	Compression of bronchi and parenchyma by effusion/tamponade	Dyspnea Cough	Dyspnea	
GI ENDO	2° to myxedema	Anginal equivalents: epigastric pain		TSH, T_3, T_4
MS RENAL	2° to uremia	Anginal equivalents: arm pain/neck pain		BUN/Cr
IMMUN	2° to tuberculosis, acute bacterial infection, autoimmune disorders, viral or fungal infection	Fever and chills Wt loss		Leukocyte count ESR ANA, Rheum factor PPD Blood cultures: bacterial, viral, fungal

Key Reference: Malach B: Pericardial diseases, with a focus on etiology, pathogenesis, pathophysiology, new diagnostic imaging methods, and treatment. Curr Opin Cardiol 1994, 9:379–388.

PERIOPERATIVE IMPLICATIONS

Preoperative Preparation

• Assess presence of paradoxical pulse, check baseline ECG, inquire about Sx suggestive of MI or Hx of recent infection. Listen to heart sounds for possible changing murmurs or friction rub.
• Assess displaced PMI for ventricular dilatation.

Monitoring

• ST segment analysis may not be helpful if ST segments elevated.
• ECHO may be useful if large effusion present.
• Use of arterial line recommended if effusion present.
• If myocarditis severe, PA catheter may be necessary.

Airway

• If tamponade physiology, positive pressure ventilation can induce sudden hemodynamic deterioration.

Induction

• If effusion or severe myocarditis present, agents least affecting hemodynamic integrity are preferred (e.g., ketamine, etomidate).

Maintenance

• Cardiovascular stability is only a problem in presence of large effusion.
• If a large effusion present, spontaneous ventilation preferred.

Extubation

• Coughing and breath holding on extubation may result in inordinate decreases in cardiac output and BP.
• If possible, extubate deep and allow patient to waken spontaneously.

Adjuvants

• NSAIDs may be preferred as postop analgesic to decrease inflammatory response and provide pain relief.

Postoperative Period

• Observe for signs of ischemia related to MI.
• Close monitoring of BP recommended for patients with effusion.
• Low threshold for use of ECHO if hypotension intervenes.

ANTICIPATED PROBLEMS/CONCERNS

• Incidence of postop problems directly related to etiology of pericarditis.
• Acutely following MI, patients at greatly elevated risk for death in immediate postop period.
• Ischemia may be more difficult to detect because of the ECG changes.

PERICARDITIS, CONSTRICTIVE

Stephen N. Harris, M.D.

RISK

- 1/1000 people hospitalized have diagnosis of acute pericarditis (27,000/y in US)
- Chronic constrictive pericarditis is a rare sequela of acute pericarditis (found in 2–6% of autopsies)
- Males > females
- Mean age at operation: 30–35 y with symptoms present for ≤ 2 y

PERIOPERATIVE RISKS

- 12–15% operative mortality; may be as high as 25% when due to hemothorax after CABG
- Hypotension from loss of preload during induction or intraoperative blood loss
- High incidence of arrhythmias during dissection

WORRY ABOUT

- For noncardiac surgery, extremely heart rate and preload dependent
- During pericardiectomy, arrhythmias and low-output syndrome following operation

OVERVIEW

- Occurs after initial episode of acute pericarditis with subsequent fibrin deposition leading to a pericardial effusion, which may be subclinical
- Large fibrotic thickened pericardium symmetrically encases and affects all four chambers to restrict diastolic filling with eventual equilibration of diastolic pressures and PCWP. Calcium contributes to stiffening
- Early diastolic filling owing to rapid ↑ CVP. Late diastolic filling halted owing to ↑ intraventricular pressures. Prominent "y descent" on CVP
- Intrathoracic pressures not transmitted to pericardial space and intracardiac chambers: venous and right-sided pressure ↑ during inspiration
- Severe cases—CVP ↑ with respiration (Kussmaul). Systolic function depressed owing to myocardial atrophy, fibrosis, and compression of superficial coronary arteries
- Approach for pericardiectomy through median sternotomy or left thoracotomy

- Differential diagnosis—suspect in patients with JVD, unexplained cardiomegaly, hepatomegaly, systemic edema, and ascites

ICD-9-CM Code: 423.2

ETIOLOGY

- Unknown; usually occurs after subclinical viral pericarditis
- In undeveloped countries, 25–50% of cases due to tuberculosis
- Can be a late result of mediastinal irradiation, chronic renal failure, RA, and SLE. Increasing in frequency owing to hemopericardium and after acute MI.

USUAL TREATMENT

- Early—diet and diuretics
- Late—with increasing symptoms, pericardiectomy

ASSESSMENT POINTS

SYSTEM	EFFECT	ASSESSMENT BY HX	PE	TEST
HEENT	May mimic SVC obstruction		↑ JVD, rapidly collapsing negative wave of diastolic "y descent"	
CV	Impaired ventricular filling	Cardiac cachexia	Diastolic pericardial knock, widened aortic and pulmonic heart sounds	ECHO; right and left heart catheterization
RESP	Pleural effusions, pulmonary venous congestion, left atrial enlargement	SOB	↓ Breath sounds, rales	CXR
GI	Hepatomegaly due to ↑ CVP Chronic passive congestion of liver		Pulsatile liver, ascites	↓ Albumin, ↑ globulin, ↑ conjugated and unconjugated bilirubin
HEME		Malaise		Normochromic and normocytic anemia
RENAL	↑ Venous pressure within kidney			Albuminuria and proteinuria consistent with nephrotic syndrome
MS	Venous congestion	Upper extremity wasting, gradual swelling of lower extremities	May be markedly edematous in severe cases	

Key Reference: Braunwald E (ed): Heart Disease: A Textbook of Cardiovascular Medicine, 4th ed. Philadelphia, WB Saunders, 1992, pp 1482–1489.

PERIOPERATIVE IMPLICATIONS

Preoperative Preparation

- Rehydrate to optimize filling pressures

Monitoring

- 2-lead ECG; consider arterial and CVP or PA catheters
- Consider transesophageal ECHO

Airway

- Significant venous congestion may make visualization difficult

Preinduction

- Avoid drugs and techniques that may cause bradycardia and ↓ venous return

Maintenance

- No specific agent or technique superior
- During excision of pericardium, arrhythmias and fluctuations in blood pressure common

Extubation

- Keep full; avoid anticholinesterase bradycardia

Postoperative Period

- Monitor for signs of myocardial depression due to epicardial myocardial stripping

ANTICIPATED PROBLEMS/CONCERNS

- Postop low-output syndrome seen in 14–28% of patients
- In-hospital mortality associated with preoperative NYHA class 3 or 4; severity of pericardial constriction and elevated RVEDP

PERIPHERAL VASCULAR DISEASE

Jacqueline M. Leung, M.D.

RISK

- 10–15% of those > age 50 y
- Long-term mortality increased 2–3 × in those with "overt" CAD, large vessel arterial disease, diabetes mellitus
- 5-y mortality rate 30–40%

PERIOPERATIVE RISKS

- High prevalence of coexisting CAD and carotid artery disease
- Presence of CAD increases operative mortality
- Pulmonary and renal insufficiency can cause prolonged recovery or morbidity

WORRY ABOUT

- Aortic clamping: may induce myocardial ischemia or ventricular failure; hypotension with declamping
- ↑ Risk of perioperative myocardial ischemia and cardiac complications
- Postop thrombosis in arterial grafts
- Postop delirium, esp if > 70 y or hypoxemic

OVERVIEW

- Vascular abnormalities involving extremities increase in frequency with age
- Coexisting diseases common (diabetes mellitus, COPD resulting from smoking, HTN, CAD)

ICD-9-CM Code: 443.9

ETIOLOGY

- Chronic arterial occlusive disease
- Less common: Takayasu's syndrome and thromboangiitis obliterans

USUAL TREATMENT

- Reconstitute pulsatile blood flow to distal vascular tree to allow healing of ulcerated or gangrenous tissue, relieve ischemic rest pain with the goal of salvaging a functional limb
- Most common surgical procedures are aortofemoral bypass, femoropopliteal bypass, femorotibial bypass
- Angiogenesis gene therapy now being combined with percutaneous angioplasty techniques in experimental protocols

ASSESSMENT POINTS

SYSTEM	EFFECT	ASSESSMENT BY HX	PE	TEST
CV	HTN Coronary artery stenoses MI	Usually asymptomatic Angina, may be asymptomatic	Normal if treated S_3 and/or S_4 Cardiomegaly	Vital signs ECG Exercise ECG Treadmill Pharmacologic stress test Coronary angiography ECHO Radionuclide studies
	Ventricular dysfunction	Exercise intolerance Sx of heart failure		
PERIPHERAL VASCULAR EXAM	Occlusive lesions Abdominal aortic aneurysm may coexist	Claudication Abdominal pain, may be asymptomatic	↓ Pulses Pulsatile abdominal mass	Angio Aortogram MRI
RESP	COPD (many are smokers)	DOE	↓ Breath sounds Prolonged expiration Wheezes	ABG PFTs
ENDO	Diabetes mellitus and associated effects such as angiopathy, peripheral and autonomic neuropathy, nephropathy	Attention to CV, PNS (See under Diabetes for autonomic nervous system and other evaluation)	Obesity (in adult-onset) Cardiomegaly Foot ulcers	Fasting blood sugar
CNS	Ischemic CNS disease	Scotoma CNS and mental status evaluation Absent spells	CNS exam Search for carotid bruits	Doppler or Angio (if indicated)

Key Reference: Leung J: Monitoring of patients during vascular surgery. Anesthesiol Clin North Am 1995; 13:67–81.

PERIOPERATIVE IMPLICATIONS

Preoperative Preparation

- Attention to and stabilization of concomitant medical conditions such as CAD, COPD, diabetes mellitus
- Identification of high-risk patients who may benefit from coronary angioplasty or CABG surgery prior to peripheral vascular operations

Monitoring

- ST-trending if available
- In aortic surgery, consider placement of CVP or PA catheters or TEE for monitoring preload
- Use of transesophageal ECHO may elucidate the mechanism(s) of declamping hypotension (hypovolemia vs. ventricular dysfunction) and regional ventricular function (myocardial ischemia).

Airway

- None

Preinduction/Induction

- Prevent tachycardia (use of short-acting β rb's desirable) and treat BP changes aggressively.
- Epidural anesthesia combined with epidural analgesia shown to decrease incidence of reoperation and arterial thrombosis of graft as compared with GA.

Maintenance

- See above

Extubation

- Same hemodynamic concerns as in induction
- Use of postop epidural analgesia decreases likelihood of arterial graft thrombosis.

Adjuvants

- Beta rb's and other antihypertensives useful in hyperdynamic situations
- Prophylactic nitroglycerin and Ca^{2+} channel blockers to treat myocardial ischemia not conclusively proven efficacious

ANTICIPATED PROBLEMS/CONCERNS

- Perioperative myocardial ischemia and cardiac complications, thromboembolic events of grafts, CHF, renal failure

PERTUSSIS (WHOOPING COUGH)

Vincent J. Kopp, M.D.

RISK

- Highest for children < age 5 y
- Females > males
- 95–100% of unimmunized infants, children, adults
- Immunization 80% effective
- Mortality highest for infants < age 1 mo

PERIOPERATIVE RISKS

- Pneumonia (22%), seizures (3%), encephalopathy (1%) most common complications

WORRY ABOUT

- Infectivity and contagion
- Hypoxemia and decreased pulmonary reserves
- Altered mucociliary function

OVERVIEW

- Severe disease with 1.3% case-fatality rate for infants < age 1 mo and 0.3% case-fatality rate each for infants 2–5 mo and 6–11 mo
- Immunization in childhood has decreased but not eliminated incidence
- Adolescents and adults display milder symptoms that may be indistinguishable from less serious causes of URI/LRI.
- Catarrhal stage mimics less serious URI.
- Paroxysmal stage associated with cough, cyanosis, apnea, vomiting, seizures
- Convalescent stage marked by persistent or episodic cough
- Infection of upper respiratory tree often accompanied by more severe symptoms (pneumonia, seizures) from gram-negative bacillus (Bordetella pertussis).

ICD-9-CM Code: 033.0

ETIOLOGY

- Bordetella pertussis, a fastidious, gram-negative, pleomorphic or rod bacillus
- A whooping cough syndrome also caused by B. parapertussis, Chlamydia trachomatis, and many adenoviruses

TREATMENT

- Hospitalization, with intensive care in severe cases, to support nutrition, control cough, treat hypoxemia, monitor apnea, and treat severe sequelae such as pneumonia, seizures, and encephalopathy
- Erythromycin (40–50 mg/kg/d, orally, qid, for 14 days) ameliorates catarrhal stage and ↓ bacterial transmission in paroxysmal and convalescent stages.
- TMP/SMX (8 mg/kg/d to 40 mg/kg/d, orally, bid) is unproven alternative when erythromycin not tolerated.
- Corticosteroids and β_2-agonists have an unclear role in paroxysmal stage.
- Transmission control is essential.

ASSESSMENT POINTS

SYSTEM	EFFECT	ASSESSMENT BY HX	PE	TEST
HEENT	Upper airway obstruction	Difficulty feeding Difficulty breathing Immunization Hx	Rhinorrhea Lacrimation Conjunctivitis	Nasal culture Direct fluorescent antibody (DFA)
CV	High O_2 consumption	Irritability	Tachycardia	ECG
RESP	Cough V/Q mismatch Pneumonia	Apnea, SOB Tachypnea, rales As above	Inspiratory whoop Cyanosis Rales	Culture + DFA Pulse oximetry CXR, ABGs
GI	Poor oral intake Fatty liver Post-tussive emesis Cough-induced hernias	Dehydration Inability to retain food Inguinal hernias	Altered turgor Hepatomegaly Wt loss Reducible hernias	Weigh on scale LFTs
RENAL		Oliguria		
CNS	Seizures Encephalopathy	Seizure type Immunization Hx Altered neuro status	Seizure type Neuro exam	EEG, CT, MRI LP, glucose

Key Reference: 1994 Red Book, Report of the Committee on Infectious Disease, American Academy of Pediatrics, 1994, pp 355–366.

PERIOPERATIVE IMPLICATIONS

Preoperative Preparation

- High infectivity requires isolation control precautions
- Uncomplicated disease resolves in 6–10 wks; optimize respiratory function and nutrition prior to surgery.
- Postpone elective surgery minimum of 6 wk after resolution of symptoms. Consider D and T immunization 2 wk prior to surgery.
- Emergency surgery benefits must exceed risks.
- Use disposable anesthesia circuit system.

Monitoring

- Routine monitors plus arterial catheter in emergency cases

Airway

- Nasal secretions may obstruct upper airway and increase risk of laryngospasm.

- Upper and lower airway edema plus secretions ↑ risk of V/Q mismatch and hypoxemia.
- Inspissated secretions may cause ET tube blockage, contribute to postop pneumonia

Preinduction/Induction

- Consider regional anesthesia whenever possible.
- Consider short-term topical nasal decongestant (e.g., xylometazoline) to clear upper airway.
- Ensure adequate preoxygenation and prehydration.
- Avoid respiratory depressant premedication.

Maintenance

- Keep warm and hydrated.
- Use disposable, humidified anesthesia delivery system.
- PEEP as needed only to maintain oxygenation
- Suction ET tube prn, using saline to moisten secretions.
- Control ventilation to minimize development of atelectasis.

Extubation

- Expand atelectatic lungs prior to extubation.
- Moisten and suction thickened secretions.
- Bronchodilators as needed

Postoperative Period

- Caudal or epidural analgesia for pain relief
- Apnea monitoring and ICU observation as indicated
- Aggressive pulmonary toilet as tolerated

ANTICIPATED PROBLEMS/CONCERNS

- Risk of transmission of infection to all contacts, including OR personnel
- Development of severe respiratory insufficiency at bronchoalveolar level during perioperative period.

PHEOCHROMOCYTOMA

Michael F. Roizen, M.D.

RISK

- People within USA: 0.03–0.04% (~80,000) by autopsy of nonselected individuals; 0.1–1% of individuals with sustained HTN have pheochromocytoma
- Race with highest prevalence: Caucasian

PERIOPERATIVE RISKS

- If emergency (life-threatening trauma, ruptured viscus), use α- and ß-blockers and nitroprusside and keep in ICU till most painful time has passed or adrenergic control is attained.
- ↑ Risk of hypertensive crisis with bleeding into myocardium, brain, or kidney or ischemia
- Mortality rate of 0–3% even if appropriately prepared for tumor resection and in "good" hands for adrenalectomy—may be higher for undiscovered case undergoing nonadrenal surgery.
- 25–50% of those who die in hospitals of pheochromocytoma crisis do so during induction of anesthesia, during stressful perioperative periods, or during labor and delivery.
- Associated with cholelithiasis and renal stones

WORRY ABOUT

- Pheochromocytoma (catecholamine excess) crisis with hemorrhage/infarcts in vital organs
- Major goal is to avoid pheochromocytoma crisis; pre- and intraoperative goals of management of extra-adrenal surgery are same as for adrenal surgery. If adrenergic blockade not present prior to surgery, try to delay operation until patient has appropriate degree of α rb. Judge appropriate blockade by:
  – No BP readings > 165/90 mmHg for 48 h
  – Presence of orthostatic hypotension, but BP on standing should not be < 80/45 mmHg.
  – ECG free of ST-T changes
  – Absence of other signs of catecholamine excess, and presence of signs of α rb

OVERVIEW

- Tumor of catecholamine-producing tissue (90% in adrenals). Painful (stressful) events cause exaggerated stress response if less than perfectly anesthetized or in daily living. For patients with pheochromocytoma, even small stresses can lead to blood catecholamine levels of 2000–20,000 pg/ml. However, infarction of tumor, with release of products onto retroperitoneal surfaces, or surgical or other pressure causing release of products, can result in blood levels of 200,000–1 million pg/ml—a situation that should be anticipated during tumor resection
- Endocrinopathy associated with CV disease—tachycardia, CHF, dysrhythmias (AFib)
- Need α rb prior to ß rb lest vasoconstrictive effects of latter go unopposed, thereby increasing risk of dangerous HTN. ß rb suggested if persistent arrhythmias or tachycardia not resolving with α rb or when aggravated by α rb
- If α rb, appropriately, risk of crisis diminished by >90%

ICD-9-CM Code: 194.0

INDICATIONS AND USUAL TREATMENT

- 90% are spontaneously arising and 10% familial (autosomal dominant genetics involving chromosome 17 implicated)
- Associated with MEA IIA (medullary thyroid carcinoma; primary hyperparathyroidism) and IIB (medullary thyroid carcinoma and muscosal neuromas)
- Associated with neurofibromatosis, von Hippel–Lindau disease (retinal and cerebellar hemangioblastoma), ataxia-telangiectasia syndrome, Sturge-Weber syndrome

ASSESSMENT POINTS

SYSTEM	EFFECT	ASSESSMENT BY HX	PE	TEST
HEENT		Nasal stuffness (from α adrenergic blockade)		
CV	HTN; dysrhythmias; AFib, sinus tachycardia, mitral valve prolapse; CHF, myocardial fibril necrosis or myocarditis	SOB, exercise tolerance, palpitations, HTN (50% sustained, 40% paroxysmal)	Standard exam + BP q 1 min in stressful environment + orthostatic maneuvers with BP/HR q 1 min	ECG, ECHO (if cardiomyopathy is suspected)
GI	90% of tumors adrenal or abdominal	Wt loss, diarrhea Dehydration	Palpating abdomen can trigger pheochromocytoma crisis	No different from normal
HEME		Mild polycythemia, thrombocytopenia (2° to ↓ intravascular fluid)		Hgb (↓ polycythemia way to judge volume expansion by α rb)
GU	Renal stones from dehydration			
CNS	↑ Catecholamine effects	Headache, tremor, anxiety, ↓ pain threshold, fatigue		
METAB	Associated with hyperparathyroidism	Glucose intolerance from α adrenergically induced gluconeogenesis and ↓ insulin secretion		Insulin Rx often before Dx made; Ca²⁺

Key Reference: Roizen MF: Pheochromocytoma. *In* Miller RD (ed): Anesthesia. New York, Churchill Livingstone, 1994, pp 922–925.

PERIOPERATIVE IMPLICATIONS

Preoperative Preparation

- "Prehydrate" liberally over 6–60 d if CV status will tolerate; expand with high salt/fluid diet while increasing α adrenergic blockade over 7–60 d.

Monitoring

- Temp
- Arterial line placement prior to induction difficult and painful but desired because of large variations in BP
- PA catheterization or TEE if CV system severely affected; CVP used in minority of cases

Anesthetic Technique

- No technique/group of agents associated with better or worse outcome; use of droperidol controversial; agents that block catecholamine reuptake (ketamine) or cause catecholamine release might be avoided

Induction/Maintenance

- Prehydrate liberally if CV status will tolerate
- Gentle induction with nitroprusside infusion plugged into IV line and running slowly
- Dopamine infusion in reserve for ready use
- Painful or stressful events often cause exaggerated stress response. Caused by release of catecholamines from nerve endings that are "loaded" by the reuptake process.

Postoperative Care

- See Adrenalectomy for Pheochromocytoma.
- Postop if catecholamine-producing tumor removed or if α adrenergically blocked, do not chase or force high UO with large crystalloid infusions, as patients have tendency to CHF since have been on endogenous inotrope for many years
- Early mobilization and deep breathing a must but fraught with difficulty owing to disturbed psyche that removal of catecholamines present for a long time often causes

Adjuvants

- Consider potential for drug interactions with chronic anti-adrenergic agents such as between verapamil or diltiazem and ß rb's in depressing AV nodal conduction if patient chronically or acutely receiving a ß rb or decreased clearance of phenytoin, barbiturates, rifampicin, chlorpromazine, and cimetidine

ANTICIPATED PROBLEMS/CONCERNS

- Important to interview family members and perhaps advise them to inform their future anesthesiologists about potential for such familial disease

PICKWICKIAN SYNDROME
Susan L. Polk, M.D., M.S.Ed.

RISK
- 5% to 10% of morbidly obese patients
- Usually associated with long-standing obesity

PERIOPERATIVE RISKS
- Much ↑ over that of normal patients
- 40% serious morbidity in intra-abdominal or intrathoracic procedures of >2 h duration

WORRY ABOUT
- Hypoventilation
- Hypercarbia
- Hypoxemia
- Polycythemia, thrombophlebitis, and subsequent pulm embolism
- Pulm HTN
- Hypersomnolence
- Biventricular cardiac failure

OVERVIEW
- Morbidly obese patients who hypoventilate because of sleep apnea and severe restrictive ventilatory disorder and have permanent pulm HTN, acidosis, and polycythemia because of their chronic hypoxemia and CO_2 retention.
- Usually associated with systemic HTN and compensatory increased circulating blood volume, leading to right and left ventricular failure

ICD-9-CM Code: 278.8

ETIOLOGY
- Long-standing morbid obesity with sleep apnea, restrictive ventilatory disorder, hypercarbia, hypoxemia

ASSESSMENT POINTS
(See under Morbid Obesity)

SYSTEM	EFFECT	ASSESSMENT BY HX	PE	TEST
HEENT	Difficult airway access	Snoring	Poor visualization	X-ray of neck may be helpful
CV	Biventricular failure	Dyspnea, poor exercise tolerance	Venous engorgement, S_3 and S_4, dyspnea	ECG, ECHO, CXR
	CAD	Angina, poor exercise tolerance		ECG, Stress ECHO, Angio
RESP	Hypoventilation	Dyspnea Sleeping upright Poor exercise tolerance	Rapid shallow breathing, cyanosis	ABGs, Hct, CXR

Key Reference: Reisin E, Frohlich ED. Obesity: Cardiovascular and respiratory pathophysiological alterations. Arch Intern Med 1981; 141:431–434.

PERIOPERATIVE IMPLICATIONS
(See also under Morbid Obesity)

Preoperative Preparation
- Consider pulm function tests with bronchodilator to determine if reversible restrictive component present
- Assess for bronchitis/pneumonia that can be improved with pulm toilet and antibiotic therapy
- Assess myocardial and volume status
- Consider maintaining semi-sitting position to avoid sudden shift of volume to central circulation and pulm edema (obesity sudden death syndrome)

Monitoring
- Frequent ABGs
- Resp volumes and pressures
- Consider PA catheter or transesophageal ECHO to monitor filling volumes and wall motion

Airway
- Awake intubation frequently required
- Shoulders and head elevated on bolster can sometimes facilitate entry to mouth

Induction
- Do not expect to ventilate patient adequately by mask. Establish airway first.

Maintenance
- May have to remain in reverse Trendelenburg position to allow adequate ventilation

Extubation
- In sitting position without residual sedation
- Ensure adequate volumes and preop levels of CO_2 retention

Adjuvants
- Regional anesthesia only if patient is able to maintain ventilation
- Residual sedation or narcosis may preclude early extubation.

Postoperative Period
- Consider prophylaxis for thromboembolism—early stir-up and ambulation may minimize pulm and thromboembolic complications
- May be extremely sensitive to resp depressant effects of sedatives and narcotics

ANTICIPATED PROBLEMS/CONCERNS
- All those associated with morbid obesity apply to pickwickian patients
- Early stir-up and ambulation may minimize pulm and thromboembolic complications.
- Preparation of patient for possible prolonged postop mechanical ventilation, especially after upper abdominal procedures

PIERRE ROBIN SYNDROME

Charles B. Cauldwell, M.D., Ph.D.

RISK

- 1/8500 live births
- No known sex or race predilection

PERIOPERATIVE RISKS

- Associated congenital anomalies, e.g., cardiac

WORRY ABOUT

- PA HTN, cor pulmonale, or pulmonary edema secondary to chronic airway obstruction
- Acute resp failure due to exhaustion or aspiration
- Cachexia due to feeding difficulties

OVERVIEW

- An anomaly consisting of micrognathia and glossoptosis, often associated with cleft palate, leading to varying degrees of airway obstruction and feeding difficulties
- Airway obstruction can lead to hypoxia, brain damage, or CHF
- Feeding problems may cause aspiration or malnutrition
- Obstruction often improves by several months of age, secondary to mandibular growth, if hypoxia and malnutrition are avoided

ICD-9-CM Code: 756.0

ETIOLOGY

- Congenital, found either as isolated syndrome or as part of multiple defect syndromes
- Gene location unknown as of 1/96

USUAL TREATMENT

- Prone positioning, lavage feeding
- Nasopharyngeal or oral airway, for short-term treatment
- Glossopexy or tracheostomy, if surgery necessary

ASSESSMENT POINTS

SYSTEM	EFFECT	ASSESSMENT BY HX	PE	TEST
HEENT	Airway obstruction	Sleep pattern		
CV	PA HTN Cor pulmonale			CXR
RESP	Pulm edema Aspiration pneumonitis			CXR
GI	Feeding problems	Failure to thrive	Percentile wt	
CNS	Hypoxia	Seizures Developmental delay		

Key Reference: Hollinger I: Pierre Robin syndrome. *In* Stehling L (ed): Common Problems in Pediatric Anesthesia. St. Louis, Mosby-Year Book, 1992, p. 63.

PERIOPERATIVE IMPLICATIONS

Preoperative Preparation

- Avoid sedative premedication
- Consider antisialagogue

Monitoring

- Oximeter and precordial stethoscope particularly important

Airway

- May obstruct in supine position while awake or early during inhalation induction
- Consider oral or nasopharyngeal airway
- Intubation may be very difficult
- Consider awake intubation in neonates
- Have fiberoptic bronchoscope and experienced personnel available
- Have surgeon in OR capable of performing tracheostomy when induction begins

Preinduction/Induction

- See airway issues

Extubation

- Child must be awake for extubation, may need to be prone to maintain patent airway

Adjuvants

- Do not use muscle relaxants unless absolutely sure patient can be intubated

ANTICIPATED PROBLEMS/CONCERNS

- Airway obstruction during all phases of anesthesia very common

PITUITARY TUMORS

Ira J. Rampil, M.D.

RISK

- People within USA: ?10,000/y
- Race/gender with highest prevalence: female:male 8:1

PERIOPERATIVE RISKS

- ↑ Risk due to secondary endocrine syndromes from secreting adenomas, e.g., acromegaly, Cushing's syndrome, diabetes mellitus, hyperthyroidism

WORRY ABOUT

- Angina, cardiomyopathy with evidence of CHF, lyte imbalance
- Difficult airway

OVERVIEW

- Symptoms due to hormonal dysregulation or local mass effect
- Microadenomas (secreting)
  - Prolactinoma (↑ PRL)
  - Cushing's disease (↑ ACTH)
  - Acromegaly (↑ GH)
- Macroademona (mass lesion)
  - Panhypopituitarism
  - ↑ ICP
  - Bitemporal hemianopsia

ICD-9-CM Code: 253.8
(See also under Hypothyroidism)

ETIOLOGY

- Usually a nonmalignant clonal tumor derived from Rathke's pouch
- Incidence ↑ with age, up to 20% by 80 y (most asymptomatic)
- May occur as a component of MEN I, an autosomal dominant trait associated with deletion at q13 locus of chromosome 11

USUAL TREATMENT

- Incidental (asymptomatic) microadenoma: conservative
- Prolactin-secreting microadenoma: bromocriptine (dopaminergic agonist)
- Trans-sphenoidal resection is viewed as safe, and curative in ~90%

ASSESSMENT POINTS

SYSTEM	EFFECT	ASSESSMENT BY HX	PE	TEST
HEENT	Acromegaly: prognathism, lingular and laryngeal hyperplasia, mandibular enlargement		Mallampati exam	Indirect laryngoscopy
CV	Cushing's disease: ↑ BP Acromegaly: ↑ BP, cardiomyopathy	Exercise tolerance	Volume status, BP	ECG (± stress test) ECHO
RESP		Sleep apnea		Usually not needed
ENDO	Acromegaly: diabetes mellitus Cushing's disease: hyperglycemia Prolactinoma: infertility, amenorrhea, galactorrhea, impotence (male) Macroadenoma (usually due to a glycoprotein-secreting adenoma leading to panhypopituitarism by compression/atrophy)		Truncal obesity, striae, moon facies	Serum cortisol; petrosal venous sampling of corticotropin; dexamethasone suppression test Serum GH and glucose suppression Serum prolactin, glycoprotein, TSH
CNS	Suprasellar compression of optic chiasm	Visual field cuts		Formal visual field testing
MS	Acromegaly: hypertrophy of facial bones and airway tissue Cushing's disease: osteoporosis, truncal obesity, skin fragility		Weakness	

Key Reference: Matjasko MJ: Anesthetic considerations in patients with neuroendocrine disease. *In* Cotrell JE, Smith D (eds): Anesthesia and Neurosurgery, 3rd ed. St. Louis, CV Mosby, 1994, pp 604–624.

PERIOPERATIVE IMPLICATIONS

Preoperative Preparation

- Replacement therapy for panhypopituitarism

Monitoring

- Invasive arterial pressure monitoring usually required if intercurrent disease
- Continuous end-tidal CO_2 and N_2 to detect venous air embolism
- Consider CVP in severe acromegaly

Airway

- Have variety of laryngoscope blades and small ET tubes available
- Consider awake, oral fiberoptic intubation if macroglossia is present

Maintenance

- HTN frequently associated with epinephrine infiltration of nasal mucosa and hammering of nasal speculum. Anticipate and pretreat.

Extubation

- Despite suctioning, pharynx and stomach may contain blood and irrigant. Patient should be fully awake and capable of protecting airway to prevent aspiration following extubation.

Postoperative Period

- UO should be followed to detect onset of diabetes insipidus

Adjuvants

- Esmolol and phentolamine (during epinephrine infiltration)

ANTICIPATED PROBLEMS/CONCERNS

- Patients with hypersecretion of ACTH or GH at ↑ risk of myocardial injury if tight hemodynamic control not maintained during the transient, intense stimulations associated with transsphenoidal surgery.

PLACENTA PREVIA

Paul W. Shabaz, M.D.
Karen S. Lindeman, M.D.

RISK

- Incidence: 1/345 to 1/53 deliveries
- Highest incidence: multiparous deliveries, repeat C-section, previous placenta previa

PERIOPERATIVE RISKS

- Maternal mortality: <1%
- Fetal mortality: ~20%
- Life-threatening hemorrhage of mother or fetus
- Fetal hypoxia

WORRY ABOUT

- Blood loss, hypovolemia
- Full stomach considerations due to pregnancy or recent oral intake
- Placenta accreta, increta, and percreta possibly requiring hysterectomy
- Fetal compromise from inadequate intervillous blood flow
- Preterm labor

OVERVIEW

- Placental implantation in advance of fetal presenting part; mode of delivery depends on relationship between placenta and cervical os
- Often presents as painless vaginal bleeding
- Dx confirmed by US or exam of cervical os under "double setup" conditions
- Concomitant tocolytic therapy can alter hemodynamic responses to hemorrhage

ICD-9-CM Code: 641.1

ETIOLOGY

- Unknown

USUAL TREATMENT

- Expectant management
- Delivery by C-section for persistent hemorrhage or when fetus is mature in patient with total placenta previa

ASSESSMENT POINTS

SYSTEM	EFFECT	ASSESSMENT BY HX	PE	TEST
HEENT	Airway edema	Pregnancy	Mallampati class	
CV	Hypovolemia, anemia	Amount of bleeding	Tachycardia, hypotension	Hct
RESP	Reduced FRC	Pregnancy		
GI	Full stomach, decreased lower esophageal sphincter tone	Reflux symptoms		

Key Reference: Mayer DC, Spielman FJ: Antepartum and postpartum hemorrhage. *In* Chestnut DH (ed): Obstetric Anesthesia. St. Louis, Mosby, 1994, pp 699–721.

PERIOPERATIVE IMPLICATIONS

Preoperative Preparation

- Nonparticulate oral antacid premedication
- Assess volume status
- Crossmatch blood and consider transfusion
- Large-gauge IVs (2)
- Consider regional anesthesia if hemodynamically stable

Monitoring

- Routine monitors
- Consider arterial and/or central venous catheter if hemodynamically unstable

Airway

- Airway edema may make intubation more difficult
- Full stomach

Preinduction/Induction

- Preoxygenate with four vital capacity breaths of oxygen
- Consider awake or rapid-sequence induction
- Induction with Pentothal or ketamine, depending on hemodynamics, plus succinylcholine

Maintenance

- Low-concentration inhalational agent 0.5–0.75 MAC before delivery
- Use of nitrous oxide before delivery of baby is controversial
- Can use nitrous oxide with IV opioid and consider benzodiazepine after delivery
- Restore intravascular volume

Extubation

- Extubate awake; greatest risk is pulmonary aspiration of gastric contents

Adjuvants

- Oxytocin, methylergonovine, prostaglandin $F_{2\alpha}$ to enhance uterine contraction and decrease bleeding after delivery

Postoperative Period

- None

ANTICIPATED PROBLEMS/CONCERNS

- Blood loss
- Full stomach
- Urgent induction of anesthesia
- Fetal distress

PNEUMOCYSTIS CARINII PNEUMONIA (PCP) Neal H. Cohen, M.D.

RISK

- Common resp infection in severely immuno-compromised patients
- Patients with acquired or congenital immunodeficiency syndromes
- Seen in all age groups
- >40% of all opportunistic infections in people with advanced AIDS, if no anti-*Pneumocystis* prophylaxis is provided

PERIOPERATIVE RISKS

- Resp failure necessitating mechanical ventilatory support
- Pneumothorax
- Hemodynamic instability associated with induction of anesthesia, positive-pressure ventilation

WORRY ABOUT

- Progressive resp failure
- Pneumothoraces, either spontaneous or associated with positive-pressure ventilation
- Persistent pulm function abn after recovery
- Other causes of cough, dyspnea, fevers
- Associated with other opportunistic infections
- Toxicity from treatment, including methemoglobinemia, anemia, leukopenia, and severe skin rashes

OVERVIEW

- Indolent disease that can progress to severe resp failure
- Associated with spontaneous pneumothoraces
- Extrapulmonary sites of infection rare, since institution of aerosolized pentamidine prophylaxis
- Often associated with coexisting infections (tuberculosis, bacterial, viral, fungal) and malignancies (Kaposi's sarcoma, lymphoma) in immunosuppressed patients

ICD-9-CM Code: 136.3

ETIOLOGY

- *Pneumocystis carinii*, previously thought to be parasite, now classified as fungus
- Organisms reside in lungs, usually as latent infection; activated in immunosuppressed host
- High prevalence of antibodies to *Pneumocystis carinii* in nonimmunosuppressed humans, suggesting that most are infected early in life
- Person-to-person transmission has never been documented

USUAL TREATMENT

- TMP-SMX
- Pentamidine
- Primaquine
- Corticosteroids
- Prophylactic therapy with aerosolized pentamidine, oral TMP-SMX, or dapsone
- Supportive resp care

ASSESSMENT POINTS

SYSTEM	EFFECT	ASSESSMENT BY HX	PE	TEST
HEENT	Oropharyngeal lesions	Fever, chills, sweats	Circumoral, acral, and mucous membrane lesions	
CV	Intravascular volume deficits Myocardiopathy	Fluid intake, resp rate	Hemodynamic lability Neck veins distended Heart sounds	Orthostatic BP changes
RESP		Cough Progressive dyspnea Hemoptysis	Tachypnea Breath sounds Exam often normal	ABG PFTs Transbronchial biopsy Gallium scan of lung LDH
GI	Hepatopathy Bowel lesions	Often associated with wt loss, other infections causing diarrhea, GI Sx	Hepatosplenomegaly	LFTs
HEME	Anemia, leukopenia Coagulopathy			CBC Clotting studies
RENAL	Nephropathy, oliguria	Orthostatic Sx		BUN, Cr
CNS	Encephalitis, meningitis	CNS changes	Abn mental status	

Key Reference: Cohen PT, Sande MA, Volberding PA (eds): The AIDS Knowledge Base. Boston, Little, Brown, 1994, Sections 6.14–6.17.

PERIOPERATIVE IMPLICATIONS

Preoperative Preparation

- Ensure adequacy of oxygenation, ventilation, acid-base balance
- Assess pulm function
- Review CXR for evidence of infiltrates, abscesses, cystic lesions or cavitations, bullae, pneumothorax, effusions

Monitoring

- Confirm presence or absence of methemoglobinemia
- Use pulse oximeter with caution, if MetHb present; measure SaO_2 by co-oximeter

Airway

- Minimize airway pressures
- Increased airway reactivity

Induction

- Maintain adequate PaO_2
- Minimize airway pressures, risk of pneumothorax
- Hypotension associated with myocardial depressants, vasodilators
- Ensure adequate intravascular volume

Maintenance

- Ensure adequate oxygenation, ventilation
- Minimize airway pressures

Extubation

- May be delayed
- Often require prolonged ventilatory support

Postoperative Period

- Ensure adequate oxygenation, ventilation
- Maintain intravascular volume
- Reinstitute anti-*Pneumocystis* therapy

ANTICIPATED PROBLEMS/CONCERNS

- Deterioration of respiratory status, prolonged respiratory failure
- Pneumothorax; may require surgical repair if tube thoracotomy unsuccessful
- Nosocomial infections
- Difficulty monitoring oxygenation with pulse oximeter if patient treated with dapsone, primaquine

POSTOPERATIVE ENCEPHALOPATHY — METABOLIC

Steven Roth, M.D.

RISK

• Patients undergoing any surgical procedure are at risk. Especially of concern following brain or cardiac surgery, or patients with COPD, renal or hepatic failure, lyte abnormalities
• No gender predominance

PERIOPERATIVE RISKS

• Aspiration, fluid and lyte imbalances, circulatory failure, hypoxia, insulin use

WORRY ABOUT

• Suspect in any patient who fails to awaken or awakens more slowly than expected following GA
• Evaluate for presence currently or earlier in perioperative period of severe hypotension, hypoxemia, fluid and lyte disorders, renal or liver dysfunction, thyroid abnormalities
• Seizures, ↑intracranial pressure, persistent coma may result.

OVERVIEW

• Altered state of consciousness that becomes apparent in perioperative period
• Patients may fail to awaken after GA for these reasons: (1) anesthetic-induced: narcotics, inhalational anesthetics, benzodiazepines, hypnotics may impair consciousness, (2) brain injury: direct surgical intervention (e.g., occlusion of major intracranial vessel, intracranial hemorrhage, edema) may result in impaired consciousness, (3) or embolization to a major artery may occur (e.g., during or after cardiac surgery).
• Metabolic abnormalities: circulatory failure, hypoxia, insulin use, hepatic and renal insufficiency, lyte abn can result in failure or slowness to awaken. In all cases, Dx should proceed quickly in order to treat underlying cause before severe brain injury results.

ICD-9-CM Code: 348.3 (Encephalopathy)

ETIOLOGY

• Anoxic-ischemic encephalopathy
• Hypercapnic encephalopathy ($PaCO_2$ >70 mmHg)
• Hypoglycemic encephalopathy (glucose ≤30 mg/dl)
• Hyperglycemic coma (glucose ≥450 mg/dl; Osm >319 mOsm/mm³)
• Acute hepatic encephalopathy: liver failure
• Uremic encephalopathy: renal failure
• Lyte imbalance: hypokalemia or hyponatremia, hypercalcemia
• Endocrine abn: thyrotoxicosis, hypothyroidism
• Drug/toxin exposure (search for drug/toxin exposure—drug/toxicology screen)

USUAL TREATMENT

• This depends upon the etiology—see assessment section

ASSESSMENT POINTS

ETIOLOGY	EXAMPLES	DIAGNOSIS	TREATMENT
ENDO	Hyperthyroid Hypothyroid	Thyrotoxicosis Myxedema	PTU Thyroid hormone replacement
Anoxic-ischemic	Cardiac arrest Prolonged shock Hypoxemia	Obvious from clinical course	Reverse acute event. Then, ↓ cerebral edema, maintain BP, ↓ temp??, prevent seizures
Hypercapnic	Narcotic-induced Severe COPD Sleep apnea	↑ Heart rate and BP ↑ End-tidal or arterial PCO_2	Reverse narcotic Mechanical vent to ↓ PCO_2
Hypoglycemia	Insulin overdose Ethanol ingestion Neonatal (idiopathic)	No IVF or PO ingestion From Hx and alcohol level ↓ Blood glucose	IV glucose (D50)
Hyperglycemia	Hyperosmolar nonketotic coma Ketoacidosis	Suspect in known diabetic Ketones in blood, urine Acidosis	Insulin, correct acidosis and fluid volume deficit
Ion disturbances	↓ Na⁺ ↓ K⁺	Serum Na⁺ <125 mmol/L e.g., SIADH Serum K⁺ <2.5 mEq/L Severe muscle weakness	Hypertonic saline (caution) NaCl and diuretics K⁺ replacement
RENAL	Renal failure		
Hepatic	Hepatic encephalopathy		

Key Reference: Victor M, Martin JB: Nutritional and metabolic diseases of the central nervous system. *In* Wilson JD, Braunwald E, Isselbacher KJ, et al (eds): Harrison's Principles of Internal Medicine, 12th ed. New York, McGraw-Hill, 1991, pp 2045–2055.

PERIOPERATIVE IMPLICATIONS

• Correct ion and fluid disturbances
• Normalize blood glucose
• Optimize organ function (e.g., renal, hepatic)
• Adequate hormone replacement
• Search for drug/toxin exposure (glycine from fluid used for bladder irrigation; sedative/hypnotics; ethanol and its street substitutes such as ethylene

PRADER-WILLI SYNDROME

Navil F. Sethna, M.B., Ch.B.

RISK

- Incidence 1:25,000 live births
- Gender predominance: None
- Highest prevalence (95%) in US: Caucasians, persons of European descent

PERIOPERATIVE RISKS

- 65% of infants born prematurely. Initial marked hypotonia and failure to thrive with poor resp effort
- Morbid obesity; frequently develop kyphoscoliosis: resp embarrassment, hypoventilation, arterial desaturation with RV strain and eventually failure
- Risk of gastric content aspiration due to reduced tendency to vomit combined with rumination and obesity
- Potential difficult intubation due to craniofacial abnormalities and limited mouth opening (fish mouth)
- Diabetes mellitus
- Regional anesthesia: avoid technical difficulties due to obesity and lack of cooperation of an awake patient because of behavioral problems associated with mental retardation

WORRY ABOUT

- Difficult intubation and aspiration pneumonitis
- Cardiopulmonary insufficiency

OVERVIEW

- Dx: combined clinical criteria and molecular genetic data
- Clinical features: hypotonia, hypogonadism, obesity, developmental delay, dysmorphic facial features, thermoregulatory disturbance, ↓ sensitivity to skin, hyperphagia, short stature
- Age at Dx: infantile stage of hypotonia followed by childhood obese phase
- Prognosis: morbid obesity leading to death early in adulthood due to cardiopulmonary insufficiency

ICD-9-CM Code: 759.81

ETIOLOGY

- Inheritance: sporadic and autosomal recessive
- Genetic abnormality: 50% have normal chromosomes. A common abnormality is deletion of long arm of chromosome 15 between bands 15q11–15q13. Less commonly, chromosome 15 has balanced translocation, mosaicism, or marker chromosomes containing duplicated segments

USUAL TREATMENT

- Strict dietary and behavior modification
- Diabetes mellitus type II usually responds to weight control

ASSESSMENT POINTS

SYSTEM	EFFECT	ASSESSMENT BY HX	PE	TEST
HEENT	Facial dysmorphia Poor mask fit Difficult intubation	Obstructive apnea	Small mouth (fish mouth) Micrognathia Short neck, limited cervical and mandibular mobility	
CV	Pulmonary HTN RV hypertrophy and failure Polycythemia	Orthopnea Arrhythmias Myocardial ischemia	Accentuated pulm component of S_2	CXR ECG ECHO Hct
RESP	Restrictive chest wall Hypoventilation	Orthopnea Sleep apnea	Tolerance of supine position	Sleep study
GI	Delayed gastric emptying Regurgitation	Rumination	Partially digested food in mouth	
ENDO	Nonketotic diabetes mellitus Central obesity Temp instability	Hypo-/hyperglycemia Hypothermia/hyperthermia		Glucose tolerance test

Key Reference: Sloan TB, Kaye CI: Rumination risk of aspiration of gastric contents in the Prader-Willi syndrome. Anesth Analg 1991; 73:492–495.

PERIOPERATIVE IMPLICATIONS

Preoperative Preparation

- Only a well-supervised patient should be considered NPO

Monitoring

- Temp
- Evaluation of adequacy of oxygenation in presence of advanced obesity
- Right atrial catheter to monitor RV function (in the absence of LV dysfunction) and safety of IV fluid infusion during major surgery

Airway

- Small mouth opening, micrognathia, short neck, poor anesthetic mask fit, difficult intubation

Maintenance

- Maintain normal body temp
- Avoid long-acting hypnosedatives and opioids in presence of obesity-hypoventilation syndrome
- No specific drug or combination recommended in obese patients
- Maintain adequate depth of anesthesia during induction and maintenance to avoid elevation of pulm vascular resistance

Extubation

- Morbidly obese child frequently requires ventilatory support in immediate postop period, especially after major surgical procedure

Postoperative Period

- Pain management is important to avoid pulm complication
- Epidural/peripheral nerve block as adjunct to GA whenever possible to minimize opioid requirement

ANTICIPATED PROBLEMS/CONCERNS

- Facial and airway anomalies
- Uncontrolled nonketotic diabetes
- Hyperthermia/hypothermia
- Cor pulmonale
- Morbid obesity
- Rumination and aspiration pneumonitis

PREECLAMPSIA

Andrew M. Malinow, M.D.

RISK

- 2.5–7% of all pregnancies
- Young, nulliparous, or multiparous with previous preeclampsia/eclampsia Hx
- May be increased with Hx of other microangiopathy (e.g., chronic HTN, diabetes, renal disease)
- Lower socioeconomic status; malnutrition; no prenatal care

PERIOPERATIVE RISKS

- ↑ Risk of fetoplacental or maternal deterioration necessitating (often operative) delivery
- Preeclampsia and eclampsia account for 20% of maternal and perinatal deaths.

WORRY ABOUT

- Hypertensive crisis leading to intracerebral bleed or LV failure
- ↑ Interstitial volume leading to edema
- Maternal hypotension producing placental hypoperfusion
- Thrombocytopenia may contraindicate regional anesthetic
- Eclampsia (or seizure in a severely preeclamptic patient) necessitating difficult tracheal intubation

OVERVIEW

- Marked by HTN, proteinuria, edema
- Maternal vasoconstriction: possibly leading to acute cardiorespiratory deterioration
- Proteinuria: sign of deteriorating renal function and widespread endothelial damage
- Edema: ↑ total body water, proteinuria, HTN lead to ↑ interstitial edema and ↓ intravascular volume.
- Hematologic: widespread endothelial damage often leads to thrombocytopenia, a poor prognostic sign for fetoplacental well-being.
- Epigastric pain an ominous sign of liver subcapsular edema and possible rupture. Delivery should be urgently effected. HELLP (Hemolysis, Elevated Liver enzymes, Low Platelet count) a poor fetoplacental prognostic sign
- Headache—seizure may be impending

ICD-9-CM Codes: Preeclampsia: 642.4 (mild), 642.5 (severe); 642.7 (with pre-existing hypertension); 760.0 (affecting fetus or newborn)

ETIOLOGY

- Acquired disease of unknown etiology
- Imbalance in circulating mediators of vascular tone and response (e.g., thromboxane vs. prostacyclin)
- Pregnant patients who later manifest the disease have been shown to demonstrate hyperdynamic CV response early in pregnancy compared with patients who do not go on to manifest disease.
- Microangiopathy leading to endothelial change, platelet consumption, hemolysis.

USUAL TREATMENT

- Prevention with daily low-dose aspirin beginning in 2nd trimester has had limited success.
- Delivery becomes cure.
- In hospital, therapy includes antihypertensives, seizure prophylaxis and support of maternal perfusion, with magnesium sulfate (therapeutic blood levels = 5–7 mg/dl), and intravascular rehydration.
- Analgesia, esp. epidural analgesia for labor, reduces catecholamine response to pain, increasing placental perfusion.

ASSESSMENT POINTS

SYSTEM	EFFECT	ASSESSMENT BY HX	PE	TEST
HEENT	Edema		Airway exam	
CV	Systemic vasoconstriction ↓ Intravascular volume		Rales JVD BP	ECG CXR ECHO
RESP	Pulm edema	Dyspnea Chest discomfort	Rales/rhonchi Cyanosis	SaO_2 CXR ECHO
GI	Hepatic subcapsular edema	Epigastric pain	Enlarged liver edge	LFT
HEME	Thrombocytopenia	Easy bruising		Plt count
RENAL	↑ Capillary permeability	Wt gain	Nondependent edema	Urinary protein Cr clearance Serum uric acid
CNS	Seizure Intracerebral hemorrhage Cerebral edema	Headache Blurred vision Seizure	Retinal edema CNS exam	CT scan
Placental	↓ Perfusion		FHR—lack of variability or bradycardia	FHR monitoring Doppler velocimetry

Key Reference: Cheek TG, Samuels P: Pregnancy-induced hypertension. *In* Datta S (ed): Anesthetic and Obstetric Management of High-Risk Pregnancy. St. Louis, CV Mosby, 1991, pp 423–456.

PERIOPERATIVE IMPLICATIONS

Antepartum Management

- Optimize maternal perfusion while lowering systemic diastolic BP <110 mmHg.
- Ensure therapeutic blood magnesium sulfate level
- Replete intravascular volume

Monitoring

- Consider art catheter
- Consider CVP or PA catheter for oliguria or pulm edema
- Fetal heart monitoring

Airway

- Often difficult 2° to edema
- Prepare for emergent airway

Preinduction/Induction

- Epidural analgesia/anesthesia induces venodilation. Maintain maternal perfusion with judicious use of intravascular volume (and small increments of intravenous ephedrine, prn)
- Rapid-sequence induction of anesthesia, titrating infusions of intravenous antihypertensive drugs

Maintenance

- Hemorrhage at delivery may lead to dramatic hypotension. Titrate antihypertensive agents.

Extubation

- Extubate awake, control pressor response

Adjuvants

- Magnesium sulfate; IV antihypertensive drugs (most often hydralazine, labetalol, nitroprusside or trimetaphan antepartum); rarely (but esp. in postpartum) dopamine to increase renal perfusion; finally, other inotropic support if demonstrable LV dysfunction.

Postoperative Period

- Risk for developing pulm edema due to previous (appropriate) intravascular hydration.
- Effective postcesarean analgesia beneficial in BP control

ANTICIPATED PROBLEMS/CONCERNS

- Maternal HTN causes maternal morbidity/mortality; maternal hypotension causes fetoplacental hypoperfusion
- Eclampsia (seizure in a severely preeclamptic patient) associated with CNS residua.

PREGNANCY-INDUCED HYPERTENSION
Susan K. Palmer, M.D.

RISK

- Incidence:
  - Preeclampsia: 5% of multiparous pregnancies
  - Pregnancy-induced HTN (PIH) in up to additional 20%

PERIOPERATIVE RISKS

- 12.3% of maternal mortality related to HTN in pregnancy
- May progress to preeclampsia or eclampsia
- Eclampsia associated with maternal mortality in up to 5% of cases

WORRY ABOUT

- ↓ Intravascular fluid (IVF) volume in patients with interstitial volume overload
- Very low plasma oncotic pressure, which decreases the usual drug-binding sites, making drugs more active at their receptor sites and more available for transfer to the fetus
- Decreased uteroplacental perfusion despite ↑ maternal BP
- Edema in larynx and airway

OVERVIEW

- Endothelial dysfunction occurs in placenta and other vascular beds such as liver (↑ enzymes, RUQ pain), CNS (headache, scotomata), lung (edema), kidneys (oliguria, proteinuria)
- PIH—defined as consistently ≥30 mmHg rise in systolic pressure and/or ≥15 mmHg rise in diastolic pressure before labor; may progress to preeclampsia
- Preeclampsia—above BP rise plus evidence of other organ system involvement, e.g., proteinuria, nondependent edema, ↑ liver enzymes, ↓ plt count, CNS dysfunction.
- Eclampsia—preeclampsia plus seizures

ICD-9-CM Code: 642.11
See also Preeclampsia, Eclampsia

ETIOLOGY

- Unknown causation; no animal models exist. PIH seems to result from or cause failure of normal CV adjustments to pregnancy.

USUAL TREATMENT

- Control of BP, maintenance or improvement of uteroplacental perfusion, and prevention of seizures are primary goals.
- Epidural analgesia may relieve vasospasm and improve uteroplacental perfusion.
- Seizure prophylaxis can be accomplished with $MgSO_4$, benzodiazepine, barbiturate, or Dilantin.
- Delivery of fetus and all of placenta usually followed by amelioration of symptoms.

ASSESSMENT POINTS

SYSTEM	EFFECT	ASSESSMENT BY HX	PE	TESTS
CV	Vasospasm, ↑ CO (usually)	↓ Exercise tolerance		Consider PA catheter Measure CO, PVR
	↓ IVF	↓ UO	BP	UA, 24-h output BUN, uric acid, Cr
RESP	Swelling	Voice became "hoarse"		Airway exam
HEME	↑ Hct, ↑ or ↓ plt ↓ Albumin ↑ BUN, Cr, uric acid			CBC Albumin, BUN, Cr
RENAL	Oliguria Proteinuria			UA, 24-h quantified proteinuria
HEPATIC	↑ Enzymes	RUQ pain, jaundice		Liver enzymes
CNS	Cerebral edema	Anxiety, headache Hyperreflexia (DTR) Optic disc edema		

Key Reference: James FM: Pregnancy-induced hypertension. *In* James FM (ed): Obstetric Anesthesia: The Complicated Patient, 2nd ed. Philadelphia, FA Davis, 1988, pp 411–437.

PERIPARTUM IMPLICATIONS

Preoperative Preparation

- Arterial line plus sodium nitroprusside or other reliable vasodilator can be used preinduction to lower BP and blunt response to rapid-sequence induction and intubation.
- Rapid-onset regional anesthesia may cause severe hypotension due to IVF deficit.

Monitoring

- Arterial line in moderate/severe or malignant accelerating cases
- CVP/PA catheter in severe cases or when cardiac output may be low rather than high
- Mg^{2+} blood levels or repeated exam of DTRs necessary to prevent overdosage in patients who may develop renal failure during labor

Airway

- Edema may obscure normal structures, making rapid-sequence intubation difficult or impossible
- Mask ventilation may be difficult if face, lips, tongue also swollen
- Awake, surface anesthetized, fiberoptic endotracheal tube placement recommended if airway is swollen or looks difficult.

Maintenance

- Pregnancy lowers MAC by 30% for all inhalation agents.
- All inhalation anesthetics cause uterine relaxation. May require greater than normal oxytocin infusion to contract uterus after delivery.

Extubation

- Extubate only when awake and strong, since half of maternal aspirations occur during emergence.

Adjuvants

- Nerve stimulator can be used to monitor Mg^{2+} potentiated effects of nondepolarizing muscle relaxants.

Post Delivery

- Diuresis after delivery
- Still at risk for severe complications and may need intensive care for several days

PREGNANCY, INTRA-ABDOMINAL

Richard J. Palahniuk, M.D.

RISK

- 11/100,000 live births in USA
- Higher incidence in African-Americans, Asians, and immigrant populations from Third World countries
- Higher incidence following in vitro fertilization procedures
- Maternal mortality 100× that of intrauterine pregnancy

PERIOPERATIVE RISKS

- Usually misdiagnosed at the time of laparoscopy or exploratory laparotomy
- Exsanguinating hemorrhage possible pre-, intra-, or postoperatively

WORRY ABOUT

- Hemorrhage

OVERVIEW

- Correct diagnosis is made preoperatively in only 10% of cases
- Differential diagnosis includes abruptio placentae, placenta previa, pelvic inflammatory disease, and bowel obstruction
- Patient usually has a normal early pregnancy and presents with midtrimester abdominal pain, nausea and vomiting, weakness, and vaginal bleeding
- Exsanguinating intra-abdominal bleeding can occur at any time

ICD-9-CM Code: 761.4

ETIOLOGY

- Intra-abdominal pregnancy always results from a missed ruptured tubal ectopic pregnancy
- Fertilized ovum may implant anywhere in the peritoneal cavity, including uterine surface, adnexae, and bowel

USUAL TREATMENT

- Volume resuscitation
- Emergency diagnostic laparoscopy or exploratory laparotomy with delivery of the fetus and excision of the placental implantation site

ASSESSMENT POINTS

SYSTEM	EFFECT	ASSESSMENT BY HX	PE	TEST
CV	Hemorrhage	Postural dizziness	Hypovolemia, hypotension	Hct
GI	Bowel obstruction GI bleed if bowel implantation	Nausea/vomiting	GI bleed	Abdominal x-ray, CT, MRI, abdominal ultrasound falsely negative
CNS			Decreased consciousness if massive hemorrhage	

Key Reference: Atrash HK, et al: Abdominal pregnancy in the United States: Frequency and maternal mortality. Obstet Gynecol 1987; 69:333–337.

PERIOPERATIVE IMPLICATIONS

Preoperative Preparation

- Assess volume status
- Fluid/blood resuscitation

Monitoring

- Arterial and central venous lines valuable if diagnosis known

Airway

- Rapid-sequence induction

Induction

- Rapid-sequence using ketamine or etomidate
- Two or three large venous access lines prior to induction

Maintenance

- Ensure vascular stability

Extubation

- May need to delay extubation for postoperative care
- Extubate awake

Adjuvants

- None

Postoperative Period

- May require intensive care if large fluid shifts or perioperative severe hypotension/hypoxia

ANTICIPATED PROBLEMS/CONCERNS

- Hemorrhage

PREGNANCY: MATERNAL PHYSIOLOGY

Ronald P. Chavez, M.D.

RISK

- All pregnant females: ~3.8 million/y in USA deliver children.

PERIOPERATIVE RISKS

- Maternal mortality: 1/14,000 live births for women 20–24 y; 1/2000 live births for women >40 y
- Perinatal mortality: 15.9/1000 live births. Higher in socioeconomically deprived and minorities.
- PT/PTT ↓ ; ↑ incidence of thrombotic complications during first 3–5 d post partum
- Risk of severe hypotension after pharmacologic sympathectomy 2° to dependence on sympathetic nervous system for maintaining hemodynamic stability

WORRY ABOUT

- Risk of aortocaval compression and impairment of uteroplacental perfusion
- Difficult airway due to wt gain, breast and capillary engorgement, swelling of nasal oral pharynx, larynx, trachea
- Hypoxia occurs more quickly owing to ↓ FRC and ↑ O_2 consumption
- ↑ Incidence of gastric reflux, silent regurgitation, active vomiting, aspiration

OVERVIEW

- Every body system affected by pregnancy
- ↑ Risk of hypoxia due to ↓ FRC, ↑ A-a gradient, ↑ O_2 consumption
- Airway management more challenging
- Incidence of failed ET intubation 1:280 vs 1:2230 in nonpregnant patients
- Risk of aortocaval compression due to gravid uterus, which may result in signs of shock and ↓ uterine blood flow
- Pseudocholinesterase activity ↓ , but recovery from succinylcholine usually not prolonged
- Concentrations of plasma proteins (e.g., albumin, α_1-acid glycoprotein) decreased, affecting pharmacokinetics.
- ↑ Plt turnover, clotting, fibrinolysis
- Bile concentrates with slowing of gallbladder emptying predisposing to gallstones
- Increased GFR results in glucosuria, ↓ serum creatinine and BUN
- Blood glucose may be elevated 2° to a reduced tissue sensitivity to insulin
- Response to anesthetics different owing to ↓ MAC and ↓ FRC, which results in faster induction and risk of anesthetic overdose
- More rapid onset and longer duration of spinal anesthesia compared with nonpregnant females

ICD-9-CM Code: V22.2 (Pregnancy)

ETIOLOGY

- Fetal and maternal hormone production combined with size of the uterus

USUAL TREATMENT

- Delivery

ASSESSMENT POINTS

SYSTEM	EFFECT	ASSESSMENT BY HX	PE	TEST
HEENT	Capillary engorgement/swelling of nasal and oral pharynx, larynx, trachea	Epistaxis Voice changes Difficult nasal breathing	Exam of airway TMD, Malampatti class	
CV	CO, SV, HR, ejection fraction ↑ SVR ↓ , 3rd and 4th heart sounds, grade I–II midsystolic murmur		Auscultation of heart, pulse, pulse pressure	ECHO, ECG, PA catheter (all rarely needed)
RESP	Tidal volume ↑ , FRC ↓ Minute and alveolar ventilation ↑ , diaphragm excursion ↓	Dyspnea		PFTs (rarely needed)
GI	Reduction in tone of lower esophageal high pressure zone ↑ Gastric reflux ↑ Intragastric pressure	Heartburn Sx		
HEME	↑ Hgb, ↑ coag factors (I, VII, VIII, IX, X, XII), ↑ plt turnover, PMN function impaired	↑ Incidence of infection		Hgb, Hct, Plt concn
GU	GFR ↑ , Cr clearance ↑			

Key Reference: Chestnut DH: Obstetric Anesthesia Principles and Practice. St. Louis, Mosby-Year Book, 1944, pp 17–35.

PERIOPERATIVE IMPLICATIONS

Preoperative Preparation

- Large-bore IV
- Non-particulate antacid (e.g., Bicitra) administration within 1 h prior to surgery
- Transport patient in left uterine displacement
- Good oral pharynx exam to determine if larynx difficult to visualize
- Preoxygenate if GA

Monitoring

- Routine

Airway

- Consider short-handled blade
- Have plan for management of difficult intubation
- Avoid manipulation of nasal airway

Preinduction/Induction

- If GA, preoxygenate with 100% O_2 high-flow rates, prevent aspiration with cricoid pressure and rapid sequence
- Maintain left uterine displacement
- Maintain normal maternal ventilation and oxygenation (hyperventilation may result in fetal hypoxemia and acidosis)

Maintenance

- If GA, maintain normal maternal ventilation and oxygenation; can use low-dose inhalational agent and nitrous oxide concentration of 50%
- Muscle relaxants titrated to effect

Extubation

- Awake without residual muscle relaxant blockade

ANTICIPATED PROBLEMS/CONCERNS

- Airway more challenging; incidence of failed intubation greater and obvious anatomic features consistent with difficult intubation may not be present
- CV instability if regional or general anesthesia due to volume shifts (aortocaval compression, blood loss), usually increased cardiac output and HR
- Pain control desirable to maintain uterine perfusion

PROSTATE CANCER

RISK

- In US men: 2nd leading cause of cancer death
- 244,000 new cases are estimated and 40,400 deaths estimated in US in 1995
- Very uncommonly diagnosed < age 50 y
- African-Americans 2/1 Caucasian
- 9% of men will develop prostate cancer (clinically evident), and >20% have on autopsy

PERIOPERATIVE RISKS

- Perioperative mortality <0.3%
- Complications include intraoperative hemorrhage; injury to obturator nerve, ureter, or rectum; DVT; pulmonary emboli (2.7%); wound and urinary tract infections; postop serious urinary incontinence; impotence

WORRY ABOUT

- Increased prevalence of age-related, multiple concomitant disease and a decline in basic organ function in these elderly men

OVERVIEW

- Heterogeneous tumors (usually acinar adenocarcinomas) composed of hormone-sensitive and hormone-insensitive cells
- Natural Hx unpredictable; often assumed localized disease; in most cases will probably have little or no effect on quality or duration of life—Degree of malignancy based on grading of various stages: A1, A2 and B1, B2 confined in thin capsule; C1 extension beyond capsule; C2 involving seminal vesicle; D1 metastatic disease in regional lymph nodes; D2 metastatic disease in bone or other organ
- Dx by (1) digital rectal exam and finger-guided biopsies, (2) transrectal US-guided biopsies, (3) prostate-specific antigen (PSA) monitoring

ICD-9-CM Code: 185

ETIOLOGY

- Genetic predisposition, hormonal influences, dietary and environmental carcinogenic influences, infectious agents

USUAL TREATMENT

- Watchful waiting (especially if other diseases present or age >80 y)
- Radical prostatectomy (retropubically or perineally)—in selected patients with clinically confined prostate cancer usually for those <70 y. Rate of radical prostatectomy has increased > fivefold over past decade because of PSA testing and development of nerve-sparing technique (preservation of the cavernosal neurovascular bundles responsible for erectile potency) to reduce the sexual impotence universally associated with older techniques
- External-beam radiotherapy or cryosurgery, or interstitial radiotherapy
- For metastatic cancer: (1) estrogens, (2) orchiectomy, (3) LH-RH agonists, (4) anti-androgens, (5) combined androgen blockade, (6) cytotoxic chemotherapy, (7) CT, MRI, pelvic lymphadenectomy to delineate lymph node involvement
- Symptomatic patients with metastatic disease: options of active surveillance vs. orchiectomy alone or combined androgen blockade

ASSESSMENT POINTS

SYSTEM	EFFECT	ASSESSMENT BY HX	PE	TEST
RESP	Lung metastases			CXR—lung metastases (uncommon); osteoblastic metastases to spine or ribs
HEME	Low Hgb and/or azotemia and uremia in advanced stages		Anemia in extensive metastases	Serum alkaline phosphatase ↑ Serum acid phosphatase ↑ in 75% with bone metastases
GU	Uncommon signs: hematuria, obstructive urinary retention, urinary infection	Pathologic finding in prostate tissue in TURP for BPH	Hard-rock nodule in digital rectal exam	Digital rectal exam with needle biopsy
METAB	Malnutrition		Wt loss in extensive metastases	
CNS	Metastases to spine		Neurologic deficits in lower limbs	
MS	Metastases to spine	Bone pain (commonly in lumbosacral area)	Pathologic fracture (uncommon)	Radionuclide bone scans

Key Reference: Perinchery N: Neoplasms of the prostate gland. *In* Tanagho EA, McAninch JW (eds): Smith's General Urology. Norwalk CT; Appleton & Lange, 1995, pp 392–433.

PERIOPERATIVE IMPLICATIONS

Preoperative Preparation

- Use of Allen stirrups
- Leg pumps or compression stockings or low-dose Coumadin to reduce DVT
- Autologous blood donation

Monitoring

- Routine

Preinduction/Induction

- None

Adjuvants

- Increased risk of adverse drug effects in elderly patients
- ↑ Liver metabolism abnormal with hormonal therapy

ANTICIPATED PROBLEMS/CONCERNS

- Air embolism from prostatic fossa during surgery in Trendelenburg position
- Intraoperative hemorrhage—less with perineal than retropubic approach

- If prostate surgery: Injury to obturator nerve, ureter, or rectum < 1%; immediate postop DVT and pulmonary embolism, symptomatic pelvic lymphocele, wound or urinary tract infections; perioperative main CV complications—MI and postop arrhythmias; long-term surgical complications—incontinence (0.5–11%) and impotence
- For nonprostate surgery: worry about effects of chemotherapeutic agents, hormones, or radiation on hematologic, liver, renal, and vascular systems

PROTEIN C DEFICIENCY

Charles Weissman, M.D.

RISK

• Congenital deficiency: heterozygote ~ 1/200–1/300
• Homozygote is estimated at 1/160,000–1/360,000
• Acquired deficiency also occurs

PERIOPERATIVE RISKS

• Patients with protein C deficiency are at risk for venous thrombosis and pulm embolism (immobility, endothelial damage, and ↓ blood flow during perioperative period may be triggers)

WORRY ABOUT

• Increased incidence of thrombophlebitis and pulm embolism
• Thrombosis of other vessels, such as intracerebral and coronary arteries, can occur.

OVERVIEW

• Protein C is a vitamin K–dependent protein found in blood and synthesized in liver.
• Inhibits blood coagulation by proteolytic inactivation of factors V and VIII
• Protein S is a cofactor of protein C
• Stimulates fibrinolysis possibly by neutralizing plasminogen activator inhibitors
• Deficiency causes hyperthrombotic state
• Skin necrosis can occur after warfarin therapy begun

ICD-9-CM Code: 286.9 (Coagulation factor deficiency)

ETIOLOGY

• Inherited—autosomal dominant with variable expressivity
• Homozygotes develop life-threatening visceral vessel thrombosis or purpura fulminans (massive cutaneous necrosis) in early neonatal period

• Heterozygotes may develop venous thrombosis and thromboembolism.
• Acquired causes: hepatic dysfunction, vitamin K deficiency, DIC

USUAL TREATMENT

• Heterozygotes:
  – With acute thrombosis should initially be heparinized
  – Long-term anticoagulation with warfarin in patients with Hx of thrombosis. (Heparin therapy should be continued until warfarin is at therapeutic levels to prevent skin necrosis.)
  – With acute thrombosis may need transfusions of FFP to increase protein C levels
• Homozygotes:
  – Periodic FFP transfusions to provide protein C
• Acquired:
  – Vitamin K deficiency—parenteral vitamin K
  – DIC—treatment of underlying cause

ASSESSMENT POINTS

SYSTEM	EFFECT	ASSESSMENT BY HX	PE	TEST
CV	MI Angina Peripheral arterial disease	Hx of MI, angina Peripheral vascular thrombosis	Peripheral pulses	ECG
RESP	Pulm embolism	Hx of previous pulm embolism		
GI	Mesenteric thrombosis	Hx bowel infarction		
HEME	Thrombophlebitis	Hx thrombophlebitis, pulm embolism	Exam of veins in legs	
RENAL	Renal vein and artery thrombosis	Hx renal problems		BUN/Cr Urine protein
SKIN	Necrosis	Cutaneous necrosis after warfarin begun	Cutaneous necrosis	
CNS	Intracerebral artery thrombosis	Hx CVA, TIA	Neurologic exam	

Key Reference: Nachman RL, Silverstein R: Hypercoagulable states. Ann Intern Med 1993; 119:819–827.

PERIOPERATIVE IMPLICATIONS

Preoperative Preparation

• In homozygotes and symptomatic heterozygotes, FFP can be administered to increase protein C levels.
• Warfarin can be stopped a few days before surgery to allow PT to return to normal range and heparin administered until surgery.
• Intermittent pneumatic compression stocking can be placed prior to induction of anesthesia.

Airway

• Some have suggested that the ET tube cuff not be inflated so as to prevent tracheal venous thrombosis.
• In neonates, there should be an audible leak.

Preinduction/Induction

• Regional anesthesia may be preferable, if possible.

Maintenance

• Special attention can be paid to positioning to reduce venous and arterial stasis.
• FFP should be given to patients with prior thrombotic manifestations and for prolonged operations.

Adjuvants

• Intermittent pneumatic compression stockings can be used.
• Postop heparinization should be started as soon as deemed safe.

ANTICIPATED PROBLEMS/CONCERNS

• Increased risk of thrombosis, esp. thrombophlebitis and pulm embolism
• When switching from heparin anticoagulation to warfarin, heparin can be continued until warfarin has achieved therapeutic effect to decrease risk of skin necrosis.

PULMONARY ATRESIA

James F. Arens, M.D.

RISK

- 1.5% of normal births
- 0.5% of all congenital heart disease

PERIOPERATIVE RISKS

- RV failure
- Hypoxemia
- Metabolic acidosis
- Deterioration in 1st days of life

WORRY ABOUT

- Progressive metabolic acidosis
- Maintaining a patent ductus arteriosus
- RV hypoplasia—50% incidence
- Maintaining prostaglandin infusion
- High risk: >50% do not survive 1st year

OVERVIEW

- Associated with other cardiac lesions, e.g., patent foramen ovale, patent ductus arteriosus, possible VSD
- High-risk infant
- Resuscitation—anesthetic technique

ICD-9-CM Code: 424.3

USUAL TREATMENT

- Prostaglandin E$_1$ infusion
- Systemic to pulm shunt
- Infective endocarditis prophylaxis
- Palliative therapy

ETIOLOGY

- Congenital

ASSESSMENT POINTS

SYSTEM	EFFECT	PE	TEST
CV	RV failure Hypoxemia Metabolic acidosis Patent foramen ovale	Cyanosis Metabolic acidosis	ECG—right atrial enlargement CXR—left- or right-sided arch CXR— ↓ pulm vascular markings ABGs
RESP	↓ Pulm blood flow	Tachypnea	ECHO, cardiac catheter
Systemic	Signs of RV failure		

Key Reference: Kambaun J: Cardiac Anesthesia for Infants and Children. St. Louis, CV Mosby, 1994.

PERIOPERATIVE IMPLICATIONS

Preoperative Diagnosis

- Pulm atresia vs. pulm valve stenosis at cardiac cath, a Rashkind balloon septostomy was likely attempted

Preoperative Considerations

- Palliative surgery initially
- Type of shunt to be performed
- Which systemic artery is to be used for shunt? Don't stick it during CVP attempts
- May surgically create a VSD
- Degree of hypoxemia, metabolic acidosis

Monitoring

- Routine
- A-Line
  - Umbilical artery if good trace
  - Radial artery—opposite side of shunt
  - Could clamp (partially) subclavian artery—same implication for pulse oximeter placement
- CVP for resuscitation drugs
- Temp

Airway

- Endotracheal

Preinduction/Induction

- Do not be rushed
- Prostaglandin infusion to keep baby alive (0.03–0.1 µg/kg/min)
- Intubation—smooth and quick by experienced individual
- Hypoxemia, bradycardia disastrous
- Avoid increased pulm vascular resistance:
  - Coughing, bucking; ↑ PEEP; ↑ CO_2; ↓ PO_2
  - ↓ systemic vascular resistance
  - Air in all lines

Maintenance

- Hemodynamically stable anesthetic, e.g., ketamine plus low-dose narcotic or inhalational agent
- Normal heart rate—avoid bradycardia, tachycardia
- Normothermia
- Normal filling volumes
- Normal myocardial contractility
- Aiming for early extubation

Extubation

- As early as reasonably safe

Postoperative Care

- Provided in the area where the most MDs and RNs are thoroughly experienced in pediatric care
- Prostaglandin infusion maintained

ANTICIPATED PROBLEMS/CONCERNS

- Palliative surgery only
- Definitive procedure later, e.g., Fontan, Rastelli
- Hypoxemia progressing—inadequate shunt/ductus closing
- Tachypnea worsening—hypoxemia, laryngeal swelling, pneumothorax (small chest tube easily occluded)

PULMONARY EMBOLISM

Ronald G. Pearl, M.D., Ph.D.

RISK

- People within US: 600,000/y
- No racial predilection
- Increased incidence in women

PERIOPERATIVE RISKS

- Risk for hypoxemia and right heart failure
- Perioperative mortality of ~90% for acute thromboendarterectomy, of ~10% for chronic thromboendarterectomy
- Postop pulm embolism in up to 1% of surgical patients

WORRY ABOUT

- Recurrent pulm embolism
- Right heart failure and CV collapse
- Hypoxemia
- Hemorrhage in patients on anticoagulants or thrombolytics

OVERVIEW

- Pulm embolism noticed in ~20% of autopsied patients
- Clinical presentation may range from asymptomatic to chest pain and hypoxemia to CV collapse
- Most patients have DVT
- Dx involves a combination of clinical suspicion, ventilation-perfusion lung scan, evaluation of the deep venous system of the legs, and pulm angiogram

ICD-9-CM Code: 415.1

ETIOLOGY

- Acquired disease
- Risk factors present in almost all patients: age >40 y, obesity, malignancy, recent surgery, trauma, pregnancy, immobilization, estrogen use, prior Hx of DVT

USUAL TREATMENT

- Therapy decreases mortality from 35% to <5%
- Heparin followed by warfarin sodium for most patients
- Thrombolytic therapy for massive pulm embolism
- Vena caval filter if massive pulm embolism or if cannot receive anticoagulants
- Surgical thromboendarterectomy in selected cases

ASSESSMENT POINTS

SYSTEM	EFFECT	ASSESSMENT BY HX	PE	TEST
CV	RV failure	Syncope Dyspnea Palpitations	↑ JVP; RV heave Hypotension Tachycardia Hepatojugular reflux	ECG ECHO
RESP	Pulm infarction V/Q abn Pain from pleural irritation	Hemoptysis Chest pain Shoulder pain	Tachypnea	CXR, SaO_2 ABG Pulm Angio
CNS	Syncope	Syncope		
MS	Phlebitis	Hx DVT Leg edema, pain	Leg edema Inflammation Palpable cord	Doppler US Impedance plethysmography Venography

Key Reference: Goldhaber SZ, Morpurgo M: Diagnosis, treatment, and prevention of pulmonary embolism. JAMA 1992; 268:1727–1733.

PERIOPERATIVE IMPLICATIONS

Preoperative Preparation

- Preop Rx with heparin, warfarin, sequential compression devices decreases incidence of perioperative DVT and PE
- If active DVT, consider preop vena caval filter

Monitoring

- Consider PA catheter
- TEE may demonstrate RV dysfunction and PA thromboembolism

Airway

- None

Preinduction/Induction

- May develop hypotension due to RV failure

Maintenance

- Adequate preload essential to RV function

Extubation

- None

Adjuvants

- None

ANTICIPATED PROBLEMS/CONCERNS

- RV failure may be initial presentation of PE or may develop with recurrent PE

PURPURA, IMMUNE THROMBOCYTOPENIC (ITP)

Evan G. Pivalizza, M.D.

RISK

- Rare
  - Children M/F 1/1
  - Adults M/F 2–4/1 (pregnancy 1–2/1000 deliveries)

PERIOPERATIVE RISKS

- Hemorrhage
- Infection and thrombocytosis post splenectomy

WORRY ABOUT

- Preop corticosteroids, immunosuppressives
- Splenectomy
- Hemorrhage (surgical and "anesthetic" related)

OVERVIEW

- Acute, intermittent, or chronic immune-mediated thrombocytopenia (accelerated destruction with appropriate megakaryocyte response) with dermal, mucosal, and CNS hemorrhage (most critical).
- Obstetric implications include risk of transient neonatal thrombocytopenia

ICD-9-CM Code: 287.3

ETIOLOGY

- "Immune" in title (previously "idiopathic") reflects presence of antiplatelet IgG autoantibody (majority plt-associated with some in plasma)
- Postulated action against plt membrane glycoproteins

USUAL TREATMENT

- Corticosteroids: initial therapy (1 mg/kg/d) with 30–60% response rates (up to 80% initially)
- IV immunoglobulin: 0.4 g/kg for 3–5 d, esp. with severe bleeding, immunocompromise, or infection (complex immunomodulatory effects)
- Splenectomy: not in acute disease. Indicated if steroids cannot be tapered, poor response to medical therapy, and chronic disease: complete response rates of 70–90%
- Other: azathioprine, vincristine, danazol (synthetic androgen), and recombinant interferon

ASSESSMENT POINTS

SYSTEM	EFFECT	ASSESSMENT BY HX	PE	TEST
HEENT	Airway manipulation—potential hemorrhage	Oral bleeding		
CVS	Vascular access			
HEME	Thrombocytopenia	Hemorrhage	Petechiae	Plts <20–80,000 × 10³/mm³ (depending on author), megakaryocytes, anti-platelet antibody
CNS	Hemorrhage in acute disease			Radiology if indicated
Obstetric	Controversy predicting neonate at risk (10–15%) and mode of delivery			

Key Reference: Tardio DJ, McFarland J, Gonzalez MF: Immune thrombocytopenic purpura: current concepts. J Gen Intern Med 1993; 8:160–163.

PERIOPERATIVE IMPLICATIONS

Preparation

- Steroid supplement
- Premedication: Avoid IM injection
- Pneumococcal vaccine if splenectomy

Monitoring

- Routine
- Protect pressure points and mucosal surfaces

Airway

- Avoid nasal ET intubation
- Careful instrumentation, esp. plt count <50,000 × 10³/mm³

Induction

- Avoid hypertensive response to ET intubation, esp. with plt count <20,000 × 10³/mm³

Maintenance

- Theoretical disadvantage of volatile agents (see also TTP)

Fluids

- If plt required, transfuse after splenic pedicle ligation. Intraoperative thromboelastography and Sonoclot analysis of plt function and clot formation may be useful guide to replacement therapy.

Extubation

- As above: care of mucous membranes and hemodynamic response

Adjuvants

- Individual analysis of risk-benefit for neuraxial technique, esp. in parturient (report of use of TEG and Sonoclot in addition to BT in decision-making)

Postoperative Period

- Risks of thrombocytosis not as crucial as in TTP and initial reports of laparoscopic splenectomy may herald decreased risk of postop pulm complications

ANTICIPATED PROBLEMS/CONCERNS

- Massive surgical hemorrhage
- CNS and airway hemorrhage

PURPURA, THROMBOTIC THROMBOCYTOPENIC (TTP)

Evan G. Pivalizza, M.D.

RISK

- Rare (1/1 million) but 20% fatality rate

PERIOPERATIVE RISKS

- Patient for splenectomy has not responded to medical therapy; hence, risks of multiorgan impairment (microthrombi) and thrombocytopenia

WORRY ABOUT

- Preop drugs and therapies
- CNS, renal dysfunction
- Thrombocytopenia (although usual quantitative plt triggers do not apply)

OVERVIEW

- Severe microvascular occlusive disease characterized by thrombocytopenia, microangiopathic hemolytic anemia, multisystem organ involvement, particularly CNS and kidney

ICD-9-CM Code: 446.6

ETIOLOGY

- Combination of abnormal PAF and plt aggregation, von Willebrand factor consumption, suppression of prostacyclin production, and endothelial damage, all leading to arteriole/capillary occlusion with microthrombi

USUAL TREATMENT

- Parity of controlled studies and usually a combination of therapies:
  - Plasmapheresis: of primary importance (platelet-poor FFP)
  - Plt aggregator inhibitors: aspirin, dipyridamole, dextran, ticlopidine
  - Immunosuppression: corticosteroids, vincristine (risk of neurotoxicity and abnormal ADH secretion), γ-globulin (strict asepsis required)
  - Splenectomy: often in failed medical responses or to prevent relapse

ASSESSMENT POINTS

SYSTEM	EFFECT	ASSESSMENT BY HX	PE	TEST
HEENT	Airway manipulation with potential hemorrhage			
CV	Rare conduction pathway involvement		Baseline MAP for perfusion of CNS/kidney Vascular access	ECG
RESP	Rare infiltrates causing hypoxemia			CXR
RENAL	Azotemia rare			BUN, serum Cr, urine sediment
HEME	Thrombocytopenia	Hemorrhage	Petechiae Jaundice	Plts 8000–44,000 × 10³/mm³; PT, PTT, fibrinogen usually normal Fragmented RBCs (Hgb 8–9g/dl); ↑ LDH, bilirubin
CNS	Diagnostic fluctuating course	Spectrum—headache, seizures, coma		Lumbar puncture, EEG, neuroradiology studies rarely performed
OBSTETRIC	May precipitate episode or relapse	Differentiate from HELLP/PIH	Termination of pregnancy not as crucial	

Key Reference: Rose M, Rowe JM, Eldor A: The changing course of thrombotic thrombocytopenic purpura and modern therapy. Blood Rev 1993:7;94–103.

PERIOPERATIVE IMPLICATIONS

Preparation

- Steroid supplement
- Premedicatioution: Not IM injection; caution with CNS dysfunction
- Pneumococcal vaccine (splenectomy)

Monitoring

- Protect skin and mucous membrane (NIBP cuff, esophageal probe, pressure points)
- Usually have central access for plasma exchange. If CVP required, avoid subclavian (difficulty in compressing hematoma)
- Theoretical risk of radial arterial line with thrombotic process

Airway

- Avoid nasal ET tube. Careful instrumentation, especially if plt count <50,000 × 10³/mm³

Induction

- Avoid sympathetic intubation response (risk of intracranial hematoma), but maintain MAP >CNS, renal autoregulatory thresholds (>50–60 mmHg)

Maintenance

- Theoretical advantage of inhibitory effect of volatile anesthetics on plt aggregation (halothane>isoflurane>enflurane)

Fluids

- Do not transfuse plts: reports of deterioration due to further plt thrombi
- Bleeding managed with RBCs (>48 h old to avoid active plts) and FFP (platelet-poor)

Extubation

- As above: care of mucous membranes and hemodynamic response

Adjuvants

- Individual analysis of risk-benefit for neuraxial technique in thrombocytopenic patient (if in remission)

Postoperative Period

- Mobilize early because of precipitous increase in plt count and viscosity with risk of thrombotic events
- Risk of atelectasis from LUQ incision and dissection

ANTICIPATED PROBLEMS/CONCERNS

- Hemorrhage due to thrombocytopenia
- Microthrombi with CNS dysfunction

PYLORIC STENOSIS

John Peder Erickson, M.D.

RISK

- Incidence 1/300–1/1,000 of all live births
- Children of affected parents have higher incidence (3–5%)
- Male predominance

PERIOPERATIVE RISKS

- Similar to other abdominal procedures in patients of same age
- Some association with other GU anomalies
- Some have elevated unconjugated bilirubin: related to decreased glucuronyl transferase activity; returns to normal after correction of stenosis

WORRY ABOUT

- Potential of full stomach
- Dehydration from recurrent emesis leads to alkalosis

OVERVIEW

- Reduced size of gastric outlet impedes emptying of contents, which can cause abnormal nutrition, repeated vomiting, and dehydration
- Onset of symptoms 3–6 wk of age
- Usually surgically cured

ICD-9-CM Code: 750.5 (Congenital)

ETIOLOGY

- Almost exclusively genetic in infants
- Can be acquired in adults

USUAL TREATMENT

- Normalize fluid/electrolyte status—this is not a surgical emergency
- Surgical: pyloromyotomy can usually be undertaken within 2–24 h of admission (unless fluid derangements are severe)
- Short procedure (<1 h)

ASSESSMENT POINTS

SYSTEM	EFFECT	ASSESSMENT BY HX	PE	TEST
GI	Small bowel obstruction	Projectile emesis	Pyloric "olive" palpable in upper abdomen	Contrast study

Key Reference: Katz J, Steward D (eds): Anesthesia and Uncommon Diseases. Philadelphia, WB Saunders, 1987, pp 226–227.

PERIOPERATIVE IMPLICATIONS

Preoperative Preparation

- Correct fluid and acid-base deficits
- Pyloric stenosis is not a surgical emergency

Monitoring

- Routine

Airway

- Potential of full stomach

Preinduction/Induction

- Some will pass orogastric/nasogastric tube to suction stomach (still does NOT guarantee empty stomach)
- Consider IV rapid-sequence induction

Maintenance

- No technique is absolutely contraindicated by pyloric stenosis alone

Extubation

- Potential of full stomach

Adjuvants

- Consider potential of associated liver and GU abnormalities

Postoperative Period

- Pain score: 2–5

ANTICIPATED PROBLEMS/CONCERNS

- Potential of full stomach
- Need to correct fluid/electrolyte imbalances preop

RAYNAUD'S PHENOMENON

Stephan J. Cohn, M.D.

RISK

- 1.9% of population (based on reporting of color changes on exposure to cold)
- Almost all with disease in ages 15–40 y; almost all with secondary phenomenon over age 40 y
- Often associated with scleroderma, systemic lupus erythematosus, and/or primary pulm HTN

PERIOPERATIVE RISKS

- Rare morbidity

WORRY ABOUT

- Arterial thrombosis
- Low blood flow states (e.g., prolonged hypotension or use of tourniquet) can lead to gangrene of extremities

OVERVIEW

- Abnormal sensitivity of small arteries and arterioles to vasoconstrictive stimuli
- Often manifested in a bilateral symmetric pattern, with hands being affected more often than feet
- Patients exhibit triphasic color pattern in affected areas: pallor, then cyanosis due to small arterial occlusion, followed by erythema and edema as vessels suddenly reopen

ICD-9-CM Code: 443.0

ETIOLOGY

- Unknown
- Likely hypothesis: hyperactive sympathetic nervous system with excess neurotransmitter and/or little or no inactivation of norepinephrine

USUAL TREATMENT

- Prevention is most effective—avoid prolonged exposure to cold, avoid cigarette smoking
- IV regional blocks with lidocaine at regular intervals. Reserpine, bretylium, and guanethidine all used as additives to lidocaine in IV regional blocks
- In severe cases, surgical sympathectomy an option but not always beneficial
(See also Systemic Lupus Erythematosus in Diseases section

ASSESSMENT POINTS

SYSTEM	EFFECT	ASSESSMENT BY HX	PE	TEST
RESP	Associated with primary pulmonary HTN	Chest discomfort DOE Weakness	JVD Pulmonic ejection click	CXR—right cardiomegaly Dilated pulmonary artery ECG—right atrial enlargement, renal vascular hypertension
MS	Impaired joint mobility due to pain or scleroderma	Joint mobility		
VASC	Small arterial occlusion	Triphasic color pattern	Often associated with numbness and diaphoresis	

Key Reference: Stoelting RK, et al: Anesthesia and Co-Existing Disease, 2nd ed. New York, Churchill Livingstone, 1988, pp 182–183.

PERIOPERATIVE IMPLICATIONS

Preoperative Preparation

- Keep warm
- Assess for coexisting disease

Monitoring

- Assess risk:benefit ratio if considering arterial cannulation because of danger of thrombosis
- Monitor patient's temp and check pressure points and distal pulses frequently

Airway

- ↓ TMJ mobility if associated with scleroderma

Induction

- General or regional anesthetic options acceptable

Maintenance

- Use of tourniquet controversial

Adjuvants

- When using regional anesthetic, consider avoiding epinephrine

Postoperative Period

- Keep as warm as possible
- Check pulses in all extremities

REFLEX SYMPATHETIC DYSTROPHY
(COMPLEX PERIPHERAL PAIN SYNDROME)

Lloyd R. Saberski, M.D.
Jerry M. Calkins, M.D., Ph.D.

RISK

• People within US: 1–6 million? (under-estimated)
• 1.5% of total peripheral nerve injuries
• No racial predilection

PERIOPERATIVE RISKS

• Heightened postop pain if operation on involved extremity
• Frequently hypertensive, and with ↑ incidence of CAD

WORRY ABOUT

• Pain can be augmented by adrenergic agonists
• Avoid vascular access in involved extremities
• Position involved extremity carefully and document

OVERVIEW

• Neuropathic pain after injury, characterized as burning associated with severe allodynia and hyperpathia
• Dx made on clinical basis from major criteria (burning pain, allodynia, hyperpathia, edema, temp changes) and minor criteria (nail and hair growth changes, skin changes). Considerable ambiguity as to who is afflicted
• Dx primarily of exclusion
• Regional sympathetic dysfunction may be present
• Operations upon involved extremities can lead to further postop neuropathic pain with significant sympathetic discharge
• HTN and tachycardia
• No correlation between severity of injury and incidence, severity, and course of symptoms
• Often classified into 3 stages and 3 grades, although new nomenclature proposed

ICD-9-CM Codes: 337.20 (reflex sympathetic dystrophy—unspecified site); 337.21 (reflex sympathetic dystrophy—upper limb); 337.22 (reflex sympathetic dystrophy—lower limb); 337.29 (reflex sympathetic dystrophy—other specified site)

ETIOLOGY

• Unknown, although involves altered peripheral and CNS response thresholds to afferent impulses
• Sympathetic dysfunction may be present. No specific diagnostic test available.
• Associated with antecedent trauma, iatrogenic causes (amputation, tight casts), and visceral, neurologic, and musculoskeletal diseases

USUAL TREATMENT

• Some cases spontaneously subside
• Desensitization therapy
• Neuropathic pain medications
• Sympatholytic medication
• Sympathectomies rarely
• Multiple therapeutic regimens

ASSESSMENT POINTS

SYSTEM	EFFECT	ASSESSMENT BY HX	PE	TEST
GI	Slow peristalsis	Constipation	↓ Bowel sounds	
SKIN	Dry, shiny skin Vasomotor and sudomotor disturbances		Dry, shiny, cool skin Nails brittle ↓ Hair growth	Abn galvanic skin reflex
PNS	Pain, allodynia, Hyperalgesia Hyperesthesia	Pain to touch		
MS	Weakness, atrophy Trophic skin changes in skin, bones, joints	Weakness	Joints sclerosed	

Key Reference: Bonica JJ: The Management of Pain. Philadelphia, Lea & Febiger, 1990.

PERIOPERATIVE IMPLICATIONS

• Avoid tourniquets, BP cuffs, and vascular punctures of involved extremity.
• Carefully position patient and protect involved extremity.
• Consider plexus infusion of local anesthetic 24–72 h before surgical procedure.

Monitoring

• Routine

Induction

• Consider regional anesthetic infusion that can be continued postop; can be combined with GA (without succinylcholine)
• Consider avoiding sympathomimetic agents such as ketamine.
• Pressors can aggravate sympathetic responsive pain and should be titrated incrementally
• Avoid Bier blocks since exsanguination and compression with tourniquet can be painful.

Maintenance

• Consider combining conduction anesthetic with sedation or nonsympathomimetic GA.
• Keep affected extremity warm.

Adjuvants

• IV phentolamine can decrease sympathetic responsive pain.
• Neuropathic medications such as lidocaine, phenytoin, and clonidine may decrease pain and anesthetic requirements.

Postoperative Period

• Balanced analgesia: plexus infusion with local anesthetic, adjuvants, opioid

SPECIAL CONSIDERATIONS

• Conduction anesthetics along with neuropathic medication may decrease plasticity (wind-up) of CNS and decrease postop pain.

RENAL FAILURE, ACUTE (ARF)

Robert N. Sladen, M.D.

RISK

- People within USA: 1% of all hospital admissions (community-acquired), 5% of all general hospital patients (hospital-acquired), 10–30% of ICU patients
- Population with highest prevalence: elderly (>65 y)

PERIOPERATIVE RISKS

- Overall mortality of perioperative ARF: 60–90%
- Acute pulm edema, electrolyte abn, arrhythmias
- Aspiration
- Bleeding (plt dysfunction)

WORRY ABOUT

- Difficult IV and arterial access
- Intolerance of hemodialysis
- GI symptoms
- Clinical signs of coagulopathy
- Hyperkalemia and arrhythmias

OVERVIEW

- Elective surgery is contraindicated with new-onset ARF; procedures are urgent or emergency.
- Underlying disorder may still be present.
- Repeated hemodynamic insults markedly impair renal recovery.
- Dialysis partially controls thrombocytopathy and enteropathy, but does not decrease risk of sepsis and poor wound healing.

ICD-9-CM Codes: 584 (acute); 977.5 (due to procedure)

ETIOLOGY

- ATN (ischemic, nephrotoxic)
  - Sepsis in 70% of all cases, multiple system failure in 80% of ICU patients
- Vascular injury (thromboembolism, occlusion, intra-abdominal HTN)
- Systemic disease (atherosclerosis, vasculitis, sickle cell)
- Acute interstitial nephritis, acute glomerulonephritis

USUAL TREATMENT

- Medical therapy
  - Fluid and electrolyte restriction, loop diuretics
  - Hyperkalemia: hyperventilation, bicarbonate, Ca^{2+}, insulin-glucose, Kayexalate enema
- Dialysis—peritoneal dialysis, intermittent hemodialysis, continuous arteriovenous or venovenous dialysis

ASSESSMENT POINTS

SYSTEM	EFFECT	ASSESSMENT BY HX	PE	TEST
HEENT	Edema		Airway edema	
	Coagulopathy	Epistaxis		See HEME
CV	VTach, VFib	Syncope, cardiac arrest		Serum K^+, Mg^{2+}
	Pericardial effusion	Dyspnea, pleuritic chest pain	Muffled heart sounds	ECG, CXR, ECHO
RESP	Pulm edema	Dyspnea, orthopnea	Rales	CXR
GI	Impaired motility	Reflux	Abdominal distention	NG, stool guaiac
	Ileus	GI bleeding	Tenderness, guarding	KUB series
	Serositis	Abdominal discomfort	Absent bowel sounds	Endoscopy
	Ulceration	Constipation, diarrhea		CT scan
HEME	Plt dysfunction	Excessive bleeding	Petechial hemorrhages	Bleeding time
RENAL	ARF	Oliguria, anuria	Edema	Urinalysis, BUN, Cr, Cr clearance Renal US, scintigraphy
CNS	Encephalopathy	Confusion, disorientation		EEG
		Coma		CT scan
MS	Rhabdomyolysis	Crush injury, limb ischemia	"Red urine"	Urine myoglobin Serum CPK

Key Reference: Prough DS, Foreman AS: Anesthesia and the renal system. *In* Barash PG, Cullen BF, Stoelting RK (eds): Clinical Anesthesiology, 2nd ed. Philadelphia, JB Lippincott, 1992, pp 1125–1155.

PERIOPERATIVE IMPLICATIONS

Preoperative Preparation

- Dialysis to control fluid overload, hyperkalemia, metabolic acidosis, acute uremia
- Consider metoclopramide, H_2-blocker to reduce reflux risk
- Consider DDAVP 0.3 µg/kg to enhance plt function (effective 8–12 h)
- Regional techniques may be contraindicated by coagulopathy
- DDAVP, insulin-glucose, Kayexalate can complicate perioperative care

Monitoring

- ECG for arrhythmia detection
- Consider PA catheter for large fluid shift operations with or without LV dysfunction
- Avoid arterial catheters and blood pressure cuffs in limbs with AV shunts

Airway

- Consider awake intubation with airway edema
- Avoid nasal intubation (epistaxis)

Preinduction/Induction

- Manage fluids as if renal function were normal (risk of hypovolemia)
- Treat as for full stomach: head up, cricoid pressure
- Succinylcholine is relatively contraindicated (avoid if K^+ concn $\geq$ 5.0 mEq/L)

Maintenance

- Restrict maintenance fluids, but replace losses appropriately guided by hemodynamic monitoring
- Avoid morphine, meperidine, pancuronium
- Increase minute ventilation to compensate for metabolic acidosis; sedative-hypnotic administration may lead to acidosis by decreasing resp rate in spontaneously breathing patient

- Anticipate increased volume of distribution but decreased clearance of most drugs
- Check ABGs, serum K^+

Extubation

- Anticipate delayed emergence
- Treat as for full stomach

Postoperative Period

- Careful assessment of CV, resp status: check ABGs, serum K^+
- Morphine, meperidine have active metabolites that are renally excreted: use with caution
- May require ultrafiltration for excess fluid removal in early postop period

ANTICIPATED PROBLEMS/CONCERNS

- Ventricular arrhythmias may occur without premonitory ECG signs. Rapid K^+ flux more ominous than high serum K^+ itself.
- Dialysis preferred 24 h preop to avoid dysequilibrium during anesthesia

RENAL FAILURE, CHRONIC

Donald S. Prough, M.D.

RISK

- People within US: >100 cases of end-stage renal disease (ESRD)/ 1 million population
- Racial prevalence: African-Americans ~200 cases/1 million; Hispanics ~100/1 million; Caucasians ~50/1 million

PERIOPERATIVE RISKS

- Overall perioperative mortality of patients with ESRD: 4%
- Overall perioperative morbidity of patients with ESRD: 50% (hyperkalemia, infections, hypotension/HTN, bleeding, dysrhythmias, clotted fistulas)

WORRY ABOUT

- Perioperative progression from chronic renal insufficiency (CRI), not requiring dialysis, to dialysis-dependent ESRD
- Hypovolemia and hypokalemia (esp. if recently dialyzed)

- Hypervolemia, metabolic acidosis and hyperkalemia (esp. if not recently dialyzed)
- Autonomic dysfunction (excessive hypotensive responses)
- Exaggerated hypertensive responses to noxious stimuli
- Prolonged responses to renally excreted drugs and metabolites (e.g., vecuronium, pancuronium, narcotics)
- Impaired immune status

OVERVIEW

- ↓ Excretory and other functions of kidney related to long-standing disease—with dialysis, a disease that can persist for many years.
- Associated with multiple complications of failed renal excretory function, including volume overload, accumulation of products of catabolism (e.g., potassium and hydrogen ions), plt dysfunction, and side effects of dialytic therapy, including hypovolemia
- Associated with complications of concurrent diseases (e.g., diabetes mellitus, HTN)

- Volume status and electrolyte balance related to recency of dialysis

ICD-9-CM Code: 585

ETIOLOGY

- HTN (15% Hispanics; 20% Caucasians; 40% African-Americans)
- Diabetes mellitus (20% Causasians; 30% African-Americans; 37% Hispanics)
- Glomerulonephritis (12% African-Americans); 22% Hispanics; 25% Caucasians)
- Other causes: polycystic disease, collagen-vascular disease, pyelonephritis

USUAL TREATMENT

- CRI: Fluid restriction, protein restriction, diuretics, antihypertensives
- Peritoneal dialysis or hemodialysis; continuous venovenous hemofiltration or continuous venovenous hemodialysis while hospitalized
- Renal transplantation (often combined with pancreatic transplantation in diabetics)

ASSESSMENT POINTS

SYSTEM	EFFECT	ASSESSMENT BY HX	PE	TEST
CV	CHF LVH Dysrhythmias	Exercise intolerance HTN Palpitations	Crackles; S_3, S_4 Pulse, auscultation	CXR ECG
GI	N/V, anorexia GI bleeding	N/V, anorexia Melena, rectal bleeding	Malnutrition	Positive occult blood
HEME	Plt dysfunction Anemia	Easy bruising Fatigability	Ecchymoses Pallor	Bleeding time Hgb
RENAL	↓ Concentrating ability (CRI)	Nocturia, frequency		Urine osm BUN, Cr
CNS	Encephalopathy Autonomic dysfunction	↓ Mental acuity, disorientation Postural hypotension	Mental status "Tilt" test: ↓ BP, ↑ HR when tilted	
PNS	Peripheral neuropathy	Paresthesias, burning, itching of lower extremities	Excoriations	

Key Reference: Kellerman PS: Perioperative care of the renal patient. Arch Intern Med 1994; 154:1674–1688.

PERIOPERATIVE IMPLICATIONS

Preoperative Preparation

- Assess adequacy of dialytic therapy, volume and acid-base status, Hgb concentration, CV status, serum K+
- If not dialysis-dependent, assess renal reserve, CV status

Monitoring

- Temp, ECG (rhythm, rate, hyperkalemia)
- Pulse oximeter, capnometer, peripheral nerve stimulator
- Consider arterial catheter if chronically hypertensive; consider PA catheter for high-risk surgery in patients with cardiac dysfunction

Airway

- Gastroparesis precautions if diabetic

Preinduction/Induction

- Reduce dose of thiopental
- Exaggerated response to benzodiazepines
- Consider avoiding renally excreted neuromuscular blockers (vecuronium, pancuronium)
- Use narcotics cautiously
- If not dialysis-dependent, avoid sevoflurane and enflurane for prolonged cases
- Exaggerated BP swings with induction and intubation
- Reduce dose of local anesthetics if metabolic acidosis present or if sedatives will cause resp acidosis

Maintenance

- Precise volume management; titration of agents

Extubation

- Ensure adequate reversal of neuromuscular blockers
- Evaluate airway reflexes

Adjuvants

- Avoid renally excreted neuromuscular blockers

Postoperative Period

- Dialyze if necessary
- Monitor for frequent causes of postop morbidity (see above)

ANTICIPATED PROBLEMS/CONCERNS

- Hyperkalemia—treatment with $CaCl_2$, insulin/glucose, or $NaHCO_3$ may be necessary; intraoperative dialysis occasionally required
- Balancing intraoperative volume requirements with need for postop fluid removal
- Exaggerated drug effects

RESPIRATORY DISTRESS SYNDROME
T. James Gallagher, M.D.

RISK

- People within USA: up to 400,000/y
- Race/gender predominance: None

PERIOPERATIVE RISKS

- ↑ Risk in patients with generalized septic conditions including perforated colon and pancreatitis
- May develop following large-volume fluid resuscitation and blood replacement

WORRY ABOUT

- ↓ Oxygenation
- ↓ Pulm compliance

OVERVIEW

- Patients rarely die directly of respiratory distress syndrome
- Contributes to prolonged mechanical ventilation and increased stay in ICU
- May last from 3 d to several wk
- Complicated by bacterial or yeast pneumonia
- Primarily results from generalized sepsis, which increases pulm vascular permeability

ICD-9-CM Code: 518.5 (following trauma and surgery)

ETIOLOGY

- Represents a symptom or sign of generalized sepsis
- A vascular disease with altered permeability
- Alterations of permeability result from endotoxin release and stimulation of other cytokines, including TNF
- Lymphatic drainage usually overwhelmed resulting in ↑ water accumulation in interstitial spaces
- ↑ Intravascular volume and ↓ colloid oncotic pressure can contribute to severity

USUAL TREATMENT

- Ventilatory support
- PEEP and CPAP to improve oxygenation
- Elimination of septic source
- Appropriate antibiotic therapy
- Inhaled nitric oxide may improve oxygenation or reduce need for mechanical ventilatory support

ASSESSMENT POINTS

SYSTEM	EFFECT	ASSESSMENT BY HX	PE	TEST
CV	Decreased O_2 delivery ↑ Intravascular volume	SOB ↓ Peripheral perfusion	Tachycardia S_3, S_4 Ischemia	ECG BP PCWP Cardiac output
RESP	↓ Oxygenation, CO_2 accumulation	Dyspnea Tachypnea	Rales Nasal flaring	CXR ABGs
CNS	Agitation Confusion	Disorientation		Level of consciousness

Key Reference: Kollef MH, Schuster DP: The acute respiratory distress syndrome. N Engl J Med 1995; 332:27–37.

PERIOPERATIVE IMPLICATIONS

Preoperative Preparation

- Avoid surgery if possible
- May require mechanical ventilator used in ICU rather than a standard anesthesia ventilator because of high airway pressures

Monitoring

- Oxygenation guided by pulse oximetry and blood gas analysis
- Peak inflation pressures
- PA catheter to judge fluid status, cardiac function frequently indicated

Airway

- Maintain intubation
- High FIO_2

Preinduction/Induction

- May develop hypoxemia
- Avoid agents requiring supplemental gases
- Anesthetic agents may blunt hypoxic PA vasoconstriction and reduce cardiac output

Maintenance

- ↓ Oxygenation may appear as a reduction in O_2 saturation or PaO_2
- ↓ Lung function may be evidenced by increase in peak inflation pressure or a decrease in tidal volume
- Once the abdomen has been opened, compliance may improve; tidal volumes may become excessively high.
- Closure of abdomen may result in extraordinarily high pressures and inability to ventilate

Extubation

- The patient should almost always remain intubated at end of procedure

Adjuvants

- Muscle relaxation may improve gas exchange
- It may be necessary to maintain paralysis in postop period

Postoperative Period

- Oxygenation and ventilation should be monitored in ICU in the postoperative period
- Ventilator changes should be based on x-ray and blood gas analysis
- If paralysis required, sedation also necessary

ANTICIPATED PROBLEMS/CONCERNS

- Oxygenation will almost always worsen following surgery.
- If pulm parenchymal changes deteriorate or worsen, patients may have difficulty with CO_2 elimination.

RETT SYNDROME

Catherine R. Bachman, M.D.

RISK

- Exclusively females
- 1/10,000 girls birth–14 y
- Incidence in severely developmentally delayed females may be up to 25%

PERIOPERATIVE RISKS

- Abnormal control of ventilation, with periods of apnea and hyperventilation
- May have GE reflux
- Multiple orthopedic and motor movement disorders

WORRY ABOUT

- Risk of perioperative apnea unknown
- Risk of succinylcholine-induced hyperkalemia unknown
- Aspiration due to GE reflux
- Intraoperative positioning because of spasticity and contractures

OVERVIEW

- Girls normal for first 6–18 mo of life, then rapidly lose acquired cognitive, verbal, and motor skills, eventually severely impaired in all areas.
- Loss of purposeful hand movements; exhibit typical hand washing or hand wringing behavior
- Abnormal EEG in almost 100% (nonspecific). Seizures in 75%
- Abnormal control of breathing with apnea intermixed with hyperventilation only when awake
- Orthopedic motor movement disorders such as ataxia, spasticity, muscle wasting, scoliosis
- Vasomotor disturbances with cool mottled extremities
- Cachexia

ICD-9-CM Code: 330.8

ETIOLOGY

- Unknown
- Possibly x-linked dominant (? lethal in males)
- Progressive deterioration suggests metabolic cause
- No specific diagnostic test available
- Dx made by Hx and physical exam (inclusion and exclusion criteria established)

USUAL TREATMENT

- Supportive only
- One case report discusses improvement with L-carnitine (SMJ 86(12):1993)

ASSESSMENT POINTS

SYSTEM	EFFECT	ASSESSMENT BY HX	PE	TEST
HEENT	Nonspecific Spasticity may make airway difficult		Neck ROM Normal face	Neck x-rays if indicated
CV	No primary heart involvement Peripheral vasomotor disturbances	? Exercise tolerance (patients inactive) Extremities cool, trophic changes	Secondary cardiac changes only Cool extremities	As indicated by Hx and physical findings
RESP	Abn control of ventilation with hyperventilation, apnea, cyanosis, desaturation Lung changes due to scoliosis or aspiration	Hx of apnea, cyanosis Hx of scoliosis, aspiration	Observation Chest exam	O₂ saturation CXR PFTs unlikely (poor cooperation)
GI	GE reflux swallowing difficulties, constipation Growth failure	Hx of GE reflux, feeding difficulties	Thin, small for age	X-ray studies for GE reflux
CNS	Severe developmental delay Seizures Ataxia Abn control of ventilation Abn sleep characteristics	Developmental level seizure activity Presence of apnea, cyanosis	Assessment of cognitive and movement disorders	EEG Resp studies, sleeping and awake
MS	Hypotonia (early); spasticity (late); ataxia Secondary orthopedic manifestations: scoliosis, joint contractures	Progress and extent of MS abnormalities	Chest exam re scoliosis Limb and joint positions	X-rays

Key Reference: Maguire D, Bachman C: Anaesthesia and Rett syndrome: A case report. Can J Anaesth 1989; 36:478–481.

PERIOPERATIVE IMPLICATIONS

Preoperative Preparation

- Optimize respiratory status
- Assess respiratory control
- Minimize aspiration risk

Monitoring

- Routine

Airway

- Normal face
- Spasticity may make positioning difficult

Preinduction/Induction

- Risk of hyperkalemia following succinylcholine unknown
- Aspiration risk due to GE reflux

Maintenance

- Respiratory control abnormal; unknown if spontaneous ventilation under anesthesia associated with significant apneas
- Attention to body temp because of thin body habitus and peripheral vasomotor disturbances

Extubation

- Aspiration risk

Postoperative Period

- Respiratory control abnormal
  - Effect of anesthetic agents
  - Duration of respiratory monitoring
  - Effect of narcotics vs local anesthetics for pain control

Adjuvants

- None

ANTICIPATED PROBLEMS/CONCERNS

- Respiratory control abnormalities not well understood. Therefore, effect of anesthetic agents intra- and postoperatively on respiration not known. Need for postop monitoring for apnea unknown.

REYE'S SYNDROME

Mary A. Keyes, M.D.

RISK

• Incidence prior to 1990 was 0.3–0.6/100,000 <16 y
• During early 1980s, association between aspirin and Reye's syndrome was recognized and incidence dramatically declined

PERIOPERATIVE RISKS

• Surgery (all but life and death emergencies) contraindicated during Reye's syndrome. Following recovery evaluate liver function tests

WORRY ABOUT

• Recurrent liver dysfunction
• Permanent neuropsychologic deficits

OVERVIEW

• An acute encephalopathy with hepatic dysfunction predominantly in children; typically starts several days after unremarkable viral illness.
• Encephalopathy heralded by protracted, severe vomiting, with abnormal behavior and combativeness that progress to coma.
• Dx made by unexplained encephalopathy with one or more of following: serum transaminases elevated to at least 3× normal; blood ammonia levels at least 3× normal; or hepatic microvesicular fatty infiltration on liver biopsy. CSF is normal.
• Most children have moderate illness that does not progress to deep coma.
• Prognosis depends on severity and duration of cerebral dysfunction. Severe disease may lead to subtle neuropsychologic defects.

ICD-9-CM Code: 331.81

ETIOLOGY

• Multifactorial; abnormal reaction to viral illness modified by exogenous toxin in susceptible host.
• Most frequently linked with influenza A and B and varicella. Exogenous toxin is aspirin in majority of cases.

USUAL TREATMENT

• Early recognition of mild cases and control of ICP.
• Management varies with severity of illness: fluids should be restricted in patients with cerebral edema. ICP monitoring aids in improving cerebral perfusion pressure and decreasing ICP.
• Mannitol to induce cerebral dehydration and barbiturates to ↓ cerebral metabolic demand
• Coagulopathies treated with vitamin K and/ or FFP

ASSESSMENT POINTS

SYSTEM	EFFECT	ASSESSMENT BY HX	PE	TEST
GI	Hepatic dysfunction	Severe vomiting	Hepatomegaly	Hepatic transaminases Ammonia levels Liver biopsy PT, PTT
CNS	Delirium Combative behavior Seizures Lethargy Coma	Alteration in mental status	No focal signs	CT scan ICP monitor

Key Reference: Hall SM: Reye's syndrome and aspirin: A review. Symposium Supplement. Br J Clin Pract, 1990; 70:4–11.

PERIOPERATIVE IMPLICATIONS

• Surgery not undertaken except in life-death emergencies.

Adjuvants

• Early recognition of mild cases and control of ICP
• Management varies with severity of illness: Fluids should be restricted in patients with cerebral edema. ICP monitoring aids in improving cerebral perfusion pressure and decreasing ICP.
• Mannitol to induce cerebral dehydration and barbiturates to ↓ cerebral metabolic demand
• Coagulopathies treated with vitamin K and/ or FFP

ANTICIPATED PROBLEMS/CONCERNS

See Overview above

RHEUMATOID ARTHRITIS

Stephen F. Dierdorf, M.D.

RISK

- 1% of US population
- Male:female 1:2–3

PERIOPERATIVE RISKS

- Increased risk for new neurologic disturbances 2° to occult cervical spine damage
- Myocardial damage insidious and may not be clinically evident
- Increased perioperative pulm complications 2° to pulm fibrosis and restrictive lung disease.

WORRY ABOUT

- Laryngoscopy and tracheal intubation may be difficult 2° to rheumatoid damage to cervical spine.
- Hx of previous tracheal intubation not predictive of current conditions.

- Cervical cord damage during laryngoscopy and tracheal intubation.
- Occult pericarditis and myocardial dysfunction.
- Difficult to determine exercise tolerance because of limitation of movement 2° to joint dysfunction.

OVERVIEW

- Chronic inflammatory disease affecting multiple joints and organ systems.
- Systemic effects include anemia, pericarditis, cardiac tamponade, myocarditis, aortitis, peripheral nerve compression, and renal dysfunction.
- Renal failure common cause of death.

ICD-9-CM Code: 714

ETIOLOGY

- Autoimmune disorder triggered by an antigen in genetically susceptible individuals
- Variability in clinical course may be due to differences in triggering antigens and/or immune response
- Pathologic changes: cellular hyperplasia of synovium and synovial invasion by lymphocytes, plasma cells, and fibroblasts with ultimate destruction of cartilage and articular surfaces

USUAL TREATMENT

- First-line drugs include aspirin and NSAIDs: ibuprofen, indomethacin, naproxen, piroxicam, sulindac, and tolmetin.
- Second-line drugs that alter immune response include hydroxychloroquine, methotrexate, sulfasalazine, azathioprine, penicillamine, and gold.
- Significant side effects of long-term corticosteroid therapy, limit them to patients failing second-line response.

ASSESSMENT POINTS

SYSTEM	EFFECT	ASSESSMENT BY HX	PE	TEST
HEENT	Edematous mucosa Arthritis of larynx	Epistaxis Hx of voice change	Friable muscosa Voice, airway exam	Direct laryngoscopy
CV	LV dysfunction	Dyspnea Orthopnea Reduced exercise	S_3 Rales	ECG Stress ECG ECHO
	Aortitis Pericarditis	Reduced exercise Dyspnea	Diastolic murmur (AL) Distant heart sounds Friction rub	ECHO ECHO
RESP	Fibrosis	Dyspnea	Dry rales	CXR, PFTs
GI	Peptic ulcer	Epigastric pain, N/V		
RENAL	Renal dysfunction	Drug induced		Cr
CNS	Spinal cord compression Neurologic dysfunction	Neck pain Numbness	Sensory deficits Motor deficits ROM of neck	Radiography MRI
MS	Arthritis	Joint pain	Swelling Pain with motion Restricted motion	Radiography

Key Reference: Macarthur A, Kleiman S: Rheumatoid cervical arthritis—a challenge to the anaesthetist. Can J Anaesth 1993; 40:154–159.

PERIOPERATIVE IMPLICATIONS

Preoperative Preparation

- Mobility of cervical spine and TMJ. Check cervical spine films and/or MRI if available; ROM of shoulders, elbows, wrists, hips, and knees
- Review treatment drugs and their effects

Monitoring

- Routine for procedure and comorbidities of patient

Airway

- Poor cervical spine mobility may necessitate awake tracheal intubation

- Smaller than predicted tracheal tube (laryngeal arthritis)

Preinduction/Induction

- No specific contraindications to common induction agents
- Greater decreases in BP 2° to myocardial dysfunction
- ↑ Risk of aspiration pneumonitis
- Careful positioning to avoid aggravation of major joint dysfunction

Maintenance

- Drug-induced hepatic dysfunction; potential for halothane hepatitis
- Exaggerated CV effects of volatile anesthetics

Extubation

- Postextubation laryngeal edema and stridor more common

Adjuvants

- Neuraxial anesthesia difficult because of spinal arthritis
- Drug interactions between anesthetics and antiarthritic drugs (see under drug in Drugs section, or in Goodman and Gilman)

ANTICIPATED PROBLEMS/CONCERNS

- Difficult tracheal intubation
- Increased neurologic deficits 2° to cervical spine degeneration
- May need perioperative corticosteroid supplementation

RICKETTSIAL DISEASES/Q FEVER

Paul R. Knight III, M.D., Ph.D.
James Foster, M.B.B.S., F.R.C.P.C.

RISK

- Mortality low—2.4% in untreated cases
- HIV-positive patients more likely to be infected and symptomatic
- Normally not transmitted between humans

PERIOPERATIVE RISKS

- ↓ Respiratory reserve 2° to pneumonia
- ↓ Myocardial reserve 2° to endocarditis and cardiac valve dysfunction
- Development of chronic Q fever 2° to immune suppression
- ↑ Hepatocellular damage in presence of liver involvement

WORRY ABOUT

- Respiratory complications
- ↓ Myocardial performance
- Thromboembolic phenomenon
- ↑ Hepatic or neurologic injury

OVERVIEW

- Usually presents as self-limited acute febrile illness with chills, headache, fatigue, and myalgia. Additional symptoms reflect severity of involvement of other organs, usually lung
- Chronic forms include endocarditis, hepatitis, and osteomyelitis and are associated with inability to clear the bacterium, resulting in monocytic inflammation
- *Coxiella burnetii* infections in immuno-compromised patients and infants produce variant syndromes of Q fever
- Multisystem disease associated with Q fever can resemble HIV infection, and false positive tests for HIV have been reported
- Elderly patients may have prolonged illness

ICD-9-CM Code: 083.9

ETIOLOGY

- *Coxiella burnetii* is an intracellular parasite usually transmitted by inhalation of small particles containing the bacterium.
- The spore stage of this bacterium can withstand harsh environmental conditions for prolonged periods
- Occupational disease affect those in constant contact with domestic ungulates
- Sheep and cattle infected by arthropod ectoparasites
- Transmission via blood products has been reported
- Chronic immune response results in an immune-complex vasculitis

USUAL TREATMENT

- Tetracyclines for treating pneumonia and hepatitis
- Chloramphenicol or erythromycin plus rifampicin also used
- Endocarditis requires prolonged, combination-antibiotic therapy
- Heart valve replacement may be necessary

ASSESSMENT POINTS

SYSTEM	EFFECT	ASSESSMENT BY HX	PE	TEST
CV	Endocarditis Immune-complex vasculitis Microthromboembolism	Rash, ↓ exercise tolerance	Clubbing, rash, murmurs, petechiae	ECHO ECG, blood cultures (negative for subacute bacterial endocarditis)
RESP	Atypical pneumonia, asymptomatic pneumonia, rapidly progressive pneumonia, interstitial pulmonary fibrosis	Pleuritic chest pain, cough, dyspnea	Consolidation, rales, pleural effusions	CXR Sputum cultures
GI	Acute hepatitis	N/V, fatigue, diarrhea, sweats and chills	Hepatomegaly or hepatosplenomegaly	SGOT, SGPT, bilirubin, granulomas on liver biopsy
HEME	Hyperglobulinemia, anemia, thrombocytosis-cytopenia	Easy fatigue, bleeding tendency	Pallor; purpuric eruptions	Sedimentation rate, Hct/Hgb, Plt
RENAL	Immune-complex vasculitis			Microscopic hematuria
REPRODUCTIVE	Q fever complications 2° to reactivation of infection during pregnancy	↑ Spontaneous abortions		Isolation of *C. burnetii* from placenta
CNS	Meningoencephalitis Optic neuritis	Weakness, seizures, meningismus, blurred vision, headache	Focal deficits, sensory loss	↑ Monocytes and protein in CFS; normal glucose
MS	Immune-complex vasculitis, vertebral osteomyelitis	Myalgia	Point tenderness	X-ray

Key Reference: Walker DH, Raoult D: *In* Mandell GL, Bennett JE, Dolin R (eds): Principles and Practice of Infectious Diseases. New York, Churchill Livingstone, 1994, pp 1721–1727.

PERIOPERATIVE IMPLICATIONS

Preoperative Preparation

- Continue or initiate antibiotic therapy and optimize any organ system dysfunction
- Only emergency surgery during acute Q fever
- Assess respiratory and cardiac reserve and hepatic and neurologic status, with chronic Q fever
- Subacute bacterial endocarditis prophylaxis may be appropriate

Monitoring

- Arterial line may be necessary if pneumonia present
- Myocardial valvular disease may require PA line or other invasive hemodynamic monitors

- Risk of complications of an arterial line may be increased with vasculitis

Airway

- None

Induction

- Pneumonia may cause rapid desaturation.
- Hypotension and CV instability if cardiac valvular injury present

Maintenance

- If acute hepatitis, avoid drugs that require hepatic metabolism or decrease blood flow to liver

Extubation

- Respiratory status and CV stability need to be considered

Adjuvants

- Depends on hepatic/renal impairment

Postoperative Period

- Respiratory/myocardial status carefully followed and may require ICU monitoring
- Liver enzymes followed if hepatic involvement

ANTICIPATED PROBLEMS/CONCERNS

- Since the development of chronic Q fever is associated with immune suppression, patients who present with acute infection and require emergency surgery might receive extended antibiotic therapy and be assessed for development of persistent infection and chronic sequelae

ROCKY MOUNTAIN SPOTTED FEVER

Paul R. Knight III, M.D., Ph.D.
Eileen Watson, M.D.

RISK

- Incidence ranges from 0.53 to 14.59/100,000 in endemic areas of USA
- Mortality ~20% in untreated cases
- Mortality higher in nonwhites, males, and patients >30 y

PERIOPERATIVE RISKS

- Increased mortality 2° to CV instability and noncardiogenic pulm edema
- Increased risk of organ injury due to compounded insults
- Increased bleeding tendency

WORRY ABOUT

- Severe intravascular volume depletion leading to shock
- Electrolyte disturbances
- Cardiac arrhythmias
- Microvascular hemorrhage
- Consumptive coagulopathy
- Intraoperative respiratory and renal failure

OVERVIEW

- An infectious disease that causes endothelial cell injury leading to edema, ↓ intravascular volume, hypoalbuminemia
- May present as an acute abdomen
- May present as multiple system failure
- Perivascular lesions in skin lead to rash that typically involves wrists and ankles first
- Monocytic responses to bacterium associated with interstitial pneumonia, myocarditis, glial nodules in CNS, and vascular lesions in abdominal viscera and skeletal muscles
- Severe microvascular injury may lead to skin necrosis or gangrene
- Thrombocytopenia and coagulation defects occur in ~50% of patients, although DIC is rare.
- Meningoencephalitis may lead to focal neurologic deficits

ICD-9-CM Code: 082.0

ETIOLOGY

- *Rickettsia rickettsii* transmitted in saliva of ticks, 6–10 h after feeding or by exposure to infected tick hemolymph
- Obligatory intracellular bacteria that replicate in endothelial cells causing direct cell injury with loss of vascular wall integrity
- Immune response to bacterium causes a monocytic inflammation in infected organs

USUAL TREATMENT

- Clinical Dx difficult because of varying symptoms; Rx initiated prior to confirmation of Dx
- Tetracycline
- Correct hypovolemia, coagulation defects, thrombocytopenia
- Provide intensive, supportive care for various organ system failure

ASSESSMENT POINTS

SYSTEM	EFFECT	ASSESSMENT BY HX	PE	TEST
CV	Extensive microvascular leak; interstitial myocarditis	Rash, swelling	Rash, edema, arrhythmias	ECG, CXR Lytes, BP
RESP	Noncardiac pulm edema; interstitial pneumonitis	↓ Exercise tolerance, dypsnea	Rales by auscultation	CXR, Spirometry
GI	Gastroenteritis; liver, spleen, and pancreatic microvascular hemorrhage and edema	N/V, pain, diarrhea	Abdominal tenderness Hepatosplenomegaly	SGOT, bilirubin
HEME	Thrombocytopenia, anemia	Easy bleeding, malaise	Rash	Hct/Hgb, Plt/PT, PTT
RENAL	Microvascular hemorrhage and edema, interstitial nephritis, prerenal azotemia	Lumbar pain		BUN, Cr Lytes
CNS	Meningoencephalitis	Focal defects, deafness, meningismus, photophobia		CSF: ± ↑ WBC, ↑ protein
MS	Microvascular hemorrhage and edema	Myalgia	↓ ROM	

Key Reference: Walker DH, Raoult D: In Mandell GL, Bennett JE, Dolin R (eds): Principles and Practice of Infectious Diseases. New York, Churchill Livingstone, 1994, pp 1721–1727.

PERIOPERATIVE IMPLICATIONS

Preoperative Preparation

- Antibiotic therapy and correction of underlying organ system dysfunction
- Surgery only for emergency
- Assess volume, respiratory, renal status

Monitoring

- Consider PA catheter, arterial line, UO
- Intraoperative ABGs and Lytes
- Plt and other coagulation variables

Airway

- Severe edema of oropharynx and ↑ bleeding tendency can lead to difficult intubation

Induction

- Hypovolemia can cause hypotension.
- Microvascular leak in lung can cause rapid desaturation.
- ↑ Cardiac arrhythmias

Maintenance

- Owing to CV instability, volume status is key.
- Possibility of resp failure and constant volume resuscitation should be anticipated when selecting anesthetic technique

Extubation

- Oropharyngeal edema and ↑ bleeding tendency may make reintubation very difficult

Adjuvants

- Vasoactive drugs used in acute resuscitation should be readily available
- Lidocaine for treatment of cardiac arrhythmias

Postoperative Period

- Intravascular volume shifts, coagulation defects, respiratory failure, CV instability, renal failure.

ANTICIPATED PROBLEMS/CONCERNS

- Owing to the possibility of multisystem failure, prolonged postop ICU management may be required
- Since early treatment with antibiotics is curative and highly successful in preventing complications, high index of suspicion, particularly in endemic areas, is needed

SARCOIDOSIS

Andrew D. Rosenberg, M.D.

RISK

- Varies: ≤1–80/100,000 with highest incidence in Sweden; in US 30/100,000
- Presenting ages 20–40 y in US
- More common in African-Americans than Caucasians
- Females > males (2:1)

PERIOPERATIVE RISKS

- Severity depends on degree of airway, lung, cardiac, and CNS involvement

WORRY ABOUT

- Airway granulomas distorting and obstructing anatomy
- Degree of lung involvement and pulm fibrosis
- Cardiac involvement, heart block, arrhythmia, CHF
- CNS involvement

OVERVIEW

- Multisystem granulomatous disorder with widespread noncaseating epithelioid cell granulomas
- Lung most frequently affected organ
- Airway abn 2° to granulomas
- Local organ distortion can result in symptoms
- Mononuclear inflammatory cells: T-helper cells + mononuclear phagocytes lead to formation of granulomas

ICD-9-CM Code: 135.0

ETIOLOGY

- Unknown disease due to exaggerated cellular immune response involving mononuclear phagocytes and T-lymphocytes

USUAL TREATMENT

- Steroids: prednisone 30–40 mg/d, tapered to 10–15 mg qod; also chloroquine

ASSESSMENT POINTS

SYSTEM	EFFECT	ASSESSMENT BY HX	PE	TEST
HEENT	Involvement of nares, polyps with distorted anatomy; larynx granulomas, epiglottis, arytenoid involvement	Dyspnea Breathing difficulty	Nasal stuffiness, wheezing, hoarseness, stridor	Laryngoscopy
CV	Heart block Cor pulmonale 2° to RV enlargement	Palpitations	Arrhythmia Rales	ECG
RESP	Pulm granulomas, airway obstruction	Dyspnea	Dry rales	CXR
	Bilateral hilar lymphadenopathy (eggshell calcifications of hilar nodes); pulm fibrosis; interstitial disease	Wheezing, cough	Wheezes	PFTs ($\downarrow$ vital and diffusing capacities) ABGs
GI	Liver involvement			$\uparrow$ LFTs; $\uparrow$ alkaline phosphatase
ENDO	Diabetes insipidus	Thirst		
RENAL	$\uparrow Ca^{2+}$ resorption			BUN/Cr
CNS	Nerve involvement Diabetes insipidus	Space-occupying lesions	Focal nerve deficits	

Key Reference: Sharma OP: Sarcoidosis. Disease-a-Month 1990; 36:470–535.

PERIOPERATIVE IMPLICATIONS

Preoperative Preparation

- Adequate steroid coverage

Airway

- Distortion or obstruction 2° to granulomas
- Hypoxia 2° to lung disease

Monitoring

- Observe for heart block
- Arrhythmia

ANTICIPATED PROBLEMS/CONCERNS

- Airway problems 2° to distorted anatomy
- Pulm problems 2° to lung involvement

SARCOMA

Stephan P. Nebbia, M.D.
Douglas Bacon, M.D.

RISK

- Osteosarcoma: 1:100,000; 2000 new cases/y in US; 2nd decade (mean age 15)
- Soft tissue sarcoma: >20 types, 5500 new cases/y in US, peak incidence in children and adults age 45–50 y
- Equal in male/female, all races

PERIOPERATIVE RISKS

- Morbidity and mortality related to surgical procedure
- Metastatic vital organ involvement, esp. pulm, hepatic
- Mass effect, direct compression of organs, vascular structures

WORRY ABOUT

- Adriamycin-induced cardiotoxicity (global LV hypokinesis)

- Mitomycin-induced acute pulm toxicity, pulm fibrosis, ARDS with increased FIO_2
- Immunosuppression, hemorrhagic cystitis, renal failure induced by antineoplastic chemotherapeutic agents

OVERVIEW

- Malignant tumors derived from embryonic mesoderm
- Multiple types in connective tissue, muscle, fat, vasculature, neural and other tissues
- Spread aggressively by local invasion and early hematogenous spread, esp. to lung

ICD-9-CM Code: 171 (depends on type)

ETIOLOGY

- Genetic factors, high-dose radiation, carcinogens (dibenzanthracene, methylcholanthrene), Maloney sarcoma virus may predispose to sarcoma
- von Recklinghausen's disease: 10–12% develop neurofibrosarcomas
- Paget's disease: 0.9% develop osteosarcoma
- Kaposi's sarcoma in AIDS patients and immunodeficient

USUAL TREATMENT

- Wide surgical resection
- Antineoplastic chemotherapeutic agents
- Radiation

ASSESSMENT POINTS

SYSTEM	EFFECT	ASSESSMENT BY HX	PE	TEST
CV	Atrial myxoma — ball-valve effect	Sx CHF, pulm edema	Rales S_3	CXR ECHO
	Vena caval obstruction	RV failure, CV collapse	Possible caput medusae, venous engorgement, edema	Angio
	SVC syndrome	Head, airway edema ↑ICP	Venous congestion of head and neck	Angio V/Q scan
RESP	Pulm embolus	Dyspnea		CXR, Angio
GI	Gastroparesis	Early satiety		
	Bowel obstruction	Vomiting	Abdominal distention	Plain film of abdomen
	Hepatic metastases	Obstructive jaundice	Jaundice	EGD, bilirubin
	Sarcoma of ampulla of Vater	Hepatic dysfunction		
HEME	Hypercoagulable			PT/PTT
	Immunosuppressive chemotherapy	Alopecia		CBC
	Anemia, due to GI hemorrhage		Gross rectal bleeding	Guaiac
RENAL	Compression of ureters by retroperitoneal tumor	Sx uremia		BUN/Cr Renal US
CNS	CN compression	Various symptoms Dysphagia Loss of sensation, motor function	Neurologic exam	EMG
MS	Bone sarcomas	Hypercalcemia	Chvostek's	Blood Ca^{2+}
	Limb loss		sign	Albumin

Key Reference: DeVita V, et al (eds): Cancer, Principles and Practice of Oncology, 3rd ed. Philadelphia, JB Lippincott, 1989.

PERIOPERATIVE IMPLICATIONS

Preoperative Preparation

- Metoclopramide, sodium citrate, ranitidine in patients with gastroparesis
- Assess end-organ impairment 2° to antineoplastic chemotherapeutic agents

Monitoring

- Arterial line and CVP or PA catheter for resection of large tumors

Airway

- Risk of aspiration with large abdominal mass, or brainstem compression

Induction

- Cautious: with cardiac involvement, caval compression may have hemodynamic instability

Maintenance

- Potential CV instability

Extubation

- Awake, if at risk for aspiration

Adjuvants

- Altered pharmacokinetics with hepatic or renal involvement

Postoperative Period

- Pulm embolism, coagulopathy

ANTICIPATED PROBLEMS/CONCERNS

- Adverse effects of chemotherapeutic agents (see in Drug section)
- Resp compromise due to pulm metastases
- Mass effect/organ compression and functional impairment
- Effects of prolonged anesthesia
- In prolonged abdominal cases; hypothermia, complications of massive transfusion

SCHIZOPHRENIA

Michael Ho, M.D.

RISK

- Incidence in USA: 2.5–4.75 million
- Estimated lifetime prevalence: 0.5–1.0%, constant worldwide
- Gender predominance: none
- First-degree biologic relative: 10× risk

PERIOPERATIVE RISKS

- Marked deterioration of function and self-care
- Surgery does not necessarily exacerbate, but rate of postop complications may be greater

WORRY ABOUT

- Uncooperative, combative, or catatonic patient
- Previously undiagnosed or poorly controlled coexisting disease
- Drug side effects and interactions

OVERVIEW

- DSM-IV: One of several psychotic disorders, all of which are delusional
- Dx based on strict criteria: hallucinations, disorganized speech, grossly disorganized or catatonic behavior, negative symptoms (decreases in affect, speech, action)
- No protection from systemic disease, including cancer, diabetes, allergies (except possibly arthritis)
- High lifetime mortality, primarily by accidents and suicide (10% of all schizophrenics complete suicide; 2–3% of all patients completing suicide are schizophrenic)
- Most devastating psychiatric illness

ICD-9-CM Code: 295.9

ETIOLOGY

- Functional hyperactivity of dopamine transmission, perhaps due to increase in D_2 receptors; evidence: dopamine antagonists treat while agonists exacerbate, disease
- Genetic vs. environmental factors controversial.

USUAL TREATMENT

- First-line: dopamine antagonist antipsychotics (phenothiazines, butyrophenones, thioxanthenes, dihydroindolones, dibenzoxazepines)
- Side effects: extrapyramidal, anticholinergic, sedation, neuroleptic malignant syndrome (NMS)
- Prevent/Rx extrapyramidal side effects: anticholinergics, amantadine, bromocriptine, antihistamines, benzodiazepines, clonidine
- Clozapine: new atypical antipsychotic (dibenzodiazepines); fewer extrapyramidal side effects, but agranulocytosis possible
- Adjuvants: benzodiazepines, lithium, antidepressants, propranolol

ASSESSMENT POINTS

SYSTEM	EFFECT	ASSESSMENT BY HX	PE	TEST
HEENT	Possible high-arched palate		Careful airway assessment	
CV	Orthostatic hypotension (α-blockade), dysrhythmias, and rare sudden death from antipsychotics	Dizziness Palpitations	Orthostasis Dysrhythmias	ECG: T wave inversion, QT or PR prolongation, ST segment depression
GI	Elevation of LFTs from antipsychotics			LFTs
HEME	Leukopenia from antipsychotics			CBC
NEURO	Extrapyramidal side effects: 1. Parkinsonism 2. Acute dystonia 3. Akathisia 4. Tardive dyskinesia 5. Anticholinergic delirium 6. Sedation		1. Catatonia, rigidity, akinesia 2. Slow, sustained contractions of neck, jaw, tongue, extraocular muscles, larynx, face, body 3. Subjective discomfort leading to agitation, pacing, restlessness 4. Choreoathetoid movements of head, limbs, trunk 5. Confusion plus other anticholinergic symptoms	
GENERAL	Neuroleptic malignant syndrome	Chronic antipsychotic use	Hyperthermia, autonomic lability, dysrhythmias Tachypnea, cyanosis, impaired consciousness	LFTs, WBC (leukocytosis), CPK, UA (myoglobinuria)

Key Reference: Black DW, Andreasen NC: Schizophrenia, schizophreniform disorders, and delusional (paranoid) disorder. *In* Hales RE, Yudofsky SC, Talbott JA (eds): The American Psychiatric Press Textbook of Psychiatry. Washington, DC, American Psychiatric Press, 1994, pp 411–464.

PERIOPERATIVE IMPLICATIONS

Preoperative Preparation

- Hx may be unreliable, unobtainable
- Ensure adequate control of psychotic symptoms
- Address any tachycardia, dysrhythmias, or hemodynamic instability (rule out NMS, anticholinergic toxicity)
- Acute psychotic episode may be treated with haloperidol 2 mg IV or benzodiazepines
- Informed consent from legal guardian (unless emergency)

Monitoring

- Routine

Airway

- None

Preinduction/Induction

- No specific technique clearly superior
- Avoid drugs predisposing to tachycardia or

dyshythmias if pre-existing CV instability or dopamine antagonists (droperidol, metoclopramide)

Maintenance

- With chronic antipsychotic therapy, NMS and anticholinergic toxicity do not acutely occur intraoperatively
- Antipsychotics may alter temp regulation (predisposing to hyperthermia) and lower seizure threshold (theoretically, may want to avoid enflurane, etomidate, methohexital, ketamine)

Extubation

- Usual criteria

Adjuvants

- Rx NMS: Discontinue antipsychotics, dantroline, bromocriptine, ECT, benzodiazepines, anticholinergics

Postoperative Period

- Difficulty in assessing mental status and pain
- Discharge to home under supervision of responsible adult guardian

ANTICIPATED PROBLEMS/CONCERNS

- Anticholinergic side effects: blurred vision, mydriasis, dry mouth, mucous plugging, constipation, urinary retention, hot skin, delirium. Rx anticholinergic crisis: physostigmine 1–4 mg IV/IM (careful with narrow angle glaucoma, prostatic hypertrophy). Excess physostigmine risks cholinergic crisis (N/V, bradycardia, seizures), which can be treated by atropine.
- Symptoms of NMS similar to malignant hyperthermia, except onset of NMS more insidious (occurring over days) and extrapyramidal side effects present
- With antipsychotic-induced α-blockade, epinephrine may cause paradoxical hypotension due to unopposed ß-mediated vasodilation

SCOLIOSIS AND KYPHOSIS

Ralph L. Bernstein, M.D.

RISK

- Idiopathic scoliotic curves of > 10° occur in 2–3% of children < 16 y
- Overall female:male prevalence 3.6:1
- In severe curves (30° or greater) female:male 10:1

PERIOPERATIVE RISKS

- Neurologic damage
- Massive blood loss
- Atelectasis, pneumonia
- Ileus

WORRY ABOUT

- Neurologic damage from direct trauma or from spinal cord injury during corrections as result of interference with blood supply to spinal cord, or during positioning intubation in surgery unrelated to correction
- Adequate blood and fluid replaced
- Pulmonary insufficiency

OVERVIEW

- Curves measured by Cobb method (which draws a line from superior surface of superior end vertebra of curve and a line along the inferior surface of inferior end vertebra). Intersecting perpendicular lines are drawn from these lines to give angle of curve.

- Kyphosis—abnormal dorsal curvature of spine, flexible or rigid, treated with A-P correction. Angular acute may be congenital, post-traumatic, or post-infection; may develop neurologic impairment. Treated by decompression and fusion in situ.
- In idiopathic scoliosis with curves diagnosed before age 10 y there is high risk (88%) of progression.
- Progression related to growth potential, onset of menarche in girls, and skeletal age.
- In patients with neuromuscular scoliosis (cerebral palsy, Friedreich's ataxia, poliomyelitis, muscular dystrophy) there are problems with swallowing, aspiration, pulm infection, poor cough, CV disease (muscular dystrophy), poor nutrition.
- Progression of scoliosis may lead to cardiorespiratory problems and painful back in adulthood.
- Neuromuscular patients may not be able to sit because of pelvic obliquity.

ICD-9-CM Code: 737.39
See Surgery for Scoliosis and Kyphosis in Procedures section

ETIOLOGY

- Idiopathic scoliosis from upper and lower motor neuron diseases and from myopathic causes.
- Kyphosis (Scheuermann's type) may be metabolic, with different types of collagen in affected end-plates, and may result from juvenile osteoporosis.

USUAL TREATMENT

- Bracing for mild curves
- Surgery for progressive curves involving fusion instrumentation, correction of curve, and fusion with bone grafts
- In some instances anterior (thoracolumbar) correction and fusion combined with posterior instrumentation and fusion
- In kyphosis, pain treated first with bracing, then surgery if needed
- AP fusion, acute angular decompression, and fusion in situ

ASSESSMENT POINTS

SYSTEM	EFFECT	ASSESSMENT BY HX	TEST
HEENT	Pharyngeal dysfunction Swallowing problems Poor cough in neuromuscular patients	Regurgitation on feeding, spitting Choking	
CV	Cardiomyopathy in muscular dystrophy	Dilated cardiomyopathy	ECG, ECHO,CXR ECG—Abn ECG, tall R: right precordial leads Deep Q: left precordial lead
RESP	Frequent pneumonias from aspiration		CXR, PFTs in neuromuscular dystrophy
GI	Poor nutrition Underweight	Poor feeding	Serum protein, albumin measurements
HEME	Antiepileptic medication can interfere with coagulation (especially valproic acid)	Prolonged bleeding time	Bleeding time Change medication to control seizure prior to surgery

Key Reference: Bernstein RL, Rosenberg AD: Scoliosis. *In* Manual of Orthopedic Anesthesia and Related Pain Syndromes. New York, Churchill Livingstone, 1994.

PERIOPERATIVE IMPLICATIONS

Preoperative Preparation

- Idiopathic scoliosis
  - Pre-donation of autologous blood
- Neuromuscular scoliosis
  - Nutritional preparation—may need gastrostomy feedings to establish adequate serum protein levels. Treat resp problems. If vital capacity <30–35% of predicted, may need ventilatory assistance postop

Monitoring

- Somatosensory evoked potentials (SSEPs), motor evoked potentials

Airway

- May need fiberoptic scope

Maintenance

- Position patient so that chest and abdomen are free without pressure, and no tension on spine.

Extubation

- In patients with idiopathic scoliosis, extubation when extubation criteria met
- In patients with neuromuscular scoliosis, ventilatory support may be needed
- Weaning important as soon as possible to avoid prolonged ventilatory support—this may lead to further muscle weakness. Check neurologic status immediately.

Adjuvants

- Valproic acid may interfere with coagulation.

SEIZURES — EPILEPSY

W. Andrew Kofke, M.D.

RISK

• Incidence of epilepsy 0.5–2%; 25%–30% of epileptics have seizures more often than 1/mo
• 300,000 people have medically uncontrolled epilepsy
• About 13% are candidates for epilepsy surgery, and about 1% actually undergo surgery

PERIOPERATIVE RISKS

• Many rare syndromes are associated with epilepsy, which can involve disturbances in major organ systems
• Various psychiatric disorders
• Sudden death syndrome reported with epilepsy, but incidence unknown

WORRY ABOUT

• Proconvulsant and anticonvulsant properties of anesthetics

• Antiepileptic drug therapy–induced resistance to NMBs and fentanyl
• Anticonvulsant-induced blood dyscrasia and hepatitis

OVERVIEW

• Poorly controlled epilepsy results in inability to maintain normal lifestyle. Intellectual and social deficits can result from brain-damaging effect of uncontrolled recurrent seizures, negative attitudes of society, or side effects of antiepileptic drug therapy
• Seizures are categorized as partial (simple, complex, or with generalization) or generalized (inhibitory, excitatory), pseudoseizures, or unclassified

ICD-9-CM Code: 345

ETIOLOGY

• *Congenital* often associated with other syndromes such as tuberous sclerosis, neurofibromatosis, multiple endocrine adenomatosis, Jervell–Lange-Nielsen syndrome
• *Acquired* often associated with trauma, stroke, or idiopathic causes

USUAL TREATMENT

• Antiepileptic drugs such as phenytoin, phenobarbital, clonazepam, carbamazepine, and many others
• 13% of epileptic patients are thought to be candidates for epilepsy surgery, but only about 1% actually undergo surgery

ASSESSMENT POINTS

SYSTEM	EFFECT	ASSESSMENT BY HX	PE	TEST
HEENT	Gingival hyperplasia	Phenytoin use		
CV	Cardiac tumors with tuberous sclerosis ↑ Incidence of sudden death with epilepsy (anesthetic implications unknown)	Tuberous sclerosis	Murmur possibly	ECHO
RESP	Pulm involvement with neurofibromatosis	Neurofibromatosis Exercise tolerance	Cor pulmonale	CXR ECG
GI	Anticonvulsant-induced hepatitis	Anticonvulsant use	Icterus Tender RUQ	LFTs if symptomatic
ENDO	Hyponatremia	Carbamazepine use (rare)		Na^+
CNS	Tolerance to fentanyl Psychiatric disturbances	Anticonvulsant use		Assess effects of preop sedatives
MS	Tolerance to NMBs	Anticonvulsant use		Train-of-four monitoring in OR

Key Reference: Kofke WA, Templehoff R, Dasheiff, RM: Anesthesia for epileptic patients and for epilepsy surgery. *In* Cottrell JE, Smith DS (eds): Anesthesia and Neurosurgery, 3rd ed. St. Louis, CV Mosby, 1994, pp 495–520.

PERIOPERATIVE IMPLICATIONS

Preoperative Preparation

• Assess neuropsychiatric status
• Determine antiepileptic drug history
• Assess for murmur suggestive of myocardial tumor (tuberous sclerosis) or stigmata of neurofibromatosis

Monitoring

• For seizure surgery EEG may be placed intraoperatively

Airway

• Routine considerations

Preinduction/Induction (for epilepsy surgery)

• GA ultrafast-acting thiobarbiturate such as thiopental. If intraoperative EEG, etomidate or methohexital suitable alternative
• For conscious analgesia craniotomy: position determined with protection of pressure points. O_2 delivered by nasal prongs with capnography and impedance resp monitor. Fentanyl 0.5–0.75 µg/kg and droperidol 0.15 mg/kg. Local anesthetic injected before surgical incision

Maintenance

• If intraoperative EEG not planned, use an anticonvulsant anesthetic maintenance regimen such as isoflurane with or without nitrous oxide or moderate-dose opioid
• For GA with intraoperative EEG, N_2O-narcotic techniques with avoidance of both isoflurane and halothane. Enflurane produces high-voltage spikes on EEG; has been used to synchronize and activate epileptogenic foci. Methohexital, 25–50 mg, alfentanil, 50–100 µg, have been used as activating agents
• For conscious analgesia continued titrated sedation during painful parts of procedure anticipated with fentanyl

Extubation

• NMB agents and narcotics may not last as long as expected, with unanticipated coughing as procedure comes to close

Adjuvants

• Muscle relaxants: ↓ effect with antiepileptic drugs
• Opioids: tolerance with antiepileptic drug therapy
• Most anesthetics have potential to precipitate seizures during or *after* surgery

• Antiepileptic drug levels can be significantly affected by anesthetics, changes in body physiology, and prolonged NPO status

Postoperative Period

• Blood levels of antiepileptic drugs can be unpredictable, and parenteral antiepileptic drugs such as phenytoin or phenobarbital may be required
• Numerous case reports of postop seizures with a variety of anesthetics suggest concern for this possibility.

ANTICIPATED PROBLEMS/CONCERNS

• Blood levels of antiepileptic drugs can be significantly affected by anesthetics, changes in physiology, and prolonged NPO status
• Opioid tolerance may result in increased need for pain medication

SEIZURES — GRAND MAL (TONIC-CLONIC) — Marek A. Mirski, M.D., Ph.D.

RISK

- 500,000–1,000,000 in USA with recurrent tonic-clonic seizures
- 10–20 million at risk to have one tonic-clonic seizure 2° to alcohol withdrawal, febrile convulsions (in children), CNS pathology, metabolic disturbances

PERIOPERATIVE RISKS

- Intraoperative and postop seizures
- Status epilepticus (unrecognized intraoperatively)
- Delayed awakening
- Todd's paralysis
- Pulmonary aspiration
- Transient hypoxemia, tachycardia, HTN
- ↑ ICP

WORRY ABOUT

- Check serum anticonvulsant levels preop, consider free vs. total serum phenytoin levels in nutritionally depleted patients. May be best to normalize low serum levels preop.
- Caution with intraoperative IV phenytoin

(hypotension, 50 µg/min limit) or phenobarbital (somnolence)
- Prudent to avoid drugs that may lower seizure threshold: tricyclics, ?etomidate, ketamine

OVERVIEW

- Although typically a benign event, trauma to head or extremities is common if precautions not taken (padded hospital bed). May lead to status epilepticus, a life-threatening condition requiring active and immediate intervention to terminate attack before cerebral injury results (30–60 min). Subtherapeutic anticonvulsant serum levels and alcohol withdrawal most commonly provoke status epilepticus.
- During seizures and post-ictally, airway reflexes are typically preserved—intubation *not* indicated unless aspiration is strongly suspected
- Post-ictally, enhancement of previous neurologic motor deficit is common (Todd's paralysis) for hours after seizure.

ICD-9-CM Code: 345.3

ETIOLOGY

- Leading cause (30%) is idiopathic; undetermined fraction have genetic predisposition
- Acquired—2° to congenital defects, perinatal asphyxia, trauma, CNS infection, drug withdrawal (alcohol most common), metabolic pathology resulting in low Na^+, Ca^{2+}, Mg^{2+}, or ↑ BUN.

USUAL TREATMENT

- For one seizure, no therapy required. Check serum anticonvulsant levels.
- For recurrent or prolonged seizures: IV midazolam 1–3 mg, diazepam 5–10 mg. Alternatively, thiopental 50–100 mg/70 kg, propofol 1 mg/kg. Ventilatory assistance should be available for greater dosage requirements.
- To prevent recurrence, IV phenytoin should be considered to reach serum target level of 10–20 µg/dl (15–20 mg/kg load in patient not currently taking phenytoin).

ASSESSMENT POINTS

SYSTEM	EFFECT	ASSESSMENT BY HX	PE	TEST
HEENT	Gingival hyperplasia (phenytoin) Seizure-induced oral trauma		Oral exam	
CV	Drug-induced SIADH (carbamazepine) Thrombocytopenia (several drugs)			CBC, electrolytes
RESP	Aspiration pneumonia	SOB, fever, supplemental O_2	Auscultation	CXR, O_2 sat ABGs, sputum culture
GI	Poor absorption of anticonvulsant Drug-induced increase of hepatic P450 Drug-induced transaminase elevation	Low serum levels Increase dosage requirement of various drugs		Drug levels
CNS	Post-ictal somnolence Possible multiple CNS abnormalities	Developmental Hx	Cognitive, motor	
MS	Seizure-induced focal injury			

Key Reference: Resor S Jr, Kutt H: The Medical Treatment of the Epilepsies. New York, Marcel Dekker, 1992.

PERIOPERATIVE IMPLICATIONS

Preoperative Preparation

- Ensure therapeutic anticonvulsant levels
- Provide protection from injury should seizure occur

Monitoring

- Routine
- EEG postop if poor emergence observed

Airway

- Evaluate for past seizure-induced oral trauma
- Gingival hyperplasia (phenytoin)

Induction

- Standard induction drugs provide anticonvulsant action
- Benzodiazepines useful adjunct

Maintenance

- CV changes may be indicative of seizure

Extubation

- Extubate awake if possible
- Delayed emergence could signal post-ictal state or status epilepticus—EEG suggested

Adjuvants

- Anticonvulsants for acute seizure: IV benzodiazepines, propofol, barbiturates
- Load with phenytoin or barbiturate; oral drugs less reliable absorption

- Muscle relaxant doses altered by some anticonvulsants

Postoperative Period

- Check serum anticonvulsant levels
- EEG indicated if postop level of arousal not as expected

ANTICIPATED PROBLEMS/CONCERNS

- Clinical seizure preinduction—injury and aspiration risk if sedative drugs given
- Intraoperative seizure with consequent delayed emergence
- Subclinical or convulsive status epilepticus

SEIZURES — INTRACTABLE

René Tempelhoff, M.D.

RISK

- People within US: 600,000 epileptics/y have uncontrolled seizures
- Racial predominance: None

PERIOPERATIVE RISKS

- Sudden death
- Status epilepticus
- Seizure-mediated cardiac dysrhythmias

WORRY ABOUT

- Liver toxicity from anticonvulsants
- Perioperative trauma from convulsions
- Sudden death
- Status epilepticus postoperatively
- Altered pharmacologic responses due to chronic drug therapy

OVERVIEW

- Neurologic disease associated with birth, congenital malformation, trauma, CNS pathology, idiopathic
- Perioperative risks increased for acquired seizure disorder, but furthermore some epilepsy/congenital malformations carry their own anesthetic risks
- Check type of seizures, clinical manifestations, duration, frequency
- Anticonvulsant therapy and side effects (liver function, level of consciousness)

ICD-9-CM Code: 780.3 (Seizure, recurrent)

ETIOLOGY

- Congenital (e.g., tuberous sclerosis/infantile seizure)
- Idiopathic
- CNS pathology: trauma, tumor, hemorrhage

USUAL TREATMENT

- Anticonvulsant and diet
- Surgery for ablation of foci
- GA regarded as a last resort for seizure that is unresponsive to sedative-hypnotics and resulting in decrease in consciousness or significant (<7.28) metabolic acidosis

ASSESSMENT POINTS

SYSTEM	EFFECT	ASSESSMENT BY HX	PE	TEST
HEENT	Tongue biting/swallowing		Airway assessment	
CV	Cardiac dysrhythmias	Syncope Tachycardia		ECG ECHO Holter
RESP	Hyperventilation due to metabolic acidosis			ABG
GI	Altered liver function Anticonvulsant toxicity Tuberous sclerosis		Jaundice	LFTs Anticonvulsant levels
ENDO	Associated multiple endocrine adenomatosis			Glucose Ca^{2+}, thyroid function tests
RENAL	Renal dysfunction Tuberous sclerosis			Cr
CNS	Psychiatric problems CNS pathology			
MS	Occult trauma from seizures		Check joints, bones Examine tongue	

Key Reference: Kofke WA, Tempelhoff R, Dasheiff RM: Anesthesia for epileptic patients and epileptic surgery. *In* Anesthesia and Neurosurgery, 3rd ed. St. Louis, CV Mosby, 1994, pp 495–520.

PERIOPERATIVE IMPLICATIONS

Preoperative Preparation

- Usual anticonvulsant regimen

Monitoring

- Routine monitors
- End tidal CO_2: increase in CO_2 production could be indirect sign of seizure
- Consider EEG monitoring

Induction

- Have sodium thiopental and/or benzodiazepines to treat possible seizures
- Significantly higher requirement for nondepolarizing muscle relaxants and narcotics

Maintenance

- Avoid proconvulsants (ketamine, etomidate, enflurane)
- Continue scheduled anticonvulsants
- GA is sometimes used as treatment for status epilepticus

Extubation

- To be delayed in case of doubt or situation such as:
  - High end tidal CO_2 despite adequate ventilation can be a sign of active seizure
    - Patient nonresponsive
    - Obvious convulsions
- Consider adding anticonvulsant (benzodiazepines) and ordering EEG

Adjuvants

- See specific anticonvulsant used

Postoperative Period

- Watch end tidal CO_2 on awakening, as high production may indicate seizure activity
- Resume anticonvulsants
- Treat seizures ad lib

ANTICIPATED PROBLEMS/CONCERNS

- Seizures on induction and awakening are treated with first-line benzodiazepine Rx (e.g., Ativan) rather than long-acting drugs (e.g., phenytoin)
- Evolution to status epilepticus: GA?
- Sudden death (ventricular arrhythmias?)

SEIZURES — PETIT MAL ABSENCE

Marek A. Mirski, M.D., Ph.D.

RISK

- Approximately 75,000–100,000 in USA
- Pure cases almost exclusively a risk in children, with age at onset 4–10 y

PERIOPERATIVE RISKS

- Few. Risk of transition of petit mal absence seizures into tonic-clonic seizures or status epilepticus is exceedingly low.

WORRY ABOUT

- Maintenance of serum anticonvulsant levels
- Inducing seizures with hyperventilation

OVERVIEW

- Relatively common seizure of childhood
- Seizure typified by brief absence (5–20 sec) with impairment of consciousness, 3/sec spike-wave EEG, mild facial motor manifestations
- Attacks may be few or occur >100/d
- Hyperventilation and bright flickering lights are common triggers
- "Atypical absence" seizures may have more motor features and be of longer duration
- Trauma from seizures rare, axial posture almost never affected
- No post-ictal sequelae; EEG and level of awareness return immediately.
- Spontaneous resolution frequent in adolescence (25–30%); ~ 50% go on to develop tonic-clonic seizures.

ICD-9-CM Code: 345.2

ETIOLOGY

- Strong genetic predisposition in otherwise normal children
- Structural lesions in adults

USUAL TREATMENT

- Valproic acid (VPA) or ethosuximide (ESM) is drug of choice.
- No emergent therapy required unless other seizure type present

ASSESSMENT POINTS

SYSTEM	EFFECT	TEST
CV	Mild thrombocytopenia (VPA) Pancytopenia (ESM)	CBC with platelet count
RESP	Hyperventilation may induce seizure	
GI	↑ Liver enzymes (ESM, VPA) GI upset (VPA) Hepatotoxicity (VPA—rare > age 2 y)	ALT, AST
CNS	EEG typically normal between seizures Normal development is rule	EEG
MS	Mild myoclonic movements	

Key Reference: Niedermeyer E: The Epilepsies; Diagnosis and Management. Baltimore, Urban & Schwarzenberg, 1990.

PERIOPERATIVE IMPLICATIONS

Preoperative Preparation

- Continue anticonvulsant therapy.
- Verify adequate anticonvulsant levels: ESM 40–100 µg/ml, VPA >50 µg/ml (variable)

Monitoring

- No issues

Airway

- No issues

Preinduction/Induction

- Avoid bright flashing lights and hyperventilation.

Maintenance

- Normocarbia unless otherwise indicated

Extubation

- Normocarbia

Adjuvants

- Muscle relaxant action is affected by some agents used to treat petit mal seizures.

Postoperative Period

- Pain management beneficial if it results in avoidance of stress-induced hyperventilation

ANTICIPATED PROBLEMS/CONCERNS

- Major perioperative morbidity rare
- Major concern is to document if other seizure types, such as tonic-clonic seizures, occur, which *would* affect perioperative risk.

SEPTIC HYPERDYNAMIC SHOCK; SYSTEMIC INFLAMMATORY RESPONSE SYNDROME (SIRS)

Myer H. Rosenthal, M.D.

RISK

- Incidence in USA: unknown but reported in 1987 at 250,000/y
- All ages; more frequent and less well tolerated in elderly
- Males = females

PERIOPERATVE RISKS

- Splanchnic circulatory insufficiency leading toqbowel permeability and resultant endotoxemia
- Organ hypoperfusion and release of variety of cytokines causing ARDS and multiorgan dysfunction syndrome (MODS)

WORRY ABOUT

- Worsening hypotension, perfusion
- Development of ARDS or MODS from release of variety of cytokines, including TNF, prostaglandin metabolites, PAF, and others, which leads to capillary permeability, intravascular hypovolemia, and cell death; ATN and hepatic, myocardial, and cerebral insufficiency 2° to oxygen free radical destruction of vital tissue

OVERVIEW

- Failure of heart to pump blood into aorta in sufficient quantity and under sufficient pressure to maintain adequate tissue perfusion and aerobic metabolism
- Initiating pathophysiologic response is reduction in SVR, often accompanied by compensatory rise in cardiac index, in an attempt to maintain satisfactory systemic perfusion pressure.
- Initial reduction in SVR complicated by impaired preload (hypovolemia), due to vasodilation, ↑ vascular permeability, and hypocontractility (cardiac failure), due to coronary hypoperfusion, β-adrenergic receptor hyporesponsiveness, direct negative inotropic effect of bacterial toxins and humoral mediators, including polypeptide, myocardial depressant factor (MDF)

ICD-9-CM Code: 785.59

ETIOLOGY

- Any microorganism may initiate sepsis leading to SIRS and septic shock
- SIRS produced by septic process with liberation of a variety of vasoactive humoral factors, including histamine, kinins, complement, and prostaglandins.
- Common with splanchnic circulatory insufficiency that can accompany major abdominal, vascular or bowel surgery or pathology. Failure of bowel or hepatic perfusion and low oxygen tension in bowel wall lead to ↑ bowel permeability and reticuloendothelial dysfunction with resultant endotoxemia. Bowel and hepatic ischemia associated with other forms of shock (hypovolemic, cardiogenic) may result in complicating pathophysiologic changes similar to that seen with hyperdynamic shock—a decrease in SVR

ASSESSMENT POINTS

SYSTEM	EFFECT	ASSESSMENT BY HX	PE	TEST
CV	Vasodilation ↑ Capillary permeability Hypoperfusion, hypovolemia, hypocontractility	Edematous, yet signs of organ hypoperfusion, cold extremities, infection	BP lying and standing Degree of vasoconstriction, HR, obtundation, tachypnea	PCWP, CVP, CO, ECHO
GI	Hepatic/GI insufficiency Vomiting Diarrhea, melena	Bowel habits		Gastric mucosal pH, temperature
HEME	Infection; hemodilution; hemolysis; thrombocytopenia; DIC	Immunocompromised bleeding, febrile	Warm, full pulses; petechiae; bleeding	WBC with differential, Hct, cultures, coagulation studies
RENAL	ATN, oliguria, anuria	UO		↑ BUN, Cr, inactive excretion of Na$^+$
METAB	Acidosis 2° to inadequate tissue perfusion		Tachypnea Mottled extremities	ABGs Lactate

PERIOPERATIVE IMPLICATIONS

Preoperative Preparations

- Ensure optimal perfusion to organs—possible within context of removing infective (and possibly causative) agent
- Aggressive invasive hemodynamic monitoring
- Evaluate and optimize oxygenation
- Verify ventilator settings and line positions prior to and after transport

Monitoring

- Consider need to assess preload, vascular resistance, and cardiac index (PA catheter or TEE) and arterial (and perhaps mixed venous) blood gas tensions
- Consider Foley catheter

Airway

- None

Induction

- If MAP <65 mmHg, consider fluids if PAOP <15 mmHg, or inotropes if PAOP >15 mmHg, or vasoconstrictor if PAOP >15 mmHG and cardiac index (CI) >4.50L/min/m^2

Maintenance

- Selection of optimal inotropic therapy controversial with support for dopamine (DA), epinephrine (EPI) and dobutamine (DOB)
- Factors including ↓ enzymatic conversion of DA to EPI, β-receptor hyporesponsiveness, and pre-existing vasodilation favor a predictable potent β-adrenergic agonist without vasodilator properties, namely EPI at a dose range 20–100 ng/kg/min. Routine therapy to produce supranormal values for oxygen delivery (DO$_2$) = CO × CAO$_2$—and CI for management of SIRS based on anecdotal reports of favorable results. However, studies in septic patients have shown inconsistent results with one report using DOB to increase CI resulting in ↑ mortality compared with controls not treated to supranormal levels. Adequate oxygen delivery must guide therapy

- Consider avoiding agents with vasodilator and negative inotropic properties

Extubation/Postoperative Period

- Consider hemodynamic and acid-base stability
- Verify infusion rates/ventilator/lines prior to and after transport

Adjuvants

- Consider renal functional status before administering drug substantially dependent upon kidney for pharmacokinetic profile

ANTICIPATED PROBLEMS/CONCERNS

- Necessity for aggressive surgical drainage of infected foci may require anesthetic administration to a patient with hyperdynamic shock. To minimize worsening hypotension and hypoperfusion, continued management as outlined above must be followed in OR and into postop period.

SHY-DRAGER DISEASE

Lisa A. Caramico, M.D.

RISK

- More common in men than women
- Symptoms begin in 5th–7th decades

PERIOPERATIVE RISKS

- Autonomic dysfunction with CV collapse
- Aspiration risk

WORRY ABOUT

- Orthostatic hypotension
- Obstructive sleep apnea—found in advanced stages
- Vocal cord paralysis—found in advanced stages

OVERVIEW

- A parkinsonism plus syndrome
- Clinical manifestations include orthostatic hypotension, parkinsonian symptoms, urinary and bowel dysfunction, impaired potency and libido, and decreased sweating
- Pathologic changes include widespread degeneration of CNS
- Irreversible progressive neurodegenerative disease
- Death often occurs 7–8 y after onset of symptoms
- Difficult to treat the parkinsonian symptoms as dopaminergic drugs may exacerbate orthostatic hypotension

ICD-9-CM Code: 333.0

ETIOLOGY

- Unknown

USUAL TREATMENT

- Symptomatic relief of orthostatic hypotension
- Liberal salt intake
- Fludrocortisone
- Elastic stockings
- Midorine—peripheral α adrenergic agonist
- Sympathomimetics—ephedrine
- Prostaglandin inhibitors—Indocin, ibuprofen
- MAO inhibitors
- Common to also receive antiparkinsonian drugs

ASSESSMENT POINTS

SYSTEM	EFFECT	ASSESSMENT BY HX	PE	TEST
HEENT	Vocal cord paralysis Obstructive sleep apnea	Obstruction; stridor; snoring	Bilateral abductor paralysis	Direct laryngoscopy Nasoendoscopy
CV	Orthostatic hypotension Fixed HR	Syncope; dizziness	Postural changes in BP	TILT test ECG
RESP	Irregular resp			
GI	Gastroparesis Fecal incontinence, diarrhea, constipation	Early satiety	Loss of rectal sphincter tone	
GU	Urinary incontinence	Nocturia Sexual impotence Atonic bladder		
CNS	Parkinsonian symptoms Anhidrosis Heat intolerance		Cogwheel rigidity Shuffling gait	
MS	Osteoporosis Aseptic necrosis			

Key Reference: Bawa R, Ramadan H, Wetmore S: Bilateral vocal cord paralysis with Shy-Drager syndrome. Otolaryngol Head Neck Surg 1993; 109:911–914.

PERIOPERATIVE IMPLICATIONS

Preoperative Preparation

- Reduce venous pooling; increase peripheral vascular resistance; increase plasma volume. Care must by taken using these techniques in the attempt to decrease postural hypotension, as fluid overload can occur.

Monitoring

- Arterial and central venous catheters if fluid shifts likely to guide fluid replacement
- Temp—reduced sweating may lead to elevations in temp

Airway

- Vocal cord paralysis and dysautonomia with gastroparesis may make awake intubation the more desirable choice

Preinduction/Induction

- Consider steroid supplementation if on fludrocortisone
- Consider effects of MAO inhibitors
- Avoid agents that may cause a decrease in cardiac output, decrease in HR, or vasodilatation, as profound hypotension may occur.

Maintenance

- IPPV may cause a decrease in venous return and exaggerate hypotension.
- Norepinephrine stores at the nerve endings may be reduced. Therefore, the response to adrenergic drugs may be reduced or exaggerated: Use direct-acting drugs in small doses titrated to effect.
- Atropine may not increase the HR owing to parasympathetic deficiency.

Extubation

- Awake

Postoperative Period

- Autonomic dysfunction

ANTICIPATED PROBLEMS/CONCERNS

- Autonomic dysfunction with CV collapse
- Aspiration risk

SICK SINUS SYNDROME (SSS)

John L. Atlee, M.D.

RISK

- Acquired condition resulting from aging in association with CAD or cardiomyopathies
- Incidence unknown, causes 50% of new pacemaker implants (USA)
- Gender or racial predominance: None
- Usually develops in 6th–7th decades but can occur sooner

PERIOPERATIVE RISKS

- Circulatory compromise 2° bradycardia, SA or AV heart block, or escape rhythms
- Paroxysmal atrial tachycardias: AFib > atrial flutter >> ectopic atrial tachycardia or SVT

WORRY ABOUT

- Possible associated CV disease, esp. coronary heart disease or cardiomyopathies
- Thromboembolism with SSS and AFib (stroke, coronaries, systemic, pulm)

OVERVIEW

- Sx due to bradycardia or tachycardia (brady-tachy syndrome)
- Thromboembolism risk with paroxysmal AFib
- Antiarrhythmic drugs used to control tachyarrhythmias may aggravate bradycardia or asystolic sinus pauses following spontaneous termination of tachycardia.

ICD-9-CM Code: 427.81

ETIOLOGY

- Due to fibrous degeneration of pacemaker cells, autonomic nerves/ganglia, atrial wall
- Extrinsic sinus node dysfunction from reflex stimulation (e.g., oculocardiac reflex), hypothermia, or drugs
- In absence of sinus node dysfunction, anesthetics alone should not cause severe sinus bradycardia.

USUAL TREATMENT

- Chronotropes (atropine, ephedrine, isoproterenol) to increase sinus rate
- Temporary or permanent pacing for bradycardia and to suppress tachyarrhythmias
- Systemic anticoagulation for patients with chronic AFib (Coumadin, heparin), better than aspirin

ASSESSMENT POINTS

SYSTEM	EFFECT	ASSESSMENT BY HX	PE	TEST
CV	Arrhythmias	Palpitations, dizziness, syncope, fatigue, lethargy	Pulse too slow, fast, or irregular	ECG, Holter monitoring Electrophysiologic studies
	ASCVD	Exercise intolerance, dyspnea, fatigue, angina	S_3, rales, wheezes	ECHO Reperfusion scintigraphy Coronary Angio
	Pacer (perm)	Sx of arrhythmias suggest pacemaker malfunction	Vagal maneuvers to check function, magnet to inhibit	Pacemaker clinic consult, pacing system analyzer, pacemaker programmer
RESP	CHF, COPD	Dyspnea, orthopnea, cough	S_3, rales, wheezes	CXR
GI	Hypoperfusion	GI distress, diarrhea		
RENAL	Hypoperfusion	Polyuria		BUN/Cr
CNS	Ischemia/stroke	Syncope episodes, paralysis, dementia	Neurologic or mental deficits	See CV assessment

Key Reference: Atlee JL: Arrhythmias and Pacemakers. Philadelphia, WB Saunders, 1996.

PERIOPERATIVE IMPLICATIONS

Preoperative Preparation

- Symptomatic bradycardia requires prophylactic perioperative pacing.
- Permanent pacemaker: check function and inactivate/reprogram if electrocautery to be used
- If acute onset AFib/flutter (≤ 3 d), consider cardioversion and anticoagulation.
- Optimize ventricular rate with chronic AFib (digitalis, β rb's or Ca²⁺ channel blockers)

Monitoring

- ECG with ST-T trending; strip-chart recorder
- Consider arterial and PA catheter monitoring if BP instability, LV dysfunction
- Arterial pulse waveform (oximetric, direct) if permanent or temporary pacer

Induction

- LV dysfunction and AFib/flutter increase risk of hypotension during induction
- Caution with agents such as thiopental or propofol
- Desflurane, ketamine, and pancuronium may accelerate ventricular rate with AFib
- Increased circulatory lability due to bradycardia or paroxysmal tachycardia

Maintenance

- With associated CV disease and LV dysfunction, less tolerance of large fluid shifts or blood loss
- No anesthetics especially contraindicated, but caution with drugs that slow sinus rate

Extubation

- Possibly ↑ risk for paroxysmal tachyarrhythmias due to catecholamine surge
- With paroxysmal AFib, ↑ risk of thromboembolism with hyperdynamic circulation

- Use drugs and other means to reduce/avoid circulatory effects of airway stimulation

Adjuvants

- Do not rely on atropine to increase sinus rate; direct-acting β adrenergic agonists are more reliable.
- Best drugs to control ventricular rate with AFib are β rb's or edrophonium (5–10 mg, ×2).

Postoperative Period

- Susceptibility to bradycardia and escape rhythms, or paroxysmal tachycardia does not decrease.

ANTICIPATED PROBLEMS/CONCERNS

- Chronotropes used to treat bradycardia may be ineffective or cause paroxysmal tachycardias.
- Perioperative pacemaker malfunction in patients with permanent or temporary pacemakers

SICKLE CELL DISEASE
William A. McDade, M.D., Ph.D.

RISK

- Affects persons with ancestors from areas endemic for falciparum malaria: Greeks, Turks, Italians, Arabs, Asian Indians, Africans
- In USA, 1/500 African-Americans (0.2%) have sickle cell anemia
- Early mortality—median age of death in men is 42 y and women is 48 y

PERIOPERATIVE RISKS

- Patients have 30% overall complication rate; risk decreases with increased levels of fetal Hgb
- Complications include anemia, stroke, acute chest syndrome, myonecrosis, heart failure, MI, hepatic or splenic sequestration, retinal hemorrhage, hematuria, renal failure, atelectasis and pneumonia, new-onset tonic-clonic seizure, intraoperative stasis and hypotension, wound infection, urinary tract infection, unexplained death

WORRY ABOUT

- Degree of anemia, dehydration, sepsis, stress, acid-base status, hypoxemia
- Percentage of HbSS-containing cells
- Postop atelectasis and pneumonia
- Previous renal or heart failure

- Precipitation of vaso-occlusive crisis
- Risk of hemolytic transfusion reaction due to alloimmunization

OVERVIEW

- Lifelong cause of painful vaso-occlusive episodes
- Average rate of painful episodes per patient year is 0.8
- 5.2% of patients with 3–10 episodes/y account for 33% of all episodes
- Mortality positively correlates with increased pain rate in adults
- Only Hct and percentage of fetal Hgb have predictive value in defining risk of painful crisis
- End-organ damage due to vaso-occlusion causes morbidity and mortality. Key conditions are pregnancy, heart failure, MI, CVA, acute chest syndrome, sequestration crisis, and severe anemia
- Enhanced O_2 delivery by sickle Hgb causes rightward shift (P50 = 31 mmHg) of oxyhemoglobin dissociation curve
- Inherited hemoglobinopathy permits deoxygenated Hgb molecules to polymerize into rigid insoluble intraerythrocytic fibers, resulting in sickled cells

- Organ damage is due to vaso-occlusive ischemia, which occurs because the sickled cells are unable to traverse narrow capillary beds, leading to distal blood flow impairment. Also, there is an enhanced tendency for sickle cells to adhere to the endothelium and cause release of vasoactive substances

ICD-9-CM Code: 282.60
See also under Sickle Cell Trait

ETIOLOGY

- Molecular lesion is on ß-chain of Hgb at position 6 glu→val
- Sickle erythrocytes are more fragile with shortened life span, which leads to chronic hemolysis and anemia

USUAL TREATMENT

- Vaccines against pneumococcus and *H. influenzae* type b, and prophylactic penicillin therapy both effective in autosplenectomized patients
- Palliative care for painful crisis
- Simple and exchange transfusions
- Hydroxyurea to increase fetal Hgb

ASSESSMENT POINTS

SYSTEM	EFFECT	ASSESSMENT BY HX	PE	TEST
HEENT	Hypoxemia due to sleep apnea	Snoring or sleep apnea Hx	Tonsillar hypertrophy	ABG
CV	MI; LV and RV dysfunction; CHF	Angina Sx; exercise tolerance; dyspnea	Displaced PMI S_3, S_4	ECG, exercise ECG; ECHO, Hct
RESP	Acute chest syndrome; lung and rib infarction; pneumonia	Previous acute chest syndrome; dyspnea	Point tenderness over rib; rales; crackles	CXR
GI	Gallstones; sickle girdle syndrome (mesenteric ischemia); hepatic sequestration crisis	RUQ pain; abdominal pain	Jaundice; RUQ tenderness	Bilirubin
HEME	Sickle pain crisis; asplenia or splenic sequestration crisis; anemia; infection	Pain in affected areas; fatigue; sepsis	Pallor; splenic enlargement; flank tenderness; fever	Hgb, Hct, WBC, % HbSS Electrophoresis
RENAL	Renal failure and insufficiency	Hematuria; hemodialysis Hx		UA, BUN, Serum Cr
REPROD	Preterm labor and delivery; perinatal mortality; placenta previa; abruptio placentae	Vaginal bleeding		US
CNS	Stroke; intracranial hemorrhage; pneumococcal meningitis; retinopathy and hyphema; seizure	Previous CNS Sx (weakness, TIA, or neurologic dysfunction); headache; vomiting or altered mental status	Focal deficits, stupor or coma; nuchal rigidity	Head CT; EEG
MS	Leg ulcers; myonecrosis; myofibrosis; infant hand-foot syndrome; shoulder or hip avascular necrosis; osteomyelitis	Pain in affected areas	ROM; skin changes; fever	WBC, UA, x-ray

Key Reference: Vichinsky EP, et al: A comparison of conservative and aggressive transfusion regimens in the perioperative management of sickle cell disease. NEJM 1995; 333:206–213.

PERIOPERATIVE IMPLICATIONS

Preoperative Preparation

- Latest data suggest there is no benefit in exchange transfusion preop. Rather, transfuse to a Hgb of 10 g/dl, independent of HbSS percent, with HbAA erythrocytes using extended matched transfusions (minor group E, K, C, Fya)
- Alkalinization has no benefit
- Autotransfusion—predonated units and Hgb-based O_2 carriers remain of unestablished efficacy
- Venous access may be difficult and a central line or implantable reservoir is useful
- Preop hydration for 12 h preceding surgery

Monitoring

- Routine
- If PA catheter indicated due to comorbidity and

surgical setting, an oximetric catheter is useful in providing continuous mixed venous blood PO_2 sat for assessment of oxygen utilization and delivery

Airway

- None

Induction

- Avoid oversedation, which may decrease respiration and lead to hypoxemia
- Avoid hypovolemia
- Retrobulbar blocks appear safe
- No differences in morbidity or mortality shown among various anesthetic agents or between regional and GA techniques

Maintenance

- Cardiopulmonary bypass presents special problems causing dilutional anemia, mechanical hemolysis, hypothermia, low-flow state, and plt activation

- Tourniquet use is relatively contraindicated, but unproven to show ↑ risk for sickle patients

Extubation

- Analgesic-induced resp depression at extubation may contribute to atelectasis, pulm infections, and hypoxemia

Postoperative Period

- Adequate hydration; analgesia; pulmonary toilet, including incentive spriometry; supplemental oxygen therapy for 12-48 h postop

ANTICIPATED PROBLEMS/CONCERNS

- All blood transfusions in these patients carry high risk for hemolytic reaction due to previous exposure
- Avoid all situations leading to hypoxemia, hypovolemia, or stasis

SICKLE CELL TRAIT

Michael F. Roizen, M.D.

RISK

- People within USA: 2.5 million
- Race with highest prevalence: African-American

PERIOPERATIVE RISKS

- Increased risk of complications following CABG
- Perioperative mortality rate in published cases of SA trait is 0.8%
- Some increased risk of CVA and pulmonary infection but not well quantified

WORRY ABOUT

- Increased risk of vaso-occlusive phenomenon with hypoxia and stress

OVERVIEW

- Is not a disease
- Is not a cause of abnormalities in blood count
- Does not produce vaso-occlusive symptoms under physiologic conditions—painful crisis not a hallmark or concomitant of condition
- Does not adversely affect individual's life expectancy
- Dx established by Hgb electrophoresis

ICD-9-CM Code: 282.5
See also Sickle Cell Disease in Diseases section

ETIOLOGY

- Heterozygous in which individual has one beta S and beta A globin gene (SA disease)

USUAL TREATMENT

- None, except iron supplementation (debated)

ASSESSMENT POINTS

SYSTEM	EFFECT	ASSESSMENT BY HX	TEST
RESP	Pulm embolism		
HEME	Hgb level usually 13–15 g/dl	Hx SOB: Exercise tolerance 10–40% of Hgb S—same cells as Hgb A	Hgb
GU	Painless hematuria and bacteriuria; pyelonephritis (especially with pregnancy)		UA (culture if prosthesis planned)
CNS	Stroke	Migraine headache	

Key Reference: Kark JA, Posey DM, Schumaeker HR, Ruehle CJ: Sickle cell trait as a risk factor for sudden death in physical training. N Engl J Med 1987; 317:781–787.

PERIOPERATIVE IMPLICATIONS

Preoperative Preparation

- Warm room
- Consider prehydration

Monitoring

- Temperature

Airway

- Occasionally distorted anatomy 2° to extra-medullary erythropoiesis
- Sinusitis possible
- Prehydrate liberally if CV status will tolerate

Induction

- Routine

Maintenance

- Keep warm
- Keep vasodilated
- Keep without stasis
- High O_2 content

Extubation

- Keep warm

Adjuvants

- Vary if hepatic or renal insufficiency exists

Postoperative Period

- Aggressively prevent pain, hypovolemia, and hypothermia

ANTICIPATED PROBLEMS/CONCERNS

- Stroke and/or pulm emboli or infection have been reported after CPB. Five of 544 patients in literature of SA disease died perioperatively.

SILICOSIS

Karen B. Domino, M.D.

RISK

• Occupational exposure to respirable dust containing crystalline free silica or crystalline quartz
• Males >> females
• No racial predominance
• Potential number of exposed workers: 1.2 to 3 million people, but with use of protection devices, disease is rare

PERIOPERATIVE RISKS

• Increased risk of hypoxemia, bronchospasm, pneumothorax, atelectasis, chronic bronchitis, pneumonia, mycobacterial and fungal pulm infection, and perioperative resp failure.
• Pulmonary HTN and cor pulmonale

WORRY ABOUT

• Resp failure and increased risk of pulm infection, especially after abdominal and thoracic surgery
• Cor pulmonale

OVERVIEW

• Pulm fibrosis (silicosis) develops after chronic occupational exposure.
• Primarily restrictive changes in pulm function (stiff lungs with reduction in lung volumes); obstructive changes may be present. In late stages, ventilatory failure, pulmonary HTN, and cor pulmonale develop.
• Increased risk of postop resp failure, especially following thoracic and abdominal procedures.

ICD-9-CM Codes: 502 (Nodular); 503 (non-nodular)

ETIOLOGY

• Major occupational exposures include mining, stone cutting, abrasive industries, foundry work, packing silica flour, and quarrying, particularly of granite, causing dose-related pulm fibrosis.
• Progressive pulm fibrosis (silicosis) occurs after many (15–20) years of exposure.

• In some cases of intense exposure (e.g., sand blasting), acute silicosis may occur after <1 y of exposure.
• Pathogenesis involves phagocytosis of silica by macrophages, rupture of phagolysosomes, cellular lysis, collagen production, and interstitial fibrosis.
• Initial lesions are pulm nodules containing silica dust. Massive fibrosis results when nodules coalesce. Bleb and bulla formation and distortion of airways and vascular bed by these nodules complicate advanced disease.

USUAL TREATMENT

• Discontinue occupational exposure
• Supportive therapy
• Prophylaxis for complicating infections (pneumococcal and influenza vaccines, tuberculosis)
• Sometimes corticosteroids used

ASSESSMENT POINTS

SYSTEM	EFFECT	ASSESSMENT BY HX	PE	TEST
CV	Pulm HTN Cor pulmonale	Dyspnea Exercise tolerance Leg swelling	S_3 Peripheral edema Distended neck veins	ECG CXR
RESP	Pulm fibrosis Bulla/bleb formation	Cough Sputum production Dyspnea Exercise tolerance	Rales, rhonchi, wheezing Cyanosis Use of accessory muscles of resp Resp rate	CXR ABGs PFTs Inspiratory force Diffusing capacity Lung biopsy
GI	Weight loss			
MS	Generalized weakness			
IMMUNO	Hilar adenopathy (eggshell calcification) ↑ Susceptibility to infection, especially pulm	Cough Fever Sputum production		CXR Sputum culture and sensitivity

Key Reference: Weill H, Jones RN: Occupational pulmonary diseases. *In* Fishman AP (ed): Pulmonary Diseases and Disorders, 2nd ed. New York, McGraw-Hill, 1988, pp 819–860.

PERIOPERATIVE IMPLICATIONS

Preoperative Preparation

• Treat bronchitis and pulmonary infection
• Treat bronchospasm if obstructive component present

Monitoring

• Consider repetitive ABGs and lung mechanics (forced vital capacity, tidal volume, inspiratory force, resp rate) especially postop
• Consider PA catheter if pulm HTN and fluid shifts expected

Airway

• Routine

Preinduction/Induction

• Caution with IV agents that depress ventilation and regional techniques that affect accessory muscles of respiration (e.g., high subarachnoid block, interscalene block)
• Maintain adequate preload and cardiac output. Avoid hypoxemia, hypercapnia, and metabolic acidosis, as these may increase PA pressures and worsen cor pulmonale.

Maintenance

• Controlled ventilation preferred during GA.
• Ventilation may require increased airway pressures because of poor lung compliance.
• Observe for spontaneous pneumothorax, especially in severe disease.

Extubation

• Consider temporary postop mechanical ventilation, especially after upper abdominal and thoracic surgery, until stringent criteria met.

Postoperative Period

• Pain management critical to avoid ↑ pulm HTN

Adjuvants

• Bronchodilators, supplemental O_2, incentive spirometry may improve ability to wean

ANTICIPATED PROBLEMS/CONCERNS

• Increased risk of resp failure and complications especially after upper abdominal and thoracic surgery
• Patients with cor pulmonale at increased risk for cardiac complications

SINGLE (Including Common) VENTRICLE

Daniel Nyhan, M.D.

RISK

- One of the less common congenital cardiac anomalies
- Racial/gender predominance: unknown

PERIOPERATIVE RISKS

- Increased risk of infective endocarditis
- Increased risk of paradoxical emboli
- Additional cardiac risks proportional to presence and severity of associated anomalies and their effects on cardiac function and arterial oxygenation

WORRY ABOUT

- Impaired growth and development
- Signs of congestive cardiac failure
- L→R shunting and cyanosis

OVERVIEW

- The term single ventricle describes all situations with double-inlet ventricular morphology, irrespective of dominant ventricle
- The term common ventricle describes a rare form of single ventricle in which both RV and LV inlets are well developed and ventricle(s) have in effect a large VSD.
- Clinical picture variable, depending on degree of associated cardiac anomalies and the level of pulmonary blood flow
- Always has mixed shunt of varying degree and thus cyanosis
- Cyanosis severe if pulm stenosis/atresia
- If there is no pulmonary stenosis/atresia, the clinical picture may be dominated by features of CHF. Extent of cardiac failure determined by level of excess pulm blood flow which is determined by ratio of SVR to PVR

ICD-9-CM Code: 745.3

ETIOLOGY

- May occur as part of a syndrome
- Majority of cases have multifactorial inheritance due to genetic-environmental interactions.

USUAL TREATMENT

- If amenable, palliative and/or definitive surgical repair

ASSESSMENT POINTS

SYSTEM	EFFECT	ASSESSMENT BY HX	PE	TEST
CV	CHF vs. cyanosis	Dyspnea Tachypnea Cough Feeding difficulty Cyanosis Failure to thrive	S_3 Rales Wheezing Cyanosis Bruit of pulm stenosis or no bruit (if pulm atresia)	CXR ECG
HEME	Polycythemic; long Hx of cyanosis	See above	See above	Hgb; Hct

Key Reference: Elliott LP, Anderson RH, Bargeron LM Jr., et al: Single ventricle or univentriular heart. *In* Adams FA, Emmanoculides GC, Riemenschneider TA (eds): Moss' Heart Disease in Infants, Children and Adolescents, 4th ed. Baltimore, Williams and Wilkins, 1989, pp 485–503.

PERIOPERATIVE IMPLICATIONS

Monitoring

- Oximetry indicating adequate pulmonary blood flow and oxygenation
- Indicators of adequate forward systemic flow (e.g., A-line).

Induction/Maintenance

- Risk of paradoxical air emboli when using venous access
- Agents causing depression of myocardial contractility should be used judiciously in patients with cardiac failure.
- Anesthetic agents (both volatile and fixed) and vasoconstrictive agents can be administered without causing deterioration in SVR to PVR relationship

SLEEP APNEA, CENTRAL AND MIXED

Andreas M. Ostermeier, M.D.
Michael F. Roizen, M.D.

RISK

- People within USA: 1–2% of adult population with sleep apnea, most believed to be obstructive or mixed
- Risk increases with male sex, old age, obesity, Hx of snoring with impaired daytime performance.
- Race with highest incidence: not known

PERIOPERATIVE RISKS

- Increased risk of central and mixed (central and obstructive) apnea
- Risk for respiratory depression also in intubated and tracheostomized patients
- Increased risk with sedative hypnotic narcotics, postoperatively with any form of pain relief

WORRY ABOUT

- See medical records for previous problems
- Look for related medical disorders (e.g., cor pulmonale, cardiac arrhythmias, erythrocytosis)

- Apnea even several hours postoperatively possible, especially after epidural anesthesia
- When administering O_2, think of possible dependence of ventilation on hypoxic drive

OVERVIEW

- Central implies failure of resp rhythmogenesis.
- Obstructive sleep apnea relates to a failed or inadequate respiratory activation of upper airway muscles resulting in lack of airflow.
- In central apnea, hypoventilation persists despite relief of obstruction
- Central apnea is unaccompanied by any respiratory effort, in contrast to obstructive sleep apnea
- Related to central alveolar hypoventilation syndrome (CAHS), also known as Ondine's curse

ICD-9-CM Code: 306.1 (Psychogenic apnea)
See also under Sleep Apnea, Obstructive

ETIOLOGY

- Central: Hereditary influence not clear; possible relation to neurologic disorders (e.g., encephalitis in childhood, damaged respiratory centers, autonomic neuropathy in diabetes)
- Mixed: has obstructive component. Upper airway narrowing superimposed on coexistent abnormality of neurologic control or function of upper airway muscle tone or ventilatory control
- Associated with obesity, nasal obstruction (polyps, rhinitis, deviated septum, acromegaly, hypothyroidism, HTN)

USUAL TREATMENT

- Continuous positive airway pressure (CPAP)
- Tracheostomy and mechanical ventilation at night
- Diaphragmatic pacing, especially at night
- Surgery to remove obstruction: uvulopalatopharyngoplasty (UPPP)
- For central/mixed apnea, additional medical treatment with protriptyline, progesterone
- For mixed apnea, also wt loss and physical aids

ASSESSMENT POINTS

SYSTEM	EFFECT	ASSESSMENT BY HX	PE	TEST
HEENT	Obstructive apnea	Snoring, partner gives Hx of patient's awakening at night with grunts	Visualization of uvula and tonsillar pillars	
CV	HTN	Dyspnea at rest, DOE Poor exercise tolerance, angina	Cardiomegaly S_3/S_4 murmur	ECG, ECHO
RESP	Right heart dysfunction, snoring, resp dysfunction, DOE	Awakening at night with grunts	Venous engorgement Rapid resp rate Cardiomegaly	Pulse oximetry on room air when supine ECG, CXR, ABGs, Hct Polysomnogram
GI	Hepatic dysfunction Full stomach NIDDM	Jaundice, bleeding disorders, ascites, heartburn, hiatus hernia, polydipsia, polyuria	Hepatomegaly, ascites, spider nevi, jaundice	LFTs, PT, PTT Fasting glucose
ENDO	Obesity Hypothyroidism Acromegaly		Mental function reflexes BMI	Free T_4 estimate TSH, GH levels
HEME	Polycythemia		Plethora, clubbing, cyanosis	Hypoxemia, Hct
CNS	Disturbed sleep, impaired daytime performance, morning headache, memory problems, irritability	Daytime sleepiness, complaints of disrupted sleep Ask for encephalitis, autonomic neuropathy, brainstem damage		Polysomnogram

Key Reference: Lamarche Y, Martin R, Reiher J, Blaise G: The sleep apnea syndrome and epidural morphine. Can Anaesth Soc J 1986; 33:231–233.

PERIOPERATIVE IMPLICATIONS

Preoperative Preparation

- Take sleep Hx, if possible from bed partner
- Avoid preop sedation with benzodiazepines and narcotics
- Examine airway carefully
- Consider metoclopramide 10 mg, cimetidine 300 mg PO the night before and IV preop
- Assess myocardial and volume status
- Consider regional anesthesia, if possible

Monitoring

- Routine; consider arterial line
- UO, possible CVP or PA catheter if volume status likely to be significantly altered

Airway

- Airway control necessary if prominent central component and sedation mandatory
- Awake, sitting, fiberoptic intubation may be indicated if difficulty anticipated

- Consider elevation of shoulders and head on bolster (facilitates insertion of laryngoscope)

Induction

- Patient may need to remain semi-sitting if Sao_2 drops when supine. Preoxygenation should be complete.

Maintenance

- Oxygenation may deteriorate with upper abdominal surgery or increased intra-abdominal pressure
- Minimize postop sedation

Extubation

- Extubate as soon as patient maintains normocapnia and responds to command
- Consider close monitoring after extubation

Adjuvants

- Initial dose of induction agent and narcotics calculated on a mg/kg basis and muscle relaxants calculated on estimated lean body mass

- Subsequent doses of sedatives, hypnotics, relaxants, and narcotics calculated on estimated lean body mass
- Regional anesthesia if physically possible and if patient can use accessory muscles to help with breathing

Postoperative Period

- Some think epidural or any narcotic indicated and others think they are relatively contraindicated unless patient continuously monitored
- Extended respiratory monitoring is mandatory
- Stabilize ABGs to levels adequate for the individual patient
- Pain control necessary. PCA acceptable in sleep apnea, but not in continuous mode

ANTICIPATED PROBLEMS/CONCERNS

- Resp insufficiency and pneumonia postop
- Postop thromboembolic phenomena

SLEEP APNEA, OBSTRUCTIVE

Charles Ahere, M.D.
Claude Brunson, M.D.
Michael F. Roizen, M.D.

RISK

- People within USA: 0.5–3% of whole population
- Gender predominance: males > females: 2/1
- Race with highest prevalence: not known

PERIOPERATIVE RISKS

- Increased risk of pulm HTN, RV failure, systemic HTN
- Some patients may be polycythemic and have an increased risk of CVA
- Complications associated with obesity
- Increased risk in supine position of sudden arrest postop

WORRY ABOUT

- Airway obstruction with sedating drugs: need for awake, sitting intubation without sedation if obstructs when supine
- Increased sensitivity to sedating drugs
- Difficult airway management: mask ventilation and intubation
- Aspiration risk in morbidly obese
- Postop airway obstruction or resp depression
- Nasal obstruction from NG tubes, e.g., may lead to resp compromise

OVERVIEW

- Apnea refers to cessation of airflow at the mouth for >10 sec.
- Sleep apnea: repetitive episodes of upper airway occlusion during sleep, often with oxygen desaturation to 85%, nearly always associated with loud snoring. Episodes of apnea often terminate with a snort or gasp.
- Upper airway obstruction from relaxation of muscles of orophanyx.
- Frequent periods of apnea lead to hypoxia and hypercarbia, which could lead to cor pulmonale.
- Polycythemia may result from chronic hypoxia.
- Nocturnal cardiac arrhythmias are common.
- Monitoring of depth and quality of sleep along with cardiopulmonary variables in those with severe symptoms.
- Other name is pickwickian syndrome associated with morbid obesity (see also under Morbid Obesity).

ICD-9-CM Codes: 780.57, 278.0 (Morbid obesity)

ETIOLOGY

- Cessation of airflow due to complete obstruction of upper airway
- Narrowing due to enlarged tonsils, adenoids, uvula, low soft palate, or craniofacial abn superimposed upon coexistent abnormalities of upper airway muscle tone and/or neurologic control
- Obesity exacerbates upper airway obstruction.
- Structural abn such as tonsillar hypertrophy, enlarged tongue, and micrognathia may contribute to airway obstruction

USUAL TREATMENT

- Weight loss in overweight patients
- Avoidance of alcohol and sedatives before sleep
- Nasal CPAP
- Physical aids such as devices to detect and prevent snoring, keep patient off back while sleeping (e.g., tennis ball sewn on nightshirt)
- Nasopharyngeal or oropharyngeal airway
- Uvulopalatopharyngoplasty
- Tracheostomy in extreme cases
- Electrophrenic pacing for central sleep apnea

ASSESSMENT POINTS

SYSTEM	EFFECT	ASSESSMENT BY HX	PE	TEST
HEENT	Obstructive apnea	Snoring; partner gives Hx of patient's awakening with grunts at night	Visualization of uvula and tonsillar pillars	
CV	HTN	Dyspnea at rest and on exertion Poor exercise tolerance	Rapid respiratory rate ↑ BP, cardiomegaly	ECG; ECHO
RESP	Right heart dysfunction Restrictive dysfunction	Snoring; partner gives Hx of patient's awakening with grunts at night DOE	Venous engorgement, rales: S_3 and S_4, cardiomegaly	Pulse oximetry on room air while supine ECG, CXR, ABGs, Hct, polysomnogram
GI	Hepatic dysfunction Full stomach NIDDM	Angina Jaundice, bleeding disorders, ascites Heartburn; hiatus hernia Polydipsia, polyuria	Hepatomegaly, ascites, spider angiomas, jaundice	LFTs, PT, PTT Fasting glucose
ENDO	Obesity Hypothyroidism Acromegaly		Mental function Reflexes BMI	Free T_4 estimate TSH level; GH eval
HEME	Polycythemia		Plethoric clubbing; cyanosis	Hypoxemia Hct
CNS	Disturbed sleep Memory problems Irritability	Daytime sleepiness Complaints of disrupted sleep		Polysomnogram

Key Reference: Connolly LA: Anesthetic management of obstructive sleep apnea patients. J Clinical Anesth 1991; 3(6) pp 461–469.

PERIOPERATIVE IMPLICATIONS

Preoperative Preparation

- Avoid sedatives
- Assess CV status
- Histamine H_2 blockers, metoclopramide, and antacids for morbidly obese patients
- Regional anesthesia if possible

Monitoring

- Routine
- Volume status if RV dysfunction present
- Consider arterial catheter if BP cuff doesn't fit or takes too long to inflate

Airway

- Airway obstruction with induction—see HEENT

- Awake intubation in those with potentially difficult airway
- Consider elevating shoulders on bolsters

Induction

- Airway obstruction
- Exacerbation of pulm HTN by hypoxemia and hypercarbia

Maintenance

- Volume status may change precipitously with position change
- Oxygenation may deteriorate with upper abdominal surgery or increased abdominal pressure

Extubation

- Only when patient fully awake
- Airway obstruction from residual anesthetics
- Avoid opioids and sedatives

- Monitor for airway obstruction and apnea.

Adjuvants

- Very sensitive to CNS depressant drugs.

ANTICIPATED PROBLEMS/CONCERNS

- Airway obstruction at induction and after extubation
- 13% risk of perioperative complications especially of pneumonia; avoided by minimal sedation, appropriate pain control, early ambulation
- Worsening pulm HTN and right heart failure
- Aspiration risk in morbidly obese
- Postop thromboembolism
- Poor motivation resulting in poor ambulation. Avoided by intensive preop teaching and postop coaching

SPASMODIC TORTICOLLIS

Peter S. Staats, M.D.

RISK

- Incidence within US: 1/100,000
- Race with highest prevalence: Caucasian
- Affects young women more frequently than men: 1.6/1.0
- Average age of onset between 40–50 y

PERIOPERATIVE RISKS

- Morbidity related to airway difficulty

WORRY ABOUT

- Airway difficulties due to hypertrophy of sternocleidomastoid and splenius capitis muscles
- Associated with jaw dystonia leading to involuntary jaw closure (trismus), jaw opening, lateral deviation of vocal cords (adductor spasmodic torticollis)
- Associated with cervical spine injuries or toxicities from various drugs
- Theoretical risk of increased K^+ release with depolarizing muscle relaxants if Rx with extensive botulism toxin injections due to denervation injury

OVERVIEW

- Second most common dystonia, characterized by sustained muscle contractions causing twisting and repetitive movements or abnormal posture resulting in sustained abnormal head postures.
- May result from basal ganglia dysfunction

ICD-9-CM Code: 333.83

ETIOLOGY

- Idiopathic
- Status post cervical trauma
- Drug-induced, e.g., neuroleptics, antiemetics (metoclopramide)
- Brain lesions, metabolic and neurodegenerative disorders

USUAL TREATMENT

- Medical: anticholinergic drugs, benzodiazepines, muscle relaxants, anticonvulsants
- Intervention: botulinum toxins (provides 3–4 mo relief), and neurosurgical stabilization and/or ablative procedures
- Avoid inciting agents

ASSESSMENT POINTS

SYSTEM	EFFECT	PE
HEENT	Hypertrophy of neck muscle	ROM of neck Abnormal phonation
RESP	Associated adductor spasmodic torticollis Restrictive lung disease	Have patient phonate
GI	Liver dysfunction: associated Wilson's disease	
ENDO	Can be associated with thyroid dysfunction (both hypo- and hyperthyroid reported) or Wilson's disease	
CNS	Wilson's disease	Kayser-Fleischer rings Serum ceruloplasmin
MS	Impaired joint mobility due to development of contractures Associated hemidystonia in ipsilateral arm	

Key Reference: Jankovic J, Brin MF: Therapeutic uses of botulinum toxin. NEJM 1991; 324:1186–1194.

PERIOPERATIVE IMPLICATIONS

Preoperative Preparation

- Consider perioperative botulinum toxin injection

Monitoring

- Placement of invasive lines can be difficult because of associated hemidystonia

Airway

- Assess ability to ventilate and intubate
- Rule out cervical spine pathology

Preinduction/Induction

- Routine

Maintenance

- Nondepolarizing muscle relaxants can lead to improved ability to ventilate and secure an airway

Extubation

- Consider inability to clear secretions from associated cranial nerve pathology

Adjuvants

- Avoid use of neuroleptics in patients who have demonstrated a hypersensitivity.

Postoperative Period

- Routine

ANTICIPATED PROBLEMS/CONCERNS

- Development of contractures from longstanding dystonia. After patient is maximally relaxed, ability to ventilate and visualize cords during intubation can be compromised.
- Associated cervical spine instability
- Inability of patient to communicate concomitant disorders
- Can be confused with akinetic disorders (parkinsonian syndromes) or other hyperkinetic movement disorders (tremor, choreoathetosis, myoclonus, asterixis)
- Placement of monitors can be compromised owing to dystonia.

SUBCLAVIAN STEAL SYNDROME

Jackie Martin, M.D.
Dolores Njoku, M.D.

RISK

- Uncommon entity with a variably reported clinical significance
- 3:1 male:female preponderance

PERIOPERATIVE RISKS

- Stroke from a plaque originating from vertebral artery system

WORRY ABOUT

- Worsening neurologic symptoms

OVERVIEW

- Variant of cerebrovascular insufficiency
- Occlusion of subclavian or innominate artery proximal to vertebral artery results in reversal of flow from ipsilateral vertebral artery into distal subclavian
- Left subclavian involved more than right
- Frequently asymptomatic
- CNS ischemia precipitated by exercise of ipsilateral arm or plaques from vertebral artery system
- Arm claudication precipitated by exercise of ipsilateral arm
- Symptoms may be obscured by concomitant carotid insufficiency

ICD-9-CM Code: 435.2

ETIOLOGY

- Atherosclerosis, primarily
- Rare causes include congenital atresia of first portion of left subclavian, or stenosis of left subclavian at old suture site of a coarctation repair

USUAL TREATMENT

- Surgical
  – Common carotid to subclavian artery bypass
  – Subclavian to subclavian artery bypass graft
  – Axillary to axillary artery bypass graft

ASSESSMENT POINTS

SYSTEM	ASSESSMENT BY HX	PE	TEST
CV	Claudication	Bruit	Difference in brachial systolic BP of at least 30 mmHg. Bruit at base of neck or supraclavicular area on affected side.
CNS	Vertigo Rarely cortical visual disturbances, ataxia, syncope, dysarthria		Retrograde catheter Angio
MS	Paresis/paresthesias		See CV

Key Reference: Mannick J: Subclavian steal syndrome. *In* Sabiston D (ed): Textbook of Surgery, 14th ed. Philadelphia, WB Saunders, 1991, p 1584.

PERIOPERATIVE IMPLICATIONS

Preoperative Preparation

- Bilateral upper extremity BP in patients undergoing surgery characterized by large variations in hemodynamic status or in patients with previous internal mammary-coronary bypass grafts

Monitoring

- Consider arterial catheterization since BP maintenance may be essential for cerebral perfusion
- Consider CVP monitoring and/or PA catheterization if contributing factors in patient

Maintenance

- Consider maintaining arterial BP and heart rate near preop levels to facilitate cerebral perfusion

Extubation

- None

Postoperative Period

- Neurologic evaluation at end of surgery

ANTICIPATED PROBLEMS/CONCERNS

- Patients with internal mammary grafts may experience a similar syndrome of coronary-subclavian steal: there is a gradient in systolic brachial blood pressure of 60 mmHg. Myocardial ischemia occurs in such situations that is refractory to medical management. Assessment points and perioperative implications are as stated above but also include myocardial protection concerns

SUBPHRENIC ABSCESS

Duane K. Rorie, M.D.
Ronald P. Kufner, M.D.

RISK

- Prior abdominal surgery
- Blunt trauma
- Immunocompromised patient
- Malignancy

PERIOPERATIVE RISKS

- Developing or impending sepsis
- Multiorgan failure
- Coagulopathy
- High morbidity and mortality (>30% mortality in some series) associated with multiorgan failure

WORRY ABOUT

- Resp compromise, including ARDS
- High cardiac output state leading to LV failure
- Septic shock
- Renal insufficiency or failure
- Electrolyte and acid/base disturbances
- High capillary permeability
- Hyper- or hypoglycemia

OVERVIEW

- Suspect with unexplained fever
- May be left-sided, right-sided, or both; above or below the liver or spleen
- Associated findings include atelectasis, pleural effusions, elevated diaphragm; ipsilateral shoulder pain or hiccups may reflect diaphragmatic irritation
- Fistulas may form to any abdominal or thoracic organ, including pericardium or bronchi
- Classic findings of fever, leukocytosis, and abdominal pain may be attenuated by antibiotic or immunosuppressive therapy
- Severity of disease may range from mild to moribund

ICD-9-CM Code: 567.2

ETIOLOGY

- *Primary:* Associated with perforated viscus such as in duodenal ulcer, diverticulitis, appendicitis, primary liver abscess, immunocompromised state
- *Secondary:* Following surgical procedure or blunt abdominal trauma
- *Causative Organisms:* Often mixed flora, usually anaerobic bacteria

USUAL TREATMENT

- Broad-spectrum antibiotics
- Percutaneous or surgical drainage of abscess
- Supportive therapy

ASSESSMENT POINTS

SYSTEM	EFFECT	ASSESSMENT BY HX	PE	TEST
CV	*Early:* Hyperdynamic state, high cardiac output associated with low SVR *Late:* Septic shock, low output associated with high SVR, LV dysfunction		Tachycardia Bounding pulses Warm, ruberous skin Tachycardia Diminished pulses Cool integument Peripheral cyanosis	ECG CVP *or* PA catheter ECG PA catheter ECHO
RESP	Atelectasis, elevated diaphragm, pleural effusion, abdominal distention, pain, or ARDS ↓ Diaphragm excursion	Dyspnea Ipsilateral shoulder pain	Tachypnea Cyanosis ↓ or abnormal breath sounds, dullness to percussion	CXR; fluoroscopy ABGs
HEME	Anemia due to suppressed marrow Coagulopathy associated with sepsis	Lack of energy	Pallor Oozing around old incisions or IV sites Petechiae Ecchymoses	Hgb, Hct Plt count PT/APTT Fibrinogen, FSPs, D-dimer Thromboelastogram
GU	↓ Perfusion due to hypovolemia or sepsis		↓ UO	BUN, Cr Lytes Acid/base
CNS	Mental status changes associated with sepsis		Range from mild confusion to coma	Must exclude other possible causes (e.g., CVA, CNS infection)

Key Reference: Van der Sluis RF: Subphrenic abscess. Surg Gynecol Obstet 1984; 158:427.

PERIOPERATIVE IMPLICATIONS

Preoperative Preparation

- Antibiotics
- Restore intravascular volume
- Optimize resp function—consider PEEP, thoracentesis, bronchodilators
- May require vasopressors or inotropes

Monitoring

- Tailor to severity of illness

Airway

- Rapid-sequence induction or awake fiberoptic intubation

Preinduction/Induction

- Titrate agents to severity of disease

Extubation

- May require prolonged mechanical ventilation

Postoperative Period

- Monitor progress; may be recurrent, drainage may have been incomplete
- Analgesia will be important for adequate resp function

SUPRATENTORIAL BRAIN TUMORS

Robert F. Bedford, M.D.

RISK

- 35,000 US adults diagnosed with primary brain tumors annually (increasing in rate considerably since 1950)

PERIOPERATIVE RISKS

- Presenting symptoms: seizures, neurologic deficit/dementia
- Endocrinopathy/visual deficits if pituitary tumor

WORRY ABOUT

- Seizure medications: Dilantin, Tegretol
  - Need adequate levels to avoid postop seizures

- Brain edema: may lead to herniation
  - Dexamethasone Rx may lead to hyperglycemia
  - Hyperglycemia may cause more retractor-induced ischemic injury to adjacent brain tissues
- Endocrinopathy, particularly diabetes insipidus if near pituitary

OVERVIEW

- Portion of brain superior to tentorium cerebelli
- Majority of intracranial surgeries
- Frequently metastatic lesions; pulmonary and GI most common

ICD-9-CM Code: 239.6 (Tumor, brain)

ETIOLOGY

- Many supratentorial tumors are lung or GI tumor metastases
- Brain edema surrounding malignant tumors causes initial Sx; often improve initially after corticosteroids
- Seizures due to local neuronal irritation

USUAL TREATMENT

- Dexamethasone for initial Sx
- Diagnostic extirpation/biopsy
- Radiation/gamma knife
- Chemotherapy
- Surgery

ASSESSMENT POINTS

SYSTEM	EFFECT	ASSESSMENT BY HX	PE	TEST
CV	CHF, ASCVD Age effect	DOE, edema, angina	Gallop, rales, jugular distention	CXR, ECG, ECHO, scan
RESP	COPD, primary tumor with cerebral metastases	Dyspnea, cough, sputum	Signs of COPD	FEV_1, FVC (if indicated) ABGs CXR
ENDO	Iatrogenic Cushing syndrome due to Decadron	Improved level of consciousness	Cushingoid appearance	Glucose levels
HEME	Anemia	Occult GI bleeding caused by tumor	Pale conjunctiva, positive occult fecal blood	Hct, Hgb
CNS	Seizures Somnolence	Headache, confusion	Papilledema Hemiparesis	MRI, CT
PNS	Hemiparesis	Clumsiness	Weakness	Nerve transmission

Key Reference: Bedford RF: Supratentorial tumors. *In* Smith DC, Cottrell JE (eds): Anesthesia and Neurosurgery, 3rd ed. St. Louis, Mosby-Year Book, 1994, pp 307–321.

PERIOPERATIVE IMPLICATIONS

Preoperative Preparation

- Level of consciousness evaluation: Is patient candidate for awake stereotaxic surgery?
- Is there elevated ICP to start with?
- Dexamethasone: May lower ICP initially, but ICP on knee of curve at time of operation
- Head scan report:
  - Temporal lobe lesion with impending herniation?
  - Massive peritumor edema with shift of midline?
  - May want to treat more as a head-trauma case than an elective case
- Antiseizure meds adequate? Beware postop seizure

Monitoring

- Consider arterial line: BP control, frequent ABGs, glucose
- End tidal CO_2 as rough guide only, rely on $PaCO_2$
- ICP:
  - If lumbar CSF drains are used, connect to transducer
  - Fiberoptic ICP monitors for postop measurement
  - Optimize hyperventilation, mannitol Rx
  - Diagnostic if patient slow to awaken from anesthetic
- NMB: ↑ receptor density in paretic extremities gives false twitch data: use nonparetic arm/leg

Airway

- None

Preinduction/Induction

- Induction with agents that act to ↓ cerebral blood flow
- Opioids prn to avoid hemodynamic responses early on
- Avoid ↑ BP with intubation/head pins
- Avoid brain swelling due to venous outflow occlusion: do not permit overflexion or rotation of neck
- Goggles: Eye protection while face covered by drapes, instruments

Maintenance

- Recheck $PaCO_2$, especially with COPD
- Mannitol: 0.5–1 mg/kg: empirical or prn?
- No painful structures below dura: Minimal anesthetic requirement with brain manipulation; low-dose inhalation agent and/or propofol infusion
- N_2O:
  - Suspected antiprotective effect
  - ↑ CBF can usually be overridden by hyperventilation
- Allow temp to ↓ spontaneously to ~34°C.

Extubation

- Awake: Normocarbia, early neuro assessment
  - Risk of coughing, straining, possible hematoma formation
  - Perhaps ↑ postop HTN
- Deep: Avoids coughing, maybe HTN
  - Transient $PaCO_2$ about 50 mmHg until patient awakens
  - Use only if no brain edema during craniotomy

Adjuvants

- Muscle Relaxants
  - Profound paralysis: may minimize need for inhalation agents
  - Monitor NMB on nonparetic extremity to avoid confusion due to increased cholinergic receptor density
- Regional Drugs
  - Expect hemodynamic effects from epinephrine in local infiltrated into scalp incision site
- Drug Interactions
  - Expect to use more nondepolarize NMB if patient taking Dilantin, most other antiseizure medications
- Vasoactive Compounds
  - Postop HTN common
  - Consider treatment with labetalol, enalaprilat
  - Consider avoiding cerebral vasodilators: hydralazine, sodium nitroprusside

ANTICIPATED PROBLEMS/CONCERNS

- Postexcision brain swelling; seizures
- Postop arterial HTN

SUPRAVENTRICULAR TACHYCARDIA (TACHYARRHYTHMIAS)

John L. Atlee, M.D.

RISK

- SVT has a paroxysmal (PSVT) or gradual onset/termination (sinus tachycardia, automatic and multiform atrial tachycardia—AAT, MAT). Distinction important for treatment.
- Aside from congenital heart disease or mitral valve prolapse, no special predilection to PSVT
- AAT ($\pm$ AV block) rare in adults, except with digitalis toxicity, hypokalemia, alkalosis
- AAT causes up to 20% of SVT in children but has no special associations.
- MAT is common in critically ill patients with chronic pulmonary disease.

PERIOPERATIVE RISKS

- Circulatory compromise or myocardial ischemia with tachycardia
- Frequent episodes of sustained PSVT/AAT/MAT can cause irreversible cardiomyopathy.

WORRY ABOUT

- Status of CV, pulm, other major systemic disease with MAT.
- Status of digitalization, K^+ and Mg^{2+} balance, and alkalosis in patients with AAT

OVERVIEW

- Aside from adverse effects of tachycardia, PSVT confers no special perioperative risks.
- Sudden AFib/flutter and very rapid ventricular rates (> 250 bpm) with Wolff-Parkinson White (WPW) or Lown-Ganong-Levine (LGL) syndrome
- With AAT/MAT, concern is with associated cardiomyopathy and other systemic disease.

ICD-9-CM Code: 427.89

ETIOLOGY

- PSVT, especially WPW or LGL syndromes, may have a congenital predilection.
- Most (80–90%) PSVT due to AV node $\pm$ accessory pathway re-entry; SA node and atrial re-entry account for 10–15% and ~5%, respectively; structural heart disease is required.
- AAT and MAT are acquired automatic or triggered arrhythmias, except for AAT in children.

USUAL TREATMENT

- PSVT: drugs that increase conduction/refractoriness in atrioventricular node, atria, or accessory pathways
- AAT: amiodarone, sotalol, and class 1C antiarrhythmics (flecainide) may suppress some AAT.
- MAT: β-blockers and Ca-channel blockers may suppress MAT; other antiarrhythmics mostly ineffective.
- Cardioversion or pacing will terminate PSVT but not AAT or MAT.

ASSESSMENT POINTS

SYSTEM	EFFECT	ASSESSMENT BY HX	PE	TEST
CV	Arrhythmia	Palpitations, dizziness, fatigue, failure to thrive (infants/young children), dyspnea, angina, syncope	Regular pulse (PSVT, AAT), irregular pulse (MAT), signs of CHF, diaphoresis	ECG, Holter monitoring Exercise ECG, cardiac electrophysiologic study
	LV function	Exercise intolerance, CHF	S_3, rales, wheezes	CXR, ECHO,
	Ischemia	Sx of angina		scintigraphy, coronary angio
RESP	CHF, COPD	Dyspnea, orthopnea, cough	S_3, rales, wheezes	CXR, PFT
GI	↓ Perfusion	GI distress, diarrhea		
RENAL	↓ Perfusion	Polyuria		BUN/Cr

Key Reference: Atlee JL: Arrhythmias and Pacemakers. Philadelphia, WB Saunders, 1996.

PERIOPERATIVE IMPLICATIONS

Preoperative Preparation

- PSVT: adenosine, esmolol, or edrophonium on hand; also procainamide if WPW or LGL patient
- AAT: check for digitalis toxicity; is there K^+, Mg^{2+}, or acid-base imbalance?
- MAT: optimize cardiopulmonary and metabolic status, treat infections or other pathophysiology

Monitoring

- ECG with ST-T trending; strip-chart recorder
- Consider direct arterial and PA catheter monitoring

Induction

- With cardiomyopathy or LV dysfunction, there is added risk of hypotension during induction.
- AAT and MAT: caution with drugs that increase heart rate (ketamine, pancuronium, desflurane)

Maintenance

- Volatile anesthetics should oppose PSVT but have little effect on AAT/MAT.
- Prophylactic β-blockers may be useful in patients with AAT/MAT during surgical stimulation.

Extubation

- At ↑ risk for tachyarrhythmias during emergence as a result of sympathetic hyperactivity
- Use drugs/means to reduce/avoid effects of airway stimulation and hyperdynamic circulation
- Consider prophylactic use of β-blockers (if tolerated) for patients with AAT and MAT

Adjuvants

- With AAT or MAT, avoid or use caution with sympathomimetic or histamine-releasing drugs.

Postoperative Period

- Attention to adequate sedation and pain control will reduce likelihood of PSVT
- AAT and MAT are suppressed by treatment of precipitating condition and with β-blockers.

ANTICIPATED PROBLEMS/CONCERNS

- In patients with WPW or LGL syndrome, be prepared to treat AFib/flutter with rapid ventricular rate or ventricular fibrillation (DC cardioversion/defibrillation).
- DC cardioversion is not effective for treatment of AAT/MAT and may cause worse arrhythmias.

SWALLOWING DISORDERS

Shiroh Isono, M.D.

RISK

- 10+% of elderly individuals have an absent gag reflex
- Patients with bulbar paralysis of any etiology

PERIOPERATIVE RISKS

- Malnutrition and dehydration due to inadequate oral intake
- Presence of pneumonia due to chronic aspiration
- ↑ Risk of aspiration pneumonia postop
- ↑ Retained bronchial secretions

WORRY ABOUT

- Aspiration pneumonia

OVERVIEW

- Condition usually associated with impairment of any part of swallowing reflex arc, such as sensory receptors in pharynx and larynx, afferent nerves, CNS, efferent nerves, muscles
- High risk for aspiration pneumonia pre- and postop can be evaluated by video fluoroscopy
- Associated with abnormal hygiene of upper and bronchial airways

ICD-9-CM Code: 787.2 (Dysphagia)

ETIOLOGY

- Depressed CNS by sedation, sleep, coma, or light anesthesia
- Neuromuscular disorders such as polymyositis, progressive muscular dystrophy, multiple sclerosis, myasthenia gravis, Eaton-Lambert syndrome
- Regional anesthesia to upper airway
- Tracheostomy or prolonged ET intubation; surgery on the head and neck
- Precurarization
- Peripheral nerve disorders such as Guillain-Barré syndrome, acute porphyria, laryngeal nerve injury; parkinsonism; advanced age

USUAL TREATMENT

- Control for underlying disorders if possible
- Cricopharyngeal myotomy sometimes indicated
- Nasogastric balloon tube reported useful

ASSESSMENT POINTS

SYSTEM	EFFECT	ASSESSMENT BY HX	PE	TEST
HEENT	Aspiration	Cough	Check gag reflex Chest exam	Videofluoroscopy
CV	Dehydration		Skin, orthostatic vital signs	UO
RESP	Pneumonia	Dyspnea, sputum production	Fever	CXR, ABG
GI	Dysphagia GE reflux	Salivation Repeated pneumonia Heartburn	UA inspection Laryngeal movement	Fluoroscopy, manometry CT, MRI, endoscopy
CNS	Cranial nerve IX or X or others dysfunctional	Eating/swallowing pattern	Cranial nerve examination	

Key Reference: Nishino T: Swallowing as a protective reflex for the upper respiratory tract. Anesthesiology 1993; 79:588–601.

PERIOPERATIVE IMPLICATIONS

Preoperative Preparation

- Control underlying disorders and complications (pneumonia, dehydration)
- Correct malnutrition and dehydration by tube feeding, gastrostomy, or parenteral alimentation
- Consider metoclopramide or domperidone as a part of preop medication to Rx prolonged retention of stomach contents
- H_2 blocker to decrease effects of silent regurgitation due to use of anticholinergic drug
- Avoid deep sedation

Monitoring

- Routine

Airway

- Tracheal intubation with cuffed ET tube
- Suction of secretions above the tracheostomy tube
- Do not apply local anesthetics to upper airway

Preinduction/Induction

- Rapid induction/intubation of trachea after cricoid pressure
- Avoid precurarization, possibly leading to severe dysphagia or pharyngeal obstruction

Maintenance

- Minimize NMB

Extubation

- Aspirate stomach contents and clear the oronasal cavity before extubation
- Eliminate or reverse residual anesthetics and muscle relaxants before extubation
- Check recovery of swallowing reflex

Possible Drug Interactions

- Light sedation may impair swallowing reflex
- Precurarization and residual muscle relaxants can severely impair swallowing
- Possible synergetic effect of low concentration of enflurane and vecuronium on impairment of upper airway muscles
- Regional anesthesia impairs other upper airway protective reflex (closure of the larynx, cough reflex)

Postoperative Period

- Fowler position if possible
- Prophylax and/or treat N/V
- Evaluate for presence of aspiration pneumonia

ANTICIPATED PROBLEMS/CONCERNS

- Aspiration pneumonia (chemical or infectious)

SYNDROME OF INAPPROPRIATE ANTIDIURETIC HORMONE SECRETION (SIADH)

Philippa Newfield, M.D.

RISK

• Increased in patients who have cancer, pneumonia, intracranial disorders

PERIOPERATIVE RISKS

• Increased risk of neurologic dysfunction: altered level of consciousness, seizures, coma from hyponatremia and cerebral swelling
• Risk of volume overload and CHF

WORRY ABOUT

• Volume overload
• Hyponatremia
• Changing level of consciousness, seizures, coma
• Neurologic complications of overly rapid correction of hyponatremia (central pontine myelinolysis or osmotic demyelination syndrome, cerebral hemorrhage) with behavioral disturbances, seizures, pseudobulbar palsy, quadriparesis

OVERVIEW

• ADH normally released in response to 1–2% ↑ in serum osmolality or 7% ↓ in intravascular volume
• SIADH is characterized by sustained endogenous release of ADH or ADH-like substances in the absence of physiologic stimuli to ADH release
• Serum sodium is reduced, urinary sodium is increased, and urine is hyperosmolar relative to plasma
• Results primarily in water retention with excretion of non–maximally dilute urine in the face of hyponatremia
• Patients reach a volume-expanded steady state in which output equals input
• ADH is released in cranial disorders because of direct hypothalamic stimulation

ICD-9-CM Codes: 259.3 (Ectopic); 259.6 (neuro-hypophysial)

ETIOLOGY

• Disease states
  – Pulmonary disease
  – Cancer
  – Cranial disorders (head trauma, skull fractures, subdural hematomas, brain tumors, infections of CNS)
  – Myxedema
  – Acute intermittent porphyria
  – Stress situations (emotional upheaval)
• Drug-induced ADH release
• Drug-induced enhancement of ADH effect on collecting ducts
• Drugs that mimic action of ADH in renal tubules
• Exogenously administered ADH
  – DDAVP for perioperative hemostasis
• Postop with impaired water secretion and hypervolemia

USUAL TREATMENT

• Water restriction to 800–1000 ml/d for plasma [Na⁺]>120–125 mEq/L
• Diuretics (furosemide)
• Replace urinary sodium losses with 0.9% saline
• 3.0% hypertonic saline if [Na⁺] < 115–120 mEq/L at a rate of 1–2 ml/kg/h to increase [Na⁺] by 1–2 mEq/L/h and to bring [Na⁺] to 125 mEq/L (or ≤ 12 mEq/L in 24 h or 25 mEq/L in 48 h)
• Hemodialysis
• Demeclocycline (dimethylchlortetracycline) and lithium
• Thyroid hormone replacement

ASSESSMENT POINTS

SYSTEM	EFFECT	ASSESSMENT BY HX	PE	TEST
CV	CHF	Dyspnea on exertion, Paroxysmal nocturnal dyspnea	Peripheral edema, gallop JVD, weight gain	
RESP	CHF	Dyspnea on exertion, Paroxysmal nocturnal dyspnea	Bibasilar rales	CXR
GI	Hyponatremia	Nausea, anorexia, vomiting		
RENAL	Dilutional hyponatremia ↓ Serum osmolality ↑ Urine osmolality ↓ Urine output Normal hydration	↓ Urine output	No edema	Urine osmolality >300–400 mOsm/kg Urine [Na⁺] >25–30 mmol/L Plasma [Na⁺] <130 mEq/L Serum Osm <280 mOsm/kg Low Cr, albumin Low BUN, uric acid
CNS	Brain swelling from ↑ extracellular and intracellular brain water Depletion of brain electrolytes	Lethargy, weakness, somnolence Mental confusion, seizures Personality changes Coma	Areflexia, weakness, altered level of consciousness	[Na⁺] <120 mEq/L
MS	Hyponatremia→changes in action potential	Cramps Muscle weakness	Skeletal muscle weakness	

Key Reference: Matjasko MJ: Multisystem sequelae of severe head injury. *In* Cottrell JE, Smith DS (eds): Anesthesia and Neurosurgery, 3rd ed. St. Louis, Mosby, 1994, pp 697–698.

PERIOPERATIVE IMPLICATIONS

Preoperative Preparation

• Correction of hyponatremia
• Discontinuation of drugs enhancing or mimicking action of ADH or increasing secretion of ADH
• Treatment of underlying disorder (e.g., hypothyroidism, pneumonia)

Monitoring

• PA or CVP catheter for large fluid shift operations or patients who have signs of LV dysfunction
• Intraoperative serum sodium concentration and osmolality
• Urinary output

Airway

• None

Preinduction/Induction

• May develop volume overload with fluid administration
• Avoid drugs known to lower seizure threshold

Maintenance

• Avoid hypotonic fluids
• Limit stress response, which may increase ADH secretion
• Limit drugs that induce ADH release (morphine, barbiturates, β-adrenergics)
• Limit total fluids if patient has received DDAVP or other ADH analogues

Extubation

• Period of risk for patients who have CHF

Adjuvants

• 0.9% saline, 3.0% saline, furosemide

Postoperative Period

• Monitor serum sodium concentration and osmolality closely, especially in day-surgery patients who have received DDAVP
• Monitor urine sodium concentration and osmolality
• Monitor volume status and urinary output
• Treat postop hypervolemia and hyponatremia

ANTICIPATED PROBLEMS/CONCERNS

• Symptoms of acute hyponatremia are more severe than those of chronic hyponatremia for same plasma sodium concentration
• Free water losses (renal, skin, GI) must exceed free water intake to ↑ serum sodium concentration
• Acute water intoxication is a medical emergency

SYNDROME X

Jonathan Moss, M.D., Ph.D.

RISK

- True incidence unknown, but occurs commonly in Europe
- Postmenopausal or posthysterectomy women most often at risk
- Most common cause of chest pain in women with angiographically normal coronary arteries

PERIOPERATIVE RISKS

- Acute withdrawal of sex hormone replacement for reasons of ↑ coagulation (thrombophlebitis risk) can potentially lead to coronary vasospasm

WORRY ABOUT

- Women on hormone replacement may be subject to acute vasospasm upon withdrawal
- Estrogen patches or therapy may be useful in alleviating chest pain

OVERVIEW

- Clinical example relating chronic sex hormone status to acute vascular responsiveness to estrogen.
- First described by Kemp (1973) but includes exertional angina, positive exercise test, and angiographically normal coronary arteries.

ICD-9-CM Code: 413.9

ETIOLOGY

- Impairment of vasodilator reserve in peripheral and coronary vessels due to estrogen deficiency
- Estrogen appears to act as Ca^{2+} channel antagonist at high doses and facilitates nitric oxide effects on coronary endothelial cells at low doses
- Acute withdrawal of estrogen appears to be more significant factor than chronic withdrawal.

USUAL TREATMENT

- Estrogen patch has been found to significantly improve exercise tolerance

ASSESSMENT POINTS

SYSTEM	EFFECT	ASSESSMENT BY HX	PE	TEST
CV	Myocardial ischemia	Exertional angina, prior hysterectomy, acute withdrawal of estrogen, physical examination, and flushing		Normal coronary angiogram in presence of chest pain without Prinzmetal's angina or valvular heart disease
SKIN	Vasodilation seen during menopause also seen in this syndrome. Migraine headache may occur coincidentally.		Flushing	17ß-estradiol levels are lowest and angina most frequent and severe during luteal phase of menstrual cycle.

Key Reference: Egashira K, et al.: Evidence of impaired endothelium-dependent coronary vasodilation in patients with angina pectoris and normal coronary angiograms. N Engl J Med 1993; 328:1659–1664.

PERIOPERATIVE IMPLICATIONS

Perioperative Preparation

- Estrogens are withdrawn because of possible thrombophlebitis. Patients with this syndrome may experience significant angina upon such withdrawal.
- Distinguish chest pain due to this syndrome from chest pain due to coronary insufficiency from other causes.

Monitoring

- ST segment analysis

Preinduction/Induction

- Contingent upon type of surgery; may consider maintaining estrogen therapy. No data as to effects on preinduction and induction and maintenance of anesthesia

ANTICIPATED PROBLEMS/CONCERNS

- Occurs most commonly in postmenopausal or posthysterectomy women (4× greater incidence than that of age-match population); successfully treated with exogenous estrogen. A major concern may be that acute discontinuation of estrogen may lead to coronary vasoconstriction. Vessels may still dilate in presence of IV nitroglycerin, but with a Hx of menopausal flushing and coincident chest pain clinicians should weigh risks and benefits of continued estrogen therapy versus withdrawal.

SYSTEMIC LUPUS ERYTHEMATOSUS
David M. Robinson, M.D.

RISK

- Average incidence 1/1000; 1/250 high-risk populations
- Females >> males
- African-American >> Caucasian
- Majority diagnosed at age 30–40: 20% diagnosed as children

PERIOPERATIVE RISKS

- N/V, abdominal pain
- Vasculitis, pancreatitis, lupoid hepatitis
- Endocarditis (nonbacterial), myocarditis, thrombophlebitis
- Precipitation of relapse related to surgery not uncommon

WORRY ABOUT

- Pituitary-adrenal chronic steroid suppression

- Antibiotic prophylaxis if valvular disease present
- Restrictive PFTs with A-a gradient and effusions
- Lupus nephritis and renal insufficiency
- Splenomegaly, thrombocytopenia
- Lupus anticoagulant may be present
- Thrombosis and hemorrhage
- Neuropathy, confusion, psychosis

OVERVIEW

- Multisystem disease requiring evaluation of each organ system
- 10 y survival is 90%
- Fibrinoid substances are deposited in multiple tissues, causing inflammation. Development of thrombocytopenia, anemia, leukopenia, and decreased complement heralds relapses.

- Drugs that can precipitate relapse include procainamide, hydralazine, phenytoin, penicillin, isoniazid

ICD-9-CM Code: 710.0

ETIOLOGY

- Unknown
- Autoimmune process possibly following trauma to mast cells and association with an X chromosome factor

USUAL TREATMENT

- Aggressive treatment limited to therapy during relapses and prevention of exacerbations. Treatments include rest, steroids, salicylates, azathioprine, cyclosporine, plasmapheresis

ASSESSMENT POINTS

SYSTEM	EFFECT	ASSESSMENT BY HX	PE	TEST
CV	Pericarditis Endocarditis Myocarditis CHF, conduction blocks	Chest pain Palpitations	Pericardial friction rub Murmur Effusion Diastolic noncompliance	ECG CXR ECHO
RESP	Infiltrates Restrictive PFTs ↑ A-a gradient Atelectasis	Pleuritic chest pain Dyspnea Cough Hemoptysis	Friction rub Effusion Cyanosis Normal peak flow	CXR PFTs ABGs
GI	Perforated viscus Pseudo-obstruction Liver congestion Lupoid hepatitis	N/V Peritonitis and pancreatitis Abdominal pain Ileus	Dilated loops of bowel Peritoneal free air Hepatomegaly Jaundice	GI series LFTs Bilirubin A/G ratio
HEME	Hemorrhage infrequent Thromboembolism Anemia	Bruising Thrombosis	Lymphadenopathy Splenomegaly Anemia	CBC Plt count PT/PPT
RENAL	Glomerulitis Nephrotic syndrome Renal insufficiency Renal failure	Polyuria Oliguria Hematuria Fever	Costophrenic tenderness Edema	Urinalysis Renal US Renal scan BUN, Cr, TP, albumin
CNS	Confusion Hallucinations Psychoses Seizures	Paranoid states Hyperirritability Numbness Hemiparesis	Psychosis Nystagmus, ptosis, diplopia Aphasia Peripheral neuropathy	EEG CT scan Neuro and psychiatry evaluations
MS and SKIN	Vasculitis and ulceration Symmetric arthritis Joint immobility Aseptic necrosis	Photosensitivity Atrophic or scarred area Ecchymosis or purpura Joint pain or immobility	Malar or butterfly rash Perioral ulcerations Reduced ROM Hip pain	Hip x-rays ANA

Key Reference: Peck M: The patient with systemic lupus erythematosus. *In* Frost EAM (ed): Preanesthetic Assessment 3. Boston, Birkhauser, 1991, pp 179–189.

PERIOPERATIVE IMPLICATIONS

Preoperative Preparation

- Stress steroid dose if on chronic steroid therapy. Hydrocortisone 100 mg IV q 6–8 h prior to induction and tapered as stress reduces over several days

Monitoring

- Consider arterial line for blood gases; consider PA catheter for pulmonary HTN
- Consider arterial line and PA line if evidence of CHF
- Foley cather and careful titration of fluid replacement (consider CVP/PA catheter) if renal involvement

Airway

- Occasionally reduced TMJ ROM and narrowed larynx with immovable arytenoids
- Consider fiberoptic intubation

Maintenance

- No specific agents indicated or contraindicated. Regional acceptable if no coagulopathy.
- If renal insufficiency present, avoid renally excreted drugs and renal toxins.

Adjuvants

- Corticosteroids, supplemental O_2, careful titration of fluids with renal involvement.

Extubation/Postoperative Period

- Reassess respiratory, renal, CV status prior to extubation

ANTICIPATED PROBLEMS/CONCERNS

- Pituitary-adrenocortical axis suppression
- CHF and arrhythmias
- Resp insufficiency and nephritis
- Renal function and volume management
- CNS dysfunction, seizure, neuropathy
- Thrombosis and abnormal coagulation tests
- Vasculitis injury, especially GI tract
- Fulminant hepatitis

TETANUS

Roy D. Cane, M.B., B.Ch.

RISK

- Incidence in US: 60–80 cases/y
- Female of any age; males >50 y and African-Americans from rural South

PERIOPERATIVE RISKS

- Focal/generalized muscle spasms occurring spontaneously or in response to external stimuli
- Autonomic nervous system instability
- Case mortality rate in USA is 30%

WORRY ABOUT

- Autonomic nervous system instability
- Toxic myocarditis
- Resp failure due to muscle spasms or treatment
- Inadequate bronchial hygiene

OVERVIEW

- An exotoxin, tetanospasmin, produced by *Clostridium tetani,* enters CNS by intraneuronal transport via peripheral nerves and inhibits release of γ-aminobutyric acid and glycine, resulting in disinhibition of motor and autonomic nervous system
- Characterized by muscle rigidity with intermittent, usually generalized, spasms; localized spasms of muscle groups close to site of skin penetration

ICD-9-CM Code: 037

ETIOLOGY

- Infection of deep penetrating wounds with anaerobic spore–producing organism, *C. tetani.*

USUAL TREATMENT

- Primary infection treated by debridement of wound and high-dose penicillin therapy (tetracycline or erythromycin if penicillin-allergic)
- Neutralization of circulating toxin by single dose of human tetanus immune globulin
- Spasms controlled by heavy sedation and/or neuromuscular relaxation or blockade
- Ventilatory and nutritional support as needed

ASSESSMENT POINTS

SYSTEM	EFFECT	ASSESSMENT BY HX	PE	TEST
HEENT	Rigidity of masseter and cervical muscles	Dysphagia, excessive salivation, drooling	Limitation of mouth opening and ROM of neck	
CV	Toxic myocarditis		Hypotension	ECG
RESP	Hypoventilation, diminished bronchial hygiene	Poor cough, SOB	Limited chest excursion, ↓ breath sounds, rhonchi	ABG, CXR
CNS	Autonomic nervous system overactivity	Flushing, palpitations	Fluctuating BP with episodic HTN arrhythmias	ECG
MS	Generalized or localized rigidity and spasms	Stiffness, painful muscle spasms	Rigidity, spasm leading to opisthotonos and risus sardonicus	

Key Reference: Groleau G: Tetanus. Emerg Med Clin 1992; 10:351–360.

PERIOPERATIVE IMPLICATIONS

Preoperative Preparation

- Adequate sedation with benzodiazepines or control of generalized spasms by NMB with vecuronium or atracurium
- Consider avoiding pancuronium because of potential for ANS stimulation

Airway

- Masseter and cervical muscle rigidity and spasms can make intubation difficult. If patient not already intubated, consider fiberoptic intubation
- Elective tracheostomy recommended for long-term support of ventilation and bronchial hygiene

Induction

- None. Most patients will already be heavily sedated or intubated with NMB

Maintenance

- Usually GA with inhalational anesthetic agents and NMB has been described
- Monitor for ANS overactivity. Consider adding continuous spinal/epidural anesthesia for controlling ANS overactivity.

Postoperative Period

- Usually managed in ICU. Maintain intubation, NMB, sedation, mechanical ventilatory support
- Provide nutritional support via nasoenteric feeding
- Continue surveillance and therapy of ANS overactivity
- Observe for toxic myocarditis manifesting as S-T segment and T-wave changes on ECG and hypotension due to drug therapy
- Hypotension with bradycardia, indicative of brainstem involvement, associated with very poor prognosis

ANTICIPATED PROBLEMS/CONCERNS

- Extremes in BP, arrhythmias, cardiac arrest may occur
- Morphine, magnesium sulfate, β-blockers are used to control ANS overactivity
- Propranolol and [?] labetalol associated with ↑ risk of sudden cardiac arrest

TETRALOGY OF FALLOT

Winnie Y. Ruo, M.D.

RISK

- 2/10,000 live births
- 15% of infants with congenital heart disease
- Race with highest prevalence: equal

PERIOPERATIVE RISKS

- Risk of "Tet spell" if unrepaired
- Mortality in tetralogy of Fallot (TOF) repair: 6–8%
- ↑ Mortality if coexisting PA hypoplasia

WORRY ABOUT

- Avoid increases in PVR resulting in ↑ right-to-left shunt
- Avoid ↓ in SVR resulting in ↑ right-to-left shunt
- Crying and agitation leading to "Tet spell" resulting in more hypoxemia, hypercarbia, acidosis
- Air bubbles in IV tubing
- Polycythemia and associated thrombocytopenia
- RV failure after inadequate repair
- Residual VSD causing difficulty in separation from CPB
- May need temporary pacemaker after repair because of AV conduction system injury

OVERVIEW

- Anatomy
  - RV outflow tract obstruction
  - Infundibular narrowing
  - Pulm valve stenosis
  - PA hypoplasia
  - VSD: May be single or multiple
  - Overriding aorta
  - RV hypertrophy
  - 5% have anomalous origin of LAD from right coronary artery
- Degree of right-to-left shunting determined by fixed factors (degree of infundibular obstruction, size of pulmonary valve annulus, size of PA) and reactive factors (PVR and SVR)
- Avoid hypoxia, acidosis, high airway pressures, excitement, agitation
- 96% 10 y survival after complete repair
- Dx by ECHO and cardiac catheterization

ICD-9-CM Code: 745.2

USUAL TREATMENT

- Palliative shunts to increase pulmonary blood flow (Blalock-Taussig shunt, aortopulmonary shunts)
- Surgical repair consists of RV outflow tract enlargement, closure of VSD, PA conduits
- β-blockers to decrease infundibular spasm
- Treatment of "Tet spell"
  - 100% O_2
  - Propranolol
  - Bicarbonate to correct metabolic acidosis
  - Phenylephrine to ↑ SVR
  - Sedation
  - Squatting to ↑ SVR
  - Aortic compression by abdominal pressure to ↑ SVR

ASSESSMENT POINTS

SYSTEM	EFFECT	ASSESSMENT BY HX	TEST
CHEST			CXR with dominant RV, concave PA segment
CV	See Overview: Anatomy	Frequency and severity of "Tet spells"	ECHO/cath ECG-RVH, RA
HEME	Polycythemia from chronic hypoxemia Plt count may be low from polycythemia		Hct, plt count

Key Reference: Lake CL: Pediatric Cardiac Anesthesia, 2nd ed. Norwalk, CT, Appleton & Lange, 1993, pp 243–252.

PERIOPERATIVE IMPLICATIONS

Preoperative Preparation

- Heavy premedication to avoid agitation, crying

Monitoring

- Arterial line to monitor blood gases
- Central line for drugs and right-sided pressures
- TEE to assess adequacy of repair

Airway

- None

Induction

- Avoid ↑ in PVR and ↓ in SVR
- Consider IM ketamine if no IV present

Maintenance

- Avoid high-dose inhalational agents to maintain stable SVR
- Narcotics may be used

Separation from CPB after Tetralogy Repair

- Measure ratio of RV to LV pressures to judge adequacy of repair. If ratio <0.8, repair adequate. If RVP > LVP, need RV patch
- Ventilation
  - Avoid high airway pressures
  - Keep Pa_{CO_2} 30–35 mmHg
  - Keep pH 7.5
- May need to ↓ PVR pharmacologically (nitroglycerin, dobutamine, amrinone, phentolamine, PGE_1)
- May need temporary pacemaker if AV conduction system injury

ANTICIPATED PROBLEMS/CONCERNS AFTER COMPLETE REPAIR

- Intraoperative "Tet spell"
- RV failure
- Residual VSD
- Arrhythmias

THALASSEMIA

David Francisco, M.D.
Ronald S. Litman, D.O.

RISK

- People in USA with severe disease: 1000
- 3–5% incidence among people of Mediterranean, African, or Asian descent

PERIOPERATIVE RISKS

- High-output CHF common with severe anemia
- Iron loading from chronic therapy can result in diabetes, adrenal insufficiency, liver dysfunction, coag abn, hypothyroidism, hypoparathyroidism, arrhythmias, intractable cardiac failure
- Hypersplenism can result in thrombocytopenia and ↑ risk of infection

WORRY ABOUT

- Difficult airway 2° to maxillary deformation
- Cardiac arrhythmias or CHF
- Coagulopathy

OVERVIEW

- Diverse group of microcytic anemias characterized by absence or ↓ synthesis of normal globin chains of Hgb (α, β, δ and γ). Decrease or absence of α or β chains most common.
- Beta thalassemia major, Cooley's anemia (homozygous)
  – Absent β chain synthesis. Results in severe anemia requiring aggressive intervention. Median survival 31 y
- Beta thalassemia minor (heterozygous)
  – Clinical manifestations range from asymptomatic to mild anemia, depending on severity of β chain deficiency. Usually does not require intervention.
- Thalassemia intermedia (heterozygous)
  – Results in milder from of anemia than homozygous type. May require transfusion therapy for aplastic crisis or folate deficiency or when hypersplenism occurs
- Alpha thalassemia
  – Four α genes: two on each chromosome 16
  – One gene deletion = silent carrier
  – Two gene deletion = α thalassemia minor—mild microcytic anemia

– Three gene deletion = α thalassemia major—severe hymolytic anemia due to formation of unstable β globin tetramer (Hgb H). Most complications 2° to iron overload, which results from compensatory GI absorption and chronic transfusion therapy
– Four gene deletion = hydrops fetalis—incompatible with life. Absent Hb F replaced with Hb Barts (γ tetramer). Intrauterine death from high-output CHF and tissue anoxia

ICD-9-CM Code: 282.4

ETIOLOGY

- Deletions of point mutations of one or all of the α and/or β globin genes.

USUAL TREATMENT

- Supportive transfusions and folate replacement for mild forms
- Chronic transfusions and iron chelation therapy for major forms
- Splenectomy when indicated
- Bone marrow transplantation in selected patients

ASSESSMENT POINTS

SYSTEM	EFFECT	ASSESSMENT BY HX	PE	TEST
HEENT	Prominent maxilla and malar eminences, frontal bossing		Airway examination	
CV	CHF, arrhythmias, pericarditis, effusion	DOE Orthopnea PND Palpitations	Rales Rub S₃ gallop	ECG ECHO
RESP	Restrictive defects, small airway obstruction	Poor exercise tolerance	Wheezing	CXR
GI	Liver dysfunction cholelithiasis	RUQ pain	Hepatomegaly	LFTs
ENDO	Diabetes, hypothyroid, hypoparathyroid	Polyuria, polydipsia, cold intolerance, growth retardation		Glucose Ca²⁺ TSH
HEME	Coagulopathy, mild to severe anemia	Bleeding or bruising	Splenomegaly	Plt count Hgb, PT/PTT
RENAL	Enlarged kidneys	Dark brown urine (heme products)		UA

Key Reference: Giardina PJ, Hilgartner MW: Update on thalassemia. Pediatr Rev 1992; 13:55–62.

PERIOPERATIVE IMPLICATIONS

Preoperative Preparation

- Search for coexisting conditions
- Careful airway evaluation

Monitoring

- Routine
- Consider invasive hemodynamic monitors if CHF

Airway

- May have distorted anatomy 2° to extramedullary hematopoiesis; may need awake and/or fiberoptic intubation

Preinduction/Induction

- Hemodynamic compromise with induction agents if low cardiac reserves

Maintenance

- Routine care; depends on organ system involvement

Extubation

- Awake if difficult intubation

Adjuvants

- Will depend on organ system involvement (e.g., hepatic insufficiency)

ANTICIPATED PROBLEMS/CONCERNS

- Difficult intubation
- Regional anesthesia contraindicated if coagulopathy exists
- Potential cardiac disease including pericardial effusion

THROMBOCYTOPENIA

Nauder Faraday, M.D.

RISK

- Common in both adults and children, especially in critical illness
- Often associated with systemic illness and pathologic conditions of pregnancy

PERIOPERATIVE RISKS

- May lead to massive bleeding

WORRY ABOUT

- Excessive perioperative bleeding
- Concurrent anemia or hypovolemia
- Concurrent hemodynamic instability from hypovolemia or infection
- Implications of specific drug therapies and potential for anesthetic interaction
- Implications of pregnancy
- Concurrent liver disease

OVERVIEW

- Definition: <150,000 plt/mm^3
- Spontaneous bleeding does not generally occur unless the plt count <20,000/mm^3

- Adequate surgical hemostasis achieved with plt counts between 50,000–100,000/mm^3, depending upon site and extent of procedure
- Generalized petechiae, purpura, and bleeding from mucous membranes denotes high risk of bleeding from other sites
- Dx of cause of thrombocytopenia is key to successful treatment; begins with CBC, PT/PTT, fibrinogen, and D-dimer
- Bleeding time has not been shown to correlate with risk of surgical bleeding

ICD-9-CM Code: 287.5

ETIOLOGY

- ↑ Plt destruction, immune: drug-induced, idiopathic thrombocytopenia purpura (ITP), rheumatologic disorders, post-transfusion purpura, neonatal immune thrombocytopenia
- ↑ Plt destruction, nonimmune: infection with or without overt DIC, preeclampsia/HELLP syndrome, thrombotic thrombocytopenic purpura (TTP), hemolytic-uremic syndrome (HUS)

- ↓ Plt production
- Marrow failure: cancer infiltration, chemo- or radiation therapy, ethanol
- Hypersplenism: cirrhosis, portal or splenic vein thrombosis
- Dilution: generally plt counts maintained until intravascular replacement >1.5–2 blood volumes

USUAL TREATMENT

- Treat underlying cause:
  – Discontinue offending drug, antibiotics for infection, splenectomy
  – Immunologically mediated syndromes generally respond to corticosteroids and IgG therapy
  – TTP and HUS may respond to plasmapheresis or to corticosteroids and IgG
- Decision to transfuse plts depends on etiology of thrombocytopenia and relative risks of bleeding vs risks of transfusion
- Each unit of transfused plts should raise count ~10,000/mm^3 if there has not been immediate plt destruction, sequestration, or dilution, but increases risk of future thrombocytopenia (alloimmunization occurs in 50% of patients transfused with plts)

ASSESSMENT POINTS

SYSTEM	EFFECT	ASSESSMENT BY HX	PE	TEST
HEENT	Mucosal hemorrhage		Petechiae, purpura, and ecchymoses of skin, oral mucosa, and conjunctiva	
CV	Hypovolemia, anemia, hemorrhagic pericardial effusion	Lightheadedness, syncope, palpitations	Vital signs, orthostasis, pericardial friction rub, pulses paradoxus	ECG, CXR
RESP	Pulm hemorrhage	Cough, hemoptysis		CXR
GI	GI bleeding	Hematemesis, hematochezia, melena		Stool guaiac
RENAL	Potential prerenal or renal azotemia, glomerulonephritis with specific disease entities	UO		BUN, Cr, urinalysis
CNS	Intracranial hemorrhage	Change in mental status	Neuro exam: mental status, focal findings	Head CT

Key Reference: Warkentin TE, Kelton VG: In Colman RW (ed): Hemostasis and Thrombosis. Basic Principles and Clinical Practice, 3rd ed. Philadelphia, JB Lippincott, 1994, pp 469–488.

PERIOPERATIVE IMPLICATIONS

Preoperative Preparation

- Assess volume status and Hct
- Qualitative assessment of bleeding risk from physical exam, extent of thrombocytopenia, type of surgical procedure
- Ensure that blood bank has adequate cross-matched PRBCs and plts available
- Plt transfusion immediately prior to surgical procedure for plt count <50,000/mm^3
- dDAVP 0.3 μg/kg IV beneficial only in patients with concurrent renal failure or von Willebrand's disease

Monitoring

- Routine
- Plt count

Airway

- ↑ Risk of mucosal bleeding demands gentle laryngoscopy—lubrication of ET and laryngoscope blade may be helpful
- Nasal intubation relatively contraindicated

Induction

- None

Maintenance

- ↑ Risk of blood loss makes vigilance to volume status and replacement essential

Extubation

- Airway trauma/bleeding can occur with extubation

Adjuvants

- Regional: Epidural and spinal anesthetics can be safely administered with plt counts ≥100,000/mm^3. Risk of bleeding increases as the plt count falls below this level, although relationship is not linear. A few dozen cases of epidural anesthesia in patients with plt counts <100,000/mm^3 have been reported by retrospective review without neurologic sequelae

ANTICIPATED PROBLEMS/CONCERNS

- Excessive perioperative bleeding
- Physical exam, plt count, type of surgical procedure are best predictors of bleeding risk

THYROID NEOPLASMS

Alisa C. Thorne, M.D.

RISK

- In the US: 11,300 new thyroid cancer cases/y; 8300 female; 3000 male
- Hispanics, African-Americans—lower rate; Caucasians—moderate rate; Japanese, Chinese, Hawaiian, Filipinos—higher rate
- Overall incidence 2–3 times higher in women than in men, but varies with age group

PERIOPERATIVE RISKS

- Large thyroid mass may produce airway compression, deviation, or vocal cord paralysis
- ↓ BP, ↓ HR, asystole with manipulation carotid sinus
- Postop complications: phrenic n. injury, pneumomediastinum, pneumothorax, tracheomalacia and tracheal collapse post extubation, hematoma or laryngeal edema→airway compromise; bilat laryngeal n. injury→tracheostomy; superior laryngeal n. injury→aspiration
- Accidental removal/injury of parathyroid glands causes ↓ Ca^{2+}

WORRY ABOUT

- Occult pheochromocytoma: bilateral lobe medullary thyroid cancer is associated with MEN IIA and IIB

OVERVIEW

- 4 types—papillary, follicular, medullary, undifferentiated
- Prognosis of well-differentiated papillary cancer excellent, especially for age <40 y with small tumors
- Prognosis worsens for large tumors with poorly differentiated, anaplastic histology
- Age at Dx and distant metastases: important prognostic factors

ICD-9-CM Code: 193

ETIOLOGY

- Factors include previous radiation, dietary iodine deficiency, goitrogens (chemical or dietary), pre-existing benign thyroid disease, and genetic factors (Gardner's syndrome, Cowden's disease)
- Increased incidence thyroid cancer found in women with breast cancer but relationship unclear

USUAL TREATMENT

- Surgery initial therapy of choice
- Lobectomy with or without isthmectomy, near-total or total thyroidectomy as indicated
- Radical debulking procedure (palliative) for large tumors invading airway and causing esophageal obstruction and bleeding
- Combined chemo- and radiation therapy for poor prognosis cases
- Doxorubicin: only agent with activity; medullary thyroid cancer responds poorly

ASSESSMENT POINTS

SYSTEM	EFFECT	ASSESSMENT BY HX	PE	TEST
HEENT	Vocal cord dysfunction Tracheal obstruction	Dysphonia SOB, DOE Wheeze/stridor	Neck mass	Indirect laryngoscopy CXR
CV	Mediastinal mass	SOB, DOE Wheeze, may be asymptomatic	Facial swelling	CXR CT/MRI
RESP	Lung metastases Lower airway obstruction	SOB, DOE Wheeze, hemoptysis		CXR CT/MRI
GI	Esophageal obstruction Liver metastases	Dysphagia		LFTs
ENDO	MEN IIA/IIB Pheochromocytoma	HTN, especially episodic Flushing Palpitations, episodic Sweating		CT/MRI 24 h urine epinephrine ↑ epinephrine/norepinephrine
	Hyperparathyroidism			↑ Ca^{2+} Hypercalciuria
	Ganglioneuromatosis	Colic Cramping Diarrhea Obstruction	Mucosal neuromas in tongue, subconjunctival areas, or GI tract Thickened lips Marfanoid features	Provocative test for calcitonin release
MS	Bone metastases PTH-induced bone disease	Bone pain		Bone scan

Key Reference: Falk SA (ed): Thyroid Disease: Endocrinology, Surgery, Nuclear Medicine, and Radiotherapy. New York, Raven Press, 1990, Ch 28, 29.

PERIOPERATIVE IMPLICATIONS

Preoperative Preparation

- Assess thyroid gland/tumor size
- Assess larynx/trachea compression
- May need smaller or armored ETT to prevent kinking
- Record description of voice preop
- Correct abnormal Ca^{2+}, TFTs prior to surgery
- Check serum calcitonin level if medullary cancer suspected; rule out pheochromocytoma

Monitoring

- Routine

Airway

- Anticipate difficult airway

Induction

- Consider awake fiberoptic intubation for large thyroid masses

Maintenance

- No one agent or technique shown superior
- CV instability may occur with manipulation of carotid sinus

Extubation

- May develop tracheomalacia
- May require reintubation owing to hematoma

Postoperative Period

- Metabolic: ↓ Ca^{2+}, hypoparathyroidism
- Nonmetabolic: unilateral or bilateral n. injury, hemorrhage, airway obstruction

Adjuvants

- May be performed under local anesthesia with IV sedation in selected cases

ANTICIPATED PROBLEMS/CONCERNS

- Patients with medullary thyroid cancer: rule out occult pheochromocytoma

TRANSFUSION-RELATED ACUTE LUNG INJURY

Christine Rinder, M.D.

RISK

• All patients receiving packed RBC, plt, FFP, CRYO, or whole blood
• Incidence probably <1%, but being recognized with increasing frequency, probably because of greater awareness by clinicians

PERIOPERATIVE RISKS

• Noncardiogenic pulm edema within 2–6 h after transfusion
• Mortality reported, but rare

WORRY ABOUT

• Oxygen toxicity
• Barotrauma
• Should be suspected from signs of pulm edema after transfusion when little clinical suspicion of volume overload

OVERVIEW

• Classic presentation is acute development of respiratory compromise indistinguishable from ARDS 2–6 h after transfusion. Sx include acute hypoxemia, bilateral pulm edema (noncardiogenic), fever, possible hypotension.
• Dx one of exclusion (rule out fluid overload, CHF, sepsis)

ICD-9-CM Code: 999.8 (transfusion, complication)

USUAL TREATMENT

• Supportive care: oxygen, pressure support. No clear indications for steroids. Generally resolves within 1–4 d with appropriate care and no supervening complications

ASSESSMENT POINTS

SYSTEM	EFFECT	ASSESSMENT BY HX	TEST
CV	Normal		PA catheter, ECHO
RESP	Pulm edema	Recent transfusion	CXR—bilateral infiltrates
HEME	Leukoagglutination		Agglutination of recipient leukocytes by donor plasma: contact blood collection agency

Key Reference: Popovsky MA, Chaplin HC, Moore SB: Transfusion-related acute lung injury: A neglected, serious complication of hemotherapy. Transfusion 1992; 32:589–592.

PERIOPERATIVE IMPLICATIONS

Perioperative Concerns

• Acute respiratory compromise that may occur shortly after transfusion in healthy patient, but more typically 2–4 h after transfusion

Monitoring

• PA catheter may aid in the exclusion of cardiac etiology

Airway

• Most require ventilatory support for several days
• Ventilator management appropriate for ARDS

ANTICIPATED PROBLEMS/CONCERNS

• Oxygen toxicity and barotrauma

TRANSVERSE MYELITIS

John A. Ulatowski, M.D.

RISK

- Incidence 1–1.7/1 million population

PERIOPERATIVE RISKS

- Few data available (usually grouped with multiple sclerosis)
- Anesthetic effect (worsening) unknown
- Sequelae of hypotension or HTN (dysautonomia)
- Urinary retention and UTI

WORRY ABOUT

- Autonomic dysfunction (midthoracic and above)
  - Acute: hypotension from spinal shock
  - Chronic: HTN, bradycardia from mass reflex
- Hyperkalemia from succinylcholine

OVERVIEW

- Inflammatory disease of spinal cord causing demyelination/necrosis
- Ascending paralysis and sensory level usually T8–12 associated with pain and urinary retention
- Spinal cord swelling; ↑ CSF protein, WBC 10–200 (higher if culture positive)
- Onset over hours to days
- Antecedent febrile illness (33%)
- Variable recovery
- Multiple sclerosis (other demyelinating lesions) occurs in 5–10% cases

ICD-9-CM Code: 323.9 (Encephalitis, unspecified cause)

ETIOLOGY

- Viral (polio, HSV, HIV)
- Bacterial, fungal, parasitic
- Noninfectious (postinfectious, postvaccine, lupus)

USUAL TREATMENT

- High-dose steroids
- Long-term antibiotics if frequent UTI

ASSESSMENT POINTS

SYSTEM	EFFECT	ASSESSMENT BY HX	PE	TEST
HEENT	Eyes (MS, Devic's syndrome)	↓ Visual acuity	Optic neuritis, ophthalmoscope	Visual EPs
CV	↑ BP, ↓ BP	Syncope, headache	BP changes	Orthostasis
RESP	Pulm embolism	Dyspnea, tachycardia	DVT, cord sign	Doppler, V/Q scan
GI	Gastric atony	N/V, dyspepsia, early satiety	Tympany, CXR	Stomach bubble
CNS	Brain Spine	Encephalitis presenting symptoms	Mental status changes Paraplegia	MRI MRI, LP
RENAL	Bladder paralysis	Retention, oliguria	Palpation, catheterization	UA, residual

Key Reference: Jones RM, Healy TEJ: Anaesthesia and demyelinating disease. Anaesthesia 1980; 35:879–884.

PERIOPERATIVE IMPLICATIONS

Preoperative Preparation

- Relieve gastric ileus

Monitoring

- Routine

Airway

- Avoid succinylcholine

Induction

- Adequate hydration because of dysautonomia

Maintenance

- GA or epidural; spinal with caution, possible toxicity with usual doses

Extubation

- Return of airway reflexes if demyelinating lesions in brain/brainstem

Adjuvants

- Resistance to nondepolarizing muscle relaxants

ANTICIPATED PROBLEMS/CONCERNS

- Unstable hemodynamics
- Possible hyperkalemia following succinylcholine

TREACHER COLLINS SYNDROME

Daniel Siker, M.D.
James Armstrong, M.D.

RISK

- People within USA: 1/8000–10,000 live births

PERIOPERATIVE RISKS

- Difficult airway management from mandibular dysostosis

WORRY ABOUT

- Difficult intubation
- Risk of obstructive sleep apnea or death postop
- Difficult mask induction of anesthesia

OVERVIEW

- Form of mandibulofacial dysostosis characterized by hypoplasia of mandible, maxilla, and malar bones as well as bilateral deformities of pinnae and lateral downward sloping of palpebral fissures
- Pharyngeal hypoplasia, esp. in lateral diameter and to lesser extent in AP dimension
- Dimensions of pharynx are reduced by hypoplastic facial bones. Base of tongue may have narrowest opening.
- Hyoid bone displaced anteriorly and inferiorly

ICD-9-CM Code: 756.0

ETIOLOGY

- Autosomal dominant with variable expressivity
- First branchial arch defect (Franceschetti syndrome) caused by loss of blood supply to area during 3rd and 5th wk of development

USUAL TREATMENT

- Operations include tympanoplasty, cleft lip and palate repair, palatoplasty

ASSESSMENT POINTS

SYSTEM	EFFECT	ASSESSMENT BY HX	PE	TEST
HEENT	Limited airway	Inspiratory stridor Coughing during feeding Diaphoresis during feeding Snoring	Narrow pharynx	
CV	Cor pulmonale ↑ Association with congenital heart defects	Easy fatigability Chest discomfort	S_3, hepatomegaly ↑ Jugular venous pulsations Heart murmur	ECG: RAE P waves in II, IIIa, VF RAO CXR: RVH ECHO
RESP	Obstructive sleep apnea	Loud nasal snoring Frequent arousal during sleep Daytime hypersomnolence		Polysomnography
CNS	Usually intellectually normal May have learning disability			

Key Reference: Rasch RK, Browder F, Barr M, Greer G: Anesthesia for Treacher Collins and Pierre Robin syndromes: A report of three cases. Can Anaesth Soc J 1986; 33:364–370.

PERIOPERATIVE IMPLICATIONS

Preoperative Preparation

- Preoperative sedation may cause upper airway obstruction
- Antisialagogue may be of benefit

Monitoring

- Communication between surgeon and anesthesiologist

Airway

- Mask ventilation may be difficult. Consider large, clear pliable facial mask
- Consider fiberoptic bronchoscope or Bullard laryngoscope or laryngeal mask airway, tactile guides, or retrograde techniques
- Airway may become more difficult to secure following pharyngeal surgery
- Tracheostomy may be considered for patient requiring multiple procedures

Preinduction/Induction

- Avoid sedatives if obstructive symptoms
- Consider direct laryngoscopy if obstructive symptoms
- Consider deep inhalation induction or ketamine induction with maintenance of spontaneous ventilation during laryngoscopy

Maintenance

- Avoid heavy use of opioids because of postop resp depression

Extubation

- Extubate when fully awake
- Risk of upper airway obstruction and negative pressure pulm edema

Adjuvants

- IV steroids for treatment of edema

Postoperative Period

- Possibility of hypersomnolent state
- Monitor for airway obstruction
- Obstructive sleep apnea
- Post palatoplasty, airway obstruction may be ameliorated by suture through tongue to relieve airway obstruction

ANTICIPATED PROBLEMS/CONCERNS

- Failure to thrive
- Significant hearing loss may be present
- Obstructive sleep apnea
- Cor pulmonale
- Removal of all oral packing

TRICUSPID ATRESIA

Susan C. Nicolson, M.D.

RISK

- Occurs in ~1/10,000 live births
- Third most common cause of cyanotic congenital heart disease
- Slight male predominance

PERIOPERATIVE RISKS

- Sequelae of chronic hypoxemia
- Surgical shunt complications
- Issues unique to patients with univentricular heart undergoing staged reconstructive surgery

WORRY ABOUT

- Associated CV anomalies
- Extracardiac anomalies (GI, musculoskeletal systems)

OVERVIEW

- Congenital cardiac malformation with agenesis of the tricuspid valve resulting in no communication between right atrium and hypoplastic RV
- Survival depends on interatrial communication and L →R shunt at ventricular (VSD) or great vessel (PDA) level
- Types of tricuspid atresia (frequency)
  - Type I—normally related great vessels (70%)
  - Type II—D-TGA (transposition of the great arteries) (30%)
  - Type III—L-TGA (rare)
  Each type further subdivided depending on presence of pulmonic stenosis/atresia and the absence or size of VSD
- Clinical presentation and treatment depend on associated cardiac anomalies that are responsible for pulm blood flow being increased, decreased, or normal

ICD-9-CM Code: 746.1

ETIOLOGY

- Postulated to result from malalignment between ventricular loop and atria

USUAL TREATMENT

- Palliative surgery usually within 1st year of life intended to
  - increase pulm blood flow when it is diminished (small VSD, pulmonary stenosis [PS]) via systemic to PA shunt or systemic venous to pulm anastomosis or
  - decrease pulm blood flow when it is excessive (large VSD) via PA band and/or
    - eliminate major interatrial obstruction
- Ultimate physiologic correction via modification of Fontan's operation

ASSESSMENT POINTS

SYSTEM	EFFECT	ASSESSMENT BY HX	PE	TEST
CV	↓ Pulm blood flow – Hypoxemia – Acidosis ↑ Pulm blood flow		Cyanosis	ABG/ SpO$_2$
	Heart failure	Poor weight gain, frequent URIs	Tachycardia, tachypnea Hepatosplenomegaly	
	Endocarditis Dysrhythmias			ECHO ECG
RESP	Pulm vascular obstructive disease			ECHO ECG SpO$_2$
HEME	Polycythemia			Hgb; Coag tests
CNS	Stroke Brain abscess	Hemiplegia		CT/ MRI

Key Reference: Okanlami O, Nichols DG, Nicolson SC, et al: Tricuspid atresia and the Fontan operation. *In* Nichols DG, Cameron DE, Greely WJ, et al (eds): Critical Heart Disease in Infants and Children. St. Louis, Mosby-Year Book, 1995, pp 737–769.

PERIOPERATIVE IMPLICATIONS

Preoperative Preparation

- PGE$_1$ infusion in neonate with ductal dependent pulm circulation
- Anticongestive measures for rare infant presenting with CHF
- Preanesthetic medication appropriate for age and physical status

Monitoring

- Routine
- Consider intra-arterial and/or central venous catheter when patient condition or procedure indicates

Airway

- Meticulous attention to maintain patency

Preinduction/Induction

- Carefully titrated anesthetic appropriate for age and procedure, taking into consideration physiology of individual patient

Maintenance

- Keep warm
- Maintain euvolemia

Adjuvants

- Consider heparin (100 U/kg) prior to systemic to pulm artery shunt placement

ANTICIPATED PROBLEMS/CONCERNS

- Manipulating physiology through appropriately timed and precisely executed palliative procedures to maximize the potential for the child to ultimately be good candidate for Fontan's procedure

TRIGEMINAL NEURALGIA (TIC DOULOUREUX) Rajakumari V. Asrani, M.D.

RISK

• Trigeminal neuralgia (TN) is a symptom and not a disease.
• 15/100,000 of population are affected. 1–3% of multiple sclerosis (MS) patients have TN.
• 45% of patients are male.

PERIOPERATIVE RISKS

• Carbamazepine and phenytoin used in treatment of TN may cause enzyme induction
• Patients on baclofen requiring GA may have severe bradycardia and hypotension due to unknown mechanism
• Potential for drug abuse with anxiolytic and opioid preparations

WORRY ABOUT

• Side effects of drug therapy
• Worsening MS after surgery
• Airway problems due to associated cranial nerve involvement
• Associated sensory or motor deficits of eyes, face

OVERVIEW

• TN is a common painful condition of the face; peak occurrence in 6th decade. The most common division of cranial nerve V involved, in order of frequency, is mandibular, or 3rd division; combination of mandibular and maxillary, or 2nd division; maxillary and rarely ophthalmic, or 1st division. Pathognomonic features of TN are

– *Pain:* Abrupt onset of paroxysmal, sharp, electric shock–like, brief lancinating pains lasting a few seconds to 1 min. In between flashes, patient is pain-free, 50% have remission lasting 6 mo. TN with MS rarely has spontaneous remission. Pain is unilateral, confined to anatomic pathways of cranial nerve V, brought about by non-noxious stimuli (light touch, cold breeze, talking, vibrations). Pain bilateral in 5% of cases, right > left, and seldom at night. Pain is of burning type, when chronic, and supersedes tic.
– *No neurologic findings*—(NF) in idiopathic TN. Symptomatic TN—abnormal NF. CT scans or MRI yields <5% positive results. 45% of patients show structural abnormalities on posterior cranial fossa surgery (PCFS). Patients with previous ganglion neurolysis may show areas of sensory deficits or other cranial nerve involvement.
– *No pathologic findings post mortem*
– *Trigger zones:* Trigger zones are present on same side of facial pain in 91%. Trigger zones are present in more than one division of the trigeminal nerve, predominantly in central part of face.
• *Recurrence:* In similar areas of face with intervals decreasing over time.

ICD-9-CM Code: 350.1

ETIOLOGY

Idiopathic

• Degeneration of myelin sheath of Vth nerve root over petrous temporal bone
• Compression by aberrant vessel

Symptomatic

• Cancer of maxillary antrum or nasopharynx, tumors of cranial nerves, vascular anomalies, and mass lesions
• Painful paroxysm of TN caused by combination of ↑ afferent activity and ↓ segmental inhibition in delta and C fibers, resulting in excessive response of wide dynamic range neurons to tactile stimulation.

USUAL TREATMENT

• *Pharmacologic*—Carbamazepine (Tegretol), phenytoin (Dilantin), baclofen (Lioresal) are used for TN. Chlorphenesin and mephenesin less commonly used
• *Anesthesiologic*—Mandibular and/or maxillary nerve blocks under fluoroscopy. Glycerol chemical or percutaneous radiofrequency lesioning of trigeminal ganglion under CT scan.
• *Surgical*—Microvascular decompression (MVD) involving posterior cranial fossa surgery.

ASSESSMENT POINTS

SYSTEM	EFFECT
CNS	Assess other cranial nerve involvement and sensory deficit in face, cornea, and areas of dysesthesia; sensory Sx

Key Reference: Barry J, Sessle S: Trigeminal pain: Nociceptive pathways and mechanisms. Pain Digest 1991; 1:78–91.

PERIOPERATIVE IMPLICATIONS

Preoperative Preparation

• Patients on baclofen requiring GA may have severe bradycardia and hypotension due to unknown mechanism. Potential for drug abuse with anxiolytic and opioid preparations

Monitoring

• Monitored anesthesia care for anesthesiologic procedures. For posterior cranial fossa surgery, A-line, CVP, Doppler US, esophageal stethoscope, and end-tidal CO_2 monitor may aid detection and treatment of air embolism and hypotension.

Airway

• Caution if patient has other cranial nerve involvement or MS (assess for intraoperative airway obstruction due to brainstem stimulation)

Induction

• Avoid succinylcholine in patients with MS

Maintenance

• Sitting posture associated with hypotension, air embolism, and hemodynamic instability intraoperatively with posterior cranial fossa surgery. Prevention, early detection, and treatment of hypotension, airway obstruction, and air embolism

Extubation

• Consider for loss of protective reflexes

Adjuvants

• Be prepared to treat bradycardia, hypotension, or air embolism efficiently.
• Carbamazepine and phenytoin used in treatment of TN may cause enzyme induction. These agents may increase dosage requirements of drugs metabolized by cytochrome P-450 such as NM blockers (see under Carbamazepine and Phenytoin)

Postoperative Period

• Consider ventilator support if difficult posterior cranial fossa craniotomy.

TRUNCUS ARTERIOSUS

Chandra Ramamoorthy, F.F.A.R.C.S.
Jeffrey P. Morray, M.D.

RISK

- Rare anomaly, 2.8% of all congenital heart defects
- No gender predilection

PERIOPERATIVE RISKS

- Thrombosis if prolonged NPO
- CHF
- Myocardial depression by volatile anesthetic agents
- Infective endocarditis
- Risks of CPB with 5–25% incidence of neurologic deficits

WORRY ABOUT

- Difficult intubation
- Heart failure
- Hypocalcemia
- Air embolus

OVERVIEW

- Common trunk is the only great artery arising from heart
- Main problems due to pulm overcirculation, volume overload of LV, and pressure overload of RV
- VSD always present
- Obligatory mixing of systemic and pulm venous blood at level of VSD and truncal valve. Degree of cyanosis inversely related to PVR
- Abnormal truncal valve, with regurgitation in 50%, stenosis in a third. Anomalies of coronary artery and aortic arch may be present. These lead to early heart failure
- Early development of pulm vascular obstructive disease due to excessive pulm blood flow
- Stenosis of PA branches limits L→R shunt, limiting CHF and pulm vascular disease
- 26% have DiGeorge anomaly (congenital absence of thymus, parathyroid hypoplasia, great vessel anomaly, micrognathia, low-set ears, short philtrum)

- Without surgical correction, truncus is usually fatal (50% die by 1 m and 80% by 1 y of age)

ICD-9-CM Code: 745.0

ETIOLOGY

- Congenital heart defect arising from partial or complete absence of truncoconal septum. Embryonic truncus fails to separate into a pulm and aortic trunk
- Maternal diabetes predisposes to truncoconal abnormalities

USUAL TREATMENT

- Medical therapy is supportive (digoxin, loop diuretics, afterload reduction) to treat CHF
- Surgical repair is definitive treatment, usually done within 2 m. On CPB, pulm trunk is separated from truncal artery. VSD is closed and an RV-to-PA (Rastelli) conduit is placed.

ASSESSMENT POINTS

SYSTEM	EFFECT	ASSESSMENT BY HX	PE	TEST
HEENT	Difficult laryngoscopy and intubation		Small mandible, small mouth	
CV	CHF—truncal valve regurgitation Pulm HTN	Difficulty feeding Sweating during feeds Failure to thrive	Cyanosis ± single S_2 Murmur—systolic or diastolic	Pulse oximeter, ECG, ECHO
RESP	CHF—excessive pulm blood flow	Difficulty breathing	Tachypnea Retraction	CXR (↑ pulm markings, cardiomegaly)
ENDO	Parathyroid hypoplasia	Seizures, tetany		Serum Ca^{2+}, parathyroid hormone level
IMMUNE FUNCTION	Cellular immunodeficiency	Recurrent infections Chronic diarrhea		CBC, T cell function
MS	Dysmorphic facies		Hypertelorism, low-set ears	

Key Reference: Lake CL: Pediatric Cardiac Anesthesia. Norwalk, CT, Appleton and Lange, 1993, pp 360–363.

PERIOPERATIVE IMPLICATIONS

Perioperative Preparation

- Avoid long NPO as ↑ risk of thrombosis
- Treat CHF with digoxin, afterload reduction, diuretics
- If intubated, adjust to normocapnia and normoxemia unless problems with pulm HTN
- Check electrolytes and Ca^{2+}

Monitoring

- Arterial catheter and CVP
- TEE valuable to assess truncal valve function, VSD patch leak, assess ventricular function, pulm blood flow
- Intraoperative placement of LA line to monitor LV function

Airway

- Laryngoscopy, intubation may be difficult

Preinduction/Induction

- Meticulous air bubble exclusion
- Antibiotic prophylaxis for bacterial endocarditis
- SVR decrease with anesthetic induction may result in hypotension with stenotic truncal valve; SVR decrease in regurgitant truncal valve will ↑ systemic blood flow
- Monitor for myocardial ischemia due to PA runoff; temporary PA band may help

Maintenance

- Narcotic relaxant technique usual
- Deep hypothermia and circulatory arrest or low-flow CPB

Extubation

- Postop ventilation required (resp acidosis will affect pulm blood flow and heart function)

Postoperative Period

- Cardiac failure: poor RV function (right ventriculotomy and Rastelli conduit placement); LV dysfunction (circulatory arrest, long bypass, myocardial ischemia)
- Increased PVR and pulm hypertension (low CO and low SaO_2) responds to hyperventilation, metabolic alkalosis, vasodilators (amrinone, PGE_1, NO), sedation (analgesia, paralysis)
- AV block requiring pacemaker
- Bleeding, tamponade

ANTICIPATED PROBLEMS/CONCERNS

- CHF
- Truncal valve regurgitation and stenosis
- Pulm HTN
- Infective endocarditis

TUBERCULOSIS (TB)

Karen B. Traber, M.D.

RISK

- 8 million cases/y
- Increased risk of exposure to infected adult in homeless, the elderly (especially in nursing homes), minorities, immigrants (especially from Asia and Latin America), and prisoners
- Increased likelihood once infection occurs in HIV co-infection, immunosuppressive therapies, malnutrition, and body wt ≥10% below ideal, infants, and with certain medical (silicosis, diabetes mellitus, carcinoma)

PERIOPERATIVE RISKS

- Depends on pulmonary and systemic dysfunction and type of surgery.
- CDC recommends delay of elective surgery until infected individual has had adequate course of chemotherapy.

WORRY ABOUT

- Co-morbidities of patient, extent of organ system impairment, toxicity of TB therapy

OVERVIEW

- *Mycobacterium tuberculosis* is one of most significant worldwide pathogens, causing estimated 8 million new cases and 3 million deaths each year.
- Number of cases in USA declined prior to 1985 but is now on the rise (poverty, drug and alcohol abuse, HIV infection, immigration of infected persons).

ICD-9-CM Codes: 013-017

ETIOLOGY

- Transmitted by droplet nuclei produced by coughing, sneezing, talking
- Primary and exogenous reinfection now more common than reactivation, especially with HIV.

USUAL TREATMENT

- Six mo of isoniazid plus rifampin, supplemented by pyrazinamide for first 2 mo
- Same therapy used for HIV-positive patients with TB, but for longer duration (at least 9 mo or 6 mo after negative cultures)
- Streptomycin and ethambutol can be used in resistant patients

ASSESSMENT POINTS

SYSTEM	EFFECT	ASSESSMENT BY HX	PE	TEST
GENERAL		Night sweats, wt loss	Fever	PPD (purified protein derivative [tuberculin])
CV	Pericardial effusion, myocarditis, heart block		Muffled heart sounds, friction rub	ECHO, ECG, biopsy
RESP	Apical infiltrates, caseation necrosis, hilar adenopathy	Cough, possible hemoptysis	Often normal	CXR, sputum culture
GI	Peritonitis, enteritis, colitis	Diarrhea, hematochezia	Ascites	Endoscopy, biopsy
GU	Chronic cystitis and epididymitis, pyelonephritis	↑ Urine frequency and urgency when advanced Painless hematuria		Urinalysis and culture
CNS	TB meningitis	Headache, dizziness, confusion		Lumbar puncture for CSF and culture
MS	Long bone and vertebral involvement	Pain		X-ray, bone scan

Key Reference: Bass JB: Tuberculosis. Med Clin North Am 1993; 77:1–447.

PERIOPERATIVE IMPLICATIONS

Preoperative Preparation

- Evaluate for possible toxic response to anti-TB therapy (hepatitis, thrombocytopenia, ototoxicity, optic neuritis, nephrotoxicity, peripheral neuropathy) and extent of organ system involvement
- Restrict spread of organism by removing unnecessary OR equipment, limiting traffic to OR, using disposable equipment, and wearing protective clothing including special surgical mask with tight face seal that prevents penetration of aerosolized particles in 1–5 μm range.
- Use ultraviolet lights (often in old orthopedic OR) as *M. tuberculosis* sensitive to UV radiation

Monitoring

- Depends on extent of systemic involvement and surgical procedure

Extubation

- Restrict exposure of perioperative personnel to aerosolized TB

Adjuvants

- Isoniazid may increase defluorination of volatile anesthetics. Increased plasma fluoride levels in patients on isoniazid after exposure to enflurane anesthesia has been reported.

ANTICIPATED PROBLEMS/CONCERNS

- TB a contagious disease with significant consequence to general public. Drug resistance and patient noncompliance to therapy are major public health problems. Universal infection precautions should be taken when managing patients in high-risk groups.

ULCERATIVE COLITIS, CHRONIC

Jeffrey Dodd-o, M.D.

RISK

• Prevalence in US: 45–80/100,000, with static incidence of 5–10/100,000/y
• Incidence in two peaks: first at age 20–30 y and again at age 60 y
• More common in Caucasians than African-Americans
• Jews > non-Jews
• Nonsmokers > smokers
• About 5–10% have family Hx

PERIOPERATIVE RISKS

• Adrenal insufficiency if preop corticosteroid use
• Infection and delayed wound healing, especially with stress steroids
• Resp compromise from abdominal incision, malnutrition, or associated seronegative spondyloarthropathy (ankylosing spondylitis)

WORRY ABOUT

• If surgery for Sx unresponsive to medical management, more likely to be anemic, dehydrated, malnourished, and with lyte imbalance

OVERVIEW

• Inflammatory reaction limited to mucosal layers of all or part of colon. Results in impaired intestinal absorption, bleeding, and colonic dilation
• Can lead to diarrhea and its complications (dehydration, hypokalemia, metabolic acidosis, malnutrition, hypoalbuminemia), anemia, and impaired colonic motility resulting in distention and perforation
• Pharmacologic adjuncts include sulfasalazine and steroids. Sulfasalazine can lead to hemolytic anemia (which worsens anemia from GI bleeding) and hepatitis. Corticosteroids can lead to uremia and adrenal insufficiency

ICD-9-CM Code: 556.9

ETIOLOGY

• Unknown, though genetics may be contributory

USUAL TREATMENT

• Mild disease—sulfasalazine. Begun at 500 mg bid and increased over 1–2 wk to 2–4 g/d. Can be continued indefinitely. Steroid retention enemas for 4–6 wk may help proctosigmoiditis
• Severe disease—corticosteroids, lyte repletion, parenteral nutrition. Corticosteroids may make abdominal exam unreliable
• Uncontrolled symptoms or threat of malignancy—surgery to remove colon and rectum. Panulcerative colitis has ↑ risk of dysplasia, with malignancy risk as high as 10% per decade

ASSESSMENT POINTS

SYSTEM	EFFECT	ASSESSMENT BY HX	PE	TEST
HEENT	Difficult positioning if associated ankylosing spondylitis	Ankylosing spondylitis		
CV	Hypovolemia Sepsis Aortic regurgitation		Orthostatic vital signs	BUN/ Cr
RESP	Apical fibrosis associated ankylosing spondylitis	Exertional dyspnea		CXR
GI	Bowel obstruction/perforation	Constipation, vomiting		Abd x-ray
HEME	Anemia	Bloody stools	Pale conjunctiva	Hgb
RENAL	Diarrhea	Diarrhea Muscle cramps		Lytes BUN/Cr

Key Reference: McGill DB, Hoffman HN II: Gastroenterology. *In* Kochar M (ed): Concise Textbook of Medicine, 2nd ed. Norwalk, CT, Appleton & Lange, 1990, pp 320–323.

PERIOPERATIVE IMPLICATIONS

Preoperative Preparation

• Fluid resuscitation; consider stress steroids
• Anticholinergics may ↑ risk of toxic megacolon

Monitoring

• Routine; consider UO
• Consider CVP catheter for fluid management

Airway

• Consider full stomach

Maintenance

• If surgery for uncontrolled symptoms, expect large intraoperative fluid requirements
• Technically difficult surgery if abdominal adhesions from prior surgeries
• Potential for progression of underlying sepsis
• Avoid nitrous oxide if intestinal obstruction

Extubation

• Keep warm

Postoperative Period

• Early parenteral nutrition and postop neuraxial analgesia may be beneficial

ANTICIPATED PROBLEMS/CONCERNS

• If prior steroid use, may be addisonian and require supplemental steroids

URINARY LITHIASIS

Terri G. Monk, M.D.

RISK

- Annual incidence of stone disease: 16.4/10,000
- 12% of all individuals will experience calculous disease
- Male:female ratio is 3:1
- Race with highest prevalence: Caucasians. Rare in North American Indians and African-Americans
- Peak incidence: 3rd to 5th decade of life

PERIOPERATIVE RISKS

- Morbidity/mortality very low

WORRY ABOUT

- ↓ Renal function from partial or complete renal obstruction
- Sepsis, possibly septic shock, if surgical procedure performed in presence of UTI
- Perinephric hematoma if bleeding diathesis
- Pregnancy testing of women of child-bearing age because urologic procedures often utilize radiation, and lithotripsy is contraindicated during pregnancy

OVERVIEW

- Urolithiasis refers to abnormal concretions occurring anywhere along collecting system of urinary tract
- Most stones seen in industrialized countries contain calcium oxalate (75%); remainder are composed of uric acid, struvite, or cystine
- If properly treated, urolithiasis does not adversely affect life expectancy
- Calculi <4 mm in diameter usually pass without intervention
- ~20% of stones cause enough symptoms to require surgical removal

ICD-9-CM Codes: 592.0 (Calculus of kidney); 592.1 (calculus of ureter)

ETIOLOGY

- Intrinsic factors: renal tubular acidosis, cystinuria, primary hyperparathyroidism
- Lesch-Nyhan syndrome
- Extrinsic factors: ↑ environmental temperatures resulting in ↑ perspiration and hyperconcentration of urine (Southeast and Southwest regions of U.S.), low-intake drinking habits resulting in low UO, diet rich in calcium, animal fat (uric acid), or leafy vegetables (oxalate), immobility including sedentary occupations

USUAL TREATMENT

- Observation and symptomatic pain Rx until spontaneous passage
- If surgical intervention necessary (20%), choice based on stone size and location

ASSESSMENT POINTS

SYSTEM	EFFECT	ASSESSMENT BY HX	PE	TEST
CV	↑ Heart rate or BP 2° to pain		Tachycardia HTN	
RESP	Grunting respiration during renal colic		Normal chest exam	
GI	Abdominal pain	N/V "Moving irritation" in abdomen	Tenderness to deep palpation of abdomen	
RENAL	Renal colic characterized by pain localizing to affected flank; pain may radiate to groin or abdomen	Sudden onset of flank pain	Flank tenderness to palpation over affected kidney	UA (hematuria)
				Abdominal film (KUB)

Key Reference: Drach GW: Urinary lithiasis: Etiology, diagnosis and medical management. *In* Walsh PC, Retik AB, Stamey TA, Vaughan ED Jr (eds): Campbell's Urology, 6th ed. Philadelphia, WB Saunders, 1992, pp 2085–2156.

PERIOPERATIVE IMPLICATIONS

Perioperative Preparation

- If obese, require acid aspiration prophylaxis and airway evaluation

Monitoring

- Routine
- Temp monitoring during immersion lithotripsy essential because water temp may produce hyperthermia or hypothermia
- Shock waves synchronized to ECG to avoid dysrhythmias

Preinduction

- Adequate padding to avoid nerve damage

Induction

- Many anesthetic techniques employed, but sedation adequate for lithotripsy and minor ureteroscopy procedures

Maintenance

- Central blood volume increases
- May become hypotensive 2° to warm water ↓ SVR
- Vital capacity ↓ and work of breathing ↑
- Pleural effusion or hydropneumothorax may occur during percutaneous renal procedures

Adjuvants

- Visualization of stone may require iodine-containing contrast material
- Anticholinergic agents (atropine) occasionally given to shorten lithotripsy treatments; however, tachycardia can occur, resulting in myocardial ischemia in high-risk patients
- Most patients receive prophylactic antibiotics prior to urinary tract procedures

ANTICIPATED PROBLEMS/CONCERNS

- Allergic reactions in 5% receiving IV contrast media
- Steinstrasse, ureteral obstruction by fragmented calculi, may cause ureteral colic following lithotripsy
- HTN may occur following lithotripsy
- Septic complications occur in 1% after lithotripsy
- Ureteral injury occurs in 9% of ureteroscopy procedures, with 1.6% requiring further surgical intervention

URTICARIA, COLD

Richard R. Bartkowski, M.D., Ph.D.

RISK

• Prevalence is very low (<1/100,000)
• Appears in all races and genders, reported between ages 3 mo–74 y but seen typically at 18–25 y.

PERIOPERATIVE RISKS

• Can develop urticaria or angioedema with skin cooling and rewarming
• Shocklike reactions can occur with whole-body cold exposure
• Cooling with cardiopulmonary bypass can induce symptoms

WORRY ABOUT

• Cold exposure of patient (e.g., cold room, cold fluids, cold instruments or devices to cool skin)

OVERVIEW

• Characterized by appearance of urticaria or angioedema after cold exposure
• Usually acquired condition—seen typically by 18–25 y
• Can be primary or 2° to underlying disease such as malignancy or infection
• Symptoms often last 5–9 y and undergo remission or recede with primary disease
• Diagnosis by cold stimulation test
• Not related to cold serum factors

ICD-9-CM Code: 708.2

ETIOLOGY

• Primary cold urticaria appears related to skin mast cells sensitized to cold by a serum factor, very likely antibodies
• Sensitized skin mast cells (not blood basophils) release histamines on interaction with cold
• Similar activation by cryoglobulins appears in secondary cold urticaria

USUAL TREATMENT

• Antihistamines, both H_1 and H_2, successful at reducing occurrences even for hypothermic cardiopulmonary bypass

ASSESSMENT POINTS

SYSTEM	EFFECT	ASSESSMENT BY HX
SKIN	Urticaria or angioedema	Hx of cold reactions
RESP	Angioedema	Hx of swelling on cold exposure

Key Reference: Wanderer AA: Cold urticaria syndromes: Historical background, diagnostic classification, clinical and laboratory characteristics, pathogenesis, and management. J Allergy Clin Immunol 1990; 85:965–981.

PERIOPERATIVE IMPLICATIONS

Preoperative Preparation

• Antihistamines H_1 and H_2 only if a cold challenge anticipated during surgery

Monitoring

• Temperature, skin condition

Maintenance

• IV fluids; keep room and patient warm

ANTICIPATED PROBLEMS/CONCERNS

• Localized areas of urticaria/angioedema not of great concern, but serious widespread edema can compromise the airway or lead to fluid extravasation or shock
• Maintain temperature
• Pretreatment with antihistamines if cold is unavoidable

UTERINE RUPTURE

Judith Ruiz-Lachica, M.D.

- Reported incidence varies: 1/1280–1/3000 of vaginal deliveries
- Incidence of uterine rupture in women with prior C-section 0.2–0.8%, in two recent series
- Incidence may increase as more women with previous C-section are undergoing trial of labor for subsequent pregnancies.
- May develop as result of pre-existing injury or anomaly; may complicate labor in a previously unscarred uterus

PERIOPERATIVE RISKS

- Uncommon but potentially catastrophic for mother and fetus: In USA, maternal morbidity ~0.1% when rupture occurs vs. 1/12,000 in all deliveries. Uterine rupture usually found at site of previous operation or injury.
- In traumatic or spontaneous rupture with no uterine scar, maternal mortality significantly higher (22 and 66% in two recent studies), likely because of low index of suspicion, inadequate resuscitation, delayed laparotomy

WORRY ABOUT

- Massive bleeding in mother
- Lack of blood/oxygen supply to fetus

OVERVIEW

- Split in walls of uterus, often due to separation of a C-section scar in trial of labor with uterine scar along most of its length, with rupture of fetal membranes so that uterine and peritoneal cavity communicate; bleeding often massive.
- If dehiscence of previous scar, fetal membranes not ruptured, peritoneum overlying defect intact, bleeding is usually minimal. Dehiscence may take place gradually, whereas rupture takes place suddenly and is symptomatic.
- Advantages of vaginal delivery over repeat C-section include ↓ maternal blood loss, ↓ incidence of febrile morbidity, earlier ambulation after delivery.
- ACOG publishes specific guidelines on trial of labor after C-section; currently recommended that all with low transverse uterine scan be considered candidates for trial of labor; ACOG guidelines specifically exclude patients who have prior classic C-section.
- Normally, lower uterine segment at term consists mostly of connective tissue and does not contain placental tissue. Dehiscence does not usually produce maternal or fetal compromise

ETIOLOGY

- Separation of scar from previous C-section, often during trial of labor
- Rupture of myomectomy scar due to precipitous or tumultuous labor
- Prolonged labor with excessive oxytocin stimulation or CPD
- Weak or stretched uterine muscles such as in grand multipara, multiple gestations, polyhydramnios
- Traumatic rupture (iatrogenic) from intrauterine manipulations, difficult forceps application, excessive suprafundal pressure, intra-amniotic fluid instillation

- Sx include vaginal bleeding, severe lower abdominal pain, ± shoulder pain from diaphragmatic irritation with blood, severe maternal hypotension/shock, disappearance of fetal heart tones (FHTs)

ICD-9-CM Code: v22.2 (Pregnancy)

USUAL TREATMENT

- Emergent delivery with repair or hysterectomy is only treatment
- Most common finding is fetal distress: occasionally, loss of intrauterine pressure or cessation of labor.

ASSESSMENT POINTS

SYSTEM	EFFECT	ASSESSMENT BY HX	PE	TEST
CV	Shock with massive blood loss		BP, HR Orthostatic VS if slow	
RESP	Difficulty breathing due to diaphragmatic irritation			
GU	Vaginal bleeding Fetal distress Rupture	Lower abdominal pain followed by severe abdominal pain, absence of contractions, and shoulder pain	Rigid abdomen if not receiving epidural anesthesia	Hct

Key Reference: Cunningham, MacDonald, Gant: Williams Obstetrics, 19th ed. Norwalk, CT, Appleton & Lange, 1993, pp 543–553.

PERIOPERATIVE IMPLICATIONS

Preoperative Preparation

- If trial of labor for patient with previous C-section, monitor FHR, uterine tone and pattern prior to initiation of epidural analgesia using lowest effective concentration of local anesthetic
- Epidural for labor advantageous and may be used for surgical anesthesia if trial of labor fails and repeat C-section required
- If no epidural, GA indicated for emergent repeat C-section in case of suspected uterine scar, rupture, fetal distress, or other
- Anesthetic management similar to management of actively bleeding, acutely hypovolemic parturient:
  - Preparation includes nonparticulate oral antacid, oxygen, 2 large-bore peripheral IV catheters, blood warmer
  - Preinduction: crystalloid, colloid and packed red blood cells infused as rapidly as indicated to treat hypovolemia (uterine blood flow at term—

~700 ml/min). Do not delay to obtain vital sign stability as it will not occur in a living patient in most emergent cases of rupture

Monitoring

- Consider arterial and central venous catheters if time permits or as soon as aortic/bleeding control obtained.

Induction/Airway

- ET intubation with cricoid pressure
- If severely hypovolemic, peripheral vasoconstriction already maximal, direct cardiac depressant effect of ketamine may contribute to hypotension. In severe situations consider intubation with succinylcholine only.

Maintenance

- 100% predelivery; consider low-dose halogenated agents if hemodynamically stable until delivery to ↓ incidence of maternal recall
- Restore blood volume based on BP, UO (CVP?)
- After delivery, when blood volume restored, consider narcotics, muscle relaxants as indicated

- Neonate may require intensive resuscitation at birth.

Extubation

- Awake

Postoperative Period

- EBL: 3000–6000 ml
- Pain score: 6–8; consider postop epidural or epidural PCA

ANTICIPATED PROBLEMS/CONCERNS

- Other more common causes of antepartum hemorrhage: placenta previa and placental abruption
- Symptoms may be misleading; high index of suspicion critical to preventing morbidity and mortality
- Rupture of classic scar much more likely to result in severe hemorrhage

VARICELLA ZOSTER

Lee A. Fleisher, M.D.

RISK

- Prevalence: <10% of adults seronegative
- Usually contracted during childhood

PERIOPERATIVE RISKS

- Minimal additional risk to patient unless immunocompromised host
- Risk of infection to caregivers

WORRY ABOUT

- Encephalitis in immunocompromised host
- Potential nosocomial transmission
- Acyclovir-induced nephrotoxicity
- Transmission to pregnant woman

OVERVIEW

- Viral cause of varicella (chickenpox) and herpes zoster (shingles)
- Both nosocomial transmission and direct contact
- Development of herpes zoster common in immunocompromised host and may be fore-runner of AIDS
- Zoster is reactivated form of varicella from neural ganglion cells
- May lead to congenital abnormalities if contracted during 1st trimester of pregnancy

ICD-9-CM Code: 053.9

ETIOLOGY

- Herpes group of viruses

USUAL TREATMENT

- Varicella immune globulin
- Vaccine currently available but controversial
- Acyclovir decreases severity if initiated within 24 h of herpes zoster
- Corticosteroid controversial for postherpetic neuralgia

ASSESSMENT POINTS

SYSTEM	EFFECT	ASSESSMENT BY HX	PE	TEST
RESP	Pneumonia	Dyspnea	Rhonchi	CXR
HEME	Thrombocytopenic purpura	Bleeding		Plts
SKIN	Rash		Erythematous macules, papules, vesicles	
RENAL	Acyclovir nephrotoxicity			Cr
CNS	Encephalitis Optic neuritis; transverse myelitis	MS changes Vision changes		CT scan
PNS	Zoster shingles		Shingles in single dermatome Multiple dermatomes in immunocompromised	
IMMUNE	Associated with AIDS			HIV tests; CD4 titer

Key Reference: Dunkle LM, et al: A controlled trial of acyclovir for chickenpox in normal children. NEJM 1991; 325:1539–1544.

PERIOPERATIVE IMPLICATIONS

Preoperative Preparation

- Consider isolation precautions

Monitoring

- Routine

Airway

- Routine

Induction/Maintenance

- Routine

Extubation

- Routine

ANTICIPATED PROBLEMS/CONCERNS

- Multiple dermatomes may indicate immunocompromised individual
- Avoid exposure to pregnant individuals

VENTRICULAR FIBRILLATION

Randy H. Steadman, M.D.

RISK

- Most frequent rhythm in sudden cardiac arrest
- At risk are the 1.5 million/y in USA who have acute MIs: about 540,000 will die, 350,000 before they reach hospital (this includes death from dysrhythmia and myocardial failure)
- 1 y mortality in near–sudden death survivors: 20–30% if nonresponsive to antidysthythmics (20–50% of near–sudden death survivors)

PERIOPERATIVE RISKS

- Primary VFib if acute infarction, when treated promptly with defibrillation, may not affect prognosis
- Secondary VFib (preceded by pump failure or hypotension) associated with 75–80% mortality during hospitalization

WORRY ABOUT

- Hypoxemia, hypercarbia, hypokalemia, hypomagnesemia, digitalis toxicity, acid-base abnormality
- Antidysrhythmic drug levels
- Availability of defibrillator, myocardial ischemia

OVERVIEW

- Asynchronous, chaotic contraction of ventricles characterized by no organized ventricular depolarization and therefore no QRS; no cardiac output
- Coarse VFib indicates recent onset, readily correctable with prompt defibrillation
- Fine VFib ("coarse asystole") indicates delay since collapse; successful resuscitation more difficult

ICD-9-CM Code: 427.41

ETIOLOGY

- Usually ischemic, often associated with LV aneurysm
- Idiopathic cardiomyopathy
- Coronary spasm
- Hypothermia
- Long QT syndrome is associated with VTach, esp. torsades de pointes (one type of polymorphic VTach; other types not associated with long QT)

USUAL TREATMENT

- Definitive emergency Rx is <u>always</u> electrical defibrillation: external—either manual or automatic (AEDs)—or internal; internal may be implanted (ICDs)
- Speed of defibrillation major determinant of survival with chances of success reduced by 10% each min
- Antidysrhythmics prevent recurrent VFib, reduce incidence of primary VFib after MI (this action of lidocaine may not be associated with a decreased in-hospital mortality); fibrillation threshold may be elevated
- Antidysrhythmic for acute Rx of VFib after unsuccessful defibrillation is lidocaine; bretylium and procainamide are the 2nd and 3rd line drugs; epinephrine improves coronary and cerebral perfusion pressures and makes VFib more susceptible to countershock; amiodarone long-term drug of choice for prevention of sudden death
- ICDs offer similar long-term prevention
- Surgical ablation techniques for near-death survivors of VT/VF include subendocardial excision, cryoablation, laser photoablation, electrical shock ablation, partial encircling endocardial ventriculotomy

ASSESSMENT POINTS

SYSTEM	EFFECT
HEENT	Right radical neck dissection assoc with increasing QT interval
CV	No effective cardiac output
RESP	Apnea should be anticipated
CNS	Glucose administration may worsen CNS outcome

Key Reference: American Heart Association: Textbook of Advanced Cardiac Life Support. Dallas, American Heart Association, 1994.

PERIOPERATIVE IMPLICATIONS

Preoperative Preparation

- Antidysrhythmic drug levels in optimal therapeutic range
- If for EPS, ablation, or ICD, antidysrhythmic medication should be withdrawn on ECG monitoring.
- Avoid anticholinergic premedication or sympathetic stimulation
- For patients with prolonged QT syndrome consider ß rb's or prophylactic left stellate ganglion block

Monitoring

- Consider ECG en route to OR
- Consider arterial catheter and pulse oximeter for transport and in OR

Airway

- Apnea expected with acute VFib; ventilation should be supported with 100% O_2
- Airway secured with ET tube if 3 successive countershocks fail to restore perfusing rhythm

Induction

- Avoid ketamine; intubate after adequate depth of anesthesia

Maintenance

- Suppress sympathetic responses to stimulation

Extubation

- Suppress sympathetic stimulation; extubate when spontaneous ventilation with oropharyngeal reflexes has been restored
- Reversal of NMBs acceptable
- Regional: Serum levels of local anesthetics given epidurally may affect intraoperative defibrillation threshold testing during ICD placement
- Defibrillator should be available with sterile defibrillator paddles on surgical field; pharmacologic therapy for dysrhythmia conversion/maintenance, for treating HTN and tachycardia, which frequently follow defibrillation; bradycardia may require pacing capabilities

Postoperative Period

- Cardiac monitoring; resumption of preop antidysrhythmics, maintaining oxygenation
- Avoid lyte abnormalities
- Pain control, post defibrillation: 1–3 from chest wall and psychic disturbances
- Psychiatric counseling if disturbed by shock or "out of body" experience

ANTICIPATED PROBLEMS/CONCERNS

- PA catheter insertion may induce VTach or VFib in dysrhythmia-prone patients; if PAC necessary consider central venous placement with advancement after ventricular dysrhythmia procedure completed
- For patients with prolonged QT syndrome avoid drugs that prolong the QT interval (class Ia antidysrhythmic drugs such as quinidine and procainamide)
- Psychic disturbances from defibrillation in "aware state"

VENTRICULAR PRE-EXCITATION
John L. Atlee, M.D.

RISK

• Incidence of Wolff-Parkinson-White (WPW) syndrome, short PR interval with ventricular pre-excitation and tachyarrhythmias: 1–3/1000 persons
• While WPW patients have accessory AV pathways, other types of anomalous pathways may cause pre-excitation or participate in re-entry tachycardia, but these are rarely diagnosed
• Lown-Ganong-Levine (LGL) syndrome, short PR and tachyarrhythmias, much rarer than WPW; chief significance is capacity for rapid AV conduction during AFib/flutter

PERIOPERATIVE RISKS

• WPW per se carries no added risk, but danger of misdiagnosis-mistreatment of tachyarrhythmias with potentially devastating consequences
• Antidromic (pre-excitation) AV reciprocating tachycardia or AFib easily mistaken for VTach
• Drugs used to slow the ventricular rate with AFib/flutter may dangerously accelerate rate in WPW (> 300 bpm)

WORRY ABOUT

• Hyperadrenergic states and other imbalance that might precipitate or aggravate tachyarrhythmias
• Drugs can accelerate AV pathway as conduction. Since accessory pathways are strands of atrial muscle, their refractoriness is shortened by cholinergic interventions or drugs as well as ↑ adrenergic tone
• Fast AFib/flutter suddenly deteriorating into VFib or being mistaken for VFib

OVERVIEW

• 90% of AV reciprocating tachycardia in WPW patients orthodromic; ventricles activated via normal (AV node) pathway and atria retrogradely via AP, so that QRS is narrow
• 10% of AV reciprocating tachycardia antidromic; ventricles activated via AP and atria retrogradely via normal pathway, so that QRS widened and often bizarre
• Orthodromic and antidromic AV reciprocating tachycardia account for 70–80% of all paroxysmal tachycardia with WPW syndrome, AFib for 15–25%, and atrial flutter for 5–10%. VT-VF rare
• Incidence of paroxysmal tachycardia with WPW is 10% ≤ 40 y, and ≥ 35% over 60 y

ICD-9-CM Codes: WPW-426.7; LGL-426.81

ETIOLOGY

• WPW may be an autosomal dominant trait, with 60 to 70% male preponderance; 1% of patients with congenital heart disease; 30–40% of pediatric patients with WPW have associated congenital heart disease
• Possible association between mitral valve prolapse and ↑ incidence of left free wall accessory pathway.
• Prolonged tachycardia bouts can cause reversible/irreversible cardiomyopathy

USUAL TREATMENT

• AV reciprocating tachycardia: vagal maneuvers, drugs that increase refractoriness in AV node (ß rb's, Ca channel blockers, adenosine) and/or AP(procainamide)
• AFib/flutter: procainamide or amiodarone best available IV drugs for slowing ventricular rate; oral drugs include these and class 1Cs; digitalis, diltiazem and verapamil may accelerate ventricular rate
• Symptomatic patients will have had catheter or surgical ablation of accessory pathway

ASSESSMENT POINTS

SYSTEM	EFFECT	ASSESSMENT BY HX	PE	TEST
CV	Arrhythmia	Palpitations, dizziness, syncope or near-syncope, angina, chest pain, cardiac arrest; sometimes asymptomatic	Monitor BP; variable S_1-pulse amplitude; fast regular, irregular, and/or weak pulse; S_3; rales	12-lead ECG, Holter ECG, cardiac evoked potential study
	LV function	Weakness, lassitude, exercise intolerance, CHF		ECHO and possible further study

Key Reference: Atlee JL: Arrhythmias and Pacemakers. Philadelphia, WB Saunders, 1996.

PERIOPERATIVE IMPLICATIONS

Preoperative Preparation

• Consult to cardiology re patient's status, type-risk of arrhythmias, management goals
• Assemble drugs for tachycardia; cardioverter-defibrillator on hand

Monitoring

• ECG monitoring (strip-chart recorder) and arterial line if patient at high risk for tachycardia

Induction

• Patient with cardiomyopathy from recurrent bouts of tachycardia may not tolerate usual doses of thiopental or propofol; etomidate (not ketamine) preferred
• Drugs that increase or maintain vagal tone (esp. opiates, vecuronium, anxiolytics) may reduce likelihood of tachycardia, and ß rb's may be useful prior to laryngoscopy

Maintenance

• Volatile anesthetics ↑ AP/AV node refractoriness; droperidol and fentanyl ↑ accessory pathway refractoriness

Extubation

• ß rb's may be useful prior to emergence/extubation; try to avoid adrenergic hyperactivity

Adjuvants

• Drugs that directly or indirectly ↑ adrenergic tone–heart rate should be used with caution.

Postoperative Period

• Adequate pain control reduces likelihood of paroxysmal tachycardia

ANTICIPATED PROBLEMS/CONCERNS

• Possibility of dangerous ventricular rates with AFib/flutter, with early deterioration into VFib
• Mistaking antidromic (pre-excited) reciprocating tachycardia or pre-excited AFib for VTach-VFib and leading to incorrect Rx

VENTRICULAR SEPTAL DEFECT (CONGENITAL) David L. Reich, M.D.

RISK

- Incidence is ≈ 2/1000 live births
- Prevalence is 1/1000 school-age children
- 10% of congenital heart disease in adults

PERIOPERATIVE RISKS

- Mortality higher in patients >5 y, PVR >7 Wood units, and surgery complicated by CHB
- RV or LV failure postoperatively related to preop status

WORRY ABOUT

- Worsening of L-R shunt with hyperventilation and increased FIO_2
- Paradoxical embolization
- Hypothermia
- Post-CPB pulmonary HTN and RV failure

OVERVIEW

- Small defects asymptomatic, present with murmur, usually close spontaneously
- Larger defects result in CHF symptoms, poor weight gain, URIs beginning at 3–12 wk of age as decreases in PVR cause massive L→R shunting
- Untreated massive L→R shunting results in fixed pulmonary HTN (Eisenmenger syndrome) by 2–6 y

ICD-9-CM Code: 745.4 (Ventricular septal defect)

INDICATIONS/USUAL TREATMENT

- 75% of small defects close spontaneously and require only antibiotic prophylaxis
- Large defects usually result in hospitalization for CHF by 2–4 mo of age
- Medical therapy includes digoxin and furosemide
- Cardiac catheterization only for measurement of pulmonary arterial pressure when not possible by ECHO
- Surgery when CHF not amenable to medical treatment, or if failure to thrive
- Surgical repair contraindicated if PVR >10 Wood units

ASSESSMENT POINTS

SYSTEM	EFFECT	ASSESSMENT BY HX	PE	TEST
CV	Low forward cardiac output due to L→R shunt Pulmonary HTN due to excessive flow	CHF symptoms, failure to thrive Age of patient	Loud holistic murmur and thrill Cyanosis	Auscultation, ECHO ECHO, cardiac cath
RESP	Congestion/edema due to L→R shunt	Frequent URTI or URI	Rhonchi	CXR
HEME	Anemia in massive L→R shunt; polycythemia in R→L shunt	Pallor or cyanosis	Paleness or plethora	Hct
MS	Chronic hypoxemia due to late reversal of shunt flow (Eisenmenger syndrome)	Cyanosis	Clubbing of digits	Pulse oximetry

Key Reference: Kidd L, Driscoll DJ, Gersony WM, et al: Second natural history study of congenital heart defects. Results of treatment of patients with ventricular septal defects. Circulation 1993, 87 (2 Suppl):I38–51.

PERIOPERATIVE IMPLICATIONS

Preoperative Preparation

- May withhold digoxin and furosemide on day of surgery
- May not be possible to delay operation until free of upper respiratory symptoms

Anesthetic Techniques

- Limit FIO_2 to minimum necessary prior to CPB to restrict excessive pulmonary blood flow
- Maintain normal to slightly high $Paco_2$ to restrict excessive pulmonary blood flow
- High-dose opioid anesthetic in neonatal repairs
- Older patients may receive inhalational, IV, or combined techniques
- Avoid nitrous oxide to prevent sequelae of paradoxical air embolization

Monitoring

- Intra-arterial line (cutdowns often required when patient is <5 kg)
- Secure peripheral IV or central venous line (ultrasonic vessel finder desirable)
- Pulse oximetry, capnometry, multiple-site T monitoring
- Transesophageal ECHO

Induction/Maintenance

- IV, mask, IM, rectal inductions all possible

Surgical Stages

- Pre-CPB
  - Low FIO_2, normal to high $Paco_2$
  - Maintain intravascular volume using crystalloid/colloid
  - Vfib and nodal tachycardia with minor heart manipulation (even during sternotomy)
- CPB
  - Washed blood usually necessary for pump prime under 15–20 kg
  - Prevent movement and intraoperative awareness during rewarming by supplementing anesthetic and NMB
- Post-CPB
  - Rule out residual shunting by transesophageal ECHO or direct measurement of arterial saturation "step-up" between SVC (or right atrium) and PA

- Maintain Hct >25–30% using residual CPB reservoir blood or fresh whole blood <48 hr old (platelets in fresh whole blood improve hemostasis)

Postoperative Considerations

- Mechanically ventilate, sedate, and maintain intense analgesia using opioids in neonates and older children prone to pulmonary hypertensive crises (e.g., Down syndrome)
- Indefinite infective endocarditis prophylaxis
- EBL: 200–800 ml

ANTICIPATED PROBLEMS/CONCERNS

- Imbalance in pulmonary to systemic blood flow ratio:
  - Excessive pulmonary blood flow results in high arterial saturation but with diminished tissue perfusion and metabolic acidosis
  - Diminished pulmonary blood flow results in good tissue perfusion but with cyanosis and potential injury due to hypoxia
- Postop ventricular dysfunction, coagulopathy, renal/hepatic dysfunction, CNS dysfunction

VENTRICULAR SEPTAL RUPTURE (DEFECT), POST MYOCARDIAL INFARCTION

David L. Reich, M.D.

RISK

- Occurs in 1–3% of acute MIs
- Majority occur within 1 wk; 20–30% in first 24 h post MI
- Rarely occurs >2 wk post MI

PERIOPERATIVE RISKS

- Accounts for 5% of MI-related deaths
- Nearly 100% die without surgery
- Surgical short-term survival 42–75%
- Results worse with inferior MI or RV/septal dysfunction

WORRY ABOUT

- Associated papillary muscle rupture
- Poor systemic perfusion and end-organ dysfunction
- Pulm congestion with massive L→R shunt

OVERVIEW

- Sudden onset of holosystolic murmur with thrill and hemodynamic deterioration (hypotension and pulmonary congestion)
- Associated with high morbidity and mortality because emergency surgery after extensive recent MI
- Prolonged postop ventilation and ICU stay

ICD-9-CM Codes: 429.71 (acquired cardiac septal defect); 410.00–410.92 (associated MI)

USUAL TREATMENT

- Repair of new VSD with hemodynamic deterioration using pericardial or prosthetic patch material
- Support preop with inotropic agents/nitroprusside/intra-aortic balloon counterpulsation

ASSESSMENT POINTS

SYSTEM	EFFECT	ASSESSMENT BY HX	PE	TEST
CV	Low forward cardiac output due to massive L→R shunt	Sudden onset of hypotension and shock	Loud holosytolic murmur and thrill Auscultation	ECHO, cardiac catheterization
RESP	Congestion/edema	Resp distress	Rales	CXR
RENAL/ HEPATIC	Dysfunction due to hypoperfusion	Anuria		ABG Foley catheter

Key Reference: Held AC, Cole PL, Lipton B, et al: Rupture of the interventricular septum complicating acute myocardial infarction: A multicenter analysis of clinical findings and outcome. Am Heart J 1988; 116:1330–1336.

PERIOPERATIVE IMPLICATIONS

Preoperative Preparation

- Consider elective tracheal intubation and PEEP
- Support cardiac output using inotropic agents
- Lower resistance to forward cardiac output using nitroprusside (if not already hypotensive) and/or intra-aortic balloon counterpulsation

Anesthetic Technique

- High-dose opioid muscle relaxant technique common
- Prior to CPB, use minimal FIO_2 (maximizes pulm vascular resistance) to decrease L→R shunt across VSD

Monitoring

- Intra-arterial line and PA catheter
- Thermodilution cardiac outputs falsely elevated
- Step-up in saturation between right atrium and PA indicates shunting
- Transesophageal ECHO (TEE) to define anatomy, diagnose associated papillary muscle rupture, monitor ventricular function, assess adequacy of surgical repair

Airway

- Frequent suctioning if pulm edema

Induction

- Avoid vasodilation associated with benzodiazepine/opioid combinations

Maintenance

- Titrate low doses of benzodiazepines if HTN

Surgical Stages

- Pre-CPB
  - Median sternotomy with aortic and biatrial cannulation
  - May require vein or internal mammary artery harvest for concomitant myocardial revascularization
  - Lowest FIO_2 consistent with adequate oxygenation
- CPB
  - Maintain Hct using hemofiltration and transfusion
- Post-CPB
  - Inotropic support almost universally required for LV failure
  - RV failure common
  - Assess ventricular repair using TEE or right atrial-to-pulm O_2 saturation ratio
  - FIO_2: 1.00 to minimize pulm vascular resistance

Blood Loss/Volume Concerns

- Plt and FFP may be necessary owing to DIC-like syndrome
- Aprotinin and antifibrinolytic therapy (beginning pre-CPB) controversial
- Pain score: 7–9

Postoperative Considerations

- Postop renal/hepatic/neurologic dysfunction
- Postop LV, RV, or biventricular failure

ANTICIPATED PROBLEMS/CONCERNS

- Cardiogenic shock
- Prolonged ventilatory dependency and ICU stay

VENTRICULAR TACHYARRHYTHMIAS

John L. Atlee, M.D.

RISK

- 3 to 5% of survivors of MI will have uniform sustained ($\geq$ 30 sec) VTach (USVT) within 1 y
- 90% due to CAD but also due to hypertrophic or dilated cardiomyopathies.
- Polymorphic VTach (PMVT) due to ischemia or class 1A antiarrhythmics (~8% of patients)
- Torsades de pointes VTach (TDP): adrenergic-dependent TDP (congenital long QT syndrome); pause- or bradycardia-dependent TDP (acquired QT prolongation)
- Nonsustained VTach (NSVT): acute MI (50% of patients) and idiopathic dilated (40%) or hypertrophic cardiopathies (20%)

PERIOPERATIVE RISKS

- Thiopental potentiates sensitization with all volatile anesthetics; halothane most sensitizing
- Volatile anesthetics tend to oppose USVT induction, but effects on other VTach unknown.

WORRY ABOUT

- Is cardiopulmonary function optimal? What about acid-base, lyte and metabolic balance?
- Sympathomimetics and drugs that $\uparrow$ QT interval (many antiarrhythmic drugs, antidepressants)

OVERVIEW

- VTach hemodynamic impact minimal or profound: rate is most important determinant; others are LV function, AV dissociation, degree of mitral regurgitation, ventricular activation pattern
- VTach and VFib often due to proarrhythmic effects of type 1A and C drugs, amiodarone, sotalol
- R-on-T or complex ventricular extrasystoles (VES) do not cause VTach in absence of acute MI

ICD-9-CM Codes: 427.1 (Ventricular tachycardia); 427.41 (Ventricular fibrillation)

ETIOLOGY

- Except for adrenergic TDP, most VTach is result of acquired, structural heart disease
- Structural heart disease provides substrate for re-entry or initiates triggered or automatic VTach
- Since VTach is due to multiple mechanisms, there can be no uniform treatment

USUAL TREATMENT

- USVT: cardioversion with hemodynamic compromise, lidocaine for VTach with acute MI, otherwise procainamide; chronic therapy includes EP study-guided antiarrhythmic drugs; ablation, intracardiac defibrillation.
- TDP: adrenergic-dependent (β-blockers, sympathectomy, pacemaker, ICD); pause-dependent (eliminate cause, $MgSO_4$, pacing to $\uparrow$ rate, drugs that do not $\uparrow$ QT, use cardioversion only if necessary, since it may precipitate fibrillation).
- PMVT: therapy for ischemia and CAD; lidocaine, class I or III drugs; avoid cardioversion.
- NSVT: none unless unstable hemodynamics (β-blockers, lidocaine, 1As, amiodarone)

ASSESSMENT POINTS

SYSTEM	EFFECT	ASSESSMENT BY HX	PE	TEST
CV	Arrhythmia	No symptoms, palpitations, dizziness, syncope or near-syncope, cardiac arrest	Monitor BP, cannon A waves with AVD, variable S_1 and pulse amplitude, regular or weak irregular pulse,	12-lead ECG (if possible), Holter ECG, cardiac electrophysiologic studies
	LV function	Weakness, lassitude, exercise intolerance, CHF	S_3, rales, findings of specific heart disease	ECHO, exercise ECG, MRI
	Ischemia	Symptoms of angina, CHF		Scintigraphy, cardiac catheter, Angio
RESP	CHF, COPD	Dyspnea, orthopnea, cough	S_3, rales, wheezes	CXR, PFTs
CNS	Ischemia	Syncope, near-syncope	Altered mental status	See CV assessment

Key Reference: Atlee JL: Arrhythmias and Pacemakers. Philadelphia, WB Saunders, 1996.

PERIOPERATIVE IMPLICATIONS

Preoperative Preparation

- USVT, NSVT: adequate treatment for underlying heart disease, optimize hemodynamic function
- TDP: adrenergic-dependent (β-blockers, stellate ganglion block); pause-dependent (off drugs that $\uparrow$ QT, correct other imbalance, Mg^{2+} and K^+ status, temporary antibradycardia pacing)
- MFVT: usually acute manifestation of CAD, so provide Rx for ischemia, reperfusion injury

Monitoring

- ECG, ST-T trending, strip-chart recorder and that indicated for underlying heart condition

Induction/Maintenance

- Use drugs compatible with patient's CV status; control exaggerated sympathetic responses with airway or surgical manipulation; avoid sympathomimetic, sensitizing, or QT-prolonging drugs

Extubation

- Consider using β-blockers and/or vasodilators to control circulatory lability

Adjuvants

- Caution with chronotropes and sympathomimetic drugs or long-acting local anesthetics such as bupivacaine in patients with acquired long-QT interval

Postoperative Period

- Adequate sedation and pain control, maintain as near normal physiology as possible; be mindful of VTach etiology and conditions, factors, or interventions that might trigger or worsen it

ANTICIPATED PROBLEMS/CONCERNS

- Do not treat VES or NSVT based on appearance: complex VES or NSVT does not cause VTach in absence of ischemia, digitalis toxicity, or catecholamine excess. Overtreatment may harm patient
- With pause-dependent TDP or PMVT, cardioversion further increases tachycardia instability, is often ineffective, and may cause myocardial injury. Do not withhold defibrillation if required

VENTRICULAR TACHYCARDIA

Edelberto Perez, M.D.
Kenneth J. Tuman, M.D.

RISK

- Structural heart disease (most commonly chronic phase of MI)
- Most common cause of mortality with CHF

PERIOPERATIVE RISKS

- Endogenous or exogenous catecholamines trigger VT in susceptible patients
- Central venous and pulmonary artery catheters and intubation can trigger VT
- Hyperventilation may ↓ serum K+
- Precipitation of polymorphic VT with agents that alter QT interval

WORRY ABOUT

- Possible effect of antiarrhythmics on cardiac and pulm function
- Perioperative ventricular dysfunction and/or ischemia
- Progression of VTach to VFib
- Reduction of LV function due to IV antiarrhythmic

OVERVIEW

- Defined as 3 or more consecutive ventricular beats (usually at a rate >100 bpm)
- Sustained VT persists for >30 sec or requires an intervention for termination
- Nonsustained VT is ≤6 consecutive beats terminating spontaneously within 30 sec
- Possible signs of VT include a wide QRS (>140 msec), presence of fusion beat, AV dissociation, LBBB morphology
- Must rule out SVT with aberrant conduction or pre-existing bundle branch block
- Torsades de pointes refers to VTach characterized by polymorphic QRS complexes that undulate in a regular fashion about baseline. Often associated with prolonged QT interval

ICD-9-CM Code: 427.42

ETIOLOGY

- CAD—acute myocardial ischemia or MI or old MI with LV scar or aneurysm
- Cardiomyopathies, esp. with ventricular dilation/enlargement
- Myocarditis
- Mechanical irritation (catheters)
- Metabolic (hypokalemia, hypomagnesemia)
- Hypertrophic cardiomyopathy or mitral valve prolapse may present with VTach
- Acquired polymorphic VTach (torsades) may result from lyte imbalances (K+, Mg2+), or drugs that prolong repolarization (phenothiazines, tricyclic antidepressants, class Ia antiarrhythmics, erythromycin, pentamidine, terfenadine, astemizole)

- Congenital QT prolongation may be associated with left-sided cardiac sympathetic dominance
- Rare association with right radical neck dissection

USUAL TREATMENT

- Removal or manipulation of catheter if patient hemodynamically stable
- Chronic PO therapy includes: Ia—quinidine, procainamide, disopyramide; Ib—mexilitene, tocainide; Ic—propafenone; II—ß rb's; III—amiodarone, sotalol
- Intravenous therapy includes procainamide, phenytoin, lidocaine, amiodarone, bretylium (less commonly quindine) as well as Mg2+ and/or K+ when necessary
- Digoxin antibodies if digitalis-induced VTach
- Class I antiarrhythmics generally contraindicated in presence of polymorphic VT (torsades de pointes)
- Electrical cardioversion for VTach with hemodynamic instability
- Nonpharmacologic management includes ablative techniques, myocardial revascularization, implantable cardioverter-defibrillators
- Treatment of torsades includes withdrawal of offending agent, correction of lyte abnormality (K+, Mg2+) and/or electrical defibrillation to terminate episode. Accelerating HR with isoproterenol or cardiac pacing may terminate rhythm. Empirical Mg2+ treatment may be lifesaving
- Treatment of congenital QT prolongation includes ß rb's to blunt sympathetic activity, Mg2+, and/or left cervicothoracic sympathectomy

ASSESSMENT POINTS

SYSTEM	EFFECT	ASSESSMENT BY HX	PE	TEST
CV	Myocardial ischemia Hypotension Cardiac arrest	Angina/anginal equivalent (syncope, SOB, palpitations and exercise intolerance) CHF	Cardiomegaly, JVD Cannon A waves; S₃, S₄	ECG, CXR Electrophysiologic studies Ambulatory ECG
RESP	Pulm edema Amiodarone effects (fibrosis)	Shortness of breath	Rales (wet or dry)	CXR, PFTs (A-a)O₂ gradient
CNS	Syncope	Dizziness or loss of consciousness		

Key Reference: Shenasa M, Borggrefe M, et al: Ventricular tachycardia. Lancet 1993; 341:1512.

PERIOPERATIVE IMPLICATIONS

Preoperative Preparation

- Ascertain etiology of VTach and associated problems
- Evaluate for Hx of palpitations, SOB, VTach, dizziness, syncope, chest pain
- Evaluate ECG for morphology of PVCs, QT interval, underlying BBB (important for Dx and therapy of wide complex tachycardia)
- Review electrophysiologic studies to determine optimal treatment of VTach
- Assess K+ and Mg2+ levels, digoxin level if indicated
- Pulmonary and thyroid function tests may be indicated for chronic amiodarone therapy
- Continue PO antiarrhythmic therapy
- Have defibrillator immediately available (nearby) whenever inserting central venous catheters

Monitor

- ECG for ischemia or QT prolongation
- Consider invasive hemodynamic monitor if suspect serious concomitant cardiac disease and major anesthetic/surgical intervention

Induction/Maintenance

- Avoid myocardial ischemia (maintain O₂ supply and minimize O₂ demand)
- Minimize surgical stimulus response and subsequent catecholamine release
- Avoid sympathomimetics, which may aggravate ventricular dysrhythmias
- Avoid hypokalemia, excessive hyperventilation

Postoperative Period

- Consider continuous arrhythmia monitoring
- Continue parenteral antiarrhythmics until able to resume PO
- Treat Mg2+ and K+ deficits (common postop, esp. after major surgical procedures)

VITAMIN B$_{12}$/FOLATE DEFICIENCY
Donald D. Koblin, Ph.D., M.D.

RISK

- 5–20% of elderly
- Predisposed by prolonged exposure to N$_2$O, ICU patients, ileal resections, chemotherapy with antifolates, ethanol abuse, AIDS, pregnancy

PERIOPERATIVE RISKS

- Worsening of pre-existing megaloblastic anemia and neuropathies after exposure to N$_2$O (infrequent)
- Anemia and limited oxygen-carrying capacity
- Limb (positioning) injuries associated with pre-existing neuropathy

WORRY ABOUT

- Delayed onset of hematologic and neurologic abn after N$_2$O exposure—several weeks may pass before Sx develop
- Untoward outcomes (e.g., death, infection) in critically ill patients with megaloblastic anemia undergoing anesthesia and surgery

OVERVIEW

- Folate metabolism requires vitamin B$_{12}$-dependent enzyme methionine synthase, which converts methyltetrahydrofolate and homocysteine to free tetrahydrofolate and methionine and is rapidly inactivated (T$_{1/2}$ ~ 1 h) by N$_2$O
- Vitamin B$_{12}$ required for two enzymes in humans: methionine synthase and methyl-malonyl-CoA mutase (which converts L-methylmalonyl-CoA to succinyl-CoA)
- Tetrahydrofolate (in its free form and derivatives) needed for many metabolic processes, including pyrimidine, purine, DNA synthesis; amino acid metabolism; formate elimination
- Vitamin B$_{12}$/folate required for synthesis and maturation of blood cells, integrity of CNS, GI function, growth of fetus and child
- Associated with ↑ serum homocysteine levels and atherosclerosis

ICD-9-CM Codes: 281.0–281.2

ETIOLOGY

- Pernicious anemia (antibodies to gastric cells and lack of intrinsic factor) is most common cause
- Impaired nutritional intake, malabsorption (e.g., ileal resection), ↑ folate demand (e.g., pregnancy), treatment with antifolate drugs (e.g., methotrexate, prolonged N$_2$O exposure)

USUAL TREATMENT

- Daily oral supplements of folate/weekly IM injections of vitamin B$_{12}$
- Folate treatment alone may produce partial hematologic remission due to vitamin B$_{12}$ deficiency but mask vitamin B$_{12}$ deficiency and result in irreversible neurologic abnormality
- Deficiencies associated with N$_2$O exposure have been successfully treated with IM injections of vitamin B$_{12}$, IV administration of folinic acid, oral methionine

ASSESSMENT POINTS

SYSTEM	EFFECT	TEST
HEENT	Glossitis and painful tongue (infrequent)	
CV	Angina and palpitations 2° to anemia DOE 2° to anemia	
GI	Anorexia, diarrhea	Schilling test for malabsorption of vitamin B$_{12}$.
HEME	Megaloblastic anemia	Serum levels of vitamin B$_{12}$ and folate. RBC folate considered better indicator of tissue folate levels than serum folate. ↑ Urinary levels of methylmalonic acid in vitamin B$_{12}$ deficiency. Hematologic variables may be normal or abnormal; anemia, ↑ mean corpuscular volume Hypersegmented neutrophils may be present
GU	Impotence	
CNS	Subacute combined degeneration of spinal cord Gait ataxia Romberg sign, memory deficits, psychosis	
PNS	Diminished vibratory sense, proprioception, and sensation; paresthesias, loss of deep tendon reflexes	

Key Reference: Chanarin I, Deacon R, Lumb M, Perry J: Cobalamin and folate: Recent developments. J Clin Pathol 1992;45:277–283.

PERIOPERATIVE IMPLICATIONS

Preoperative Preparation

- If elective procedure, postpone to correct vitamin deficiencies and hematologic/neurologic abnormalities

Monitoring

- Myocardial ischemia may occur with anemia and is associated with ↑ homocysteine levels

Airway

- Large and painful tongue may be present

Induction/Maintenance

- Avoid nitrous oxide if patient known to be vitamin B$_{12}$/folate–deficient and has hematologic/neurologic abnormalities

Adjuvants

- Regional: Documentation of pre-existing neurologic deficits is required before proceeding with regional anesthesia

Postoperative Period

- Worsening of hematologic and neurologic abn may not occur until several weeks after N$_2$O exposure

ANTICIPATED PROBLEMS/CONCERNS

- Anemia may result in impaired oxygenation of tissues and be associated with myocardial ischemia
- CNS and PNS abnormalities may exist
- Nitrous oxide may exacerbate pre-existing hematologic/neurologic abnormality associated with vitamin B$_{12}$/folate deficiency

VITAMIN K DEFICIENCY

Ronald P. Chavez, M.D.

PERIOPERATIVE RISKS

• ↑ Risk of bleeding

WORRY ABOUT

• Prolongation of prothrombin time
• Inadequate surgical hemostasis
• May need to give FFP
• Vitamin K administered to correct problem may take several hours to days to take effect

OVERVIEW

• Major Sx: ↑ bleeding tendency: GI bleeding, epistaxis, hematuria, ecchymoses, intracranial hemorrhage, operative bleeding

ICD-9-CM Code: 286.7

ETIOLOGY

• Inadequate intake of vitamin K
• Prolonged use of drugs that inhibit intestinal bacterial growth
• Inadequate absorption due to intra- or extrahepatic biliary obstruction
• Inadequate utilization due to hepatocellular disease
• Drug-induced owing to anticoagulants such as warfarin
• Malabsorption syndromes such as sprue or ulcerative colitis, or induced by Olestra
• Newborn infants: due to inadequate dietary intake and unestablished normal intestinal flora

USUAL TREATMENT

• Administration of vitamin K; poor liver function may have inadequate response
• Phytonadione (vitamin K_1, AquaMEPHYTON) is the only natural form available for therapeutic use. (Oral and IM routes are less likely than IV routes to cause side effects such as allergic reactions or bronchospasm)
• Menadione (vitamin K_3) (water-soluble) is an artificial provitamin converted to menaquinone (vitamin K_2) by liver. Does not require presence of bile salts for systemic absorption, useful when malabsorption of vitamin K is due to biliary obstruction
• Dosage
  – Vitamin K deficiency induced by warfarin: 2.5–10 mg po or slow IV (1 mg/min)
  – Hyperalimentation: 10 mg IM or IV q wk
  – Vitamin K deficiency in newborn: 0.5–1 mg phytonadione to infant immediately after delivery
  – Preoperative: If immediate treatment needed, give 10 mg sc qd for 3 d; response should be seen within 24 h

ASSESSMENT POINTS

SYSTEM	EFFECT	ASSESSMENT BY HX	PE	TEST
HEENT	Bleeding	Epistaxis		PT/PTT
GI	GI bleeding	Hematemesis Melena Hematochezia	Tenderness Masses Ascites/hepatomegaly	UGI endoscopy
HEME	↑ Bleeding 2° to ↓ Factor VII, IX, X, prothrombin	Easy bruising Bleeding gums Drug use such as warfarin		
RENAL	Hematuria			Urinalysis
CNS	Intracranial hemorrhage	Injury	CNS exam	CT scan

Key Reference: Vermeer C, Hamulyak K: Pathophysiology of vitamin K deficiency and oral anticoagulants. Thromb Haemost 1991; 66:153–159.

PERIOPERATIVE IMPLICATIONS

Perioperative Preparation

• If immediate surgery is obligatory, consider transfusing 2–4 U FFP and follow PT/PTT
• Factor VII has $T_{1/2}$ of 6–12 h and is metabolized quickly; repeat treatment may be needed 6–12 h later. Begin treatment with vitamin K 10 mg sc qd for 3 d; response should be seen after 24 h. (Liver disease may have poor response to vitamin K)

Monitoring

• Routine

Airway

• ↑ Risk of bleeding trauma with direct laryngoscopy
• Potential difficult airway 2° to bleeding

Maintenance

• Observe for clot in surgical field

Extubation

• Watch for blood in oropharynx

ANTICIPATED PROBLEMS/CONCERNS

• ↑ Bleeding and problems associated with decreased RBC mass
• Trauma to oropharynx with direct laryngoscopy may obscure vision during laryngoscopy and result in difficult intubation

VON WILLEBRAND'S DISEASE
Thomas M. McLoughlin, Jr., M.D.

RISK

- People within US: 1 million (severe disease 1:10,000–1 million)
- Race/gender with highest prevalence: equal

PERIOPERATIVE RISKS

- ↑ Risk if hepatic or immune dysfunction from prior plasma product transfusions
- Significant risk of bleeding if untreated

WORRY ABOUT

- Excessive perioperative hemorrhage
- Adverse reactions to desmopressin therapy (seizures due to hyponatremia, hypotension, anaphylaxis)

OVERVIEW

- Coagulopathy characterized by quantitative/qualitative alterations in von Willebrand factor (vWF), which molecularly bridges plts and vascular subendothelium and prolongs $T_{1/2}$ of circulating factor VIII
- Presents as defect in primary hemostasis—mucocutaneous hemorrhage
- Highly variable severity
- Classified by band pattern of radiolabeled vWF after gel electrophoresis (multimeric analysis)
- Type I: quantitative decrease in vWF of all sizes; type II: quantitative/qualitative alterations primarily in largest molecular weight vWF multimers (many type II subtypes exist depending on abnormality); Type III: severe quantitative reductions or absence of vWF

ICD-9-CM Code: 286.4

ETIOLOGY

- Autosomal dominant trait; variable penetrance and expression leads to unpredictable clinical severity; most severe disease in homozygotes
- Rarely, acquired disorder due to autoimmune disease or induced alterations in vWF function

USUAL TREATMENT

- *Must* know disease subtype prior to therapy
- Desmopressin acetate (DDAVP), 0.3 µg/kg IV, stimulates release of endothelial vWF, variably effective in types I and II disease
- Desmopressin absolutely contraindicated in type IIB
- Pasteurized pooled factor VIII concentrates that preserve vWF (Humate-P) are mainstay of therapy
- Cryoprecipitate best alternative if Humate-P unavailable
- Antifibrinolytics often useful adjuncts

ASSESSMENT POINTS

SYSTEM	EFFECT	ASSESSMENT BY HX	TEST
HEENT		Epistaxis	
GI	GI bleeding	Melena, hematochezia	Stool guaiac
HEPATIC	Requirement for transfusion therapy	Random donor exposures	LFTs, hepatitis panel
HEME	Coagulopathy, principal defect in primary hemostasis	Easy bruising, menorrhagia, dental extractions, epistaxis	Prolonged bleeding time PT, PTT, Plt count often normal; quantitative vWF antigen; ristocetin cofactor activity; multimeric analysis

Key Reference: Cameron CB, Kobrinsky N: Perioperative management of patients with von Willebrand's disease. Can J Anaesth 1990; 37:341–347.

PERIOPERATIVE IMPLICATIONS

Preoperative Preparation

- Collaboration with consultant hematologist and blood bank
- Desmopressin 1 h preop in all but IIB subtype
- Antifibrinolytics for dental procedures

Monitoring

- Bleeding time/vWF activity periodically in prolonged procedures; $T_{1/2}$ of administered vWF about 8–12 h

Airway

- Laryngoscopy can lead to tissue trauma
- Nasotracheal route best avoided

Induction

- No specific recommendations

Maintenance

- Meticulous surgical hemostasis

Extubation

- Avoid coughing if possible; gentle orotracheal suction best performed under direct vision

Adjuvants

- Consider regional anesthetics with caution
- Repeat desmopressin doses likely to be less effective than initial; reaccumulation of endothelial stores takes time

ANTICIPATED PROBLEMS/CONCERNS

- Excessive intra- and postoperative blood loss
- Increased likelihood of infectious blood-borne disease

WALDENSTRÖM'S MACROGLOBULINEMIA
Kamla K. Prasad, M.D.

RISKS

- Incidence in USA: 1/100,000
- Racial preponderance: none
- Males > females 3/2
- 100% fatality rate; median survival 5 y

PERIOPERATIVE RISKS

- Hyperviscosity syndrome
- Hemorrhage

WORRY ABOUT

- Hyperviscosity syndrome
- Multifactorial coagulopathy
- Pre-existing peripheral neurologic deficits
- Difficulties in evaluation and treatment of anemia

OVERVIEW

- Plasma cell dyscrasia characterized by neoplastic proliferation of clone of IgM-producing B cells
- Pathology from excessive monoclonal IgM production
- Potentially severe adverse neurologic, hemostatic, CV problems perioperatively
- Anesthetic concerns similar to those in multiple myeloma except that hypercalcemia and bone lesions are rare; renal failure; Bence Jones proteinuria less common

ICD-9-CM Code: 273.3
See also Multiple Myeloma

ETIOLOGY

- Cause unknown; possible genetic predisposition

USUAL TREATMENT

- Alkylating agents and prednisone
- Plasmapheresis prior to transfusion and to treat hyperviscosity syndrome

ASSESSMENT POINTS

SYSTEM	EFFECT	ASSESSMENT BY HX	PE	TEST
CV	Hyperviscosity syndrome (microvascular sludging)	Angina Fatigue CHF	Venous thrombosis	Serum viscometry
RESP	Pulm involvement	Dyspnea	Pleural effusion	CXR (pleural effusion, diffuse pulm infiltrates)
HEME	Impaired plt aggregation Inhibition of factors V, VII, VIII Impaired clot formation	Episodic epistaxis Episodic mucosal and gum bleeding		Bleeding time PT, PTT, TT
	Normocytic/normochromic anemia	Fatigue	Pallor	CBC
	Cryoglobulinemia	Cold intolerance Raynaud's syndrome Arthralgia	Purpura	Cryoglobulin assay
RENAL	Glomerulonephritis			BUN/Cr
CNS	Leukoencephalopathy Abnormal cerebral vascular permeability		Mental status changes	
PNS	Demyelinating peripheral neuropathy		Symmetric peripheral neuropathy, legs > arms	

Key Reference: Dimopoulos MA, Alexanian R: Waldenstrom's macroglobulinemia. Blood 1994; 83:1452–1459.

PERIOPERATIVE IMPLICATIONS

Preoperative Preparation

- Consider plasmapheresis and transfusion

Monitoring

- Normothermia to prevent cryoglobulin precipitation

Airway

- Macroglossia if amyloidosis (5%)

Adjuvants

- All drugs: theoretical unpredictable pharmacokinetics due to alterations of relative proportions of globulins and albumin in blood; unpredictable pharmacodynamics due to increased cerebrovascular permeability

Postoperative Period

- Transient postop paresis due to disease rather than anesthetic management

ANTICIPATED PROBLEMS/CONCERNS

- Hyperviscosity syndrome (20% incidence perioperatively)
  – Develops from markedly increased concentration of large, asymmetric IgM molecule
  – Capillary blood flow impaired, reducing O_2 delivery through microcirculation
  – Expanded plasma volume, ↑ ICP and ↑ cerebrovascular permeability
  – Findings include fatigue, dizziness, headache, visual blurring, mucosal bleeding, impaired mentation, CHF, dilated, segmented retinal and conjunctival vessels
  – Plasmapheresis mainstay of therapy
- Anemia
  – Hgb value may be artificially reduced by as much as 2 g/dl because of increased plasma volume
  – Transfusion may precipitate CHF or hyperviscosity syndrome (by increasing serum viscosity) and actually decrease O_2 delivery
  – Consider plasmapheresis before transfusion
- 5% at risk for cryoglobulinemia. At cold blood temp, cryoglobulins precipitate, triggering complement activation, causing immune complex vasculitis, and resulting in ischemia of skin, nerve, and renal tissues. Raynaud's syndrome, arthralgia, purpura, peripheral neuropathy, hepatic dysfunction, and renal failure may ensue

WOLFF-PARKINSON-WHITE (WPW) SYNDROME

Jeffrey R. Balser, M.D., Ph.D.

RISK

- Prevalence: 3/1000 in general population

PERIOPERATIVE RISKS

- Paroxysmal supraventricular tachycardia (PSVT): rapid heart rate impairs LV filling. May cause hypoperfusion if LV failure, LV hypertrophy, aortic stenosis, or mitral stenosis
- AFib occurs in 10–35% of patients with WPW, with ↑ incidence with age. Major concern is rapid ventricular response due to antegrade conduction over accessory pathway (AP) and induction of VFib

WORRY ABOUT

- Perioperative hypotension in patients with LV failure (systolic or diastolic dysfunction)
- Ischemia in patients with CAD if PSVT or AFib occurs
- Induction of VFib

OVERVIEW

- Accessory pathway (AP) is congenital auxiliary electrical connection between atria and ventricles. WPW present when this AP is manifested on surface ECG and when it participates in PSVT. Other patients may have concealed APs (not apparent on surface ECG) that also underlie PSVT and ↑ tendency to develop AFib
- APs may conduct antegrade or retrograde. During sinus rhythm, antegrade conduction through AP may produce ventricular pre-excitation on ECG with a short PR interval (<0.12 sec), a slurred QRS upstroke (delta wave), and wide QRS complex. These abnormalities in QRS complex may vary in magnitude and depend on relative contribution of normal AV nodal system and AP to ventricular depolarization
- PSVT results from re-entrant circuit involving AV node AP. QRS complex during PSVT matches the usual QRS morphology when conduction is antegrade through AV system and retrograde over AP (orthodromic). 5–10% of time, conduction over AP is antegrade (antidromic), producing wide QRS complex. This rhythm may be confused with VTach

- AFib/flutter more common in patients with WPW. Usually, but not always, AFib precipitated by episode of PSVT. Rapid (≥300 beats/min) ventricular rates may occur in patients with APs with short refractory periods. These patients at risk for developing VFib and hemodynamic collapse

ICD-9-CM Code: 426.7

See also Paroxysmal Supraventricular Tachycardia and Ventricular Tachycardia in Diseases section

USUAL TREATMENT

- With severe hemodynamic compromise: DC cardioversion (50–100 J)
- PSVT: usually terminated by vagal maneuvers or adenosine. Small incidence of induction of AFib with adenosine therapy for PSVT in WPW has been described
- AFib: IV procainamide is drug of choice, effective in converting AFib to sinus rhythm and blocks conduction over AP. Disopyramide may be effective. Avoid digoxin, Ca channel blockers, ß rb's, adenosine. These AV nodal blockers may reduce accessory tract refractory period, thereby increasing ventricular rates, and raising risk of VFib

ASSESSMENT POINTS

SYSTEM	EFFECT	ASSESSMENT BY HX	PE	TEST
CV	Tachycardia, hypotension	Palpitations, diaphoresis, angina, vague chest discomfort, neck pounding	Prominent jugular venous pulsations due to atrial contraction against closed tricuspid valve	12-lead ECG Electrophysiologic study and catheter ablation
RESP	CHF exacerbation if PSVT + poor LV function	Dyspnea, orthopnea	Rales, wheezing, S_3	CXR
CNS	Lightheadedness			

Key Reference: Wellens HJJ, Smeets JLRM, Todriguez LM, Gorgels APM. Atrial fibrillation in Wolff-Parkinson-White syndrome. *In* Falk RH, Podrid PJ (eds): Atrial Fibrillation: Mechanisms and Management. New York, Raven Press, 1992, pp 333–344.

PERIOPERATIVE IMPLICATIONS

Preoperative Preparation

- If pre-excitation on ECG a Hx of WPW, consider cardiology evaluation
- If symptomatic, consider electrophysiologic study and catheter ablation

Monitoring

- ECG for detection of perioperative PSVT or AF
- Consider arterial line and CVP catheter if LV dysfunction or valve disease because of high dependence on preload and atrial kick

Induction/Maintenance/Extubation

- Avoid tachycardia, light anesthesia, hypoxia, and lyte abnormalities

Adjuvants

- Limit use of vagolytic agents such as pancuronium and atropine

Postoperative Period

- Pain management to avoid catecholamine excess

ANTICIPATED PROBLEMS/CONCERNS

- Digoxin, Ca channel blockers, and ß rb's may shorten refractoriness in AP and thereby provoke VFib in WPW patients with AFib
- Hemodynamic collapse may occur when verapamil or ß rb's used in VTach mistaken for antidromic (wide complex) PSVT in patient with WPW

SECTION II

PROCEDURES

ABDOMINAL AORTIC ANEURYSM REPAIR

Garry V. Walker, M.D.
Charles Beattie, Ph.D., M.D.

RISK

- Incidence: 3% of males aged >55 y, autopsy incidence of 1.8–6.6%
- Most Dx in 6th, 7th decades
- Male:female, 4:1
- Predominantly caused by atherosclerosis, HTN, tobacco abuse

PERIOPERATIVE RISKS

- Depends on patient condition, level of aortic occlusion
- Mortality: 1.5–8%, elective; 25–60% emergent/ruptured
- Morbidity: strongly depends on level of aortic cross-clamp: infrarenal, suprarenal, supraceliac
- Nonlethal MI 4–15%
- Resp 5–10%
- Renal insufficiency 2–5% (infrarenal), 17% (suprarenal)
- Bowel complications 3–4%
- Paraplegia <1% (infrarenal), 1–5% (supraceliac)

WORRY ABOUT

- Myocardial ischemia/MI with aortic clamping; postop MI
- Renal failure/insufficiency
- Blood loss, hypothermia, acid-base abnormal with supraceliac clamp release

OVERVIEW

- High incidence of coexisting HTN (40–60%), CAD (30–40%), carotid bruits (10–30%)
- Emergent repair has much higher associated mortality
- Significant cardiac stress can occur with aortic cross-clamp
- Anesthesia goals are to keep normal intrachamber cardiac size; optimize coronary, renal, cerebral O_2, esp during aortic cross-clamp

ICD-9-CM Code: 441.4

INDICATIONS AND USUAL TREATMENT

- Asymptomatic aneurysms of less than 5 cm may be followed by quarterly exams
- Elective repair for aneurysms >5 cm
- Evidence of leak or rupture; documented recent ↑ in size
- Prompt repair of all aneurysms that become symptomatic (sudden severe abd pain that may radiate to back associated with faintness or syncope)

ASSESSMENT POINTS

SYSTEM	EFFECT	ASSESSMENT BY HX	PE	TEST
CV	Previous MI, CAD with poss ventricular dysfunction	>70 y, angina, ventricular arrhythmia, Q-wave, PND	Pedal edema, S_3	Stress ECG, ECHO, dipyridamole thallium or dobutamine ECHO
RESP	COPD, pulm edema	Dyspnea	Barrel chest, bronchospasm	CXR, ABG, ?PFTs
RENAL	Renal insufficiency	Renal vascular HTN		Cr
CNS	Carotid/vertebral disease	TIA, stroke	Neuro deficits, carotid bruits	Neuro assessment, carotid Doppler

Key Reference: Beattie C, Frank SM: Anesthesia for major vascular surgery. *In* Rogers, Tinker, Covino, Longecker (eds): Principles and Practice of Anesthesiology. St. Louis, CV Mosby, 1993.

PERIOPERATIVE MANAGEMENT

Preoperative Preparation

- Assess coexisting morbidities, prepare to maintain homeostasis
- Consider epidural placement for pre-emptive, perioperative analgesia

Monitoring

- Invasive arterial pressure monitoring, large-bore vascular access essential
- A-line, CVP for all, PA cath for suprarenal and supraceliac aortic cross-clamps and those with infrarenal who have cardiac disease (LVEF <35%, and/or significant CAD-ischemia on preop Holter, coronary stenosis >70%)
- Consider intraoperative TEE for patients with significant LV dysfunction

Anesthetic Technique/Induction

- Stable induction technique essential
- All variations of carefully conducted general or regional-supplemented general anesthesia
- Influence of anesthesia technique on perioperative morbidity unestablished

SURGICAL STAGES

Dissection

- Ability to transfuse blood products must be immediate and blood scavenging is indicated
- For suprarenal and supraceliac consider establishing brisk UO; mannitol (25 g) well before aortic cross-clamping, or dopamine 3 µg/kg/min for suprarenal and supraceliac, and infrarenal with pre-existing renal dysfunction
- Consider heparin 100 U/kg 5 min prior to aortic cross-clamping

Aortic Clamping

- Control BP with nitroprusside, nitroglycerine, and/or inhalation agent
- Consider fluid loading at end of aortic cross-clamping to prep for clamp release
- Cerebral, renal, myocardial protection depend on adequate perfusion pressure, maintaining nml cardiac chamber size during operation

Aortic Unclamping

- Normalize preload, discontinue vasodilators before unclamping to effect stable hemodynamics

- Acidosis with supraceliac aortic cross-clamping release can be profound; consider treating with bicarbonate during clamp period, esp. if >1h; may need Ca^{2+} Rx for blood transfusion, if liver is "out of circ" during aortic cross-clamping
- EBL: 600–4000 ml

Postoperative Considerations

- BP and HR control
- Many routinely extubate at end of case, but postop fluid shifts/requirement may be significant
- Pain score: 6–9; depends on incision type
- Postop analgesia: epidural or IV—PCA

ANTICIPATED PROBLEMS/CONCERNS

- Combined regional/general can be associated with hypotension
- Desirable to maintain body temperature, but not with lower extremity warming during aortic cross-clamping
- Controversies include need for renal protection; use of nitroprusside for supraceliac aortic cross-clamping; prompt extubation; need for routine ICU care

ABDOMINOPERINEAL RESECTION
Randolph B. Gorman, M.D.

RISK

- Rectal cancer: 40,000 cases/y; abdominoperineal resection used in~10% of operations for condition; remainder, low anterior resection, sparing anus, sphincter
- Males/females: 1.4:1
- Racial predominance: none

PERIOPERATIVE RISKS

- Perioperative mortality 2–3%
- Mortality mostly related to cardiopulm issues, older patients
- Morbidity mainly urol, pulm, wound dehiscence

WORRY ABOUT

- Perioperative fluid deficit (bowel prep, leaky capillaries)
- Poss, blood loss during pelvic dissection
- Poss ureteral, bladder injury
- Patient position in lithotomy or jackknife position
- Coexisting disease in elderly

OVERVIEW

- Surg involves removal of distal colon, rectum; closure of anus, creation of permanent colostomy

ICD-9-CM Code: 154.1

INDICATIONS AND USUAL TREATMENT

- In curative, palliative resections of tumors of middle and lower 3rd of rectum, some tumors of anus
- Poss occasionally used for severe inflammatory bowel disease
- Use of operation ↓ in favor of low ant resection or local excision in absence of invasive lesion
- Chemo/radiotherapy may be employed pre- or postop

ASSESSMENT POINTS

SYSTEM	EFFECT	ASSESSMENT BY HX	PE	TEST
CV	Impairment due to advanced age	CP, SOB, Exercise tolerance	CV exam	ECG
RESP	Metastasis	Cough, SOB	Auscultation	CXR, CT
GI	Hepatic metastases Bowel obstruction	Pain N/V	Palpation Distention, pain	CT Abd x-ray
ENDO	Malnutrition	Wt loss	Cachexia	Lytes, albumin
HEME	Bleeding	Weakness	Pallor, tachycardia	CBC
GU	Obstruction	Pain, oliguria		BUN, Cr IVP

Key Reference: Rothenberger DA, Wong WD: Abdominoperineal resection for adenocarcinoma of the low rectum. World J Surg 1992; 16:478–485.

PERIOPERATIVE IMPLICATIONS

Preoperative Preparation

- Worry about occult dehydration, consider H_2 blockers if bowel obstruction

Anesthesia Technique

- Performed with general anesthesia or combined regional/general

Monitoring

- Routine monitors
- Consider arterial line in patients with CV or pulm disease
- Monitor UO for volume status, indicator of bladder, ureter injury

Airway

- If bowel obstruction, consider rapid-sequence induction

Induction

- Replace volume deficit from bowel prep, NPO, esp. in patients admitted on the day of surgery

SURGICAL STAGES

- Dissection: 2 stages: abd, perineal patients usually in lithotomy position

Definitive Surgery

- Abd phase 1st; mobilization of rectum, sigmoid colon, creation of descending colostomy
- Perineal phase: dissection beginning with elliptical incision from perineum to coccyx; dissection in posterior, lateral planes for 270°; specimen then pulled through perineal wound, final dissection done
- Abd perineal wounds closed; colostomy is matured
- EBL: 1000 ml

Postoperative Considerations

- Pain score: 7–8
- Pain management: PCA IV; epidural
- Morbidity: Urol (bladder/ureter injury, sexual dysfunction), wound dehiscence/infection, blood loss, adhesions (late)

ANTICIPATED PROBLEMS/CONCERNS

- Hypovolemia from bowel prep, capillary leak
- Ureter/bladder injury
- Surg technically more difficult in males (narrow pelvis) with ↑ morbidity

PATHOLOGY

- Dukes' classification:
  - A — limited to bowel wall
  - B — invading through bowel wall
  - C — B plus node involvement
  - D — distant metastasis (liver, lung)
- 5-y survival:
  - A — >90%
  - B — 60–80%
  - C — 20–50%
  - D — <5%

ADRENALECTOMY FOR PHEOCHROMOCYTOMA

Michael F. Roizen, M.D.

RISK

- People within USA: 0.03%–0.04% (~80,000) by autopsy of nonselected individuals; 0.1%–1.0% of individuals with sustained HTN have pheo
- Race with highest prevalence: Caucasian

PERIOPERATIVE RISKS

- Major goal to avoid pheo crisis; pre-, intraop goals of management of extraadrenal surgery no different from those of adrenal surgery; if α blockade not present before surg, try to delay operation until appropriate degree of α blockade judged appropriate by:
  – No BP >165/90 mmHg for 48 h
  – Presence of orthostatic hypotension, but BP on standing should not be <80/45 mmHg
  – An ECG free of ST-T changes due to cardiomyopathy
  – Absence of Sx of catecholamine excess; and signs of α blockade (such as nasal stuffiness)
- If emergency use α rb, ß rb, nitroprusside; keep in ICU till most painful time has passed or adrenergic control attained

- ↑ Risk of HTN crisis with bleeding into myocardium, brain, kidney or ischemia
- Mortality rate to 3% even with appropriate preparation for tumor resection, in "good" hands
- 25%–50% of those who die in hospitals of pheo crisis do so during induction of anesthesia/stressful periop periods, or in labor, delivery
- Associated with cholelithiasis, renal stones

WORRY ABOUT

- Catecholamine crisis with hemorrhage/infarcts in vital organs, hypotension due to ↓ levels of catecholamines postop (uncommon more than 3 d postop if all pheo tissue removed)

OVERVIEW

- Tumor of catecholamine-producing tissue (90% in adrenals): painful (stressful) events often cause exaggerated stress response
- For patients with pheo, even small stresses can lead to blood catecholamine levels of 2000–20,000 pg/ml; infarction of tumor, with release of products on retroperitoneal surfaces, surgical, or other pressure causing release of products, can result in blood levels of 200,000–1 million pg/ml.
- Need α rb before ß blockade lest vasoconstrictive effects of latter go unopposed, causing ↑ risk of dangerous HTN. ß rb suggested if persistent arrhythmias or tachycardia not resolving α adrenergic effects or when aggravated by α adrenergic effects
- If appropriate, α blockade preop can lower risk of crisis by >90%

ICD-9-CM Code: 194.0

INDICATIONS AND USUAL TREATMENT

- 90% spont arise; 10% familial (autosomal dominant genetics involving chromosome 17 implicated)
- Assoc with MEA IIA (medullary thyroid cancer, primary hyperparathyroidism), IIB (medullary thyroid cancer, mucosal neuromas; assoc with neurofibromatosis, von Hippel–Lindau syndrome, and retinal and cerebellar hemangioblastoma, ataxia-telangiectasia, Sturge-Weber syndrome
- "Prehydrate" liberally over 6–60 d if CV status tolerates; expand with high salt/fluid diet while ↑ α rb over 7–60-d period

ASSESSMENT POINTS

SYSTEM	EFFECT	ASSESSMENT BY HX	PE	TEST
HEENT		Nasal stuffiness (from alpha adrenergic blockade)		
CV	HTN, dysrhythmias, AFib, sinus tachycardia, mitral valve prolapse, CHF, myocardial fibril necrosis or myocarditis	SOB, exercise tolerance, palpitations, HTN (50% sustained, 40% paroxsymal)	Standard exam plus measurement of BP q1min in stressful environment plus orthostatic maneuvers with BP/HR measurement q1min	ECG, ECHO (if cardiomyopathy suspected)
GI	90% tumors adrenal or abdominal Wt loss, diarrhea, dehydration		Be careful on palpating abdomen not to trigger pheo crisis	No different from normal
HEME		Mild polycythemia (?2° ↓ IVF), thrombocytopenia		Hgb (↓ of polycythemia way to judge volume expansion by α rb)
CNS	↑ Catecholamine effects	Headache, tremor, anxiety, ↓ pain threshold, fatigue		
METABOLIC	Assoc with hyperparathyroidism	Glucose intolerance due to α adrenergic gluconeogenesis, ↓ insulin secretion		Glucose often ↑ (insulin Rx prescribed before correct Dx of cancer made)

Key Reference: Roizen MF: Pheochromocytoma in anesthetic implications of concurrent disease. *In* Miller's Anesthesia. New York, Churchill Livingstone, 1994, pp 922–925.

PERIOPERATIVE MANAGEMENT

Monitoring

- Temperature
- Arterial line placement before induction difficult
- Consider PA cath and/or TEE if CV system severely affected; CVP used in minority of cases

Anesthetic Care/Technique

- No technique assoc with better or worse outcome; use of droperidol controversial. Agents that block catecholamine reuptake (ketamine) or cause catecholamine release should be avoided

Induction/Maintenance

- Prehydrate liberally if CV status will tolerate
- Gentle induction with nitroprusside available
- Dopamine infusion in reserve
- Painful or stressful events often cause exaggerated stress response caused by release of catecholamines from nerve endings "loaded" by reuptake

SURGICAL STAGES

Initial Dissection

- Transabdominal incision preferred if localization studies do not exclude bilateral tumors; flank/post approach with nephrectomy/jacknife positioning if unilateral adrenalectomy w/o paraganglionoma exploration planned

Adrenal Removal

- Dissection to secure venous drainage, double ligature with transection between; then arterial supply; then complete mobilization, liberation
- After predominant tumor removed, palpation of paraganglionic chain with observation to monitor for sudden ↑ in BP or HR
- Goal in tumor resection is securing venous supply from tumor(s). Surgical or other pressure on tumor causing release of products can result in blood levels of 200,000–1 million pg/ml (ask for temporary stay of surgery, if poss, while rate of nitroprusside infusion ↑)
- Good communication between surgeon, anesthesiologist essential

- Relative hypotension often develops after venous drainage of tumor or its removal. If perfusion adequate can let BP stay at 80/40. Massive infusions of catecholamines occasionally required since patients have often been on endogenous inotropes for many y
- EBL: 100–400 ml; cell saver use not advised (possible to infuse high levels of catecholamines)
- Often hypovolemic if < 2–3 weeks has been allowed for ↑ titration of α rb drugs; guide volume replacement with PCWP or TEE vol estimates

POSTOPERATIVE CONSIDERATIONS

- Postop, do not force high UO with large, crystalloid infusions, as patients have tendency to CHF
- Postop, ~50% remain hypertensive for 1–3 d, when all but 25% become normotensive
- Usually use epidural, PCA, IV narcotics for 2–4 d postop; then wean to NSAID

ANTICIPATED PROBLEMS/CONCERNS

- Pheo crisis a life-threatening illness in patients, manifested by hyperpyrexia, tachycardia, striking alterations in consciousness

ADVANCED CARDIAC LIFE SUPPORT (ACLS)

Stanley J. Glowacki, M.D.
Alan Jay Schwartz, M.D., M.S.Ed.

RISK

- People within USA: 1000 cardiac arrests/d
- Risk factors: male sex, HTN, cigarette smoking, older age, elevated blood cholesterol, diabetes mellitus, Hx of premature artherosclerosis
- No racial predominance

PERIOPERATIVE RISKS

- 1.7 cardiac arrests/10,000 anesthetics
- Associated pathology: ischemic, valvular, or hypertensive heart disease; congestive cardiomyopathy
- Uncommon associated conditions: pre-excitation syndromes, hereditary or acquired prolonged QT disorders, metabolic abnormalities, adverse drug reactions

WORRY ABOUT

- Cardiac pathology
- Perioperative ischemic changes, metabolic abnormalities
- Subsequent episodes postresuscitation
- Postresuscitation end-organ ischemic damage

OVERVIEW

- Morbidity and mortality decreased when ACLS initiated promptly
- Outcome dismal if initiation of ACLS is delayed >8 min or lasts >30 min
- Other factors associated with decreased survival: age >70 y, unwitnessed, sepsis, cancer, renal failure, prearrest hypotension
- Survival rate for in-hospital cardiac arrest is 14%

ICD-9-CM Code: 997.1 (Resulting from procedure)

INDICATIONS/USUAL TREATMENT

- ACLS indicated for treatment of potentially life-threatening dysrhythmias and fatal dysrhythmias or cardiac arrest, e.g., supraventricular bradycardias and tachycardias, ventricular fibrillation, bradyasystole and electrical mechanical dissociation.
- Treatment depends on the dysrhythmia or cause of cardiac arrest and the hemodynamic stability of the patient. (Spinal anesthetics associated with hypotension and bradycardia.)

ASSESSMENT POINTS

SYSTEM	EFFECT	ASSESSMENT BY HX	PE	TEST
CNS	Dysrhythmia may cause hypotension	Syncope	CNS exam	ECG, MRI
CV	Dysrhythmia, HTN, valvular disease	CV status, Hx angina, SOB, palpitation	CV exam	ECG, ECHO
RESP	Pulmonary edema	SOB, orthopnea	Chest exam	SaO_2, CXR

Key Reference: Textbook of Advanced Cardiac Life Support, Dallas American Heart Association, 1994.

INTRAOPERATIVE MANAGEMENT

Monitoring

- Routine, with SpO_2 and end tidal CO_2 encouraged
- Invasive monitoring as indicated by the patient's condition.

Management

- Dependent upon type of rhythm and hemodynamic status
- Emergency drugs, including epinephrine, lidocaine, and atropine, must be immediately available.
- Cardiac defibrillator and means of cardiac pacing must be available.
- Initiate BLS with attention to maintenance of airway, ventilation, and circulation via chest compressions until definitive treatment established.
- Supraventricular Bradydysrhythmias
  – Treat if significant decrease in BP or cardiac output or in the presence of PVCs; atropine 0.5 mg to 1 mg IV, repeat 3–5 min, if needed, to total of 0.03–0.04mg/kg; transcutaneous or transvenous pacing; dopamine or epinephrine infusion; isoproterenol infusions used with extreme caution as last resort.
- Supraventricular Tachydysrhythmias
  – Paroxysmal supraventricular tachycardia (PSVT) with severe hypotension and atrial fibrillation or flutter with hemodynamic compromise.

  – If stable in PSVT, vagal maneuvers followed by adenosine 6mg IV, then adenosine 12mg IV after 1–2 min if PSVT persists. If PSVT recurs and BP remains stable, verapamil 2.5–5.0mg IV.
  – If stable in AFib or atrial flutter, consider diltiazem, β-blockers, or verapamil.
  – If unstable, cardioversion with 100, 200, 300, and 360J may be used in succession until converted.
  – Atrial flutter responds to lower energy (25J).
- Ventricular Bradydysrhythmias
  – CHB with slow idioventricular escape rhythm treated with transvenous or external pacing
  – Atropine or isoproterenol tried until pacing instituted. Beware of precipitating VTach or VFib.
- Premature Ventricular Beats
  – Look for treatable cause.
  – Suppress with lidocaine 1.0–1.5mg/kg IV; may repeat 0.5–0.75mg/kg every 5–10 min to total 3 mg/kg, then procainamide and bretylium.
- Ventricular Tachycardia
  – If stable, lidocaine 1.0–1.5mg/kg IV; may repeat 0.5–0.75mg/kg every 5–10 min to total of 3mg/kg; then procainamide and bretylium.
  – If unsuccessful or hemodynamically unstable, cardioversion with 100, 200, 300, and 360J in progressive increments
- Ventricular Fibrillation (VFib)
  – Rapid defibrillation with 200, 300, and 360J shocks in rapid sequence if VFib persists.

  – If persistent, intersperse defibrillation with epinephrine 1.0mg IV, then lidocaine 1.0–1.5mg/kg IV followed by bretylium 5mg/kg.
- Bradyasystole
  – High mortality, suspect hypoxia
  – Consider immediate transcutaneous pacing.
  – Epinephrine is drug of choice along with atropine.
  – Defibrillation may be tried with asystole as unrecognized VFib is alternative diagnosis.
- Pulseless Electrical Activity
  – Caused by acute derangements in preload (hypovolemia, cardiac tamponade, tension pneumothorax), afterload (pulmonary embolism), myocardial performance (acidosis, hypoxemia)
  – Treatment dependent on cause
  – Epinephrine and atropine may be given.

ANTICIPATED PROBLEMS/CONCERNS

- Following resuscitation continued support of vital organ function often required: CNS insult may cause increase in ICP or seizures; myocardial damage may result in persistent dysrhythmias or decreased contractility; renal damage may result in acute renal failure.

AMPUTATION, ABOVE-KNEE — AKA Candidad Bravo-Fernandez, M.D.

RISK

- 22/100,000 people undergo amputations, 49% above knee
- Mean age 70 y
- Male/Female 3–9:1
- Cause: vascular insufficiency, DM, malignant neoplasm, trauma
- HTN dominant underlying medical condition

PERIOPERATIVE RISKS

- Operative mortality 5%–30% (within 30 d)
- Morbidity includes myocardial ischemia, infarction, CHF, arrhythmias
- Pulmonary emboli: 6–10%
- Nonhealing, infection common surgical problems

WORRY ABOUT

- Underlying disease→AKA
- Associated infection, gangrene
- CVD
- Perioperative pulmonary emboli
- Flexion contractures of involved limb
- Decubiti
- Phantom limb pain

OVERVIEW

- Associated with high operative mortality
- Vascular insufficiency to limb limits viability, ↑ risk of sepsis and complications of immobility, viability evaluated by Doppler, blood flow studies to determine level of amputation
- Preop epidural narcotics to eliminate rest pain
- Regional anesthesia, postop analgesia frequently used; contraindicated in patients receiving anti-coags

- Rehabilitation less optimal than with below-knee amputation; AKA avoided if possible

ICD–9-CM Codes: 747.64 (PVD); 897.2 (Trauma)

INDICATIONS AND USUAL TREATMENT

- Amputations for trauma done early to ↓ contamination
- Control infection, sepsis with antibiotics
- Control blood sugar with regular insulin in diabetic patients
- Smoking should be discontinued 1 wk before operation
- Consider limited revascularization to improve changes for good results
- Below-knee amputation preferred for better rehabilitation

ASSESSMENT POINTS

SYSTEM	EFFECT	ASSESSMENT BY HX	PE	TEST
CV	CAD, HTN	CV status, chest pain, previous MI, SOB	CV exam	ECG, stress test
RESP	Emphysema	SOB, smoking, exercise tolerance	Chest exam	O$_2$ sat, CXR, ABGs
ENDO	DM	Polyuria, polydipsia Cardiomyopathy, neuropathy Autonomic neuropathy Delayed gastric emptying	Sensory exam	Glucose, orthostatic BP
HEME	Thrombophlebitis, bleeding	Pain, bruising, bleeding	Ulcerations, ecchymosis	PT, PTT
RENAL	Renal insufficiency/failure			BUN/Cr
CNS	CVA, TIA	CNS deficits	CNS exam	Carotid studies
PNS	Poor circulation	Claudication	Peripheral pulses	Doppler, flow studies, Angio
INFECTION	Malaise, swelling, gangrene	Fever, chills	Extremity ulcers, swelling, calor, rubor	T, cultures for organism

Key Reference: Lee CS, et al: Changing patterns in the predisposition for amputation of the lower extremities. Am Surg 1992; 58:474–477.

INTRAOPERATIVE MANAGEMENT

- Volume status monitoring—blood loss without tourniquet

Preoperative Preparation

- Antibiotics for trauma
- Ensure availability of blood products

Anesthetic Technique

- Either regional or GA appropriate

Monitoring

- Routine monitors including ST segment analgesia
- Consider arterial, CVP, or PA line if long surgery, depending on CV status

Airway

- In trauma, consider "full stomach"

SURGICAL STAGES

Induction

- Spinal or epidural acceptable in patients with normal coagulation profile
- If GA, worry about myocardial ischemia and ventricular dysfunction

Skin Incision

- Circular incision at the level of amputation
- Observe blood loss; need for ligation of large vessels

Dissection

- Identify femoral artery, vein for clamping, division, ligation; sciatic nerve for ligation
- Assessment of viability of tissue by observing blood loss

Definitive Surgery/Closure

- Femur is divided with a saw, filed
- Wound closed in 2 layers

- Sterile dressing applied
- Immediate postop prosthesis can be applied
- Approximate duration: 1–2 h
- EBL w/o tourniquet: 250–500 ml

POSTOPERATIVE CONSIDERATIONS

- Blood loss may continue; replace as indicated by Hct
- Venous thrombosis associated with prolonged hosp, immobilization, venous stasis
- Aggressive pulmonary toilet to prevent atelectasis, pneumonia
- Phantom limb sensation in 100% of patients; usually resolves in 1 y
- Pain score: 5–10
- Pain relief by PCA if epidural not contraindicated

ANTICIPATED PROBLEMS/CONCERNS

- CV morbidity, mortality common

AMPUTATION, LOWER EXTREMITY
Robert H. Bode, Jr, M.D.

RISK

- 100,000 patients undergo LEAs annually
- Racial/gender predominance: none
- 40%–70% of patients diabetic

PERIOPERATIVE RISKS

- Mortality 3%–15%; usually CV-related
- ↑ Risk of MI, CHF, cardiac ischemia
- Survival in diabetic amputees <50% at 3 y
- Postop phantom limb pain common

WORRY ABOUT

- Perioperative cardiac morbidity/mortality
- Phantom limb pain
- Blood glucose control in diabetic patient

OVERVIEW

- Vast majority of LEAs performed for vasc insufficiency complicated by secondary infections and/or chronic pain
- Below-knee/above-knee amputations in USA 20:1
- >70% of patients undergoing below-knee amputations can be rehabilitated vs only 30% of patients receiving above-knee amputations
- Postop phantom limb pain may ↓ with use of continuous regional anesthesia/analgesia techniques
- High incidence of assoc cardiac morbidity, mortality
- Coexisting diseases common, e.g., CAD, CHF, ↓ LV function, sepsis, diabetes

ICD-9-CM Code: 433.9 (PVD)

INDICATIONS/USUAL TREATMENT

- Most common condition requiring LEAs: vasc insufficiency with lower extremity infections and/or chronic pain (other indications include severe trauma, malignancy, congenital deformities)
- Preservation of knee joint important for rehab; creation of adequate stump flap essential
- Circumferential guillotine amputations are used in cases of severe infection/gangrene and battlefield injuries; guillotine amputations require extensive revision

ASSESSMENT POINTS

SYSTEM	EFFECT	ASSESSMENT OF HX	PE	TEST
CV	Coexisting CAD, CHF Autonomia neuropathy	SOB, angina	Rales S_3 JVD	ECG, stress test, vs Holter, ECHO
RESP	Diabetes/difficult intubation	Chart review	Airway exam Prayer test (see Diabetes, Type I in Diseases section)	
	Coexisting COPD	SOB/bronchospasm	Auscultation	CXR
GI	Diabetes/gastroparesis	Vomiting, early satiety		
ENDO	Diabetes			Blood sugar, urinalysis
HEME	Patients on antithrombotic agents or aspirin	Bleeding		?Bleeding time
GU	Diabetes/nephropathy			BUN/serum Cr
MS	Infections/sepsis	Chart review	VS	WBC with differential, Blood/wound cultures

Key Reference: Humphrey, et al: The contribution of non-insulin-dependent diabetes to lower-extremity amputation in the community. Arch Intern Med, 1994; 154:885–892.

PERIOPERATIVE MANAGEMENT

Preoperative Preparation

- CV assessment for all
- If patients diabetic consider need to control blood glucose, preserve renal function, provide prophylaxis against aspiration
- Regional anesthesia may be contraindicated if patients septic and/or on antithrombotic Rx

Anesthetic Technique

- Can be performed with regional, GA, or combined anesthetic techniques

Monitoring

- Rare need for arterial line, CVP, and/or PA line, except in patients with active and significant heart disease

Airway

- Consider possibility of difficult airway in diabetics

Induction/Maintenance

- Vigilant control of hemodynamic variables and limiting fluids indicated in patients with heart disease

SURGICAL STAGES

Definitive Surgery

- Min. blood loss during dissection (100 to 200 ml)
- Procedure <2 h

Postoperative Considerations

- Both early and late postop pain problems common
- Pain scores: 6–10
- Continuous regional anesthesia/analgesia techniques assoc with less phantom limb pain. Other modalities include PCA, TENS, TCA
- If significant CAD, consider need for postop monitored care for 24–48 h
- Blood glucose control in diabetic patients may be difficult to achieve; keep <200 ml/dl to preserve renal, CNS autoregulation, <250 mg/dl for WBC phagocytic function

ANTICIPATED PROBLEMS/CONCERNS

- ↑ Incidence of CV morbidity/mortality
- Phantom limb pain common after LEAs; may be ↑ with continuous regional anesthesia/analgesia

ANTERIOR CERVICAL FUSION

Laurel E. Moore, M.D.

RISK

- 10,000–80,000 procedures/y (underestimated in literature); 12,000 deaths/y from cervical spine disease in USA
- Racial predominance: none
- Gender predominance: male > female (3/2)

PERIOPERATIVE RISKS

- <1% 30 d mortality
- Recurrent nerve injury: 5%

WORRY ABOUT

- Airway management
- Risk of injury to esophagus, carotid artery, jugular vein
- Postop tracheal edema, recurrent laryngeal nerve injury, ↑ radicular pain or myelopathy, dysphagia

OVERVIEW

- Repair of degenerative, congenital, or traumatic injury to cervical spine or discs
- Anterior approach permits supine position with neutral head position
- Anterior approach provides good access to vertebral bodies, transverse processes of C2–C7
- Generally low blood loss procedure
- Good fusion rate at 12 wk postop

INDICATIONS AND USUAL TREATMENT

- Central herniated disc or spur
- Degenerative hypermobility or subluxation
- Radiculopathy with foraminal stenosis
- ↓ AP diameter of spinal canal
- Compressive myelopathy
- Degenerative kyphoscoliosis
- Alternative Rxs include posterior cervical approach and conservative care with NSAID, rest

ASSESSMENT POINTS

SYSTEM	EFFECT	ASSESSMENT BY HX	PE	TEST
HEENT	Access limited 2° pain, anatomy, prior fusion, neurologic Sx	↑ Neurologic Sxs or pain with movement	Oral opening, cervical ROM, neuro exam	Review of cervical x-ray studies
PNS	Radicular Sxs, myelopathy	Onset of pain, numbness, weakness, bowel or bladder Sx	Motor, sensory assessment, ? single root vs. cord compression	Review of cervical x-ray studies (MRI, CT, myelogram)

Key Reference: Miller JI, Parsa AT: Neurosurgical disease of the spine and spinal cord: surgical considerations. *In* Cottrell JE (ed): Anesthesia and Neurosurgery, 3rd ed. St. Louis, Mosby, 1994, pp 543–567.

PERIOPERATIVE IMPLICATIONS

Anesthetic Technique

- General endotracheal due to surgical traction on trachea, esophagus

Monitoring

- Generally routine
- If multiple levels with instrumentation, consider invasive monitoring
- Arms, neck inaccessible during procedure, so invasive monitoring placed prospectively
- Consider neurologic monitoring (somatosensory or MEP)

Airway

- Consider awake intubation based on presence, absence of neurologic Sx with cervical motion
- Radiologic evidence of cord compression
- Frequently position requires greater neck extension than for direct laryngoscopy

Maintenance

- Consider narcotic-based anesthesia, particularly if neurologic monitoring
- Muscle relaxation assists in distraction of cervical spine
- Generally not stimulating procedure except with placement of vertebral spreading retractor; removal of iliac bone for interbody fusion graft

Emergence

- Rapid awakening for neurologic assessment optimal

SURGICAL STAGES

- 10–15 lb traction applied by Gardner-Wells tongs or head brace for cervical distraction
- Combination of weighted traction, muscle paralysis, vertebral spreading retractor gives access to disc space

Exposure

- Trachea and esophagus retracted medially
- Carotid artery retracted laterally
- Recurrent laryngeal nerve retracted inferiorly
- Sup laryngeal, hypoglossal nerves retracted superiorly
- Vertebral artery ascends via foramina of transverse processes
- Disc space cleaned; interbody fusion performed with autologous (iliac crest) or cadaveric bone graft
- EBL, 3rd space losses generally small

POSTOPERATIVE CONSIDERATIONS

- Pain at iliac graft site (pain score: 6–8), can be attenuated with local anesthetic injection pre-emergence
- Dysphagia common postop 2° traction on esophagus
- Complic include
  - recurrent largyngeal nerve injury
  - ↓ HR, BP with carotid sinus manipulation
  - ↑ radicular pain or myelopathy
  - postop hematoma formation
  - transient tracheal or esophageal edema, dysmotility from prolonged retraction
  - nonunion of fusion

ANTICIPATED PROBLEMS/CONCERNS

- Airway management
- Vital structures close to operative site causing hemodynamic changes intraoperatively or nerve injury postoperatively
- Fusions involving >1–2 levels have ↑ risk of non-union or pseudarthrosis

AORTIC VALVE REPLACEMENT

Jonathan G. Latour, M.D.
James G. Ramsay, M.D., F.R.C.P. (C).

RISK

- Number of operations in USA/y: 26,000 (1991)
- Gender predominance: M/F: 8/5

PERIOPERATIVE RISKS

- 2–6% perioperative mortality
- Heart block—disruption of the bundle of His (may require permanent pacemaker)
- CVA—associated with atherosclerotic disease, manipulation of ascending aorta, incomplete evacuation of air at end of CPB

WORRY ABOUT

- Reason for replacement (stenosis vs. regurgitation)

- ↓ LV function preop, especially with AR
- Coronary perfusion pressure: diastolic BP minus LVEDP (especially with AS)
- Arrhythmias: significant change in HR or loss of atrial contribution may cause severe ↓ CO
- LV distention with initiation of CPB before aortic cross-clamping if AR present
- De-airing before to discontinuation of CPB

OVERVIEW

- Operative mortality for isolated AVR <5%, ↑ mortality with ↑ age, ↓ LV function, coexisting CAD, and ↓ exercise tolerance
- Patients with AS generally have better prognosis than those with AR especially when ↓ LV function present

- Arrhythmias/heart block—atrial contribution to CO very important after AVR, especially in hypertrophied heart. Bundle of His prone to injury; atrial, ventricular pacing wires often used

ICD-9-CM Codes: (AS) 424.1; (AR) 424.1; 35.22 (AVR—other)

INDICATIONS AND USUAL TREATMENT

- AS Sx of syncope, angina, CHF
- Asymptomatic AS with aortic valve area <0.7 cm^2 or pressure gradient >50 mmHg at rest (with normal LV function)
- AR Sx of CHF, DOE, angina
- Asymptomatic AR with evidence of LV dysfunction

ASSESSMENT POINTS

SYSTEM	EFFECT	ASSESSMENT BY HX	PE	TEST
HEENT	Coexisting dental infection Rx before AVR to ↓ incidence of postop endocarditis	Oral hygiene	Oral exam	
CV	Chronic AS or AR may →impairment of LV systolic, diastolic function (especially AS), dysrhythmia; coexisting CAD may be present Other valvular abnormality possible	CV status (NYHA class) Chest pain, orthopnea, PND palpitations, syncope Exercise intolerance, DOE, SOB	CV exam rhythm	ECG ECHO Cardiac cath
RESP	Pulmonary vascular congestion from ↑ LVEDP	DOE, orthopnea, PND, SOB	Resp exam	CXR SaO$_2$
GU	Impairment 2° to age			BUN/Cr
CNS	CNS Hx if 1) patients in chronic AFib, 2) elderly patient with poss co-existing carotid vascular disease, 3) patients with valvular vegetations	CNS Hx Hx palpitations Hx SBE prophylaxis	CNS exam CV exam	Carotid Doppler TEE to evaluate for atrial thrombus, valve vegetations

Key Reference: Ross J Jr: Afterload mismatch in aortic and mitral valve disease: Implication for surgical therapy. J Am Coll Cardiol 1985; 5:811.

INTRAOPERATIVE MANAGEMENT

Preoperative Preparation

- Light premed; prevent anxiety but avoid heavy premed that may significantly ↓ preload, afterload
- Supply O$_2$ after premed

Anesthetic Technique—AS

- Perioperative hemodynamic goals: (1) maintain preload, afterload, (2) avoid ↓ BP (coronary perfusion pressure essential with LVH), (3) maintain sinus rhythm, normal rate, (4) aggressive Rx for dysrhythmias (loss of atrial click/rapid rate poorly tolerated) may require synchronized cardioversion

Anesthetic Technique—AR

- Perioperative hemodynamic goals: (1) maintain preload, (2) maintain arterial dilation (nitroprusside, nicardipine), (3) avoid significant myocardial ↓, (4) maintain high normal HR (90–100/min); bradycardia results in ↑ regurgitation LVEDP, (5) inotropic support frequently required postbypass if ↓ LVEF
- IABP contraindicated in presence of AR

Monitoring

- Large-bore IVs, arterial line, 5-lead ECG

- PAC vs. CVP (CVP may grossly underestimate LVEDP, but placement of PAC has potential for dysrhythmias, heart block)
- Consider TEE; monitor vol status, contractility, regional wall motion abnormality, other coexisting valvular disease, adequacy of de-airing and postop valve function
- Consider external defibrillation pads with capability of transthoracic pacing
- Consider esophageal stethoscope with atrial pacing capacity

SURGICAL STAGES

Induction/Prebypass

- Opioid-based induction recommended in presence of ↓ LVEF
- CV instability 2° to alteration in preload, afterload, HR, myocardial contractility. Aggressively Rx for hypotension; determine cause later (hypovolemia vs. dysrhythmia)
- Cardiac surgeon, perfusionist present at induction prep for emergency CPB
- Avoid ↑ PaCO$_2$, associated ↑ PVR
- Consider antifibrinolytic drug

Cardiopulmonary Bypass

- In AR prevent LV distention at initiation of CPB by maintaining sinus rhythm: (1) IV

esmolol 1–2 mg/kg, (2) IV lidocaine 1–2 mg/kg; urgent aortic cross-clamping/LV venting poss necessary
- Consider thiopental (to flat EEG) to ↓ incidence/severity of CVA (↑ inotropic support, postop ventilation may be required)
- Evacuation of air before discontinuing CPB; TEE may evaluate adequacy of de-airing, valve function

Postoperative Considerations

- Blood loss: check ACT, platelets, fibrinogen. Maintain Hct of 25–30
- Arrhythmia/heart block—Atrial, ventricular pacing wires recommended; bundle of His prone to injury, permanent pacemaker poss required
- Extubate when normothermic
- Anti-coag—mech valves only—Coumadin usually begun 2–3 d postop
- Consider low-dose β rb to prevent arrhythmias

ANTICIPATED PROBLEMS/CONCERNS

- ↓ Preop LV function may require inotropic support and/or IABP (especially AR)
- AFib/AF poorly tolerated with LVH
- Heart block can develop on 1st d postop

AORTOPULMONARY WINDOW

Howard Alan Zucker, M.D.

RISK

- 0.2–0.6% of congenital HD
- Associated with secundum ASD, PDA, VSD, aortic origin of right PA, type A interrupted aortic arch, tetralogy of Fallot, anomalous origin of coronary arteries
- No gender predilection

PERIOPERATIVE RISKS

- Perioperative mortality rate <3%

WORRY ABOUT

- ↑ Pulmonary flow 2° to L→R shunt preop
- Development of preop CHF
- Pulmonary HTN with associated reactive pulmonary vascular bed; of concern if repaired later in life

OVERVIEW

- Manifests similarly to VSD or PDA with overcirculation of pulmonary vascular bed
- Sx of CHF include failure to thrive, diaphoresis, dyspnea

ICD-9-CM Code: 745.0

INDICATIONS AND USUAL TREATMENT

- Surg correction indicated in all cases using CPB with patch closure (Dacron or glutaraldehyde-treated pericardium)
- Associated congenital heart lesions may result in postop problems unrelated to the aortopulmonary window repair
- Eisenmenger vs physiologic changes from long-standing L→R shunting only contraindication to surg closure

ASSESSMENT POINTS

SYSTEM	EFFECT	ASSESSMENT BY HX	PE	TEST
CV	CHF, Pulmonary HTN, Eisenmenger's	Exercise tolerance, dyspnea, cyanosis	CV exam	ECG ECHO CXR
RESP	Reactive pulmonary vascular bed	Tachypnea	Auscultation	O$_2$ sat

Key Reference: Brooks M, Heyman M: Aortopulmonary window. *In* Emmanouilides, Allen, Riemenschneider, Gutgesell (eds): Moss' Heart Disease in Infants, Children and Adolescents, 5th ed. Williams & Wilkins, 1995, pp 764–768.

PERIOPERATIVE IMPLICATIONS

Anesthetic Technique

- General anesthesia with narcotic-based technique
- Avoid extubation in neonatal patient or those with reactive pulmonary vascular bed

Monitoring

- Arterial line
- Two peripheral IVs
- Right and left atrial lines placed by surgeon at conclusion of CPB

Airway

- No associated airway anomalies

Induction

- If IV access available can use opioids, ketamine, or etomidate
- If patient w/o IV access, halothane mask induction acceptable
- Use principles applied to VSDs, PDAs, other L→R shunting lesions

SURGICAL STAGES

Dissection

- Under CPB through midline sternotomy

Definitive Surgery

- Involves placement of pericardial or Dacron patch
- Performed under moderately hypothermic conditions
- Deep hypothermic circulatory arrest used in certain situations
- Modifications of reconstruction may occur in situations of patients with associated coronary anomalies

Postoperative Considerations

- Significant postop pain
- Use of duramorph in caudal space to control pain with associated postop monitoring for respiratory compromise may be helpful
- Pain score: 6–8
- Reactive pulmonary vascular bed with associated pulmonary HTN; often seen with tube suctioning
- Postop blood loss 2° to CPB
- Packed RBC, platelets, cryoprecipitate, and/or FFP replacement as indicated

APPENDECTOMY

Joseph Rosa III, M.D.

RISK

- Consider in any patient with abd pain
- Rare in infants, more common in childhood; max incidence, teens, 20s; thereafter declines; 1 in 7 sometime in their lifetime (15% of USA population)
- M/F 3:2
- Etiology: 60% hyperplasia of submucosal lymphoid follicles; 35%, fecal stasis (fecalith); 4%, other foreign bodies; 1% tumors

PERIOPERATIVE RISKS

- Mortality: overall <1/100,000; in acute but not gangrenous, <0.1%; gangrenous, 0.6%; perforated, 5%.
- Morbidity: pelvic, intra-abd, subphrenic abscess with perforation, ≈20%; wound abscess, <5%; fecal fistula, <1%; wound hematoma, <0.5%; ileus, variable.
- Greater morbidity and mortality in peds, 2° to absence of fully developed omentum, subsequent spread of infection, with development of peritonitis after perforation.

WORRY ABOUT

- Intravascular vol status 2° to poor oral intake, ± vomiting, 3rd spacing with peritonitis
- Aspiration—ileus, full stomach
- Electrolyte abnormalities
- Perioperative sepsis
- If laparoscopic, usual concerns with pneumoperitoneum, CO_2 insufflation
- Differential Dx: consider more catastrophic etiologies of abd pain, incl rupturing aneurysm, intestinal ischemia, acute pancreatitis
- Postop infection, sepsis

OVERVIEW

- Obstruction of appendiceal opening
- Perioperative infection a concern with perforated appendix, peritonitis
- ↑ Morbidity, mortality with perforation.
- Fewer normal appendixes removed since US, laparoscopy used for Dx

ICD-9-CM Code: 540

INDICATIONS AND USUAL TREATMENT

- Suspected appendicitis
- Differential Dx in young children: acute gastroenteritis, mesenteric lymphadenitis, pyelitis, Meckel's diverticulitis, intussusception pneumonia.
- Differential Dx in teenagers and adults depends on gender: in F, ruptured ectopic pregnancy, mittelschmerz, endometriosis, salpingitis, regional enteritis; in M, regional enteritis, renal calculi, testicular torsion, acute epididymitis.
- Differential Dx, older adults: diverticulitis, perforated ulcer, acute cholecystitis, pancreatitis, intestinal obstruction, perforating cecal cancer, torsion of ovarian cyst, mesenteric vascular occlusion, rupturing abd aortic aneurysm

ASSESSMENT POINTS

SYSTEM	EFFECT	ASSESSMENT BY HX	PE	TEST
CV	Age-related considerations; dehydration 2° to fever, emesis; ↓ PO intake	CV status, Hx CP, SOB, exercise tolerance	CV exam	ECG if indicated, orthostatics to assess vol
RESP	Resp impaired 2° to abd pain/splinting in elderly; tachypnea, hyperpnea may suggest perforation/sepsis; full stomach considerations		Chest exam	CXR if indicated
HEME	Leukocytosis, with left shift hemoconcentration; 4% of patients have normal WBC, differential			CBC with differential
RENAL/CNS	Mental status changes associated with dehydration; electrolyte abnormalities, early sepsis; ↓ UO 2° to ↓ IV vol	Hx UO; Hx mental status	CNS exam	UA

Key Reference: Sabiston DC, Jr: Textbook of Surgery: The Biological Basis of Modern Surgical Practice, 14th ed. Philadelphia, WB Saunders, 1991, p 884.

PERIOPERATIVE MANAGEMENT

Preoperative Preparation

- Restore IV vol/T management.

Anesthetic Technique

- General ET with rapid-sequence intubation with Sellick's maneuver or awake if difficult airway
- Regional: spinal vs. epidural if no absolute contraindications; patient adequately hydrated, cooperative; high abdominal exploration unlikely

Monitoring

- Routine—continue monitoring prn

Airway

- Usual considerations apply

Induction

- Consider IV volume status when choosing induction agents
- Consider possibility of myopathy in children if choosing succinylcholine

Maintenance

- Usually volatile agent ± N_2O, narcotic, relaxant

SURGICAL STAGES

- Skin incision: McBurney's incision (RLQ)
- Dissection: extent depends on appendix location, degree of inflammation; 3rd space volume a consideration
  - retrocecal position, 65%
  - 30% tip in pelvis
- Closure: perforated ± skin closure, if abscess present, surgeon may place drain; minimal if laparoscopic
- EBL: <75 ml
- Vol requirements: replace deficit and 5–8 ml/kg/h with normal saline or lactated Ringer's solution

Postoperative Considerations

- Pain score: 5–7; PCA for postop pain

ANTICIPATED PROBLEMS/CONCERNS

Complications

- Sepsis, paralytic ileus, atelectasis
- Aspiration risk
- Prolongation of NMB drugs 2° to interaction with antibiotics, esp aminoglycosides

ATRIAL SEPTAL DEFECT, REPAIR OF
Charles W. Hogue, Jr., M.D.

RISK

- Ostium secundum occurs in 7% and 40% of all congenital heart disease in children and adults, respectively
- Female/male ratio 2:1, except for ostium primum ASD, for which ratio is 1:1

PERIOPERATIVE RISKS

- Risk dependent on age, degree of reversibility of ↑ PVR; mortality usually <1%
- Supraventricular arrhythmias including atrial flutter, AFib
- AV conduction block possible if ASD close to AV node

WORRY ABOUT

- Paradoxical venous embolism
- Right heart volume overload with RV dysfunction
- MVP, regurgitation with ostium secundum
- Partial anomalous pulmonary venous drainage with sinus venosus
- Cleft anterior mitral valve leaflet with ostium primum defect
- Endocarditis prophylaxis

OVERVIEW

- Classified by location: *ostium secundum* (70% of ASDs) involves midseptal fossa ovalis; *sinus venosus,* high in RA, close to RA/SVC junction; *ostium primum,* in inferior septum, is an endocardial cushion defect
- Unless heart murmur heard, usually not diagnosed until symptomatic in 3rd–4th decade of life
- Degree of L→R shunting dependent on size of ASD, relative compliance of ventricles, relative SVR, PVR
- MVP in 10%–30% of patients; may be 2° shift of I-V septum from RV volume overload; usually reversed with closure of ASD
- RV diastolic dimensions ↑, interventricular septum shifted; normal resting but ↓ LVEF with exercise possible

ICD-9-CM Code: 745.5

INDICATIONS AND USUAL TREATMENT

- Surgical closure for uncomplicated ASD with pulmonary-to-systemic flow ratio >1.5
- Optimal age of repair may be <5 y
- PVR at rest >8 U/m² that fails to ↓ to <7 U/m² with pulmonary vasodilators usually contraindication to surgery
- Lung Tx considered with correction of ASD or heart and lung Tx for irreversibly ↑ PVR
- Transcatheter closure possible in some centers

ASSESSMENT POINTS

SYSTEM	EFFECT	ASSESSMENT BY HX	PE	TEST
CV	Pulmonary HTN, RHF	SOB, DOE, fatigue	↑ RV impulse, JVD Fixed split S₂, hepatomegaly, ascites, edema	CXR, ECHO Cardiac catheterization
RESP	Infection	Cough, sputum	Rhonchi, wheezing, consolidation	CXR, CBC, Cultures
HEPATIC	Passive edema		Hepatomegaly, jaundice, ascites	Liver enzymes, albumin, PT, PTT

Key Reference: Skorton DJ, Garson A: Congenital heart diseases in adolescents and adults. Cardiol Clin 1993; 11:717–720.

PERIOPERATIVE IMPLICATIONS

Anesthetic Technique

- General

Monitoring

- CVP
- Arterial line
- Consider TEE with color-flow Doppler, LAP

Induction/Maintenance

- Anesthetic technique guided by preferences, age, condition; extubation early after surgery in most patients

SURGICAL STAGES

- Median sternotomy, but anterior lateral thoracotomy, cosmetic submammary incision appropriate at times
- Cardioplegic arrest
- Direct suture closure if ASD small, pericardial patch closure otherwise. Dacron graft, Gore-Tex CV patch suitable substitutes for pericardial patch in some cases
- Anomalous pulmonary venous drainage repaired with pericardial patch "baffle," redirecting pulmonary venous flow into LA

Postoperative Considerations

- LAP/PCWP may be high, 2° MR, LV diastolic dysfunction from coexisting disease or shift of IV septum
- RV dimension, hemodynamics improve shortly after surgery
- Supraventricular arrhythmias including AFib/flutter
- Reoperation uncommon, but occasional dehiscence of atrial baffle
- Pulmonary and peripheral thromboembolism with AFib (Coumadin commonly started 2nd d after surg for 8–12 wk)

AV GRAFT FOR HEMODIALYSIS
Anthony J. Cunningham, M.D.

RISK

- End-stage renal failure with Cr clearance of <10 ml urine almost certain to need hemodialysis in 3 mo
- Population on hemodialysis in 1985: 373/10 in USA
- M:F predominance: none

PERIOPERATIVE RISKS

- Minimum mortality depends on associated risk factor present with ESRD: cardiac decompensation, lyte-caused arrhythmias
- 10%–15% technical failure
- Other possible periop complications in order of risk: thrombosis, infection, no venous outflow, venous aneurysm, venous HTN, arterial steal, CHF

WORRY ABOUT

- Adequate preop management of HTN, CAD, diabetes, hyperkalemia

- Adequate hydration, maintenance of BP to protect patency of AV graft

OVERVIEW

- Of all patients receiving Rx for ESRD, 71% in USA dependent on dialysis
- Causes of ESRD: glomerulonephritis, diabetes, HTN, pyelonephritis
- Associated conditions: PVD, CAD, electrolyte abn
- Patients often have Adams-Stokes attacks grade III, IV
- Local infiltration—i.e., monitored anesthesia care or regional anesthesia advantageous due to ↓ number of drug effects, but contraindicated if coagulopathy, residual heparin effect, postrenal dialysis, or hyperkalemia (made worse with hypoventilation)—worry about hypoventilation with sedatives

ICD-9-CM Code: 585 (Chronic renal failure)

INDICATIONS/USUAL TREATMENT

- Dialysis timed to begin when renal failure advanced but before severe deterioration in well-being
- Biochem indications: Cr clearance ≤5 ml/min or serum Cr >1200 μmol/L
- Choice of dialysis: hemodialysis or CAPD, based on assessment of general condition
- Contraindications to hemodialyis: psychosis, severe mental retardation, carcinomatosis
- Adverse factors: CHF, widespread vascular disease, multiple nonrenal complications—e.g., blindness, neuropathy of DM
- CAPD: preferred method in young children, diabetics, elderly

ASSESSMENT POINTS

SYSTEM	EFFECT	ASSESSMENT BY HX	PE	TEST
RESP	Pneumonia, pulm edema, uremic pleuritis	SOB, orthopnea, PND	Resp	CXR
GI	↓ Gastric emptying GI bleeding	Regurgitation; N/V; early satiety		
HEME	Anemia, bleeding diathesis	SOB, bruising		Plts
GU/ENDO	Oliguria/anuria, uremia, electrolyte/acid-base imbalance; diabetes	Wt (baseline & high), hiccoughs, anorexia, N/V/diarrhea, diabetes	CV, resp	Cr, BUN, HCO$_3^-$, glucose
CNS	Encephalopathy, seizures, neuropathy	MS	CNS	

Key Reference: Marx AB, Landmann F, Harder FH: Surgery for vascular access (Review). Curr Prob Surg 1990; 27:1–48.

PERIOPERATIVE MANAGEMENT

Anesthetic Technique

- Monitored anesthetic care; regional or GA
- Regional anesthesia—pronounced sympatholytic vasodilation useful in patient with sparse venous network
- GA & MAC: must remember ↓ protein binding, acid-base, electrolyte disturbances

Monitoring

- Avoid IV, pulse oximeter, BP cuff placement on operated arm
- End-tidal CO$_2$ esp for MAC if resp drive depressants given
- Careful fluid monitoring, non-K$^+$-containing fluid given

Induction/Maintenance

- Renal failure ↓ protein binding→prolonged, exaggerated effects of highly protein-bound drugs
- Acidemia: ↑ proportions of agent in nonionized, unbound state, so active portion of drug also mostly non-ionized
- Uremia: ↑ permeability of BBB
- Local anesthetics have ↓ duration of action in patients with renal failure due to ↓ elimination; also acidosis, hyperkalemia in patients with CHF ↑ myocardial susceptibility to bupivacaine toxicity

- Avoid succinylcholine if K$^+$ concn ≥ 5.5 mmol/L
- Pancuronium, d-tubocurarine have delayed excretion, ↑ duration of action (atracurium, vecuronium duration not significantly affected)
- Biotransformation: organic fluoride production not an issue in dialysis patients
- Opioids produce ↑ magnitude, duration of effect
- ↑ Accumulation of morphine glucuronides, prolonged respiratory depression
- Normeperidine, an accumulated metabolite of meperidine, can cause Sz; fentanyl better choice

Surgical Considerations

- Vasc access requirement
  – Blood flow >200 ml/min allows completion of dialysis within 3–4 h
  – Shunt must be easily accessible
  – If possible, shunt should be on nondominant arm for self-cannulation for patients on home dialysis
- Location
  – wrist: "snuff box"/antebrachium-cephalic vein to radial art
  – forearm: radial/ulnar/brachial art to antecubital/brachial vein
  – upper arm: brachial art above elbow to basilic/ax vein
- Access: natural:
  – fistulas (e.g., Brescia-Cimino)
  – vasc substitutes—prosthetic: (e.g., polytetrafluoroethylene (Teflon) graft

- EBL: 25–100 ml; depends on type of access fashioned
- Surg, 1–2 h

Postoperative Considerations

- Pain score: 1–2
- Pain management: PO analgesia
- Operated arm must remain elevated several d to minimize swelling at surgical site
- Venipuncture, BP measurements not allowed on surgical arm; pt must also avoid wearing wristbands or constrictive clothing on that arm
- Always monitor AV fistula/graft for adequate blood flow by palpating thrill + auscultation, Doppler

ANTICIPATED PROBLEMS/CONCERNS

- Blood flow in autogenous AV fistula ↑ with time; resulting venous wall thickening prevents venous tears, infiltration during dialysis; maturation time varies from 3–6 wk; fistula not to be used for 3 wk to avoid aneurysm formation
- In graft fistulas, infection rate depends on material used, site of access

PROGNOSIS

- Renal transplantation: optimal Rx for ESRD; waiting time varies considerably
- As AV access for hemodialysis has finite lifespan, revising or replacing AV fistulas/grafts usual

BLALOCK-TAUSSIG (BT) SHUNT

Richard D. Alessi, Jr., M.D.

RISK

- For patients (usually neonates or infants) with severely ↓ pulmonary blood flow due to congenital heart disease
- Including infants with tetralogy of Fallot, pulm atresia, pulmonary stenosis, tricuspid atresia, some cases of TGV

PERIOPERATIVE RISKS

- 30-d mortality: 5.5% for all cases, probably closer to 2% for tetralogy of Fallot
- Other complications include Horner's syndrome, chylothorax, phrenic nerve damage, acute arm ischemia when subclavian arterial flow is diverted

WORRY ABOUT

- Maintain saturation prerepair by continued prostaglandin E_1 or physiologic ↑ pulmonary blood flow, avoiding hypoxemia, hypercarbia, hypotension, acidosis
- Possible severe hypoxemia while PA clamped
  - (see Postoperative Period)

OVERVIEW

- One of multiple types of systemic pulm shunts to ↑ pulmonary blood flow
- Familiarity with underlying anatomy and physiology is essential to management, including ductal patency, VSD, ASD
- Subclavian (opposite side of arch to limit kinking) to PA anastomosis performed directly (classic), or using Gore-Tex tube graft (modified)
- Goal: adequate but not excessive pulmonary blood flow
- Followed by mechanical or pharmacologic closure of ductus, if still open
- Nonconfluence of pulmonary arteries or distal pulmonary artery stenosis may require bypass, more extensive surgery

ICD-9-CM Code: 745.2 (Tetralogy of Fallot)

INDICATIONS AND USUAL TREATMENT

- Palliatively for cyanotic congenital heart defects not surgically correctable or in infants as part of a staged procedure to allow development of pulmonary vasculature or heart: including tetralogy of Fallot, pulm atresia, pulmonary stenosis, tricuspid atresia, some cases of TGV

ASSESSMENT POINTS

SYSTEM	EFFECT	PE	TEST
HEENT	↑ Incidence of craniofacial defects	Airway	
CV	Congestive heart disease		ECHO or angio
RESP	↓ Pulmonary blood flow	Cyanosis	O_2 sat ABG

Key Reference: Arciniegas E, Farooki ZQ, Hakimi M: Classic shunting operations for cyanotic congenital heart defects. J Thorac Cardiovasc Surg 1982; 84:88–96.

PERIOPERATIVE MANAGEMENT

Preoperative Preparation

- Patients often already intubated due to cyanosis, acute or chronic
- Maintain ↓ PVR to max pulmonary blood flow (hyperventilate, high FIO_2)
- Arterial line usually should be placed to monitor contralateral upper extremity, femoral, umbilical pressures

Intraoperative Period

- May use inhalation induction but effect may be delayed with ↓ pulmonary blood flow (despite faster rise in Fa/Fi)
- Lateral thoracotomy classic, but CPB possible, median sternotomy may be used
- Heparin sometimes used (1 mg/kg)
- Anticipate worsened hypoxia with PA clamping
- Transfusion not usually required

Postoperative Period

- Goal is adequate but not excessive pulmonary blood flow; shunt should be slightly restrictive to avoid CHF; check, compare pressure in subclavian or aortic artery with PA (should be almost equal), or flows compared with ECHO Doppler (usually aim for 3:1 Qp/Qs ratios)
- Cyanosis or clotting possible if shunt too small or systemic vessel kinks
- CHF or pulmonary edema possible (may be unilateral) if pulmonary blood flow is too great
- Shunt flow usually restricted by shunt orifice, therefore adequate pulmonary blood flow, oxygenation require normal pressure (i.e., avoid hypotension)
EBL: 50–100 ml
Pain score: 8–10

PROGNOSIS

- Ultimate prognosis depends on underlying congenital defects
- Recent advances, techniques in surgery allow many patients to undergo primary (complete) repair, avoiding BT shunts

BLOOD COMPONENTS

Linda Stehling, M.D.

RISK

- Estimated utilization in USA: 22 million
- RBC: 12; Plt 7; FFP 2; CRYO 1 (million)

PERIOPERATIVE RISKS

- Overtransfusion
- Undertransfusion

WORRY ABOUT

- Transfusion-transmitted disease (e.g., HIV, hepatitis)
- Hemolytic reaction due to RBC incompatibility
- Nonhemolytic reactions (fever, urticaria)
- Immunosuppression (infection, cancer recurrence)

OVERVIEW

- RBC: To increase oxygen-carrying capacity in chronic anemia and acute blood loss
- Plt: To prevent or treat bleeding due to thrombocytopenia or impaired platelet function
- FFP: To prevent or treat bleeding due to coagulation factor depletion
- CRYO: For bleeding due to hypofibrinogenemia or dysfibrinogenemia; also used in treating some patients with von Willebrand's disease and hemophilia; used in preparing fibrin glue

DOSE

- RBC: 3 ml/kg ↑ hematocrit 3% (Hgb 1g)
- Plt: 1 concentrate/10 kg [1 apheresis unit = ± 6 concentrates]
- FFP: 10–15 ml/kg
- CRYO: 1 unit/7–10 kg

ASSESSMENT POINTS

COMPONENT	EFFECT	ASSESSMENT BY HX	PE	TEST
RBC	Oxygen delivery	Anemia; blood loss; cardiopulmonary reserve, oxygen consumption	Pallor; blood loss	Hgb, Hct, O_2 extraction ratio
Plt	Coagulation	Petechiae, mucosal bleeding; disease, drugs affecting Plt function	Microvascular bleeding	Plt count
FFP	Coagulation	Ecchymoses, bleeding into joints; liver disease	Microvascular bleeding	PT, PTT
CRYO	Coagulation	von Willebrand's disease, hemophilia, congenital fibrinogen disorders	Microvascular bleeding	Fibrinogen

Key Reference: Stehling L, Luban NL, Anderson KC, et al: Guidelines for blood utilization review. Transfusion 1994; 34:438–448.

PERIOPERATIVE IMPLICATIONS

Preoperative Preparation

- RBC: Hct/Hgb may be indicated
- Plt, FFP, CRYO: Labs not required in absence of positive Hx

Induction/Maintenance

- RBC: Inability to ↑ cardiac output in response to lower O_2 delivery can cause myocardial ischemia.
- Plt: Clinically significant thrombocytopenia (Plt count < 50 × 10^9/L) may occur with ≥1 blood volume replacement.
- FFP: Bleeding may occur if PT, PTT > 1.5 × mean normal value and/or ≥1 blood volume replacement.
- CRYO: Bleeding may occur with fibrinogen <100 mg/dl and with von Willebrand's disease unresponsive to DDAVP.

Regional Anesthesia

- RBC: Hypotension may further impair O_2 delivery
- Plt, FFP, CRYO: Epidural hematoma can occur in patients with coagulopathy.

Postoperative Period

- Continued bleeding may necessitate additional component therapy.

ANTICIPATED PROBLEMS/CONCERNS

- Indications for transfusion should be documented.
- Fear of tranfusion-transmitted disease should not lead to withholding of necessary transfusion.

BLOWOUT ORBITAL FRACTURE

Kathryn E. McGoldrick, M.D.

RISK

- Rare
- Patients subjected to blunt trauma with a nonpenetrating object (e.g., fist)
- Racial predominance: none

PERIOPERATIVE RISKS

- In absence of serious associated injuries, rare perioperative mortality (<0.1%)
- Postop risk of visual disturbances, including blindness, infection, and cosmetic deformity

WORRY ABOUT

- Intraocular damage (ruptured globe rare in isolated orbital blowout fracture owing to release of compressive forces into the maxillary sinus)

- Associated nonophthalmic injuries (intracranial injury, cervical spine fracture or subluxation, Le Fort fractures with basilar skull fracture)
- Prolapse and incarceration of orbital soft tissues
- Preop systemic steroids (to distinguish neuromuscular edema or related motility disturbance from true entrapment, unmask enophthalmos, and reduce discomfort) predispose to sinus-orbital infections
- Hemostasis for delicate surgery

OVERVIEW

- Fractures of orbital floor are repaired by various surgical approaches.
- Intraoperative infiltration with lidocaine with 1:100,000 epinephrine for hemostatic effect

- Entrapped tissues freed with care taken to avoid infraorbital neurovascular tissue trauma
- Autologous or alloplastic implant material placed over fracture site

ICD-9-CM Code: 802.6

SURGICAL INDICATIONS/USUAL TREATMENT

- The three standard indications for surgical intervention are enophthalmos, motility disturbance secondary to entrapment, hypoophthalmos.
- Timing of surgical intervention depends on associated injuries and patient's age, general health, and preference; preferable to delay in order to permit some resolution of edema and bleeding; technical ease and functional result typically enhanced by surgery within 5–14 d

ASSESSMENT POINTS (in addition to evaluation of coexisting disease)

SYSTEM	EFFECT	ASSESSMENT BY HX	PE	TEST
EYE	Trauma may produce orbital subcutaneous emphysema, restriction of globe motility, globe ptosis, enophthalmos, retinal or choroidal injury		Inspection Palpation Funduscopic exam	CT scan
CNS	Trauma may produce head injuries	CNS Hx	CNS exam	CT scan
MS	Trauma may produce assorted MS and organ injuries	Pain	Palpation	Plain films as indicated

Key Reference: Mead MD: Evaluation and initial management of patients with ocular and adnexal trauma. In Albert DM, Jakobiec FA (eds): Principles and Practice of Ophthalmology. Philadelphia, WB Saunders, 1994, pp 3362–3382.

PERIOPERATIVE IMPLICATIONS

Preoperative Preparation
- None

Anesthetic Technique
- GA usual; also local

Monitoring
- Routine

Airway
- Other facial injuries may complicate airway management.

Induction/Maintenance
- Without associated injuries, few hemodynamic perturbations
- Avoid HTN (to minimize bleeding)
- Adequate depth of anesthesia to prevent patient movement during delicate surgery
- Consider antiemetic prophylaxis

SURGICAL STAGES

Dissection
- Minimal blood loss

Definitive Surgery
- Minimal blood loss (<100 ml) and fluid shifts
- Approximate duration: 2 h

Postoperative Considerations
- Mild postop pain
- IV-PCA usually not necessary
- Without other injuries, discharge on day of surgery

ANTICIPATED PROBLEMS/CONCERNS

- Blindness
- Infraorbital paresthesia
- Implant extrusion
- Diplopia and delayed extraocular muscle restriction
- Obstructive sinus disease
- Infection
- Return to potentially violent environment

BONE MARROW TRANSPLANTATION (HARVEST PROCEDURE)

Charles D. Boucek, M.D.

RISK

- Autologous: patients with malignancies that respond to chemotherapy (9740 cases 1989–93, North American Autologous Bone Marrow Transplant Registry)
- Allogeneic: HLA-matched healthy donors for (usually related) recipient with malignancy or marrow failure (16,905 cases worldwide 1964–93, International Bone Marrow Transplant Registry)

PERIOPERATIVE RISKS

- Postop morbidity high 2° to underlying malignant disease (autologous donor)
- Life-threatening complications extremely rare (0.27%) for allogeneic (healthy) donor

WORRY ABOUT

- Volume status/blood loss
- Position related injuries (prone)
- Anesthetic drug interactions with prior ChemoRx ↓ adrenal reserve
- Puncture of intrathoracic structures if sternal harvest necessary

OVERVIEW

- Multiple needle aspirations of marrow from post iliac crest (occasionally other sites) made to obtain stem cells for reinfusion following marrow ablative chemotherapy for malignancy
- Operating physician usually hematologist (not surgeon)

(See also Chemotherapeutic Agents and individual chemotherapeutic agents [e.g., Bleomycin Sulfate, Alkylating Agents] in Drugs section)

INDICATIONS AND USUAL TREATMENT

- Marrow failure, hematologic malignancy, selected chemotherapy-responsive solid tumors
- Recipient anticipates prolonged hospitalization in major medical center, aggressive support for anemia, thrombocytopenia, neutropenia, GVHD
- Autologous transplantation may follow first or subsequent remission for hematologic malignancy or be performed prior to chemotherapy for solid tumor of sites remote from bone marrow stores

ASSESSMENT POINTS

(applies primarily to autologous donors)

SYSTEM	EFFECT	ASSESSMENT BY HX	PE	TEST
CV	CHF, dysrhythmias	Doxorubicin, pericardial effusions	CV exam	ECG, consider ECHO/MUGA
GI	Electrolyte imbalance	Vomiting, melena	Edema, orothostasis	Na^+, K^+, Ca^{2+}
HEME	Blood loss, infection	Recent ChemoRx	Petechiae, ecchymosis	CBC, platelets

Key Reference: Armitage JO: Bone marrow transplantation. N Engl J Med 1994; 330:827–838.

INTRAOPERATIVE MANAGEMENT

Monitoring

- Large-bore IV (×2)
- Consider CVP, if access difficult
- Check availability of irradiated blood
- Urinary cath may be necessary (large fluid shifts)
- Arterial access may result in hematoma (thrombocytopenia); useful if BP is labile
- Pulse oximetry may guide O_2 requirements: acutely reduced end-tidal CO_2 may indicate embolism from marrow space

Induction

- ↓ Dose of induction agent if there is Hx of cardiotoxic chemotherapy

SURGICAL STAGES

- Establishment of adequate venous access
- Induction of general anesthesia (spinal/epidural possible for homologous donors)
- Establish prone position
- Supine to prone position change requires minimum of 4 persons
- Wt supported on chest/pelvis with arms extended on armboards
- Avoid pressure on eyes, throat, genitals
- Abd position for free excursion
- Aspiration of marrow
- Cell count of marrow determines volume needed (1–4×10^8 cells/kg recipient body wt frequently > 1000 ml)
- Return to supine position
- Approximate duration 2–4 h
- Postop pain score 1–4; usually PO meds (Tylenol with codeine) adequate

ANTICIPATED PROBLEMS/CONCERNS

- Familiarity with patient's specific chemotherapy protocols
- Volume replacement with irradiated RBCs, crystalloid, albumin
- Avoid starch (interferes with processing of marrow)
- Avoid nonirradiated RBCs (potential engraftment of random donor nucleated cells)
- Prior steroid Rx may result in ↓ adrenal reserve
- Avoid unnecessary O_2 enrichment if prior chemotherapy included bleomycin
- Air/O_2 may be used (N_2O inhibits methionine synthetase resulting in marrow toxicity)

BOWEL RESECTION

Kevin Stierer, M.D.

RISK

- Incidence: colon cancer: 30/100,000; Crohn's: 1–6/100,000
- Gender predominance: 1.3:1 male/female for colon cancer

PERIOPERATIVE RISKS

- Perioperative mortality of 0.5–5% due mainly to underlying disorder
- Perioperative morbidity: prolonged ileus: 5%–10% with small-bowel resection; small bowel obstruction: 5%–10% with large-bowel resection; anastomotic leak: 2-4%; wound dehiscence: 1–2%; bleeding: 1%; splenic injury: 1%

WORRY ABOUT

- Preop bowel preparation leading to hypovolemia, hypokalemia
- ↑ Risk for pulmonary aspiration
- Bowel obstruction, especially small bowel, at risk for bowel necrosis, perforation, septic shock

OVERVIEW

- Removal of bowel: Performed for a variety of malignant, nonmalignant processes
- Small-bowel resection involves varying amounts of mesentery; may include regional lymph nodes if malignancy suspected with primary anastomosis
- Large-bowel resection involves mobilization prior to resection
  - ureter possibly transected during mobilization of pelvic colon
  - primary anastomosis via creation of colostomy depends on number of factors (local ischemia, inflammation, unprepped bowel)

ICD-9-CM Codes: 153.9 (Neoplasm, large intestine); 555.9 (Crohn's disease)

INDICATIONS AND USUAL TREATMENT

- Small-bowel resection: intestinal obstruction, volvulus, intussusception, Crohn's disease, small-bowel tumors, trauma
- Large-bowel resection: colon cancer, diverticulosis, Crohn's disease, ulcerative colitis, lower GI bleed, trauma
- Usual medical Rx varies. Depends on underlying cause (see Diseases section)

ASSESSMENT POINTS

SYSTEM	EFFECT	ASSESSMENT BY HX	PE	TEST
CV	Hypovolemia	Lightheadedness	Orthostatic VS, capillary refill	BUN/Cr, ABG (acidosis)
RESP	Aspiration risk Hypoventilation or hypoxemia 2° to intra-abdominal process	N/V Splinting (due to pain)	Abdominal exam Observation, auscultation	SpO_2, ABG
RENAL	Electrolyte abnormality			ECG, serum electrolytes

Key Reference: Greenfield L: Complications in Surgery and Trauma, 2nd ed. Philadelphia, JB Lippincott, 1984, pp 471–475.

PERIOPERATIVE MANAGEMENT

Preoperative Preparation

- Volume replacement before induction due to bowel preparation and/or 3rd space fluid loss with intra-abdominal process
- Consider H_2 antagonist for aspiration prophylaxis
- Metoclopramide contraindicated if bowel obstruction/perforation suspected

Anesthetic Technique

- General anesthesia may combine technique with epidural for postop analgesia

Monitoring

- Routine
- Consider Foley catheter if of long duration

Airway

- High incidence of gastric aspiration
- Consider secure airway with rapid-sequence or awake technique

Induction

- Hemodynamic instability 2° hypovolemia

SURGICAL STAGES

Dissection

- Hypotension after peritoneum opened, especially if intra-abd bleeding tamponaded
- Hypotension, ↑ airway pressure may be encountered during surgical manipulation of secretory small-bowel tumors
- Hypotension during manipulation of strangulated or perforated small bowel

Definitive Surgery

- Anticipate large 3rd space fluid loss, depending on degree of bowel exposure, amount resected (10–15 ml/kg/h of crystalloid)
- Additional fluid requirements if suction enterostomy of obstructed bowel performed
- Monitor for ureteral injury during pelvic dissection
- EBL usually <500 ml but may ↑ significantly for reoperation or inflammatory bowel disease
- Maintain normothermia

Postoperative Considerations

- Significant postop pain: Pain score 5–8
- Epidural analgesia or IV PCA
- Pulmonary dysfunction 2° to splinting with inadequate analgesia
- Paralytic ileus usually related to amount of bowel manipulation, not narcotic analgesia

ANTICIPATED PROBLEMS/CONCERNS

- Preop hypovolemia with hemodynamic instability unless proper volume resuscitation instituted before induction

BRAIN CORTEX RESECTION (FOR EPILEPSY) Patricia H. Petrozza, M.D.

RISK

- 75,000 patients in USA with drug-resistant epilepsy
- 1500 ablative operations/y
- Racial predilection: none

PERIOPERATIVE RISKS

- Depends on procedure
- Combined morbidity, mortality rates <5% for epileptogenic focus resection, <20% for corpus callosotomy, <50% functional hemispherectomy
- Blood loss diathesis (functional hemispherectomy)
- Risk of craniotomy includes hypercoagulable state (PE, thromboembolism)

WORRY ABOUT

- Status epilepticus
- Aspiration
- Tailoring anesthetic technique for appropriate intraoperative testing, responsiveness
- Favorable cranial conditions
- N/V
- Blood loss diathesis

OVERVIEW

- Used for intractable seizures
- Requires discussion with surgeons, concerns about intraoperative electrocorticography, patient responsiveness
- Concerns about seizures, possible status epilepticus
- Concerns about craniotomy, including blood loss, adequate operating conditions, postop responsiveness

- Patient may have comorbid conditions—e.g., psychiatric disorders, tuberous sclerosis, neurofibromatosis
- Patients on anticonvulsants often require larger doses of narcotics, muscle relaxants than expected

ICD-9-CM Code: 345.91

INDICATIONS AND USUAL TREATMENT

- Patients recommended for cortical resection for epilepsy have met these criteria:
  - have focal seizure not responding to adequate trial of anti-epileptic agents
  - seizures significantly interfere with patient's overall function
  - surgery appears to offer reasonable opportunity for improvement of overall function.
- Medical Rx is first-line Rx with max Rx with 1 drug before multiple-drug Rx, then surgery

ASSESSMENT POINTS

SYSTEM	EFFECT	ASSESSMENT BY HX	PE	TEST
HEENT	Gum hypertrophy related to phenytoin		Airway exam	
GI/LIVER	Hepatitis	Rx with ethosuximide, mephenytoin, phensuximide, valproic acid	Hepatomegaly, jaundice	LFTs, bilirubin, AST, ALT
HEME	Blood dyscrasias related to anti-epileptic drugs	Weakness, fatigue, Rx with carbamazepine, ethosuximide, mephenytoin, methsuximide, phensuximide, phenytoin	Petechiae, rash	CBC
RENAL	Nephritis	Methsuximide, clonazepam therapy		BUN, Cr
NEURO	Lethargy, depression, etc., related to anticonvulsants		MS exam	

Key Reference: Kofke AW, Tempelhoff R, Dasheiff RM: Anesthesia for epileptic patients and epilepsy surgery. *In* Cottrell J, Smith DW (eds): Anesthesia and Neurosurgery, 3rd ed. St. Louis, Mosby-Year Book, 1994; pp 495–518.

PERIOPERATIVE MANAGEMENT

Intraoperative Electrocorticography/ Awake Craniotomy

- Discussion by surgeon, anesthesiologist about specific patient's suitability
- Patients position themselves as comfortably as possible; O_2 delivered by nasal prongs

Monitoring

- Capnography by nasal prongs
- Urinary cath
- 1 large-bore IV line
- Consider arterial line

Airway

- Careful inspection mandatory: difficult intubation anticipated in lateral position with pre-existing airway abn

Induction

- If intraoperative electrocorticography, general anesthesia chosen, induction can be with ultra–short-acting barbiturate—e.g., thiopental, maintenance with N_2O, narcotic technique supplemented with low-dose isoflurane

- NMB used
- anesthesia maintenance with fentanyl infusion often satisfactory for intraoperative electrocorticography recording
- Fentanyl, NMB agent requirements may be ↑
- During closure of craniotomy, care must be taken to avoid HTN, movement by patient
- For craniotomy, monitoring under local anesthesia, 2 generally accepted techniques: (1) fentanyl 0.5–0.75 µg/kg, droperidol 0.15 mg/kg with additional fentanyl boluses 25–100 µg IV or (2) propofol, initial bolus 1 mg/kg IV followed by infusion at 75 µg/kg/min
- Infusions discontinued ~15 min before patient needs to be responsive
- Local infiltration of scalp by surgeons (careful attention to local anesthesia overdose)

SURGICAL STAGES

- Scalp incision: Should be comfortable with adequate local anesthesia
- Removal of bone flap: Patient may be bothered by drilling (should be warned)
- Stripping of dura: May cause N/V

- Meningeal vessel manipulation: May cause pain
- Blood loss: While usually not large, replaced to avoid hypovolemia
- N/V: Can be controlled with metoclopramide 5–10 mg or droperidol 1.5–2.5 mg
- Patient at risk for seizures
  - May require therapy with IV methohexital 0.5–1.0 mg/kg if electrocorticography anticipated; following electrocorticography, benzodiazepines acceptable

Postoperative Considerations

- Fluctuating blood levels of anticonvulsants
- Monitoring for seizure activity
- Control of hemodynamics, possibility of recurrent seizures

ANTICIPATED PROBLEMS/CONCERNS

- Difficulties with seizure control
- Possible brain swelling or intracranial hematoma related to resection
- Patient anxiety related to lengthy operation time
- Intraoperative N/V

BRONCHOSCOPY, FIBEROPTIC

Andranik Ovassapian, M.D.

RISK

- Technique for evaluation of tracheobronchial tree
- Has virtually replaced rigid bronchoscopy

PERIOPERATIVE RISKS

- Depends on nature of disease for which bronchoscopy performed

WORRY ABOUT

- Coughing, breath holding, hypoxemia
- ↑ Airway resistance when performed through endotracheal or tracheostomy tube
- Postbronchoscopy airway irritation, coughing, airway obstruction, hypoxemia if not treated with O_2

OVERVIEW

- Fiberoptic bronchoscopy enables endoscopist to go deeper into bronchial tree for evaluation, biopsy of lesions not commonly accessible to rigid bronchoscopy
- Fiberoptic bronchoscopy associated with repeated coughing, HTN, tachycardia often due to inadequate topical or general anesthesia
- Hypoxemia common when performed without supplemental O_2 Rx
- Blood loss from biopsy site of lower airway lesions can be troublesome
- Tracheal and sometimes bronchial intubation, separation of lungs possibly necessary for major hemoptysis

ICD-9-CM Code: 162.9 (lung cancer)

INDICATIONS AND USUAL TREATMENT

- Evaluation of upper, lower airway problems, Dx of pulm disease
- Rx of acute atelectasis performed by saline lavage, aspiration of thick secretions
- Transbronchoscopic bronchial biopsy, brushing cytology, transbronchial needle aspiration biopsy, bronchoalveolar lavage performed
- Absolute contraindications include acutely unstable CV system, current life-threatening cardiac arrhythmias, severe hypoxemia

ASSESSMENT POINTS

SYSTEM	EFFECT	ASSESSMENT BY HX	PE	TEST
HEENT	Airway compromise	Wheezing, stridor	Lung, airway exam	CXR
CV	Hx of CV disease	Exercise intolerance, angina	S_3, rales	ECG Stress test
RESP	Hx of smoking	Wheezing Exercise tolerance impairment	Clubbing, cyanosis, wheezing	PFT ABG CXR

Key Reference: Prakash UBS: Bronchoscopy. New York, Raven Press, 1994, pp 53–89.

PERIOPERATIVE MANAGEMENT

- Usually done as outpatient with patient in sitting or supine position
- Antisialagogue (glycopyrrolate 0.2 mg IV or 0.4 mg IM) to minimize secretions, enhance topical anesthesia of airway
- Appropriate size bronchoscope, ancillary equipment should be available

Monitoring

- Routine

Anesthetic Technique

- Usually done under sedation, topical anesthesia
- Lidocaine 10% spray of oropharynx followed by translaryngeal injection of 3 ml 4% lidocaine provides excellent topical anesthesia
- Spray-as-you-go technique used to anesthetize rest of bronchial tree
- For GA, large ET tube is placed
- Laryngeal mask airway can provide passageway for fiberoptic bronchoscopy
- Short-acting IV drugs used during fiberoptic bronchoscopy
- Jet ventilation can be applied through fiberscope but not commonly practiced

Postoperative Concerns

- Hypoxemia treated with supplemental O_2 Rx
- Irritable airway, coughing, tachycardia, HTN common during early recovery

ANTICIPATED PROBLEMS/CONCERNS

- Inadequate ventilation, hypoxemia when sedation heavy
- Airway obstruction, hypoxemia, barotrauma of lungs possible
- Consider precautions to minimize fire hazards during laser surgery

BRONCHOSCOPY, RIGID

Andranik Ovassapian, M.D.

RISK

• Performed for removal of foreign body, massive hemoptysis, to dilate tracheobronchial strictures, laser bronchoscopy, endoscopy, and lesion biopsy

PERIOPERATIVE RISKS

• Depends on nature of disease
• Incidence of reintubation reported at 0.39% when panendoscopy performed for upper airway path.

WORRY ABOUT

• Ventilation, oxygenation in patients with chronic pulm disease, airway pathology
• Endoscopist, anesthesiologist share airway, complicating ventilatory management

OVERVIEW

• Associated with severe CV response manifested with tachycardia, HTN
• Bleeding from biopsy site could be troublesome
• Level of the lesion critical
• Ventilation performed through side arm
• Requires communication with surgeon throughout procedure

ICD-9-CM Code: 146.9 (Oropharyngeal cancer)

INDICATIONS AND USUAL TREATMENT

• Removal of foreign bodies
• Management of major hemoptysis
• Dilation of tracheobronchial stricture
• Laser surg
• Bronchoscopy in infants, small children
• Bronchoscopy, esophagoscopy, laryngoscopy for staging of oropharyngolaryngeal malignant lesions
• Biopsy of endobronchial lesion
• Establishing emergency airway

ASSESSMENT POINTS

SYSTEM	EFFECT	ASSESSMENT BY HX	PE	TEST
HEENT	Limited neck flexion/extension Rule out unstable C-spine	Pain upon neck movement	ROM of neck, opening of mouth, pain on motion	C-spine x-ray
RESP	Hx smoking	Wheezing; coughing; SOB; exercise tolerance	Wheezing, cyanosis	CXR PFTs with flow-volume loop

Key Reference: Prakash UBS: Bronchoscopy. New York, Raven Press, 1994, pp 53–89.

PERIOPERATIVE MANAGEMENT

• Observe patients with lower airway obstruction, preferably in ICU
• Communicate with endoscopist; as airway shared with anesthesiologist
• Check size of bronchoscope, ventilating side port attachment

Monitoring

• Routine

Anesthetic Technique

• Consider maintaining spontaneous ventilation if signs and symptoms of compromised airway are present
• Short-acting IV analgesics attenuate CV response to rigid bronchoscopy
• For jet ventilation, patient often totally paralyzed
• Surgical blood loss negligible, unless patient with hemoptysis, bleeding endobronchial lesions
• For laser operation, low concentration O_2 (<30%) in combination with N or He, special laser ET tube cuff inflated with saline used to minimize danger of fire; patient paralyzed to avoid movement

Surgical Stages

• Patient supine with head and neck extended
• Bronchoscope is entered through right side of the mouth going midline to visualize the larynx
• Biopsy may be taken through bronchoscope
• Steroid considered if airway is compromised or if manipulation was extensive

Postoperative Concerns

• Continue observation of airway

ANTICIPATED PROBLEMS/CONCERNS

• Postbronchoscopy hypoxemia common; supplemental O_2 Rx recommended
• Coughing, secretions, SOB common
• Severe limitation of cervical spine precludes extension
• Contraindicated if unstable CV system
• Manipulation of the foreign body carries the risk of total airway obstruction
• Removing the bronchoscope and foreign body together endangers control of the airway

BURR HOLE

Jonathan D. Halevy, M.D.

RISK

- 470,000 people/y sustain traumatic brain injury in USA
- 15% die before reaching a medical facility
- 10% have severe brain injury
- Average age: 30 y
- M:F ratio 2:1

PERIOPERATIVE RISKS

- Mortality 25%–30%
- Clinical good outcome in only 60%

WORRY ABOUT

- Complex injury presentation
- Establishment of airway may be complicated by associated cervical spine injury (~10%)
- Hemorrhagic shock related to other injury
- Air embolism, esp if burr hole over/near major sinus
- Intracranial pressure

OVERVIEW

- Types of head injuries include:
  – skull fractures
  – intracranial lesions (56% diffuse vs 42% focal injury)—e.g., subdural hematoma (in 24% of closed head injuries, CT shows high density crescent-shaped lesion); *epidural hematoma* (in 6% of closed head injuries, often temporal [91% with skull fractures], CT shows biconvex hyperdense lesion); *intracranial hematoma* (in 3% of closed head injuries, often frontal or temporal lobes, poss delayed Dx on CT scan); *diffuse brain injury* (no focal mass lesion, 60% with diffuse axonal injury if duration of unconsciousness >6 h)
- Anesthetic techniques: local with monitored anesthesia care with or w/o IV sedation according to patient's LOC
- On Glasgow Coma Scale, >12 is rough guide for tolerating some sedation; otherwise GA

ICD-9-CM Codes: 851–854

INDICATIONS/USUAL TREATMENT

- For evacuation and/or drainage of subdural/epidural/intracranial hematoma
- May be Dx as well as Rx: —brain biopsy
  – ICP monitoring—implantation of ventricular catheter/reservoir or EEG electrodes
  – stereotactic surgery
  – brain cyst/abscess

ASSESSMENT POINTS

SYSTEM	EFFECT	ASSESSMENT BY HX	PE	TEST
HEENT	Cervical spine injury in 10%; full stomach in most cases; ↑ blood alcohol levels in 50%	Based on cause of injury; usually patient not good source of info	Airway exam; assume unstable, not cooperative	C-spine series
CV	Autonomic dysfunction, blunt chest trauma concerns		Auscultation VS	CXR
RESP	Resp distress issues, neurogenic pulm edema, blunt chest trauma concerns	Neuro dysfunction	Auscultation	ABGs, pulse oximetry, CXR
ENDO	Hyperkalemia, hyperglycemia, hyponatremia, diabetes insipidus			Na^+, K^+, glucose Serum, urine osmolality
HEME	May have large blood loss from many causes; watch for DIC			CBC, PT, FSP, plts
GU	ARF due to hypotension			BUN, Cr
CNS	Impaired LOC	Glasgow Coma Score assessment	Neuro exam	CT, MRI scan
MS	Special positioning concerns in OR, look for long bone fractures			Radiologic evaluation

Key Reference: Gopinath SP, Robertson CS: Management of severe head injury. *In* Cottrel JE, Smith DS (eds): Anesthesia and Neurosurgery, 3rd ed. St. Louis, Mosby-Year Book, 1994, pp 661–684.

PERIOPERATIVE MANAGEMENT

Preoperative Preparation

- Look at CT/MRI scans (if available) to confirm side of lesion
- Consider need for preop steroids, anticonvulsants, antiemetics, H_2 antagonists, and/or antibiotics

Anesthetic Technique

- Local anesthesia with monitored anesthesia care or GA

Monitoring

- Consider large-bore IV access, art line, central line
- Consider ICP monitoring, Foley catheter (esp if osmotic diuretics to be used)
- Nasal end-tidal CO_2 monitoring with anesthesia care technique
- Blood glucose levels (keep <250 mg/dl; >50 mg/dl)

Airway

- Patient often already intubated
- Assume C-spine injury if post trauma (motor vehicle accident)
- Secure ET tube well

Induction/Maintenance

- Consider ↑ ICP issues
- Neuro prep/drape time possibly lengthy; watch for low BP during minimal stimulation period

SURGICAL STAGES

Dissection

- Definite risk for complications during drilling—e.g., plunging into, through dura
- If hit major sinus, watch for air embolism

Definitive Surgery

- Hemodynamic changes if brain-stem herniation
- May need intraop ICP monitoring early instead of late (CPP >90 mmHg; higher Glasgow Coma Score → better neuro outcome)
- Observe surgical site for excessive brain swelling (impending disaster)

Closure/Postoperative Considerations

- Goal to have patient as awake as possible
- May require intubation postop to assess CNS status (esp if starting from poor LOC)

- Postop pain difficult to assess due to MS problems
- Neuro exam of paramount importance to assist in management in neuro ICU
- Use vasoactive medications to control BP/HR at end of procedure
- Pain Rx: Codeine and/or narcotic; PCA not appropriate due to CNS derangement
- EBL: 50–100 ml (may be more)

ANTICIPATED PROBLEMS/CONCERNS

- Outcome depends on severity of injury, presence of focal lesion, duration of unconsciousness, ICP course
- Goal to avoid secondary neuronal insults (48% of comatose patients postop)
- Expect impaired autoregulation of cerebral vasculature
- Assess realistic postop LOC in view of preop condition
- Intensive management of hemodynamic/metabolic/neuro/other issues required in neuro ICU

BYPASS — FEMORAL-FEMORAL

Alexandru Gottlieb, M.D.

RISK

• An average of 8000 femoral-femoral by-passes per year performed in USA

PERIOPERATIVE RISKS

• Mostly related to diffuse atherosclerosis CV disease
• Perioperative MI as high as 10%
• Mostly geriatric patients with age-related risk factors
• Potential for indefinite improvement and/or more distal occlusion with risk of amputation

WORRY ABOUT

• Thrombosis of graft
• Embolic phenomena to legs
• Groin considered "dirty" location, rendering prosthetic graft infection common

OVERVIEW

• Femoral-femoral bypass suggested for patients for whom another procedure is too risky
• Femoral-femoral bypass mostly done with prosthetic graft—a nonanatomic graft possibly "fed" by non-optimal vessel
• Regional anesthesia can be beneficial in effect on coag, graft patency
• Procedure can also be performed under monitored anesthesia care

INDICATIONS AND USUAL TREATMENT

• Extra-anatomic procedure
• Performed in patients with lower extremity ischemia, gangrene, or severe short-distance claudication; in 1 limb more than another
• Replace standard anatomic bypass of aorto-iliac or aorto-femoral anastomosis in patients with following conditions:
  – Patients with previous abdominal procedure
  – Status post–extensive abdominal radiation
  – Patients with intestinal stoma
  – Patients with infected abdominal wall
  – Patient with poor medical condition

ASSESSMENT POINTS

SYSTEM	EFFECT	ASSESSMENT BY HX	PE	TEST
CV	High incidence of CAD, myocardial ischemia and/or infarction	Angina, MI, CHF, dysrhythmia, PTCA, CABG, exercise tolerance, activity level	Chest auscultation, VS	ECG stress test: dipyridamole thallium imaging, dobutamine; cardiac cath;
	Chronic HTN	BP Rx, drug interaction, myocardial hypertrophy	BP	ECG CXR, retinal
RESP	High incidence of lung disease that could have selected this procedure	Smoking, chronic cough, dyspnea	Clubbing	CXR, ABG Spirometry
ENDO	High incidence of DM	Infection, stress-related DM, gestation DM	Skin infection, polydipsia, polyuria, diabetic coma, hypoglycemic stupor	CNS exam UO Serum glucose
HEME	Some patients on perioperative heparin or aspirin	Petechiae, nasal blood loss	Petechiae or clinical blood loss	PT, PTT, clotting time, ACT
GU	High incidence of renal insufficiency 2° to age, arteriosclerosis, multiple dye studies	Edema, intolerance to NaCl load	Edema Anuria	Cr, urea, electrolytes
CNS	Possibly carotid disease	Syncope, stroke, TIAs	CNS Carotid bruit? Rule out conductive heart disease	Carotid angio CT, MRI

Key Reference: Roizen MF, Ellis JE: Anesthesia for vascular surgery. *In* Barash PG, Cullen BF, Stoelting RK (eds): Clinical Anesthesia. Philadelphia, J.B. Lippincott, 1992, pp 1059–1094.

PERIOPERATIVE MANAGEMENT

Perioperative Evaluation

• Detailed Hx, PE of CV (system)
• Dysrhythmias, CAD, CHF
• HTN heart disease, valvular heart disease
• Noninvasive, invasive cardiac evaluation—e.g., cardiac cath, if needed

Anesthetic Technique

• GA, regional anesthesia, or monitored anesthesia care; regional anesthesia preferred by some clinicians because of lack of systemic effect on resp, CV, GI systems; some positive effect of regional anesthesia on coagulation, preserving fibrinolysis, graft patency

Monitoring

• HR, arterial line BP, UO
• Consider CVP or PA line in patients with severe CAD or LV impairment
• Monitoring for myocardial ischemia; ECG with continuous 3-lead ST-T segment analysis, PA cath, or TEE
• Vol replacement; CO, PA cath, or TEE?

Surgical Stages

• Thoroughly prep, drape groin area (procedure can be 2–4 h, but with min. 3rd space, controlled blood loss)
• Avoid ↓ in BP; femoral-femoral bypass can thrombose easily with lack of flow

Postoperative Period

• Mild postop pain: 5–7
• Ischemic leg pain should improve postop
• Epidural, if used during, can be extended for postop pain control

ANTICIPATED PROBLEMS/CONCERNS

• High incidence of perioperative cardiac, pulmonary complications
• Inappropriate blood flow from donor site tends to make bypass not functional
• Infection of prosthetic graft at groin relatively frequent compared with other prosthetic graft sites

BYPASS GRAFT PROCEDURE — INFRAINGUINAL

Rose Christopherson, M.D., Ph.D.

RISK

- Operations/y: 300,000
- Risk factors for atherosclerotic vascular disease include smoking, HTN, diabetes
- Demography: no known racial predominance; slightly more prevalent among males than females

PERIOPERATIVE RISKS

- Death: 0–5%
- Major cardiac morbidity, including MI, unstable angina, ischemic pulm edema, significant dysrhythmias: 6–33%

WORRY ABOUT

- Perioperative cardiac morbidity
- Concomitant diseases, including COPD, diabetes, HTN, vascular disease

OVERVIEW

- ↓ Graft failure associated with regional and/or regional-supplemented GA, with optimization of cardiac performance using PA cath
- ↓ Myocardial ischemia, major cardiac morbidity reported when patient's Hct maintained >28–29% in nonrandomized studies
- Workup, monitoring, Rx appropriate for patients at high risk for CAD

ICD-9-CM Code: 440.2 (Atherosclerosis)

INDICATIONS AND USUAL TREATMENT

- Severe claudication, ischemic pain at rest, nonhealing foot or leg ulcers if due to poor circulation
- At some institutions, laser endarterectomy performed as alternative to infrainguinal bypass grafting
- Graft materials including native vein, Gore-Tex, other artificial grafts; vein considered superior except for femoral-femoral bypass grafting; vein may be used either in situ or reversed

ASSESSMENT POINTS

SYSTEM	EFFECT	ASSESSMENT BY HX	PE	TEST
CV	Associated CAD	MI, CHF, angina, palpitations	CV	ECG ECHO Holter, dipyridamole thallium imaging, or dobutamine ECHO if indicated
RESP	COPD 2° to smoking	Dyspnea, wheezing	Chest auscultation	PFT if indicated CXR
ENDO	Diabetes	Hx of diabetes		Glucose
RENAL	Renal insufficiency	Renal failure		Cr/BUN
CNS	Associated conditions	TIA, CVA	CNS	Carotid Doppler (if indicated)

Key Reference: Christopherson R, et al: Perioperative morbidity in patients randomized to epidural or general anesthesia for lower extremity vascular surgery. Anesthesiology 1993; 79:422–434.

PERIOPERATIVE MANAGEMENT

Anesthetic Technique

- Performed under spinal, epidural, general, or combined techniques; evidence supports ↓ neuraxis blockade for improved surgical outcome, but not for ↓ cardiac morbidity

Monitoring

- Routine
- ST segment analysis (computerized if possible)
- Intra-arterial cath in most cases
- CVP or PA cath, depends on CV workup

Induction/Maintenance

- GA—depends on cardiac, other medical status
- Regional—block at T8-T10 adequate, but good sacral blockade necessary. If pure regional, motor blockade necessary
- Maintain normothermia

Surgical Stages

- Vein harvest: if previous CABG, vein sometimes from dorsum of leg; patient may be turned prone, then supine for arterial surgery
- Heparin usually given (~70 U/kg) before clamping femoral artery
- Cross-clamp
- Blood loss usually controlled by pressure on or clamping of femoral artery
- Patency of graft tested intraoperatively with Doppler and/or angio
- EBL ~500 ml, but highly variable
- 3rd spacing minimal
- Hypovolemia may be conducive to clotting of graft

Postoperative Considerations

- Not extremely painful: pain score 3–6
- Routinely admitted to PACU, step-down ICU, or intermediate care unit for 18–24 h for pulse, cardiac monitoring, especially if diabetic with autonomic neuropathy (see Diabetes, Type I (Insulin Requiring) in Diseases section)
- Body T <35°C immediately after surgery associated with ↑ cardiac morbidity

ANTICIPATED PROBLEMS/CONCERNS

- Continuing epidural may ↓ early graft occlusion
- Perioperative MI, ischemia, CHF common
- Low Hct possibly associated with ↑ cardiac morbidity; advise transfusing to Hct 30

CARCINOID, EXCISION OF

Randy H. Steadman, M.D.

RISK

- Incidence: 1.5 cases/100,000/y; 1/300 appendectomies; 1/2500 proctoscopic exams
- Race/gender predominance: none
- Age with highest incidence: 5th or 6th decade; range: 10 y–ninth decade.
- Indications for operation: ability to identify; primary should be treated with resection regardless of metastases; local complications—e.g., obstruction, intussusception—frequent

PERIOPERATIVE RISKS

- CV collapse due to release of vasoactive peptides
- Severe bronchospasm
- 1.5–10% perioperative mortality reported before use of somatostatin analogue

WORRY ABOUT

- Crisis consisting of flushing and hemodynamic changes, usually hypotension, but rarely HTN
- Severe bronchospasm

- Midgut (ileal, jejunal) carcinoids associated with fibrosis of mesentery (can result in short-gut syndrome if too extensive resection)
- Tricuspid, pulmonic valve regurgitation, stenosis, right heart failure

OVERVIEW

- Slow-growing malignancies capable of metastases, derived from APUD cells of embryonic neuroectoderm originating in GI tract 85% (most commonly, appendix; next, rectum, ileum); 10% from lung
- Release vasoactive peptides; in 10% these peptides access systemic circulation due to hepatic metastases (or primary tumor when drainage not portal); carcinoid syndrome can develop
- The peptides include serotonin, bradykinin, histamine, others; common Sx include facial flushing (94%), watery diarrhea (78%), asthma (19%); right heart involvement can also result in tricuspid insufficiency, pulmonic valve stenosis or insufficiency requiring valve replacement. Dx made as incidental finding during appendectomy, upper GI endoscopy, proctoscopic exam
- Even without carcinoid syndrome, serotonin metab 5-HIAA may be elevated in 50% of patients with GI carcinoid tumors

- Prognosis related more to location, size of primary than to pathologic findings
- Patients with noninvasive appendiceal, rectal tumors <2 cm have 5-y survival rates near 100%; if tumor is >2 cm, survival declines to 40%; with liver metastases, 5-y survival 21–42%.

ICD-9-CM Codes: 199.1 (tumor); 259.2 (syndrome)

INDICATIONS AND USUAL TREATMENT

- Surgery only potentially curative Rx
- With distant metastases, cure by resection of all tumor
- When resection not possible, palliative procedures may be needed for obstruction or to debulk tumor ↓ quantity of vasoactive peptides released, or to replace heart valves
- Medical Rx for symptomatic relief from flushing, diarrhea with advanced disease
- Octreotide (Sandostatin), a somatostatin analogue, inhibits synthesis, release, binding of vasoactive peptides; can control Sx, retard tumor growth, and prolong survival by as much as 3 years

ASSESSMENT POINTS

SYSTEM	EFFECT	ASSESSMENT BY HX	PE	TEST
CV	Carcinoid crisis, right heart valve involvement	Hx carcinoid syndrome, fatigue, ascites, edema	Hemodynamic collapse; JVD, murmur	ABG ECHO
RESP	Bronchospasm	SOB	Wheezing	O_2 sat
GI	Diarrhea	Abd pain, wt loss	Flushing	Electrolytes, 5-HIAA
ENDO	10% MEN (hyperplasia of parathyroid, pancreas, pituitary) associated with carcinoid	Ulcers, renal calculi	Lipomas	Glucose Ca^{2+}, PO_4^{2-}, prolactin, gastrin
CNS	Postop sedation			
NUTRITION	Pellagra due to niacin deficiency if large amt serotonin produced	Diarrhea	Dermatitis, dementia	None Rx niacin

Key Reference: Loftus J, van Heerden J: Surgical management of gastrointestinal carcinoid tumors. Adv Surg 1995; 28:317.

OPERATIVE MANAGEMENT

Preoperative Preparation

- Adequate sedation to avoid sympathetic stimulation resulting in carcinoid crisis
- Pretreatment for 24 h with subcutaneous octreotide

Monitoring

- Arterial catheter
- Consider CVP cath for vol monitoring (substitute PA cath or TEE if valvular lesions)

Airway

- Gastric emptying may be delayed
- Occasional laryngeal tumors

Anesthesia Technique

- Attempt to avoid histamine-releasing drugs (thiopental, succinylcholine, atracurium, morphine) although they have been used without incident
- Adrenergic agonists—e.g., epinephrine, norepinephrine—stimulate release of vasoactive substances

- Etomidate or propofol appropriate for induction, maintenance with volatile agent (isoflurane), narcotic (fentanyl)
- Succinylcholine may, by causing fasciculations of abd wall, cause mechanical compression of tumor with release of vasoactive peptides
- Epidural techniques controversial since hypotension may lead to sympathetic stimulation, precipitating a carcinoid crisis, which may be difficult to treat without use of sympathomimetics

SURGICAL STAGES

Skin Incision

- Site varies according to location
- Sympathetic and/or mechanical stimulation with skin preparation has caused crisis

Dissection

- May be extensive if small-bowel fibrosis has occurred
- Manipulation of tumor may release vasoactive substances

Definitive Surgery

- En bloc resection of ileal carcinoids justified due to freq presence of multiple tumors

Closure and Postoperative Considerations

- About 1/3 of patients with advanced (hepatic) disease require blood transfusions intraoperatively
- Postop PCA usual
- Subcutaneous octreotide resumed with IV supplement for hypotensive episodes
- Pain score depends on location: abd 4–7

ANTICIPATED PROBLEMS/CONCERNS

- Carcinoid crisis can result in abrupt CV collapse or severe bronchospasm
- Sympathomimetics should not be used; IV octreotide (somatostatin analogue), miracle drug for aborting or prophylaxis of CV, bronchospastic effects
- HTN may be treated by IV ketanserin (a 5-HT antagonist)

CARDIOPULMONARY BYPASS
Marvin L. Appel, M.D., Ph.D.

RISK

- 300,000 open heart operations/y in North America.

PERIOPERATIVE RISKS

- Heavily dependent on patient's underlying condition requiring bypass
- Stroke occurred in 0–13% in different studies
- Neuropsychiatric deficits common perioperatively, but 0–5% of patients have persistent deficits 6 mo postop (bubble membrane oxygenator)

WORRY ABOUT

- Underlying HD may make it difficult to maintain patient until CPB can start; may predispose to difficulty separating from bypass
- Condition of arterial cannulation site; aneurysmal, calcified, severely atheromatous areas may be unsuitable (evaluate with CXR, ECHO, catheterization)

- Dilutional anemia from 2 L fluid to prime pump; may obligate RBC transfusions in small patients
- Air embolism
- Clot formation in pump, with arterial embolization
- Awareness during bypass, especially during rewarming
- Protamine reaction (H_2-mediated hypotension, anaphylaxis, pulmonary HTN)
- Coagulopathy post-bypass
- Spontaneous recooling of patient post-bypass

OVERVIEW

- CPB involves passively draining blood from venous system into pump, forcing it through oxygenator, back into patient's arterial circulation. Bypass machine assumes functions of heart and lung.
- Safety features include air detectors to prevent pumping air into arterial circ, continuous measurement of patient's mixed venous O_2 sat to detect inadequate tissue O_2 delivery, continuous monitoring of hydrostatic pressure within pump circuit to detect obstruction, prevent rupture of circuit
- Bypass associated with post-bypass myocardial dysfunction, lung injury, hematologic derangements, usually reversible in perioperative period
- Significant 3rd space fluid shifts during bypass and for several days post-bypass

INDICATIONS

- CAB, valve surg, heart TX, some lung TX, removal of intracardiac tumors or those involving great vessels, rewarming from severe hypothermia, resection of some intracranial aneurysms

ASSESSMENT POINTS

SYSTEM	EFFECT	ASSESSMENT BY HX	PE	TEST
CV	Underlying cardiac disease dictates anesthetic management pre-, post-bypass, affect ability to separate from bypass	Angina, CHF, arrhythmias, etc	Cardiac	ECG, ECHO, cath, CXR
ENDO	CPB elicits hormonal stress response; glucose control may worsen in diabetics	diabetes		May choose to check glucose during CPB
HEME	Preop plt dysfunction (including ASA use) or coagulopathy may obligate transfusion post-CPB	Bleeding problems, anticoagulation Aspirin use	Skin: bruises, petechiae	PT, PTT, Plt count, bleeding time
RENAL	Preop renal dysfunction predisposes to postop problems Preop diuretic use may require diuresis during CPB to maintain UO	Renal dysfunction, diuretic use		BUN, Cr, UA
CNS	Prior CVA ↑ risk of intraop CVA	CVA, TIA	Neuro exam	Carotid US

Key Reference: Kaplan JA (ed): Cardiac Anesthesia, 3rd ed., Philadelphia, WB Saunders, 1993, pp 919–956.

INTRAOPERATIVE MANAGEMENT

- Arterial line mandatory: CPB flow is insufficiently pulsatile for BP cuff; maintain mean arterial BP from 40–80 mmHg using anesthesia, pressors, vasodilators as needed
- Periodically sample ABG to treat acidosis, abnormal K^+, Ca^{2+} values
- Foley cath: keep UO at least 1 ml/kg/h using mannitol, diuretics, dopamine as needed
- If PA line present, pull back during CPB to prevent its drifting into wedge position
- Ventilation and/or pulse oximetry mandatory during partial bypass (i.e., when some of venous return allowed to pass through lungs instead of all going to pump)
- Consider priming pump with FFP to correct pre-existing coagulopathy
- Consider giving antifibrinolytics (e.g., ε-ACP, aprotinin) for patient at high risk for bleeding complications (long pump runs, redo ops)

SURGICAL STAGES

- Dissection
- Heparinization
- ECHO of proposed aortic cannulation site
- Arterial cannulation—site chosen should be free of atherosclerosis
- Venous cannulation
- Bypass
- Cross-clamp, cardioplegia (if used)
- Circulatory arrest (if used)
- Rewarming
- Separation from bypass
- Reversal of anticoagulation (usually with protamine)

Anesthesia During Bypass

- Opiates, benzodiazepines, nondepolarizing muscle relaxant, potent inhalational agent (delivered into pump oxygenator with a standard vaporizer).

- Anticoagulation: Heparin or LMW heparins common.

Checklist Before Separation from Bypass

- Venous reservoir volume sufficient to fill heart (usually > 1 L)
- Acceptable lab values (Hb > 7, K^+ > 4.0, Ca^{2+} > 1.0)
- SVR: 800–1600
- ECG with rate of 60–120, with sinus rhythm, pacing, or Afib, and free of ischemia
- Myocardial contractility acceptable (inotropes and/or mechanical assistance as needed)
- Patient warm (rectal or bladder temp > 34°C, nasal temperature > 36°C)

CARDIOVERSION

Ross H. Zoll, Ph.D., M.D.

RISK

- Electively usually performed for AFib
- Incidence 2% over 20 y
- Occasional urgent or emergent; also routine with other diseases or surgery—e.g., acute MI or CV surgery

PERIOPERATIVE RISKS

- Greatest risk is embolization from stagnant blood in atria (2%)
- ↑ In presence of mitral valve disease
- Long duration of arrhythmia or left atrial size >4.5 cm indicates poor response to conversion—either failure to convert or rapid recurrence

WORRY ABOUT

- Coag status, poss presence of clot with duration of arrhythmia >24 h
- NPO status, presence of CHF or ischemia
- Poss arrhythmias—e.g., VF, asystole, or presence of permanent pacemaker wires (poss damaged by defibrillation)
- Poss of recall
- Digitalis toxicity may predispose to refractory VF; synchronized shock ↓ risk of shock during vulnerable phase of recovery of ventricles; ↓ risk of VF. In WPW, Dig, Ca channel blocker contraindicated

OVERVIEW

- Term *cardioversion* applied to synchronized shock for AF, AFib, SVT, VT
- Cardioversion of AF, VT usually easy; requires small energy
- Cardioversion of AFib, like VFib, requires depolarizing significant no. of muscle fibers at once and large dose of electrical current. Reasonable therapeutic ratio exists, but actual delivered current (dose) unpredictable. Defibrillators store a set amount of energy, and most delivered to patient, but current delivered to the heart is relevant variable, depending on geometric factors, impedance that varies widely, etc
- Underdosing ineffective
- Overdose may cause myocardial damage, dysfunction, persistent arrhythmia. Rx should begin at low energy (50 J) but may proceed to 400 J unless complications evident or current is known to be adequate by measurement
- To obtain a reasonably uniform current density in atria, AP paddle placement preferred

ICD-9-CM Code: 427.31(AFib)

INDICATION/USUAL TREATMENT

- AFib
- Many patients tolerate AFib well and may need rate control with digoxin, ß-blocker or Ca channel blocker
- 5% yearly incidence of stroke; therefore anti-coag indicated if tolerated; if atrium small, so that cardioversion likely successful, it is preferable
- Cardioversion with drugs such as quinidine or procainamide often attempted while anti-coag being established
- Cardioversion indicated if rate control difficult (often exercise rate response not well controlled); hyperthyroidism, HTN, CHF, lyte disturbances, COPD all predispose to AFib; Rx before cardioversion likely successful, NSR sustained
- Atrial contribution to contractility may be needed to prevent CHF

ASSESSMENT POINTS

SYSTEM	EFFECT	ASSESSMENT BY HX	PE	TEST
CV	Valve disease CHF	SOB Palpitations Chest pain	Ausculation Edema	ECG ECHO
HEME	Anticoag			PT, PTT
CNS	CVA TIA	Duration of abn rhythm Coag status	Neuro	Cardiac ECHO

Key Reference: Miles W, Zipes DP: Cardioversion and defibrillation: Clinical aspects. *In* El-Sherif N, Samet P (eds): Cardiac Pacing and Electrophysiology. Philadelphia, WB Saunders, 1991, pp 727–736.

PERIOPERATIVE MANAGEMENT

Anesthetic Technique

- Usually brief; requires only IV induction agent titrated to LOC; propofol, benzodiazepines, thiopental, methohexital, etomidate, ketamine, etc, may be used
- If ET intubation indicated for preventing aspiration or because of difficult mask fit, succinylcholine may be added
- In CHF or ischemia, short-acting narcotic may be added; inhalation agents not useful (may predispose to arrhythmias; are longer acting)

Postoperative Considerations

- Pain: minimal

ANTICIPATED PROBLEMS/CONCERNS

- Recall can be a problem, esp in severely compromised patient or in emergency cardioversion when adequate anesthesia not well tolerated
- CNS function should be assessed on waking
- Ischemia or HTN may be induced by electrical stimulation
- Arrhythmias can be induced by shock or absence of atrial electrical activity
- Hypotension, ↓ CO poss from anesthetic drugs or effect of electrical shock on myocardium; atrial mechanical systole may not be effective immediately after a period of fibrillation

CAROTID ENDARTERECTOMY

John A. Youngberg, M.D.

RISK

- TIAs in ~0.5/1000 population
- ~91,000 procedures in 1992; 200,000, 1987; 70,000, 1990; ↑ due to establishment as most beneficial Rx for TIAs, nonsymptomatic >70% carotid atherosclerosis
- Asymptomatic bruit in ~4%–5% of patients >40 y
- Smoking, DM, HTN, male, high cholesterol, high triglycerides, obesity, family Hx, stress, plt function, alcohol use all risk factors

PERIOPERATIVE RISKS

- Periop mortality 0–2.6%
- Periop permanent neuro deficit 0–6.3%
- Risk of periop MI
- Risk of associated nerve injury

WORRY ABOUT

- Coexisting CAD
- CBF/oxygenation during carotid clamping/shunting

- HTN/hypotension postop
- Associated nerve injury
- Postop hematoma
- Postop CNS assessment
- Hyperperfusion syndrome

OVERVIEW

- Plaque removed from carotid artery
- Significant risk of embolization of plaque debris
- Significant risk of cerebral ischemia/hypoxia during surgery from both surgical and anesthetic techniques
- Significant percentage of patients have known, unknown CAD
- Periop mortality highest from cardiac event, followed by cerebrovascular event
- Regional anesthesia does not appear to lower cardiac or CNS event rate
- Regional anesthesia may be associated with shorter period of HTN postop, shorter ICU/hosp stay

ICD-9-CM Code: 443.1 (arteriosclerosis of carotid artery)

INDICATIONS/USUAL TREATMENT

- Patients who have experienced RIND, TIA, or stroke are candidates
- According to ACAS data, asymptomatic patients with stenosis >60%–70% are candidates if surgeon has low periop risk of morbidity/mortality (<3%)
- Surgical removal of plaque in carotid artery by endarterectomy with or w/o vein patch graft
- Intravascular removal of plaque by mechanical device—e.g., Simpson's atherectomy cath
- Stroke risk 1–2%/y in asymptomatic patient vs 6%–10% if patient has TIAs; stroke risk ↑ significantly in asymptomatic patient if stenosis >75%
- Significant ↓ in stroke rate in "at risk" patients following surgery

ASSESSMENT POINTS

SYSTEM	EFFECT	ASSESSMENT BY HX	PE	TEST
CV	Patients often have known or unknown CAD HTN	Chest pain, MI, CHF, SOB, dyspnea, exercise tolerance	HR & BP, both arms, lying, standing murmur, S_3 or S_4 dysrhythmia	ECG, ECHO, stress test, Holter
RESP	Often smoker with COPD	SOB, cough, exercise tolerance	Auscultation	CXR
ENDO	Often coexisting DM	Ketoacidosis, diet/insulin control		Glucose
CNS	Reversible ischemic neurologic deficit, TIAs, stroke, asymptomatic, bruit	RIND, TIA, stroke, ringing in ears, dizziness, changes in vision, weakness, slurred speech, paralysis	Bruit, evidence of weakness	CT EEG Angio

Key Reference: Garrioch MA, Fitch W: Anaesthesia for carotid artery surgery. Br J Anaesth 1993; 71:569–579.

INTRAOPERATIVE MANAGEMENT

Monitoring

- Art line in nondominant arm for ABGs, glucose, BP measurement
- ECG leads II, V_5
- Monitor CNS well being:
  - awake patient: mentation, speech quality, motor function
  - asleep patient: Raw or processed EEG, SSEP, near infrared monitoring, transcranial Doppler, JV O_2; stump pressure usually not helpful
- Monitoring as indicated for patients with coexisting CAD

CNS Protection

- Avoid exogenous glucose unless indicated by serum hypoglycemia
- Maintain normocarbia
- Maintain patient's usual BP; in HTN patients, cerebral autoregulation curve has shifted to RT
- Consider use of barbiturates, hypothermia, etc, to ↓ $CMRO_2$

Anesthetic Technique

- Regional: local, superficial with or w/o deep cervical plexus block, epidural, etc
- Avoid oversedation of patient due to loss of cooperation and inability to assess CNS status
- General: few to no outcome data to recommend one technique over another; isoflurane can ↓ critical CBF from 20 ml/100 g/min to 8–10 ml/100 g/min, but may not be achievable in clinical setting

SURGICAL STAGES

Induction

- CV instability due to possible coexisting CAD
- EBL usually not of major concern
- Cross-clamping of carotid
  - assess adequacy of cerebral perfusion in awake patient or by changes in monitors in asleep patient
  - consider use of shunt
  - consider use of barbiturates, etc, for CNS protection
  - maintain patient's normal BP, CO_2 levels
- EBL <200 ml, keep vol replacement <1 L to avoid postop HTN

Postoperative Considerations

- HTN
- Hypotension (from hyperactive carotid sinus)
- Hematoma formation (possible airway compromise)
- Associated cranial nerve injury (hypoglossal, recurrent, etc)
- Phrenic nerve block in regional anesthesia in patient with COPD
- Hyperperfusion syndrome, esp in patients with high-grade stenosis
- CNS deficit (ischemia, emboli, intimal flap, thrombosis, etc)

ANTICIPATED PROBLEMS/CONCERNS

- HTN/hypotension postop
- Ability to assess neuro deficit vs residual anesthetic effects
- Myocardial ischemia in patients with coexisting CAD
- Associated nerve injury or residual from regional anesthesia

CARPAL TUNNEL SYNDROME

Scott Mittman, M.D., Ph.D.

RISK

- 1.5% of adults in US
- Racial predominance: white > African-Americans
- Gender predominance: female > male

PERIOPERATIVE RISKS

- Morbidity very rare
- Perioperative exacerbation of median neuropathy

WORRY ABOUT

- Flexion of the wrist during long procedures
- ↑ Risk of exacerbation with cannulation of neighboring radial artery

OVERVIEW

- A compression neuropathy of the median nerve at the wrist

ICD-9-CM Code: 354.0

ETIOLOGY

- Numerous factors→compression of median nerve in the carpal tunnel or ↑ susceptibility of nerve to compression:
  - decrease in size of the carpal tunnel (e.g., bony abnormalities of the carpal bones, thickening of transverse carpal ligament)
  - ↑ volume of contents of carpal tunnel (e.g., neuroma, lipoma, pregnancy, hemodialysis, myxedema)
  - ↑ susceptibility (e.g., diabetes, alcohol abuse)
  - Position and use of the wrist (e.g., flexion of wrist during sleep, repetitive use injuries)

USUAL TREATMENT

- Treatment of any underlying medical condition
- Avoidance of exacerbating wrist positions or repetitive movements; splinting
- Steroid injections
- Release of the transverse carpal ligament

ASSESSMENT POINTS

SYSTEM	EFFECT	ASSESSMENT BY HX	PE	TEST
PNS	Median neuropathy	Sensory or motor symptoms in median nerve distribution	Sensory and motor function of median nerve distribution	Phalen's and Tinel's tests Nerve conduction velocities

Key Reference: Szabo RM, Madison M: Carpal tunnel syndrome. Orthop Clin North Am 1992; 23:103–109.

PERIOPERATIVE IMPLICATIONS

Anesthetic Technique

- Can be performed under axillary block, Bier block, MAC, or GA techniques

Monitoring

- Routine
- For non–carpal tunnel decompression surgery, consider sites other than the radial artery of an affected hand for arterial catheters

Positioning

- Avoid flexion of either wrist (bilateral disease is common)

Airway

- No special considerations

Induction

- No special considerations

Surgical Stages

- EBL: minimal
- Minimal fluid shifts

Postoperative Considerations

- Pain score: 2–4
- Oral medications usually adequate

ANTICIPATED PROBLEMS/CONCERNS

- Exacerbation of median neuropathy

CATARACT ± IOL

Kathryn E. McGoldrick, M.D.

RISK

- >1.5 million cataract operations/y in US
- Gender predominance: None
- Advanced age
- Direct trauma
- Response to other intraocular conditions, including chronic uveitis, glaucoma, retinal detachment
- Systemic diseases (diabetes mellitus, myotonic dystrophy, galactosemia)
- Chronic use of topical or systemic corticosteroids
- Congenital (idiopathic, familial, associated with prenatal infection)

PERIOPERATIVE RISKS

- Perioperative mortality exceedingly rare
- Surgical morbidity: bleeding into anterior chamber; capsule rupture; posterior dislocation of lens into degenerative vitreous; loss of vitreous, producing retinal detachment and macular edema; expulsive hemorrhage

WORRY ABOUT

- Anesthetic morbidity following retrobulbar block
  - retrobulbar hemorrhage (1–3%)
  - perforation of globe (0.1% or less)
  - central spread of local anesthesia that may affect brainstem (0.1%)
  - intra-arterial injection with immediate seizures (<0.1%)
  - optic nerve injury (<0.1%)

OVERVIEW

- Removal of cloudy lens with small incision(s), with aspiration or ultrasonic fragmentation
- Associated with extremely low mortality, although complications of retrobulbar block (e.g., brainstem anesthesia) can be life threatening
- Morbidity can include blindness in operated eye.
- Topical anesthesia for selected patients (cooperative and able to control eye movements, not photophobic, appropriate-size pupil) avoids potentially serious complications of regional anesthesia

ICD-9-CM Code: 366.9

INDICATIONS AND USUAL TREATMENT

- Based on degree of visual impairment in relation to visual needs of the individual, as well as anticipated visual improvement and risk of serious complications
- With congenital cataracts, risk of amblyopia dictates that surgery be performed within the first few months of life

ASSESSMENT POINTS

SYSTEM	EFFECT	ASSESSMENT BY HX	PE	TEST
OCULAR	Determination of lens power of intraocular implant			Ultrasonic measurement of axial length of eye; optical measurement of corneal curvature
CARDIOPULM	Impaired ability to lie flat; chronic coughing	SOB, orthopnea	Inspection Auscultation	
CNS	Impaired ability to follow instructions and remain motionless because of age, anxiety, claustrophobia, deafness, tremors	CNS Hx	CNS exam	

Key Reference: McGoldrick KE, Mardirossian J: Ophthalmic surgery. In McGoldrick KE (ed): Ambulatory Anesthesiology: A Problem-Oriented Approach. Baltimore, Williams & Wilkins, 1995; pp 507–535.

PERIOPERATIVE IMPLICATIONS

Preoperative Preparation
- None

Anesthetic Technique
- Can be performed under regional (peribulbar or retrobulbar), general, sub-Tenon's, or topical anesthesia

Monitoring
- Routine
- Invasive monitoring seldom indicated

Regional Techniques
- Eye in neutral gaze to minimize risk of optic nerve injury
- Small-gauge needle, no longer than 31 mm (1¼ inch) to ↓ risk of globe perforation
- Consider general or topical anesthesia if high risk (e.g., extreme myopia; severe enophthalmos; staphyloma; previous ocular complications of regional anesthesia; severe vascular disease; bleeding diathesis; one-eyed patient) for complications associated with retro- or peribulbar block
- Avoid deep orbital penetration
- Avoid heavy sedation

General Anesthesia
- Meticulously secure endotracheal tube to prevent intraoperative extubation
- Neuromuscular paralysis with appropriate monitoring to avoid coughing or bucking that can cause loss of intraoccular contents
- Consider prophylactic antiemetic

SURGICAL STAGES

- Two basic techniques of cataract extraction — intracapsular and extracapsular.
- Majority extracapsular because an intact posterior capsule may reduce posterior segment complications: retinal tear, retinal detachment, macular edema.

Incision for Extracapsular Procedure
- With the pupil fully dilated, an anterior capsulotomy is performed

Definitive Surgery
- Central anterior capsule removed, with expression or irrigation of lens nucleus through wound. Alternatively, nucleus may be fragmented ultrasonically (phacoemulsification) behind iris plane to avoid corneal epithelial damage
- Incision partially closed and every precaution taken to maintain normal anterior chamber depth (by air infusion, fluid infusion, or injection of viscoelastic solution) to prevent corneal endothelial damage during intraocular lens insertion
- Supporting loops of posterior chamber lens inserted into capsular bag or ciliary sulcus
- EBL: negligible
- Minimal hemodynamic disturbance
- Approximate duration: 1 h or less

Postoperative Considerations
- Minimal postop pain
- Patients instructed to avoid bending, lifting, straining

ANTICIPATED PROBLEMS/CONCERNS

- Ptosis
- Postop wound dehiscence
- Iris prolapse
- Infectious endophthalmitis
- Retinal tear or detachment
- Cystoid macular edema
- Delayed posterior capsule opacification

CENTRAL VENOUS OXYGEN

John F. Schweiss, M.D.

RISK

- Misinterpretation
- Error with pulmonary art reflection oximetry; wedging in distal pulmonary art; drift, loss of calibration (recalibration every 24 h recommended); damage to fiberoptic bundles; blood coagulum on tip of catheter; changing Hgb level (with 2-wave systems, Baxter)

OVERVIEW

- SvO_2 is O_2 saturation of venous blood in PA (%)
- Determined by
  - transmission spectroscopic measurement of a pulmonary arterial blood sample in a hemoximeter (e.g., OSM-3 Radiometer), or
  - reflection oximetry with indwelling oximetry PA catheter (Abbott, Baxter, Spectromed) or
  - PvO_2 determination with calculation of SvO_2 based on PvO_2, pH (computer derivation from mixed venous blood gas determination)

ICD-9-CM Code: 89.66

INDICATIONS

- Represents balance of Hgb level (g/100 ml), art O_2 saturation, O_2 extraction by body (metabolic demand), perfusion/min (CO) based on following formulas: under normal physiological conditions, arterial O_2 content based on a Hgb of

$$15 \text{ g} \times (1.34 \text{ ml/g}) = 20 \text{ ml } O_2/100 \text{ ml}$$

$$SvO_2 = \frac{\text{mixed venous } O_2 \text{ content}}{\text{arterial } O_2 \text{ content}}$$

$$= \frac{A(20 \text{ vol\%}) - (A-V) \text{ diff. } (5 \text{ vol\%})}{20}$$

$$= \frac{15}{20} = 75\% \text{ (nml)}$$

- Interplay among Hgb level, O_2 consumption, arterial O_2 sat, CO responsible for value of SvO_2; body attempts to maintain SvO_2 >60%, ideally 75%

USES

- Evaluation of O_2 delivery
- Evaluation of cardiorespiratory efficiency

ABNORMALITIES INDICATE

- ↓ Can be caused by fall in SaO_2 (art O_2 sat), ↓ in CO, ↑ in O_2 consumption [normal (A–V) O_2 difference is 5 vol percent], a fall in Hgb level, or any combination of the above
- ↑ Occurs with >normal CO, as in sepsis, with hyperdynamic circulation (liver disease), with A→V venous shunt, with ↓ metabolism (hypothermia), hyperoxia (FiO_2=1.0), or with poisoning of metabolic processes (rare)
- During anesthesia when Hgb levels are stable, art O_2 content is normal (ideally), O_2 consumption ↓, SvO_2 changes parallel changes in CO

Implications

- When SvO_2 at 60%, some compromise of O_2 delivery exists. When SvO_2 falls below 60%, concern over compensatory forces, early system failure should lead to initiation of corrective measures. Below 50%, compensation is failing; below 40%, hypoxemia of tissues is striking; below 30%, O_2 delivery so compromised as to lead to death unless reversed
- A low Hgb level, especially less than 8 g/dl in presence of normal (A–V) O_2 difference (global), ↑ CO results in lower than normal SvO_2 without evidence of compromise of patient, if CO appropriately ↑

OPERATIVE IMPLICATIONS

- If SvO_2 low (<60%) or falling rapidly:
  - Check for arterial desaturation, ↑ in A-V difference; 5–6 vol% A-V difference normal
  - Check CO, evaluation for hypovolemia (CVP). Negative inotropy and an ↑ in systemic vascular resistance freq associated with low CO
  - Check Hgb level
  - Check for evidence of elevated O_2 consumption (↑ metabolism, fever, shivering, ↑ work of breathing)

INDICATIONS AND USUAL TREATMENT

- Improve arterial O_2 sat by ↑ FiO_2, expand lungs for atelectasis (shunting). Add PEEP, determine best PEEP, check peak inspiratory pressure, respiratory rate, and tidal/min vols
- ↑ CO with inotropes—e.g., dobutamine, $CaCl_2$ pacing (for bradycardia), vasodilators, (nitroprusside, nitroglycerin, hydralazine), volume expansion with fluids or blood products
- ↑ Hgb level by transfusion if indicated (packed RBCs)
- ↓ Metabolic demand by decreasing body T if latter is elevated; induce NM paralysis for shivering; Rx malignant hyperpyrexia, if Dx (rare)

Key Reference: Krafft P, Steltzer H, Hiesmayr M, et al: Mixed venous oxygen saturation in critically ill septic shock patients. The role of defined events. Chest 1993; 103:900.

CEREBRAL ANEURYSM CLIPPING
Frederick E. Sieber, M.D.

RISK

- Prevalence: 2–5% of general population
- ~28,000 cases/y of subarachnoid hemorrhage, only 18,000 surviving to receive medical attention
- Gender predominance: M:F ratio, 3:2

PERIOPERATIVE RISKS

- Perioperative morbidity, mortality for unclipped aneurysms <5%; bleeding aneurysms ~20% mortality
- Leading causes of death and disability vasospasm, CNS effects of initial subarachnoid hemorrhage

WORRY ABOUT

- Intraoperative aneurysmal rupture
- CNS ischemic episodes

OVERVIEW

- Congenital aneurysmal dilation, usually at branch points of circle of Willis
- Surgical position technique may vary according to location, configuration of aneurysm
- Most aneurysms managed by placement of metal clip on aneurysm base
- Use of temporary clip modifies intraoperative management

ICD-9-CM Codes: 437.3; 430 (A-V, ruptured)

INDICATIONS AND USUAL TREATMENT

- Unruptured aneurysms >5 mm in diameter in patients with life expectancies justifying expected surgical risks
- Ruptured cerebral aneurysms with Hunt-Hess grade 1, 2, or 3 subarachnoid hemorrhage
- Controversial whether clipping of aneurysms with grade 4 or higher subarachnoid hemorrhage should be performed because of poor CNS outcome
- Nimodipine-induced hypertension may be used to reduce risk of vasospasm

ASSESSMENT POINTS

SYSTEM	EFFECT	ASSESSMENT BY HX	PE	TEST
CV	ECG changes	Rule out angina		Lytes ECG, ECHO, CK.MB (rarely required)
RESP	PE	Dyspnea SOB	Rales, rhonchi on auscultation	CXR Consider ABG
CNS	Hydrocephalus ↑ICP	↓ Consciousness	Neuro	CT scan

PERIOPERATIVE IMPLICATIONS

Anesthetic Technique

- Performed under GA, deliberate hypotension may be required
- Mild hypothermia may be cerebroprotective

Monitoring

- Arterial line
- CVP to direct fluid mx
- Consider EEG, SSEP

Airway

- Routine

Induction

- Aneurysm rupture rare, but can follow sudden BP ↑ during laryngoscopy

SURGICAL STAGES

Dissection

- BP control to prevent aneurysm rupture
- Brain relaxation to assist visualizing aneurysm
- Spinal fluid drainage possibly required to assist visualizing aneurysm

Definitive Surgery

- Temporary clip placement may require CNS monitoring, administration of cerebral metabolism depressants—i.e., barbiturates, etomidate, or propofol
- Aneurysmal rupture may require induced hypotension
- Confirmation of correct placement of aneurysm clip may require intraoperative angiography

Postoperative Considerations

- Significant risk of vasospasm requires Rx with Ca channel blockers and hypervolemic, hypertensive, hemodilutional Rx
- If aneurysm unclipped, significant risk of rebleed exists
- Rapid emergence from anesthesia desired to assess immediately CNS status
- EBL: 200–500 ml

ANTICIPATED PROBLEMS/CONCERNS

- Cerebral ischemia possible during temporary clip placement, with inadequate maintenance of CPP, or with incorrect clip placement

CEREBRAL AVM REPAIR

Armin Schubert, M.D.

RISK

- ~2000–3000/y
- More common in middle-aged adults
- Risk of hemorrhage higher in small (5%/y) than in large (2%/y) lesions
- Racial predominance: none

PERIOPERATIVE RISKS

- Preop embolization attempts to ↓ risk by ↓ AVM flow; 30-d morbidity 20–40% (disability significantly improves over time)
- 30-d mortality <5%
- Unique complication: normal perfusion pressure breakthrough syndrome; overall risk = 1–18%; at highest risk are high-flow lesions, border-zone AVM location, large AVMs (19–37% risk); lesions with severe hypoperfusion or steal around AVM; severe CNS deficit (may significantly improve over time)
- Postop CNS deficits may predispose to airway obstruction, aspiration

WORRY ABOUT

- Blood availability
- Effects of recent CNS radiologic interventions
- Emergence: to allow early CNS assessment
- Massive brain swelling
- High-dose barbiturate Rx to prevent edema, intracranial HTN
- Tight BP control on emergency, early postop

OVERVIEW

- Rare congenital lesions
- Associated with cerebral aneurysms in 5–10%; in neonates, infants, shunt usually causes high-output heart failure. Excision can be associated with substantial blood loss
- After extirpation of nidus, may get hyperemic brain swelling

ICD-9-CM Code: 747.81 (Cerebral AVM)

INDICATIONS AND USUAL TREATMENT

- Surg excision: small surface AVMs; large AVM if resectable with low risk of deficit; progressive Sx; refractory seizures; <40 y
- Alternate Rx (stereotactic radiosurg with linear accelerator or by proton-beam irradiation): older population; location in eloquent area; symptomatic therapy, embolization only palliative

ASSESSMENT POINTS

SYSTEM	EFFECT	ASSESSMENT BY HX	PE	TEST
CV	Hyperdynamic CHF in small children, failure to thrive	Recurrent respiratory failure, prolonged ventilatory support Diaphoresis with feeding	Auscultation	CXR, ECHO
RESP	May aspirate during seizure, hemorrhage	Review with family; records from ER, ICU	Auscultation, hepatomegaly, JVD, diaphoresis	CXR, pulmonary compliance, ABG, oximetry
GU	Dehydration and/or mild renal insufficiency from multiple CNS imaging	Chart review		BUN, Cr
CNS	Seizures, chronic ischemia of brain surrounding AVM; hydrocephalus, intracranial HTN	LOC, headache, diplopia, nausea; family to describe Sz	MS CNS exam (esp hemiplegia, cranial nerves)	EEG, CT; Angio

Key Reference: Dodson BA: Interventional radiology and the anesthetic management of patients with arteriovenous malformations. *In* Cottrell JE, Smith DS (eds): Anesthesia and Neurosurgery. St. Louis, Mosby-Year Book, 1994, pp 407–424.

INTRAOPERATIVE MANAGEMENT

Preoperative Preparation

- Avoid premedication if mental status impaired or ICP high;
- Determine risk of normal perfusion pressure breakthrough

Anesthetic Technique

- Requirements include brain relaxation, BP control, early emergence (or in patients at high risk for normal perfusion pressure breakthrough, high dose barbiturates)
- Hyperventilation to $PaCO_2$ of 25–30 mmHg
- Avoid glucose-containing fluid

Monitoring

- Routine
- Consider art line, central venous or PA catheter
- Consider EPs
- Consider EEG for barbiturate effect
- ICP for emergence and postop

SURGICAL STAGES

Induction

- Avoid succinylcholine with hemiplegia, ↑ ICP
- Maintain BP control; avoid coughing

Skeletal Fixation

- Avoid BP spike during fixation

Skin Incision

- Avoid HTN; may see effects of local anesthesia, epinephrine
- Consider beginning mannitol 0.5–1.0 g/kg

Dissection

- Arterial supply resected 1st; severe episodic bleeding, especially if dural sinuses involved
- Consider high-dose barbiturates to prevent normal perfusion pressure breakthrough Rx vs. mild hypothermia, diuretics

Definitive Surgery

- May develop brain swelling as soon as nidus occluded

Closure/Postoperative Period

- EBL: 300–2000 ml; depends on AVM size, location; no need for 3rd space allowance
- Control BP, often to <130 systolic
- Assure normal coag status
- Pain score: 3–5
- Rx small doses of IV opioid, if CNS status OK

ANTICIPATED PROBLEMS/CONCERNS

- Intraoperative concerns: bleeding, brain volume control; CNS assessment at end of procedure
- Normal perfusion pressure breakthrough (hematoma, hydrocephalus, etc.), Rx regimens (barbiturate Rx, mild hypothermia) after AVM surg essential

CESAREAN SECTION, EMERGENT

Gertie Marx, M.D.

RISK

- 1992: total USA C-sections 964,000/y
- Emergent CS: 5–10%
- Racial predominance: none

PERIOPERATIVE RISKS

- Anesthesia-related mortality: 0.6/100,000 live births
- Most maternal deaths from anesthesia occur during emergent C-sections
- Most freq causes: failed intubation, pulmonary inhalation of gastric contents, drug misuse
- Nonanesthetic perioperative risks: amniotic fluid embolism, PE, preeclampsia-eclampsia

WORRY ABOUT

- Limited time for preanesthetic evaluation
- Airway
- Recent solid food intake
- Hypovolemia
- Coagulopathy

OVERVIEW

- Truly emergent C-sections—threatening life or essential functions of mother, fetus—are performed immediately, within min after recognition of complications
- True emergencies immediately threaten life or essential functions of mother, fetus
- Regional block safer for mother, less depressant for fetus than GA
- Incision-delivery interval:
  – skin incision to delivery interval: with appropriate uterine displacement, admin of suppl O_2—no bearing on fetal outcome
  – uterine incision to delivery interval: deterioration of 1-min Apgar score after 189 seconds with regional anesthesia vs. 90 seconds with GA

ICD-9-CM Code: 656.31 (Fetal distress resulting in delivery)

INDICATIONS AND USUAL TREATMENT

- Maternal: massive hemorrhage (placenta previa, abruptio placentae, trauma) associated with deteriorating maternal and/or fetal VS, uterine rupture, nonabating uterine tetany (cocaine overdose)
- Fetal: severe distress, prolapsed umbilical cord, associated (usually) with late decelerations (often prolonged), sometimes preceded by loss of beat-to-beat variability

ASSESSMENT POINTS

SYSTEM	EFFECT	ASSESSMENT BY HX	PE	TEST
HEENT	Engorged oropharynx		Airway exam	
CV	↓ MAP ↑ HR, ↑ CO		CV	ECG monitor
RESP	Compensated respiratory alkalosis ↑ Minute ventilation, ↓ FRC		Tachypnea	SaO_2
GI	Gastroesophageal reflux	Heartburn		
HEME	Dilutional anemia			Hb, Hct

Key Reference: Marx GF, Luykx WM, Cohen S: Fetal-neonatal status following caesarean section for fetal distress. Br J Anaesth 1984; 56:1009–1013.

PREOPERATIVE PREPARATION

- Administer oral antacid (e.g., 30 ml cooled, pH-adjusted sodium citrate)
- Position mother with uterine displacement
- Maintain fetal HR monitoring until onset of surgery

Anesthetic Technique

- Hemorrhage: GA
- Uterine rupture: GA or extension of epidural block
- Uterine tetany: GA
- Fetal distress: spinal block, extension of epidural block, GA
- Prolapsed umbilical cord: GA or extension of epidural block

Monitoring

- Routine unless significant blood loss

Airway

- Consider full stomach, edematous oropharynx

Induction/Maintenance

- Spinal anesthesia: give IV preload of crystalloid solution rapidly but do not delay block because of as yet insufficient amount of solution; continue IV infusion; use moderate-size needle—i.e., 22-gauge—to obtain CSF readily
  – inject hyperbaric bupivacaine for average duration of surgery or hyperbaric lidocaine for duration of less than 1 h.
  – treat falling BP immediately with ↑ IV fluid, ↑ uterine displacement, ephedrine 5–10 mg doses: if no improvement, use phenylephrine 50 μg
- Epidural anesthesia: extend pre-existing block with 3% 2-chloroprocaine or 2% pH-adjusted lidocaine for fast action; can supplement with 10-mg doses of ketamine IV; for incomplete analgesia, have obstetrician perform local infiltration with 1% 2-chloroprocaine or 0.5% lidocaine
- GA: Rapid-sequence IV induction with ketamine, 0.75–1.0 mg/kg, or ketamine, 0.5 mg/kg, followed by thiobarbiturate, 2.0 mg/kg, except in uterine tetany when barbiturate preferable (ketamine thought less cardiodepressant than barbiturates, especially in hypovolemia)
  – maintenance until birth with at least 60% but preferably 100% O_2 + low concentration (½ MAC) of halogenated agent

SURGICAL STAGES

- Uterine incision (2 techniques):
  – horizontal (lower segment)—stronger scar, less blood loss, less infection, T4 blockade required
  – vertical (classic)—faster delivery of fetus, T6 blockade sufficient
- EBL: 800–1200 ml
- Volume concerns: Patients freq hypovolemic

Postoperative Pain Management

- Pain severity: varies; Rx 24–48 h: IM, IV, or epidural opioid bolus injections or IV or epidural opioid infusion, PCA
- Postpartum depression more likely to develop if emergent C-section vs vaginal delivery

ANTICIPATED PROBLEMS/CONCERNS

- After GA: pulmonary inhalation of gastric contents, HTN, arrhythmia, awareness
- After regional anesthesia: hypotension, failed block, high block, systemic toxicity

CESAREAN SECTION, PLANNED

Andrew P. Harris, M.D., M.H.S.

RISK

- 1993 total USA C-sections 921,000/y
- Racial predominance: none

PERIOPERATIVE RISKS

- Perioperative pulmonary morbidity varies by type of anesthesia: GA associated with ↑ pulmonary morbidity
- Low mortality, but anesthesia (5–24/100,000) significant contributor to mortality

WORRY ABOUT

- Embolism—thromboembolism, air embolism, amniotic fluid embolism
- Unintentional high regional block
- Inability to intubate
- Unanticipated blood loss
- Spinal HA
- Postop endometritis

OVERVIEW

- "Significant other" frequently accompanies patient to OR
- Hysterotomy usually through lower uterine segment
- Occasional uterine atony after delivery Rx with oxytocic agents, occasionally progressing to cesarean hysterectomy
- Exteriorization of uterus during closure associated with greater intraoperative discomfort if regional anesthesia
- Regional anesthesia preferred to avoid risk of airway mishaps, postop pulmonary morbidity

ICD-9-CM Code: V22.2 (Pregnancy)
(See also Maternal Physiology in Diseases section and Nonobstetric Surgery in Pregnant Patient in Procedures section)

INDICATIONS AND USUAL TREATMENT

- Conditions which would result in ↑ perinatal morbidity for mother or fetus if vaginal delivery attempted; most common examples include: Hx of classic C-section, macrosomia, Hx of CPD, twin gestation
- May also be emergent (see emergency C-section)
- Vaginal birth after C-section may be attempted in lieu of elective repeat C-section

ASSESSMENT POINTS

SYSTEM	EFFECT	ASSESSMENT BY HX	PE	TEST
CV	↑ CO, ↑ dilutional anemia, vena caval obstruction	Cardiac failure, supine hypotensive syndrome	Edema	Hct
RESP	Engorged vessels, breast development ↑ minute ventilation, ↑ O_2 consumption	SOB	Airway Mallampati's classification	
GI	Delayed gastric emptying	Regurgitation		
MS	↑ Back pain	Back pain, sciatica		

Key Reference: Reisner LS, Lin D: Anesthesia for cesarean section. *In* Chestnut DH (ed): Obstetric Anesthesia Principles and Practice. St. Louis, Mosby–Year Book, 1994, pp 45–486.

PERIOPERATIVE MANAGEMENT

Preoperative Preparation

- Antacids and/or H_2-blocker/metoclopramide
- Left uterine displacement

Anesthetic Technique

- Any: general, local, spinal, epidural, but regional preferred due to potential airway problems

Monitoring

- Fetal HR monitoring preop
- Consider air embolism monitoring

Airway

- Engorgement leads to easy bleeding, difficult intubation
- ~1/300 unanticipated difficult intubation

Induction/Maintenance

- 1/3 less local anesthesia required for regional anesthesia
- T4 level during regional anesthesia desirable
- If GA, discontinue halogenated agents (if possible) after delivery to ↓ blood loss
- Prophylactic antibiotic after cord clamp

Surgical Stages

- Skin incision to delivery: venous air embolism, amniotic fluid embolism possible
- Closure: uterine atony or hemorrhage possible
- EBL: 750–1000 ml normal; can be much greater with uterine atony

Postoperative Considerations

- Uterine atony possible
- Pain score: typically 4–8
- IV-PCA or epidural PCA for 1–2 d

ANTICIPATED PROBLEMS/CONCERNS

- Inability to intubate
- High block with hypotension, sudden bradycardia
- Hemorrhage
- Postop headache

CHOLECYSTECTOMY, LAPAROSCOPIC

Sorin J. Brull, M.D.

RISK

- 20 million in USA with gallstones
- 600,000 cholecystectomies/y
- Prevalence ↑ with age; higher incidence in women, 17%; men, 8%
- Among Pima Indian women, 75% affected
- Incidence in African-Americans higher than in Caucasians

PERIOPERATIVE RISKS

- Perioperative mortality ~0.1%, morbidity 4–6 × lower than in open procedure (2–9%)
- Most benefits derived from avoidance of large abdominal incision

WORRY ABOUT

- Intraoperative hemorrhage
- Visceral damage
- Bacterbilia, sepsis
- PE, arrhythmias (CO_2 absorption)
- SC emphysema from improperly placed CO_2 insufflating needle
- Hemodynamic consequences of pneumoperitoneum
- CO_2 absorption, position changes; CO_2 embolism

OVERVIEW

- Laparoscopic procedure ↑ in freq
- Lower incidence of complications than with open
- Freq short stay; OP procedure in appropriate patients

ICD-9-CM Code: 574.0 (Cholelithiasis)

INDICATIONS AND USUAL TREATMENT

- Indications: chronic cholecystitis, symptomatic cholelithiasis
- Early contraindications: large stones in common bile duct, acute inflammation, pregnancy, obesity, but now used in acute cholecystitis and pregnancy
- Considered technique of choice in octogenarians
- Alternative Rx: open procedure, stone/contact dissolution, biliary lithotripsy, cholecystolithotomy

ASSESSMENT POINTS

SYSTEM	EFFECT	ASSESSMENT BY HX	PE	TEST
CV	Likely comorbidities: PVD, CAD		CV	ECG
RESP	Comorbidity likely: COPD (elderly)		Chest	CXR O_2 sat
HEME	Intraoperative blood loss (cystic artery liver laceration)	Preop dehydration (N/V, elderly)	Orthostasis	Hct, electrolytes
GU	Impairment secondary to age, comorbidity	CNS Hx	CNS	BUN/Cr

Key Reference: Cunningham AJ, Brull SJ: Laparoscopic cholecystectomy: Anesthetic implications. Anesth Analg 1993; 76:1120–1133.

INTRAOPERATIVE MANAGEMENT

Monitoring

- Routine, UO (Foley catheter)
- End-tidal CO_2 not good substitute for arterial P_{CO_2}

Airway

- Change in position from head-up to head-down may displace ET tube into endobronchial position

Anesthetic Technique

- GA, controlled ventilation with cuffed ET tube (prevent aspiration during pneumoperitoneum); regional (axial) anesthesia not advocated

SURGICAL STAGES

Induction

- CV instability if coexisting disease, elderly
- Trocar insertion: injury to viscera
- Trendelenburg position:
  – CV effects: improves venous return, CO, BP; pulmonary effects: reduced VC, atelectasis, shunting

- Pneumoperitoneum creation:
  – subcutaneous emphysema from poorly placed insufflating needle
  – CV effects: intra-abd pressure <15 mmHg associated with minimal CV changes (slight increase in MAP, no change in CO)
  – pulmonary effects: hypoventilation, respiratory acidosis, hypoxemia, tension pneumothorax (via patent pleuroperitoneal canal), atelectasis, shunting; exogenous CO_2 insufflation—rapid absorption, necessitating controlled ventilation; arrhythmias, catecholamine release; poss CO_2 pulmonary embolism, especially at release of pneumoperitoneum

Definitive Surgery

- Postop N/V high (42%); prophylaxis recommended: metoclopramide, droperidol, ?ondansetron
- Avoiding neostigmine, ↓ narcotic requirements by using NSAIDs (ketorolac) also effective
- Narcotic-induced sphincter of Oddi spasm reversed with narcotic antagonists, local anesthetic infiltration, glucagon

- Use of N_2O controversial due to ? bowel distention, ? postop N/V
- Pre-emptive/adjuvant anesthesia with local anesthetic infiltration of skin, gallbladder bed may reduce postop pain
- Blood loss min. ~surg duration: 1–3 h
- Fluid shifts: minimal
- Pain score: 2–5; same day or next day hospital discharge

ANTICIPATED PROBLEMS/CONCERNS

- Intraoperative: tension pneumothorax, CO_2 absorption, arrhythmias, hemodynamic compromise from pneumoperitoneum, visceral damage from surgical trocar, CO_2 embolism
- Conversion to open procedure (1–7% incidence) due to technical factors
- Gasless (traction) laparoscopic techniques under trial

CHOLECYSTECTOMY, OPEN
Sorin J. Brull, M.D.

RISK

- 20 million in USA have gallstones
- 600,000 cholecystectomies/y
- Prevalence ↑ with age; in women incidence is 17%, in men 8%
- Pima Indian women, incidence is 75%
- African-Americans affected more often than Caucasians

PERIOPERATIVE RISKS

- Perioperative mortality: 0–0.5% (0.1% in patients <50 y
- In elderly: up to 10%
- Morbidity: 5–25%, especially 2° to impairment of pulmonary mechanics (abdominal incision)

WORRY ABOUT

- Intraoperative hemorrhage
- Hepatic failure
- Bacterbilia, sepsis

OVERVIEW

- Becoming less frequent mode of cholecystectomy
- Antibiotic prophylaxis; midline, paramedian, or subcostal surg incision
- Identification of cystic duct, common hepatic duct, common bile duct, cystic artery
- Operative cholangiogram performed for choledocholithiasis
- US ~98% sensitivity, specificity

ICD-9-CM Code: 574.0 (Cholelithiasis)

INDICATIONS AND USUAL TREATMENT

- Chronic cholecystitis and symptomatic cholelithiasis
- Biliary colic treated with parenteral narcotics; antibiotic therapy for patients over age 60 with chronic cholecystitis, and for patients with acute cholecystitis or with concomitant common duct stones
- Nasogastric suction and low-fat diet not proven beneficial.
- Other Rx: gallstone dissolution; percutaneous shock wave lithotripsy; contact dissolution; percutaneous cholecystolithotomy; laparoscopic cholecystectomy

ASSESSMENT POINTS

SYSTEM	EFFECT	ASSESSMENT BY HX	PE	TEST
CV	Rule out angina vs. cholecystitis ECG changes & arrhythmias	Rule out CAD Relief by nitroglycerin (relieves both angina, biliary colic)		ECG coronary angio; exercise tolerance test if unable to differentiate
RESP	Comorbidity likely: COPD (elderly)	Pulmonary reserve Exercise tolerance	Auscultation	CXR
GI	N/V	N/V		

Key Reference: Nahrwold DL: The biliary system. *In* Sabiston DC Jr (ed): Textbook of Surgery, 14th edition, Philadelphia, WB Saunders, 1991, pp 1042–1075.

PERIOPERATIVE MANAGEMENT

Perioperative Evaluations

- Assess CV system, CAD

Anesthetic Technique

- GA
- Regional (axial) anesthesia may not be appropriate due to high level of sensory denervation required (at least T4)
- Local anesthesia for cholecystostomy
- Adjunct techniques: interpleural cath, intercostal nerve block
- Prophylaxis for postop N/V

Monitoring

- Routine

Airway

- Consider rapid-sequence induction if preop N/V

Induction

- Narcotic-induced sphincter of Oddi spasm reversed with narcotic antagonists, injection of local anesthesia, or glucagon
- Use of N_2O controversial because of nausea, bowel distention

Surgical Stages

- Skin incision: large, usually subcostal

Dissection

- Possible bleeding from cystic artery, liver laceration/damage
- Possible pneumothorax if diaphragmatic or pleural damage

Definitive Surgery

- Exposure, bowel manipulation/traction may lead to hypotension (release of vasoactive substances from gut and/or ↓ venous return)
- Approximate duration: 0.5–3.0 h
- Fluid shift: can be marked if bowel exposed for long periods
- Hypothermia a concern if prolonged procedure, esp in elderly
- EBL: 50–150 ml

Postoperative Considerations

- N/V: consider prophylaxis
- Pain score: 6–10; narcotic requirements ↓ by "preemptive analgesia," adjunct techniques (interpleural cath, intercostal nerve block), local anesthetic infiltration of gallbladder bed

ANTICIPATED PROBLEMS/CONCERNS

- Severe postop pain (incisional) may lead to ↓ ambulation; splinting; ↓ cough, mobilization; atelectasis, pulmonary infection

CIRCUMCISION

Stanley W. Stead, M.D.

RISK

- ~2 million/y
- Most common surgical procedure in USA
- Generally performed in neonatal period

PERIOPERATIVE RISKS

- Considered minimal 0.2% (aspiration, bleeding, hematoma, malignant hyperthermia reported 1 series (2/476), postop fever); complications from local anesthesia rare
- Local skin necrosis after dorsal penile nerve block (<0.5%)

WORRY ABOUT

- Complicated preop neonatal course: sepsis, hypospadias, immaturity

OVERVIEW

- Most common surg procedure; as many as 76.9% of boys circumcised neonatally
- ↑ From 1985–1992; largest increment following 1989 American Academy of Pediatrics stating "potential benefits and advantages" of procedure
- From 1975–1984, rate among newborn boys ↓ significantly, from 88%–70%
- Risk from UTI ↑ 5–89 times in uncircumcised during same period

ICD-9-CM Codes: V50.2 (Circumcision [no medical indication, ritual, routine]); 605 (phimosis); 607.1 (balanitis)

INDICATIONS AND USUAL TREATMENT

- Parental choice
- Coincidence with other surg
- Recurrent balanoposthitis
- UTIs
- True phimosis (obstruction of urine flow)
- Difficulty retracting foreskin

ASSESSMENT POINTS

SYSTEM	EFFECT	PE	TEST
GU	Hypospadias	Urethra ventral surface of penis	
	Balanoposthitis, phimosis	Nonretractile prepuce or tight ring	
	Urinary tract infections		UA, microscopic
Overall	Immaturity, sepsis		

Key Reference: Niku SD, Stock JA, Kaplan GW: Neonatal circumcision. Urol Clin North Am 1995; 22:57–65.

INTRAOPERATIVE MANAGEMENT

- In neonate commonly performed without anesthesia. Recently, dorsal penile nerve block, topical anesthesia with Emla cream have been proposed
- In older individuals, local anesthesia infiltration of prepuce or dorsal penile nerve block
- GA may be preferred in children

Monitoring

- Routine

Airway

- Routine: mask, laryngeal mask airway, intubation

SURGICAL STAGES

Skin Incision/Definitive Surgery

- Two methods "sleeve" or "freehand" in which ring incision made around prepuce, or using a clamp (Plastibell, Gomco, or Mogen). In either, maximum surgical stimuli at this point; no dissection. Bleeding controlled with compression or electrocautery; suture placement rare
- Commonly, petrolatum-based gauze used to dress wound edges, which are brought together

Postoperative Considerations

- Pain score: 2–4
- Pain relief by rectal acetaminophen in neonates
- Older individuals may require opiates

ANTICIPATED PROBLEMS/CONCERNS

- Newborn infants experience pain manifested by physiol changes (↑ in BP, HR, sweating, ↓ oxygenation), behavioral changes, which persist for at least 22 h; physiol, behavioral effects attenuated by local or regional anesthesia
- Pain often undertreated
- Infection remains a possibility in neonates, since hygiene may be compromised

CLEFT LIP REPAIR

Andrei Cernea, M.D.

RISK

- ~1/1000 live births
- Racial predominance: Caucasian, 2:1: black infants
- More frequently male than female
- Very frequently associated with cleft palate
- Associated with maternal phenytoin or alcohol ingestion

PERIOPERATIVE RISKS

- Extremely low morbidity/mortality; no deaths reported in recent literature with cleft lip repair alone
- When associated with cleft palate repair, the most significant risk is postop airway obstruction

WORRY ABOUT

- Difficult airway when associated with syndromes—e.g., EEC, Mohr's, Shprintzen's, 4P, or Pierre Robin's
- UnDxed associated congenital heart, renal disease
- Intraoperative dysrhythmias caused by surgical infiltration of epinephrine in presence of halothane
- Timing of surgery coinciding with physiologic anemia of infancy
- Postop airway obstruction by forgotten pharyngeal pack
- Associated with cleft palate, risks of: preop anemia due to poor feeding; intrainduction laryngospasm due to chronic otitis media, URI; intrainduction airway obstruction due to tongue wedged in cleft palate; postop airway obstruction due to lingual edema

OVERVIEW

- Congenital condition by 7th wk intrauterine life
- Strong genetic influence; ¼ cases bilateral cleft lip
- Traditionally done at ~3 mo, but recently done neonatally

ICD-9-CM Code: 749.10

INDICATIONS AND USUAL TREATMENT

- If in good health, cheiloplasty electively performed
- Primary indications are aesthetic: early repair encourages maternal bonding
- Should be done by 18 mo to assure normal speech, social integration

ASSESSMENT POINTS

(inclusive for associated cleft palate)

SYSTEM	EFFECT	ASSESSMENT BY HX	PE	TEST
HEENT	Otitis media Clear rhinorrhea, difficult airway	Ear pain Snore, grunt	TM Airway exam	
CV	Associated CHD	SOB, cyanosis, poor growth	CV exam Club feet	ECG, ECHO
RESP	URI aspiration	Cough/fever SOB, cyanosis	Auscultation Chest exam	CXR, ABG
GI	Impaired deglutition Malnutrition	Nasal regurgitation Poor growth		Observe feeding Albumin
HEME	Anemia	Malnutrition	Pallor	Hgb/Hct
GU	Associated congenital defects	UTI	Club feet	UA, BUN/Cr

Key Reference: Stehling L: Common Problems in Pediatric Anesthesia, 2nd ed. St. Louis, Mosby–Year Book, 1992, pp 87–91.

PERIOPERATIVE IMPLICATIONS

Preoperative Preparation

- During neonatal period ascertain associated birth defects
- Establish postconceptual age to exclude premature neonates

Anesthetic Technique

- GA, anticholinergic agent usual
- Oral intubation using appropriate-sized RAE tube well secured to mandible
- Maintenance with inhalational agent; NMB not usual

Monitoring

- Well-placed precordial stethoscope especially important since intraoperative access to airway severely limited
- If neonate, aggressively prevent heat loss

SURGICAL STAGES

- Placement of pharyngeal pack
- Local anesthetic and epinephrine infiltration
- Minimal tissue mobilization, direct closure of defect
- Procedure time usually brief
- EBL: usually minimal

Postoperative Considerations

- Check that pharyngeal pack removed before extubation
- If patient premature continue apnea monitoring for at least 24 h postop
- Pain score: 2–5
- Oral or rectal Tylenol usually sufficient
- Oral feeding can start after ~2 h with clear liquids

ANTICIPATED PROBLEMS/CONCERNS

- Undiagnosed cardiac anomalies in neonate
- Postop airway obstruction due to forgotten pack or airway edema

CLEFT PALATE REPAIR

C. Dean Kurth, M.D.

RISK

- Incidence of cleft palate is about 1/1000 live births
- Repaired before speech develops, usually at age 3–18 mo

PERIOPERATIVE RISKS

- Perioperative mortality rare in pediatric centers

WORRY ABOUT

- Associated deformities, their risks: congenital heart disease (SBE prophylaxis, cyanosis, CHF), micrognathia (difficult intubation), retroglossia (difficult mask airway), upper airway congestion (laryngospasm)
- Tracheal tube: difficult intubation; tube occlusion, extubation, endobronchial during surgery
- Intraoperative arrhythmias and HTN.
- Postoperative airway obstruction.

OVERVIEW

- Usually isolated deformity; it can also be part of syndrome (e.g., Pierre Robin)
- Repaired to separate oral, nasal cavities; improve feeding, speech; prevent middle ear disease, hearing loss
- Surgical position: supine, head extended, mouth open, pharyngeal packs in
- Before incision, palate is infiltrated with epinephrine for hemostasis
- Surgery involves undermining tissues around defect to create flap to cover it; soft palate edema; opioid administration may contribute to postop obstructive apnea

ICD-9-CM Codes: 749.0, 749.2

INDICATIONS/USUAL TREATMENT

- Defects are surgically repaired if life expectancy reasonable
- Bottle-fed with special nipple before defect closed; caloric intake, growth monitored
- Otitis media often occurs; antibiotic prophylaxis common preop
- Myringotomy tubes frequently placed concomitantly with repairs

ASSESSMENT POINTS

SYSTEM	EFFECT	ASSESSMENT BY HX	PE	TEST
HEENT	Palate defect, other deformities, rhinorrhea	Apnea, known syndrome	Defect size, airway exam, nasal secretions	
CV	Cardiac defect	Slow feeding, diaphoresis	Murmur, liver size, cyanosis, HR, RR	ECG/CXR ECHO
RESP	Bronchitis, chronic aspiration	Cough, fever, feeding problem	Rhonchi, wheeze	O_2 saturation CXR
HEME	Anemia	Age 3–9 mo	Pallor	Hct

Key Reference: Randall P: Cleft of the alveolus and palate. *In* Serafin O, Georgiade N (eds): Pediatric Plastic Surgery. St Louis, Mosby, 1984, p 290.

PERIOPERATIVE MANAGEMENT

Preoperative Preparation

- Premedication: Atropine only for young infants, those with obstructive apnea
- Consider cross-match, depending on surgeon, patient's Hct

Anesthetic Technique

- No special techniques

Monitoring

- Routine

Airway

- Secure tracheal tube at midline, flat against chin, bend of tube at lip; use water-resistant tape; oral RAE tube
- Flex, extend head to check for bronchial intubation or inadvertent extubation

Surgical Stages

- Palate infiltrated with epinephrine before incision; keep dose <10 µg/kg
- Tissue on both sides of defect mobilized to create flap
- During dissection, observe wound for bleeding, but transfusion rarely required
- After defect, check palate for edema, gauge airway caliber
- At end, heavy ligature may be placed through tongue, or NP airway may be inserted
- Wound may be injected with bupivacaine for postop analgesia; keep dose < 2mg/kg
- Surgical duration: 2–4 h
- EBL variable

Emergence

- Before extubation, ensure that the pharyngeal pack is gone and that the oral cavity is dry
- Extubation best done when patients are awake
- Restrain arms to prevent child from pulling at oral suture line

POSTOPERATIVE CONSIDERATIONS

- Analgesia with acetaminophen or opioid; careful with opioid dose (obstructive apnea)
- Pulse oximetry, cardiorespiratory monitoring recommended for 24–48 h

COLOSTOMY

Kevin C. Limp, M.D.

RISK

- Approximately 70,000/y in USA
- Racial predominance: colostomy for colon cancer: none; Crohn's/ulcerative colitis: white > African-American
- Gender predominance: colostomy for colon cancer: M:F, 3:1; Crohn's: M ≤ F; ulcerative colitis: M ≤ F; trauma: M:F, 3:1; diverticulitis: M:F, 1:1

PERIOPERATIVE RISKS

- Perioperative morbidity related to concurrent medical diseases, associated surgical procedure(s)
- Colostomy performed to ↓ perioperative complications
- Specific periop mortality rare (<0.5%)
- Specific periop morbidity: infection (<5%), stomal ischemia/necrosis (<2%), stomal retraction, parastomal fistula, stomal stenosis, parastomal hernia, stomal prolapse, bleeding

WORRY ABOUT

- Malnutrition, hypoproteinemia, lyte disturbances

- Intravascular volume depletion (bleeding, npo status, vomiting, bowel prep, 3rd spacing, poor PO intake)
- Anemia (bleeding, chronic disease)
- Aspiration risk (obstruction, npo status, urgent surgery, pain, debilitation)
- Complications, metabolic derangements of hyperalimentation
- Perioperative corticosteroid supplementation (inflammatory bowel disease)
- Associated trauma lesions
- Extracolonic manifestations of inflammatory bowel disease (IBD) (e.g., arthritis, anemia)

OVERVIEW

- A type of enterostomy that creates an opening in the colon, the proximal end of which is exteriorized and fashioned as a stoma to form an abdominal anus
- Patients present electively (e.g., inflammatory bowel disease), urgently (e.g., colon cancer with obstruction), or emergently (penetrating abdominal trauma)

- Performed in association with surgical procedure(s) for patient's underlying condition (e.g., large bowel resection for ulcerative colitis, abdominoperineal resection for colon cancer)

ICD-9-CM Codes: 555–569

INDICATIONS AND USUAL TREATMENT

- General indications: to replace anus as distal opening of GI tract, to divert fecal stream from more distal pathologic process, to decompress obstructed colon
- Specific indications: colon cancer, Crohn's disease, ulcerative colitis, abdominal trauma, diverticulitis, Hirschsprung's disease
- Usual Rx: colon CA: primary resection (chemotherapy, radiation therapy 2°)
  - Inflammatory bowel disease: sulfasalazine, corticosteroids, bowel rest, resection
  - Penetrating abdominal trauma with bowel injury: laparotomy, resection

ASSESSMENT POINTS

SYSTEM	EFFECT	ASSESSMENT BY HX	PE	TEST
HEENT	Ankylosing arthritis of IBD can affect ability to intubate	Spine immobility	Airway exam	Spine imaging
CV	Intravascular volume depletion	Bleeding, vomiting, diarrhea, npo, bowel prep, poor PO intake	VS Cardiac exam	ECG
RESP	Pulm metastases (colon CA)	Cough, hemoptysis, dyspnea	Chest exam	Chest imaging
GI	Potential for aspiration	Obstruction, npo status	Abd exam	Abdominal imaging
HEME	Anemia (hemorrhage, chronic disease)	Orthostasis, ↓ exercise tolerance	Cardiac exam	Hct

Key Reference: McGinnis LS: Surgical treatment options for colorectal cancer. Cancer 1994; 74:2147–2150.

PERIOPERATIVE MANAGEMENT

Preoperative Preparation

- Restoration of intravascular volume; correction of electrolyte, metabolic disturbances
- Corticosteroid supplementation if appropriate
- Consider H₂ blocking agents, antacids

Anesthetic Technique

- Balanced GA with ET intubation provides protection from aspiration of gastric contents; allows use of muscle relaxants for optimal surgical conditions
- Combined general, epidural anesthesia may facilitate rapid extubation, excellent postop analgesia, early return of bowel function, ↓ intraoperative blood loss, ↓ incidence of postop DVT, pulmonary emboli

Monitoring

- Consider Foley catheter
- Consider CVP based on volume status, anticipated bleeding, 3rd spacing, need for postop access
- Consider arterial line for coexisting disease or hemodynamic instability

Airway

- ET intubation preferred

Induction

- If at risk for aspiration, rapid-sequence induction with cricoid press, or awake intubation
- In combined epidural/GA, administer epidural drug slowly if intravascular volume repletion not assured

Maintenance

- Prudent to avoid N₂O until wound closure
- Anticipate large 3rd space losses, potential bleeding if other procedures planned

Emergence

- For patients at risk for aspiration, extubate after full recovery of airway reflexes

Postoperative Considerations

- ICU for coexisting disease, extensive surgery, hemodynamic instability
- Corticosteroid supplements for inflammatory bowel disease,
- Ongoing fluid shifts, hemodynamic instability
- Pain score: 5–8 (for laparotomy)
- EBL: <100 ml for stoma creation; often 200–300 ml for primary surgical procedure
- Anticipate significant 3rd space fluid shifts, possible blood loss

ANTICIPATED PROBLEMS/CONCERNS

- None

CORONARY ARTERY BYPASS GRAFT

Daniel M. Thys, M.D.

RISK

- 360,000 CABG operations/y
- Risk factors for CAD: cigarette smoking, HTN, diabetes, ↑ cholesterol, high LDL, low HDL, age, male sex, family Hx

PERIOPERATIVE RISKS

- 30-d mortality: 1.5–5%
- Risk factors for poor outcome: age, reop, disaster/emergent surg, EF <30%
- Cardiac outcomes: cardiac failure, MI, arrhythmias, cardiac death
- Severe perioperative morbidity: stroke (1%–25%) dependent upon condition of aorta, degree of neuropsychiatric testing

WORRY ABOUT

- Perioperative ventricular function
- Myocardial protection, perioperative ischemia
- Completeness of surg revascularization
- Bleeding with reoperations

OVERVIEW

- Occluded or severely diseased coronary arteries bypassed with venous or arterial grafts
- Anesthesia technique, monitoring, postop ventilatory care affected by patient's physical condition
- Early extubation, discharge goal if good preop condition, but safety of "fast-tracking" effects of rapid temperature normalization upon stroke rate under investigation

ICD-9-CM Code: 414.0

INDICATIONS AND USUAL TREATMENT

- High-grade (>75%) stenosis of left main coronary artery
- Severe angina with multivessel disease, poor LV function
- Angina after failed medical therapy, PTCA, or previous CABG

ASSESSMENT POINTS

SYSTEM	EFFECT	ASSESSMENT BY HX	PE	TEST
CV	Cardiac failure	Exercise tolerance	Auscultation	Radionuclide stress test, ECHO
	Atheromata bruits	Asymptomatic, TIA, etc.	Auscultation	ECHO, Doppler, angio
	HTN	None to SOB	BP measurement	ECG for LVH, ECHO, radionuclides for diastolic function
ENDO	Diabetes (see in Diseases section)	Medical Rx, autonomic dysfunction: gastroparesis, etc.	BP lying, standing	Glucose BUN/Cr
HEME	Bleeding diathesis	Bleeding, bruising	Ecchymosis	PT, PTT, Plt(s)

Key Reference: O'Connor JP, Ramsay JG, Wynands JE, Kaplan JA: Anesthesia for myocardial revascularization. *In* Kaplan JA (ed): Cardiac Anesthesia, 3rd ed. Philadelphia, WB Saunders, 1993, pp 587–628.

INTRAOPERATIVE MANAGEMENT

Preoperative Preparation

- Maintain all preop meds, including IV heparin

Anesthetic Technique

- Narcotics, relaxants, amnesics in patients with poor physical condition
- Hypnotics, volatile agents, ↓ narcotic doses in patients with good physical condition

Monitoring

- Multilead ECG for detection of ischemia
- Invasive arterial pressure in all patients because of nonpulsatile CPB flow
- Central venous access for assessment of CVP, drug administration
- Activated clotting or heparin levels to assess adequate coag paralysis, reversal with protamine
- PA cath and/or TEE if ↓ LV function, high risk of intraop ischemia, or associated cardiac disease (e.g., ischemic mitral regurgitation)

Induction

- Minimize imbalance between myocardial O_2 supply, demand
- Avoid intraoperative awareness

SURGICAL STAGES

Skin Incision

- Large, midline chest incision

Graft Dissection

- During dissection of internal mammary art, potential for occlusion of an ipsilateral radial artery line

Heart Cannulation

- Cannulation of aorta associated with HTN, ischemia, emboli
- Cannulation of right atrium with arrhythmias

Cardiopulmonary Bypass (CPB)

- Concerns are:
  - Potential for awareness
  - Management of acid-base status to optimize cerebral perfusion
  - Management of anticoagulation
  - Management of perfusion press flow
  - Temperature control

Termination of CPB

- Inotropes, vasoactive agents, IABP may be needed to optimize ventricular function
- Post-CPB ventricular function determined by preop ventricular function, myocardial protection during CPB, completeness of revascularization; mech assist devices (e.g., IABP) will often be used

Postoperative Consideration

- Less severe than after other chest incisions
- Use of regional analgesic techniques (spinal or epidural) not widespread due to potential for complications with heparinization

ANTICIPATED PROBLEMS/CONCERNS

- Presence of myocardial ischemia, MI suggests incomplete revascularization or inadequate protection during CPB
- In reoperations, antifibrinolytics, aprotinin, other drugs that influence coagulation under intense evaluation

CRANIOTOMY

Robert McPherson, M.D.

RISK

- Head trauma
- Intracranial tumors
- Vascular lesions

PERIOPERATIVE RISKS

- Periop risk of poor CNS outcome highly depends on disease process
- Underlying risk in all processes is hypoperfusion of neural tissue

WORRY ABOUT

- Perfusion pressure = inflow pressure (usually MAP) less outflow resistance (can be ICP, cerebral venous pressure, or tissue pressure caused by tumor or brain retractor)
- Blood gases: avoid hypoxia, hypercapnea (even mild)

OVERVIEW

- Craniotomies performed for variety of lesions, both space-occupying and vascular
- Nervous system accommodates well to chronic processes, even mild CNS Sx indicate exhaustion of compensatory mechanisms in patients with chronic diseases
- Decompensation can occur from ↑ ICP, hypoxia, hypercapnia, ↓ venous return or ↓ MAP

ICD-9-CM Code: 239.6 (Brain tumor)

ETIOLOGY

- Brain tumor: benign, malignant
- Vascular lesion, aneurysm, AVM, HTN, hemorrhage
- Head trauma, epidural hematoma, subdural hematoma

INDICATIONS AND USUAL TREATMENT

- Debulking of malignant tumors
- Complete removal of benign lesions
- Ablation of aneurysm
- Ablation, removal of AVM

ASSESSMENT POINTS

SYSTEM	EFFECT	ASSESSMENT BY HX	PE	TEST
CV	Head injury, Intracranial HTN, subarachnoid hemorrhage, ECG/changes	?Hx of CV disease	Peak acid output usually within normal limits	PA cath ECHO
RESP	Brain stem pressure causes apnea	Cushing's response	Pupils dilate	
GI	Arterial bleed 2° to steroids	Hx of steroid use	Blood in stool, gastric ulcer	
CNS	Change in consciousness	Acute vs. chronic	Depends on location	MRI

PERIOPERATIVE IMPLICATIONS

Preoperative Preparation

- Emergency/trauma: maintain MAP
  —control airway to prevent hypoxia/hypercapnia
  —if Cushing's response present, do not let MABP ↑ until hyperventilation established

Elective

- Preop steroids
  – preop diuretics (mannitol, Lasix)
- Evaluation for midline shifts
  —indicates ↑ sensitivity to ↓ MABP

Monitoring

- Pupillary responses
- Hemodynamic response (Cushing's response)
- Invasive art pressure
- Consider CVP/PA catheter, depending on surg procedure
- UO
- EEG/EPs
  – establish ASAP
  – IV agents usually not very depressant
  – volatile anesthetic gases, N_2O depressants

Airway

- Trauma victims may have associated neck injury

Preinduction/Induction

- Avoid premedication
- IV induction with barbiturate, narcotics
- Support with phenylephrine

Maintenance

- Support until any compression relieved
- Low-dose volatile agent
- ± N_2O (may interfere with EP monitoring if waves small)
- Preincision mannitol (0.5–1.0 g/kg)
- Hyperventilation to $PaCO_2$ until beginning of dural closure

Extubation

- Prompt awaking important
- If level of arousal less than anticipated, immediate study (CT scan, MRI) frequently indicated
- Patient with posterior fossa surg may have loss of airway reflexes despite ability to respond to commands

CRANIOTOMY — SITTING POSITION

Thomas J. Toung, M.D.

RISK

- Patients with infratentorial tumors (pineal, floor of 4th ventricle, pontomedullary junction, vermis, cerebellopontine angle)
- Trend ↓, but still used in 50% of US institutions

PERIOPERATIVE RISKS

- Periop mortality rare (<1%)
- Venous and/or paradoxical air embolism
- Pneumocephalus
- Airway swelling, cervical spinal cord ischemia
- Macroglossia

WORRY ABOUT

- Subdural hematoma due to major brain shift (excessive CSF drainage)
- Venous and/or paradoxical air embolism
- Brainstem, lower cranial nerve injury
- Poor cerebral venous drainage with acute flexion of head on neck

OVERVIEW

- Acoustic neuroma most common infratentorial tumor in adults
- 2 mmHg reduction in cerebral BP with every inch of elevation above heart
- Head, neck markedly flexed for better exposure
- Operation is performed around brainstem centers vital to respiration and circulation
- N_2O avoided during closure of dura
- Muscle relaxant avoided by some because of facial nerve monitoring; when used, 2–3 twitches of train-of-four usually maintained

ICD-9-CM Code: 239.6 (Brain tumor)

INDICATIONS/USUAL TREATMENT

- Supracerebellar infratentorial approaches to pineal region, midline/4th ventricular lesions, cerebellopontine angle
- Following conditions beneficial:
  - Good general health; no known cardiac instability or patent foramen ovale; no existing ventriculoatrial shunt; no hydrocephalus; no autonomic dysfunction
- With coexisting disease, use alternative positions: prone, park bench

ASSESSMENT POINTS

SYSTEM	EFFECT	ASSESSMENT OF HX	PE	TEST
HEENT	Dysphagia, facial paralysis	Choking, hoarseness	ENT exam	CineXR
CV	Patent foramen ovale predisposes to paradoxical air embolism	Easy fatigability	Auscultation	CXR Cardiac cath
RESP	Aspiration	Coughing	Auscultation	CXR
CNS	Ventriculoatrial shunt predisposes to shunt surgery Venous air embolism Hydrocephalus to tension pneumocephalus		CNS exam	Head CT scan

Key Reference: Majasko J, Petrozza P, Cohen M, et al: Anesthesia and surgery in the seated position: analysis of 554 cases. Neurosurgery 1985; 17:695–702.

PERIOPERATIVE IMPLICATIONS

Preoperative Preparation

- Antishock trouser (MAST suit)
- Precordial Doppler
- Multiorificed RA catheter
- Adequate hydration

Anesthetic Technique

- General with controlled ventilation

Monitoring

- Arterial catheter
- PA catheter can provide useful information
- End tidal CO_2
- Precordial Doppler or TEE

Airway

- ETT may be kinked by acute flexion of neck
- Allow at least 2 fingerbreadths between chin, sternum

Induction/Maintenance

- Isoflurane-N_2O-low-dose fentanyl most common technique
- Use of long-acting NMB limited if facial nerve function monitored

SURGICAL STAGES

Dissection

- Sudden onset of tachycardia/bradycardia, PVCs, hypotension

Definitive Surgery

- Except for extra-axial lesions in cerebellopontine angle, surgery for pathological Dx, and/or to reduce mass effect
- Blood loss usually not significant
- Chemo/radiation Rx

Postoperative Considerations

- Pain score: 0–5
- Minimize coughing, straining on ETT
- Cranial nerve dysfunction
- Extubation determined by extent of surgery
- Postop HTN possibly caused by brainstem compression

ANTICIPATED PROBLEMS/CONCERNS

- CV complications resulting from venous air embolism
- Tension pneumocephalus
- Cranial nerve paresis
- Macroglossia
- Failure to awaken from anesthesia: ? brainstem or subdural hematoma

ECMO (EXTRACORPOREAL MEMBRANE OXYGENATION)

Brent A. Graham, M.D.

RISK

• Primarily used in newborns for reversible respiratory failure.
• The most common causes of respiratory failure requiring ECMO include meconium aspiration syndrome, respiratory distress syndrome, congenital diaphragmatic hernia, and persistent pulmonary hypertension of the newborn.

PERIOPERATIVE RISKS

• Depends upon the underlying condition. Survival rate with congenital diaphragmatic hernia was 61.6%; with meconium aspiration syndrome, 92.7%.
• Overall survival rate for 3876 patients was 82.5%.
• Mortality rate high without ECMO.

WORRY ABOUT

• Cause of respiratory failure
• Persistent pulmonary hypertension of the newborn
• Intracranial hemorrhage

OVERVIEW

• Provides total respiratory support with venovenous and venoarterial bypass
• Venoarterial bypass also provides total hemodynamic support.
• Patient is anticoagulated to maintain an activated clotting time (ACT) of ~200 seconds.

ICD-9-CM Code: 756.6 (Congenital diaphragmatic hernia)
RDS: 769

INDICATIONS AND USUAL TREATMENT

• Criteria vary between institutions.
• Contraindications: congenital abnormalities not compatible with meaningful life, profound neurologic impairment, irreversible lung disease, or prolonged ventilatory support (>7–10 d).
• Relative contraindications: estimated gestational age <35 wk or evidence of intracranial hemorrhage.

ASSESSMENT POINTS

SYSTEM	EFFECT	ASSESSMENT BY HX	PE	TEST
CV	Persistent pulmonary hypertension of the newborn	Hypoxemia, acidosis Right to left shunting through PDA and foramen ovale	CV exam	ABG ECHO
NEURO	Hemorrhage	Intracranial hemorrhage	Neuro exam	Cranial US

Key Reference: Bartlett RH: Extracorporeal life support for cardiopulmonary failure. Curr Prob Surg 1990; 27:667–677.

INTRAOPERATIVE MANAGEMENT

Monitoring

• IV lines must be free of air.
• Umbilical artery and venous line are frequently in place.
• Patients with a patent ductus arteriosus can have different preductal (right arm) and postductal (lower body) oxygen saturations.

SURGICAL STAGES

Anesthetic Choice

• Performed in ICU with local infiltration, supplemented with narcotics and muscle relaxants.

Initiating ECMO

• Right internal jugular vein (RIJ) is used for venovenous bypass.
• Venoarterial bypass utilizes RIJ and right common carotid artery.
• Heparin is given (100–150 units/kg).
• The vessels are ligated distally and cannulated proximally.
• Bypass is initiated slowly by increasing extracorporeal flow rate.
• After reaching full flow rates, ventilator settings are decreased to nontraumatic settings.

ECMO MANAGEMENT

• Heparin is given to maintain an ACT of 200 seconds. If there is bleeding the ACT is lowered to 180 seconds.
• Platelets are transfused to maintain a count of 100,000/mm^3.
• Hct kept between 40–50%.
• As pulmonary function improves, the pump flow is decreased. Prior to decannulation the patient is given a trial off ECMO.
• After decannulation the vessels are ligated proximally.

ANTICIPATED PROBLEMS/CONCERNS

• Hypoxia and hemodynamic instability prior to bypass.
• Bleeding associated with anticoagulation.
• Renal insufficiency may be treated with dialysis or ultrafiltration.
• Mechanical problems.

ELECTROCONVULSIVE THERAPY (ECT)

Laurel E. Moore M.D.

RISK

- Prevalence of major depression: 3.2% of males, 4.5–9.3% of females
- 4% of all psychiatric admissions are for ECT

PERIOPERATIVE RISKS

- Perioperative mortality rare
- Dysrhythmias, HTN common

WORRY ABOUT

- Sympathetic stimulation producing myocardial ischemia
- Risk of dysrhythmia as result of parasympathetic, sympathetic stimulation
- Confusion, short-term memory loss from Rx
- Adequate medical Hx frequently difficult to obtain

OVERVIEW

- Induced seizures produce multiple neuroendocrine changes (↑ ACTH, cortisol, epinephrine, norepinephrine) effective in Rx of depression; but exact mechanism unclear

- Seizure time may be related to clinical response: <25–<120 sec/Rx; patients undergo ~6–10 ECT Rx (200–1000 sec of cumulative seizure time).
- Seizure induces sympathetic response, ↑ myocardial O_2 requirements in elderly
- Use of antidepressants complicates anesthesia management:
  – TCAs block reuptake of serotonin, norepinephrine, causing acute release, depleting central adrenergic stores, causing unpredictable response to indirect-acting sympathomimetics. Direct-acting sympathomimetics may cause exaggerated response; most TCAs have anticholinergic effects.
- MAOIs form irreversible complex with MAO, preventing breakdown of intraneuronal norepinephrine, serotonin, dopamine; use of an indirect-acting sympathomimetic can produce HTN crisis; direct-acting agents may also produce exaggerated response.
- Lithium may prolong effects of depolarizing, certain nondepolarizing relaxants, sedatives (barbiturates). It may also ↑ incidence of confusion, memory loss from ECT; is generally discontinued before ECT.

ICD-9–CM Codes: 296.2 (Major depression, single episode); 296.3 (Major depression, recurrent episode); 311 (Depressive disorder, not elsewhere classified)

INDICATIONS AND USUAL TREATMENT

- Clinical indications:
  – failure to respond to conventional pharmacologic Rx
  – medical contraindication to pharmacologic Rx (e.g., cardiac conduction defect)
  – profound depression if delay in Rx places patient at unacceptable risk for suicide
  – controversial indications include forms of schizophrenia, mania, eating disorders, catatonia
- Relative contraindications include intracranial space–occupying lesion, recent MI, recent CVA, pheochromocytoma, long-bone fractures, pregnancy
- Alternative therapies include use of antidepressants, psychotherapy

ASSESSMENT POINTS

SYSTEM	EFFECT	ASSESSMENT BY HX	PE	TEST
CV	CAD	Angina, prior MI		ECG as indicated
	↓ LV function	↓ Exercise tolerance	Enlarged heart	ECG/ECHO
		PND, orthopnea,	JVD	as indicated
	Conduction defect	syncope or near-syncope	Rales	Holter as indicated
			? Rhythm	
GI	GE reflux	Reflux Sx		
MS	Fracture or vertebral collapse	Pain or trauma	Palpation	X-ray of back
NS	Confusion/delirium	?Clear prior to ECT	CNS exam	Routine work-up for change in MS
PSYCHIATRIC	Competent for consent			Determined by psychiatric exam

Key Reference: Selvin BL: Electroconvulsive therapy—1987. Anesthesiology 1987; 67:367–385.

ANESTHETIC MANAGEMENT

Monitoring

- Routine
- EEG to determine adequacy, duration of seizure
- In high-risk patients consider invasive monitoring, esp for 1st few Rx

Induction/Maintenance

- GA, usually by mask
- IV induction with methohexital (↓ seizure threshold, rapid awakening), thiopental (↑ seizure threshold, delayed awakening), or propofol (↓ seizure duration, rapid awakening)
- Muscle relaxation achieved with small dose of succinylcholine (0.5 mg/kg) to ↓ potential for injury from seizure

- Hyperventilation with 100% O_2 by mask before stimulus ↓ seizure threshold, possibly prolongs seizure
- Stimulus produces initial parasympathetic stimulation assoc with bradycardia, hypotension; asystole possible
- Subsequent sympathetic stimulation assoc with ↑ HR, ↑ BP, ↑ CO, ↑ myocardial O_2 consumption
- Other physiol effects include ↑ $CMRO_2$, ↑ CBF, ↑ ICP, ↑ intragastric pres, ↑ IOP
- Vasodilators (sodium nitroprusside, nitroglycerin) and β rb, esmolol effective
- Bradycardias rarely require Rx

ECT Management

- Waveform, frequency, duration of stimulus adjusted to produce desired seizure
- Bilat Rx, prolonged seizure associated with ↑ memory loss

- Place, inflate BP cuff on extremity before succinylcholine admin to monitor seizure
- Seizures ideally 25–120 seconds but controversial whether clinical efficacy related to seizure duration
- Patients may complain of headache or myalgias post-ECT

ANTICIPATED PROBLEMS/CONCERNS

- Elderly patient in whom thorough preop interview difficult if not impossible
- Repetitive short anesthetics require efficient system to record medical Hx, allergies, drug dosages, complications, etc
- Rx produces sympathetic activation in patient population deemed medically unfit to tolerate conventional pharmacologic Rx

ENDOSCOPIC SINUS SURGERY (ESS)

Daniel Chou, M.D.
Michael Peck, M.D.

RISK

- Common procedure
- M:F ratio of 1:1

PERIOPERATIVE RISKS

- 1.1% incidence of major complications including orbital hematoma, blindness, diplopia, CSF leak, CNS infection, stroke, carotid arterial injury, death
- 5.4% incidence of minor complications including periorbital emphysema, ecchymosis, lip pain or numbness, bronchospasm, epistaxis

WORRY ABOUT

- Asthma control preop
- Bronchospasm
- Aspiration of blood, secretion
- Blood vessel injury/bleeding
- Postop N/V

OVERVIEW

- Procedure aims to eliminate chronic infection of sinuses, allowing aeration, restoring mucociliary flow, clearance
- Major complications may result from:
  - perforation of ethmoid sinus roof
  - dehiscence or breaking of lamina papyracea
  - injury to optic nerve or carotid artery during sphenoidectomy
- Advantage of MAC:
  - possibility of early discharge
  - maintain sensation of orbit, base of skull as warning signals
  - ↓ Blood loss

ICD-9-CM Code: 473.9 (Chronic sinusitis)

INDICATIONS AND USUAL TREATMENT

- Recurrent sinusitis refractory to medical Rx
- Chronic hyperplastic sinusitis with obstructive nasal polyposis
- Chronic sinusitis with mucocele formation except frontal sinus mucocele (laterally placed)
- Fungal sinusitis in immunocompromised patients including diabetics; Dx of neoplasm, orbital cellulitis (abscess unresponsive to medical Rx)
- Usual medical treatments
  - identify and control the suspected allergen
  - steroid
  - antihistamine
  - antibiotics
  - decongestant

ASSESSMENT POINTS

SYSTEM	EFFECT	ASSESSMENT BY HX	PE	TEST
HEENT	Postnasal drip	Cough/aspiration in A.M.	Airway	Direct laryngoscopy
CV	Impairment due to age Toxicity from medication (e.g., theophylline)	SOB; exercise tolerance Hx of chest pain, palpitation	CV	Theophylline level ECG
RESP	40–50% of patients with Hx of asthma, 30% with multiple allergy Laryngotracheal bronchitis from chronic drip	Wheezing, allergen, systemic steroid Hx of intubation Hx of hospitalization, ER visit Voice strength and hormone history	Chest; listen to voice	Spirometry
GI	Theophylline toxicity	NVD, epigastric pain		Theophylline level
CNS	Rule out meningitis from sinusitis	Headache, fever, N/V, double/blurred vision, mental status change	Neuro	Spinal tap
	Theophylline effect	Headache, irritability, reflex hyperexcitability, muscle twitching, convulsion		Theophylline level

Key Reference: Levin HL, May M: Endoscopic Sinus Surgery. Thieme Medical Publishers, New York, 1993.

PERIOPERATIVE MANAGEMENT

Preoperative Preparation

- Continue bronchodilator, antihypertensive medication
- Consider stress steroid
- Cocaine-soaked pledgets before lidocaine and epinephrine injury

Anesthetic Technique

- MAC or general ET anesthesia
- Supine position with shoulder roll, head extended

Monitoring

- Routine

Airway

- Oropharyngeal packing before surgery; removal after extubation

Induction/Maintenance

- Ketamine may potentiate effects of cocaine, epinephrine
- Avoid histamine-releasing medications
- Achieve deep anesthesia before intubation to prevent bronchospasm
- Controlled normotension to avoid excessive blood loss

Surgical Stages

- Lidocaine, epinephrine injection may cause arrhythmia, tachycardia, HTN
- Nasal septoplasty may be needed to gain access to osteomeatal complex
- Orbit palpated to prevent injury to orbit from maxillary sinus ostium seeker
- Roof of ethmoid sinus may be perforated when mucosa removed from posterior ethmoid cell
- Lamina papyracea may be breached during exposure
- Sphenoidotomy associated with injury to brain, optic nerve, carotid artery

Closure and Postoperative Considerations

- Nasal packing placed after surgery
- Remove oropharynx packing; suction oropharynx, stomach before extubation
- EBL: 100 ml
- Pain score: 4–5
- Oral opiates, NSAIDs

ESOPHAGECTOMY

RISK

Esophageal Carcinoma

• Squamous cell more common among African-Americans, M (3:1), tobacco abusers (4:1), alcohol abusers (6:1), Hx of achalasia, caustic burns to esophagus, Paterson-Kelly syndrome (iron-deficiency anemia, esophageal webs, glossitis)
• Adenocarcinoma more common among M; associated with Barrett's esophagus

PERIOPERATIVE RISKS

• Operative mortality less than 5%.
• Periop complication rate of 10–27% including anastomotic disruption (leading to sepsis), pulmonary insufficiency, delayed emptying of intrathoracic stomach, diaphragmatic herniation of abdominal viscera, chylothorax, massive aspiration, pancreatitis, delayed splenic rupture.

WORRY ABOUT

• Aspiration risk
• Hemodynamic effects of blunt dissection
• Consequences of N_2O technique if colonic interposition performed
• Recurrent laryngeal nerve injury if cervical anastomosis performed
• Consequences of perioperative TPN (hypoglycemia, $\uparrow CO_2$ production)

OVERVIEW

• Midline laparotomy to explore for metastases
• Mobilization of stomach (Kocher's maneuver), pyloromyotomy
• Mobilization of esophagus: depends on site of lesion, surgeon's preference; may occur via transhiatal approach, right (Ivor-Lewis) or left thoracotomy
• Reconstruction: stomach is preferred conduit, but colon or jejunum may be used
• Endoscopic resection still experimental

ICD-9-CM Code: 150.9 (Esophageal carcinoma)

INDICATIONS AND USUAL TREATMENT

• Surgery only curative treatment (5-y survival as high as 70% if limited to stage I disease)
• At presentation disease is usually advanced with overall 5-y survival of only 10–15%
• Palliative Rx includes chemotherapy, combined chemo-radiation, or radiation alone
• Postop chemotherapy has not resulted in improved survival
• Preop (neoadjuvant) chemotherapy with irradiation may downstage tumors before resection; role in possible improved survival not clearly established

ASSESSMENT POINTS

SYSTEM	EFFECT	ASSESSMENT BY HX	PE	TEST
HEENT	Aspiration risk, esophagorespiratory fistula	Dysphagia, heartburn, N/V		Barium swallow
	Tracheal compression			CT, flow loops
CV	Chemotherapy-induced cardiomyopathy	DOE, PND, orthopnea, exercise tolerance	Auscultation JVD, edema, hepatojugular reflex	CXR, ECHO, MUGA
RESP	Chronic aspiration	Wheezing, dyspnea	Auscultation	CXR, spirometry
GI	Malnutrition	Wt loss, fatigue	Cachexia	Serum protein Albumin, pre-albumin
Renal	Dehydration Electrolyte wasting Renal failure (nephrotoxic chemotherapy)		Orthostatic VS	BUN/Cr Serum electrolytes
Hematologic	Anemia Impaired immune function			CBC

Key Reference: Livstone EM: General considerations of tumors of the esophagus. *In* Bockus JE (ed): Bockus Gastroenterology, 4th ed. Philadelphia, WB Saunders, 1985, pp 818–840.

PERIOPERATIVE MANAGEMENT

Anesthetic Technique

• General or combined technique
• If transhiatal or left thoracotomy approach, single-lumen ETT is adequate. Right thoracotomy approach requires placement of a double-lumen tube or bronchial blocker.

Monitoring

• Large-bore intravenous access
• Consider arterial catheter
• Consider central venous catheter

Airway

• Full stomach precautions
• Possibility of tracheal compression if significant mediastinal lymphadenopathy
• Possible esophagorespiratory fistula (may need to maintain spontaneous ventilation)

Induction

• Potential for significant hypotension if dehydrated
• If esophagorespiratory fistulae: avoid positive pressure ventilation, vent stomach if necessary, isolate fistula with appropriate double-lumen ETT

SURGICAL STAGES

Dissection

• Initial laparotomy
• Depending on approach may have right or left thoracotomy
• Cervical incision if cervical anastomosis to be performed (necessary with transhiatal approach)

Definitive Surgery

• Blunt dissection during transhiatal approach may result in compression of vena cava or heart with resultant hypotension or dysrhythmias
• Impaired gas exchange may occur during 1-lung ventilation if required
• EBL: ~2L

Postoperative Considerations

• High perioperative mortality due to cardiorespiratory complications, sepsis
• Significant postop pain, espcially with approaches employing thoracotomy
• Pain management may include IV PCA, epidural PCA, epidural and subarachnoid narcotics, intrapleural techniques
• High likelihood of disruption of cervical anastomosis if reintubation required immediately postop; consider delayed extubation of selected high-risk patients

ANTICIPATED PROBLEMS/CONCERNS

• Possibility for unrecognized pneumothorax with transhiatal approach

ESWL (EXTRACORPOREAL SHOCK WAVE LITHOTRIPSY)

Christopher D. Beatie, M.D.

RISK

- Incidence of urolithiasis: 1.5/1000

PERIOPERATIVE RISKS

- Shock waves can trigger cardiac dysrhythmias if not delivered during ventricular refractory period
- Shock waves can damage kidney resulting in renal hematoma, parenchymal injury with loss of renal function, hematuria, new onset HTN
- Shock waves can cause pancreatic, hepatic injury resulting in elevations in amylase, lipase, bilirubin, lactic dehydrogenase, transaminases, CK; changes are usually mild, transient
- Hemodynamic changes associated with immersion in water bath may precipitate myocardial ischemia, MI in high-risk patients

WORRY ABOUT

- Cardiac dysrhythmias
- Cardiopulmonary derangements resulting from immersion
- Electrical safety
- Renal insufficiency
- Platelet dysfunction

OVERVIEW

- Shock waves propagated through body to pulverize urinary stones. Older lithotriptors require immersion in water bath, which complicates monitoring, airway management; regional (usually epidural) anesthesia preferred for procedures in these machines. Immersion also induces changes in cardiac/pulmonary physiology, which may be detrimental to patients with concurrent cardiac and/or pulmonary disease
- Newer, 2nd-generation (dry) lithotriptors eliminate these problems, generate less powerful shock waves, so lighter planes of anesthesia or sedation combined with topical anesthesia may be effective
- Newest (3rd-generation) lithotriptors use piezoelectric crystals, are essentially painless; may also be used to pulverize gallstones

ICD-9-CM Codes: 592.0 (kidney stones); 592.1 (ureteral stones); 592.9 (urinary stones)

INDICATIONS AND USUAL TREATMENT

- Rx of choice for upper urinary tract stones. Contraindicated in presence of morbid obesity, pacemakers, pregnancy, coagulopathy; in patients with orthopedic implants in lumbar/pelvic areas, those with intra-abd calcific processes—e.g., AAAs
- Urolithiasis may also be Rx by adjustments in urinary pH using weak bases such as sodium bicarbonate or weak acids such as ammonium chloride
- Urinary stones can be extremely painful; Patients may be taking variety of analgesic drugs including NSAIDs, opioids

ASSESSMENT POINTS

SYSTEM	EFFECT	HX ASSESSMENT	PE	TEST
GI	Delayed gastric emptying, gastritis, PUD	Reflux Sx, dyspepsia, abdominal pain		Hgb, endoscopy, upper GI x-ray Stool heme
HEME	Anemia (due to renal failure, GI losses)	Fatigue	Pallor	Hct
	Platelet dysfunction (due to analgesia or uremia)	Bruising, bleeding	Ecchymoses, petechiae	Bleeding time
GU	Obstructive uropathy, analgesic nephritis	Oliguria, anuria, CHF Sx	Rales, edema	BUN/Cr UA, CXR

Key Reference: London RA, et al: Immersion anesthesia for extracorporeal shock wave lithotripsy. Review of two hundred twenty treatments. Urology 1986; 28:86–94.

INTRAOPERATIVE MANAGEMENT

Preoperative Preparation

- Evaluate renal function
- Evaluate platelet function
- R/O anemia

Anesthetic Technique

- Regional anesthesia usually preferred for immersion-type lithotriptors
- Platelet dysfunction may influence decision to use regional anesthesia
- If GA used, small TV should be used to keep stone at focal point of shock wave
- Patient position in gantry requires care to avoid peripheral nerve damage
- Local anesthesia, topical anesthesia (e.g., Emla) and/or IV sedation may be used with newer (dry) lithotriptors

Monitoring

- Easier if patient's arms not immersed
- Cover ECG leads with waterproof tape; usually lead placed on each shoulder with 3rd on left arm or high on chest wall
- If BP cuff to be immersed, use clip-type cuff (Velcro will not work)
- Pulse oximetry probes may be placed on ear or nose if fingers immersed

Airway

- Intubation or LMA indicated for GA if immersion required

Induction/Maintenance

- T4–6 level required for regional block
- Cover epidural cath with waterproof dressing; avoid air bubbles under dressing and foam tapes (attenuate shock wave energy)
- Euthermic water bath to prevent hyperthermia or hypothermia/shivering
- 1000–4000 shocks/Rx
- Since shock waves synchronized to ECG, bradycardia can prolong Rx
- HR higher than lithotriptor's max firing rate also prolongs Rx by forcing shock waves to be triggered by every other QRS complex

EBL/Volume Concerns

- Effects of immersion in water bath
  - ↑ venous return due to hydrostatic pressure, resulting in ↑ CO
  - afterload, FRC, TV ↓
  - ↓ renin, ADH secretion result in diuresis, kaliuresis, natriuresis
- Hypotension possible on emergence from water bath
- Diuretics, hydration may be used to encourage passage of stone fragments

Postoperative Considerations

- Pain scale: 1–3; NSAIDs usually sufficient
- Hematuria frequent postop—usually resolves spontaneously over several d

ANTICIPATED PROBLEMS/CONCERNS

- Lithotripsy suite often noisy, dimly lit: use caution to maintain adequate monitoring, patient safety

EYE ENUCLEATION

Nader El-Gamal, M.D.

RISK

- 7,000–10,000 operations/y in USA
- Racial predominance: none
- More common in older age group, males

PERIOPERATIVE RISKS

- Morbidity, mortality 0.1%, mortality rate related to patient's other diseases
- Oculocardiac reflex may result in bradycardia, asystole

WORRY ABOUT

- Other associated diseases of patient (DM, HTN)
- Postop N/V, pain

OVERVIEW

- Age, comorbidity of patient
- Age of patient varies with disease of eye but common in older group

INDICATIONS

- Tumor (melanoma, retinoblastoma)
- Blind painful eye
- Trauma

ASSESSMENT POINTS

SYSTEM	EFFECT	ASSESSMENT BY HX	PE	TEST
HEENT		Snoring	Airway exam	
CV	Associated diseases			
RESP	Co-existing diseases	SOB, exercise tolerance		O_2 sat

Key Reference: Blanc VF, Hardy J-F, Milot J, Jacob J-L: The oculocardiac reflex: A statistical analysis in children. Can J Anaesth 1983; 30:360.

INTRAOPERATIVE MANAGEMENT

Anesthetic Technique
- General anesthesia

Monitoring
- Routine

SURGICAL STAGES

Induction/Dissection
- ECG monitoring for oculocardiac reflex during dissection of eye muscles
- Deep level of anesthesia needed during dissecting, cutting optic nerve
- Recovery/extubation: avoid bucking, coughing which leads to venous congestion, bleeding (fentanyl, lidocaine, deep extubation an option)

Postoperative Considerations
- Postop N/V, pain
- Psychologic issues
- Pain score: 3–5

ANTICIPATED PROBLEMS/CONCERNS

- Bradycardia, asystole: treat by stopping surgical stimulation with atropine; lidocaine to nerve beforehand
- Postop N/V

PROCEDURES **385**

GAS EMBOLISM

Richard E. Moon, M.D.
Bryant W. Stolp, M.D., Ph.D.

RISK

- Accidental injection of gas into a blood vessel during diagnostic or therapeutic procedures: cardiopulmonary bypass, cardiac catheterization, angiography, hemodialysis, pressurization of an IV bottle using air
- Entrainment of air into a vein during surgical procedures in which venous pressure at the wound site is subatmospheric (wound higher than heart): sitting craniotomy, spine surgery, total hip replacement, dental implant surgery, C-section
- Surgery in which gas is injected into tissues: intrauterine laser surgery, laparoscopy, arthroscopy
- Other forceful instillation of air into tissues: injury due to industrial compressed air, blowing air intravaginally during oral sex in pregnancy
- Pulmonary overexpansion, in which gas enters the pulmonary capillaries: breath-holding or regional gas-trapping during ascent from a scuba dive, positive pressure ventilation

PERIOPERATIVE RISKS

- Gas in blood vessels or tissues can expand if N_2O used to 2–4 times its original volume

$$\frac{V_{new}}{V_{old}} = \frac{1}{1-F_{N_2O}}$$

compounding the original injury.

WORRY ABOUT

- Stroke
- Myocardial infarction
- Pulmonary edema

OVERVIEW/ETIOLOGY

- Immediate effect: obstruction of blood flow and tissue ischemia; pulm HTN if venous gas
- Secondary: increased permeability of vascular endothelium, tissue edema (pulm edema from venous gas)
- Tertiary effect: leukocyte accumulation on vascular endothelium, resulting in release of mediators and late reduction in blood flow
- While small venous gas emboli are prevented by the pulm capillary network from entering the arterial circulation, large volumes of gas can exceed its filtration capacity. Air can also enter the left heart via intracardiac R→L shunts.
- Venous gas embolism can cause sudden hypotension, hypoxemia, pulm HTN, or cardiac arrest. Awake individuals may experience dyspnea, tachypnea, or cough.
- Arterial gas embolism is manifested by altered consciousness, acute onset of focal neurologic deficit, arrhythmias, and ST segment elevation or depression
- Venous gas embolism is suggested by a sudden change in cardiac sounds on precordial Doppler monitor or abrupt reduction in end-tidal CO_2. If inspired gas contains no air, venous gas emboli may manifest as nitrogen in expired gas, detectable by mass spectrometer or Raman gas analyzer. Bubbles can be detected using transthoracic or transesophageal ECHO and transcranial Doppler.
- Rarely, a "mill-wheel" murmur (a "whoosh" in both systole and diastole) can be heard by precordial stethoscope.

ICD-9-CM Codes: 958.0; 999.1

USUAL TREATMENT

- If possible, prevent further ingress of gas
- If surgical gas embolism:
  - Flood surgical field with fluid
  - Lower surgical site with respect to heart
  - Elevate venous pressure (application of PEEP may augment R→L shunt if patient has an intracardiac defect, e.g., patent foramen ovale)
- 100% inspired O_2 to enhance oxygenation of ischemic tissues and increase nitrogen diffusion gradient from bubble into blood
- IV fluid administration to maintain intravascular volume
- Hyperbaric O_2 to effect reduction in size and rapid resolution of bubbles. Hyperbaric O_2 may inhibit endothelial leukocyte adherence. Immediate recompression treatment is most efficacious; delayed treatment can also be effective.

ASSESSMENT POINTS

SYSTEM	EFFECT	ASSESSMENT BY HX	PE	TEST
CV	Filling of cardiac chambers with air		Hypotension Mill-wheel murmur	ECG, ECHO, precordial Doppler, $ETCO_2$, ETN_2, Brain CT
	↑ Permeability of vascular endothelium Tissue edema		↑ Third-space fluid requirement cerebral edema	
RESP	Pulm HTN Pulm edema	Dyspnea Tachypnea Cough	↑ P_2 heart sound Crepitations on auscultation of chest	PA pressure CXR
CNS	Arterial gas embolism or transpulmonary/transcardiac passage of venous gas emboli	Mental status Acute onset of focal neurologic deficits	Neuro exam	

Key Reference: Moon RE, Camporesi EM: Clinical care at altered environmental pressure. *In* Miller RD (ed): Anesthesia. New York, Churchill Livingstone, 1994, pp 2277–2305.

PERIOPERATIVE IMPLICATIONS

- Consider in patients at high risk for venous gas embolism: Direct arterial pressure monitoring, precordial Doppler or continuous mass spectrometry (ETN_2 and $ETCO_2$), TEE
- If gas embolization occurs, immediately discontinue N_2O
- Avoid N_2O in individuals requiring surgery who have recently suffered gas embolism due to scuba diving or decompression sickness (in situ gas formation due to nitrogen supersaturation)

GASTRECTOMY

RISK

- Incidence of gastric cancer in USA: 8/100,000
- Male predominance (3:1)
- ↓ Incidence secondary to ↓ incidence of gastric cancer, and to medical Rx of Zollinger-Ellison syndrome

PERIOPERATIVE RISKS

- Mortality in hospital from 0–11.7% for early cancer to 25% for advanced cancer at esophagogastric junction
- Pulmonary complication: 15%
- High mortality, complication rate result from poor nutritional status of patient

WORRY ABOUT

- Malnutrition (see Diseases section)
- Anemia
- Perioperative hypovolemia
- Large 3rd space losses

OVERVIEW

- Resection of all or part of stomach for malignant or benign conditions is common
- Periop hypovolemia from N/V, diarrhea or GI bleeding
- Anemia may be masked by dehydration
- Regional anesthesia as an adjuvant to GA, postop epidural analgesia offers potential benefits in pulmonary mechanics, ↓ periop catabolism, effects of stress on immune system

ICD-9-CM Codes: 151.9 (Gastric cancer); 531 (Gastric ulcer)

INDICATIONS AND USUAL TREATMENT

- Total gastrectomy
  - gastric cancer
  - hemorrhagic gastritis
  - Zollinger-Ellison syndrome; medical management more common using H_2 blocker, misoprostol
- Partial gastrectomy
  - gastric cancer
  - gastric ulcers

ASSESSMENT POINTS

SYSTEM	EFFECT	ASSESSMENT BY HX	PE	TEST
CV	Hypovolemia	N/V, diarrhea Poor oral intake	Low BP, UO, orthostatic hypotension	
GI	Pulmonary aspiration	N/V	Abdominal exam	Radiologic studies
HEME	Anemia	GI bleeding	Pallor	Hct
GU	Prerenal vs renal	↓ UO	Hydration status	BUN, Cr
MS	Malnutrition	Weight loss	Muscle wasting	Albumin

Key Reference: Heberer G, Teichmann RK, Krämling HJ, Günther B: Results of gastric resection for carcinoma of stomach: The European experience. World J Surg 1988; 12:374–381.

PERIOPERATIVE MANAGEMENT

Preoperative Preparation

- Aspiration prophylaxis with H_2 blocker, nonparticulate antacids, metoclopramide
- Preop rehydration
- Consider preop transfusion to maintain Hct at 30 if CV disease

Anesthetic Technique

- General anesthesia
- Consider adjuvant Rx intra/postoperatively; may include epidural local anesthesia/opioids or intrathecal opioids

Monitoring

- Volume status monitoring important concern 2° to periop hypovolemia, large intraoperative 3rd spacing, potential blood loss
- Consider CVP or PA catheter depending on coexisting disease
- Foley catheter for urine output
- Consider arterial line

Airway

- Intubation awake or using rapid-sequence induction with cricoid pressure if there is aspiration concern

Induction/Maintenance

- Prevention of hypothermia by forced warm air, warming IV fluids, using warmed humidified gas
- Epidural anesthesia/analgesia is placed preferably in low thoracic region, tested prior to induction to ensure correct placement

Surgical Stages

- Exploration of abdomen before removal of malignant tumor to search for hepatic, serosal, pelvic implants; dictates procedure of choice: palliative vs curative
- Palliative surgery indicated for pyloric stenosis, bleeding, impending perforation
- Incision upper midline, unilateral or bilateral subcostal
- Left lobe of liver retracted for exposure; ↑ peak airway pressures may occur during retraction, packing
- Omentum resected
- Splenectomy performed in total gastrectomy
- Vessels supplying stomach ligated first; stomach then resected
- Intestinal continuity restored
- Drains inserted before closure
- EBL: >500 ml for total gastrectomy
- 3rd space losses: ~10 ml/kg/hr

Postoperative Considerations

- Pain score: 8–9
- Consider postop mechanical ventilation 2° to diaphragmatic impairment following abdominal procedure, severe abdominal discomfort, hypothermia, CV instability
- Consider ICU postoperatively
- IV PCA or epidural analgesia

ANTICIPATED PROBLEMS

- Pulmonary complications from ↓ functional residual capacity (general anesthesia, abdominal surgery), poor nutrition: 15%
- Reoperation 0–5%

GASTRIC BYPASS STAPLING FOR MORBID OBESITY

John C. Alverdy, M.D., F.A.C.S.

RISK

- 30,000/y undergo procedure
- Gender predominance: F > M (2:1)

PERIOPERATIVE RISKS

- In mild to moderate obesity (250–350 lbs), risks depend on medical comorbidities; procedure itself does not impose any greater risk
- In the severely obese (>400 lbs) significant cardiopulmonary problems arise intraoperatively and postop, including fluid shifts, abd closure under tension, high peak airway press, prolonged ventilator dependence due to need for complete muscle relaxation
- Severe sleep apnea
- Pulmonary HTN
- Cardiomyopathy of obesity
- Morbidity (~10% with 1 of following): anastomotic leak; dilation of bypassed stomach; bleeding; wound dehiscence; obstruction; postop apnea from combination of underlying sleep apnea, narcotic use
- Mortality: ~0.5%

WORRY ABOUT

- Positioning patient
- Proper OR table
- Airway
- Adequate relaxation
- Adequate anesthesia

OVERVIEW

- Gastric bypass is surgical Rx of morbid obesity designed to limit food intake, also limits desire for food
- Medical Rx of obesity in USA has recidivism rate of 98%
- Americans spend ~30 billion dollars/y trying to lose weight
- Accumulated data with 10-year follow up demonstrate that gastric bypass achieves sustained weight loss (>50% excess wt lost) in ~75% of patients

ICD-9-CM Code: 278.0

INDICATIONS AND USUAL TREATMENT

- Patients 100 lbs over ideal body wt who have one or more of following medical comorbidities:
  – wt-bearing osteoarthritis, stress urinary incontinence, pseudotumor cerebri, sleep apnea syndrome, pulmonary insufficiency, cardiomyopathy, gastroesophageal reflux, HTN, diabetes mellitus, thromboembolism

ASSESSMENT POINTS

SYSTEM	EFFECT	ASSESSMENT BY HX	PE	TEST
HEENT	Tight airway	Snoring, hoarseness	Airway exam	
CV	CAD, HTN	Angina	BP	ECG, stress test
RESP	Restrictive lung disease	SOB	CV	PFTs
Peripheral VASC	DVT	PE	None	

Key Reference: NIH Consensus Development Conference Proceedings: Gastrointestinal surgery for severe obesity. Am J Clin Nutr 1992; 55:478s–619s.

INTRAOPERATIVE MANAGEMENT

- Patient position: Check position of all extremities; do not hyperabduct arms; elevate arms on cushions so AP position physiologic
- If shoulders fall back during muscle paralysis, brachial plexopathy likely; problem in superobese when shoulders, arms very anterior to trunk
- Venodynes must be fitted preop and work before induction

Monitoring

- 1 large-bore IV for induction
- Consider central line after induction in superobese
- Consider PA cath if cardiopulmonary problems such as sleep apnea
- CO in superobese ranges from 10–18 L/min
- Arterial cath due to unreliable pneumatic devices

Airway

- Intubate; most intubations straightforward as airway is usually widely patent
- Fiberoptic intubation sometimes difficult due to large tongue, bulky hypopharynx

SURGICAL STAGES

- Induction: watch for inadequate anesthesia/muscle relaxants shortly after induction (tendency to underestimate dose requirements)
- Skin incision: midline incision from xyphoid to umbilicus
- Dissection: stomach mobilized along greater curvature to GE junction; large self-retaining retractors used; can press on RV at diaphragm; watch for ectopic ventricular beats. Spleen injury can cause sudden blood loss. Following evisceration, tendency to volume load; but upon closure CVP may be elevated
- Definitive surgery: stomach stapled; small (30-ml) pouch created; ~100–200 cm of small intestines bypassed. Jejunojejunostomy performed to reestablish continuity; total operation usually 3 h

- Watch for mesenteric traction syndrome as cause of sudden hypotension
- Closure/postop considerations: because of fluid shifts, extensive volume expansion may be necessary. On closure of abdomen significant ↑ in intra-abdominal pressure may impose restrictive elements to pulmonary circulation. Under these circumstances it is recommended that patient be transported to recovery facility, intubated, anesthetized
- EBL: <500 ml
- Pain score: 6–8

ANTICIPATED PROBLEMS/CONCERNS

- Thromboembolism, infection/prophylaxis routine
- Epidural analgesia, narcotic use, sleep apnea syndrome can result in unanticipated postop apnea/respiratory arrest
- Prolonged postop ventilation needed in select cases

GASTROSCHISIS SURGERY

Peter J. Davis, M.D.

RISK

- Rare abdominal wall abnormality
- Occurs in 1/20,000 births

PERIOPERATIVE RISKS

- Increased risk of infection
- 90–100% survival reported

WORRY ABOUT

- Large fluid requirements
- Temperature instability
- Cardiopulmonary compromise 2° to ↑ intra-abdominal pressure
- Postop ventilation
- Postop nutrition
- Postop infection

OVERVIEW

- Extrusion of abdominal contents through a defect *TO THE RIGHT* of the umbilical cord. Must be differentiated from omphalocele
- True surgical emergency
- Abdominal contents not covered by sac
- Abdominal viscera matted together and thickened 2° to amniotic fluid exposure and chemical peritonitis
- 60% of patients are premature
- Associated abnormalities (other than GI) rare
- GI abnormalities include intestinal atresia and stenosis

ICD-9-CM Code: 756.7 (Congenital)

USUAL TREATMENT

- Medical management
  - Wrap exposed viscera in saline-soaked gauze
  - NG tube to decompress abdominal contents
  - Antibiotics
  - Treat CV and resp instability
- Increased fluid requirements, large third-space fluid losses
- Temperature instability
- Surgery definitive treatment

ASSESSMENT POINTS

SYSTEM	EFFECT	ASSESSMENT BY HX	PE	TEST
CV	Impaired transitional circulation	Cyanosis and acidosis	Poor capillary refill Poor perfusion	CXR, ECHO SaO$_2$
	Hypotension 2° to hypovolemia	Poor UO Poor tissue perfusion		BP ABGs
			Poor UO	
	Hypotension 2° to ↑ intra-abdominal pressure	Poor UO Poor tissue perfusion; cold lower extremities; vascular congestion; Cyanosis		
RESP	Surfactant deficiency 2° to prematurity Restrictive lung disease 2° to ↑ abdominal pressure	Tachypnea Hypoxemia	Auscultation	ABGs ↓ Pulm compliance
METABOL	Large third-space requirements Hyper/hyponatremia	Review of volume replacement	Skin perfusion UO	BP Electrolytes
TEMP	Hypothermia 2° to large heat loss from large third-space fluid requirements			

Key Reference: Yaster M, Buch JR, Dydgeon DL, et al: Hemodynamic effects of primary closure of omphalocele/gastroschisis in human newborns. Anesthesiology 1988; 69:84–88.

PERIOPERATIVE IMPLICATIONS

Anesthetic Technique

- GA
- Endotracheal intubation
- Avoid nitrous oxide

Monitoring

- Pulse oximeters on both the right upper extremity and a lower extremity
- Adequate venous access preferably above the diaphragm
- Consider arterial catheter
- Consider central venous catheter
- Foley catheter

Airway

- Expect usual neonatal variants
- Endotracheal intubation
- Avoid distention of bowel by bag and mask ventilation
- Muscle relaxation required

Induction

- CV instability 2° to hypovolemia
- Avoid N$_2$O

SURGICAL STAGES

Dissection

- Care in bowel manipulation
- Blood loss 2° to adhesions
- Hypotension from bowel manipulation, blood loss, and large third-space fluid requirements

Definitive Surgery

- Three surgical options:
  - primary fascial closure,
  - skin closure, *or*
  - prosthetic silo with delayed closure
- All options associated with ↑ intra-abdominal pressure. With abdominal closure: if intragastric pressure >20 mmHg and CVP changes by >4 mmHg, consider silo. If intragastric pressure <20 mmHg and CVP changes <4 mmHg, consider primary repair.

- All surgical closure options associated with ↑ risk of sepsis

POSTOPERATIVE CONSIDERATIONS

- Need for mechanical ventilation
- Need for hyperalimentation
- In patients with silo, gradual reduction of abdominal contents, ↑ risk of sepsis, and prolonged ventilatory requirements

ANTICIPATED PROBLEMS/CONCERNS

- Hypovolemia 2° to large third-space fluid requirement
- Instability 2° to ↑ intra-abdominal pressure following abdominal wall closure
- Decrease in lung compliance 2° to impaired diaphragmatic movement from reduced abdominal contents and ↑ intra-abdominal pressure
- Prolonged postop pain relief may be required

GERIATRIC SURGERY

Timothy M. Bittenbinder, M.D.
Charles H. McLeskey, M.D.

RISK

- 13% of USA population >65 y, 17–20% by 2030

PERIOPERATIVE RISKS

- Multiple concomitant diseases are rule, not exception
- Atherosclerosis, HTN, renal disease, mental dysfunction most common concomitant diseases

WORRY ABOUT

- ↑ Risk for perioperative morbidity/mortality, more dramatic in emergent surgery

- Physiologic changes with aging result in ↑ pharmacologic sensitivity of elderly to many anesthetic drug classes

OVERVIEW

- Most commonly refers to patients >65 y
- Aging changes important in perioperative period including cardiac, pulmonary, CNS, renal, hepatic decrement in function, loss of physiologic reserve
- Age-related disease combines with age-related ↓ in basic organ function to contribute to ↑ risk for perioperative complications, death

ETIOLOGY

- Birth a long time ago
- Degree of management of environmental exposure, resulting in ↑ or ↓ physiologic age (Real Age) in relation to chronologic age

USUAL TREATMENT

- None specific other than specific disease-related Rx and age-reduction strategies such as keeping BP at 115/75, physical fitness, strength, dietary fat restriction; antioxidant or vitamin E, C, folate, and D use still somewhat experimental

ASSESSMENT POINTS

SYSTEM	EFFECT	ASSESSMENT BY HX	PE	TEST
HEENT	Inadequate mask fit, difficult laryngoscopy	Presence of dentures	State of dentition ROM of cervical spine and TMJ, facial contour changes	
CV	↑ Systolic BP, concentric hypertrophy of LV, mild aortic dilation, ↑ SVR, ↑ PAP, ↓ max HR, ↓ responsiveness to atropine and sympathomimetics Incidence of concomitant CAD very high in elderly; many subclinical Age dependent ↓ in CO, cardiac reserve found in all but active, healthy geriatric patients; CO maintained in "healthy" elderly patients but at cost of ↑ filling pressure	Exercise tolerance, CAD Hx, Sx of CAD		ECG Stress test as indicated
RESP	Reduction in vital capacity, total lung capacity, max breathing capacity, ↓ FVC Age-induced parenchymal changes mimic emphysema, creating V/Q mismatch, age-related ↓ in resting PaO_2 Ventilatory response to hypoxia or hypercapnia ~½ that seen in young patients Above physiologic changes of aging greatly affected by concomitant pulm disease	Exercise tolerance		Consider CXR, PFT Anticipated: PaO_2 = 100 − [0.4 × age (y)] mmHg
GI	↓ Hepatic size, blood flow			
RENAL	Age-related ↓ in glomerular filtration, tubular function			BUN Small elevations in serum Cr may represent large ↓ in renal function in elderly due to age-related reduction in muscle mass, Cr production
CNS	↓ Requirement for anesthetic agents, both inhalation, IV Greater sensitivity to inhalation agents, benzodiazepines, opioids due to pharmacodynamic changes Risk of postop delirium ↑ with ↑ age	Preop mentation		"Test dose" of pentothal before induction

Key Reference: McLeskey CH: Anesthesia for the geriatric patient. *In* Barash DG, Cullen BF, Stoelting RK (eds): Clinical Anesthesia, 2nd ed. Philadelphia, JB Lippincott, 1992, pp 1353–1387.

PERIOPERATIVE IMPLICATIONS

Preoperative Preparation

- Light or no sedative premed

Monitoring

- Generally should be more intense
- Individual patient assessment critical

Airway

- Laryngeal, pharyngeal, airway reflexes less effective in older patients
- Optimal head position important because laryngoscopy is more difficult, and vertebrobasilar insufficiency more common

Induction

- Consider regional anesthesia (reduce dose 4–5%/decade)
- All common induction agents require smaller dose (4–5%/decade of Real Age) for induction of GA; injecting IV induction agents slowly permits titration of dose for required effect

Maintenance

- MAC of inhalational agent ↓ in elderly (4–5%/decade after 20 y)
- Keep warm: periop hypothermia more common due to ↓ BMR, ↓ shivering threshold

Extubation

- ↑ Risk for hypothermic complications
- At ↑ risk for passive aspiration
- Consider supplemental O_2

Adjuvants

- Muscle relaxants: initial dosing is same as with younger patients; duration of action longer with all agents other than atracurium

ANTICIPATED PROBLEMS/CONCERNS

- Starting low, going slow with all drugs critical to safe perioperative care

GIFT PROCEDURE

Bernard Wittels, M.D., Ph.D.

RISK

- Infertility affects 3 million couples in USA
- Age (years) Live delivery (%)

Age (years)	Live delivery (%)
<25	0
25–29	30
30–34	29
35–39	21
40–45	10
>45	0

PERIOPERATIVE RISKS

- Perioperative mortality nil
- Anesthetic morbidity:
  - local: none
  - spinal: headache   2–37%
  - epidural: headache   0.5–5%
  - general: nausea   18–78%
    emesis   16–92%
- Failed fertilization   70%
- Successful fertilization   30%
  - ectopic pregnancy   5%
  - spontaneous abortion   19%
  - multiple delivery   8%
  - chromosomal abnormality 2%
  - congenital anomaly   3%

WORRY ABOUT

- Drug effects on oocyte fertilization, implantation, growth, development
- CO_2 insufflation requires hyperventilation
- Residual peritoneal CO_2 causes diaphragmatic, subscapular pain
- CO_2 can be insufflated/injected into unintended areas: air embolism possible

OVERVIEW

- Young, female outpatients have ↑ risk of postop N/V
- ↑ Ventilatory demands with regional, GA

ICD-9-CM Code: 628.9 (Infertility, female)

INDICATIONS

- Primary or 2° infertility:
  - endometriosis
  - ovulatory disorders
  - male factor infertility
  - unexplained infertility
- Criteria:
  - ovulation (serum LH, US)
  - adequate luteal phase (serum progesterone)
  - normal endometrium (biopsy)
  - normal TSH, T_4, prolactin
  - tubal patency (laparoscopy or hysterosalpingogram)
  - normal semen analysis

USUAL TREATMENT

- Clomiphene, hCG, Gn-RH analogues
- Chromotubation, tuboplasty

ASSESSMENT POINTS

SYSTEM	EFFECT	ASSESSMENT BY HX	PE	TEST
RESP	↑ Workload	Asthma, smoking, obesity	Auscultation	Oximetry
GI	Adhesions	Previous abdominal surgery	Scar survey	
GU	Tubal patency	Previous infection, surgery		Hysterosalpingogram

Key Reference: Medical Research International, Society for Assisted Reproductive Technology, The American Fertility Society: In vitro fertilization-embryo transfer (IVF-ET) in the United States: 1990 results from the IVF-ET Registry. Fertil Steril 1992; 57:15–24.

PERIOPERATIVE MANAGEMENT

Anesthetic Technique

- Local anesthetic with US
- Spinal, epidural or GA for laparoscopy or laparotomy

Monitoring

- Routine

Induction/Maintenance

- Consider avoiding benzodiazepines, N_2O due to potential teratogenicity, inhibition of DNA synthesis

SURGICAL STAGES

Trocar Introduction

- Adhesions of intestines to anterior abdominal wall ↑ risk of bowel perforation
- Traumatic trocar placement may perforate bowel, bladder, blood vessel

CO_2 Insufflation

- ↑ Intragastric pressure, ↑ CO_2 absorption requires ↑ ventilation (↑ rate to avoid barotrauma with ↑ PIP)

Postoperative Considerations

- Mild abdominal pain after laparoscopy
- EBL: minimal
- Pain score: 2–4
- Residual peritoneal CO_2 may cause subdiaphragmatic or subscapular discomfort
- Ibuprofen may suffice

ANTICIPATED PROBLEMS/CONCERNS

- Excessive postop pain warrants evaluation for peritoneal trauma

Leonard Firestone, M.D.

RISK

- ~14,000 candidates/y with end-stage heart disease (HD) in USA; most common Dx ischemic cardiomyopathy
- ~1800 orthotopic procedures/y in USA, limited by suitable donor organ availability
- Overwhelmingly male; no unambiguous racial predominance for end-stage HD

PERIOPERATIVE RISKS

- Early (30-d) mortality: ~8% due to surgical technique complications; fulminant rejection or infection; reperfusion injury
- Early morbidity from nosocomial bacterial infection (*Pneumococcus* pneumonia, *Pseudomonas* sepsis); later opportunistic infection with *Pneumocystis carinii, Candida* spp, CMV

WORRY ABOUT

- *Recipient heart* usually compromised by low cardiac index; ventricular irritability; mediasti-nal adhesions from prior cardiac surgery; chronic pulmonary HTN (but transpulmonary gradient [= MPAP – MLAP] must be < 15 mmHg)
- *Donor heart* (allograft) function may be compromised after CPB by transient pulmonary vasospasm, reperfusion injury, prolonged ischemia, atypical drug responses (see Anticipated Problems)
- Mural thromboembolism before CPB or systemic air embolism after CPB from completely "open" heart
- Allograft dysfunction from prolonged ischemia (function ↓ after 4–6 h); may be due to technical problems or poor coordination of donor-recipient teams
- Hyperacute rejection (rare with ABO matches)
- Pulmonary gastric aspiration (all procedures emergencies)

OVERVIEW

- Transplantation markedly improves survival of end-stage heart disease patients
- In standard midatrial orthotopic procedure, native heart (except for post atrial walls) replaced by donor heart in normal anatomic location
- Rejection, infection, reperfusion injury, hemorrhage are major causes of perioperative morbidity/mortality
- Stroke from air or thromboembolism may also occur

ICD-9-CM Code: 425.40 (cardiomyopathy)

INDICATIONS AND USUAL TREATMENT

- *Specific indication:* End-stage heart disease (NYHA Class IV = severely compromised status with guarded prognosis) unimproved by maximal medical Rx
- *Maximal medical Rx* usually includes oral inotropes, ACE, PDE-III inhibitors, diuretics, antiarrhythmics.
- Only *absolute contraindication:* irreversible pulmonary HTN (transpulmonary gradient >15 mmHg)

ASSESSMENT POINTS

SYSTEM	EFFECT	ASSESSMENT BY HX	PE	TEST
CV	Biventricular failure	Exercise intolerance Orthopnea PND	JVD Liver edge ↓	R & L heart cath
RESP	Pulmonary edema	Orthopnea	Rales	CXR
RENAL	Prerenal azotemia	PND, nocturia		BUN/Cr
CNS	Poor perfusion	Confusion?	Mental status	
HEPATIC	Chronic congestion	RUQ fullness/pain	Liver edge	LFTs

Key Reference: Firestone L: Heart transplantation. *In* Firestone L, Firestone S (eds): Transplantation, Anesthesia and Critical Care Medicine Procedures at the University of Pittsburgh. Boston, Butterworth, 1996.

INTRAOPERATIVE MANAGEMENT

Monitoring

- PA cath with long sheath (to facilitate withdrawal during cardiac anastomoses, use of caval snares); placement may be complicated by AF, TR, RV dilation, low CO; RIJ vein appropriate location
- TEE useful to optimize vol; rule out mural thrombus pre-CPB; assist in de-airing during CPB; rule out mediastinal tamponade postop

Airway

- To minimize nosocomial pneumonia risk, bacterial filter placed in anesthesia circuit

Blood Products

- Only CMV-neg blood products used for seroneg recipients, to avoid CMV sepsis
- Leukocyte-filtered or γ-irradiated blood unnecessary to avoid alloimmunization during transplant
- FFP and/or vit K may be required if on chronic warfarin
- Bleeding may be profuse, lead to coagulopathy, if transplant follows a prior cardiac procedure

Anesthetic Technique

- IV premed judiciously
- Azathioprine infused ASAP after arrival in OR
- GA regimen should be least perturbing to precarious CV status; also, full-stomach precautions essential during induction
- Phenylephrine, inotrope, judicious vol infusion may then be required to optimize CO

SURGICAL STAGES

Dissection

- Cardiomegaly and/or prior cardiac surgery ↑ risk of RV or innominate vein laceration
- Epicardial irritability can lead to VFib
- Redo surgery is associated with protracted pre-CPB interval
- With LV mural thrombus, cardiac manipulation can lead to systemic embolism

Definitive Surgery

- Bicaval cannulation for CPB mandatory due to atrial anastomoses; SVC pressure must be scrupulously monitored to avoid intracranial HTN
- Cardiectomy not performed until just before donor organ arrival
- After atrial, great vessel anastomoses, aortic cross-clamp removed ASAP to end ischemia; methylprednisolone 500 mg IV used to prevent hyperacute rejection

Weaning/Post-CPB Considerations

- Inotrope usually required to support HR (due to denervation, contractility (due to mild reperfusion injury)
- Pulmonary vasospasm possibility transiently seen; treated with PGE₁ infusion (0.025–0.1 µg/kg/min)
- Typical transfusion requirement 2–4 units of packed RBCs
- Pain management same as that following CABG

ANTICIPATED PROBLEMS/CONCERNS

- Atypical responses to cardioactive drugs by denervated donor heart—e.g., indirect-acting agents (e.g., atropine) fail to produce expected cardiac effects (tachycardia); thus only direct-acting agents should be used (e.g., isoproterenol); but, denervation supersensitivity to catecholamines, a theoretical concern, is NOT clinically relevant
- Persistently slow junctional rhythms lead to need for permanent pacemakers in ~5% of recipients
- Rejection marked by low CO and arrhythmias

Pathology Findings

- Myocardial fibrosis, edema, necrosis, or (in appropriate cases) infiltration with amyloid deposits; coronary atherosclerosis
- May also see patent foramen ovale; congenital cardiac lesions leading to Eisenmenger's physiology

HEART TRANSPLANT (PEDIATRIC)

Susan Firestone, M.D.
Leonard Firestone, M.D.

See also Heart Transplant (Adult)

RISK

• ~3000 neonatal candidates/y with hypoplastic heart syndrome or equivalent; does not include older children with complex congenital end-stage heart disease, or idiopathic or viral cardiomyopathy
• ~250 orthotopic pediatric procedures/y in USA, limited by organ availability
• No unambiguous gender or racial predominance; bimodal age distribution, with peaks in those <1 y, adolescents

PERIOPERATIVE RISKS

• Early (30-d) mortality: ~25% in patients <1 y due to technical complications; ~10% in adolescents due to same factors as in adults
• Early morbidity in patients <1 y from acute rejection; viral infection (CMV, adenovirus)

WORRY ABOUT

• Pulm HTN common in neonatal recipients
• Mediastinal adhesions from prior cardiac surgery and chronic pulm HTN

• Donor heart (allograft) intrinsic rate often too slow in neonatal recipients, necessitating mech or pharmacologic chronotropic support
• Deep hypothermic circulatory arrest always needed for neonatal procedures
• Cardiac index may be compromised after CPB
• Systemic air embolism after CPB

OVERVIEW

• Treatment alternative to complete repair of complex lesions with superior early real survival (70%, vs <60% at 1 y for complex repairs)
• Standard midatrial orthotopic procedure as for adults, except aortic arch reconstruction necessary in neonates with hypoplastic left heart syndrome
• Surgical technical difficulties, hemorrhage, reperfusion injury, rejection, infection cause perioperative morbidity/mortality
• Seizures common in infant recipients, especially after circulatory arrest

ICD-9-CM Codes: 746.9 (Congenital HD); 425.40 (Cardiomyopathy)

INDICATIONS AND USUAL TREATMENT

• Specific indications: univentricular anatomy, esp hypoplastic left heart syndrome, pulm atresia with intact ventricular septum in neonates, end-stage heart disease, for adolescents with cardiomyopathy (NYHA class IV = severely compromised status with guarded prognosis) unimproved by max medical Rx
• No long-term alternative medical Rx for hypoplastic left heart syndrome; alternative surgical Rx is Norwood's procedure (neoaortic reconstruction, creation of central aortic-to-pulm artery shunt), but high mortality
• Max medical Rx for cardiomyopathy in adolescents is similar to that for adults
• Same general conditions for other organ transplant candidates apply, as in adults
• Only absolute medical contraindication is irreversible pulm HTN (transpulmonary gradient >15 mmHg); unfavorable social milieu may also contraindicate pediatric transplantation

ASSESSMENT POINTS

SYSTEM	EFFECT	ASSESSMENT BY HX	PE	TEST
Neonates with Hypoplastic Left Heart Syndrome:				
CV	Systemic hypoperfusion	Poor systemic perfusion Cyanosis rarely	Low BP, tachypnea	ECHO Cath (rare) ABG: low pH
RESP	Pulm overperfusion	Tachypneic	Rales Resp distress	CXR
GU	Prerenal axotemia	Oliguria		BUN/Cr
HEPATIC	Systemic hypoperfusion	Liver		LFTs abn

Key Reference: Firestone S, Firestone L: Pediatric organ transplantation. *In* Healey, Cohen (eds): Wylie and Churchill-Davidson's A Practice of Anesthesia, 6th ed. Chicago, Mosby, 1995, pp 1190–1204.

INTRAOPERATIVE MANAGEMENT

Monitoring

• Neonates with hypoplastic left heart syndrome require a short, high internal jugular cath (bicaval cannulation obligatory)
• Frequent ABGs to detect inadequate systemic perfusion
• Management of older children with cardiomyopathy analogous to that of adults

Blood Products

• Only CMV-neg blood products, organs used for neonates, to avoid CMV sepsis
• Plt dysfunction, clotting factor consumption may lead to profuse bleeding after hypothermic circulatory arrest

Anesthetic Technique

• Management of children with cardiomyopathy analogous to that for adults
• In neonates with hypoplastic left heart syndrome, overriding goal is to maintain proper balance between systemic and pulm perfusion. Hyperventilation, high FIO_2 must be avoided, otherwise pulm overperfusion results; admin of

hypoxic gas mixtures (FIO_2 = 0.15–0.18) with exogenous CO_2 may be necessary; targets are SaO_2 = 75%, pH = 7.3–7.4
• Azathioprine is infused ASAP after arrival in OR
• Induction, maintenance of GA is frequently accomplished with narcotics (e.g., fentanyl 25–50 µg/kg), supplemented with vagolytic muscle relaxants to avoid bradycardia

SURGICAL STAGES (with hypoplastic left heart syndrome)

Dissection

• Branch PA isolated early, to allow tight control of pulmonary blood flow
• For CPB, arterial cannula placed in main PA; venous cannulation is bicaval

Definitive Surgery

• Long segment of donor aorta used to reconstruct aortic arch to level of ductal insertion
• Arterial cannula removed during circulatory arrest; after arch reconstruction, replaced in neoaorta, CPB resumed
• SVC pressure must be scrupulously monitored to avoid intracranial HTN

• After atrial and great vessel anastomoses, aortic cross-clamp removed ASAP to end ischemia; methylprednisolone 10 mg/kg IV used to prevent hyperacute rejection

Weaning/Post-CPB Considerations

• Inotrope (e.g., dobutamine 5 µg/kg/min) usually infused to support HR (due to denervation), contractility due to mild reperfusion injury
• Pulm vasospasm may be seen transiently; Rx with PGE_1 infusion (0.025–0.1 µg/kg/min)
• Typical transfusion requirement: 1–2 U pRBCs; 2 U platelets; 2 U cryoprecipitate

ANTICIPATED PROBLEMS/CONCERNS

• Donor HR commonly requires support after neonatal transplantation to preserve CO
• Atypical responses to cardioactive drugs similar to those in adults. Denervation supersensitivity to catecholamines NOT clinically relevant
• Rejection episodes (low CO, low ECG voltage) common, Rx with glucocorticoid boluses, poss OKT3
• Late morbidity from accelerated coronary atherosclerosis; lymphoproliferative disorders; nephrotoxicity from immunosuppressants

HERNIORRHAPHY

Douglas S. Snyder, M.D.

RISK

- Groin hernias: 680,000/y
- Gender predominance:
  - inguinal: M/F 9:1
  - femoral: M/F 1:3
  - abdominal: M/F 7:13

PERIOPERATIVE RISKS

- Perioperative mortality rare (<0.3%)
- Higher mortality/morbidity if strangulated bowel
- Risk related to comorbidities
- Morbidity: wound abscess, hematoma

WORRY ABOUT

- Appropriateness of surgery as outpatient
- Possible strangulated bowel, sepsis
- Vagal stimulation with retraction, resultant bradycardia
- Postop urinary retention
- Spinal headache: incidence ≤3% with 25-gauge needle

OVERVIEW

- Procedure performed for repair of abd wall (epigastric, femoral, incisional, umbilical)
- May be uncomplicated or may be with bowel contents
- Strangulated with necrotic bowel can be associated with sepsis syndrome
- May require bowel resection if necrotic
- Laparoscopic hernia repair currently performed; exact role poorly defined

ICD-9-CM Codes: 550–553.9

INDICATIONS AND USUAL TREATMENT

- Uncomplicated hernia: elective surg, binder, truss
- Incarcerated hernia: urgent surg
- Strangulated hernia: emergent surgery

ASSESSMENT POINTS

SYSTEM	EFFECT	ASSESSMENT BY HX	PE	TEST
CV	Potential of sepsis		HR, BP	Invasive monitor
GI	Reflux, obstruction	Reflux Sx, emesis		
HEME	Coagulation DIC if necrotic bowel	ASA use		PT, PTT, fibrinogen, FSP

Key Reference: Rutkow IM: A selective history of groin herniorrhaphy in the 20th century. Surg Clin North Am 1993; 73:395–411.

PERIOPERATIVE IMPLICATIONS

Preoperative Preparation

- Determine appropriateness of outpatient procedure

Anesthetic Technique

- Local, regional, GA, or combined anesthetic technique
- Local anesthesia ± sedation preferred for appropriate cases
- Local anesthesia permits patient to strain, cough during procedure if desired by surgeon
- Consider local wound or nerve infiltration for postop pain control
- Laparoscopic surgery, strangulated hernia require GA

Monitoring

- Routine
- Consider arterial line, CVP, PA cath if signs of sepsis

Airway

- Routine

Induction

- Require level of at least T8 for regional
- Local infiltration of ilioinguinal, iliohypogastric nerves

SURGICAL STAGES

Dissection

- Depends on hernia site

Definitive Surgery

- Inguinal hernia most common: transversalis aponeurosis, internal oblique fascia sutured to shelving edge of inguinal ligament
- Prosthetic mesh can be used for all sites to relieve tension
- Incisional hernia may require intraperitoneal approach
- EBL: 50–100 ml

Postoperative Considerations

- Postop pain depends on site, use of local infiltration
- Pain score: 3 (local)–6
- Important to void before discharge if outpatient
- Consider stool softener for inguinal hernias

to avoid strain

ANTICIPATED PROBLEMS/CONCERNS

- Bradycardia during peritoneal retraction
- Potential for necrotic bowel

HYSTERECTOMY, VAGINAL

Robert K. Parker, D.O.

RISK

- Hysterectomy within USA/y: 600,000, 1988; 580,000, 1992
- Vaginal hysterectomy: 133,000 (22%), 1988; 177,000 (31%), 1992
- Laparoscopy-assisted ↑ 3-fold from 1991–1993
- Cost estimated at $1.7 billion/y

PERIOPERATIVE RISKS

- Mortality very rare
- Risks: 20–30% associated morbidity with abdominal hysterectomy, 6–10% with vaginal hysterectomy
- More common risks (laparoscopy-assisted) include unintended laparotomy (1.4%), hemorrhage (1.3%), bowel or UR tract injury (0.9%)

WORRY ABOUT

- Indication for procedure (abnormal bleeding?)
- Effects of positioning
- Effects of CO_2 insufflation (laparoscopic-assisted)
- Unrecognized, underestimate of blood loss

OVERVIEW

- Laparoscopy-assisted not necessarily a replacement for vaginal hysterectomy
- Laparoscopy-assisted considered when vaginal hysterectomy contraindicated, e.g., pelvic endometriosis, PID, previous uterine suspension, nulliparity with insufficient prolapse, significant pelvic pain requiring abd-pelvic exploration

ICD-9-CM Codes: 618.1 (Prolapse); 625.3 (Dysmenorrhea)

INDICATIONS AND USUAL TREATMENT

- Uterine prolapse with other organ compromised, dysmenorrhea, dysfunctional uterine bleeding, premalignant endometrial lesion, CIN, uterine myomas, failed medical Rx of endometriosis, uterine cancer
- Usual medical Rx includes oral contraceptives, prostaglandin inhibitors, Danocrine or Gn-RH analogs

CONTRAINDICATIONS

- Multiple previous abdominal laparotomies (relative contraindication)
- Uterine fibroids exceeding size comparable to 16-wk gestation (relative contraindication)
- Significant medical problems that would be exacerbated by a lengthy procedure in dorsal lithotomy or Trendelenburg position and/or abdominal CO_2 insufflation

ASSESSMENT POINTS

SYSTEM	EFFECT	ASSESSMENT BY HX	PE	TEST
HEENT	Obesity hinders airway management	Prior difficult intubation	Airway	
CV	Obesity/CO_2 insufflation/Trendelenburg position inhibit venous return/CO	CV status Hx CHF/cardiopulmonary disease/SOB, exercise tolerance	CV	ECG Stress test if indicated
RESP	Obesity/CO_2 insufflation/Trendelenburg position inhibit respiratory excursion	Orthopnea	Chest	O_2 sat
HEME	Chronic/acute blood loss due to uterine bleeding	Orthostatic changes		Hct Tilt test

Key Reference: Nezhat F, Nezhat CH, Admon D, et al: Complications and results of 361 hysterectomies performed at laparoscopy. J Am Coll Surg 1995; 180:307–316.

INTRAOPERATIVE MANAGEMENT

Monitoring

- Routine
- End-tidal CO_2 should be followed during CO_2 insufflation under GA as end-tidal CO_2 may rise, requiring alteration in ventilation
- Peak airway pressure may rise considerably during Trendelenburg positioning, CO_2 insufflation; obesity may markedly exaggerate these changes
- Subcutaneous emphysema due to tissue extravasation of insufflated CO_2 may occur

Anesthetic Technique

- GA may be used for vaginal hysterectomy; often preferred for laparoscopy
- Regional anesthesia may be used for vaginal hysterectomy; for laparoscopy, regional anesthesia may be considered for highly motivated patients

Airway

- Risk of aspiration of gastric contents increased 2° to Trendelenburg position, CO_2 insufflation
- Laryngeal mask airway anesthesia may be contraindicated
- Orogastric tube to ↓ abdominal content may be indicated

SURGICAL STAGES

Induction

- CV instability 2° to preop blood loss
- Rapid onset of regional anesthesia (esp. if large intra-abdominal mass) may exacerbate instability
- Sensory level of T6 may need to be achieved with regional anesthesia

CO_2 Insufflation

- Observe for CO_2 extravasation—e.g., subcutaneous emphysema, sudden increase in airway pressure (laparoscopy-assisted)
- Trauma to major vessels may occur with introduction of trochar with laparoscope; unrecognized hemorrhage can occur

Positioning

- Observe, protect pressure points
- Trendelenburg position may lead to cephalad spread of local anesthetic during regional anesthesia
- Sacral anesthesia may be difficult to reestablish with epidural redosing in Trendelenburg position

Intraoperative

- Hemorrhage may occur during ovarian, uterine artery dissection

- Ureters need to be identified and isolated to avoid inadvertent ligation
- During laparoscopy, surgical stimulation variable; stimulus high during laparoscopy, low during vaginal approach; high again during repeat laparoscopy just prior to completion of procedure. Consider IV infusion to titrate to surg stimulus
- Approximate duration: 1–5 h

Closure/Postoperative Considerations

- Evacuation of CO_2 may be aided by Valsalva maneuver
- Postop nausea, shoulder pain from CO_2 irritation of diaphragm ↓ by adequate CO_2 evacuation, avoidance of early semi-Fowler position
- Blood loss generally 250–1000 ml; ~1% require transfusion. In isolated cases, traumatic injury to major vessels may cause massive, rapid blood loss
- Pain scores: 3–6 (generally lower than for abdominal hysterectomy)
- Postop pain relief plans may include PCA or epidural (if used during surgery), although most patients tolerate oral pain med in early postop period; use of NSAIDs may depend upon degree of bleeding, exposed surfaces

HYSTEROSCOPY

David Wlody, M.D.

RISK

- Performed diagnostically, therapeutically in women of all ages
- 100,000/y in USA

PERIOPERATIVE RISKS

- Overall complication rate 2%
- Anaphylactic reaction to distending medium (1/10,000).
- Serious complications: uterine perforation, hemorrhage, fluid overload, bowel or urinary tract injury, <1% combined

WORRY ABOUT

- Fluid overload, absorption of hyponatremic fluid
- Coagulopathy
- CO_2 embolization

OVERVIEW

- Direct exam of endometrial cavity to investigate uterine bleeding
- Distending medium to adequately visualize endometrium
- CO_2 used for Dx procedures; excess pressure can result in embolization
- Electrolyte solutions acceptable for non-electrical procedures
- With electrosurgery, use a non-electrolyte solutions
- Hyskon (32% dextran-70) most commonly used; rarely associated with significant complication

ICD-9-CM Code: 626.2 (Menometrorrhagia)

INDICATIONS

- Evaluation of infertility
- Evaluation of abnormal uterine bleeding
- Resection of submucous myomas, endometrial ablation, resection of uterine septae

ASSESSMENT POINTS

SYSTEM	EFFECT	ASSESSMENT BY HX	PE	TEST
HEME	Blood loss	Abn bleeding, syncope	Orthostasis	Hgb/Hct

Key Reference: Mangar D: Anesthetic implications of 32% dextran-70 (Hyskon) during hysteroscopy. Can J Anesth 1992; 39:975–979.

PERIOPERATIVE MANAGEMENT

Preoperative Preparation

- If Hx of reaction to dextran, consider alternative distending medium; alternatively, pretreatment with monovalent dextran ↓ freq of anaphylaxis

Anesthetic Technique

- Can be performed under paracervical block with sedation with less extensive surgery
- For extensive procedures, GA, epidural used

Monitoring

- Routine
- Significant cardiopulmonary disease, consider invasive monitoring because absorption of large vol of distending fluid

Airway

- Since no pneumoperitoneum, mask anesthesia or LMA acceptable

Induction/Maintenance

- Usually performed on ambulatory basis: any technique allowing rapid emergence, recovery

Postoperative Concerns

- Monitor for excess bleeding
- EBL: minimal
- Pain score: 3–5
- Postop pain can be managed with NSAID

ANTICIPATED PROBLEMS/CONCERNS

- Monitor for development of anaphylaxis
- Each ml of dextran absorbed into circulation expands blood vol by 8.6 ml; therefore, minimize pressure, limit vol infused to 500 ml
- When CO_2 used to distend, use insufflator designed for hysteroscopy (laparoscopic insufflators produce flow rates high enough to lead to gas embolization)

ILEOSTOMY

Michael S. Higgins, M.D.

RISK

- Relatively common procedure for adults 20–65 y
- Male/female predominance: equal. For cancer, men ≥ women; for inflammatory bowel disease, women > men
- Racial predominance: none
- Usually performed for intestinal obstruction (60–70%) or diseases requiring a total procto-colectomy (10–15%); often associated with intestinal adhesions, inflammatory bowel disease, abdominal cancer, trauma

PERIOPERATIVE RISKS

- Mortality: varies widely with coexistent disease, generally <1%
- Procedural morbidity: ileus 5%, wound infection <5%, intestinal obstruction 2–3%, fistula formation 1–3%, ostomy necrosis <0.5%

WORRY ABOUT

- Pulm aspiration
- Perioperative intravascular volume deficiency
- Hemorrhage
- Postop pulm atelectasis
- Sepsis

OVERVIEW

- Co-morbid diseases include malnutrition, hypovolemia, lyte abn, effects of chronic steroid therapy, effects of primary oncologic process, associated traumatic injuries
- Often ↑ risk of gastric regurgitation and pulm aspiration
- Associated with preop hypovolemia and continuing intravascular volume shift to extravascular tissues (third-spacing) perioperatively
- Intraoperative monitoring modalities determined by patient age and coexisting disease

ICD-9-CM Code: 560.9 (Bowel obstruction)

INDICATIONS AND USUAL TREATMENT

- Ileal disease: inflammatory bowel disease, small bowel obstruction, volvulus, intussusception, mesenteric vascular occlusion, radiation enteritis, intestinal fistulae, small bowel tumors, Crohn's disease, trauma (if reanastomosis contraindicated by infection)
- Large bowel disease: proctocolectomy for inflammatory bowel disease, ulcerative colitis, familial polyposis, neoplasm, trauma
- Surgical intervention for inflammatory bowel disease and Crohn's disease may follow prolonged steroid therapy
- Surgical alternatives include both incontinent and continent ileostomy (Kock pouch)

ASSESSMENT POINTS

SYSTEM	EFFECT	ASSESSMENT BY HX	PE	TEST
CV	Hypovolemia from ↓ fluid intake, bowel prep, third-spacing	PO status, vomiting, bowel prep, UO	Hypotension with tachycardia, orthostatic BP, skin turgor	BUN/Cr, urine output, electrolytes, consider ECG
RESP	Resp insufficiency from abdominal distention/splinting and reduced FRC	Dyspnea Abdominal pain	Rales Abdominal distention and rigidity	CXR Pulse oximetry Consider ABG
GI	Possible ↑ intragastric pressure, volume, acidity Possible perforation with peritonitis	Abdominal pain	Peritoneal signs	X-ray—dilated bowel
HEME/IMMUN	Hemoconcentration from dehydration DIC possibly associated with sepsis Immune suppression from chronic steroid therapy Potential malnutrition from malabsorption Bacteremia and sepsis	GI losses Abnormal bleeding Hemodynamic instability	See under CV Febrile, hypotensive	PCV, plt, PT/PTT, WBC count with differential
RENAL	Possible hypokalemic, hypochloremic metabolic alkalosis with vomiting, lyte abn from lower GI losses/bowel prep, hemoconcentration Associated renal insufficiency in elderly	Vomiting, bowel prep	See under CV	Serum lytes

Key Reference: Binderow SR, Wexner SD: Current surgical therapy for mucosal ulcerative colitis. Dis Colon Rectum 1994; 37:610–624.

PERIOPERATIVE MANAGEMENT

Premedication

- Consider H₂ antagonists and oral nonparticulate antacid
- Consider metoclopramide—contraindicated if intestinal obstruction
- Consider steroid coverage if on chronic steroid therapy (hydrocortisone 100 mg IV over 24 h)
- Consider NSAIDs to reduce incidence of mesenteric traction syndrome

Monitoring

- Consider arterial catheter if hemodynamically unstable or severe cardiopulmonary disease
- Foley catheter
- Volume status monitoring a major concern—consider CVP, PA cath, or transesophageal ECHO monitoring if renal insufficiency or significant cardiac dysfunction with intravascular volume or prolonged surgical procedure

Airway

- Routine; consider awake intubation, rapid-sequence or modified rapid-sequence intubation (aspiration risk)

Induction

- Consider peri-induction intravascular volume expansion (10–20 ml/kg) if hypovolemic

Maintenance

- May be performed under regional, general, or combined anesthetic techniques; NG tube placed to suction reduces gastric distention
- Usual blood loss <300 ml
- Consider convective air warming

Emergence

- Extubation depends on usual criteria with emphasis on volume status, body temp
- Pain score: 5–8
- Consider epidural or IV PCA
- Postop volume requirements moderate

PROCEDURES **397**

IMPLANTABLE CARDIOVERTER-DEFIBRILLATORS (ICDs) — IMPLANTATION

Paul D. Eckenbrecht, M.D.

RISK

- 300,000/y in USA suffer sudden cardiac death
- Pharmacologic Rx for *near* sudden death is ineffective in 20–50%; 1-y sudden death rate is 30%.
- 10,000 undergo ICD implantations annually, after which the 1-y sudden death rate is 2%.
- Gender predominance: 76% male.
- Associated diseases: CAD—65%; cardiomyopathy—19%; valvular disease—8%; LV dysfunction with mean LVEF 35 ± 10%.

PERIOPERATIVE RISKS

- 3.3% perioperative mortality; varies inversely with LVEF (2.3% when performed separately from cardiac surgery)
- Factors increasing perioperative mortality: LVEF <30%; concomitant cardiac surgery; postop device deactivation; preop amiodarone administration
- 72% of deaths are cardiac (24% sudden; 17% tachydysrhythmic/nonsudden; 31% cardiac, nondysrhythmic) and 28% are noncardiac.
- Perioperative cardiac morbidity: sustained VTach/VFib (5–15%); AFib (10–19%); CHF (2%); MI (1%).
- Perioperative pulmonary morbidity (with thoracotomy approach): Pleural effusions/atelectasis/pneumonia (3–27%); ARDS 2–21%
- Perioperative noncardiopulmonary morbidity: CVA (1–2%); renal failure (1%)
- Nonthoracotomy, transvenous implantation has a lower perioperative mortality (0.5–1.6%).

WORRY ABOUT

- Myocardial ischemia, low cardiac output, organ underperfusion during defibrillation threshold (DFT) testing.
- Increase DFT: antidysrhythmics (class IA, B, C—including lidocaine, propranolol, amiodarone, verapamil); halogenated hydrocarbons; hypothermia; myocardial ischemia; acidosis.
- Increased incidence of intraoperative conduction defects, atropine-resistant bradycardia, CHB, pacemaker and inotropic dependency, α-blockade with low SVR and hepatic, thyroid, and pulm dysfunction if taking chronic amiodarone.

OVERVIEW

- ICDs have two basic, interrelated functions: dysrhythmia detection and dysrhythmia therapy.
- Dysrhythmia detection may be based on morphology (electrogram shape) or rate criteria.
- For dysrhythmia therapy, the CPI Ventak AICD treats VTach and VFib with countershocks only.
- The Medtronic PCD and Ventritex Cadence have tiered therapy: VVI pacing for bradycardia, antitachycardia pacing (ATP) and low-energy cardioversion for VTach, and high-energy defibrillation for VFib.
- Surgical approaches: Left anterolateral thoracotomy—67%; median sternotomy—27%; subcostal—6%.

- A nonthoracotomy approach includes a left pectoral subcutaneous patch, and/or a transvenous sense/pace and defibrillating leads.
- DFT testing is performed after both initial lead placement and generator implantation.

ICD-9-CM Codes: 427.1 (for VTach); 427.41 (for VFib)

INDICATIONS AND USUAL TREATMENT

- Survivors of cardiac arrest, presumably due to VTach/VFib not associated with acute MI
- Patients with sustained VTach at electrophysiologic study (EPS) are: noninducible; nonsuppressed by drug or surgical therapy; intolerant of drugs
- No randomized trials demonstrate ICDs are superior to elecrophysiologic-directed, antidysrhythmic drug therapy for sustained VTach
- ICDs are considered first-line therapy for poorly tolerated VTach with impaired LV function, or VTach in patients who are not inducible at EPS.
- 80% of ICD patients receive concomitant antidysrhythmic therapy to reduce required device interventions

ASSESSMENT POINTS

SYSTEM	EFFECT	ASSESSMENT BY HX	PE	TEST
CV	Myocardial ischemia LV dysfunction Rate, mechanism of VTach	Angina symptoms Exercise tolerance, DOE	S_3, rales	ECG, Ex. thallium ECHO, MUGA, cath EPS, ambulatory ECG
RESP	Amiodarone toxicity	Exercise tolerance, DOE		CXR, PFTs, ABG
RENAL	Renal insufficiency		Edema	BUN, Cr
NEURO	CV disease	Stroke, TIAs	Bruits	Carotid duplex
ELECTROLYTES	Reversible VTach/VFib	Diuretic Rx		Serum K^+ and Mg^{2+}

Key Reference: Nacarelli GV, Veltri EP: Implantable Cardioverter-Defibrillators. Cambridge, Blackwell, 1993.

PERIOPERATIVE MANAGEMENT

Anesthetic Technique

- GA required for thoracotomy, median sternotomy, and subcostal approaches.
- Local with sedation will become more widely utilized for transvenous, nonthoracotomy implantation.
- Opioid-hypnotic-relaxant techniques used since least likely to affect hemodynamics and EPS or DFT testing.
- Halogenated hydrocarbons may increase DFT, so keep concentrations <1.0 MAC.

Monitoring

- Pulmonary artery catheters reserved for patients with LVEF <35% but may dislodge hardware positioned in SVC

Airway

- A left double-lumen tube for thoracotomy approach

- A single-lumen tube for all other approaches

SURGICAL STAGES

- Incisions depend upon surgical approach
- Implantation of sense/pace and defibrillation lead systems (may be transvenous)
- Determine R-wave amplitude from sensing and defibrillating leads (5 mV and 1 mV, respectively)
- Determine pacing threshold for ATP capable devices (<1.5 V endocardial, <2.0 V epicardial)
- DFT testing of implanted ICD leads using external cardioverter-defibrillator (≤15–25 joules).
- Creation of the ICD generator pocket in left paraumbilical area above abdominal fascia.
- Tunnel and connect leads to ICD, implant generator, and repeat DFT testing using ICD
- Inactivate ICD during closure of pocket, then reactivate at end of procedure.
- EBL and volume shifts are minimal.

Postoperative Considerations

- Significant postop pain with thoracotomy approach (pain score 6–10).

- Consider epidural/spinal narcotics
- Inappropriate device discharge due to postoperative atrial tachydysrhythmias prevented by device deactivation; however, intentional postop device deactivation increases risk of postop tachydysrhythmic death.
- An association exists between chronic, preop amiodarone administration and postop ARDS (as high as 50% in one study).

ANTICIPATED PROBLEMS/CONCERNS

- 10–20% of transvenous implants require conversion to thoracotomy owing to high DFTs (>25 joules).
- 3–18% of all implants result in high DFTs. This results in a 1-y sudden death rate 15× greater than in implants with acceptable DFTs.
- Sustained VFib during DFT testing should be promptly treated with rescue shocks and CPR/ACLS as needed. Because lidocaine raises DFT, IV bretylium, which has no effect on DFT, is drug of choice.

INGUINAL HERNIORRHAPHY

Lucinda L. Everett, M.D.
Surinder K. Kallar, M.D.

RISK

- 700,000 groin hernias/y repaired in USA
- Congenital: 1–2% of live births
- Age predominance: congenital, especially premature infants; elderly
- Sex: 80–90% of adult repairs in males; incidence in congenital hernias quoted as 4–10 × higher in males

PERIOPERATIVE RISKS

- Mortality: < 0.01% elective repairs; up to 5% in emergency cases and very elderly
- Morbidity: hematoma, 2–3%; infection, 1–2%; entrapment of ilioinguinal or genitofemoral nerve with neuralgia; ischemic orchitis, 0.03–0.5% in primary hernias; recurrence, 10–15%

WORRY ABOUT

- Straining or bucking with emergence may damage repair
- Bowel obstruction with incarcerated hernia
- Apnea risk in ex–premature infants

OVERVIEW

- Groin hernias represent defect of transversalis fascia
- Classification includes location (medial [direct], lateral [indirect], femoral) and size; also sliding, recurrent, or incarcerated
- Chronically increased abdominal pressure thought to be predisposing factor, as in obesity, COPD, prostatic hyperplasia, ascites, pregnancy, constipation, colonic stenosis
- Most inguinal hernias can be diagnosed by palpation, though clinical exam distinguishes direct from indirect with only 70% accuracy
- US exam useful in patients with symptoms but no signs

ICD-9-CM Code: 550.9

INDICATIONS AND USUAL TREATMENT

- Early elective surgery recommended to prevent incarceration/strangulation; "broad direct bulges" have lower incidence of incarceration (some manage this type conservatively, but others endorse repair in all, as preop differentiation of direct vs indirect is not absolute by clinical exam); recurrence depends on size and location
- Mesh repair indicated for multiple recurrences and bilateral hernias, particularly in elderly
- Laparoscopic repair may ↓ postop pain but may require longer surgical time

ASSESSMENT POINTS

SYSTEM	EFFECT	ASSESSMENT BY HX	PE	TEST
CV	Ischemic heart disease prevalent in elderly	Exercise tolerance Chest pain/discomfort		ECG > 50 y or with Hx Testing for myocardium at risk if Hx suggests
RESP	Obstructive pulm disease may predispose	Dyspnea, wheezing	Auscultation Forced exhalation Chest diameter Clubbing, cyanosis Periodic breathing	O_2 saturation CXR if infection suspected PFT if etiology unclear or to evaluate Rx
	Postop apnea risk in ex–premature infants	Postconceptual <56 wk Hx apnea; caffeine Rx		
GI	Bowel obstruction if hernia incarcerated	N/V	Abdominal distention	KUB Electrolytes
CNS	Ability to tolerate procedure under local anesthesia	Orientation/cooperation	Mental status exam	
SOCIAL	Most procedures done on outpatient basis	Adequate home support for elderly		

Key Reference: Schumpelick V, et al: Inguinal hernia repair in adults. Lancet 1994; 344:375–379.

PERIOPERATIVE MANAGEMENT

Preoperative Preparation

- Consider caffeine citrate, 20 mg/kg in ex-premature infants at risk for apnea
- Avoid sedatives in premature infants having procedure under spinal anesthesia

Anesthetic Technique

- Local infiltration effective for repair; potentially fewer side effects than field block/nerve block
- Spinal or epidural; T8 level
- GA by mask or LMA
- General endotracheal (especially if obstructed or if large/recurrent hernia)

Monitoring

- Routine
- Consider postop apnea monitoring for ex–premature infants

SURGICAL STAGES

Skin Incision

- Above inguinal ligament

Dissection

- To identify type of hernia and vital structures

Definitive Surgery

- Management of peritoneal sac; repair of fascial defect

Postoperative Considerations

- Minimal blood loss; minimal fluid shifts unless incarcerated hernia with bowel obstruction
- Pain management: local infiltration; nerve block; caudal (pediatric)
- Pain score: 4–5

ANTICIPATED PROBLEMS/CONCERNS

- Potential complications of laparoscopy with laparoscopic repair
- Occasional vagal response to traction
- Femoral nerve palsy with leg weakness possible after "blind" ilioinguinal block

INTESTINAL OBSTRUCTION

David A. Rosen, M.D.
Kathleen R. Rosen M.D.

RISK

- Operations counted in millions if all etiologies included
- Small bowel obstructions predominate by 60–80%
- Race and gender predilection: none

PERIOPERATIVE RISKS

- Apache II scores >8 correlate with ↑ risk
- Mortality 8–10% overall: small bowel obstruction
- ↑ Risk (bowel factors): strangulation, malignancy, high obstruction, delay in diagnosis or surgery, bowel excision
- ↑ Risk (general): sepsis, CV instability (especially hypovolemia and hypotension prior to surgery), extremes of age, coexisting disease, suboptimal nutritional state

WORRY ABOUT

- Coexisting medical conditions
- Volume status; acid-base, lytes
- Perfusion: systemic, pulmonary, regional
- Sepsis
- Physiologic problems can persist or worsen after surgery

OVERVIEW

- Indications for surgery: Strangulation of vascular supply or complete obstruction of lumen. Functional or partial obstructions may be amenable to conservative management
- Patients may need aggressive management prior to surgery (see Worry About)

ICD-9-CM Code: 560.9

INDICATIONS/USUAL TREATMENT

- Any intrinsic or extrinsic lesions that obstruct the intestinal lumen or strangulate the vascular supply require urgent surgery.
- Prophylactic surgery may be indicated if an abnormality that predisposes to obstruction is detected.
- If diagnosis is uncertain, water-soluble contrast material may be used to distinguish partial from complete obstruction.
- Hemodynamic resuscitation can occur prior to surgery in virtually all cases.

ASSESSMENT POINTS

SYSTEM	EFFECT	ASSESSMENT BY HX	PE	TEST
CV	Hypotension Tachycardia Poor peripheral perfusion Venous return impeded	Orthostasis, edema	BP (positional) Skin color Capillary refill Pulse quality, HR	As indicated by pre-existing disease and age as well as present condition
RESP	Restrictive defect	SOB (positional)	Resp rate/pattern, skin color Resp work/effort	ABG, oximetry
GI	Loss of fluids, lytes, or blood	I/O, vomiting (amount, description) BM (timing, character) Abdominal pain ± distention Prior operations	Abdominal scars Mass Rectal tenderness Abdominal girth Bowel sounds Hernias	Abdominal x-ray ± enhancement NG drainage
RENAL/ HYDRATION	↓ UO ↑ Other fluid, ↓ Electrolytes	I/O	Skin turgor Dry mouth	BUN, Cr, Na+, K+, Cl−, HCO3−, UA
IMMUN	Contamination of GI flora, sepsis or peritonitis	Fever, chills	Temperature (see above, CV and GI)	CBC with differential

Key Reference: Welch JP: Bowel Obstruction: Differential Diagnosis and Clinical Management. Philadelphia, WB Saunders, 1990.

PERIOPERATIVE IMPLICATIONS

Preoperative Preparations

- Restoration of intravascular volume
- Correction of acid-base and lyte abnormalities
- Decompression of stomach
- Antibiotic coverage

Anesthetic Technique

- Usually GA
- Hemodynamic concerns mandate careful selection of anesthetic, relaxant, and analgesic medication.

Monitoring

- Required: routine + Foley catheter
- Consider: arterial line, CVP, PAC, TEE

Induction/Maintenance

- Rapid-sequence
- CV instability 2° to volume status
- Avoidance of nitrous oxide
- Muscle relaxation
- Large-bore intravenous access

SURGICAL STAGES

- Variable according to specific etiology
- Large fluid shifts on opening of abdomen
- Tumors or mass manipulation may cause hemodynamic alterations
- Restriction of pulmonary function or cardiac performance 2° to placement of surgical retractors
- Release of hemodynamically active substances when the bowel is manipulated
- Relaxation until abdomen closed
- Body heat and fluid loss due to exposed bowel
- Blood loss ranges from minimal to significant depending on etiology
- Abdominal closure may be difficult or contraindicated

POSTOPERATIVE PERIOD

- Delay extubation if pulm and CV status in question.
- Continued fluid and lyte abnormalities
- ARDS a potential if large fluid volumes were required
- Pulmonary atelectasis, pneumonia, or aspiration
- DVT ± pulm emboli
- Infection: general or local
- Pain management may be vital to ensure deep breathing and coughing
- PCA for 3–5 days (pain score: 2–9)
- Coagulopathies
- Renal failure
- Malnutrition
- Antiemetics

ANTICIPATED PROBLEMS/CONCERNS

- Hemodynamic, fluid, lyte, pulm alterations
- Sepsis

INTRA-AORTIC BALLOON COUNTERPULSATION (IABP)

Carole Vannier, M.D.

RISK

- Used in >75,000 patients/y world-wide (1992)

PERIOPERATIVE RISKS

- Frequency of complications: 14–45% (4–9% major; 22–41% minor); vascular (9–22%); infectious (1–22%); failure to place balloon pump (5–11.7%; no difference between percutaneous and surgical); bleeding (4–10%). Rare complications include excessive bleeding, balloon catheter leak, perforation or entrapment, gas embolism, small bowel infarction, aortic dissection leading to paraplegia.

WORRY ABOUT

- Timing of balloon inflation
- Dysrhythmias including sinus tachycardia
- Bleeding at insertion site
- Distal extremity ischemia

OVERVIEW

- Cardiac assist device placed surgically or percutaneously for management of acute LV dysfunction or unstable angina
- Removes volume from central aorta prior to and during LV ejection (reduces aortic pressure and therefore LV work by decreased afterload)
- Returns volume to central aorta during diastole (increases aortic pressure and therefore improves coronary blood flow and myocardial oxygen delivery)
- IABP system consists of: drive unit; balloon catheter (30–40 ml displacement volume) placed surgically or percutaneously. Helium most effective inflating gas
- Beneficial effects: ↓ time-tension index 20–40% (reflects ↓ myocardial O_2 ventilation rate); ↑ diastolic pressure–time index (reflects ↑ myocardial blood flow); ↓ LVEDP 25–40% while maintaining CO; ↓ LV work 18–50% while maintaining perfusion; improves CO (10–100%); improves EF; improves subendocardial perfusion as assessed by endocardial viability ratio; ↑ coronary blood flow (5–100%); ↑ cerebral blood flow (56%); ↑ myocardial O_2 supply (56%); ↓ myocardial O_2 consumption; ↓ lactate production

INDICATIONS/CONTRAINDICATIONS

Indications

- LV failure or ischemia refractory to pharmacologic intervention: status post MI, precardiac transplant (bridge), postcardiac transplant, acute mitral regurgitation, unstable angina
- May also be useful in: high-risk patients undergoing PTCA, refractory ventricular dysrhythmia, high-risk cardiac patients undergoing noncardiac surgery

Contraindications

- Aortic insufficiency, aortic dissection
- Relatively contraindicated in patients with prosthetic thoracic aorta graft (may be considered if graft is >12 mo old)

ASSESSMENT POINTS

SYSTEM	EFFECT	PE	TEST
CV	Dysrhythmias	Pulse	ECG
	Volume status	BP	CVP, PCWP
	Bleeding	Inspect site	CT, Hgb (retroperitoneal bleed)
	Vascular insufficiency	Inspect distal extremities	Doppler

Key Reference: Kantrowitz A, Cardona PR, Freed P: Percutaneous intra-aortic balloon counterpulsation. Crit Care Clin 1992; 8:819.

PERIOPERATIVE MANAGEMENT

- Femoral insertion
  - Select site with greater pulse
  - Monitoring to include radial arterial pressure catheter and PA catheter
  - Heparinize if not contraindicated (LMW dextran or alternative can be used otherwise)
  - Cannulate femoral artery
  - Sheath and wire left in place, balloon advanced either under fluoroscopic guidance or to estimated level of angle of Louis. Final position should be 1cm below origin of left subclavian artery. Central lumen can be connected to pressure transducer and used for balloon pump timing. Confirm with CXR.
- Usual balloon volume approximates that of failing LV, ~20–40 ml.
- Usual balloon diameter occludes 75–90% of cross-sectional area of descending aorta during inflation (overinflation can damage intima and lead to hemodynamic compromise)
- Inflation timing is critical to ensure benefit. Improper timing can worsen hemodynamics.
- Central aortic pressure tracing is related to ECG to determine interval between R wave of ECG and aortic valve opening (pressure wave upstroke) and aortic valve closure (dicrotic notch). This is used to program drive unit.

- Usual inflation initiated at the dicrotic notch on the central aortic BP waveform.
- Deflation occurs at the end of diastole.
- Incorrect timing can be recognized by examination of assisted pressure tracings and includes:
  - Early inflation: augmented wave superimposed over systolic component of pressure trace
  - Late inflation: augmented wave initiated after valve closure
  - Early deflation: deflation occurs before isovolumetric contraction
  - Late deflation: inflation extends into systolic component
- At HR >120, balloon may not be able to fill and empty completely. Consider augmentation at alternate beats (1:2 timing).
- Dysrhythmias may cause difficult or impossible adequate timing. Treatment of underlying dysrhythmia is a must. Avoid hypovolemia.
- Assess balloon timing frequently, esp. with changes in HR. Wean vasopressors ASAP.
- Maintain APTT 1.5–2.0 × control if possible.
- Check extremities frequently for evidence of ischemia.
- Monitoring to include: HR, BP, CVP, PAP, PCWP, CO, UO, electrolytes, ABG, pH, CBC, temp. ECHO may also be useful.
- Consider weaning if CI >2.2L/min/m², PCWP <18 mmHg, BP normal, and no ongoing ischemia.

- Frequency weaning involves decreasing ratio of assisted beats to total number of beats (1:1, 1:2, 1:3, 1:4)
- Volume weaning involves decreasing balloon volume gradually (opponents of volume weaning cite risk of clot formation on balloon; proponents cite minimal risk if balloon volume maintained 10–15% stroke and this method is more physiologic)
- Prior to removing IABP, heparin should be stopped for at least 4 h. Balloon is deflated and Doppler monitoring of distal leg vessels is performed. Catheter and sheath are removed as one unit while pressure is applied distal to puncture site to prevent distal embolization. Proximal pressure applied to encourage distal back-bleeding and to flush thrombi.

ANTICIPATED PROBLEMS/CONCERNS

- Timing may be difficult in patients with changing HR. Assess frequently.

INTUSSUSCEPTED BOWEL REPAIR

David A. Rosen, M.D.
Kathleen R. Rosen, M.D.

RISK

Pediatric Population

- 80–90% of infantile bowel obstruction
- 0.3% of live births
- 50% first year of life
- Greatest incidence at 3–10 months
- Male predominance 3:2
- Usually idiopathic

Adult Population

- 2–5% of bowel obstruction
- Associated with tumor/other bowel abnormalities
- Common in underdeveloped nations (idiopathic)

PERIOPERATIVE RISKS

- Prolapse of bowel and passage of necrotic tissue are grave signs

Pediatric Population

- Mortality <1%
- Increased morbidity and mortality if delayed diagnosis
- Preoperative perforation risk if < 6 months or symptoms > 3–4 days
- Bowel perforation risk during hydrostatic reduction

Adult Population

- Site and extent of intussusception influences risk
- Ileocolic intussusception greatest risk of bowel strangulation

WORRY ABOUT

- Hydration and electrolyte status
- Sepsis
- Viral illness (URI or GI)

OVERVIEW

- Definition: Invagination of one portion of intestinal tract into adjacent portion
- Lead point: Anatomic abnormality that triggers intussusception
- Lead point is drawn into distal bowel
- Bowel lymphadenopathy (Peyer's patches) in idiopathic cases

Pediatric Population

- 90% idiopathic (no lead point)
- Lead point present in neonates < 3 months
- Seasonal peaks parallel seasonal occurrence of viral illness
- Classic triad: pain, abdominal mass, intestinal bleeding
- Currant jelly stool in 65% of those < 2 years
- Associations: Henoch's purpura, cystic fibrosis, Meckel's diverticulum, polyps

Adult Population

- Lead point in 75% (tumor most common)
- Peutz-Jeghers syndrome (pigmentation of face/oral mucosa) + acute abdominal pain = intussusception
- Malignant melanoma: Intussusception most common form of bowel obstruction
- Tumor associations: small bowel (benign = lipomas, polyps, neurofibromas, leiomyomas, fibromas, hemangiomas, hamartomas); large bowel (malignant = adenocarcinoma, carcinoid, leiomyosarcoma, lymphoma); varied location (metastatic = melanoma, renal cell carcinoma, lung carcinoma, chondrosarcoma, myeloma)
- Other associations: Meckel's, Crohn's disease, eosinophilic granuloma, foreign body, AIDS, intraabdominal adhesions
- Presentation variable: 70% crampy, recurrent or steady abdominal pain
- Intraoperative diagnosis in majority

ICD-9-CM Code: 560.0 (Intussusception)

INDICATIONS AND USUAL TREATMENT

Pediatric Population

- Primary hydrostatic reduction (barium enema with sedation and fluoroscopy)
  - General anesthesia may facilitate reduction
  - 75% successful
  - Contraindications: bowel perforation or strangulation, sepsis
  - Recurrence rate 4–10%
- Surgery
  - Neonates < 3 mo (lead point)
  - Bowel compromise
  - Failed closed reduction
  - Bowel resection uncommon

Adult Population

- Rarely amenable (idiopathic) to hydrostatic Rx
- Surgery first line of treatment
- Bowel resection likely
- Enterostomy unusual

ASSESSMENT POINTS

SYSTEM	EFFECT	ASSESSMENT BY HX	PE	TEST
GI	Bowel obstruction Bowel compromise	Nausea and vomiting Diarrhea (bloody), currant jelly stools Abdominal pain	Increased peristalsis RUQ abdominal mass Legs drawn up	X-ray Barium enema
RENAL/HYDRATION	Dehydration	I/O, vomiting	Decreased UO Decreased skin turgor	Electrolytes BUN, Cr, UA
HEME	Anemia Sepsis	Listlessness/pallor Fever	Tachycardia, hypotension (orthostasis)	Hgb, Hct CBC

Key Reference: West KW, et al: Intussusception: Current management in infants and children. Surgery 1987; 102:704–710.

PERIOPERATIVE MANAGEMENT

Preoperative Preparation

- Restore intravascular volume
- Decompression of stomach
- Antibiotics if sepsis is suspected

Anesthetic Technique

- General anesthesia is preferred
- Hemodynamics mandate careful selection of anesthetic, relaxant, and analgesics

Monitoring

- Routine plus Foley catheter
- Consider invasive monitors if septic

Induction/Maintenance

- Rapid sequence
- CV instability 2° to volume status
- Nitrous oxide can aid in reduction if bowel is not ischemic
- Relaxation usually needed

SURGICAL STAGES

Pediatric Population

- Right transverse incision
- Gentle proximal milking on nonischemic bowel
- Bowel manipulation may produce hemodynamic changes
- 25% require resection

Adult Population

- Etiology and location determine surgical approach
- Resection of lead point with primary anastomosis

Postoperative Period

- Recurrence or adynamic ileus
- Fluid shifts
- Opiates required for 2–3 days
- Pain score: 6–8
- Fever

ANTICIPATED PROBLEMS/CONCERNS

- Maintenance of intravascular volume
- Sepsis
- Decrease in body temperature
- Pediatric anesthesia

JOINT REPLACEMENT CEMENTING
(METHYLMETHACRYLATE CEMENTING)

Jonathan L. Parmet, M.D.

RISK

- Cemented knee arthroplasty >141,000/y
- Cemented hip arthroplasty >250,000/y
- Racial predominance: none
- Gender predominance: none

PERIOPERATIVE RISKS

- 30 d mortality (1–5%)
- DVT (no prophylaxis 72% and 50%, respectively, for TKR and THR; 45% and 20% with prophylaxis)
- Myocardial ischemia (31%)
- Fat embolism syndrome (10–20%)
- Pulm embolism (5%)

WORRY ABOUT

- ↑ PA pressures after cementing
- Intraoperative arterial desaturation (30%) with FIO_2 <50%

- Hypotension in 34% of hypovolemic patients. Euvolemia seems to reduce incidence of hypotension
- Fatal pulm embolism (1–5%)
- Transient third-degree heart block (?)

OVERVIEW

- An acrylic bone cement is freshly prepared and inserted into reamed bony cavities.
- Cementing associated with echogenic emboli regardless of joint (100%)
- Intraoperative CV collapse
- Hypotension due to monomer and release of emboli
- Regional anesthesia ↓ postop DVT but does not ↓ echocardiographic emboli

INDICATIONS AND USUAL TREATMENT

- Cemented joint replacement (DJD, obesity, connective tissue diseases), distal and proximal femoral fracture, revision joint replacement; rare in craniotomy
- Treatment: NSAIDs, steroids, subcutaneous heparin, LMW heparin

ASSESSMENT POINTS

SYSTEM	EFFECT	TEST
HEENT	Taste of monomer after cementing	
CV	Cardiac output (no Dx, ↓ hypovolemia), preload (↓), afterload (↓), PVR (↑), third-degree heart block, pericardial effusion Heart failure from pulm HTN	MAP, ECG, TEE CVP, PA catheterization
HEME	↑ Plt aggregation, ↑ thrombosis	Venography, duplex US, impedance plethysmography
CNS	↓ Cognitive function, stroke, confusion	
RESP	V/Q mismatch, ↑ pulm pressure, pulm emboli Atelectasis	V/Q scan, PA catheterization Pulm angio, SaO_2, ABG End-tidal CO_2, TEE, electrolytes

Key Reference: Parmet JP, et al: Echogenic emboli upon tourniquet release during total knee arthroplasty. Anesth Analg 1994; 79:940–945.

INTRAOPERATIVE MANAGEMENT

Monitoring

- Volume status: Foley catheter, CVP (revision procedures, THR lateral approach)
- Consider PA catheter or transesophageal ECHO (↓ ventricular function, pulm HTN, age >70 y, severe connective tissue disease)
- Cardiac status: continuous monitoring of BP at time of cementing (A-line or NIBP 1 min cycle), end-tidal CO_2. Consider PA catheter (as above), TEE (intravascular volume, RV function, severity of emboli released after cementing, paradoxical emboli), ECG with ST-segment trending
- Exhaled gas analysis: ↓ end-tidal CO_2 if significant pulm embolism; ↑ end-tidal N_2 if air embolus
- Pulm: blood gas analysis, pulse oximetry

SURGICAL STAGES

Pre-Cement

- THR: insidious blood loss due to irrigation
- TKR: tourniquet-induced HTN (tourniquet time >45 min)
- Maintain intravascular volume
- Upon mixing of cement and cementing, volume load with colloid, crystalloid, or autologous blood)
- Discontinue N_2O during mixing of polymer
- Have inotrope available

Cementing

- Hypotension can result from monomer-induced vasodilation, open IV fluids
- FIO_2 100% to combat ↑ PVR from emboli
- If GA, lighten anesthetic and discontinue N_2O, maintain NMB
- Give inotrope (epinephrine or dobutamine) if 20% ↓ MAP

ANTICIPATED PROBLEMS/CONCERNS

- Intraoperative hypovolemia
- Impaired cardiopulmonary function leads to ↓ tolerance to cementing
- Fat embolism syndrome (hypoxemia, petechiae, neuro change)

KIDNEY TRANSPLANTATION

Dennis W. Coalson, M.D.

RISK

- 25,000 patients with ESRD on waiting list in USA 1993
- 7000 cadaveric, 2000 living related transplants 1993
- 60% cadaveric donors and recipients are male, 80% recipients between ages 19–44 years
- Cadaveric donors 80% Caucasian, 10% African-American; cadaveric recipients 67% Caucasian, 20% African-American

PERIOPERATIVE RISKS

- 1–2% 30-d mortality
- Allograft survival: 1-y cadaveric graft survival: 83% primary grafts, 80% secondary grafts, 79% subsequent grafts
- Hyperacute rejection episode

WORRY ABOUT

- Hypovolemia or hypervolemia depending on dialysis-surgery interval
- Hyperkalemia with long interval since dialysis
- Prolonged duration of drugs excreted by kidneys
- Protection of hemodialysis access site, AV shunt or fistulas

- Noncardiogenic pulm edema with perioperative administration of OKT3
- Complications of IDDM (gastroparesis, CAD, autonomic neuropathy)
- Positioning: diabetics at increased risk for perioperative nerve injuries

OVERVIEW

- Extraperitoneal graft placement results in smaller fluid loss
- Potential for rapid blood loss
- Blood volume expansion desired to promote diuresis and early graft function

ICD-9-CM Code: 585

INDICATIONS AND USUAL TREATMENT

- Treatment of choice for patients with ESRD. Improves quality of life and increases life expectancy
- Cause of ESRD: IDDM (31%), chronic glomerulonephritis (28%), polycystic kidney disease (12%), nephrosclerosis (9%), systemic lupus erythematosus (3%), interstitial nephritis (3%), IgA nephropathy (2%), Alport's syndrome (1%)
- Most common cause by race: type I diabetes in Caucasians, hypertensive nephrosclerosis in African-Americans, and chronic glomerulonephritis in Hispanics and Asians
- Alternative therapies: hemodialysis, peritoneal dialysis

ASSESSMENT POINTS

SYSTEM	EFFECT	ASSESSMENT BY HX	PE	TEST
CV/RESP	Hypervolemia Hyperkalemia	SOB	Rales, tachypnea Irregular HR	CXR, ABG, ECG, electrolytes
HEME	Anemia		Systolic murmur, pale mucous membranes	Hct
PNS	Peripheral neuropathy, gastroparesis, autonomic neuropathy	Early satiety, nausea, postural syncope	↓ Peripheral sensation	Tilt test, gastric emptying studies
MS	Osteopenia	Fractures		Bone density

Key Reference: Suthanthiran M: Renal transplantation. N Engl J Med 1994; 331:365.

PERIOPERATIVE MANAGEMENT

- Administration of antibiotics and attention to sterile technique in catheter placement
- Volume status monitoring and potential blood loss a concern
- Consider invasive arterial and CVP measurement
- UO absent or unreliable marker of volume status
- Administration of immunosuppressives prior to graft reperfusion
- Maximize renal blood flow at time of graft reperfusion with blood volume expansion and pharmacologic promotion of diuresis with mannitol, furosemide, and dopamine (2-4 µg/kg/min)

Anesthetic Technique

- General or regional (epidural) acceptable
- Rapid-sequence induction if full stomach or gastroparesis present

Surgical Stages

- Skin incision—Adults: oblique lower abdominal incision for placement of graft in extraperitoneal iliac fossa
  - Small children: midline abdominal incision for retroperitoneal placement of graft
- Renal artery anastomosed end-to-end to recipient's artery or end-to-side to internal or common iliac artery
- Renal vein anastomosed to external iliac vein in adults and to inferior vena cava in children
- Donor ureter inserted by creating submucosal tunnel in recipient's bladder

POSTOPERATIVE CONSIDERATIONS

- Maintain normal to elevated art pressure and CVP to maximize renal blood flow
- Pain relief with PCA or epidural analgesia. If graft does not have early function, avoid prolonged use of meperidine/morphine
- Watch for fluid overload and pulm edema

ANTICIPATED PROBLEMS/CONCERNS

- Noncardiogenic pulm edema if OKT3 given intraoperatively
- Sudden BP drops with local vasodilators used by surgeon

KNEE ARTHROSCOPY

Nigel E. Sharrock, M.B., Ch.B.

RISK

- Arthroscopy of knee: in USA, >700,000/y
- Arthroscopic anterior cruciate (ligament) repair: in USA, 100,000/y
- Patients primarily <60 y—related to athletic injury
- No racial or gender predominance

PERIOPERATIVE RISKS

- Mortality rate <1:10,000
- Morbidity
  - Rare
  - Infection (esp. with allografts)
  - Deep vein thrombosis/pulm embolism in patients >40 y if tourniquet used
  - Nerve injury to superficial branches of femoral nerve resulting in neural trauma–associated sympathetically maintained pain
  - Popliteal artery injury

WORRY ABOUT

- Risk of bradycardia/asystole following tourniquet deflation or with regional anesthesia
- Risk of dural puncture in young patients
- Ability to discharge ambulatory patients
- Whether patient has an empty stomach
- Technical problems with obese or very muscular patients

OVERVIEW

- Arthroscopy is rapid ambulatory procedure in which arthroscope and repairing instruments/medications are inserted into joint; anatomic defects are viewed and recorded; and repair is initiated
- Very low perioperative mortality and morbidity
- Regional anesthesia preferred: early discharge, reduced pain, patients able to participate by viewing surgery on monitor
- Postop pain control an issue, esp. following ACL repair
- MRI diagnosis

ICD-9-CM Codes: 717.83 (Anterior cruciate ligament tear); 836.0 (medial meniscus tear)

INDICATIONS AND USUAL TREATMENT

- Meniscectomy or meniscal repair for torn medial or lateral meniscus
- Removal of loose bodies
- Reconstruction of torn ACL
- Debridement of osteochondral defects or osteoarthritis
- Synovectomy for inflammatory arthritis
- Nonsurgical treatment includes NSAIDs, physical therapy to increase strength of quadriceps, intra-articular steroids

ASSESSMENT POINTS

SYSTEM	EFFECT	ASSESSMENT BY HX	PE	TEST
CV	Risk of bradycardia/asystole due to tourniquet deflation, conduction anesthesia, emotional reaction	Hx of athletic state	Slow resting HR	ECG
HEME	Bleeding diathesis contraindication to regional anesthesia	Bleeding or bruising with injury or tooth extraction	Bruises	PT, aPTT, plt count, bleeding time as indicated by Hx
GU	Postop urinary retention	Nocturia Hx of prior catheterization	Size of prostate	
CNS	Risk of bradycardia/hypotension and nausea with sight of blood/surgery	Fainting or stress prior surgery Rx with anxiolytic medication	Visibly anxious	

Key Reference: Small NC, Sledge CB, Katz JN: A conceptual framework for outcomes research in arthroscopic meniscectomy: results of a nominal group process. Arthroscopy 1994;10:486–492.

PERIOPERATIVE IMPLICATIONS

Preoperative Issues

- Does patient want to watch procedure?
- Focus on early discharge
- Potential length of procedure

Monitoring

- Routine

Anesthetic Technique

- Local infiltration of portals + intra-articular injection of 20–30 ml 0.25% bupivacaine (often requires additional sedation). Cannot tolerate thigh tourniquet
- Femoral nerve block—limited by tourniquet and surgery in back of knee
- Epidural, spinal, or combined spinal epidural. Issues are dural puncture headache, duration of surgery, and rate of onset and resolution of blockade
- Conscious to deep sedation to GA: Issues are short-acting agents (e.g., propofol/desflurane), airway problems, N/V, orthostatic dizziness postop
- Choice depends on duration of surgery, use of thigh tourniquet, the surgeon, patient preference, ease of discharge
- Induction—infiltration, blocks, intra-articular local anesthetic usually performed 15 to 20 min before surgery
- Spinal/epidural: control hemodynamic state
- GA: airway/full stomach

SURGICAL STAGES

Incisions

- Multiple portals around knee
- Tourniquet—pain may limit use if surgery is long—advantage of epidural or combined spinal epidural
- Watch for bradycardia/hypotension with deflation of tourniquet
- Excessive bleeding can occur—observe on monitor
- Irrigation can distend soft tissues around knee
- Rotation of leg can stress hip joint or lumbar spine (figure 4 position)

POSTOPERATIVE CONSIDERATIONS

- Control of pain and side effects can lead to early discharge
- N/V and orthostatic dizziness limit discharge, esp. after deep sedation or GA, excessive sedation, or use of narcotics (less of a problem after regional anesthesia)
- Pain control—easier with regional anesthesia
- Options—intra-articular drugs, e.g., bupivacaine ± morphine
- Local infiltration of portals with bupivacaine
- Femoral nerve blocks helpful after ACL repair, synovectomy, debridement or lateral release
- IV or IM NSAIDs reduce narcotic requirement
- Narcotics—IV morphine (2 mg boluses) or oral medications every 3–4 h
- Urinary retention usually not limiting factor in young patients
- Follow-up phone call helps define and treat problems

ANTICIPATED PROBLEMS/CONCERNS

- Postop back pain (with or without regional anesthesia)
- Dural puncture headaches—should be followed and treated
- Postop pain usually controlled with oral medication
- Late urinary retention
- Bradycardia and hypotension can occur

LABOR — EPIDURAL BLOCK

Raymond S. Sinatra, M.D., Ph.D.

RISK

- ~16–17% of laboring women receive epidural analgesia
- Higher rates of use occur in hospitals with >1500 deliveries/y; placement dependent upon availability of skilled anesthesia caregivers

PERIOPERATIVE RISKS

- Hypotension 2° to sympathetic blockade; incidence as high as 17% in parturients not given adequate prehydration
- Inadequate analgesia 2° to unilateral block, dermatomal "window," rapid progression of labor
- Intravascular injection (risk of seizure and cardiotoxicity) 2° to needle insertion or catheter migration into epidural vein
- Other risks include excessive sensory, motor block, backache, transient and persistent paresthesias

WORRY ABOUT

- Reduction in uteroplacental perfusion, fetal hypoxia/acidosis.
- CV collapse/convulsions 2° to intravascular injection of local anesthetic.
- Early placement of labor epidural block (e.g., primiparas <3–4 cm cervical dilation) or use of concentrated local anesthetic may slow progress of labor and increase incidence of dystocia and C-section.
- High level of anesthesia "total spinal" with loss of airway (incidence 1/4500) related to excessive dose or to subarachnoid or subdural injections; hypoxemia and acidosis develop rapidly in parturients and cardiopulmonary resuscitation is difficult.
- Epidural hematoma/epidural abscess may occur with abnormal hemostasis (preeclampsia, abruption, ITP), underlying sepsis.

OVERVIEW

- During 1st stage of labor, combinations of dilute local anesthetics and opioids effectively block pain impulses from uterus and cervix that travel via visceral afferent fibers (T10–T12, L1).

- During 2nd stage, epidural analgesia extended caudally to block input from S2–S4, controlling pain associated with vaginal and perineal distention.

INDICATIONS

- Nearly complete pain relief with higher satisfaction than any other labor analgesia; reduces maternal stress response and may improve uteroplacental perfusion
- Facilitation of vaginal delivery of twins and preterm infants; control of catecholamine release and maternal BP in preeclampsia and cardiac disease
- Contraindications include patient refusal, infection at site of placement, uncooperative patient, ↑ ICP, coagulopathy, uncorrected hypovolemia, certain cardiac conditions. Alternatives include parenteral opioids, intrathecal opioids, distraction, TENS, hypnotherapy

ASSESSMENT POINTS

SYSTEM	EFFECT	ASSESSMENT BY HX	PE	TEST
CV	Aortocaval compression	Dizziness, syncope ↓ FHR	Hypotension in supine position	Assess UO, provide left uterine displacement
RESP	↓ FRC ↑ Minute ventilation and O₂ consumption	Rapid development of hypoxemia	Tachypnea	Avoid high spinal blockade; provide supplemental O₂
CNS	↓ MAC Epidural vein distention	Exaggerated effect of local anesthetics	Sedation; ↑ sensory and motor block	Assess dermatomal blockade frequently
COAGULATION	↓ Plt count, abnormal function	Abnormal hemostasis	Oozing at IV site Bruising	Assess plt count Fibrinogen, FSPs, check bleeding time
FETAL HEART RATE	Sensitive to maternal hypotension	Bradycardia, ↓ HR variability	↓ Movement HR variability; meconium	Phonocardiogram, fetal scalp blood sampling

Key Reference: Chestnut DH, et al: Does early administration of epidural analgesia affect obstetric outcome in nulliparous women who are receiving oxytocin? Anesthesiology 1994; 80:1193–1200.

PERIOPERATIVE MANAGEMENT

Monitoring

- Establish BP and continuous maternal/fetal HR monitoring
- Assess airway; have resuscitation drugs and equipment immediately available
- Prehydrate with 750–1000 ml Ringer's lactate

Induction

- Epidural needle and subsequent catheter insertion at the L2–3 or L3–4 interspace. Test dose 3 ml local anesthetic solution containing 5 μg/ml epinephrine (epinephrine test dose controversial in labor)

- Maintain left uterine displacement; treat maternal hypotension with small doses of ephedrine (5–10 mg IV)

SURGICAL STAGES

- Very dilute local anesthetic/opioid solutions indicated for primiparas <5 cm cervical dilation. More concentrated solutions safely provided to multiparas
- Epidural induction—bupivacaine 0.25% (8–10 ml) + fentanyl (50–75 μg), sufentanil (10–15 μg), or hydromorphone (200 μg). Lidocaine 1% may be utilized in multiparas.
- Epidural infusion—bupivacaine 0.063%–0.125% with fentanyl 1–2 μg/ml at 10–14 ml/h

- May be maintained for episiotomy repair or to facilitate removal of retained placenta
- May be extended with lidocaine 2% (15–20 ml) for C-section

ANTICIPATED PROBLEMS/CONCERNS

- Technical difficulty 2° to obesity, edema, patient movement; multiple attempts ↑ risk of dural puncture, backache, paresthesia
- Fetal hypoxia 2° to ↓ uteroplacental blood flow. Neonatal CNS depression related to opioid/local anesthetic exposure
- Motor blockade, excessive relaxation of pelvic floor, ↓ ability to push, need for oxytocin augmentation, possible ↑ length of 1st and 2nd stages of labor

LABOR — PERIPHERAL BLOCKS

Martin G. Cascio, M.D.
Sivam Ramanathan, M.D.

RISK

- Pregnant women in labor who request analgesia

PERIOPERATIVE RISKS

- Perioperative mortality from anesthetic technique: rare
- Morbidity—maternal IV local anesthetic (LA) injection: risk of seizures and cardiotoxicity
- Morbidity—fetal bradycardia

WORRY ABOUT

- IV injection
- Hypotension
- Fetal bradycardia (paracervical block)
- Nerve damage
- Infection

OVERVIEW

- Lumbar sympathetic block (LSB)—analgesia for 1st stage of labor
- Paracervical block—analgesia for 1st stage of labor
- Pudendal block—analgesia for 2nd stage of labor

ICD-9-CM Code: V22.2 (for pregnancy)

INDICATIONS AND USUAL TREATMENT

- Indications—parturient in whom regional, parenteral, or other means of analgesia are not possible
- Lumbar sympathetic block may accelerate 1st stage of labor. Avoid in patients with history of uterine hyperstimulation
- Paracervical block may produce fetal bradycardia

ASSESSMENT POINTS (potential complications)

SYSTEM	EFFECT	ASSESSMENT BY HX	PE	TEST
CV	Cardiac arrest Hypotension (LSB) Hematoma	IV injection Vessel puncture	Unresponsive peripheral vasodilation Swelling	ECG BP
CNS	Total spinal nerve damage Seizures	SA injection IV injection	Loss of consciousness Neuropathy	 EMG
FETAL	Bradycardia	Fetal absorption		FHR
INFECTIOUS	Retropsoas abscess Subgluteal abscess	Poor aseptic technique	Fever, pain	MRI

Key Reference: Norris MC: Obstetric Anesthesia. Philadelphia, JB Lippincott, 1993.

PERIOPERATIVE IMPLICATIONS

Anesthetic Technique

Lumbar Sympathetic Block

- Patient prone
- Bilateral L2 transverse processes
- Needle advanced approx. 9 cm to anterolateral surface of vertebra
- 10 ml of LA will block entire lumbar sympathetic chain
- Analgesia 2–3 h

Paracervical Block

- Blocks Frankenhäuser's plexus
- Lithotomy position
- 1st injection—lateral fornix of vagina at "4 o'clock" position 0.5 cm deep
- 3–5 ml LA each side
- Assess fetal HR
- 2nd injection at "8 o'clock" position
- Epinephrine with LA may ↑ fetal bradycardia

Pudendal Block

- Perineal anesthesia for 2nd stage of labor, episiotomy, forceps or vacuum delivery
- Transvaginal approach
- Bilateral injections 1 cm posteromedial to ischial spines
- 10 ml of LA

LAPAROSCOPY, GYNECOLOGIC

Susan Chan, M.D.

RISK

- >400,000 patients underwent laparoscopy in USA in 1994; female > male (50:1)
- Most common gyn surgical procedure

PERIOPERATIVE RISKS

- Mortality: 1.6–11/100,000
- CV complications (e.g., air embolus): 1–10/100,000
- Intra-abdominal complications—1%
- Postop pain necessitating hospitalization—0.5–2%

WORRY ABOUT

- Hypercarbia, resp acidosis, hypoxemia, pulm HTN, systemic vasodilation
- Pressure of pneumoperitoneum
- Hypothermia
- Pulm—atelectasis, ↓ FRC, high peak airway pressure, CO_2 embolus
- CV— ↓ venous return, ↓ cardiac output, cardiac dysrhythmia
- Gastric reflux—esp in patients with gastroparesis, hiatal hernia, obesity, or gastric outlet obstruction

OVERVIEW

- Endoscopic technique to visualize pelvic structure
- Adhesions and endometriosis can be treated endoscopically
- A small incision below umbilicus is made to insufflate CO_2 and 2 or more slightly larger incisions for insertion of visualization devices and instruments.
- Duration of hospital stay significantly reduced. Most performed on outpatient basis, but duration of procedure may exceed that for open technique.
- Surgical complications include misplacement of Veress needle or trocar resulting in acute hemorrhage; bowel, bladder, uterus perforation; subcutaneous emphysema

ICD-9-CM Code: 54.21

INDICATIONS

- Tubal ligation, ectopic pregnancy, vaginal hysterectomy, PID, infertility

ASSESSMENT POINTS

SYSTEM	EFFECT	ASSESSMENT BY HX	PE	TEST
CV	CV arrhythmia; ↓ venous return; ↑ level of stress hormones.	Chest pain, SOB, Hx of CAD, DM, arrhythmia	CV exam	ECG
RESP	If pre-existing lung disease, hypercarbia, acidosis, hypoxia not tolerated well	SOB, ↓ exercise tolerance	Chest exam	O_2 sat ?ABG
GI	↑ Intra-abdominal pressure; Trendelenburg position may ↑ chance of aspiration	DM, gastroparesis, hiatal hernia, obesity, gastric outlet obstruction	Airway exam	
HEME	Minimal blood loss normally	Hx of anemia, exercise tolerance	Vital signs	?Hct

Key Reference: Chi IC, Potts M, Wilkens L: Rare events associated with tubal sterilizations: An international experience. Obstet Gynecol Surv 1986; 41:7–19.

INTRAOPERATIVE MANAGEMENT

Monitoring

- Postop course more benign than in open procedure, yet intraoperative period may have much physiologic derangement
- Routine with end-tidal CO_2 waveform

Airway

- ↑ Risk of passive regurgitation and aspiration due to Trendelenburg position and ↑ intra-abdominal pressure. GA with ET intubation most common.
- Laryngeal mask airway satisfactory alternative in nonobese patients undergoing relatively short procedures.

Anesthetic Technique

- No advantage of less physiologic stress has been shown by using regional anesthesia
- With ↑ intra-abdominal pressure, ↑ ventilatory pressures required to ventilate
- Nasogastric tube recommended to minimize gastric reflux
- Complete relaxation of abdominal muscle

Postoperative Considerations

- Pain score 2–8 depending on procedure
- Potent opioid analgesics (fentanyl) most commonly used. NSAID ketorolac, 60 mg IM or IV, shown to decrease postop analgesic requirement

ANTICIPATED PROBLEMS/CONCERNS

- Hypercarbia and acidosis most common physiologic complications when CO_2 used
- Subcutaneous emphysema, pneumothorax, pneumopericardium, pneumomediastinum, gas embolism less common
- Hypothermia and cardiac arrhythmia may be due to ↑ ventricular irritability, ↓ venous return, ↓ cardiac output, hypoventilation, gas embolism, or profound vagal response
- Blind insertion of the Veress needle or trocar associated with injuries to hollow viscera, major vessels, abdominal wall vessels

LARYNGOSCOPY

Andranik Ovassapian, M.D.

RISK

- Procedure used in millions of patients, to visualize pharynx and larynx for diagnostic/therapeutic purposes
- All age groups

PERIOPERATIVE RISKS

- Depends on nature of complaint and underlying disease
- HTN and tachycardia common because of pain and stimulation of airway reflexes
- Higher incidence of postextubation airway obstruction and reintubation than without tracheal intubation
- Incidence of reintubation when laryngoscopy performed for upper airway pathology: 0.39%

WORRY ABOUT

- CV response to laryngoscopy
- Postextubation laryngeal spasm and airway obstruction
- Establishing airway in postextubation period

OVERVIEW

- Rigid laryngoscopy associated with severe CV responses and increase in plasma catecholamine concentrations.
- If difficult laryngoscopy associated with difficult mask ventilation, can cause cerebral damage and death in paralyzed patient

INDICATIONS AND USUAL TREATMENT

- Routinely applied for tracheal intubation during GA
- In combination of esophagoscopy and bronchoscopy, is applied for diagnosis and staging of oropharyngolaryngeal malignant lesions

ASSESSMENT POINTS

SYSTEM	EFFECT	ASSESSMENT BY HX	PE	TEST
HEENT	Upper airway obstruction due to tumor edema Limitation of movement	Degree of compromise Airflow pattern Snoring Stridor	Mandibular subluxation Size of tongue Head and neck anatomy Mouth opening Neck ROM	Lateral x-ray CT scan Barium swallow Flow-volume loop
CV	Ischemic CAD potential	CAD Hx: chest pain CHF Sx	Hr Rate and rhythm; S3; rales	ECG with stress
GI	Aspiration potential	GE junction integrity by Hx of regurgitation Nighttime cough Sour nighttime taste	Evaluate nutritional status	Esophagoscopy Examination of larynx
CNS	Sleep dysfunction due to obstruction	Sleep history	CNS exam	MRI
RESP	Upper airway obstruction due to tumor	Tumor Hx	Wheezing Cyanosis Clubbing	Flow-volume loop; ABG

PERIOPERATIVE MANAGEMENT

Preoperative Preparation

- Dependent on indication:
–If laryngeal tumors, evaluate for degree of airway compromise
–If stridor present, closely observe, preferably in ICU. Humidified O_2 and steroids may be given to avoid severe/complete airway obstruction
- Patient lies supine with head and neck in sniffing position when laryngoscopy performed for tracheal intubation. When performed by otolaryngologist for Dx and therapy, head and neck hyperextended.

Monitoring

- Routine

Anesthetic Technique

- Done with great caution and with spontaneous ventilation if Sx of compromised upper airway
- Secure airway with patient awake under topical anesthesia if resp failure due to airway obstruction
- Short-acting IV drugs (e.g., alfentanil, midazolam, esmolol) may provide analgesia and attenuate CV response to rigid laryngoscopy
- Surgical blood loss negligible

Postoperative Concerns

- CV hyperactivity
- Status of upper airway

ANTICIPATED PROBLEMS/CONCERNS

- Difficult mask ventilation and difficult intubation in immediate postop period common

LASER SURGERY OF AIRWAY

Ira J. Rampil, M.D.

RISK

- People within USA: 3000–5000/y
- Race/gender predominance: None

PERIOPERATIVE RISKS

- Postop airway compromise
- Airway fires (5–70 reported/y)

WORRY ABOUT

- Loss of patent airway
- Displacement or ignition of ET tube
- Postop laryngospasm
- Residual NMB
- Misdirected laser beam
- Infection of OR personnel by vaporized papillomavirus

OVERVIEW

- Focused, coherent far-infrared (CO_2) laser light can precisely vaporize superficial tissue lesions at a distance
- Shorter wavelength (i.e., Nd-YAG) laser light can coagulate and necrose deeper lesions

ICD-9-CM Code: 478.4 (Laryngeal polyp)

INDICATIONS

- Many heterogeneous conditions, including laryngeal papilloma, tracheal scarring, webs or synechiae, vascular malformations, neoplasms, idiopathic subglottic stenosis

ASSESSMENT POINTS

SYSTEM	EFFECT	ASSESSMENT BY HX	PE	TEST
HEENT	Glottic or tracheal stenosis	DOE Stridor	Mallampatti exam	Indirect laryngoscopy PFTs (flow-volume loop)
RESP	Neoplasia (V/Q mismatch)	Hemoptysis	Auscultation	CT or MRI of chest ABG

Key Reference: Rampil IJ: Anesthetic considerations for laser surgery. Anesth Analg 1992; 74:424–435.

PERIOPERATIVE IMPLICATIONS

Preoperative Preparation

- Consider antisialagogue
- Eye protection for OR personnel

Anesthetic Technique

- GA
- FIO_2 ≤40% to retard combustion, consider FIO_2 of 21%
- Avoid N_2O as it supports combustion
- Complete neuromuscular blockade

Monitoring

- Routine

Airway

- Use protected ET tubes, either commercial or smoothly wrapped with metal foil
- To allow surgical access, use smallest diameter tube consistent with adequate ventilation, i.e., 5.5 to 6.5 mm outside diameter for adults

Maintenance

- Maintain close communication with surgeon as procedure may conclude without significant lead time.
- Be ready to emergently extubate trachea and provide mask ventilation in event of airway fire.

Extubation

- Despite suctioning, pharynx may contain blood that may promote laryngospasm
- Some surgeons have strong preference for "deep" extubation following vocal cord surgery in order to avoid cough-induced injury

Postoperative Period

- Stridor, excess coughing, or bronchospasm warrants immediate investigation

Adjuvants

- Topical lidocaine ointment on ET tube and/or saline in cuff may retard ignition
- Surgeons may place moist pledgets in airway—be sure to retrieve them.

ANTICIPATED PROBLEMS/CONCERNS

- Airway fire: clamp ET tube and remove; then reintubate with new ET tube

LIVER RESECTION

Steven M. Frank, M.D.

RISK

- Primary neoplasms: 5% of hepatic tumors
- Incidence: 4/100,000
- Males > females: 2:1
- Racial predominance: Asian
- Metastatic neoplasms—95% of hepatic tumors, mostly from GI tract

PERIOPERATIVE RISKS

- 1–10% perioperative mortality, dependent on institution and co-morbidities of patient
- CV collapse from hypovolemia or vena cava crossclamp
- Morbidity: hepatic failure (5%), intra-abdominal infection (10–15%)

WORRY ABOUT

- Blood loss and proximity of blood bank
- IV access
- Need for vena cava crossclamp, and inability of liver to clear fibrin degradation products

OVERVIEW

- Surgical removal of tumors if no end-stage liver disease and potential to increase longevity or quality of life
- Potential for blood loss is increased with inexperienced surgical staff, large tumors, tumors located near porta hepatis or vena cava

- Consider intraoperative hemodilution to ↓ need for banked blood
- Consider veno-veno bypass when IVC crossclamp may be required

ICD-9-CM Code: 235.3 (Neoplasm)

INDICATIONS AND USUAL TREATMENT

- Benign tumors: liver cell adenoma, hemangioma
- Malignant
  - Metastatic—GI tract, lung, breast, esophagus
  - Primary—hepatocellular carcinoma, cholangiocarcinoma, hepatoblastoma, angiosarcoma, lymphoma

ASSESSMENT POINTS

SYSTEM	EFFECT	ASSESSMENT BY HX	PE	TEST
RESP	Restrictive lung disease due to ascites	Dyspnea		Pericentesis
GI	Ascites	Ability to lie flat	Fluid wave Abd girth	Pericentesis
HEME	Splenomegaly can ↓ plt	Bleeding Hx	Petechiae	Plt count, Hct
RENAL	Hepatorenal syndrome	UO	Uremia signs	BUN/Cr

INTRAOPERATIVE MANAGEMENT

Preoperative Preparation

- Check availability of blood in bank or blood collection bags for hemodilution
- Check availability of FFP, plt, RBCs

Monitoring

- If large blood loss expected, consider arterial, CVP, and large-bore venous lines
- Clinical suspicion for venous air embolus

SURGICAL STAGES

Induction

- Consider rapid-sequence technique if ascites

Skin Incision

- Large RUQ incision

Dissection

- Cavitron (US), scalpel, finger dissection, cautery (electro- or argon beam)
- Wedge resection: least invasive; segmentectomy: moderately invasive; lobectomy: very invasive; trisegmentectomy: most invasive

Intraoperative Problems

- Vena cava crossclamp needed for tumor invasion into cava— ↓ venous return
- Need for veno-veno bypass—from iliac vein to internal jugular
  - best accomplished through extra large-bore percutaneously placed introducer

Closure and Postoperative Considerations

- Patients often remain intubated postop if large amount of IV fluid given or if hemodynamically unstable
- Can observe for postop bleeding through drains
- Analgesia can be by IV or epidural PCA
- EBL: 500–2000 ml
- Pain score: 8–10

ANTICIPATED PROBLEMS/CONCERNS

- Blood loss/hypovolemia—ensure IV access, blood availability; titrate anesthesia
- Need for plt after ~1 blood volume transfusion
- Need for FFP after ~1–2 blood volumes

LIVER TRANSPLANTATION

Deborah M. Barron, M.D.
Simon Gelman, M.D., Ph.D.

RISK

- 2500 people within USA/y
- Estimated need of 15/1million population

PERIOPERATIVE RISKS

- Mortality decreasing with recent advances
- Morbidity: Bleeding, infection
- 90% 6-mo survival
- 82% 2-y survival
- 1 y allograft survival of >70%
- Five-year survival is 65%

WORRY ABOUT

- Massive blood loss
- Right heart failure upon liver reperfusion
- Nerve injury from positioning
- Coagulopathies
- Metabolic disturbances

OVERVIEW

- Liver removed and replaced with donor liver
- Significant blood loss associated with procedure
- Usually occurs within 24 h of removal from donor

ICD-9-CM Codes: 571.9 (for chronic liver disease); 155.0 (for primary liver neoplasm)

INDICATIONS AND USUAL TREATMENT

- Replacement of liver due to end-stage liver disease, hepatic failure or malignancy, inherited metabolic abnormality

ASSESSMENT POINTS

SYSTEM	EFFECT	ASSESSMENT BY HX	PE	TEST
CV	Vasodilatation, ↓ SVR ↑ Cardiac output, splanchnic hypervolemia, central hypovolemia, ventricular dysfunction, pericardial effusion			MUGA, ECHO, coronary Angio, ECG, radionuclide scintigraphy, cardiac stress test
RESP	ARDS, pleural effusion, pulmonary HTN, hepatopulmonary syndrome, atelectasis due to ascites, restrictive lung defect	SOB, DOE	Auscultation	CXR, PFTs, pulm Angio
GI	Ascites, GI bleeding, portal HTN Esophageal varices, delayed gastric emptying			LFTs, UGI endoscopy, mesenteric angiography
HEME	Thrombocytopenia Coagulopathies			CBC, PT, PTT, fibrinogen
RENAL	Hepatorenal syndrome Acute tubular necrosis (rare)			BUN, Cr
CNS	Encephalopathy, coma, ICP increase	Mental status changes	Pupillary findings, abnormal posturing	ICP monitor, EEG, MCA Doppler
INFECTION	Infections, sepsis			HIV test, hepatitis B vaccine Fungal, parasite, viral serologies
NUTRITION	Malnutrition			Albumin
ELECTROLYTES				Glucose, Na+, K+, Ca2+

Key Reference: Carton EG, Plevak DJ, Kranner PW, et al: Perioperative care of the liver transplant patient. Anesth Analg 1994; 78:120–133; 382–399.

PERIOPERATIVE IMPLICATIONS

Preoperative Preparation

- Correction of coagulopathies and lyte imbalances
- Drainage of pleural effusions

Monitoring

- Meticulous sterile technique as immunocompromised
- Large-bore IV lines
- Consider bilateral arterial lines—1 for hemodynamic monitoring, 1 for blood-drawing capability
- Central access—two 8.5F percutaneous sheaths, proximal for volume administration, distal for placement of PA catheter if one jugular vein is used
- Consider TEE (concern for varices) to identify and treat CV dysfunction
- Foley catheter

Induction

- Rapid-sequence induction following oral sodium citrate premedication

Maintenance

- Avoid drugs that ↓ SVR
- However, vasodilating prostagladins may be used on reperfusion
- Administration of low-dose dopamine for potential preservation of renal function

- Carefully titrate drugs because of changes in pharmacodynamics and pharmacokinetics
- Administer air/O₂ combination. Avoid nitrous oxide because of intestinal accumulation and metabolic disturbances
- Consider PEEP to optimize oxygenation
- Monitor K+ and Ca2+ carefully because of large administration of blood products

SURGICAL STAGES

- Dissection: Major bleeding associated with dissection possible because of prior surgeries, portal HTN, coagulopathies

Anhepatic Stage

- Clamping of portal vein, hepatic artery, IVC above and below liver
- Clamping of IVC causes decrease in preload, cardiac output, and BP
- Veno-veno bypass is usually utilized: femoral and portal vein catheters decompress venous system during anhepatic phase
- Blood returned to right atrium via axillary or jugular cannulas
- Consider use of vasopressors and/or inotropes to maintain hemodynamic stability

Neohepatic Stage

- Major profound, but transient, CV instability (hypotension, high ventricular filling pressures, bradycardia, significant decreases in SVR) can occur

- May be due to citrate intoxication, hemorrhage, cold hyperkalemic blood, or air or particulate emboli; require immediate treatment including epinephrine and calcium chloride
- Keep Hct <35; higher Hct ↑ risk of hepatic artery thrombosis
- Following graft perfusion, adequate function indicated by a PT of ≤16 sec

Postoperative Considerations

- Significant postop pain
- Pain relief from IV narcotics administered by medical team, then by PCA
- Observe for postop bleeding—correct coagulopathies, re-explore if necessary
- Persistent hypocalcemia, lactic acidosis, hemodynamic instability, hyperglycemia, coagulopathies indicate poor function of transplanted liver

ANTICIPATED PROBLEMS/CONCERNS

- Massive blood loss may require blood-salvaging equipment and rapid-infusion devices
- Avoid salvaged blood in transplantation for treatment of cancer
- Need for access to large amounts of packed RBC, plt concentrates, FFP
- Blood should be seronegative to minimize infection transmission
- Careful attention to positioning of patient and to minimizing hypothermia

LUMBAR LAMINECTOMY

Sally C. Palmon, M.D.

RISK

- Up to 80% of USA population have at least temporary disability from low back pain (even Michael Jordan). Majority without neurologic deficit recover with conservative therapy; <5% undergo surgery.
- Laminectomy for ruptured disk is most common major neurosurgical procedure
- Most common site of herniated nucleus pulposus is L4–L5 or L5–S1. Spinal cord ends at L2; therefore problems related to cord dysfunction are extremely rare.

PERIOPERATIVE RISKS

- Mortality rate ≤0.02%
- Continuing or recurrent pain is most common postop complication
- Life-threatening complications: hemorrhage from major vascular injury 0–1.6%; pulm embolism, thrombophlebitis, visceral injuries 0–0.5%

WORRY ABOUT

- Hemorrhage due to perforation of major blood vessel (rare)
- Positioning complications: blindness, brachial plexus injury (esp when horseshoe headset used), meralgia paresthetica or other peripheral nerve injuries, quadriplegia, and Horner's syndrome from hyperextension of neck
- Chest wall and abdominal compression: at risk for resp embarrassment or hypotension due to ↓ preload
- Spinal cord compromise by extruded intervertebral disk
- Period of "monitoring blackout" during which ECG leads and BP monitor disconnected; prone position causes ↓ right heart filling, resulting in ↓ BP

OVERVIEW

- Operative procedures: can be done in prone, lateral, or kneeling position (prone-sitting frame). Last is associated with venous pooling and may cause hypotension. In posterior approaches, midline incised to detach and mobilize paraspinous muscles through subperiosteal technique. Removal of posterior neural arch in piecemeal fashion is termed laminectomy.

ICD-9-CM Codes: 722 (Herniated disk); 724 (spinal stenosis)

INDICATIONS AND USUAL TREATMENT

- Rest, antispasmodics, NSAID
- For lumbar stenosis: a brief course of epidural steroid injections, physiotherapy, or lumbar corset
- When medical therapy fails, surgery is indicated
- Laminectomy for decompression of lumbar stenosis indicated for recurrent intolerable pain associated with leg weakness or radiculopathy that restricts or prevents activities of daily living

ASSESSMENT POINTS

SYSTEM	EFFECT	ASSESSMENT BY HX	PE	TEST
CV		↓ Exercise tolerance—difficult to assess Smoking Hx, pulm disease	Heart murmur, gallop	ECG, ?ECHO
RESP			Lung exam—signs of failure?	PFTs if severe lung disease
CNS/PNS	Peripheral neuropathy, paraplegia, myelopathy or sensory deficit, compromised by prone position	Pain, inability to ambulate, bowel or bladder dysfunction	Sensory deficit, ?motor deficit	Preop evoked potentials, EMG, or MRI/CT
MS	Skeletal metastasis from primary cancer	Primary tumor from breast, lung, kidney, thyroid, prostate Chemotherapy Hx		?CXR, electrolytes (Ca^{2+}), bone scan
PSYCH	Chronic pain, possible substance abuse (opioids)	Multiple medications (narcotics, NSAIDs, antidepressants)		

Key Reference: Bedford R: Surgery of the spine. *In* Frost EAM (ed): Clinical Anesthesia in Neurosurgery. Stoneham, MA, Butterworth-Heinemann, 1991, pp 265–276.

PERIOPERATIVE IMPLICATIONS

Preoperative Preparation

- Preload patient before turning to prone position to avoid CV effects of ↓ preload.

Anesthetic Technique

- Need to know if single- or multilevel decompressive laminectomy to estimate blood loss, monitoring, and time to awakening to obtain neurologic exam
- General ET intubation with inhalational or N$_2$O/narcotic anesthesia and muscle relaxants is preferred but spinal, epidural, or local anesthesia has been used
- If regional chosen, preop evaluation for pre-existing neurologic deficit is important
- To evaluate nerve root stimulation, no muscle relaxant used. Avoid succinylcholine if severe neurologic deficit present (paraplegia)

- If cord compromised with neurologic deficit, attempt to maintain spinal cord perfusion pressure by maintaining BP at preop level

Monitoring

- Consider intra-arterial catheter if severe spinal stenosis or neurologic deficit present

Airway

- Patient in prone position after hours of surgery for multilevel laminectomy with more than usual fluid requirements and blood loss may have airway edema and facial swelling. Be aware of coexisting cervical spine disease. Consider postop ventilation if breathing cannot occur around ET tube when cuff is down.

SURGICAL STAGES

Dissection

- Cauda equina injury (0.01–0.02%) and root injury rare during dissection

- Major vascular injury during dissection also rare (0–1.6%)

Definitive Surgery

- Hypotension may develop from unrecognized blood loss or ↓ preload in prone position
- Air embolism can occur in spinal surgery in prone position (rare)

Postoperative Considerations

- Early neurologic assessment required; consider anesthetic tailored to prompt awakening
- PCA or epidural or spinal analgesia

ANTICIPATED PROBLEMS/CONCERNS

- Problems with prone positioning
- Need for reoperation

LUNG VOLUME REDUCTION SURGERY (PNEUMOPLASTY)

Brett A. Simon, M.D., Ph.D.

RISK

- Severe, activity-limiting pulm emphysema; given prevalence of emphysema (13.5 million Americans affected), the number of potential candidates for this operation is enormous
- Average preop FEV_1 25–30% predicted
- New procedure performed in small number of centers so experience relatively limited

PERIOPERATIVE RISKS

- In-hospital mortality: 3–6%
- 25% morbidity includes prolonged air leaks, resp failure, pulm embolism, pneumonia
- Greatly increased risk of complications in patients with reactive airways disease, CAD, pulm HTN

WORRY ABOUT

- Hypotension due to air trapping with controlled ventilation
- Difficulty with ventilation and oxygenation (less so) during one-lung ventilation
- Exaggerated resp depressive effects of narcotics (IV and neuraxial)

- Minimizing airway pressures and smoothly extubating spontaneously ventilating patient in OR to avoid creating or worsening air leaks

OVERVIEW

- Palliative procedure for severe, activity-limiting emphysema with 20–30% of lungs resected to reduce lung volume and reshape diaphragm and chest wall
- Bovine pericardial strips used to reinforce staple lines and reduce air leaks.
- Variety of unilateral, bilateral, open, and thoracoscopic techniques being explored. Open, bilateral lung volume reduction via median sternotomy is original approach and has best documented results to date.
- Benefit thought to result from improving mechanical function of chest wall and diaphragm by reducing total lung volume, combined with reduction and reshaping of lung tissue; results in increase in lung recoil at this lower volume and increased expiratory flows.
- Patients typically require a great deal of attention to keep them extubated during first several hours postop

- Successful outcome requires team approach including experienced pulmonologists, pulm rehab, thoracic surgeons, anesthesiologists, pain service, chest PT, ICU physicians. Sophisticated pulm function testing and lung imaging facilities should be available

ICD-9-CM Code: 492.8 (Emphysema)

INDICATIONS AND USUAL TREATMENT

- Alternative to lung transplantation for patients with primarily pure emphysema which significantly limits their activity.
- Exclusion criteria include pulm HTN (mean PAP >35 at rest), bronchospasm, LV dysfunction, bronchitis or excessive sputum production, persistent smoking, previous thoracotomy or pleurodesis, obesity, or cachexia.
- All patients required to undergo at least 6 wk of preop pulm rehab, with supplemental O_2 if necessary. Poor results expected if cannot perform at least 800 ft in standard 6-min walk test.
- Successful procedures typically result in 60–70% increase in FEV_1 by 3 mo sustained at least 1 y, ↓ TLC and RV, improved exercise tolerance, and significant reductions in O_2 requirements at rest and during exercise. Long-term results unknown.

ASSESSMENT POINTS

SYSTEM	EFFECT	ASSESSMENT BY HX	PE	TEST
CV	LV/RV dysfunction Pulmonary HTN	CHF, PND, palpitations	Peripheral edema, JVD, S_3	MUGA, ECHO may be unreliable with COPD
RESP	Emphysema	SOB, exercise tolerance and performance with rehab, bronchospasm, sputum production	Wheezing	PFTs, CT, plethysmography, quant. V/Q scan

Key Reference: Cooper JD, et al: Bilateral pneumectomy (volume reduction) for chronic obstructive pulmonary disease. J Thorac Cardiovasc Surg 1995; 109:106–119.

PERIOPERATIVE MANAGEMENT

Preoperative Preparation

- Successful completion of pulm rehab program
- Maximize bronchodilator therapy

Anesthetic Technique

- Thoracic epidural placement at ~T4 interspace for intraop and postop use; test and verify onset of segmental block prior to induction
- Minimize narcotics because of risk of resp depression
- Goal of anesthetic is to maximize possibility of extubation in OR
- Chest tubes placed to water seal only unless suction required

Monitoring

- Arterial line required
- Consider central line for intraoperative infusions and postop fluid management

Airway

- Left-sided double-lumen tube placed for bilateral procedures

Induction/Maintenance

- Anticipate hypotension due to air trapping with chest closed
- Ventilate with low pressures and low rates; tolerate hypercapnia if necessary
- Maintain on low-dose inhaled agent
- Use of epidural depends on hemodynamic stability; consider waiting until chest open before dosing; use of straight local may require phenylephrine infusion for BP maintenance; if narcotics used, limit dose
- Continue bronchodilator therapy in OR if necessary

Surgical Stages

- Bronchoscopy: Flexible bronchoscopy
- Resection: "Better" side, usually right, resected first to improve tolerance of one-lung ventilation when second side resected
- Emergence: Switch to single-lumen tube, LMA, or mask while patient is deep to facilitate emergence
- Elevate head; optimize pain control; suctioning; bronchodilators for emergence

- Patients require 30–90 min observation, encouragement, and "fine-tuning" in OR prior to transport to ICU; first ABG in ICU has PCO_2 >70 mmHg in >50% of patients

Fluid Considerations

- Typically run "dry"
- Significant blood loss requiring transfusion unusual

Postoperative Considerations

- Make every effort to extubate in OR and avoid reintubation and ventilation; if required, use minimum pressure support without mandatory breaths if possible
- Use epidural infusion (⅛–¼% bupivacaine ± 1–3 µg/ml fentanyl) supplemented with nonnarcotic pain relievers
- Pain score 6–8

ANTICIPATED PROBLEMS/CONCERNS

- Extremely marginal patients susceptible to even mild postop insults (pneumonia, pulm embolism, oversedation, pneumothorax, bronchospasm)
- Reintubation and mechanical ventilation associated with high morbidity

MENINGOMYELOCELE REPAIR

Madelyn Kahana, M.D.

RISK

- 2/1000 live births
- Most common in lumbar and lumbosacral segments

PERIOPERATIVE RISKS

- Failure to surgically close in a timely fashion results in ↑ risk of infection
- Coexisting congenital defects largely determine operative risk

WORRY ABOUT

- Coexisting congenital abnormality
- Intraoperative temp instability
- Proper prone positioning

OVERVIEW

- Defect in closure of bony spine at any level associated with defects of meninges and spinal cord
- Associated with high frequency of other abnormalities
- Prenatal diagnosis possible with amniocentesis and US
- Gestational age important as predictor of coexisting pulm insufficiency
- Postop apnea not uncommon following GA in newborn, esp. if premature

ICD-9-CM Codes: 741.9 (without hydrocephalus); 741.0 (with hydrocephalus)

INDICATIONS AND USUAL TREATMENT

- Prompt closure of meningomyelocele with preservation of viable neural tissue after careful evaluation of infant for associated abn, esp. significant cardiac defects
- Initial resuscitation generally unnecessary; wound covered with sterile saline-soaked dressings until operative closure possible

ASSESSMENT POINTS

SYSTEM	EFFECT	ASSESSMENT BY HX	PE	TEST
CV	Associated cardiac defect		Murmur Cyanosis	ECG ECHO O_2 saturation
RESP	Possible IRDS Resp failure	Prematurity High thoracic or cervical lesion		CXR
RENAL	Associated renal anomalies	Abdominal mass		US
CNS	Varying degrees of paralysis Associated Chiari deformity Associated hydrocephalus Associated hydromyelia/ diastematomyelia		Careful neurologic exam	CT US

Key Reference: McClone DG, Dias MS: Complications of myelomeningocele closure. Pediatr Neurosurg 1991–1992; 17:267–273.

INTRAOPERATIVE MANAGEMENT

Preoperative Management

- Meticulous debubbling of lines in patients with septal defects
- Infection control—postop sepsis a major concern

Anesthetic Technique

- Performed under general anesthesia in prone position

Monitoring

- Temp maintenance can be problematic
- Consider a warming mattress and lamps
- Resp status determines need for arterial catheter
- Foley catheter indicated if preop bladder distention

Airway

- Associated proximal bowel atresias may dictate precautions for full stomach intubation

SURGICAL STAGES

Induction

- Consider coexisting cardiac and intestinal malformations in the choice of agents
- Infants prone to hypotension with deep inhalation anesthesia
- Atropine as premedication recommended by some

Dissection and Definitive Surgery

- Minimal blood loss

Postoperative Considerations

- Recovered in prone position
- Apnea a frequent problem, associated with prematurity, GA, Chiari malformation
- Pain postop influenced by sensory level associated with defect
- CSF leaks not uncommon

ANTICIPATED PROBLEMS/CONCERNS

- Associated congenital malformations, especially of heart, brain, intestinal tract
- Comorbidity of prematurity
- Eventual development of latex allergy common

MITRAL VALVE REPLACEMENT

David L. Berger, M.D.

RISK

- Majority of cases are post-rheumatic
- Associated with advancing age and myxomatous degeneration
- Ischemia increasingly a cause
- Gender predominance: none
- Age: 40–75 y

PERIOPERATIVE RISKS

- Perioperative 30-d mortality: 5–8%
- Morbidity – CNS complications: transient neurologic dysfunction 5–10%; CVA 1–2%
  - pneumonia: 10–15%
  - infection: <1%

WORRY ABOUT

- Cardiac failure
- Dysrhythmias
- Hemorrhage
- Tamponade
- Conduction defects
- AV disruption

OVERVIEW

- Mitral valve repair or replacement typically done for correction of post-rheumatic degenerative mitral insufficiency, or repair after endocarditis
- Normal valve area is 4–6 cm^2
- Symptoms occur at 50% decrease in area, with severe symptoms at 1 cm^2
- Severe symptoms if regurgitant fraction >0.6

ICD-9-CM Codes: 394.0 (Stenosis); 424.0 (Insufficiency)

INDICATIONS AND USUAL TREATMENT

- For mitral regurgitation (MR) from posterior leaflet abnormality (myxomatous degeneration, torn chordae) or pure annular dilatation, most valves can be repaired
- For severe rheumatic calcific mitral stenosis (MS), replacement with preservation of subannular structures may be necessary

ASSESSMENT POINTS

SYSTEM	EFFECTS	ASSESSMENT BY HX	PE	TEST
CV	MS: DOE, pulm edema MR: acute: CHF; chronic: DOE, paroxysmal nocturnal dyspnea	Exertional dyspnea, fatigue	Rales S$_3$	ECG ECHO
RESP	Pulm congestion, SOB	SOB	Chest exam	CXR
GI	Hepatic congestion Coagulation problems		Hepatomegaly	LFTs
HEME	May be on anticoagulants			PT, PTT
RENAL	↓ CO may lead to renal failure			BUN, Cr, electrolytes
CNS	CVA due to thrombus in AF		Neuro exam	CT scan, ECHO

Key Reference: DiNardo JA: Anesthesia for valve replacement in patients with acquired valvular heart disease. *In* DeNardo JA, Schwartz MJ (eds): Handbook of Cardiac Surgery. Norwalk, CT, Appleton & Lange, 1990, pp 98–113.

PERIOPERATIVE MANAGEMENT

Preoperative Preparation

- Assess status of ventricular function

Monitoring

- Arterial line
- CVP, PA catheter
- Urinary catheter
- ST segment analysis
- Consider TEE (help in volume management, regional wall motion, assessment of valve repair)

Anesthetic Technique

- GA with low- to moderate-dose narcotic

SURGICAL STAGES

Induction

- MS—hypotension treated with fluid; maintain SVR with phenylephrine if necessary. Avoid tachycardia and treat with increased anesthesia (esmolol if cardiac function adequate). Sinus rhythm should be maintained

- Treat new-onset AFib/flutter with defibrillation. Avoid increases in PVR
- MR—Maintain or augment preload based on response to fluid load. Inotropic agents may be necessary for contractility. Afterload reduction to improve forward flow. IABP may be useful if acute MR due to MI

Maintenance

- MS: Avoid tachycardia, exacerbation of pulm HTN; maintain preload
- MR: Maintain mild tachycardia, low SVR, adequate preload

Post-Bypass

- Patients with MR usually do well after valve replacement. Minimal inotropes necessary for separation from CPB
- Patients with MS, especially late in disease, may require significant inotropes on separation from CPB

Emergence

- Transport to ICU intubated and ventilated
- Consider continuation of hypnotic infusions into ICU
- Pain scores: 5–10
- Manage pain with small doses of opioids; hypnotic/anxiolytic infusions or small doses for sedation while intubated
- EBL 300–400 ml

ANTICIPATED PROBLEMS/CONCERNS

- Postop ventilation usually necessary; may be a candidate for "fast-tracking" if cardiac function adequate and uncomplicated operative course
- Inotropic support or vasodilator therapy may be needed
- IABP for mitral incompetence, especially with infarction-associated MR
- Postop neurologic deficit

MYRINGOTOMY AND TYMPANOSTOMY
Kenneth B. Fickling, M.D.

RISK

- Most common pediatric surgical procedure in USA requiring anesthesia
- No racial or gender predominance

PERIOPERATIVE RISKS

- Perioperative mortality extremely low (<<1%)
- Concurrent URI symptoms not associated with increased perioperative morbidity

WORRY ABOUT

- Upper airway obstruction 2° to or worsened by hypertrophied adenotonsillar tissue, lateral head positioning, nonpatent nasal airways
- Laryngospasm
- Immediate IV access usually not available
- Cardiac dysrhythmias and suppression 2° to inhalational anesthesia (usually halothane or sevoflurane)

OVERVIEW

- Procedure to remove infection potential of fluid and to allow pressure equalization
- Vast majority of procedures performed in children aged 12 mo–5 y
- May be performed on anyone 6 mo to adult
- Associated with chronic or recurrent middle ear infections (otitis media [OM]) 2° to eustachian tube dysfunction
- Eustachian tube dysfunction etiologies include viral URI infections, congenital obstruction, adenotonsillar hypertrophy
- 30–40% present with URI symptoms at time of surgery (URI not contraindication to surgery without airway intubation in absence of productive cough; may increase risk of postop airway problems)

ICD-9-CM Code: 382.9

INDICATIONS AND USUAL TREATMENT

- Pressure equalization (PE) tubes are generally placed only if:
  - Episodes of acute OM are frequent, recurrent, and poorly responsive to conventional antibiotic therapy
  - A chronic OM ensues that is refractory to antibiotic prophylaxis
  - A chronic middle ear effusion associated with hearing loss develops

ASSESSMENT POINTS

SYSTEM	EFFECT	ASSESSMENT BY HX	PE	TEST
HEENT	Ear pain, effusions, concurrent URI symptoms	Tugging at ears, hearing loss, nasal congestion or discharge, sneezing, snoring	Ear exam, adenotonsillar enlargement	Audiogram
CV		Hx of heart murmur or congenital heart disease	Murmur	
RESP	URI symptoms	Cough, wheezing	Auscultation for wheezing	CXR, O_2 sat

Key Reference: Markowitz-Spence L, Brodsky L, Syed N, et al: Anesthetic complications of tympanotomy tube placement in children. Arch Otolaryngol Head Neck Surg 1990, 116:809–812.

PERIOPERATIVE MANAGEMENT

Preoperative Preparation

- Age-appropriate NPO modifications to avoid mask induction in dehydrated child
- Potential need for preop sedation with midazolam (rectal and nasal) in extremely anxious child; best if avoided because procedure extremely brief

Monitoring

- Routine including precordial stethoscope
- IV unnecessary unless significant coexisting disease mandates use

Airway

- Mask induction with O_2, N_2O, inhalational agent
- Maintenance with mask anesthesia often easier with oral airway in place, as nasal passages are frequently obstructed. Consider LMA placement
- Lateral head positioning can compromise airway

SURGICAL STAGES

Induction

- Potential for CV instability 2° to volume status
- Deep anesthesia generally maintained until after final myringotomy

Postoperative Considerations

- Emergence generally rapid if procedure is brief
- Minimal to moderate postop pain
- Acetaminophen 30–40 mg/kg rectally prior to emergence may be helpful
- EBL: minimal

ANTICIPATED PROBLEMS/CONCERNS

- Speed and experience of surgeons inversely and duration of anesthetic directly proportional to airway complication rate
- S_pO_2 desaturation with even brief periods of airway obstruction or in presence of coexisting lung disease (e.g., former premature infants with bronchopulmonary dysplasia)
- Laryngospasm if adequate depth of anesthesia not achieved prior to myringotomy

NEPHRECTOMY/RADICAL NEPHRECTOMY   Vinod Malhotra, M.D.

RISK

- Radical nephrectomy (> half of all nephrectomies) performed for renal carcinoma. Incidence: 24,000 cases/y.
  - Male:female ratio: 2:1
  - Urban dwellers > rural dwellers
  - 3–7% of lesions extend into IVC
- Simple nephrectomy: indicated for nonfunctioning obstructed kidney, polycystic kidney, donor transplants, uncontrollable renal HTN

PERIOPERATIVE RISKS

- Perioperative mortality rare (<1%)
- Considerable risk (22%) of DVT, pulm embolism, pulm atelectasis, renal dysfunction

WORRY ABOUT

- Massive blood loss (injury to renal vein, vena cava, renal artery, liver, spleen)
- Pneumothorax in thoracoabdominal approach
- Hypotension in flank position with kidney rest (bar) up
- Preservation of remaining kidney function
- Thrombus in IVC/hepatic vein

OVERVIEW

- Kidney with its pedicle removed in simple nephrectomy
- Kidney, adrenal, perinephric fat, and Gerota's fascia removed en bloc in radical nephrectomy
- Monitoring requirements depend upon IVC involvement and patient's medical status
- Excessive bleeding may occur if IVC involved
- CPB indicated if large atrial thrombus (right heart catheterization to be avoided)
- Venous return impeded by tumor thrombus in IVC leads to hypotension and falsely ↑ CVP
- Pulm embolization may occur during mobilization of tumor thrombus
- Pneumothorax likely
- Epidural analgesia for postop pain relief preferred by many. *Note*: With vena caval obstruction, epidural veins are dilated and space is narrowed.

ICD-9-CM Codes: 593.89 (Obstructed kidney); 189.0 (renal neoplasm); V59.4 (donor kidney)

INDICATIONS AND USUAL TREATMENT

- Radical nephrectomy only effective treatment for renal carcinoma
- Pre- and postop radiation therapy as adjunct of questionable value
- Nonfunctioning, obstructed kidney must be removed to prevent sepsis, renovascular HTN, dysfunction of contralateral kidney
- Donor nephrectomies are elective and in healthy subjects

ASSESSMENT POINTS

SYSTEM	EFFECT	ASSESSMENT BY HX	PE	TEST
CV	Thrombus extending into IVC and right atrium	SOB	Lower limb edema Collateral prominent abdominal wall veins Varicocele	MRI MRA MRV
RESP	Pulm metastases Pleural effusion Pulm embolus	SOB	Auscultation	CXR CT
HEPATIC	Portal vein occlusion (Budd-Chiari syndrome)			CT Venogram
CNS	Brain metastasis	Altered neural function		CT
MS	Metastasis	Bone pain	Bone deformity in advanced cases	X-ray, bone scan CT

Key Reference: Shah N: Radical cystectomy, nephrectomy, RBLD. *In* Malhotra V (ed): Anesthesia for Renal and Genitourinary Surgery. New York, McGraw-Hill, 1996, pp 209–211.

PERIOPERATIVE MANAGEMENT

Preoperative Preparation

- US, CT, MRI, metastatic work-up
- Cardiorespiratory, renal evaluation

Anesthetic Technique

- GA with controlled ventilation
- Combined epidural/general or epidural for postop analgesia
- CPB may be required

Monitoring

- Consider arterial line and ECHO if renal vein–IVC involvement
- Consider CVP/right heart catheter (right heart catheter contraindicated if intra-arterial thrombus).
- Foley catheter

Surgical Stages

- Bleeding during renal dissection, renal vein/IVC injury, or injury to spleen/liver
- Hypotension during positioning in kidney position
- Decrease venous return during removal of IVC/intra-arterial thrombus.
- Pulmonary embolus during thrombectomy
- Pleura may be entered through diaphragm
- EBL: 500–2000 ml

Postoperative Considerations

- Pain score: 5–10
- Epidural analgesia may improve resp function, or IV PCA for 3 days
- May develop DVT or pulmonary embolism
- Atelectasis due to splinting
- Head and neck edema from head-down positioning

ANTICIPATED PROBLEMS/CONCERNS

- Blood loss, pulmonary embolism, pneumothorax

OMPHALOCELE SURGERY

Wendy B. Binstock, M.D.

RISK

- Incidence varies from 1/3200 to 1/10,000 live births
- Racial predominance: none

PERIOPERATIVE RISKS

- Significant heat losses
- Major fluid shifts
- Infection
- Complications related to associated congenital abnormalities

WORRY ABOUT

- Blood glucose, especially with possibility of Beckwith-Wiedemann syndrome
- Possibility of cardiac defects and CV compromise
- Possibility of respiratory compromise, postop ventilation difficulties
- Metabolic problems

OVERVIEW

- Congenital abdominal wall defects that result in a portion of GI tract remaining outside abdominal cavity
- Translucent avascular sac consisting of peritoneum and amniotic membrane at base of umbilical cord
- Vary in size: may contain only small bowel or may contain liver, spleen, stomach, and other abdominal organs
- 30–50% associated with other congenital anomalies: most commonly GI, CV, GU, CNS
- Often associated with other known syndromes, particularly trisomies 13 and 18, and Beckwith-Wiedemann syndrome
- Associated with prematurity in 11% of cases if omphalocele alone is present but up to 43% when there are associated congenital anomalies

ICD-9-CM Code: 756.7

ETIOLOGY

- Congenital abnormality attributed to failure of embryonic folding at level of lateral folds, or to persistent body stock in the region normally occupied by somatopleure
- Amniotic sac always present, although it may have been ruptured during birth or shortly thereafter

USUAL TREATMENT

- Prompt surgical repair, either primary or staged, depending on size

ASSESSMENT POINTS

SYSTEM	EFFECT	ASSESSMENT BY HX	PE	TEST
HEENT	Beckwith-Wiedemann syndrome: macroglossia, microcephaly		Head exam	
CV	Congenital heart disease: tetralogy of Fallot, ASD		CV exam	Transthoracic ECHO
RESP	If associated with prematurity, may have immature lungs	Gestational age	Chest exam and signs of respiratory distress	O_2 saturation If available, predelivery lecithin/sphingomyelin ratio
GI	Gastric and intestinal distention, small abdominal cavity		Size of omphalocele	
ENDO	Possibility of Beckwith-Wiedemann syndrome			Blood glucose
RENAL/HEPATIC	Immaturity of hepatic and renal systems Possibility for ↓ hepatic blood flow and impaired renal perfusion post closure			

Key References: Berry FA, Steward PJ: Pediatrics for the Anesthesiologist. New York, Churchill Livingstone, 1993, pp 103–106.

PERIOPERATIVE MANAGEMENT

Preoperative Preparation

- IV access and restoration of intravascular volume
- Fluid losses tend to be isotonic; therefore, balanced salt solutions often used
- Up to 10–15 ml/kg/h of fluid often necessary initially
- Maintain normothermia by wrapping abdomen in moist, warm, sterile dressing; lower body can be placed in plastic bag

Monitoring

- Consider arterial line depending on extent of defect and ventilatory status of patient
- Consider CVP if defect is large and closure difficult
- Adequate temp monitoring, usually rectal

Airway

- Either awake intubation or rapid-sequence intubation with cricoid pressure after gastric decompression and preoxygenation
- ET tube should be secured in a manner suitable for prolonged postop ventilation

Maintenance

- Nitrous oxide usually avoided

- A suitable mixture of O_2 and air to produce adequate oxygenation (PaO_2 50–70 mmHg, SaO_2 97–98% for term infants, 87–92% for preterm infants); will vary as surgeons attempt to replace bowel in abdomen
- Maximal muscle relaxation throughout surgery
- Increases in CVP more than 4 mmHg during surgical closure associated with reduction in venous return, cardiac index, anuria
- Ability to tolerate primary closure assessed by measuring BP in lower extremities, or by following lower extremity circulation with pulse oximeter
- If hernia is left extraperitoneally, it is gradually reduced over a period of days
- Primary closure may cause ventilatory, circulatory, and renal dysfunction and bowel necrosis if abdomen is too tense
- Placing bowel in a silo associated with higher infection rate
- If vital signs are abnormal after the expected respiratory changes associated with hernia reduction, it is usually impossible to achieve adequate ventilation and oxygenation until intra-abdominal pressure and distention diminish

Extubation

- Postop care varies with magnitude of defect, type of repair, and associated pathology
- Healthy patients treated with a silo or a small primary closure often tolerate extubation at end of procedure
- In patients with large defects (especially those with compromised circulation), postop intubation, ventilation, and maximal muscle relaxation should be continued until abdominal pressure results in little respiratory or circulatory compromise

ANTICIPATED PROBLEMS/CONCERNS

- Ventilatory care: similar to that for other neonates with respiratory distress
- Fluid requirements: may remain high until abdominal venous pressure decreases, at which time fluid restriction and diuresis probably indicated
- FIO_2: adjust to maintain a normal PaO_2
- PEEP: appropriate levels used to ↑ FRC
- Nutritional status: because bowel function is usually compromised and slow to resume, TPN requirements are often extended
- Circulatory and renal dysfunction common
- Infection: common, especially if silo used instead of primary closure

ORCHIOPEXY

W. Casey Lenox, M.D.

RISK

- Premature infants—risk is 30% for one or both testicles to be undescended
- Full-term infants—risk is 3%
- 60% of undescended testicles found in inguinal position; 8% intra-abdominal; only 24% in the easily operable low inguinal/high scrotal position
- Progressive injury occurs when testicle is left undescended: decreased sperm production after age 6 y, impaired hormonal production, ↑ risk of malignant degeneration
- Risk of malignant degeneration may not be improved following orchiopexy but self-examination becomes more reliable

PERIOPERATIVE RISKS

- Perioperative mortality rare in term infants (<0.01%)
- Risks in ex–premature children dependent upon coexisting morbidity (e.g., bronchopulmonary dysplasia, reactive airway disease, subglottic stenosis, hydrocephalus and seizure due to intraventricular hemmorhage, GI dysfunction due to necrotizing enterocolitis, malnutrition, anemia, RV hypertrophy/failure, poor IV access)
- Operative risks of testicular atrophy or hypotrophy: 8% for those beyond external ring, 13% when canicular, 26% for intra-abdominal locations

WORRY ABOUT

- Co-morbidity associated with prematurity
- Venous air embolism, aspiration, diaphragmatic embarrassment if laparoscope utilized for repair

OVERVIEW

- Testicle(s) located and spermatic cord and accompanying vasculature freed and mobilized so that testicle can be relocated within hemiscrotum. Spermatic vessels may be sacrificed, with vasculature of vas deferens supplying collaterals
- Operative laparoscope increasingly utilized for relocating intra-abdominal or high inguinal testicles
- Operative time: 1 h (open, low testicular location) to 3 h (laparoscopic)

ICD-9-CM Code: 752.5 (Cryptorchidism)

INDICATIONS AND USUAL TREATMENT

- Testicle will not descend beyond 1 year of age and ultrastructural changes have been demonstrated by 2 years, so that most repairs should occur at 12–24 months of age
- Some evidence that hCG may promote testicular descent, so this may be attempted prior to operation

ASSESSMENT POINTS (IN EX–PREMATURE INFANTS)

SYSTEM	EFFECT	ASSESSMENT BY HX	PE	TEST
HEENT	Subglottic stenosis		Stridor, wheezing, croup	CXR, bronchoscopy
CV	Pulm HTN, PDA, RV hypertrophy	Failure to thrive	↑ S$_2$, murmurs	ECG Cardiac ECHO/catheter
RESP	Bronchopulmonary dysplasia, blebs	Asthma, oxygen? Apnea monitor alarms Diuretics		CXR
RENAL	Nephrocalcinosis	HTN		BP, electrolytes, BUN, Cr
CNS	Intraventricular hemorrhage Seizures, hydrocephalus	Mental status Development Seizure type, frequency Ventriculoperitoneal shunt		Shunt evaluation, Anti-epilepsy drug levels

Key Reference: Hannallah RS, Broadman LM, Belman AB, et al: Comparison of caudal and ilioinguinal/iliohypogastric nerve blocks for control of post-orchiopexy pain in pediatric ambulatory surgery. Anesthesiology 1987; 66:832–834.

PERIOPERATIVE MANAGEMENT

Preoperative Preparation

- May have clear liquids up to 2 h before induction
- No lab work necessary if otherwise normal
- If uncomplicated, may be done as outpatient procedure .

Anesthetic Technique

- Combined general and regional anesthetic in open case
- Usually regular mask or laryngeal mask airway (LMA) and caudal injection of local anesthetic or ilioinguinal/iliohypogastric nerve block for analgesia intra- and postoperatively
- Combined technique in laparoscopic procedures but with trachea intubated (usually; LMA now being used by some)

Monitoring

- Routine

Induction

- Inhalational mask induction, then maintenance with halothane or sevoflurane and nitrous oxide
- IV, then single-injection caudal placed following induction of anesthesia

SURGICAL STAGES

Dissection

- Caudal usually not effective in blocking visceral pain that occurs with pulling on spermatic cord, may require increasing volatile anesthetic concentrations temporarily
- Possible respiratory compromise if laparoscopic procedure
- Minimal blood loss

Postoperative Considerations

- If 0.025% bupivacaine used for caudal, 4–6 h of analgesia usual
- Most children need enteral opioids for 2–3 d
- Incidence of emesis postop 45%; usually self-limited

ANTICIPATED PROBLEMS/CONCERNS

- Ex–premature children have an ↑ incidence of wheezing and desaturation intra- and postoperatively. May need to be observed overnight

ORIF OF HIP

Kevin V. Sanborn, M.D.

RISK

- 200,000/y in USA
- Predominantly elderly women
- Racial predominance: none

PERIOPERATIVE RISKS

- 7%—30-day mortality
- Anemia and hypovolemia
- Multiple trauma victims—other injuries?
- Perioperative confusion—etiology of fall in elderly: TIA, stroke, MI
- Decubitus ulcers

WORRY ABOUT

- Etiology of fracture: reason for falling—syncope
- Drug abuse, including ethanol
- Anemia, hypovolemia, hypothermia
- Pulmonary emboli

OVERVIEW

- Break in bone supporting weight with pain and fluid/blood collection in leg
- Early treatment to stabilize associated with better functional recovery and fewer perioperative complications
- Usually occurs in elderly with comorbidities; dehydration, anemia, at least mild CNS disturbances
- Both regional and general anesthesia are supported in literature. Meta-analysis failed to show any significant benefit of one vs. the other.
- With good preop assessment of medical problems, preinduction resuscitation of fluid and blood losses, and appropriate monitoring, choice of light GA or cautiously induced regional anesthesia can be based on anesthesiologist's preference and patient's condition.
- Pin fixation of hip fracture does not violate major body cavities and is not associated with massive bleeding or fluid shifts; usually reasonably well tolerated.

ICD-9-CM Code: 820.8 (Closed fracture of hip)

INDICATIONS AND USUAL TREATMENT

- Fracture of femoral neck results in pain and disability corrected by pin fixation under x-ray guidance.
- Severe fracture involving femoral head may require replacement with cemented femoral prosthesis
- In elderly patients, treatment of fracture with traction results in high morbidity and mortality due to pulmonary and septic complications.
- Coexisting chronic medical problems and acute disturbances of physiology of vital organs should be rapidly assessed and treated. Delay in surgical treatment associated with poor outcome.

ASSESSMENT POINTS

SYSTEM	EFFECT	ASSESSMENT BY HX	PE	TEST
CV	HTN, CAD, MI, heart block or AS → syncope?	Hx HTN, CAD, TIA	Chest exam, VS	ECG
RESP	Atelectasis, pneumonia, fat embolism, pulm edema	Hx CHF, ?SOB, chest pain	Chest exam	SpO_2, ABG, CXR
ENDO	Diabetes	Hx of adult-onset DM	Peripheral pulses	FBS, UA
HEME	Anemia, thrombocytopenia (2° fat embolism)	Dyspnea, GI bleeding	Pallor, petechiae	CBC
RENAL	Dehydration, electrolyte imbalance, UTI	Nursing home?, NPO × ? h	Jugular veins	BUN/Cr, electrolytes
CNS	Stroke, TIA, confusion, delirium, syncope	Previous stroke, TIA, medications	Auscultation of carotid	Neuro exam

Key Reference: Sorensen RM: Anesthetic techniques during surgical repair of femoral neck fractures. Anesthesiology 1992; 77:1095–1104.

INTRAOPERATIVE MANAGEMENT

- Early surgical treatment associated with fewer postop complications. Assessment and treatment of medical problems and fluid resuscitation can be completed within 24 h
- Spinal, epidural, or light general anesthesia
- Analgesia ± sedation needed for positioning and transfers
- Lateral decubitus position preferred for induction of spinal or epidural anesthesia

Monitoring

- Routine
- Consider arterial line, CVP, PA catheter depending on coexisting disease

Induction

- Consider fluid resuscitation, vasopressors before induction of spinal or epidural anesthesia
- Consider warming blanket, warmed fluids to offset heat losses due to advanced age and exposure
- Minimize sedation during regional anesthesia to avoid postop delirium

SURGICAL STAGES

Positioning

- Use of fracture table and x-ray image intensifier adds 30–60 min to setup
- Fracture table makes it difficult to avoid exposure to drafts → hypothermia
- Consider positioning ipsilateral arm carefully out of field

X-ray

- Consider wearing lead apron and thyroid collar

Pin or Screw Fixation

- Add 1 U of hematoma to EBL
- Minimally invasive procedure, well-tolerated even by sick patients

Replacement of Femoral Head

- Cemented femoral prosthesis—problems similar to total hip replacement

Postoperative Period

- Pain score: 3–5
- IV PCA well tolerated

ANTICIPATED PROBLEMS/CONCERNS

- Anemia, hypovolemia, hypotension, hypothermia
- Pulm edema due to too aggressive fluid replacement; may not be evident until recovery from sympathetic blockade after regional anesthesia
- Confusion, delirium
- Sensitivity to narcotics and sedatives
- Postop pulmonary complications (pulmonary embolism, pneumonia, bone marrow fat embolism, ARDS)
- Postop urinary sepsis
- Postop GI disturbances (intestinal obstruction, GI bleeding)

PACEMAKER IMPLANTATION FOR SICK SINUS SYNDROME

Carl Lynch III, M.D., Ph.D.

RISK

• Accounts for ~50% of pacemaker implantations, or about 200/1 million population/y
• Typically seen in older patients, although may be familial or follow surgery for congenital heart defects

PERIOPERATIVE RISKS

• Perioperative bradycardia (unpaced) or tachycardia, with potential for CV compromise, including pulm edema

WORRY ABOUT

• Previously undiagnosed or early disease (see Etiology), with modest early symptoms
• In the absence of pacemaker or with pacemaker dysfunction, severe bradycardia or asystole may occur, especially with ↑ vagal tone
• In the presence of pacemaker, sustained paroxysmal tachycardia may require control

OVERVIEW

• Sick sinus syndrome divided into three types: (1) simple sinus bradycardia; (2) sinus arrest or SA block with or without sinus bradycardia; (3) bradycardia with paroxysmal tachycardia ("tachy-brady syndrome")
• Tachycardia may be caused by AFib/ flutter
• Syncope or severe lightheadedness results from prolonged sinus or atrial pause following termination of tachycardia; atrial pause frequently caused by SA exit block
• Sinus or atrial pauses may be 15 sec duration
• May be associated with high-degree AV block (pan-conduction defect)
• Increased likelihood of stroke in patients who are paced ventricularly (VVI) and more prone to develop AFib

ICD-9-CM Code: 427.81

ETIOLOGY

• Usually due to degenerative (possibly familial), sclerotic, or fibrotic changes of sinus node
• May be manifestation of cardiac disease: ischemia, pericarditis, cardiomyopathy
• May be secondary to cardiac involvement by other diseases (typically infiltrative):
  – muscular dystrophy, collagen disease, hemochromatosis, amyloidosis, metastatic disease

INDICATIONS AND USUAL TREATMENT

• Permanent cardiac pacemaker placement in symptomatic patients, or in asymptomatic patients who take β blockers or antiarrhythmic drugs
• For previously undiagnosed disease, temporary transvenous pacing may be appropriate
• Sinus rate and atrial conduction may be enhanced by stimulation with β-adrenergic agonists (isoproterenol, epinephrine, ephedrine) and parasympathetic blocking agents (atropine, glycopyrrolate)

ASSESSMENT POINTS

SYSTEM	EFFECT	ASSESSMENT BY HX	PE	TEST
CV	Bradycardia, tachycardia	Pacemaker implantation	Low (or high) HR	ECG, electrophysiologic testing
CNS		Unexplained episodic lightheadedness, confusion, syncope		Holter CT scan

Key Reference: Wu D, Yeh S-H, Lin F-C, et al: Sinus automaticity and sinoatrial conduction in severe symptomatic sick sinus syndrome. JACC 1992; 19:355–364.

PERIOPERATIVE IMPLICATIONS

Monitoring
• ECG
• Monitor of perfusion if pacemaker (Doppler, SpO$_2$, ECHO, arterial line)

Airway
• None

Maintenance
• Volatile agents, especially halothane and enflurane, may suppress SA function
• If pacemaker is not implanted, high doses of fentanyl or sufentanil or maneuvers that ↑ vagal tone may worsen bradycardia, requiring treatment with atropine

Extubation/Emergence
• Emergence excitation may contribute to development of paroxysmal tachycardia

Adjuvants
• Calcium channel blockers, especially verapamil, contraindicated in the absence of pacemaking capability
• With pacemaker present, paroxysmal tachycardia may be treated acutely with IV adenosine or verapamil; digoxin may be added for longer duration control

ANTICIPATED PROBLEMS/CONCERNS

• Severe bradycardia (or tachycardia) 2° to anesthetic agents or autonomic imbalance associated with perioperative period. Since problems may arise from parasympathetic dominance, atropine or glycopyrrolate is indicated

PANCREAS TRANSPLANTATION

Dennis W. Coalson, M.D.

- 12,000–19,000 new cases of type I diabetes/y
- 555 pancreas transplants in USA in 1993
  - 86% simultaneous pancreas-kidney transplant (SPK)
  - 9% pancreas transplant after a kidney (PAK)
  - 6% pancreas transplant alone (PTA)

PERIOPERATIVE RISKS

- 30-d mortality: 1–2 %
- Combined 1-y patient survival: 91%
- 1-y pancreas graft function (insulin-independent) rate of 71%
- 1-y pancreas graft function: 75% SPK, 48% PAK, 51% PTA
- Morbidity of SPK is 15% greater than kidney transplant alone
- Rejection episodes
- Infections—2° to immunosuppressants

WORRY ABOUT

- Positioning for long surgical time (4–8 h)
- Diabetics at ↑ risk for perioperative nerve injuries
- Potential rapid blood loss
- Complications of IDDM (gastroparesis, CAD, autonomic neuropathy)
- Noncardiogenic pulm edema with perioperative OKT3
- For SPK, hypovolemia if recently dialyzed; hyperkalemia and hypervolemia if long since last dialysis. Protection of hemodialysis access site, AV shunt, or fistulas. Prolong duration of drugs renally excreted

OVERVIEW

- Only treatment of type I diabetes mellitus that establishes insulin-independent euglycemic state.

- Improvement in quality of life primary reason for transplant. Potential for favorable effect on secondary complications of diabetes is additional goal.
- Usually performed along with kidney transplant

ICD-9-CM Code: 250.01
See also Diabetes, Type I

INDICATIONS AND USUAL TREATMENT

- Usually uremic diabetic patients who need kidney transplant or have received prior kidney transplant
- For nonuremics, problems of diabetes considered more serious than potential side effects of immunosuppression therapy (diabetics with extreme lability in metabolic control and hypoglycemic unawareness)

ASSESSMENT POINTS

SYSTEM	EFFECT	ASSESSMENT BY HX	PE	TEST
HEENT	Difficult laryngoscopy Joint immobility	Hx of difficult airway Joint contractures	Airway exam Palm or prayer sign	Test palms together to estimate joint mobility
CV/RESP	CAD Hypervolemia Hyperkalemia	SOB	Rales, tachypnea	CXR, ABGs, ECG, lytes
HEME	Anemia		Systolic flow murmur, pale mucous membranes	Hct
PNS	Peripheral neuropathy, gastroparesis, autonomic neuropathy	Early satiety, nausea, postural syncope	↓ Peripheral sensation	Tilt test, RR interval with breathing or Valsalva maneuver
MS	Osteopenia	Fractures		Bone density

Key Reference: Sutherland DER: State of the art in pancreas transplantation. Transplant Proc 1994; 26:316.

PERIOPERATIVE MANAGEMENT

Preoperative Preparation

- Absence of infection, dental evaluation
- Administration of preop antibiotics

Anesthetic Technique

- Usually general or combined technique because of length of case
- Rapid-sequence induction for full stomach or gastroparesis

Monitoring

- Consider arterial and central venous catheters
- Frequent blood glucose measurements

Airway

- High incidence (30%) of difficult laryngoscopy in type I diabetics
- ↑ Risk for aspiration

Induction/Maintenance

- Blood glucose assessment as pancreatic graft function occurs rapidly; in most patients, blood glucose levels decrease to normal within several hours
- Administration of immunosuppressant agents prior to graft reperfusion.

Surgical Stages

- Preservation times up to 30 h safe for cadaveric pancreas

Dissection

- Midline incision. Mobilization of iliac artery and vein bilaterally. Intraperitoneal placement in side opposite renal graft.

Definitive Surgery

- Graft superior mesenteric and splenic arteries anastomosed to recipient iliac artery via donor iliac artery Y graft. Graft portal vein anastomosed to recipient iliac vein.
- Most commonly exocrine drainage provided by anastomosing a graft duodenal segment to bladder. Can also have enteric exocrine drainage.

Postoperative Considerations

- Pain relief with PCA or epidural analgesia
- Occasional postop anticoagulation to ↓ graft thrombosis
- Rejection after SPK transplantation determined by serum Cr and kidney biopsy
- 90% of rejection episodes: kidney dysfunction earlier than pancreatic dysfunction
- Rejection in PTA diagnosed by ↓ urine amylase activity in urinary bladder–drained pancreas grafts.
- Delayed complication with urinary drainage related to pancreatic juice in bladder, such as hematuria, UTI, chemical cystitis, metabolic acidosis, reflux pancreatitis

ANTICIPATED PROBLEMS/CONCERNS

- Positioning problems associated with long surgical time
- Noncardiogenic pulm edema with intraoperative administration of OKT3
- Early return to euglycemic state after surgery requiring ↓ in exogenously administered insulin

PARATHYROIDECTOMY

Eli Brown, M.D.

RISK

- Incidence: 0.1–0.2%
- Peak incidence 5th–6th decades
- Females > males
- Racial predominance: none

PERIOPERATIVE RISKS

- Hypercalcemia produces symptoms related mainly to renal, skeletal, neuromuscular, GI systems
- Perioperative mortality rare
- Most common postop complications are injury of recurrent laryngeal nerve(s), hematoma, eye injury, hypocalcemia

WORRY ABOUT

- Parathyroid crisis (Ca^{2+} >14 mg/dl) accompanied by marked dehydration and coma
- Positioning—presence of osteoporosis or simple diffuse osteopenia may result in pathologic fracture
- Skeletal muscle weakness
- Renal insufficiency
- Nerve injury, hematoma, hypocalcemia postop

OVERVIEW

- Low incidence of morbidity (<1%)
- 85% of primary hyperparathyroidism caused by benign adenoma in a single gland
- Major symptoms result from hypercalcemia

ICD-9-CM Code: 252.0 (Hyperplasia)

ETIOLOGY

- Hyperparathyroidism present when secretion of parathormone is increased
- Classified as primary, secondary, or ectopic

INDICATIONS AND USUAL TREATMENT

- Complete removal of gland containing adenoma with biopsy of 1 or 2 normal-appearing glands
- For known hyperplasia, 3 glands are removed and 4th gland partially excised

ASSESSMENT POINTS

SYSTEM	EFFECT	ASSESSMENT BY HX	PE	TEST
CV	Conduction disturbances (short Q-Tc; prolonged P-R intervals associated with hypercalcemia) HTN			ECG BP
GI	Disorders of stomach and pancreas Zollinger-Ellison syndrome	Vague abdominal pain	Abdominal exam	Endoscopy (if indicated)
RENAL	Calculi Insufficiency	Flank pain Polyuria Polydipsia	Flank tenderness	X-ray (if indicated) GFR (if indicated) Cr
NEUROMUSC	Peripheral muscle weakness Atrophy of muscles	Easy fatigability	Extremity exam	Ca^{2+} level
MS	Osteitis fibrosa cystica Osteopenia	Frequent fractures Bone pain	Skeletal exam	X-ray; CT (if indicated) Quantitative digital radiography (if indicated)

Key Reference: Hensel P, Roizen MF: Patients with disorders of thyroid function. Anesth Clin North Am 1987; 5:287–297.

PERIOPERATIVE MANAGEMENT

Preoperative Preparation

- Treat hypercalcemia—primarily hydration and diuresis accompanied by phosphate repletion.
- Glucocorticoids, mithramycin, calcitonin may be used if necessary
- Correct hypovolemia and electrolyte imbalance
- Check ECG for P-R, Q-T changes

Monitoring

- Routine

Airway

- None

Preinduction/Induction

- Careful positioning to avoid bone fracture
- Patient may exhibit unpredictable response to muscle relaxants
- No specific anesthetic agent or technique is advantageous or contraindicated
- Local or regional anesthesia may be appropriate for poor-risk patients or limited surgery
- Protect eyes

Maintenance

- Check ECG for prolonged P-R and short Q-Tc intervals
- Tracheal manipulation may cause bucking if patient inadequately anesthetized or partially paralyzed

Extubation

- Be aware of possibility of damage to recurrent laryngeal nerves or presence of bullous glottic edema producing airway obstruction

ANTICIPATED PROBLEMS/CONCERNS

- Airway obstruction 2° to damage to recurrent laryngeal nerves, hematoma, bullous glottic edema
- Hypocalcemia or hypomagnesemia may occur. Severe hypocalcemia may result in laryngeal spasm and seizure
- Perform serial determinations of serum Ca^{2+}, inorganic phosphate, magnesium, parathyroid hormone
- Chvostek's sign and Trousseau's sign are classic indications of latent tetany.

PATENT DUCTUS ARTERIOSUS, LIGATION OF

Eugenie Heitmiller, M.D.

(see also Patent Ductus Arteriosus in Diseases section)

RISK

- Full-term infants: 1/2500 live births
- Premature infants: 45% <1750 g; 80% <1200 g
- Overall incidence: 8/1000 live births
- Female preponderance 2–3/1 male
- High incidence in congenital rubella syndrome

PERIOPERATIVE RISKS

- Perioperative mortality rare (0.4%)
- Residual ductal patency 0.4–3.1%
- Rare complications: chest wall deformity, recurrent nerve injury, ligation of left PA or aorta

WORRY ABOUT

- Hypothermia
- Adequate venous access and blood products readily available for uncontrolled hemorrhage
- Vagal reflex with lung and vessel retraction
- Fluid status of premature infant on diuretics and fluid restriction

OVERVIEW

- Left to right shunt between aorta and PA that causes increased pulmonary blood flow with pulm edema and cardiac failure in premature infants, or cyanosis in lower half of body with R →L shunt
- Antibiotics required to prevent bacterial endocarditis in all patients
- Air embolism can occur with bidirectional shunting
- Massive hemorrhage may occur during ductal ligation

ICD-9-CM Code: 747.0 (patent ductus arteriosus)

INDICATIONS AND USUAL TREATMENT

- Premature infants: initial treatment with fluid restriction and diuretics; administration of indomethacin (a prostaglandin inhibitor) usually causes ductal closure in 24 h; surgery indicated if trial of indomethacin fails; procedure in NICU at some hospitals.
- Full-term infants and older children: ligated electively after age 6 mo if asymptomatic
- Standard surgical treatment is via open thoracotomy. Investigational procedures for closure of PDA include transcatheter device closure and a video-assisted thoracoscopic approach

ASSESSMENT POINTS

SYSTEM	EFFECT	ASSESSMENT BY HX	PE	TEST
CV	L →R shunt Diastolic runoff Heart failure	CHF Failure to grow	Rales Murmur Low diastolic BP Bounding pulses	ECHO
RESP	↑ Pulm blood	Failure to wean from ventilator		CXR

Key Reference: Rosen DA, Rosen KR: Anomalies of the aortic arch and valve. *In* Lake C (ed): Pediatric Cardiac Anesthesia, 2nd ed. Norwalk, CT, Appleton and Lange, 1993, p 347.

PERIOPERATIVE MANAGEMENT

Preoperative Preparation

- Monitor premature infants during transport
- Adequate vascular access. Blood products available prior to incision
- Warm OR prior to patient arrival
- IV lines cleared of air bubbles

Anesthetic Technique

- Combined GA with regional block for thoracotomy pain

Monitoring

- Pulse oximetry on right hand and on one lower extremity to confirm that correct vessel is ligated
- Use invasive monitors if used in ICU
- Temp closely monitored

Airway

- May have associated congenital anomalies of airway

Induction/Maintenance

- May require fluid resuscitation at induction because of fluid restriction and diuretics

Surgical Stages

- Incision
  - Usually left thoracotomy incision; can have right-sided PDA
- Dissection
  - Lung retraction can produce hypoxemia and hypercarbia
  - Vagal reflex produced by surgical traction on lung; may require atropine, since bradycardia poorly tolerated in infants
- Definitive surgery
  - Major blood loss can occur if ductal vessel injured or if clip/suture on vessel is inadequate or slips off vessel
  - Chest tube placed prior to chest closure

- Fluid shift: can have ↑ systemic volume after ductus arteriosus is ligated

Postoperative Considerations

- CXR immediately postop to check for pneumothorax
- EBL: usually minimal
- Pain score: 6–9
- Continuous regional technique or intercostal blocks with parenteral narcotics for thoracotomy pain management

ANTICIPATED PROBLEMS/CONCERNS

- Shunt predominantly L →R
- Large shunts can result in heart failure and pulm HTN
- Cyanosis of lower half of body indicative of a R →L shunt

PITUITARY RESECTION, TRANSSPHENOIDAL APPROACH

Stephen M. Rupp, M.D.

RISK

- Pituitary adenoma: 14.7/100,000
- M/F: 1:2

PERIOPERATIVE RISK

- <1% Immediate perioperative mortality
- 8–15% Morbidity (transient [1–3 d] diabetes insipidus is most frequent); hypopituitarism in large resections
- Microadenomas of all types can have up to 90% cure rates in some surgical series
- 50% of untreated acromegalics die before age 50 y
- Untreated Cushing's disease has a 50% 5-y mortality

WORRY ABOUT

- Airway in acromegalics and Cushing's syndrome
- Intraoperative injection of epinephrine-containing local anesthetics to vasoconstrict nasal mucosa (precipitate dysrhythmias or myocardial ischemia); severe HTN if ß-blocker present
- Hemorrhage intraoperatively (cavernous sinus intrusion)
- Air embolism reported
- Saddle deformity of nose postop
- Blood in airway at end of procedure
- Diabetes insipidus postop

OVERVIEW

- Pituitary microadenoma usual indication for surgery; in descending order of frequency, tissue types/most common presenting symptoms are:

   – Nonsecreting adenoma/visual field defect, headache, CN III–VI may be affected by pressure
   – Prolactin-secreting adenoma/amenorrhea; galactorrhea, lost libido
   – ACTH-secreting tumor/Cushing's disease; obesity, HTN, diabetes
   – Growth hormone–secreting tumor/acromegaly, HTN, cardiomyopathy, diabetes mellitus

ICD-9-CM Codes: 253.0 (Acromegaly); 255.0 (Cushing's syndrome)

INDICATIONS AND USUAL TREATMENT

- Bromocriptine is first line of Rx for prolactin-secreting tumors and can suppress GH tumors
- Irradiation used as single treatment and surgical adjuvant in selected cases
- Surgical treatment is choice for macroadenomas (>10 mm in diameter)

ASSESSMENT POINTS

SYSTEM	EFFECT	ASSESSMENT BY HX	PE	TEST
HEENT	Airway in acromegalics; glottic fixation or narrowing in GH excess Airway in Cushing's CN III–VI impingement	Hoarseness, sleep apnea? Tongue size, stridor/DOE? Visual disturbance, field cut	Airway Visual field	
CV	HTN in acromegaly and Cushing's	CV status Exercise tolerance Chest pain		ECG
RESP	↓ FRC in obese	SOB, DOE		ABG
ENDO	Diabetes mellitus Hypercortisolism	Glucose intolerance		Glucose
RENAL	Hypertensive or diabetic kidney disease			Cr
CNS	↑ ICP in severe suprasellar extension	Headache, N/V		Funduscopic exam

Key Reference: Klibanski A, Zervas NT: Diagnosis and management of hormone-secreting pituitary adenomas. N Engl J Med 1991; 324:822–831.

PERIOPERATIVE MANAGEMENT

Preoperative Preparation

- Evaluate for significant CAD (Hx, ECG, exercise tolerance); may suffer myocardial stress from exogenous epinephrine
- Airway assessment requires oral ET tube; plan fiberoptic intubation if indicated
- Surgeon may request lumbar subarachnoid drain to inject saline or air or N_2O intraoperatively to outline and monitor progress of suprasellar extension of adenoma. Postop, CSF catheter may be placed to drain if CSF leak anticipated

Anesthetic Technique

- GA required

Monitoring

- Routine + air embolism
- If plan to have patient in >30° upright sitting position, consider multi-orificed single-lumen CVP for air aspiration and plan Doppler monitoring/end-tidal N_2

Airway

- In acromegalics, hypertrophy of facial bones, jaw, nose, turbinates, soft palate, tonsils, epiglottis, and larynx may occur: mask fit/intubation may be difficult. Fiberoptic intubation may be indicated.

Induction/Maintenance

- Rapid-acting induction agent acceptable
- Maintain anesthetic with narcotic, volatile anesthetic (isoflurane good choice because of favorable profile of ↓ sensitivity of myocardium to exogenous epinephrine), ± N_2O and relaxant
- Aim to have patient comfortable and cooperative (awake) prior to extubation
- Mouth and pharynx packed with gauze to prevent blood in stomach or airway
- Subarachnoid drain prior to positioning

Surgical Stages

- Surgical positioning: semi-sitting 5–35° head-up
- Placement of tongs: watch for adrenergic/hypertensive response!
- Injection of epinephrine containing local anesthetic to vasoconstrict: watch for dysrhythmias and HTN
- Nasal septal and sublabial incision (blood loss)
- Placement of transsphenoidal speculum: bone work, needs fluoroscopic control to ensure midline approach (high anesthetic requirement for this stage)
- Adenoma removal under direct visualization with microscope
- If suprasellar extension, surgeon may want air injected: if so, discontinue N_2O

- If lateral extension of tumor occurs, excessive bleeding may ensue from invasion of cavernous sinus. Induced hypotension via high-concentration isoflurane may reduce venous pressure to allow adequate hemorrhage control
- Rebuilding sella turcica (part of nasal septum used)
- Pack with fat pad (abdominal wall donor site)
- Close
- EBL: 150–400 ml

Postoperative Considerations

- Pain score: 2–3

ANTICIPATED PROBLEMS/CONCERNS

- Extubate awake!
- Diabetes insipidus in 8–15%, usually transient. Dx via analysis of high volume (1–2 L/h) of dilute urine (<200 mOsm/L, specific gravity = 1.001–1.005). May require aqueous vasopressin 0.5 ml (10 U) q4–6h SQ. Replace urinary losses. If serum >320 Osm/L, replace H_2O loss.
- CSF rhinorrhea: lumbar CSF drain to reduce CSF pressure
- If excessive packing needed to control cavernous sinus bleeding, CN II, IV, or VI compression can occur. Impingement of cavernous internal carotid can result in carotid spasm.
- If air has been injected subarachnoid, tension pneumocephalus can occur.

PITUITARY TUMOR, EXCISION OF
Herman Turndorf, M.D.

RISK

- 15% of all intracranial tumors
- 30% nonfunctioning
  - Diagnosed later so tend to be larger tumors with extrasellar extension and chiasmal compression
  - Secondary compression can decrease levels of gonadotropin, growth hormone, thyroid hormone, ACTH. May require thyroid, corticosteroid replacement preop
- Functional tumors, secretory or nonsecretory, ordinarily small, can produce compressive effects, over- or undersecretion: Cushing's syndrome, acromegaly (in adult), gigantism (in youth), hyper- or hypothyroidism
- Pituitary apoplexy from tumor hemorrhage or ischemic infarction produces headache, decreased vision, adrenal insufficiency, loss of consciousness (1–3%); may require urgent decompression

PERIOPERATIVE RISKS

- Mortality <1%
- Appropriate pre- and postop hormone replacement

- ICP usually normal except with large extrasellar tumors
- CV and rhythm abn, esp. with Cushing's disease or acromegaly
- Difficult airway and intubation, esp. with acromegaly or gigantism

WORRY ABOUT

- HTN and arrhythmias after cocaine pledget application
- Significant HTN when entering sphenoidal sinus
- Cavernous sinus, carotid hemorrhage: not common, but loss can be rapid and large

OVERVIEW

- Intrasellar micro- or macroadenomas. Suprasellar extension primarily with nonfunctional tumors. Cavernous sinuses and carotid arteries may be entered. Cranial nerves III–VI and optic chiasma may be injured during resection.
- Corticosteroid replacement for Cushing's disease through perioperative period.

- Hyperaldosteronism, metabolic alkalosis, ↓ serum K+, HTN, CHF, insulin resistant DM, peptic ulcer disease common
- Acromegaly: Markedly abnormal airways from facial, soft tissue, epiglottic, tonsillar, laryngeal, and false cord engagement and deviation. LV hypertrophy, HTN, ischemic heart disease, supraventricular conduction defects, sinus bradycardia, atrial arrhythmias, and CHF common.
- Panhypopituitarism: preop replacement required depending on spectrum of hormone deficiencies

ICD-9-CM Code: 253.8

INDICATIONS AND USUAL TREATMENT

- Transseptal and/or sublabial transsphenoidal resection using video-enhanced microscopic dissection
  - Transcranial approach seldom used except for very large extrasellar masses
  - Hormonal excess or deficiency from micro- or macroscopic pituitary mass
  - Progressive chiasmal compression
  - Extrasellar extension

ASSESSMENT POINTS

SYSTEM	EFFECT	ASSESSMENT BY HX	PE	TEST
HEENT	Acromegaly: prognathism	Snoring, hoarseness, ring-size growth	Airway exam	Serum GH, laryngoscopy
CV	HTN if Cushing's syndrome or acromegaly	End-organ dysfunction Exercise intolerance	BP, 2-flight walk	Serum cortisol Serum GH
CNS	↑ ICP Suprasellar compression of optic chiasm	N/V Headache Visual field deficit	Neck flexion pain Papilledema	Visual field testing
ENDO	Depends on syndrome	see Overview above		
MS	Weakness if Cushing's syndrome	Weakness	↓ Ability to get up from chair without using arms	K+ and serum cortisol

Key Reference: Klibanski A, Zervas NT: Diagnosis and management of hormone secreting pituitary adenomas. N Engl J Med 1991; 324:822–831.

PERIOPERATIVE IMPLICATIONS

Anesthetic Technique
- GA with orotracheal intubation
- Microscope requires use of remote machine location and extension tubing
- Patient supine with head tilt
- Special eye protection

Monitoring
- Normal. Arterial line usually not needed. Doppler and CVP if head up 15°. Urine and blood osmolality and Na+ if diabetes insipidus present

Airway
- For acromegaly: detailed airway evaluation; fiberoptic-guided intubation; smaller than normal tube
- Tagged oropharyngeal gauze pack for blood absorption

Induction
- Inhalation or IV anesthesia with relaxants. ICP precautions only for large extrasellar masses
- Rapid closure after resection completed; nasal pack forces mouth breathing; may need nasal airways with nasal pack.
- Airway suction to clear blood
- Awake before extubate

SURGICAL STAGES
- Cocaine pledgets in nares for vasoconstriction
- Lidocaine and epinephrine 1/200,000 infiltration in septal mucosa
- Sphenoid dissection (↑ BP)
- CSF drain if large extrasellar mass
- Blood loss <200 ml

POSTOPERATIVE CONSIDERATIONS
- Nostrils packed—obligatory mouth breathing; rapid emergence desirable
- Hypocorticism—steroid support up to 6 mo postoperatively
- Hypopituitarism
- Hypothalamic, intracranial injury, stroke
- Transient diabetes insipidus 15–20% (generally lasts 12 h–4 d)
- CSF rhinorrhea ± 5%—may require CSF drainage or reoperation

ANTICIPATED PROBLEMS/CONCERNS
- ↑ BP and arrhythmia from cocaine pledgets, infiltration with lidocaine and epinephrine with 1/200,000
- ↑ BP marked but usually transient
- Occasional cavernous sinus or carotid hemorrhage—severe and rapid
- Cortisol and other hormonal replacement
- Diabetes insipidus management

PNEUMONECTOMY

RISK

- Cigarette smoking, radon, certain industrial exposures
- Male:female 2:1 (female proportion increasing)
- 30,000 lung resections (all types) performed annually; 19,000 lobectomies

PERIOPERATIVE RISKS

- Mortality 5–15% within 30 d
- Cardiac morbidity significant
- Morbidity/mortality higher after right pneumonectomy/more extensive resections

WORRY ABOUT

- Pulm reserve/pulm HTN after resection
- Concomitant CV disease

- Postop pain relief
- Cardiac arrhythmias common postop
- Perioperative thromboembolic events in 26%
- Pulm edema

OVERVIEW

- Untreated, mortality from non–small cell CA is 100%; nonoperative therapy ineffective
- Surgery is primary treatment for non–small cell CA of lung
- Paraneoplastic syndromes not a contraindication to definitive surgical treatment
- Lobectomy performed if disease limited to a lobe or lobar bronchus
- Pneumonectomy for complete removal of lesions involving a main bronchus, with spread or fixation of tumor to hilum, or crossing lobar fissure
- Sleeve pneumonectomy: resection of segment of trachea followed by bronchotracheal anastomosis

- Completion pneumonectomy: removal of all remaining lung following previous removal of a portion of a lung

ICD-9-CM Codes: 162.2–9 (Primary lung cancer)

INDICATIONS AND USUAL TREATMENT

- Non–small cell lung cancer (T2) with hilar involvement, no distant metastases, ± metastases to lymph nodes in peribronchial or ipsilateral hilar region
- T3 lesions: additional resection of involved structures (chest wall, diaphragm, mediastinal pleura, pericardium)
- Positive ipsilateral mediastinal nodes (N2), stage IIIA: possibly pneumonectomy with neoadjuvant radiation and/or chemotherapy (may be associated with high mortality from ARDS)

ASSESSMENT POINTS

SYSTEM	EFFECT	ASSESSMENT BY HX	PE	TEST
HEENT	Recurrent laryngeal nerve involvement	Hoarseness	HEENT exam	
CV	RV dysfunction due to PA HTN LV function, valvular disease Arrhythmias	Chest pain/SOB; Exercise tolerance, palpitations	CV exam	ECG; possible ECHO, Doppler studies, PA catheterization
RESP	Sputum, bronchospasm; ability to tolerate loss of lung	SOB, exercise tolerance, sputum, smoking Hx	Resp exam Clubbing	Chest CT; ABG; PFTs: FEV_1, DLCO, split lung function tests (VO_2 peak)
ENDO	Hypercalcemia; SIADH → hyponatremia; Cushing's syndrome	Somnolence, anorexia, N/V Wt loss, signs of water intoxication		Check Ca^{2+}, Na^+; SIADH → hypotonic plasma, relatively hypertonic urine; Cushing's: hypokalemic alkalosis
HEME	Anemia, polycythemia Migratory thrombophlebitis	Hx of thrombophlebitis		Hct
NEURO-MUSC	Eaton-Lambert syndrome (E-L) Polymyositis		May be subclinical; Polymyositis → more muscle wasting	E-L: sensitivity to nondepolarizing muscle relaxants

Key Reference: Benumof JL: Anesthesia for Thoracic Surgery, 2nd ed. Philadelphia, WB Saunders, 1995.

PERIOPERATIVE IMPLICATIONS

Preoperative Preparation

- Bronchodilators
- If sputum: antibiotics, hydration, mobilization
- Prophylactic digoxin in patients in NSR probably not warranted

Anesthetic Technique

- General ± epidural anesthesia

Monitoring

- Arterial line
- CVP not routine intraoperatively, but may be useful postop
- PA: requires placement on nonoperative side; fluoroscopy helpful; consider TEE

Airway

- If difficult airway or unable to intubate orally: bronchial blocker, nasal intubation
- Aspiration devastating

Induction/Maintenance

- Lateral decubitus positioning: check ear and eye on down side, axillary roll, arm positioning
- Potent inhalational agents bronchodilate but ↓ LV function, attenuate hypoxic vasoconstriction; ↑ in Qs/Qt not clinically significant at 1.0 MAC

- Problems with one-lung ventilation techniques: trauma, malposition, hypoxemia

SURGICAL STAGES

Dissection

- Posterolateral thoracotomy incision in 5th or 6th intercostal space for best exposure
- Venous drainage may be temporarily occluded to ↓ theoretical dissemination of tumor cells, while avoiding engorgement
- PA may be divided first to ↓ blood loss in specimen
- Closure tested with positive pressure breath
- Bronchial vessels may cause significant postop blood loss

Definitive Surgery

- Limit volume administration.
  - EBL: <500 ml
  - Capillary leak and ↑ PVR due to loss of pulm tissue → pulm edema
- Chest tube usually not on suction, but pleural pressure regulated to –4 to –10 cm/H_2O to prevent mediastinal shift

Postoperative Considerations

- Cardiac arrhythmias >20%, usually supraventricular

- Postpneumonectomy pulm edema
  - high mortality
  - commonly ascribed to excess fluid administration but frequently associated with low-normal filling pressures, little response to diuresis; may be related to ARDS
- Risk of pulm insufficiency
- Significant postop pain: epidural analgesia probably most effective

ANTICIPATED PROBLEMS/CONCERNS

- Postop bleeding due to inadequate surgical hemostasis
- Hypotension from unrecognized blood loss; cardiac tamponade; MI/ischemia with low cardiac output
- Postop pulm edema: rule out myocardial dysfunction; volume overload; correct dysrhythmias, hypoalbuminemia
- Atelectasis, pneumonitis
- Wound dehiscence and infection rare
- DVT and pulm embolism common (20%)
- Persistent air leak may occur where incomplete fissures were divided
- Bronchopleural fistula
- Empyema in 5%

PREGNANT SURGICAL PATIENT

Rhonda Zuckerman, M.D.

RISK

- 50,000 pregnant patients/y undergo nondelivery procedures in USA
- Most common: trauma-related procedures, cervical suture, appendectomy, biliary tract disease–related procedures, breast biopsy, ovarian cystectomy

PERIOPERATIVE RISKS

- ↑ Maternal anesthetic risk for hypoxemia/pulmonary aspiration due to failed ET intubation
- Potential risk to fetus
  – Preterm delivery (preterm labor incidence 8–11%, higher for pelvic procedures)
  – Teratogenicity

WORRY ABOUT

- Maternal airway precautions
- Gastric chemoprophylaxis
- Prevention and treatment of maternal hypoxemia
- Avoidance of aortocaval compression (after 20 weeks of gestation) and hypotension
- Detection and treatment of preterm labor

OVERVIEW

- If surgery must be performed during pregnancy, 2nd trimester is preferred period, since organogenesis is complete and risk of preterm delivery relatively low

- Acute exposure to anesthetic agents has not been not associated with fetal malformations at birth.
- Depressant effects of anesthetic agents are mainly of concern if fetus is delivered perioperatively.

ICD-9-CM Code: V22.2 (Pregnancy)

INDICATIONS AND USUAL TREATMENT

- Cervical suture placement for prevention of preterm delivery due to cervical incompetence (performed at 12–16 weeks of gestation).
- Other procedures performed only when risks of postponement outweigh benefits of avoiding increased maternal anesthetic risk and potential fetal harm.

ASSESSMENT POINTS

SYSTEM	EFFECT	ASSESSMENT BY HX	PE	TEST
HEENT	Engorged, fragile mucosa, difficult intubation		Airway exam	Mallampati class
CV	Supine hypotensive syndrome	Nausea, diaphoresis while supine	Assess for hypotension, bradycardia while supine	
RESP	↑ O_2 consumption; ↓ FRC ↑ PaO_2, ↓ $PaCO_2$			ABG (if indicated)
GI	Full stomach, decreased LES tone	Reflux symptoms		
CNS	↓ MAC, ↓ intraspinal local anesthetic requirements			

Key Reference: Cohen SE: Nonobstetric surgery during pregnancy. *In* Chestnut DH (ed): Obstetric Anesthesia: Principles and Practice. St. Louis, Mosby-Year Book, 1994, p 273.

PERIOPERATIVE IMPLICATIONS

Anesthetic Technique

- Regional Anesthesia: ↓ Risk of maternal airway problems, ↑ risk of hypotension (compared with GA).
- General Anesthesia: Inhalation agents are tocolytic—may prevent contractions in OR; however, preterm labor may occur in recovery period.

Monitoring

- Viable gestational age fetus: consider pre-, intra-, postoperative fetal heart tone and uterine activity monitoring.
- Nonviable gestational age fetus: pre- and postoperative fetal heart tone documentation; consider pre-, intra-, and postoperative uterine activity monitoring.
- Obstetric consultation recommended; pediatric notification indicated if delivery of a viable fetus is possible.

Airway

- Edema and engorgement: ↑ Risk of failed intubation, ↑ risk of bleeding, especially during nasal intubation
- ↑ Risk of pulm aspiration

Induction

- Regional Anesthesia: Spinal, epidural, or other block may be appropriate depending on location of surgical site
- General Anesthesia: Full stomach—awake intubation vs. denitrogenation followed by rapid-sequence induction

Maintenance

- Maintain left uterine displacement
- General Anesthesia: Inhalation agent—consider nitrous oxide, opioid, benzodiazepine (last often avoided in 1st trimester, although acute exposure not thought to be teratogenic). Muscle relaxants—minimal placental transfer.

Extubation

- After patient awake, able to protect airway

Postoperative Considerations

- Pain: Consider IV or epidural PCA (opioids should not be withheld)
- Left uterine displacement in PACU
- Document fetal viability
- Consider monitoring for preterm labor

ANTICIPATED PROBLEMS/CONCERNS

- Pulm aspiration, failed intubation
- Preterm labor
- Fetal distress

PYLORIC STENOSIS REPAIR

J. Lance Lichtor, M.D.

RISK

- 1.5–3/1000 Caucasian births
- Lower incidence in African-Americans, Puerto Ricans, Asians
- Male > female (4:1)
- Tends to run in families (children of affected parents have higher incidence [3–5%])
- 2.5–5.5: higher incidence for first-born

PERIOPERATIVE RISKS

- Hypotension due to preop hypovolemia and volume shifts common
- Hypoglycemia common with postop apnea or convulsions due to cessation of IV glucose and inadequate glycogen stores
- Mortality <1%
- Wound infection 5–20%

WORRY ABOUT

- Fluid and electrolyte deficiency (hyperchloremic metabolic alkalosis, hypokalemia)
- Not a surgical emergency

OVERVIEW

- Gross thickening at circular smooth muscle of pylorus resulting in gradual obstruction of gastric outlet
- Projectile vomiting usually 2–4 wk; can have severe dehydration and acid-base abnormality

ICD-9-CM Code: 750.5

INDICATIONS AND USUAL TREATMENT

- Persistent vomiting usually after or toward the end of a feed with inability to feed
- Pyloromyotomy is treatment of choice
- No successful medical therapy

ASSESSMENT POINTS

SYSTEM	EFFECT	ASSESSMENT BY HX	PE	TEST
GI	Pyloric thickening	Vomiting	Olive-size mass, upper abdomen	GI series with barium or US
HEME	Hemoconcentration		Volume status measures; orthostatic vital signs Vasoconstriction	Hct
ELECTROLYTES	Dehydration Acid-base abnormalities		Volume status measures; orthostatic vital signs; area with cold skin	Electrolytes
RENAL	Alkaline urine Acid urine	Persistent vomiting, volume depletion		

Key Reference: Bissonnette B, Sullivan PJ: Pyloric stenosis. Can J Anaesth 1991; 38:668–676.

PREOPERATIVE IMPLICATIONS

- Correct electrolyte and acid-base abnormalities. Gastric sections are lost; therefore, hypochloremic alkalosis results.
- Stop oral feeds, replace ECF volume, replace K+.

Monitoring

- Routine

Airway

- Risk of aspiration: evacuate stomach contents. Consider rapid-sequence induction.
- Nasogastric tube after induction.

Maintenance

- Avoid narcotics: rarely needed, prolong awakening. Local anesthetics (in addition to GA) useful.

SURGICAL STAGES

Induction

- Consider emptying stomach before induction.

Skin incision

- Abdomen opened through right transverse skin incision above liver edge or a right paramedian incision.

Dissection

- Pylorus delivered into wound; incision through serosa and extended through circular muscle the length of tumor; circular muscle spread bluntly.

ANTICIPATED PROBLEMS/CONCERNS

- Hypotension due to altered volume status.
- Hypoglycemia, apnea, and convulsions, possibly due to cessation of IV glucose and depletion of liver glycogen.
- Postop vomiting if early feeds.
- Wound infection not uncommon.
- Duodenal perforation may occur during myotomy; not a problem if recognized intraoperatively.

RADICAL NECK DISSECTION

Noel Lee Chun, M.D.

RISK

- Performed for a variety of cancers, both local and metastatic from head and thorax
- Frequency ↑ with age, peaking in 7th decade
- Male > female (3:1)

PERIOPERATIVE RISKS

- Mortality rare, related to preop medical condition
- Morbidity includes MI, CVA, cranial nerve injury (20+%), pneumothorax, chylothorax, vascular injury, venous air embolism

WORRY ABOUT

- Tumor may distort airway and cause obstruction
- Associated cigarette use affecting CV and pulmonary systems
- Associated alcohol use affecting hepatic, hematologic, neurologic systems
- Malnutrition

OVERVIEW

- A complete cervical lymphadenectomy and sacrifice of sternocleidomastoid muscle, internal jugular vein, and spinal accessory nerve (cranial nerve XI). A functional neck dissection preserves these three structures; many modifications in between attempt to preserve some of these structures (termed modified)

ICD-9-CM Code: 144 (Malignant neoplasm of floor of mouth)

INDICATIONS AND USUAL TREATMENT

- To remove neoplastic tissue. In 80%, cancer is metastatic from another site. In 85%, primary tumor is supraclavicular.
- Often performed in conjunction with an operation to remove primary tumor (glossectomy, laryngectomy)
- Often performed in conjunction with flap reconstruction or skin graft to cover surgical defect
- Patient management often includes a course of preop or postop radiation therapy.

ASSESSMENT POINTS

SYSTEM	EFFECT	ASSESSMENT BY HX	PE	TEST
HEENT	Tumor may affect airway	Dyspnea, dysphagia, dysarthria	Airway exam Headlight exam Fiberoptic exam	CXR CT/MRI Flow volume loops
CV	Smoking and alcohol related	Angina/PND/orthopnea HTN/CHF/MI Exercise tolerance	Chest exam	CXR ECG Stress test ECHO/Angio
RESP	Smoking related	SOB Cough/sputum Exercise tolerance	Chest exam	ABGs, ?PFTs CXR
HEME	Anemia, coagulopathies, cirrhosis	Fatigue Bleeding, bruisability Abdominal distention	Inspection for evidence of same	CBC PT, PTT, BT LFTs
NEURO	Alcohol withdrawal, nutritional deficiencies (see Malnutrition)	Anxiety, tachycardia, diaphoresis, seizures, peripheral neuropathy	Neuro exam	Treatment based on Hx and PE

Key Reference: Dougherty TB, et al: Anesthetic management of the patient scheduled for head and neck cancer surgery. J Clinical Anesth 1994; 6:74–82.

INTRAOPERATIVE MANAGEMENT

Monitoring

- Consider 2 major IVs at a minimum, as blood loss can be significant (esp. with flap reconstruction), and usually both arms are tucked with head 180° away
- Blood loss usually <800 ml; volume shifts usually not hemodynamically significant
- Consider precordial Doppler, end-tidal CO_2/N_2, TEE to monitor for venous air embolism (head usually elevated 30–45°)
- Consider arterial catheter and CVP/PA catheters for monitoring pressures and checking laboratory tests and monitoring volume status if CV unstable

Airway

- Head and neck tumors can compromise airway. Consider awake intubation or elective tracheostomy.
- Nasal and oral airways may be impossible to use because of airway distortion or tumor.
- Patient usually 180° away from anesthesiologist.
- Often a tracheostomy placed at beginning or end of procedure; airway control crucial at this stage.

SURGICAL STAGES

Induction

- Once airway secured, routine

Skin Incision

- Many variations of neck incisions with an apron of dermis and epidermis stripped of subcutaneous fat and reflected upward.

Dissection

- During dissection, all lymphatic tissue and fat removed en bloc and major anatomy defined.
- Large neck vessels and important structures can be damaged with significant blood loss, cranial nerve paralysis, chyle leak

Definitive Surgery

- If performed in conjunction with excision of primary, extensive flap reconstruction, microvascular reanastomosis, laryngectomy, and tracheostomy may be necessary
- If flap reconstruction, avoid peripheral vasoconstrictors
- LMW dextran or other anticoagulation with postop monitoring for ischemia/thrombosis may be desirable.
- Approximate duration: 4–10 h

- Occasionally carotid artery must be sacrificed because of tumor invasion; it may be ligated, anastomosed to external carotid, or reconstructed with graft material.

Closure and Postoperative Considerations

- Airway considerations are first concern: have tracheostomy obturator available at all times.
- Disfiguring procedure; if laryngectomy, patients often unable to communicate. Need sensitivity.
- Pain score: 2–6.

ANTICIPATED PROBLEMS/CONCERNS

- Extent of surgery and preop medical condition determine complications.
- If bilateral neck dissection performed, and both internal jugular veins are sacrificed, ↑ ICP with blindness has been reported.
- Majority, even patients in poor medical condition, tolerate procedure well.
- Postop pulm toilet and nutritional support crucial to short-term recovery, but patients must remember that they are in a marathon to get well.

RADICAL PROSTATECTOMY (RETROPUBIC) Lee A. Fleisher, M.D.

RISK

- 50,000 patients/y
- Racial predominance: none

PERIOPERATIVE RISKS

- Perioperative mortality rare (<1%)
- Increased risk of DVT, pulmonary embolism
- 25% risk of impotence with nerve-sparing procedure; 75% risk without nerve-sparing procedure

WORRY ABOUT

- Venous air embolism
- Massive blood loss
- Nerve injury from position and surgical manipulation
- Often in flexed position with head down, increasing risk of aspiration

OVERVIEW

- Prostate, bladder, and seminal vesicles are removed
- Significant blood loss associated with transection of dorsal vein
- Regional anesthesia may be associated with lower blood loss and lower incidence of DVT

ICD-9-CM Code: 185.0 (Cancer of prostate)

INDICATIONS AND USUAL TREATMENT

- The following conditions should be met:
  - Isolated and localized prostatic malignancy
    - Anticipated life expectancy of ≥10 y
    - Good general health
    - Absence of indication of metastatic disease by work-up
- If coexisting disease, orchiectomy and hormonal therapy primary treatment
- Radiation therapy has similar 5-y survival rates.
- "Smart bomb" radiation therapies also have similar 5-y survival rates with less surrounding tissue toxicity than classic radiation therapy.
- Herbal therapies are alternative—8 hydroxy compounds in green teas have effectiveness in experimental animal models

ASSESSMENT POINTS (in addition to evaluation of coexisting disease)

SYSTEM	EFFECT	ASSESSMENT BY HX	PE	TEST
RESP	Pulmonary metastases	SOB	Auscultation	CXR, CT scan
MS	Skeletal metastases	Bone pain	Palpation	X-ray, bone scan, prostate-specific antigen (PSA)
RENAL	Chronic obstruction			Cr and/or BUN

Key Reference: Shir Y, Raja SN, Frank SM: The effect of epidural versus regional anesthesia on postoperative pain and analgesic requirements in patients undergoing radical prostatectomy. Anesthesiology 1994; 80:49–56.

PERIOPERATIVE IMPLICATIONS

Anesthetic Technique

- Can be performed under regional, general, or combined anesthetic techniques

Monitoring

- Large-bore IV lines for blood loss
- Consider arterial line
- Consider CVP, PCWP, or TEE if coexisting disease
- Consider monitoring for air embolism

Airway

- None

Induction

- Requires level of at least T8 for regional
- Continuous regional techniques offer excellent pain management

SURGICAL STAGES

Dissection

- Steady blood loss during dissection

Definitive Surgery

- May have significant blood loss during control of dorsal vein complex
- Hypotension may develop from blood loss or air embolism
- Indigo carmine frequently given to facilitate repair—incidence of anaphylaxis after indigo carmine and disturbance of pulse oximetry
- EBL: 1000–2000 ml
- Moderate volume shifts

Postoperative Considerations

- Significant postoperative pain
- Epidural may lead to fewer complications
- Pain score: 4–8
- IV PCA or epidural PCA for 2–3 d; newer modalities with education are associated with discharge on postop day 2 or 3.
- May develop pulmonary embolism or DVT
- May develop peroneal nerve injury from lithotomy position

ANTICIPATED PROBLEMS/CONCERNS

- Air embolism may occur because of large open veins and patient position

RETAINED PLACENTA, REMOVAL OF

Mark C. Norris, M.D.

RISK

- Manual extraction needed in 5% of vaginal deliveries.
- Third stage of labor is complete within 10 min in 75% of women. After 10 min, risks of retained placenta, hemorrhage, and need for transfusion increase.
- If more than 30 min, >40% will require manual placental extraction.
- Preterm gestation, 2 or more previous abortions, induced or augmented labor, and nulliparity increase risk of prolonged 3rd stage of labor.

PERIOPERATIVE RISKS

- Retained placenta places patient at ↑ risk of significant blood loss, need for transfusion, and need for D&C.
- Uterine perforation is a risk with D&C.

WORRY ABOUT

- Full stomach (airway, other forms of effective analgesia present—epidural)
- Volume status
- Need uterine relaxation?
- Risk of placenta accreta/percreta

OVERVIEW

- Obstetrician requires good analgesia ± uterine relaxation
- One cause of prolonged third stage of labor is abnormal placental implantation.
- Women with a previous cesarean delivery may be at greater risk of placenta accreta. These women are at very high risk of postpartum hemorrhage and may require immediate hysterectomy to remove placental fragments and control bleeding.

ICD-9-CM Code: 666-O (Retained placenta with hemorrhage)

INDICATIONS/USUAL TREATMENT

- Most obstetricians will attempt manual removal of placenta if 3rd stage of labor lasts beyond 30 min
- Some will intervene earlier, especially if lower uterine segment contracts and will not allow placenta to pass
- Usual treatment is manual exploration and extraction

ASSESSMENT POINTS

SYSTEM	EFFECT	ASSESSMENT BY HX	PE	TEST
AIRWAY	Pregnancy-related changes: ↑ vascularity, airway edema, ↑ risk of difficult intubation	Previous difficulties	Mouth opening, oropharyngeal structures, dentition	
CV (volume status)	Significant, rapid hemorrhage possible ↑ Blood volume with pregnancy	EBL	BP, HR, tissue turgor, mucous membranes	Tilt test
GI	Delayed gastric emptying (worse during painful labor)	Last meal		

Key Reference: Combs CA, Laros RK Jr: Prolonged third stage of labor: morbidity and risk factors. Obstet Gynecol 1991; 77:863–867.

PERIOPERATIVE MANAGEMENT

Preoperative Preparation

- Prepare for IV resuscitation (if needed) including potential for blood transfusion

Anesthetic Technique

- Epidural: If present and functioning and volume status adequate
- MAC: If *minimal* sedation/analgesia/relaxation adequate. Most appropriate if placenta separated but trapped by contracted lower uterine segment
- GA: Excessive bleeding, no epidural, need for uterine instrumentation, placenta accreta

Monitoring

- Consider arterial line, CVP, Foley catheter if significant blood loss

Airway

- Consider full stomach: Rapid-sequence induction with cricoid pressure if GA

- Minimal sedation if MAC/regional anesthesia used (constant verbal contact). *Remember:* Pregnancy decreases MAC and speeds uptake of inhaled anesthetics
- Increased risk of difficult intubation: Consider awake intubation

Induction/Maintenance

- Regional requires T10 level
- May require uterine relaxation if placenta trapped by firmly contracted lower uterine segment
  - Beta-adrenergic agonists (terbutaline): slow onset, significant hemodynamic effects
  - Amyl nitrate: explosive, difficult to titrate, headache
  - Potent anesthetic agent: effective, requires general ET anesthesia
  - NTG: rapid onset, short duration, minimal hemodynamic effects; IV: 50 µg: onset 60 sec, duration 60 sec (obstetrician must be ready, hands in vagina, traction on umbilical cord); sublingual spray NTG (Nitrolingual Spray, Rhone Poulenc Rorer Pharmaceuticals Inc., Collegeville, PA): 0.8 mg (2 sprays): onset 35–65 sec; minimal maternal side effects

Surgical Stages

- Removal can be complete, partial, or unsuccessful
- Partial: May require manual exploration of uterus or curettage; will need more complete analgesia; very difficult with sedation alone; consider GA if no regional anesthesia
- Unsuccessful: If placenta accreta, will require laparotomy, possible hysterectomy (↑ blood loss due to changes associated with pregnancy)
- EBL (uncomplicated): 500 ml
- Postpartum hysterectomy: potential for severe hemorrhage 1–20 L

Postoperative Considerations

- Uncomplicated: minimal pain
- Hysterectomy: pain like that of C-section (neuraxial opioids if regional, PCA [24–48 h] if GA)

ANTICIPATED PROBLEMS/CONCERNS

- Amount of blood loss correlates with ease of extraction.

RETINAL BUCKLE SURGERY

Nader El-Gamal, M.D.

RISK

- People within USA: 20,000–30,000/y
- Racial predominance: none

PERIOPERATIVE RISKS

- Morbidity and mortality: 0.1% mortality rate related to patient-associated diseases
- Airway management
- Intravitreal injection of gas (SF_6) and N_2O

WORRY ABOUT

- Oculocardiac reflex
- Intravitreal injection of gas
- Other associated diseases (diabetes mellitus, HTN)
- Postop N/V, pain

OVERVIEW

- Age and comorbidity of patient: usually elderly with other associated diseases
- Scleral buckle then positioned over tears and sutured in place to cover every retinal tear

ICD-9-CM Code: 361.9 (Retinal detachment)

INDICATIONS AND USUAL TREATMENT

- Treatment of retinal detachment
- Cryotherapy over retinal tears

ASSESSMENT POINTS

SYSTEM	EFFECT	ASSESSMENT BY HX	PE	TEST
HEENT		Snoring	Airway exam	
RESP	Associated diseases	SOB, exercise tolerance	Chest exam	O_2 sat
HEME	Bleeding disorder			PTT
	Retrobulbar hemorrhage	Hx of easy bruising		PT
RENAL	Impairment 2° age, DM			BUN, Cr
				Glucose

Key Reference: Wong DHW: Regional anesthesia for intraocular surgery. A review. Can J Anesth 1993; 40:635.

PERIOPERATIVE MANAGEMENT

Anesthetic Technique

- Regional preferred over general
  - ↓ Incidence of oculocardiac reflex
  - ↓ Interference with body physiology
  - ↓ Incidence of postop N/V
- Contraindications to local retrobulbar block—abnormal coagulation or bleeding profile
- Infection at or near injection site
- Inability to communicate (language barrier, deafness)
  - Inability to lie flat
  - Chronic cough or tremor
  - Patient refusal
  - Open globe

Monitoring

- Routine

Airway

- In sedation cases avoid oversedation that may obstruct the airway, since intraoperative access difficult
- If using heated instrument, ensure that drapes are such that oxygen is not directed to instrument and is diluted rapidly in air

SURGICAL STAGES

Induction

- Sedation: midazolam, fentanyl, propofol
- Retrobulbar block and then titrate sedation, but avoid oversedated, disoriented, uncooperative patient
- In GA: Avoid any sudden bucking or coughing; muscle relaxation preferred

Surgery

- During isolation of muscles monitor for bradycardia, asystole
- In GA twitch monitor to make sure patient completely paralyzed
- Near end of procedure, surgeon might inject air or SF_6, so N_2O should be discontinued 15–20 min before

Postoperative Considerations

- Pain score: 3–5
- EBL: minimal

ANTICIPATED PROBLEMS/CONCERNS

- Airway obstruction, respiratory depression from oversedation
- Oculocardiac reflex
- Inappropriate level of sedation (disoriented, confused, oversedated patient or anxious, hypertensive, lightly sedated patient)
- Postop N/V

ROTATOR CUFF SURGERY

Noel Lee Chun, M.D.

RISK

- People within USA: ~50,000/y; almost all >40 y; some younger athletes
- Fluoroscopic examination of 6061 random asymptomatic people revealed cuff calcification in 2.7%
- 20–30% incidence of rupture of supraspinatus tendon in cadavers >60 y
- Males >> females (3:1)

PERIOPERATIVE RISKS

- Risks associated with interscalene block (ISB) anesthesia include spinal, epidural, and IV injection of local anesthetic, recurrent laryngeal nerve block, and pneumothorax

- Infections 1–5%
- Limitation of motion 5%
- Nerve damage 1–5%
- Mortality—minimal and related to preop conditions

WORRY ABOUT

- Whether to use regional or general anesthesia
- Airway management critical, as head is often only partially accessible

OVERVIEW

- Rotator cuff composed of subscapularis tendon anteriorly and supraspinatus, infraspinatus, and teres minor tendon insertions posteriorly.

- Most common injury is tear of supraspinatus insertion; however, any of the tendons may be involved.
- Associated surgical findings include biceps tendon rupture, glenohumeral arthritis, and labral fraying, resulting in shoulder pain and variable degrees of loss of function and ROM.

ICD-9-CM Codes: 727.61 (Nontraumatic); 840.4 (Traumatic)

INDICATIONS AND USUAL TREATMENT

- Cuff tears are repaired primarily when possible; however, sometimes hardware and special techniques necessary owing to poor quality of tissue involved.
- Arthroscopic evaluation and debridement often performed prior to repair.

ASSESSMENT POINTS

(see Rheumatoid Arthritis [RA] if appropriate)

SYSTEM	EFFECT	ASSESSMENT BY HX	PE	TEST
HEENT	If RA or connective tissue disease, may have limited ROM of head/neck	Limited ROM Head/neck or neck	Airway exam	C-spine X-ray
CV	If RA or connective tissue disease, may have valvular heart disease/conduction defects	Angina/PND/orthopnea Palpitations/CHF Exercise tolerance	Chest exam Exam of peripheral pulses and vital signs	ECG ECHO
RESP	If RA, may have pulm fibrosis or pleural effusion	SOB Exercise tolerance	Chest exam	CXR ABGs PFTs
HEME	Hx NSAID use—may affect coagulation	Hx medications, bleed/bruise	Inspection for evidence of same	
IMMUNE	If RA, may be immunocompromised	Hx medications, infectious disease		CBC and differential

Key Reference: Brown AR, et al: Interscalene block for shoulder arthroscopy: Comparison with general anesthesia. J Arthroscop Rel Surg 1993; 9:295–300.

INTRAOPERATIVE MANAGEMENT

Monitoring
- Routine
- Precordial Doppler/end-tidal N_2 or TEE to monitor for venous air embolism in sitting position
- Pad pressure points, and protect eyes to avoid corneal abrasion

Airway
- Lateral decubitus or sitting position with restricted access to head
- Securing airway management crucial

SURGICAL STAGES

Induction
- For GA, routine
- For interscalene block (ISB) 40 ml of local.
  – With ISB, 100% incidence of phrenic nerve paralysis, and significant incidence of recurrent laryngeal nerve paralysis and cervical plexus blockade
- Technique contraindicated if advanced pulm disease or contralateral vocal cord paralysis

- Field blocks or SQ local infiltration may be used for skin of shoulder (C3–C4) and medial upper arm (T2).
- Muscular relaxation important to help mobilize cuff; this can be provided by regional anesthesia or NMB

Skin Incision
- Rotator cuff approached via oblique incision over acromion

Dissection
- Part of overlying deltoid muscle detached and then divided to reach rotator cuff. Care must be taken in reattaching deltoid to acromial bone edge to avoid avulsion and loss of function. If splitting of deltoid is carried more than 5 cm anteriorly, axillary nerve may be damaged with loss of function of all or part of deltoid.
- Supraspinatus tendon should not be dissected and elevated from contiguous bone floor for a distance exceeding 2 cm medial to superior glenoid rim; otherwise, suprascapular nerve injury with additional weakening of external rotator muscles may result

Definitive Surgery
- Ruptured tendons sewn together primarily if possible; sometimes necessary to dissect additional length of muscle and anchor it to head of humerus with suture or hardware.

Closure and Postoperative Considerations
- Arm is placed in sling or abduction pillow prior to awakening; usually no active motion for several weeks to avoid possibility of disruption of repair.
- Pain score: 3–8. Pain can be significantly mitigated by use of long-acting local anesthetics in an interscalene block.

ANTICIPATED PROBLEMS/CONCERNS

- Preop medical condition determines anticipated complications; majority of patients, even those in poor medical condition, tolerate this procedure well
- Postoperative pain management with IV PCA or interscalene block.

SEIZURE SURGERY

Barbara A. Dodson, M.D.

RISK

- 0.5–2% of general population with recurrent seizures (szs)
- ~300,000 patients have medically refractory szs

PERIOPERATIVE RISKS

- ↑ or ↓ sz threshold with anesthetics
- Adverse drug reactions from anticonvulsants themselves and interactions with anesthetic adjuvants

WORRY ABOUT

- Status epilepticus, loss of airway during conscious sedation, ↑ICP in patients with mass lesions

OVERVIEW

- Szs, of both epileptic and nonepileptic origin, classified as partial or generalized. Partial szs have focal origins (but may progress to bilateral). Simple partial sz implies undetectable change in consciousness and limited EEG distribution. Sz focus spreads in complex partial szs to multiple areas and alters consciousness. Generalized szs simultaneously involve both hemispheres and are subdivided into inhibitory (absence and atonic) and excitatory (clonic, tonic, and myoclonic).

ICD-9-CM Code: 790.3

ETIOLOGY

- Szs may be secondary to multiple neurologic conditions, including post-traumatic injuries, tumors, AVM, and idiopathic epilepsy
- Other causes include psychiatric disorders, neurofibromatosis, tuberous sclerosis, drug and alcohol abuse

INDICATIONS

- Primary goal to render patient seizure-free with minimal toxicity using variety of anticonvulsants
- Szs arising from discrete foci may be amenable to surgical resection (e.g., temporal lobectomy)

ASSESSMENT POINTS

SYSTEM	EFFECT	ASSESSMENT BY HX	PE	TEST
HEENT	Gingival hyperplasia, facial trauma		Facial fracture, broken or missing teeth, gingival hyperplasia	
RESP	Aspiration during szs	Hx of pneumonia	Rales, ↓ breath sounds	CXR
GI	Liver toxicity 2° to medications			LFTs
ENDO	Bone marrow suppression and thrombocytopenia 2° to medication	Bleeding	Petechiae, ecchymoses	CBC, plt count, PT, PTT
CNS	Seizures, both partial and generalized Personality disorders	Preseizure auras, automations	Neurologic exam	CT, MRI, EEG telemetry, Wada test (to determine dominant hemisphere for memory and speech)
MS	Injury during szs		Signs of trauma	

Key Reference: Kofke WA, Tempelhoff R, Dasheiff RM: Anesthesia for epileptic patients and for epilepsy surgery. *In* Cotrell JE, Smith D (eds): Anesthesia and Neurosurgery, 3rd ed. St. Louis, Mosby, 1994, pp 495–524.

PERIOPERATIVE IMPLICATIONS

Preoperative Preparation

- Determine baseline neurologic status
- Evaluate cooperativeness if conscious sedation planned
- Determine type and frequency of szs; anticonvulsant medications, and whether tapered preop
- Review results of preop neurologic evaluation, esp. hemispheric dominance and relationship of surgical field to speech, motor, and memory areas
- Avoid premedication with drugs such as benzodiazepines that could ablate seizure foci even temporarily.

Monitoring

- Consider arterial catheter and Foley catheter
- End-tidal CO_2 via nasal cannula during conscious analgesia

Airway

- Obvious airway difficulties may preclude use of conscious analgesia technique

Maintenance

- NO_2-narcotic technique with low-dose isoflurane and/or propofol can be used for GA if electrocorticography (ECOG) is not planned. Anticonvulsant medications will ↑ both opioid and muscle relaxant requirements. Hyperventilation should be avoided. If ECOG is planned, a NO_2-narcotic technique should be used and benzodiazepines, volatile anesthetics, and muscle paralysis should be meticulously avoided
- Fentanyl and/or alfentanil infusion, droperidol, and benadryl can be used for conscious sedation. Effect of low-dose propofol on ECOG controversial.

Extubation

- Facilitate rapid emergence and avoid HTN and coughing

Postoperative Period

- Anticonvulsant blood levels can both ↑ and ↓ postop

Adjuvants

- Low-dose methohexital and etomidate can be used to ↑ activity at sz focus to aid in location and evaluation of area for resection during surgery
- Benzodiazepine and higher dose methohexital to ↓ sz activity

ANTICIPATED PROBLEMS/CONCERNS

- New neurologic deficits, seizures, anticonvulsant toxicity, status epilepticus

SPINAL FUSION

Madelyn Kahana, M.D.

RISK

- Prevalence: 4/1000 in North America
- Female predominance: 8:1

PERIOPERATIVE RISKS

- Perioperative mortality rare (0–0.5%)
- Venous air embolism (VAE) can occur and produce CV collapse
- Postop neurologic deficit in 0.7–5%
- Massive blood loss possible (1–5%)
- Pneumothorax 1–5%

WORRY ABOUT

- Etiology (? syndrome or tumor rather than idiopathic)
- Large intraoperative blood loss
- Potential for VAE
- Problems of prone position
- Postop resp insufficiency, hyponatremia

OVERVIEW

- Scoliosis is rotational abnormality of spine and ribs
- Dx of idiopathic scoliosis one of exclusion
- May be significant restrictive lung disease
- Evoked potential monitoring can limit choice of anesthetic technique
- An intraoperative "wake-up" may be requested by operating surgeon
- Intraoperative VAE is possible

ICD-9-CM Code: 737.30

INDICATIONS AND USUAL TREATMENT

- Surgical correction absolutely indicated if curve > 60° or if a lesser curve with resp compromise, pain, or likelihood of progression to 60°
- Most patients with curve <40° do not need surgical correction
- Medical management with proven efficacy includes a variety of bracing techniques but is generally used if curve 20–45°
- Failure to correct significant curve results in a doubling of mortality for age, potential for progressive back pain, and progressive pulmonary dysfunction

ASSESSMENT POINTS

SYSTEM	EFFECT	ASSESSMENT BY HX	PE	TEST
CV	Cor pulmonale possible if significant lung disease	Exercise tolerance		ECG ECHO
RESP	Pulm dysfunction occurs with significant thoracic curves		Exercise tolerance	PFTs corrected for height
CNS	Preop neurologic dysfunction unusual; should lead to further assessment and diagnostic tests		Complete neurologic exam	?CT ?MRI
MS		Careful exam may lead to an alternative dx, e.g., Marfan's, Ehlers-Danlos, Goldenhar's syndrome; syrinx		

Key Reference: Kafer E: Respiratory and cardiovascular functions in scoliosis and the principles of anesthetic management. Anesthesiology 1980; 52:339–351.

PERIOPERATIVE IMPLICATIONS

Anesthetic Technique

- Performed utilizing general ET anesthesia in prone position
- Controlled hypotension used to limit blood loss
  – Potential for interference with evoked potential monitoring influences anesthetic agent choice

Monitoring

- Arterial line useful
- Consider CVP line to monitor volume and perhaps to treat VAE
- Foley catheter may facilitate adequate volume resuscitation

Induction/Maintenance

- Narcotics do not interfere with SSEPs or MEPs
- <1 MAC inhalation agent exerts only minimal effect on potential monitoring
- Anticipate need for midprocedure wake-up test

- Controlled hypotension accomplished with ß-blockade and IV vasodilators

Preoperative Management

- Large-bore IV lines because of anticipated blood loss

SURGICAL STAGES

Positioning

- Patient positioned prone on a frame that allows abdomen to be free from external compression to reduce venous pressure
- Pressure points padded carefully
- There must be no pressure on ocular structures or ear cartilage

Dissection/Definitive Surgery

- Prior to skin incision, surgical field is often infiltrated with dilute solution of epinephrine
- Steady bleeding during dissection
- Steady bleeding during decortication
- Hypotension may be due to blood loss or VAE
- After instrumentation in place, distraction is performed

- After distraction complete, a wake-up test is often performed
- Approximate duration: 4–8 h

Postoperative Considerations

- Pain score: 6–9
- Postop resp failure unusual but should be considered a possibility in patients with pre-existing restrictive lung disease
- New neurologic injury is an emergency and requires urgent removal of all hardware

ANTICIPATED PROBLEMS/CONCERNS

- Potential for massive blood loss and rapid development of hypotension
- Modest risk of VAE because of open epidural veins and prone position
- Perioperative neurologic injury in 0.7–5%; generally occurs during distraction
- Occasional reports of neurologic injury in spite of normal evoked responses support considering continued use of wake-up test
- Be confident that patient has idiopathic scoliosis (vs. neurologic/spine abn or other etiology)

SPLENECTOMY

Wendy K. Bernstein, M.D.
Lee A. Fleisher, M.D.

RISK

- No age or sex predilection

PERIOPERATIVE RISKS

- Mortality rate 0–3%
- Overall complication rate is 11.8% associated with pulm complications, DVT

WORRY ABOUT

- Potential for major blood loss requiring transfusion

OVERVIEW

- Spleen most commonly injured organ in blunt trauma
- Splenic trauma frequently associated with other intra-abdominal injuries

ICD-9-CM Codes: 865.10 (splenic trauma); 289.4 (hypersplenism)

ETIOLOGY

- S/P blunt or penetrating abdominal trauma requiring emergency operation (14%)
- Idiopathic thrombocytopenic purpura
- Hodgkin's lymphoma (27%)
- Hereditary spherocytosis
- Felty's syndrome
- Myeloid metaplasia
- Sickle cell disease
- Thalassemia
- Chronic leukemia

USUAL TREATMENT

- Depends upon indication
- Splenorrhaphy for splenic salvage after trauma

ASSESSMENT POINTS

SYSTEM	EFFECT	ASSESSMENT BY HX	TEST
CV	Cardiotoxicity Dysrhythmias, CHF	Chemotherapeutic agents—doxorubicin (dose >550 mg/m^2)	ECG, ECHO, MUGA → determine LV function
RESP	Pleural effusions; left lower lobe atelectasis if splenomegaly; pulm fibrosis	Chemotherapeutic agents—bleomycin, methotrexate, cytarabine	CXR
GI	Hepatotoxicity	Chemotherapeutic agent—methotrexate	LFTs
HEME	Splenomegaly Cytopenia	Hematologic disease	CBC with differential Plt count Bleeding time
GU	Renal insufficiency	Chemotherapeutic agents—methotrexate, cisplatin	BUN, serum Cr UA, electrolytes
CNS	Neurologic deficits Peripheral neuropathies	Chemotherapeutic agents—vinblastine, cisplatin	

Key Reference: Feliciano DV, et al: A four year experience with splenectomy vs. splenorrhaphy. Ann Surg 1985; 201(5): 568–575.

PERIOPERATIVE IMPLICATIONS

Preoperative Implications

- Polyvalent pneumococcal vaccine (7 d prior to surgery, if possible)
- Nasogastric decompression
- Stress steroids (100 mg hydrocortisone q8h), if received in past

Monitoring

- Routine

Airway

- Trauma patients—rule out cervical instability

Induction

- Routine

Maintenance

- Prevent hypothermia

Extubation

- Routine

Adjuvants

- Combined general/epidural (1.5–2% lidocaine with 1:200,000 epinephrine)
- Muscle relaxants required
- Minimize sedatives: ↑ likelihood of postop resp depression

Postoperative Period

- Postsplenectomy sepsis—due to encapsulated organisms (i.e., pneumococci)

ANTICIPATED PROBLEMS/CONCERNS

- Bleeding
- Atelectasis (left lower lobe)

SPLIT-THICKNESS SKIN GRAFT

Robert Gaiser, M.D.

USES

- To cover granulating wound:
  - Burns: 2 million people injured/y
  - Wounds: trauma, diabetic foot ulcers, postradiation skin breakdown, sacral decubitus, melanoma excision

PERIOPERATIVE RISKS

- Perioperative mortality: rare
- 40% BSA burns have 40% mortality in 60–75 y (90% survival in <45 y)
- Large areas may involve significant blood loss

WORRY ABOUT

- Airway involvement in burns that may make intubation difficult

- Blood loss if large areas to be debrided and grafted
- Hypotensive shock, electrolyte abn, sepsis, arrhythmias, myoglobinemia, ATN, compartment syndromes
- Nutritional status of patient
- Cleanliness of donor and recipient sites
- Suitable locations for application of monitors and IV access
- Loss of joint mobility due to scarring

OVERVIEW

- Split-thickness skin graft (STSG) consists of epidermis and only a portion of dermis. STSGs categorized as thin (0.005–0.012 in), medium (0.012–0.018 in), or thick (0.018–0.028)

- Must consider both donor and recipient sites: Addition of epinephrine will decrease bleeding at donor site without affecting survival of STSG

ICD-9-CM Codes: 707.0 (decubitus ulcer); 707.1 (ulcer of LE); 873.4 (wound face); 884 (UE); 891 (LE); 941 (burn face); 942 (trunk); 944 (UE); 945 (LE)

INDICATIONS AND USUAL TREATMENT

- Used to cover granulating wound: tolerates less vascularity than full-thickness skin graft
- Disadvantage: lack of growth in children, abnormal pigmentation, contraction
- Donor site: any area of body including scalp and extremities; depends on resulting skin match and appearance of the donor scar

ASSESSMENT POINTS

SYSTEM	EFFECT	ASSESSMENT BY HX	PE	TEST
SKIN	Donor/recipient site	Discussion with surgeon		
HEENT	Burns or radiation	Review medical record	Airway exam	
CV	Hypotensive shock, arrhythmias, myocardial contractile depression	Dyspnea, orthopnea, chest pain	Vital signs, chest exam	CXR, ECG, orthostatic vital signs
RESP	ARDS	Dyspnea, SOB, chest pain, mental status change	Chest exam	CXR, ABGs
GI	Debilitated patient	Bed bound		Albumin
HEME	Possible large blood loss			Hct
RENAL	ATN, myoglobinemia	Massive tissue destruction, Prolonged hypotension	Oliguria, anuria	BUN, serum Cr, Cr clearance; serum/urine myoglobin
NEURO	Paresis of lower extremity, Compartment syndromes	Functional limitations, Hx of circumferential extremity burns	Neuro exam, Weak pulses	Transduce compartment pressures

Key Reference: Skouge JW: Techniques for split-thickness skin grafting. J Dermatol Surg Oncol 1987; 13:841.

PERIOPERATIVE MANAGEMENT

Preoperative Preparation

- Determine donor/recipient sites
- Stabilize hemodynamically first
- IV access: large-bore IVs if anticipate large blood loss
- Warm room and all fluids

Monitoring

- Donor/recipient sites limit locations available for application of monitors: secure leads and pulse oximeter to sites used
- May use lower extremity for BP monitoring
- Temp monitoring

Airway

- For burn or postradiation patient, determine if airway involved. Involvement of face may make intubation more difficult: Consider fiberoptic intubation/consider consultative, collaborative airway management

Induction/Maintenance

- Avoid succinylcholine as may precipitate hyperkalemic response
- No generally accepted preferred agent or technique
- If using local anesthetic, keep amount within recommended limits

- Acute phase: anticipate hemostatic problems; electrolyte abn, hypovolemia
- Chronic phase: scarring causing loss of function and positioning problems, infection, poor nutritional status, NMB resistance

SURGICAL STAGES

- Variety of dermatomes available to cut STSG. In general, air- or electric-powered dermatomes and free hand knife are used to cut lengthwise on extremity; drum dermatomes used sidewise across extremity.
- Width of graft determined by width setting on dermatome.
- If Betadine is used to prep donor area, it must be washed off to prevent sticking.
- Skin thoroughly lubricated with sterile mineral oil to facilitate graft cutting.
- Advancing the dermatome flat across the skin with gentle downward pressure.
- Wound cleaned with saline or Betadine solution
- Surgical debridement may cause bleeding; hemostasis important for graft survival.
- Graft placed on the wound, sutured around the periphery, and dressed. Main object of the dressing is to ensure contact between graft and host bed. Dressing left in place for ~7 d, at which time sutures can be removed.

- Reasons for graft failure: inadequate graft bed (poor vascularity), hematoma, movement, infection, technical errors
- EBL: depends on extent of grafting, minimal to 250–500 ml

POSTOPERATIVE CONSIDERATIONS

- Pain score: 4–6
- Activity level kept at a minimum for the first 2 days after surgery.
- Monitor CV status
- Heat loss in transfer to/from OR

ANTICIPATED PROBLEMS/CONCERNS

- Blood loss may be difficult to assess and may be high; assess Hct and volume status frequently
- Malnutrition may lead to unexpected amounts of edema
- Hypothermia common if not assiduously avoided pre- and intratransport

STRABISMUS SURGERY

Karen Jaranowski, M.D.
Ronald S. Litman, D.O.

RISK

- 5% of the population have malalignment of visual axes
- Strabismus repair is the most commonly performed pediatric ocular operation
- Gender/race prevalence: none

PERIOPERATIVE RISKS

- Mortality: extremely rare
- Probably higher than average incidence of masseter muscle rigidity (MMR) and malignant hyperthermia (MH)

WORRY ABOUT

- Oculocardiac reflex (trigeminal-vagal)
- Postop nausea/vomiting (PONV)
- Development of malignant hyperthermia

OVERVIEW

- Can be congenital anomaly or acquired defect
- Congenital strabismus due to innervation abnormalities
- Acquired strabismus has multiple potential etiologies including restrictive disease (e.g., orbital mass), ocular myopathy, myasthenia gravis
- Strabismus can be sign of an as yet undiagnosed underlying myopathy
- High incidence of strabismus in patients with CNS disease (e.g., meningomyelocele with hydrocephalus, cerebral palsy, congenital myopathies)

ICD-9-CM Codes: 368.01 (Amblyopia); 378.60 (mechanical)

INDICATIONS AND USUAL TREATMENT

- Surgical correction within the first 4 months of life will help ensure proper development of stereoscopic vision.
- Strabismus repair in the older child is performed for cosmetic reasons.

ASSESSMENT POINTS

SYSTEM	EFFECT	ASSESSMENT BY HX	PE	TEST
CV	Myopathies (e.g., Duchenne) can cause conduction abn and myocardial dysfunction	Palpitations, exercise tolerance	S_3, irregular rhythm	ECG, ECHO if central myopathy exists
RESP	Cerebral palsy patients may have chronic lung disease Congenital myopathies may affect oropharyngeal and esophageal muscles.	Prolonged intubation, reactive airway disease, frequent aspiration	Rhonchi, wheezing	Baseline SpO_2 Consider CXR if recent change in pulm status

Key Reference: Woods AM, Berry FA, Carter BJ: Strabismus surgery and postoperative vomiting: clinical observations and review of the current literature; a medical opinion. Pediatr Anaesth 1992; 2:223–229.

PERIOPERATIVE IMPLICATIONS

Preoperative Preparation

- IM atropine decreases incidence of oculocardiac reflex from 90% to 50%

Anesthetic Technique

- Possible masseter muscle rigidity with use of succinylcholine—use with caution
- Oral RAE tube required in most instances
- Narcotics increase incidence of PONV
- Consider PONV prophylaxis

SURGICAL CONSIDERATIONS

- Oculocardiac reflex can be induced by traction on extraocular muscles, pressure on eyeball, eye pain
- Hypercapnia increases incidence of bradycardia
- First step in treatment is to stop surgical stimulation. If necessary, follow with IV atropine

Postoperative Considerations

- Pain score: 2–3 (severe irritation rather than pain)
- PONV occurs in 50–80% of patients

ANTICIPATED PROBLEMS/CONCERNS

- Higher than average incidence of MMR and MH
- PONV

SURGERY FOR SCOLIOSIS AND KYPHOSIS Ralph L. Bernstein, M.D.

RISK

- 1–3% of screened adolescents with curves > 10°
- Females > males 3.6:1

PERIOPERATIVE RISKS

- Pneumonia, atelectasis, neurologic damage
- Neurologic damage—injury to spinal cord by excessive traction

WORRY ABOUT

- Extensive blood loss
- Postop atelectasis, pneumonia
- Superior mesenteric artery syndrome—when curve straightened, superior mesenteric artery occludes duodenum, may require nasogastric tube or surgery

OVERVIEW

- Thoracoabdominal approach to release vertebrae anteriorly, remove disks, apply instrumentation or bone grafts followed by posterior spinal fusion at the same operation
- In kyphosis surgery anterior release and grafting may be followed by posterior instrumentation and fusion during a subsequent operation
- Prepare for large blood loss

ICD-9-CM Codes: 737.10 (Scoliosis and Kyphosis); 737.39

INDICATIONS/USUAL TREATMENT

- Scoliosis with increasing curve in growing child or severe deformity, or pain not controlled by conservative measures such as bracing.
- In kyphotic curve that is progressing and curves causing severe back pain, in curves in which neurologic impairment is occurring from congenital, post traumatic, or infectious causes

ASSESSMENT POINTS

SYSTEM	EFFECT	ASSESSMENT BY HX	PE	TEST
HEENT	Regurgitation, aspiration in neuromuscular patients	Parents' report		
CV	Cardiomyopathy in Friedreich's ataxia and muscular dystrophy	Exercise tolerance		ECG, ECHO, CXR
RESP	Restrictive pulm disease in patients with severe deformities of thorax Paralytic or neuromuscular scoliosis may cause severe resp impairment	Exercise tolerance		Vital capacity if curves >50–60°, ABG
HEME	Preop autologous blood donation			Hgb, Hct
CNS	In neuromuscular and congenital scoliosis, evaluation of neurologic status		Neuro exam	Preop SSEP

Key Reference: Bernstein RL, Rosenberg AD. Scoliosis. *In* Manual of Orthopedic Anesthesia and Related Pain Syndromes. New York, Churchill Livingstone, 1994.

PERIOPERATIVE MANAGEMENT

Preoperative Preparation

- Instruct patient concerning possibility of wake-up test (shut off N₂O, relaxants reversed, naloxone given if needed)
- Tell patient to move the hands; if done, to move toes of both feet
- In anterior thoracolumbar approach, chest tube will be present.
- Teach patient pulm toilet and how to use PCA devices

Monitoring

- Consider arterial line
- CVP line useful to assess blood volume status; urinary catheter
- SSEP
- Blood loss—measure suction, weigh sponges, use blood salvage device

Induction/Maintenance

- Consider administering β-blockers to control heart rate if hypotensive anesthesia is used
- Inhalation agents may interfere with SSEP monitoring
- ET intubation: secure tube (double-lumen tube not required)

SURGICAL STAGES

- For anterior approach—patient placed in lateral decubitus position. Recommend adequate padding and axillary roll on down side
- Apply external warming device
- Thoracolumbar incision is made, diaphragm detached, vertebra approached
- Vascular compromise of spinal cord may occur if segmental vessels taken are major feeders to spinal cord. Disks removed, bone graft and instrumentation placed according to structural needs
- Following closure, chest tube inserted, patient placed into prone position
- Surgeon may infiltrate incision with epinephrine 1:500,000 solution
- Blood loss can be brisk, esp. as dissection is made down to bleeding bone, more in neuromuscular scoliosis. Instrumentation inserted, correction obtained, bone graft inserted
- Consider hypotensive anesthesia with MAP at 60 mmHg in normotensive patients. During correction, pressure returned to normal levels. Sodium nitroprusside infusion or labetalol commonly used
- Excessive crystalloids may cause postop edema

- Monitor SSEPs or NMEPs—if decrease in latency of 10% or decrease in amplitude of 60%. Check ETCO₂, pulse oximeter, body temp.
  – Tell surgeon to stop operation
  – Raise BP to above-normal levels to increase perfusion of cord
  – Prepare to perform wake-up test
- At conclusion of procedure patient is placed in supine position
- Consider not rushing to extubate until extubation criteria met and normothermic
- Blood loss may continue with wound drainage apparatus. Reinfusion of this blood has resulted in red-colored urine on occasion
- Make certain chest tube functioning
- Have patient awake enough for neurologic evaluation
- Consider pain relief by PCA

ANTICIPATED PROBLEMS/CONCERNS

- Pulm: atelectasis
- GI: ileus
- In patients with neuromuscular scoliosis, postoperative ventilatory support may be needed. Consider weaning these patients as soon as possible to avoid loss of muscle strength

TESTICULAR TORSION SURGERY

Ronald S. Litman, D.O.

RISK

- 1:160 males, most commonly around puberty but also in neonatal period
- 20% have antecedent trauma
- Racial predominance: none
- Left testicle affected twice as often as right

PERIOPERATIVE RISKS

- Pts are generally young and healthy—no special risks

WORRY ABOUT

- Full stomach
- Testicular ischemia
- Patient anxiety

OVERVIEW

- Manifested by acute scrotal pain and results from twisting of spermatic cord with vascular compromise of testicle
- Caused by high investment of tunica vaginalis on spermatic cord (bell-clapper deformity)
- If not surgically corrected in relatively short time (6–8 h), testicular ischemia can result
- Generally considered a surgical emergency
- Temporizing treatment involves manual detorsion by a urologist, which may alleviate ischemia, but orchidopexy still required

ICD-9-CM Code: 608.2

INDICATIONS/USUAL TREATMENT

- Emergency scrotal exploration usually indicated for any male with acute scrotal pain and swelling
- Differential Dx includes epididymitis, orchitis, appendix torsion, Henoch-Schönlein purpura (abdominal pain, hematuria, nephritis). Studies show that color Doppler US reliable for Dx of testicular torsion, which may spare majority of children with acute testicular pain (from other causes) unnecessary surgery

ASSESSMENT POINTS

Patients usually young and healthy. Testicular torsion not associated with and does not cause abnormalities in other organ systems.

Key Reference: Leape LL: Torsion of the testis. *In* Welch KJ, Randolph JG, Ravitch MM, Rowe MI (eds): Pediatric Surgery, 4th ed. St. Louis, Mosby–Year Book, 1986, pp 1330–1334.

PERIOPERATIVE IMPLICATIONS

Preoperative Preparation

- Patient should be considered to have full stomach (recent meal), pain/anxiety
- Treat with metoclopramide and oral sodium citrate
- IV opioids for preop pain and IV midazolam for anxiety and amnesia

Anesthetic Technique

- General endotracheal, spinal, epidural, or local infiltration—scrotum innervated by inferior pudendal branch (long scrotal nerve) of posterior femoral cutaneous nerve (from the sacral plexus), and the medial and lateral posterior scrotal branches of perineal nerve (from the pudendal nerve)

Monitoring

- Depends on physical condition

Airway

- No special considerations

Induction/Maintenance

- Rapid-sequence induction if GA and full stomach likely

Surgical Stages

- Scrotal incision, detorsion, bilateral orchidopexy (to prevent recurrence). No special postop considerations

Blood /Fluid Losses

- None, usually

ANTICIPATED PROBLEMS/CONCERNS

- Full stomach—risk of pulm aspiration with induction of GA
- Testicular ischemia if duration of torsion prolonged (>6–8 h)

TETRALOGY OF FALLOT (TOF), CORRECTION OF

Wendell C. Stevens, M.D.
Henry Casson, M.D.

RISK

- Congenital heart disease incidence: 6/1000 live births
- TOF: accounts for 10% of congenital heart disease

PERIOPERATIVE RISKS

- Closely related to severity of pulm outflow obstruction
- Operative mortality <5% for children without RV failure

WORRY ABOUT

- Episodic increase in right-to-left shunt
- Arterial hypoxemia
- Venous air entrainment—paradoxical embolism
- Polycythemia and thrombotic episodes

OVERVIEW

- TOF includes VSD(s), RV outflow obstruction, aorta overriding RV and LV, RV hypertrophy
- Symptoms and urgency of correction depend on degree of pulm obstruction with resultant RV failure, right-to-left shunt, and diminished pulm blood flow
- Challenge: to provide sufficient anesthesia but with little decrease in systemic arterial pressure or increase in pulm obstruction

ICD-9-CM Code: 745.2

INDICATIONS AND USUAL TREATMENT

- Cyanotic "tet" spells in first months of life may necessitate creation of palliative systemic-to-pulmonic shunt
- Increase in severity of cyanosis and polycythemia leads to early correction of TOF
- Corrections now often done in 1st year of life to avoid progressive RV failure

ASSESSMENT POINTS

SYSTEM	EFFECT	ASSESSMENT BY HX	PE	TEST
CV	Right-to-left shunt	Cyanosis, yes or no, relation to crying or exercise	Observe	ECHO
	RV failure	Exercise intolerance Syncope	Tachypnea, sweating	
	Polycythemia Prior palliative shunt	CVA	Neurologic exam Scars, absent pulse	Hct
RESP	↓ Pulm blood flow	Exercise intolerance	Tachypnea	
OTHER	Associated congenital anomalies		Observation	

Key Reference: Marnach RL, Hansen DD, Hickey PR: Anesthesia for children with heart disease. *In* Cote CJ, Ryan JF, Todres ID, Goudsouzian NG (eds): A Practice of Anesthesia for Infants and Children, 2nd ed. Philadelphia, WB Saunders, 1993, pp 291–310.

PERIOPERATIVE MANAGEMENT

Anesthetic Technique

- Less important than achieving goals; aim for quiet, rapid induction, normal or perhaps ↓ myocardial contractility and HR, patent airway at all times
- Overall goals: avoid ↑ dynamic pulm outflow obstruction and ↓ SVR

Monitoring

- Arterial catheter—has the child had a palliative shunt?
- Two IV catheters with short injection port access—scrupulous avoidance of bubbles
- CVP will be needed for postpump management

Airway

- Avoid excessive airway pressure and hyperventilation, since these may ↑ PVR

Induction

- Avoid dehydration—special risk in severely polycythemic child
- Premedication—IM/IV morphine or oral or IM/IV midazolam based on age and emotional state; consider giving in presurgical holding area
- Maintenance—combined IV and inhaled agents commonly used; quiet, controlled operating field essential

Surgical Stages

- Pre-CPB
  - Maintain cardiac output and SVR
  - Severe episodic cyanotic "tet" spells may require IV fluids to augment blood volume and ↓ Hct, 100% O_2, phenylephrine to ↑ SVR, esmolol/halothane to ↓ RV outflow obstruction
- During CPB—no unique requirements
- Post-CPB
  - Measure of successful repair will be RV pressure—ideally no more than half LV pressure
  - Inotropic and high filling pressure support of RV may be required for 1–3 days
  - Close attention to coagulation, esp. if CPB prolonged
  - RV conduction delay common, but CHB (pacemaker) rare
  - If RV pressure high and function poor, look for residual VSD; TEE of great help
- Postoperatively
  - Consider above all else: adequacy of RV performance and reduction of PVR
- EBL: Moderate
- Pain score: 7–10

ANTICIPATED PROBLEMS/CONCERNS

- Persistent pulmonary outflow obstruction or high PVR
- Persistent RV dysfunction

THORACIC AORTIC REPAIR

Christopher C. Young, M.D.

RISK

- People within US: 3.4% incidence of aortic aneurysm; 26% involve thoracic aorta
- ↑ Incidence with HTN (?African-Americans)
- Males 2–9 × > females
- Peak incidence 50–70 y

PERIOPERATIVE RISKS

- HTN, coronary and carotid vascular disease
- Untreated dissection: 25–35% mortality within 24 h, 90% in 3 mo
- Surgical repair carries 10% mortality. Causes of postop death are hemorrhage (29%); cardiac events—ischemia, MI, CHF—(26%); and multiorgan system failure (22%)
- Traumatic disruption immediately fatal in 85%

WORRY ABOUT

- Elevated HR and BP promote dissection
- Acute dissection can lead to compromised blood flow (coronary, renal, splanchnic, spinal cord), pericardial tamponade, acute aortic valvular insufficiency, or bleeding

- Associated injuries (lungs, heart, head, abdomen) with traumatic rupture
- Major blood loss; need for rapid transfusion intraoperatively
- Acute dissections frequently brought for repair with minimal preop preparation

OVERVIEW

- Primary risk factors are HTN and atherosclerosis.
- Thoracic aortic aneurysms 2–3 × more likely to dissect than abdominal
- Distribution of thoracic dissections: ascending aorta 60–70%; descending aorta 30–35%; aortic arch 5–10%

ICD-9-CM Code: 441.x

ETIOLOGY

- Aneurysm develops as vascular wall weakens from hydraulic forces (HTN) coupled with degeneration (atherosclerosis). Involves all 3 layers of aortic wall. Usually becomes symptomatic by compression of adjacent structures.

- Dissection risk factors: HTN, syphilis, Marfan's, congenital anomalies (coarctation, AS), pregnancy, bacterial infection. Intimal tear allows separation of intima from media and adventitia.

Location	DeBakey	Dailey
Ascending and descending aorta	Type I	Group A
Ascending aorta only	Type II	Group A
Distal to left subclavian	Type III	Group B

- Traumatic rupture occurs commonly at ligamentum arteriosum (aorta fixed at this point).

INDICATIONS AND USUAL TREATMENT

- Group A (types I and II) dissections are surgically repaired immediately via median sternotomy using CPB.
- Group B (type III) dissections are medically managed; when operation is indicated (>10 cm diameter, progressive enlargement, or producing symptoms), left thoracotomy and one-lung ventilation employed.
- Traumatic aortic dissections are treated surgically regardless of symptoms.

ASSESSMENT POINTS

SYSTEM	EFFECT	ASSESSMENT BY HX	PE	TEST
HEENT	SVC syndrome Recurrent laryngeal nerve compression	Dyspnea Hoarseness	JVD Edema	Flow-volume loop Indirect laryngoscopy
CV	Myocardial ischemia LV dysfunction Valvular disease Venous compression	Angina Dyspnea	S_3 gallop Friction rub Muffled heart sounds Plethora	ECG ECHO Stress testing Coronary Angio
RESP	Bronchial/tracheal compression Recurrent pneumonia Pulm compression	Dyspnea Cough	Wheezing Tracheal deviation Hemoptysis	ABG Flow-volume loop CXR Chest CT or MRI
GI	Mesenteric ischemia	Abdominal pain Bloody diarrhea	Tenderness	Colonoscopy Angio
RENAL	↓ Renal perfusion	Oliguria		Cr, Cr clearance
CNS	Spinal cord ischemia Carotid stenosis	Weakness Paraplegia		Carotid duplex
MS		Back or chest pain		Chest CT or MRI

Key Reference: Kwitka G, Kidney SA, Nugent M. Thoracic and abdominal aortic aneurysm resections. *In* Kaplan JA (ed): Vascular Anesthesia, New York, Churchill Livingstone, 1991.

PERIOPERATIVE IMPLICATIONS

Preoperative Preparation

- IV sodium nitroprusside with β-blockers; trimethaphan infusion may be used.
- Premedication to prevent anxiety and pain

Monitoring

- Invasive arterial BP—left radial for group A, right radial for group B, and femoral or dorsalis pedis for distal aortic pressure measurement during cross-clamping
- PA catheter and/or TEE
- SSEPs not consistently reliable guide to spinal cord ischemia

Airway

- Difficult airway if compression or deviation of tracheobronchial tree
- May interfere with placement of double-lumen ET tube

Induction/Maintenance

- High-dose narcotic useful to blunt intubation response
- Inhalation agent useful to ↓ myocardial contractility, provide amnesia
- Avoid N_2O during one-lung ventilation and to prevent expansion of air emboli

Extubation

- Usually keep sedated and mechanically ventilated 12–24 h until warmed and stable
- Prevent hemodynamic response to extubation

Adjuvants

- β-blockers, nitroprusside, nitroglycerin continued perioperatively
- Maintain adequate hydration
- Consider mannitol 0.5 g/kg well prior to cross-clamping; "renal dose" dopamine

- Maintenance of aortic pressure distal to crossclamp; mild hypothermia; CSF drainage; steroids, intrathecal papaverine may limit spinal cord ischemia (5–7% incidence)

ANTICIPATED PROBLEMS/CONCERNS

- Aortic cross-clamping causes ↑ LV afterload, LV wall tension, and O_2 consumption. Vasodilators useful, but distal hypotension may induce spinal cord ischemia. Vascular shunting or partial bypass during crossclamp may overcome these effects.
- Aortic unclamping results in ↑ stroke volume but profound ↓ in SVR and significant metabolic acidosis if no shunt used. Fluid management, α-agonists (phenylephrine), and sodium bicarbonate may be useful.

THYROIDECTOMY FOR HYPERTHYROIDISM Michael F. Roizen, M.D.

RISK

- People within USA: 400,000/y develop hyperthyroidism + 5% of pregnant females
- 1/1000 females, 1/3000 males; ~200,000 thyroid operations/y (1985–1989 data)
- Race with highest prevalence: not known

PERIOPERATIVE RISKS

- ↑ Risk of thyroid storm, even if patient made euthyroid prior to surgery
- Related to risk of thyroid storm
- Risk of postop airway compromise
- Occasionally late tetany (usually 2–3 days postop) due to removal of, or damage to, parathyroid glands
- Mortality <0.3%
- Hypoparathyroidism 2–3%

WORRY ABOUT

- Assessing euthyroid state
- Securing airway if large goiter or displaced trachea

- Postop risks of nerve injury (immediate stridor requires immediate reintubation); surreptitious bleeding (examine wound—prior to PACU discharge); thyroid storm (uncommon without another acute illness or after 3 days postop)

OVERVIEW

- Major goal is to avoid thyroid storm; if not euthyroid prior to surgery, try to delay operation
- If emergency operation, use beta rb's and ↓ iodides to ↓ perioperative effects of released thyroid hormones and ↓ further synthesis and release of thyroid hormones; keep in ICU until risk of thyroid storm has passed
- Done in young adults with hyperthyroidism, or normal thyroid function with a cold nodule, or with a goiter that is bothersome physiologically or psychologically
- Hyperthyroidism is an endocrinopathy with CV disease—tachycardia (commonly idiopathic if no prior Dx of hyperthyroidism), CHF, dysrhythmias (AFib)—as major manifestation

- Other target systems of hyperthroidism are resp and CNS (↓ drive to breathe, anxiety, psychoses) and metabolic
- If patient is made euthyroid prior to operation, risk of thyroid storm and perioperative CV problems diminished by > 90%

ICD-9-CM Codes: 242.9 (Hyperthyroidism [thyrotoxicosis]); 242.0 (Graves' disease); 245 (Thyroiditis); 193 (Malignant thyroid disease); 198.89 (Metastatic malignant thyroid disease)

ETIOLOGY

- Multinodular diffuse enlargement (Graves' disease)
- Thyroid adenoma—toxic multinodular goiter (firm gland) later in life and (almost never), malignant; unilateral solitary nodule with autonomous function earlier in life almost always benign
- Cold nodules associated with radiation therapy of other diseases as well as idiopathic
- Goiter previously associated with iodine deficiency

ASSESSMENT POINTS

SYSTEM	EFFECT	ASSESSMENT BY HX	PE	TEST
HEENT	Weakened tracheal rings, distorted/displaced trachea Ophthalmopathy Large tongue if associated with goiter or amyloidosis	Snoring, hoarseness, neck pain	Ask to vocalize "e"; examine airway and neck Look at eyes	CXR (PA and lat) Lat neck films CT scan of neck
CV	CHF, cardiomyopathies Sinus tachycardia, mitral valve prolapse, AFib	DOE on exertion, orthostatic SOB Palpitations; ↑ HR during sleep	Standard exam	Rhythm strip or full ECG
GI	Wt loss, diarrhea, dehydration	Dizziness on arising; Hx of diarrhea, constipation	Skin turgor, orthostatic VS	↑ Serum alkaline phosphatase
HEME		Mild anemia, thrombocytopenia Agranulocytosis 2° to propylthiouracil or methimazole	Skin/mucous membranes for infection/petechiae	CBC with plt count differential
CNS		Shaking, anxiety, emotional lability Hypothyroid goiter associated with slow thought processes	Reflex speed, tremor, nervousness, mental status	
METAB	Need to assess if euthyroid Malnourished	Refer to all other systems: esp reflex speed, tremor, heat intolerance, fatigue, weakness; wt loss, anorexia or ↑ appetite	Reflex speed, HR	Free T_4 estimate

Key Reference: Roizen MF: Implications of concurrent disease. *In* Miller: Anesthesia, 4th ed. New York, Churchill Livingstone, 1994, pp 926–928.

PERIOPERATIVE IMPLICATIONS

Anesthetic Technique

- No one technique has proved to be associated with better outcome

Airway

- Occasionally distorted anatomy 2° to goiter, tracheal ring involvement, inflammation 2° to thyroiditis
- Consider awake fiberoptic intubation
- Consider armored tube or equivalent if tracheal rings are affected

Preinduction/Induction

- Prehydrate liberally if CV status will tolerate
- Routine unless abnormal airway or CV system or noneuthyroid condition

Monitoring

- T (also place cooling blanket on OR table to treat thyroid storm if it occurs)
- Consider invasive monitoring if CV system severely affected

- If considerable head-up position, consider air embolus monitoring and therapy strategies

Induction/Maintenance/Extubation

- Extubate in situation with optimal conditions for reintubation

SURGICAL STAGES

Initial Dissection

- Transverse collar incision
- Thyroid lobe freed from strap muscles with securing of superior thyroid vessels; these are clamped after ensuring localization and preservation of recurrent laryngeal nerve and parathyroid glands

Thyroid Removal

- Following division of middle and inferior thyroid vessels, thyroid lobe is retracted medially and liberated.

Adjuvants

- Usually no requirement for NMB

- Can be done with regional: superficial and deep cervical plexus blocks and infiltration

Postoperative Considerations

- EBL: 50–150 ml
- Pain score 2–4
- Usually can be treated with NSAIDs or occasionally with PCA

ANTICIPATED PROBLEMS/CONCERNS

- Thyroid storm is life-threatening illness manifested by hyperpyrexia, tachycardia, striking alterations in consciousness
- Surreptitious bleeding can suddenly compromise airway function
- Recurrent laryngeal nerve injuries damage abductor fibers, resulting in hoarseness. Bilateral injury results in fixed narrow opening to glottis with inspiratory airflow obstruction (stridor), inability to vocalize, aspiration risk, and immediate need for tracheal intubation

TMJ ARTHROSCOPY

Stephen O. Heard, M.D.

RISK

- Up to 17% of population suffers from TMJ disorders
- Majority of patients aged 15–45 y
- Female: male—estimates vary from 3:1–9:1
- Initiating factors: trauma; adverse loading of masticatory system

PERIOPERATIVE RISKS

- Perioperative mortality exceedingly rare
- Epistaxis

WORRY ABOUT

- Coexisting diseases (e.g., rheumatoid arthritis)
- Establishing and maintaining airway
- Medications

OVERVIEW

- Used to evaluate and treat pain or lack of motion in TMJ
- TMJ anatomy: joint divided into superior and inferior articular cavities by articular disk
- Approaches: inferolateral, posterolateral, anterolateral
- Structures to watch: facial nerve, superficial temporal branch of auriculotemporal nerve, maxillary artery, superficial temporal artery and vein, parotid gland

ICD-9-CM Code: 524.6

INDICATIONS AND USUAL TREATMENT

- Diagnosis of TMJ pain
- Surgery
  - Biopsies
  - Debridement and lavage
  - Incision of adhesions
  - Restoration of disk mobility and position
  - Instillation of medication
  - Capsular or disk attachment scarification/plication
- Usual Treatment
  - Behavior modification
  - Pharmacotherapy
  - Physical therapy
  - Appliance therapy
  - Occlusive therapy

ASSESSMENT POINTS

SYSTEM	EFFECT	ASSESSMENT BY HX	PE	TEST
HEENT	Epistaxis associated with nasotracheal intubation	Epistaxis; nasal polyps; occluded nostril	Airway exam including assessment of nostril patency	
	Mouth opening	Trismus Pain on opening mouth Headache	Clicking of TMJ Muscle spasm	
CV/RESP	Arthritis can be systemic disease: restrictive pulmonary disease, cardiomyopathy	SOB Exercise tolerance	Auscultation of heart and lungs Inspection of legs	O_2 saturation, ECG or CXR (if suggested by Hx, PE)
MS	Look for other joint involvement	Arthralgias	Inspection Palpation	

Key Reference: Merrill R: Disorders of TMJ. I. Diagnosis and arthroscopy. Oral Maxillofacial Surg Clin North Am 1989; 1:1.

PERIOPERATIVE MANAGEMENT

Preoperative Preparation
- IV sedation if needed

Monitoring
- Standard

Induction/Maintenance
- After standard induction, prepare nostrils with 4% cocaine or phenylephrine and dilate with lubricated nasal airways of increasing diameter
- Nasotracheal intubation (soften NT tube in warm H_2O: may need Magill forceps)
- Cover eyes with moistened eye pads (possible laser use)
- Some surgeons request IV administration of dexamethasone (10 mg)

SURGICAL STAGES

- Injection of local anesthesia: usually 1% lidocaine with 1:100,000 epinephrine
- Incision over superior joint space, insertion of obturator/sheath, removal of obturator, camera attachment
- Use of helium or Nd-YAG laser
  - Protective eyewear for patient and staff
  - Wet towels surrounding operative area
  - Water readily available
- Complications (<1%)
  - Hemorrhage (usually superficial temporal artery or vein)
  - Joint damage
  - Perforation into middle cranial fossa
  - Damage to middle ear ossicles
  - Injury to auriculotemporal nerve
- Minimal blood loss
- Some surgeons inject intra-articular steroids or local anesthetics (bupivacaine 0.5% with 1:200,000 epinephrine) for anti-inflammatory and analgesic effects

Postoperative Considerations

- Pain score: 0–5
- IV or PO narcotics/anti-inflammatory medications in PACU

ANTICIPATED PROBLEMS/CONCERNS

- Epistaxis with intubation or extubation
- Postextubation pulm edema reported
- IV injections of local anesthetic

TONSILLECTOMY AND ADENOIDECTOMY
Helen W. Karl, M.D.

RISK

- > 340,000 procedures/y in USA
- Incidence ~120/100,000 (↓ by 23% from 1970 due to John Wennberg's work on small area variation)
- Racial/gender predominance: None

PERIOPERATIVE RISKS

- Estimates of 30-day mortality range from 1:4000 to 1:27,000, usually from hemorrhage (0.1–8% of tonsillectomies ± adenoidectomy)

WORRY ABOUT

- Indication for procedure
- Associated URI
- Perioperative fluid deficiency
- Bleeding, airway obstruction, or apnea postop

OVERVIEW

- Adenoidectomy and tonsillectomy usually performed together, but consideration given to the specific risk/benefit ratio for each procedure
- Bleeding most common about 7 d postop, but may occur in first 8–24 h
- Age and co-morbidities of patients dictate postop care

ICD-9-CM Codes: 474.0 (Chronic tonsillitis); 474.1 (Hypertrophy of tonsils and adenoids)

INDICATIONS AND USUAL TREATMENT

- Obstruction of nasal or pharyngeal airway, especially when associated with anatomic or physiologic disturbances
- Chronic or recurrent infection of adenoids (also ears or sinuses) or tonsils despite adequate antibiotic therapy
- Acute peritonsillar abscess

ASSESSMENT POINTS

SYSTEM	EFFECT	ASSESSMENT BY HX	PE	TEST
HEENT	Chronic nasal obstruction associated with abnormal facial growth	Snoring, poor feeding, speech disorders	Adenoid facies, mouth breathing	Ask child to breathe with mouth closed
CV	Chronic airway obstruction may lead to pulm HTN and right heart failure		Cardiac exam	ECHO, ECG, CXR
RESP	Tonsillar hyperplasia may result in sleep apnea and CO_2 retention	Disturbed sleep, daytime sleepiness	Airway exam, tonsil size	Polysomnography O_2 saturation
HEME	Patients with pre-existing bleeding disorders are at greater risk of postoperative hemorrhage	Patient or family Hx of bleeding, bruising, or aspirin (check OTC meds)	Multiple bruises above the knees	PT, PTT, plt count, bleeding time if positive history
NEURO	Brainstem dysfunction may amplify sleep apnea with moderate tonsillar hyperplasia	Cerebral palsy, Arnold-Chiari malformation		Polysomnography O_2 saturation
SYSTEMIC	Children with craniofacial abnormalities (e.g., trisomy 21, Treacher Collins) may have pre-existing airway narrowing		General exam	

Key Reference: Ferrari LR, Vassalo SA: Anesthesia for otorhinolaryngology procedures. *In* Cote CJ, Ryan JF, Todres ID, Goudsouzian NG (eds): A Practice of Anesthesia for Infants and Children, 2nd ed. Philadelphia, WB Saunders, 1993.

PERIOPERATIVE MANAGEMENT

Preoperative Preparation

- Avoid preanesthetic sedatives if Hx of sleep apnea or very large tonsils
- Consider moderate dose of anxiolytic to ease induction
- Evaluate for bleeding abnormalities

Monitoring

- IV prior to induction if Hx of significant airway obstruction

Airway

- Preformed RAE endotracheal tubes fit best into groove of mouth gag

Induction

- Antisialagogue usual during induction

Surgical Stages

- Placement or removal of mouth gag may dislodge ET tube
- Corticosteroid administration may decrease edema
- Local infiltration with epinephrine-containing local anesthetic decreases intraoperative blood loss but does not improve pain control
- Check that oropharynx is clear of blood packs and secretions before extubation
- Extubation and recovery in lateral position with head slightly down keeps blood away from larynx
- If trachea is extubated while patient is anesthetized, recovery personnel must be very experienced in management of airway obstruction in small children

Postoperative Considerations

- EBL: Underestimated because blood may be swallowed during or after surgery
- Bleeding most common cause of morbidity; ketorolac might be avoided
- N/V in up to 60% of patients after tonsillectomy due to blood in stomach, inflammation of posterior pharynx, early oral fluid intake, may necessitate hospital admission
- Pain score: 3–4 after adenoidectomy; managed with Tylenol alone in some patients
- Pain score: 7–9 after tonsillectomy; may require IV and PO opioids
- Children with Hx of sleep apnea should receive greatly reduced doses of opioids and be admitted for overnight monitoring
- Admission for those < 3 y and with associated anatomic or physiologic abnormalities
- Most children may be discharged day of surgery if stable, no evidence of bleeding, and free of pain and vomiting

TOTAL ABDOMINAL HYSTERECTOMY
Ferne B. Sevarino, M.D.

RISK

- ~650,000/y in USA
- ~Half of women undergo hysterectomy
- Racial predominance: none
- Age: 30+ y

PERIOPERATIVE RISKS

- Overall mortality ~0.1%; lowest mortality in women <55 y, greatest mortality in women > 75 y
- Perioperative morbidity rare; overall incidence of 7.5% (fever and wound infections most common)

WORRY ABOUT

- Femoral nerve injury
- Bladder/ureter injury
- Hemorrhage requiring transfusion

OVERVIEW

- Choice of TAH vs. total vaginal hysterectomy (TVH) made according to pelvic anatomy, uterine size, adnexal or other associated disease (i.e., malignant vs. benign)
- Technique for TAH varies according to indication for operation
- Choice of anesthetic will vary with indication for surgery as well as presence of coexisting disease

ICD-9-CM Codes: 218.9 (Uterine fibroid); 179, 180.9, 183, 219.9, 220 (Neoplasm)

INDICATIONS AND USUAL TREATMENT

- Indications for hysterectomy include
  – uterine, cervical, ovarian cancer
  – pelvic relaxation syndrome, fibroids, abnormal bleeding, endometriosis, or other benign disorders (usually via vaginal approach)
- Vaginal approach may be used unless uterine size, pelvic adhesions, or cancer requires abdominal approach

ASSESSMENT POINTS

SYSTEM	EFFECT	ASSESSMENT BY HX	PE	TEST
CV	Dehydration 2° to bowel prep Blood loss from primary problem	Menorrhagia	Orthostasis	Hgb/Hct Lytes
RESP	Rule out effusion or metastases	SOB, bronchospasm	Auscultation	CXR ABG ± PFTs as indicated

Key Reference: Dicker RC, Greenspan Jr, Strauss LT, et al: Complications of abdominal and vaginal hysterectomy among women of reproductive age in the United States. Am J Obstet Gynecol 1982; 144:841–848.

PERIOPERATIVE MANAGEMENT

Anesthetic Technique

- Regional, general, or combined techniques are options

Monitoring

- Routine
- Consider arterial line, central monitoring for extensive oncologic precedure if indicated by surgical plan/skill or by coexisting disease

Induction/Maintenance

- GA—abdominal manipulation makes ET intubation preferable to LMA or mask airway
- Regional anesthesia—dense T3–T4 level necessary

SURGICAL STAGES

Incision

- Pfannenstiel or low transverse incision—limited access to upper abdomen
- Midline incision extending from ~4 cm above symphysis pubis to umbilicus offers greater exposure

Inspection

- Avoid excessive bowel manipulation
- Self-retaining retractor may be used

Dissection

- Extrafascial hysterectomy
- Intimate proximity of uterus to ureters makes ureteral indentification and dissection important
- Bladder must be carefully advanced down off lower uterine segment
- EBL: 1500 ml

Postoperative Considerations

- Moderate–severe postop pain (VAS 5–7)
- Single-dose spinal opioid followed by IV-PCA for 36–48 h (48–72 h for oncologic procedures)
- Nononcologic patients usually taking oral medication on postop day 1

ANTICIPATED PROBLEMS/CONCERNS

- Older patients and oncology patients at risk for DVT
- Bladder/ureteral damage may prolong Foley catheterization/hospitalization
- Recognition of femoral nerve injury may be delayed by use of regional anesthesia—consider epidural opioid analgesia without local anesthetic postop

TOTAL ANOMALOUS PULMONARY VENOUS RETURN CORRECTION

William J. Greeley, M.D.

RISK

- 2–3% of all congenital heart disease
- Marked male predominance

PERIOPERATIVE RISKS

- Perioperative mortality rare (<3%)
- Symptomatic arrhythmias infrequent

WORRY ABOUT

- Total anomalous pulmonary venous return with obstruction manifesting in newborn period
- PA, venous HTN major contributors to postop morbidity, mortality

OVERVIEW

- All pulmonary veins drain abn outside LA, connect directly or indirectly to RA via remnants of cardinal or umbilical venous system
- Classification based on anatomic sight of abn connection: type 1—supracardiac defect; most commonly enters left innominate vein; type 2—cardiac defect; venous connection to coronary sinus; type 3—infracardiac defect, distal site of connection usually below diaphragm, connecting with vessel of portal system; type 4—mixed defect, 2 or more sites of anomalous venous connections
- Because oxygenated, deoxygenated blood returning to RA is mixed, R→L shunt causes systemic desaturation, cyanosis; under most circumstances, usually not severe enough to produce hypoxemia, end-organ dysfunction. If pulmonary venous obstruction, can result in PA HTN, ↓ PBF, significant R→L shunting, severe hypoxemia in newborn period.

ICD-9-CM Code: 747.41

INDICATIONS AND USUAL TREATMENT

- All require surgery, its urgency dictated by anatomy, physiology, and clinical presentation

ASSESSMENT POINTS

SYSTEM	EFFECT	ASSESSMENT BY HX	PE	TEST
CV	CHF	Tachycardia, cyanosis	Flow murmur	ECHO
RESP	PV obstruction	Tachypnea	Pulmonary edema	CXR
RENAL	Renal insufficiency	↓ UO		BUN, Cr

Key Reference: Raisher BD, Grant JW, Martin TC, et al: Complete repair of total anomalous pulmonary venous connection in infancy. J Thorac Cardiovasc Surg 1992; 104:728–735.

PERIOPERATIVE IMPLICATIONS

Anesthetic Technique

- Opioid, NMB, controlled ventilation

Monitoring

- Arterial line, IV, CVP, transthoracic PA catheter placed by surgeon during CPB; TEE very helpful

Airway

- No unique concerns

Induction

- Usually IV induction with benzodiazepine, opioid, NMB

Extubation

- Usually requires postop ventilation

Surgical Stages

- Goal to connect pulmonary venous return to LA, obliterate pathway connecting pulmonary veins to systemic venous system (requires CPB)
- Ordinarily confluence behind LA to which all pulmonary veins converge. Surgical correction involves anastomosis of this confluence to post aspect of LA, ligation of ascending or descending anomalous connection

Postoperative Considerations

- To reduce risk of pulmonary HTN if venous obstruction, hyperventilate, paralyze, maintain on high dose of narcotic in early postop period
- NM blocking agents, analgesics weaned as pressure monitoring indicates ↓ PA pressure, resistance

ANTICIPATED PROBLEMS/CONCERNS

- After correction of total anomalous pulmonary venous return with obstructed veins, ↑ risk for right and left ventricular dysfunction, failure
- RV dysfunction direct result of pulmonary HTN, can lead to dramatic reduction in CO
- LV dysfunction due to inadequate myocardial protection during surgery or inadequate "preconditioning" of LV due to predominant L→R atrial-level shunting
- Most useful pharmacologic agents for management: dopamine (5–15 µg/kg/min), epinephrine (0.03–0.1 µg/kg/min).

TOTAL HIP ARTHROPLASTY

Michael F. Roizen, M.D.

RISK

- People in USA: ?200,000/y (133,000/y in Medicare population, 1986)
- Racial predilection: none

PERIOPERATIVE RISKS

- Risks: 2–3% 30-d mortality
- CV collapse ? 2° to pulm emboli, embolization of fat, marrow, bone, or cement
- Thromboembolism (peripheral venous thrombophlebitis in 60+% of patients w/o prophylaxis—50+% ↓ with prophylaxis)—pulm emboli in 2–4% of patients who do not receive prophylaxis

WORRY ABOUT

- Causes of Fx (? CV disease)
- Perioperative fluid deficiency
- Hypoxia/hypotension on cementing
- Pulm emboli perioperatively

OVERVIEW

- Associated with high immediate morbidity, mortality 2° to volume shifts, embolization
- 1–6-d mortality associated with pulm emboli
- Age, comorbidities of patients dictate monitoring strategies
- Regional anesthesia and postop analgesia preferred by many to ↓ blood loss, risk of thromboembolism; to ↑ mobility

ICD-9-CM Code: 715.9 (Osteoarthritis)

INDICATIONS AND USUAL TREATMENT

- Replacement of hip socket (acetabulum) and/or femur with alloys of metals/plastic/porcelain for:
  - Chronic osteoarthritis
  - Hip Fx (large amounts of blood can be sequestered around Fx site). Investigate cause
  - Avascular necrosis 2° to steroids, infarction (e.g., sickle cell disease)
- Usual medical Rx includes NSAIDs, aspirin

ASSESSMENT POINTS

SYSTEM	EFFECT	ASSESSMENT BY HX	PE	TEST
HEENT	Arthritis can involve airway joints	Snoring	Airway exam	
CV	Impairment due to age; if Fx caused by CV problem—dysrhythmia, etc. Hypovolemia if Fx, bleed into leg	CV status Hx chest pain/SOB Hx palpitations Exercise tolerance	CV exam	ECG Orthostatic BP by table tilt
RESP	Arthritis can be systemic restrictive pulmonary disease/fat emboli with Fx or with replacement of hip	SOB Exercise tolerance	Chest exam Leg exam	O$_2$ sat
HEME	Blood loss 2° to Fx	Orthostatic dizziness	Leg; tilt table BP	Hct
RENAL/ CNS	Impairment secondary to age; if fracture, investigate cause: CNS Hx if cause of Fx is CVA, dysrhythmia, etc.	CNS Hx	CNS exam	BUN/Cr

Key Reference: Merli GJ: Update: Deep venous thrombosis and pulmonary embolism prophylaxis in orthopedic surgery. Med Clin North Am 1993; 77:397.

INTRAOPERATIVE MANAGEMENT

Monitoring

- Volume status monitoring of blood loss a major concern—blood loss ↓ with regional anesthesia or intentional hypotension
- Consider CVP or PA line, several large-bore IVs
- Check availability of predeposited autologous and/or homologous blood; irradiate directed donor blood
- UO, HR, BP not reliable signs of intravascular volume during anesthesia or with postop epidural pain relief
- Myocardial ischemia with ECG, ST segments, even PA cath or TEE if general anesthesia
- Patients' Sx of angina or CHF may be used, but may be distorted if "high" regional anesthesia (need T6 level for regional)

Airway

- Side operated on is usually up, so securing airway after surgical positioning may be difficult
- Airway involvement with arthritis possible
- Delayed gastric emptying of acute hip fracture with pain
- Positioning often uncomfortable after 1–2 h in patient with regional anesthesia due to pressure on side, axilla; in GA patients, pay special attention to eye-ear position
- BP can be taken in up arm (but ↓)—down arm may have altered BP

SURGICAL STAGES

Induction

- CV instability 2° to volume status
- If regional, consider slow titration

Skin Incision

- Large incision over operated hip, leg
- Can observe wound for excessive bleeding

Dissection

- During dissection down to femur, acetabulum, major blood vessel can be accidentally injured, difficult to control—esp femoral, iliac vessels
- Reaming of acetabulum, then femur
- Major blood loss 2° to bone dissection
- High-pressure lavage occasionally used to prepare surfaces: embolization of fat possible

Definitive Surgery

- Some are cemented—methacrylate produces hypotension (within 30 min)
- ↑ Pulmonary embolization (?fat, air, methylmethacrylate monomer) that results in ↑ ventilation-perfusion mismatch or shunt, ↓ O$_2$ sat, right heart dysfunction

- ↓ Myocardial contractility 2° to above
- Can anticipate, hydrate for 10–20 min prior to cementing, ↑ FIO$_2$, have ephedrine ready
- ~Duration: 2–5 h
- Fluid shift can be sizable
- ↓ Emboli by cath removal of pressure on cement insertion

Closure/Postoperative Considerations

- Blood loss of 1–2 units continues—if autotransfusion used, may have reaction to nonwashed cells immediately and may not get as great a long-term boost in Hct as planned (Hcts of 30 desirable for patients with CV disease)
- Pain score: 6–9
- Pain relief via PCA or epidural (start epidural narcotics 1 h prior to end of surgery)
- Early ambulation reduces risk of thromboembolism

ANTICIPATED PROBLEMS/CONCERNS

- Blood volume status and rapid changes due to position, onset of regional/general anesthesia
- Extreme age may make less able to tolerate resp insult and CV instability after cementing
- Thromboembolism and infection prophylaxis desirable
- Pain with early ambulation may be considerable

TOTAL KNEE ARTHROPLASTY

Michael Urban, M.D., Ph.D.

RISK

- 140,000 cases in USA
- Gender predominance: none

PERIOPERATIVE RISKS

- Mortality rare (<1%)
- Despite prophylactic Rx, highest incidence (>40%) of DVT of all orthopedic patients
- Pulmonary emboli in 1–5% of patients
- Fatal pulmonary embolism after tourniquet release rare
- Common orthopedic surgical procedure in morbidly obese patients with concomitant ↑ risk
- Age, comorbidity ↑ risk, need for more invasive monitoring
- Postop bone-cement implantation syndrome, more common with simultaneous bilateral knee arthroplasty

WORRY ABOUT

- CV collapse with tourniquet deflation
- Postop bone-cement implantation syndrome
- Pulmonary emboli perioperatively
- Postoperative bleeding

OVERVIEW

- Replacement of both tibial, femoral components of knee joint, usually with methyl-methacrylate cemented implants

ICD-9-CM Codes: 715.26 (Osteoarthritis, knee); 714.0 (Rheumatoid arthritis)

INDICATIONS AND USUAL TREATMENT

- Chronic osteoarthritis
- Rheumatoid arthritis
- Seronegative spondyloarthropathies (ankylosing spondylitis)
- Post-traumatic arthritis
- Hemophilia arthropathy of knee

TREATMENT

- NSAIDs
- Surgery

ASSESSMENT POINTS

SYSTEM	EFFECT	ASSESSMENT BY HX	PE	TEST
HEENT	Arthritis involving cervical spine, TMJ, cricoarytenoids Sleep apnea	Hoarseness, difficult intubation Pickwickian Sx	ROM of neck Morbid obesity	C-spine x-ray or CT scan
CV	Pericardial effusion, cardiac conduction abn, cardiac valve fibrosis	Dyspnea, palpitations		ECG, ECHO
RESP	Restrictive disease, pulmonary effusions	Dyspnea, cough	Lung auscultation	CXR, ABG
GI	Obesity: full stomach	Weight gain Inability to lie flat	Observation, lying flat	
HEME	Hemophiliac arthropathy of knee	Hemophilia		PTT, PT
CNS	Cervical nerve root compression	Pain on movement, paresthesias	Extremity weakness, ↓ sensation	Lateral neck x-ray

Key Reference: Parmet JL, Horrow JC, Singer R, et al: Echogenic emboli upon tourniquet release during total knee arthroplasty: Pulmonary hemodynamic changes and embolic composition. Anesth Analg 1994; 79:940–945.

PERIOPERATIVE MANAGEMENT

Preoperative Preparation

- Treat hemophilia if present
- Thromboembolism: Rx with DVT prophylaxis, stockings, early ambulation

Anesthetic Technique

- Although no clear advantage of regional over GA, regional eliminates manipulation of airway, provides vehicle for postop pain Rx; epidural anesthesia may be extremely difficult with severe arthritis, scoliosis, or ankylosing spondylitis. Consider paramedian approach

Monitoring

- Consider arterial catheter for dramatic swings in BP with tourniquet inflation, deflation

- For patients with Hx of significant cardiac disease (LV dysfunction or ischemic disease) consider PA cath or TEE; embolization of fat, cement, bone marrow debris may result in significant ↑ in PA pressure without change in PAOP

Surgery

- Positioning may be difficult
- Prolonged tourniquet inflation may result in elevated BP, myocardial ischemia and/or elevated pulmonary artery pressure in patients with ASCVD, LV dysfunction
- Tourniquet deflation: hypotension, tachycardia, pulmonary emboli with hypoxia, possible cardiac arrest. Consider hydration, ephedrine before deflation
- EBL: 100–200 ml
- Pain score: 7–10

Postoperative Considerations

- Significant blood loss over the 1st 24 h from surgical drain; if possible, consider autologous blood donation, erythropoietin preop
- Pain Rx with epidural infusion of narcotic, local anesthesia

ANTICIPATED PROBLEMS/CONCERNS

- Pulmonary emboli of cement, thrombi, bone marrow debris with tourniquet deflation
- Blood volume status postop
- DVT, thromboembolization
- Fat embolism syndrome: hypoxia, tachycardia, hyperpyrexia, thrombocytopenia, leukocytosis, mental status changes; if monitoring PA pressures, pulmonary artery diastolic to PAOP gradient present. Rx aimed at minimizing pulmonary edema while maintaining end-organ perfusion; judicious use of diuretics, O_2, blood transfusions; may progress to ARDS

TRACHEOESOPHAGEAL FISTULA REPAIR
Michael Tobin, M.D.

RISK

- 1:3000 live births
- Dx confirmed by the inability to pass a soft suction cath into stomach

PERIOPERATIVE RISKS

- Perioperative mortality low in full-term, healthy newborns; almost 100% survival
- Perioperative mortality approaches 15–60% in infants less than 1800 g
- Tracheomalacia
- Esophageal stricture

WORRY ABOUT

- Difficult ventilation/hypoxemia

- Prematurity: up to 30% associated with TEF; consider possibility of retinopathy of prematurity
- VATER syndrome: Vertebral anomalies, Anal atresia, Tracheoesophageal fistula, Esophageal atresia, Radial dysplasia
- Congenital heart disease to 25% associated with TEF (VSD, ASD, PDA, tetralogy of Fallot), causing CV instability
- CV collapse/hypotension due to gastric distention or surgical compression
- Hypothermia, consequent acidosis/metabolic dysfunction

OVERVIEW

- Primary repair including fistula ligation, esophageal anastomosis

- Staged repair includes placement of gastrostomy tube under local anesthesia, subsequent ligation of fistula, esophageal repair when more stable

ICD-9-CM Code: 750.3 (Congenital)

INDICATIONS AND USUAL TREATMENT

- Carefully define other congenital defects
- Unstable patients: consider staged procedure
- Premature infants: consider staged procedure
- Gastrostomy tube placement when gastric distention compromises ventilatory status
- Passage of Fogarty cath through gastrostomy into esophagus can occlude esophagus/fistula, thus promoting ventilation of lungs

ASSESSMENT POINTS

SYSTEM	EFFECT	ASSESSMENT BY HX	PE	TEST (If Indicated)
CV	CV decompensation, cyanosis, CHF	Cyanosis, tachypnea, resp distress	Murmur, cyanosis, enlarged liver, hypotension, bounding pulses	CXR, ECG, ECHO, cardiac cath
RESP	Pneumonia, subglottic stenosis	Resp distress, tachypnea, stridor	↓ Breath sounds, tachypnea, cyanosis	CXR, ABG (if indicated), flexible fiberoptic bronchoscopy
GI	Gastric distention, associated anal atresia or bowel obstruction	Enlarged abdomen Resp distress	Tympanic abdomen, enlarged abdomen	KUB series
RENAL	Dysplastic/dysfunction	Anuria	Palpation for kidneys	Créde, cath, or collect urine by bag appliance BUN/Cr

Key Reference: Cook DR, Marcy JH: Common surgical conditions of the newborn. *In* Cook DR, Marcy JH (eds): Neonatal Anesthesia. Pasadena, CA, Appleton Davies, 1988, pp 168–171.

PERIOPERATIVE IMPLICATIONS

Anesthetic Technique

- GA for complete repair
- Local anesthesia for gastrostomy tube placement in staged repair

Monitoring

- Large, well-functioning IV for blood loss
- Consider art line if respiratory or CV problems
- Urinary catheter

Airway

- Awake intubation/careful rapid sequence
- ET tube positioned just above carina to avoid ventilating fistula and to ensure ventilation of both lungs: intentional right mainstem intubation with subsequent slow withdrawal of ET tube until breath sounds 1st heard on left usually ensures that ET tube optimally placed
- Consider facing bevel post during intubation to avoid direct intubation of fistula
- Monitor for kinking/obstruction of trachea/ET tube by surg traction during dissection, repair
- Monitor for complete obstruction of ET tube by blood/secretions, necessitating suctioning/replacement
- Precordial stethoscope on left chest to monitor breath sounds intraoperatively; accidental advancement of ET tube into right mainstem bronchus may then be detected
- Subglottic stenosis may necessitate placement of smaller diameter ET tube than usual

- Soft Silastic cath or esophageal stethoscope most easily placed in blind esophageal pouch before final positioning

Induction

- Healthy neonates may tolerate inhalation induction with spontaneous ventilation until chest opened when a muscle relaxant is given
- Premature infants or those with significant respiratory disease may require careful mechanical ventilation, use of muscle relaxant at induction

SURGICAL STAGES

Dissection

- Blood loss usually minimal, although large blood vessels may be transected
- Recurrent laryngeal nerve damage may occur

Definitive Surgery

- Hypercarbia/hypoxemia possible from these causes: compression/retraction of right lung, kinking of trachea/ET tube from surgical traction, plugging of the ET tube, its migration into right mainstem bronchus or fistula, preferential ventilation of fistula
- Hypotension may result from cardiac compression, hypovolemia, or blood loss
- Hypothermia may result from administration of cold IV fluids, cool ambient room, anhydrous gas administration, heating pad malfunction. Metabolic acidosis may result from hypothermia

- Blood loss can be steady; apparently small losses can be clinically significant in newborn

Postoperative Considerations

- Vigorous infants may be extubated at conclusion of surg: this preferred for maintenance of repair
- Premature infants and those with significant pulmonary disease may require continued mechanical ventilation
- Suction caths marked to point at which they will contact repair

Postoperative Complications

- Pulmonary aspiration, tracheomalacia, vocal cord paralysis
- At later date, patients at risk for intubation of tracheal diverticulum that may develop at site of fistula closure
- Esophageal stricture, esophageal foreign body entrapment relatively common following repair

ANTICIPATED PROBLEMS/CONCERNS

- Pulmonary disease
- Difficulty sustaining airway, avoiding hypoxemia/hypercarbia
- CV compromise/congenital heart disease
- Hypovolemia/blood loss
- Hypothermia
- Prematurity

TRANSPOSITION OF THE GREAT VESSELS (TGV), REPAIR OF

Irene B. O'Hara, M.D.
Alan Jay Schwartz, M.D., M.S.Ed.

RISK

- Incidence: 19.3–33.8/100,000 live births; 5–7% of all congenital cardiac defects
- M>F (2–3.1:1)

PERIOPERATIVE RISKS

- Associated cardiac anomalies: VSD, LV outflow obstruction
- Systemic or pulmonary ventricular failure
- Pulmonary HTN
- Polycythemia, associated coagulopathy in cyanotic patients
- Rhythm disturbances affecting CO
- Preop ductal patency may be maintained with PGE_1 infusion

WORRY ABOUT

- Neonates with CHF, cyanosis should be evaluated for presence of TGV. In presence of intact ventricular septum, PGE_1 infusion may maintain ductal patency, blood mixing until balloon atrial septostomy performed

- Pulmonary and systemic resistance may need to be balanced to maintain optimal ratio of systemic:pulmonary blood flow
- In cyanotic patients, polycythemia may cause sludging; has been implicated in CVAs
- Thrombocytopenia, ↓ plasma clotting factors can be present

OVERVIEW

- Common cardiac defect rarely associated with other congenital anomalies; is secondary only to VSD in frequency
- Without intervention, 30% mortality in 1st w, 45% 1st mo, 90%, 1st y; anoxia, CHF primary causes of death
- Palliation vs. definitive surgery depends on associated presence of VSD or LV outflow obstruction
- Balloon septostomy, early corrective surgery have improved long-term outcome

ICD-9-CM Code: 745.10

ETIOLOGY

- Common congenital cardiac defect; accounts for 5–7% of congenital cardiac lesions
- Associated risks: possible maternal diabetes

USUAL TREATMENT

- PGE_1 infusion to maintain ductal patency
- Balloon (Rashkind-Miller) atrial septostomy
- Palliative surgery; if LV outflow obstruction, VSD present, systemic to PA shunt. If VSD, and advanced pulm vascular occlusive disease present, atrial switch (Mustard) may be performed without VSD closure
- Definitive repair: intra-atrial repair (Mustard or Senning) to connect systemic, pulm circuits at atrial level. Arterial switch (Jatene) with coronary artery reimplantation to anatomically correct circulation by anastomosing aorta to systemic ventricle and PA to the pulm ventricle

ASSESSMENT POINTS

SYSTEM	EFFECT	ASSESSMENT BY HX	PE	TEST
CV	CHF	Respiratory distress Poor perfusion	Rales, S_3, hypotension	ECHO
RESP	Pulmonary vascular occlusive disease	Dyspnea	Clubbing, cyanosis	CXR, cath
HEME	Polycythemia (if >6–9 mo) Coagulopathy, bleeding Thrombocytopenia	Bleeding		CBC Coag factor levels, plt studies
CNS	CVA	Associated with polycythemia	Focal deficit	CT or MRI

Key Reference: DiNardo JA: Transposition of the great vessels. *In* Lake CL (ed): Pediatric Cardiac Anesthesia, 2nd ed. Norwalk, CT, Appleton & Lange, 1993, pp 253–270.

PERIOPERATIVE IMPLICATIONS

Preoperative Preparation

- Maintain CO with adequate HR, contactility, preload
- Maintain ductal patency with PGE_1 (0.05–0.1 µg/kg/min)
- Atropine vs sedative premedication (usually if >6 mo old)

Monitoring

- Arterial line may be placed after induction
- Consider right atrial line (for drug infusion, pressure monitoring)

Airway

- Patient may already be intubated

Preinduction/Induction

- Avoid ↑ PVR—can ↓ PBF, intercirculatory mixing
- If pulmonary vascular occlusive disease present, use ventilatory interventions—i.e., ↑ FIO_2, ↓ $PaCO_2$ to ↓ PVR
- If ventricular outflow tract obstruction present, ↑ ventilation can ↓ PVR, ↑ pulmonary blood flow and intercirculatory mixing

- Maintain SVR relative to PVR to maintain effective pulmonary blood flow and thus adequate SpO_2
- If CHF present with VSD, ventilatory manipulations may be deleterious, due to pre-existing ↑ pulmonary blood flow, difficulty of maintaining systemic blood flow with failing heart
- Anesthetic induction may be accomplished with opioid if IV line in place, otherwise inhalation induction may be used

Maintenance

- Avoid agents that depress contractility; in infants with TGV, intact ventricular septum, O_2 delivery tenuous; with VSD, volume overload possible. Opioids preferred drugs for maintenance anesthesia (fentanyl 50–100 µg/kg or sufentanil 10–15 µg/kg); affords hemodynamic stability; does not depress myocardium; blunts reactive pulmonary HTN. Pancuronium usually relaxant of choice for vagolytic properties

Extubation

- In ICU postop when pulmonary, hemodynamic stability present, patient awake

- EBL: 200–2000 ml
- Pain score: 6–9

ANTICIPATED PROBLEMS/CONCERNS

- Atrial switch
  - interatrial baffle may result in venous obstruction (systemic or pulmonary) immediately postop with result of low CO or SVC syndrome; pulmonary venous obstruction may result in low CO, pulmonary edema
  - dysrhythmias: sinus bradycardia may require atrial pacing; junctional rhythm may require AV sequential pacing; rapid AF may require cardioversion
  - RV (systemic) dysfunction may occur if right ventriculotomy used
- Arterial switch:
  - bleeding from suture lines
  - myocardial ischemia due to coronary reimplantation (air or kinking)
  - inadequate LV function due to insufficient mass, ischemia, or inadequate preservation during CPB—inotropic support

TRANSSPHENOIDAL SURGERY

Kristy Z. Baker, M.D.

RISK

- Pituitary adenoma: 14.7/100,000/y

PERIOPERATIVE RISKS

- Mortality <1% (direct hypothalamic injury)
- Major morbidity 3.5% (stroke, visual loss, vascular injury, meningitis, CSF leak, CN palsy)

WORRY ABOUT

- Endocrine status (especially panhypopituitarism, Addison's, Cushing's, thyroid dysfunction)
- Acromegaly affecting airway
- Diabetes insipidus (DI)

- ↑ Intracranial pressure
- Venous air embolus
- Intracranial hemorrhage

OVERVIEW

- Pituitary tumor resected through sublabial, nasal septal incisions with operating microscope, fluoroscopic guidance
- Tumors can be hypersecreting (GH, acromegaly; ACTH, Cushing's; TSH, hyperthyroid; PRL, prolactinoma) or nonfunctional (mass causing headache, visual change, CN palsy, panhypopituitarism, DI, hypothyroidism, or Addison's)

ICD-9-CM Code: 227.3 (Benign pituitary adenoma)

INDICATIONS AND USUAL TREATMENT

- Pituitary tumor with no/minimal suprasellar extension, no optic nerve or hypothalamic involvement
- Alternative: transcranial approach, medical treatment (bromocriptine or somatostatin analogs), radiation

ASSESSMENT POINTS

SYSTEM	EFFECT	ASSESSMENT BY HX	PE	TEST
HEENT	↑ GH→growth of chin, tongue, soft tissues; vocal cord paralysis, subglottic stenosis	Snoring, sleep apnea, voice changes	Stridor, oral/facial anatomy, airway exam	Fiberoptic evaluation Lateral neck film
CV	↑ GH or ACTH→HTN, DM, obesity, H_2O retention, CHF, cardiomegaly, ischemic CV disease	Chest pain, SOB, exercise tolerance	CV exam	ECG, stress thallium, ECHO, CXR
ENDO	Panhypopituitarism Acromegaly (↑ GH), Cushingoid (↑ ACTH), hyperthyroid (↑ TSH)	Sluggish, cold intolerant, growth, wt gain, nervousness	Hemodynamic instability, CV collapse, obesity, striae	Cortisol level, dexamethasone suppression test, GH level, glucose, TSH, T_4
CNS	↑ ICP from mass	Changes in mental status or vision, N/V	Papilledema, neuro exam	CT/MRI
MS	↑ GH→cartilage overgrowth, nerve and artery entrapment	Weakness, pain	Peripheral neuropathy, inadequate ulnar flow	EMG, Allen test, refill
RENAL/LYTES	↑ ACTH can ↑ aldosterone→ ↑ Na, ↓ K metabolic alkalosis ↓ ADH→DI	Oliguria / Thirst, polyuria	Pulm/peripheral edema / ↑ UO, orthostatic ↓ BP	ABG, urinary/serum electrolytes Urine specific gravity Urine/serum osmolality

Key Reference: Bendo AA, Kass IS, Hartung J, Cotrell JE: Pituitary tumors. *In* Barash PG, Cullen BF, Stoelting RK (eds): Clinical Anesthesia, Philadelphia, JB Lippincott, 1992, pp 896–898.

PERIOPERATIVE IMPLICATIONS

Preoperation

- No sedation if ICP ↑

Anesthetic Technique

- GA with controlled ventilation

Monitoring

- Foley if preop DI
- Consider art line/CVP/PA cath if severe CV dysfunction (not usually necessary)
- Precordial Doppler/RA cath if >15° head up (detect venous air embolism)

Airway

- Awake fiberoptic bronchoscope (vs. tracheal) for acromegaly with airway involvement
- Oral intubation, ET tube, taped contralateral to surgeon
- Tubing secured by radiolucent means (metal obscures fluoro)

- Oropharynx packed to prevent aspiration of blood, intraoral prep

Induction/Maintenance

- Same as for any craniotomy under GA; need less brain relaxation
- Stress-dose steroids mandatory
- Antibiotics to cover nasal, oropharyngeal flora

SURGICAL STAGES

Incision

- Local infiltration with cocaine or lidocaine with epinephrine can cause HTN, tachycardia, dysrhythmias

Definitive Surgery

- DI; intracranial hemorrhage possible
- Intraoperative air study rarely used to delineate superior border; air injected into CSF drain; discontinue N_2O (tension pneumocephalus)

Postoperative Concerns

- Nasal packing necessitates mouth breathing (extubate awake)
- Steroid replacement essential
- PO analgesia sufficient
- CSF leak, DI, epistaxis, sinusitis, meningitis, intracranial hemorrhage possible
- EBL: 50–250 ml
- Pain score: 2–4

ANTICIPATED PROBLEMS/CONCERNS

- DI caused by lack of ADH, ↑ ↑ UO, ↑ serum osm; treat with fluid, add vasopressin or DDAVP if needed
- Intracranial hemorrhage from internal carotid or cavernous sinus can cause brainstem compression, herniation, death; sudden mental status change requires immediate neurosurgical evaluation
- Addisonian crisis manifested by hemodynamic instability or CV collapse; treat with steroids

TRANSURETHRAL RESECTION OF BLADDER TUMOR

Denis L. Bourke, M.D.

RISK

- USA incidence: 16.5/100,000; 50,000 new cases/y. Fourth most common cancer in men
- Gender, race: male 2:1; Caucasian, 2:1
- Risk factors: chemical exposure, cigarettes, coffee, analgesics, artificial sweeteners

PERIOPERATIVE RISKS

- Perioperative mortality low (<1%)
- Ureteral obstruction from tumor or tumor resection
- Less risk of absorption syndromes than during TURP

WORRY ABOUT

- Bladder perforation
- Occult blood loss
- Nerve injury in lithotomy position
- Obturator nerve stimulation

OVERVIEW

- Usually relatively simple, brief (15–45 min) procedure
- 70% of patients achieve 5-y survival with simple transurethral resection/fulguration
- Median age at Dx: 67–70 suggests probability of comorbidities
- Metastases in order of frequency: regional nodes, liver, lung, bone, adrenal, intestine
- Usually minimal postop pain

ICD-9-CM Code: 188.0

INDICATIONS AND USUAL TREATMENT

- Usual presenting symptom: painless hematuria
- Dx tests include: cytology of bladder washings, excretory urography, cystoscopy
- Procedure for—diagnosis; tumor staging; definitive Rx
- Tumor recurrence, repetitive procedures common
- Other Rx include: intravesical chemotherapy, intravesical immunoRx, systemic chemotherapy, photoradiation therapy, laser therapy, vitamins, cystectomy

ASSESSMENT POINTS

SYSTEM	EFFECT	ASSESSMENT BY HX	PE	TEST
CV	↓ Reserve primarily due to age	Hx of chest pain, SOB, palpitations, etc.	CV exam, auscultation	ECG, CXR
RESP	Age effects, associated with cigarettes, pulmonary metastases	Smoking, SOB, cough, sputum, hemoptysis	Auscultation	CXR, CT scan, PFTs
GU	Age, obstructive effects	Hematuria, oliguria		BUN, Cr

Key Reference: Catalona WJ: Urothelial tumors of the urinary tract. *In* Walsh PC, Retik AB, Stamey TA, Vaughan ED (eds): Campbell's Urology. Philadelphia, WB Saunders, 1992, pp. 1094–1158.

INTRAOPERATIVE MANAGEMENT

Anesthetic Technique

- Either GA or regional can be used

Monitoring

- Routine
- CVP may be considered because UO cannot be measured

Airway

- Lithotomy position: airway can be managed by mask or ET tube

Induction

- GA dictated by general health status. Resection of lateral bladder wall tumors may stimulate obturator nerve, cause leg to jump, disrupting resection; in these cases, profound muscle relaxation required, or change in electrocautery settings
- Spinal anesthesia: T10 level sufficient, higher level prevents Dx of perforation of bladder. Spinal anesthesia will not prevent obturator n. musc stimulation during resection of lateral wall tumors. Obturator n. block below pubic ramus if resection at lateral wall to be performed

SURGICAL STAGES

- Stimulation can begin, end suddenly, unexpectedly
- Painful stimulation moderate
- Large veins or artery rare, IV absorption of irrigating solution rare
- Actual resection time usually <30 min
- Blood loss is usually minimal
- Bladder wall perforation rare

Postoperative Considerations

- Pain score: 2–5
- Upper abdominal, precordial, shoulder, or back pain may indicate bladder perforation
- Observe for ureteral obstruction if resection near ureteral orifice
- Peroneal nerve injury can be caused by lithotomy position

ANTICIPATED PROBLEMS/CONCERNS

- Patient age-related CV, pulmonary complications
- Occult blood loss
- Obturator nerve stimulation during lateral wall resections

TRANSURETHRAL RESECTION OF PROSTATE (TURP)

Dorene A. O'Hara, M.D., M.S.E.

RISK

- 11–12% of male population > 65 y; most costly operation under Medicare in USA (1.4% of Medicare charges)
- Racial predominance: none; but African-American patients have higher comorbidity (stroke, COPD, DM, preop infection)

PERIOPERATIVE RISKS

- 30-d mortality 0.1–0.3% (higher in patients > 90 y, 2.6%)
- Morbidity 7–20%; TURP syndrome 2% (hyponatremia, headache, confusion, visual changes, nausea, twitching, hypotension, bradycardia), due to intravascular absorption of irrigant fluid
- Blood loss requiring transfusion, 2.5% (0.2–0.3 ml blood loss/g tissue/min resection)
- Capsule perforation 1%

WORRY ABOUT

- Concomitant CV disease
- Volume of irrigant absorbed
- Time of resection (limit to 60 min if poss)
- Sudden perforation
- Hypothermia
- Rx of benign bothersome (Sx) disease; other Rx aimed at shrinking size of prostate (meds) or watchful waiting (tolerating Sx)

OVERVIEW

- Common procedure in males > 65 y
- High incidence of cardiopulmonary disease in this population
- Preop renal insufficiency associated with poorer outcome

- Bacteremia common perioperatively
- Significant benefits with use of regional anesthesia

ICD-9-CM Code: 600 (Benign prostatic hypertrophy)

INDICATIONS/USUAL TREATMENT

- Enlarged prostate→urinary retention
- Urodynamic studies may be performed
- Size of gland estimated at < 80 g (> 80 g: consider open prostatectomy)
- Tissue may be benign or malignant
- Recent medical Rx include α-blocker, androgen-blocking agents

ASSESSMENT POINTS

SYSTEM	EFFECT	ASSESSMENT BY HX	PE	TEST
CV	Risk of MI, arrhythmias, hypovolemia	HTN, stroke, angina, CHF, SOB	BP, HR, cardiac exam	ECG, Holter
RESP	Resp difficulty during regional, cough	Smoking, cough, sputum, SOB	Chest exam	PFTs (only if Sx severe)
GI	Risk of GI bleeding, anemia	Ulcer, GI bleeding, melena		Hemoccult, Hct
HEME	Added intraoperative blood loss; regional risks	Weakness, fatigue, anticoagulant Rx	VS, pallor	Hct PT/PTT
GU	Concomitant renal failure	Hx of chronic renal failure, kidney stones		UA, BUN, Cr
CNS	Mental status and regional anesthesia, stroke risk	Visual, general CNS	Neuro, carotids	
MS	Osteoarthritis, difficult spinal/epidural	Arthritis, back problems	Back	

Key Reference: Mebust WK, Holtgrewe HL, Cockett ATK, Peters PC, et al: Transurethral prostatectomy: Immediate and postoperative complications. A cooperative study of 13 participating institutions evaluating 3,885 patients. J Urol 1989; 141:243–247.

PERIOPERATIVE MANAGEMENT

Preoperative Preparation

- As indicated by assessment above

Anesthetic Technique

- Regional (esp spinal) preferred for monitoring of CNS, early recognition of perforation, poss EBL
- General may be chosen for spinal OA, contraindications to regional, or patient preference

Monitoring

- Routine
- Light/minimal sedation to communicate with patient, monitor CNS
- Temperature (risk of hypothermia)
- Time of resection, surgeon estimate of gland size; vascularity, volume of irrigant
- Consider CVP/PA if severe coexisting disease
- Serum Na⁺ postop, if CNS changes develop

Airway

- Coughing/straining must be prevented during resection

Induction/Maintenance

- Regional requires levels T8–T10; higher level may mask Sx of bladder perforation, impede respiration
- High sympathetic block may cause undesirable bradycardia, hypotension

Surgical Stages

- Preparation, positioning (lithotomy)
- Via resectoscope, excision of prostate with electrically charged wire loop; coagulation used to control bleeding (to limit blood loss, improve surgical view)
- Continuous irrigation required; water clearest but if absorbed can cause hyponatremia, RBC hemolysis, CNS effects. Lyte solutions disperse current; nonelectrolyte solutions generally used: sorbitol, mannitol, glycine. Fluid absorption = 10–30 ml/min resection time (glycine metabolized to NH_3)

- Post-resection: supine position; observe for hypotension with legs again dependent
- Blood loss can be 2 units or more
- Volume overload major risk due to irrigant
- Hyponatremia: Lasix 40–120 mg, consider hypertonic saline 3%

Postoperative Considerations

- Postop pain generally minimal, mainly due to indwelling catheter maintained with traction, continuous irrigation

ANTICIPATED PROBLEMS/CONCERNS

- BP changes due to onset of regional anesthesia, positioning
- Development of CNS changes, esp double vision, confusion, headache (TURP syndrome)
- Sudden pain, hypotension, loss of returning irrigant (perforation)
- Transient blindness (possible glycine toxicity)

TRAUMA

Alexander W. Gotta, M.D.

RISK

- 570,000 Americans/y injured
- In USA, 175,000/y die from trauma
- Most common in young

PERIOPERATIVE RISKS

- Perioperative morbidity, mortality dependent on extent of injury
- Hemorrhage, hypovolemia, hypotension
- Specific organ damage, i.e., blunt or penetrating trauma to vital organs, brain, lungs, kidney
- Difficult airway 2° to injury to face, neck, chest
- Full stomach
- Recent drug and/or alcohol use

WORRY ABOUT

- Replacing blood volume
- Securing airway
- Ventilating traumatized lungs

OVERVIEW

- Causes loss of potential years of life; and 4th leading cause of death in USA
- Cost: $160 billion/y
- Morbidity and mortality: hemorrhage, head injury, airway disruption, fractures

ICD-9-CM Code: 959.9

ETIOLOGY

- Alcohol use ↓ but still important risk factor in automobile accidents; involved in 17,700 traffic fatalities in 1992 (45.1%); contrasted with 25,165 (57.3%) in 1982
- Drug abuse use other than alcohol; cocaine leads to manic behavior; heroin creates need for money to support habit
- Absence of gun control legislation; guns in home not protective; marker for suicide; homicide rates highest in countries without gun control legislation

USUAL TREATMENT

- Blood, fluid resuscitation, correction of acid-base abnormalities
- Mnemonic: "WOVCATH":
  - Wonder if can tolerate anesthesia
  - O_2
  - Vecuronium or pancuronium
  - Coagulation
  - Acid-base
  - Temperature
  - Hemodynamics

ASSESSMENT POINTS

SYSTEM	EFFECT	ASSESSMENT BY HX	PE	TEST
HEENT	TMJ dysfunction; basal skull fracture	Nature of trauma; location; ability to open jaw; CSF rhinorrhea	Often misleading; skeletal fracture often not related to soft tissue trauma	X-rays of face, base of skull, neck
CV	Hypotension, myocardial, depression due to hypovolemia; cardiac tamponade Cardiac contusion	Nature of injury; reported and observed blood loss

Blunt trauma to thorax | Hypotension, tachycardia, cold, sweaty, cyanotic; ↓ heart sounds with tamponade | Hb, Hct (of little value early in course) ECG, ECHO |
RESP	Hyperpnea to counter metab acidosis; labored ventilation with airway injury	Nature, location of injury	↓ Breath sounds with hemo- or pneumothorax; subcutaneous emphysema with penetrating injury of airway	CXR
GI	Ruptured viscus; torn spleen, liver; bowel disruption	Location of injury, tenseness of abdomen	Sx of shock, sepsis	CT scan; minilaparotomy
RENAL	Hypoperfusion ↓ UO	Amount of blood loss	Sx of shock, hypotension, tachycardia	UO, Na$^+$ IVP
CNS	Confusion, obtundation	Location of injury, amount of blood loss	Cranial injury, paresis, paralysis, dilated pupils	X-rays of skull, cervical spine CT scan

Key Reference: Jaffe D, Wesson D: Emergency management of blunt trauma in children. N Engl J Med 1991; 324:1477–1482.

PERIOPERATIVE IMPLICATIONS

Preoperative Preparation

- Large-bore (16-gauge or larger) IV lines, Foley, adequate blood and components for transfusion
- Consider pulmonary arterial catheter introducer or CVP

Monitoring

- Consider arterial line, CVP
- Pulmonary arterial catheter rarely acutely indicated
- Consider TEE for volume status

Airway

- May be disrupted by direct trauma; consider tracheostomy or cricothyrotomy
- In-line traction if C-spine not cleared

Preinduction/Induction

- May become hypotensive with anesthesia induction
- Attempt to correct hypovolemia as quickly as possible
- Ketamine offers no advantages if catecholamine depleted

Maintenance

- Treat severe metabolic acidosis
- Beware hyperkalemia due to tissue injury and/or acidosis
- Maintain normothermia since hypothermia associated with morbidity/mortality

Extubation

- Consider prolonged intubation, mechanical ventilation postop
- Facial edema must subside before extubation

Postoperative Period

- Pain Rx not problem until patient resuscitated, responsive
- EBL: depends on procedure

Adjuvants

- Inotropes, blood components

ANTICIPATED PROBLEMS/CONCERNS

- Hypovolemia leads to shock, inadequate organ perfusion, multiorgan failure
- Hypotension and/or release of tissue factor (especially in neurotrauma) may lead to DIC
- Hypothermia leads to coagulopathies, cardiac arrhythmias, death

TUBAL LIGATION

Gilbert J. Grant, M.D.

RISK

- 500,000 performed in 1992
- Performed post partum (minilaparotomy) or as interval procedure (laparoscopy)

PERIOPERATIVE RISKS

- Risk for serious complication <2%: hemorrhage; sepsis; embolism; cardiac arrest (2/1000)

WORRY ABOUT

- Post partum: aspiration risk; hypovolemia (hemorrhage, uterine atony)
- Interval: complications of laparoscopy: hypercarbia, adverse hemodynamics, pneumoperitoneum, Trendelenburg position
- Peripheral nerve injury from malpositioning; embolism (gas); trauma to vessel or viscus (trocar, cautery)

OVERVIEW

- Usually, choice technique for isolating uterus from ovary (sterilization) by interrupting tube with rings or by cutting tube (surgically with laser) into 2 separate sections
- With either minilaparotomy or laparoscopy, peritoneal traction painful
- Regional technique preferred post partum to reduce aspiration risk (local technique can also be used—i.e., direct injection of local anesthetic into wound, onto mesosalpinx)
- For laparoscopy, GA with controlled ventilation avoids hypercarbia from peritoneal insufflation. Laparoscopy may be contraindicated if Hx of abdominal surgery

ICD-9-CM Codes: V25.2 (Elective sterilization); 659.4 (for multiparity)

INDICATIONS AND USUAL TREATMENT

- Multiparity
- Medical contraindication to pregnancy (appropriate advance consent must be obtained with reaffirmation)

ASSESSMENT POINTS

(Post partum)

SYSTEM	EFFECT	ASSESSMENT BY HX	PE	TEST
HEENT	Airway edema		Airway exam	
CV	Hypovolemia	Hemorrhage	HR, BP (orthostatics)	Hct
GI	↑ Gastric vol, ↓ gastric pH, ↓ lower esophageal sphincter tone	Heartburn		
GU	Uterine atony, chorioamnionitis	Postpartum hemorrhage, fever, diaphoresis	HR, BP (orthostatics), foul lochia	Hct ↑ WBC, T

Key Reference: Hawkins J: Postpartum tubal sterilization. *In* Chestnut DH (ed): Obstetric Anesthesia. St Louis, Mosby–Year Book, 1994, pp 443–454.

PERIOPERATIVE MANAGEMENT

Preoperative Preparation

- If post partum, assess volume status, replace as necessary

Anesthetic Technique

- Can be performed using local, regional, or GA

Monitoring

- Routine

Airway

- If post partum, may have upper airway edema

Induction

- If post partum, use nonparticulate antacid ± H_2 antagonist, metoclopramide; induce with rapid-sequence technique
- For spinal or epidural, T6 level required; if epidural already in place, inspect catheter site; administer test dose to confirm proper position
- If laparoscopic, suction stomach before trocar insertion; use large-bore IV, hyperventilate to maintain normocarbia; reassess ventilatory variables after insufflation (peak airway pressure, minute volume)

Surgical Stages

- Post partum: small periumbilical incision
- Interval: introduction of trocar to peritoneal cavity; insufflation of CO_2 (or N_2O); insertion of laparoscope, instruments
- Interval/post partum (both)—fallopian tubes identified, incised, ligated or cauterized

Dissection

- EBL: negligible

Postoperative Considerations

- EBL: minimal
- Time <30 min
- Pain minimal (score 1–3)
- Consider local infiltration by surgeon (mesosalpinx, wound)

URETERAL STENT PLACEMENT

Denis L. Bourke, M.D.

RISK

- Common procedure performed for variety of reasons
- Gender/race predominance: M more common; no racial predilection
- Risk factors: related to coexisting disease; etiologic need for procedure

PERIOPERATIVE RISKS

- Perioperative mortality very low (<<1%)
- Ureteral perforation

WORRY ABOUT

- Nerve injury in lithotomy position
- Some urologists prefer "one leg down" position, which ↑ potential for hip dislocation or fracture, especially in debilitated patients
- Occasionally immediate open repair performed if ureter is perforated during procedure
- Occult blood loss (rare)

OVERVIEW

- Usually relatively straightforward, minimal painful, brief (5–25 min) procedure
- Usually 2° or temporizing procedure
- Patient profiles span extremes from young, healthy to old, moribund
- Procedure→minimal physiol disturbance
- Many different types of stents can be used (see Key Reference)
- Usually minimal postop pain
- Fluoroscopy may be required

INDICATIONS AND USUAL TREATMENT

- Prophylactic for potential ureteral obstruction after ureteral instrumentation
- Bypass intrinsic obstruction—e.g., stones (especially during pregnancy) or strictures
- Bypass fistulas—e.g., ureterovaginal, ureteroenteric, or ureterocutaneous
- Bypass extrinsic obstructions—e.g., tumors, hematoma, or post-traumatic (surgical or other) edema
- For ureteral identification during gynecological or pelvic cancer surgery
- To maintain reimplantation site patency following transplant

ASSESSMENT POINTS

SYSTEM	EFFECT	ASSESSMENT BY HX	TEST
CV	Depends on patient's age, diseases		
ENDO	Depends on nature of stone		Ca^{2+}
GU	Age, obstructive effects	Hematuria, oliguria	BUN, Cr

Key Reference: Saltzman B: Ureteral stents: Indications, variations, and complications. Urol Clin North Am 1988; 15:481–491.

INTRAOPERATIVE MANAGEMENT

Anesthetic Technique

- Usually monitored anesthesia care with IV sedation adequate
- Occasionally, GA or regional anesthesia required

Monitoring

- Routine monitoring
- Age, coexisting diseases may dictate more extensive monitoring
- CVP occasionally indicated if UO cannot be measured

Airway

- Patient usually awake with minimal sedation required
- Patient in lithotomy position if GA required; airway can be managed by mask or ET tube

Induction

- Commonly, no specific induction required; sedation/analgesia used
- Spinal anesthesia: T12 level usually sufficient: discomfort confined to urethra

Surgical Stages

- Like other endoscopic procedures, ureteral stent placement stimulation can begin, end suddenly, unexpectedly.
- Surgically painful stimulation minimal
- Large veins or arteries rarely encountered; IV absorption of irrigating solution rare
- Placement time usually <15 min
- Blood loss often small

ANTICIPATED PROBLEMS/CONCERNS

- Ureteral perforation rare, seldom of any immediate consequence to anesthetist unless immediate open repair required
- Nerve injury in lithotomy position

VAGINAL DELIVERY, NORMAL

Mukesh C. Sarna, M.D.
Nancy E. Oriol, M.D.

RISK

- 3.82 million live births in USA in 1988

PERIPARTUM RISKS

- Maternal mortality ↓: 7.8/100,000 live births in 1985 compared with 582/100,000 in 1935
- Perinatal mortality rate also ↓: 14.7/1000 live births, 1985
- Thromboembolism, hemorrhage, HTN disorders, infection remain common causes of maternal mortality, morbidity
- Decline in anesthetic-related causes noted (UK data)

WORRY ABOUT

- Supine hypotension syndrome
- Difficult airway
- Comorbid conditions: pre-eclampsia, DM, ante/post partum hemorrhage, multiple gestation, vaginal delivery after C-section
- Fetal well-being

OVERVIEW

- Effects of maternal interventions on fetus
- Effects of maternal intervention on course of labor
- Role of anesthesiologist:
  - labor analgesia
  - anesthetic for operative delivery
  - high-risk obstetrics
  - newborn resuscitation
  - maternal resuscitation

ICD-9-CM Code: v22.2

INDICATIONS AND USUAL TREATMENT

- Labor analgesia:
  - lumbar epidural
  - spinal
  - combined spinal/epidural
  - parenteral opioids
  - others: psychoprophylaxis, parenteral, TENS, hypnosis/inhalational analgesia
- Operative delivery
  - Spinal anesthesia
  - Epidural anesthesia
  - Continuous spinal analgesia
  - GA
  - Local anesthesia
  - Bilateral pudendal nerve block
- Neonatal resuscitation, especially in situations of nonreassuring fetal heart tracings, meconium-stained amniotic fluid

ASSESSMENT POINTS

SYSTEM	EFFECT	ASSESSMENT BY HX	PE	TEST
CV	↑ CO, ↓ SVR		BP, HR	
RESP	Edema, ↑ soft tissue	Previous GA	Airway exam	None
HEME	↑ plasma vol. > ↑ RBC mass	Sx of easy fatigability with significant anemia	None specific	CBC: occasional ↓ plt in normal preg
HEPATIC/ RENAL	Significant changes if preg complic by PIH	Epigastric pain, N/V, HA	Epigastric tenderness, hyperreflexia	BUN, Cr, LFTs, UA

Key Reference: Shnider SM, Levinson G: Anesthesia for obstetrics. *In* Miller RD (ed): Anesthesia, 4th ed. New York, Churchill Livingstone, 1994, pp 2031–2076.

INTRAPARTUM MANAGEMENT

- Parturients in active labor should consider brief interview with anesthesiologist; emphasis on airway exam, prev anes experience, comorbid conditions
- Establish fetal status by cardiotocography, relevant prenatal test
- Antacid prophylaxis before any anesthetic intervention
- Establish IV access; consider preload before regional procedure; maintain left uterine displacement at all times

Monitoring

- Baseline pulse, BP, T
- Following regional technique, monitor hemodynamics aggressively for the 1st 30 min; then at 1/2-h to 1-h intervals
- Equal attention to fetal status at induction, during maintenance of regional analgesia for labor

LABOR ANALGESIA

Lumbar Epidural

- Drugs
  - local anesthetics, opioids alone or in combination; low-dose, ultra low-dose (0.04% bupivacaine) solns; latter allow for consideration of ambulation during labor as incidence of motor blockade is low
- Complications
  - hypotension
  - inadequate analgesia
  - dural puncture headache
  - subarachnoid block
  - subdural block
  - nerve damage (rare)
- Contraindications
  - coagulopathy
  - infection
  - patient refusal

Spinal

- Intrathecal Drugs
  - of opioids, sufentanil seems most suitable (7.5–10 µg); addition of bupivacaine 2.5 mg may improve quality, duration of analgesia
- Much ↓ incidence of spinal headache since introduction of pencil-point needles

Parenteral Opioids

- Maternal N/V, sedation
- ↓ Beat-beat variability in FHR
- Risk of neonatal depression
- Despite low efficacy, remain commonest form of labor analgesia

ANTICIPATED PROBLEMS/CONCERNS

- Airway: ↑ incidence of difficult/failed intubation with resultant hypoxemia, aspiration
- Aortocaval compression
- Peripartum hemorrhage
- Effect of interventions on fetus
- Postpartum neuropathy
- 20–25% of all planned normal spontaneous vaginal deliveries go to cesarean section!

VENOUS AIR EMBOLISM

Thomas J. Toung, M.D.

RISK

- Patients with operative site–right heart gradient of >5 cm
- Patent foramen ovale in ~25% of adults
- Racial predominance: none

PERIOPERATIVE RISKS

- Perioperative mortality <1%, but depends on early detection
- Venous air embolism 40% sitting, 10% prone, 15% supine, 8% lateral
- Paradoxical air embolism (as high as 12%)

WORRY ABOUT

- Pulmonary venous outflow obstruction
- CV collapse
- Paradoxical air embolism

OVERVIEW

- Entrainment of air in venous system: can cause clinical Sx by paradoxical embolization, air lock, or change in RV function
- Multi-orificed catheter tip must be placed 2 cm below the SVC-atrial junction.
- Consider right heart catheter in all sitting cases
- 75% N_2O can increase air bubble size about 3-fold
- Sensitivity for detection: TEE > precordial Doppler > PAP and end-tidal CO_2 > CVP > BP, and ECG
- Mill-wheel murmur late, catastrophic sign
- PA catheter may provide prognostic info

ICD-9-CM Codes: 958.0; 673.0 (obstetrical)

INDICATIONS AND USUAL TREATMENT

- Operative site elevated to gain better exposure, blood drainage
- When venous air embolism occurs:
  - notify surgeon of episode
  - turn off N_2O
  - gently apply bilateral jugular vein compression
  - inflate MAST trousers
  - aspiration of air from central catheter
  - CV support
  - Left decubitus position (Durant's maneuver)

ASSESSMENT POINT

SYSTEM	EFFECT	ASSESSMENT BY HX	PE	TEST
CV	Patent foramen ovale	SOB	Auscultation	CXR, cath

Key Reference: Albin MS, Carroll RG, Maroon JC, et al: Clinical considerations concerning detection of venous air embolism. Neurosurgery 1978; 3:380–384.

INTRAOPERATIVE MANAGEMENT

Monitoring

- Precordial Doppler (or alternative, see Overview)
- End-tidal CO_2
- Consider CVP or PAP

SURGICAL STAGES

Dissection

- Venous air embolism mostly in beginning, closure

Definitive Surgery

- Depends on pathology
- When venous air embolism occurs:
  - notify surgeon of episode
  - turn off N_2O
  - gently apply bilateral jugular vein compression
  - inflate MAST trousers
  - aspiration of air from central catheter
  - CV support
  - Left decubitus position (Durant's maneuver)

Postoperative Considerations

- Possible hypoxemia from pulmonary infarction
- Possible stroke from parodoxical air embolism
- Possible cardiac arrest from massive venous air or paradoxicalaer embolism

ANTICIPATED PROBLEMS/CONCERNS

- Hypoxemia, ARDS late sequelae from massive air embolism or resuscitation

VENTRICULAR SEPTAL DEFECT, REPAIR OF   Cindy Hughes, M.D.

RISK

- Incidence: 2/1000 live births
- Isolated defect in 23% with CHD
- In combination with other cardiac anomalies 26% of time
- High incidence in premature births; most close spontaneously

PERIOPERATIVE RISKS

- Endocarditis: antibiotic prophylaxis required for any medical/dental procedure
- Worsening L→R shunting in infant with pain, hypoxia, hypothermia
- ↑ Risk of perioperative CHF, arrhythmia, shunting, paradoxic air embolism
- High surgical mortality (20%) if VSD repair necessitated before age 6 mo

WORRY ABOUT

- Paradoxical air embolism
- Poor tolerance of induction if CHF (unable to feed, sweating while feeding, FTT, irritability)
- Residual or unrecognized VSD causing failure to separate from CPB, CHF, or failure to wean from mechanical ventilation
- Arrhythmia or heart block due to damage of conducting system post repair

- Ventricular outflow obstruction post repair
- Aortic regurgitation 2° to prolapse of aortic valve leaflet post repair

OVERVIEW

- Most common congenital heart defect
- 30–40% of all small membranous VSDs close spontaneously by 1st y
- 80% of those that do not spontaneously close develop CHF by 4 mo if untreated
- Pulmonary vascular HTN can be seen by 1 y if large VSD, multiple VSDs, or PDA exists; Eisenmenger's syndrome seen in second decade of life
- Factors determining time of repair include:
  - degree of L→R shunting
  - CHF unresponsive to medical Rx
  - FTT
  - Sx of ↑ pulmonary vascular HTN

ICD-9-CM Code: 745.4

ETIOLOGY

- Interventricular septum divided into 3 parts:
  - membranous septum (part of endocardial cushion)
  - the muscular septum
  - bulbus cordis (divides outflow tract into right, left ventricles)
- Type I (8%), supracristal VSD: close to pulmonary valve, right coronary cusp of aortic valve may lack support
- Type II (75%), membranous VSD: failure of septum to grow up to cushion
- Type III (4%), endocardial cushion VSD or complete AV canal: associated with ostium primum (ASD); lies very high in septum
- Type IV (12%), muscular VSD: freq multiple VSDs; caused by excessive absorption of septal tissue

USUAL TREATMENT

- Medical Rx for control of CHF: digoxin, diuretics
- High surgical mortality (20%) if VSD repair required before age 6 mo; closure of associated PDA or palliative procedure—e.g., banding—may precede definitive repair
- Surgical mortality in children ≥2 y with slight elevations in PVR: less than 2%

ASSESSMENT POINTS

SYSTEM	EFFECT	ASSESSMENT BY HX	PE	TEST
CV *(small defect)*	L→R shunting trivial	Incidental murmur found by pediatrician	Left parasternal holosystolic murmur	CXR normal, ECG may show mild LVH
(large defect)	Significant L→R shunting, ↑ PAP	FTT, dyspnea, feeding difficulties, recurrent pulmonary infections	Harsh pansystolic murmur, systolic thrill	CXR: cardiomegaly, pulmonary congestion ECG: biventricular hypertrophy, notched P waves

Key Reference: Kambam J: Ventricular septal defects. *In* Kambam J (ed): Cardiac Anesthesia for Infants and Children. St. Louis, Mosby-Yearbook, 1993, pp 193–202.

PERIOPERATIVE IMPLICATIONS

Preoperative Preparation

- Optimal control of CHF
  - Child should be feeding, growing
- Adequate premedication for hemodynamic stability
- Antibiotic prophylaxis

Monitoring

- Arterial, central venous monitoring for tight control of hemodynamics
- Consider TEE or color flow Doppler to assist with postop Dx of residual VSD

Preinduction/Induction

- Heavy premedication, ↓ SVR to limit L→R shunting

Airway

- PPV may limit degree of L→R shunting

Maintenance

- Choice based on preference

Extubation

- If repair of VSD, extubate in ICU when hemodynamically stable (weaned from inotropes, free of arrhythmias, normothermic, etc)
- If patient with unrepaired VSD is undergoing noncardiac surgery, extubate at end of procedure if overall condition good. Avoid worsening L→R shunting (hypoxia, pain, shivering) or worsened CHF (excess fluid administration)

Adjuvants

- Oxygen, furosemide, digoxin for continued CHF

Postoperative Period

- Pain management critical

ANTICIPATED PROBLEMS/CONCERNS

- If large VSDs, CHF, or FTT, at greatest risk and difficult to wean from bypass

VENTRICULOPERITONEAL SHUNT

Aaron Lloyd, M.D.

RISK

- Elevated ICP
 –congenital (e.g., meningomyelocele, Chiari malformations)
  – aqueductal stenosis
  – traumatic
  – post fossa tumors
  – overproduction of CSF
- Normal ICP
 – associated dementia, gait disorders in elderly
- Gender predominance: none

PERIOPERATIVE RISKS

- Perioperative mortality rare
- Intracranial bleeding may occur to placement of proximal tubing

WORRY ABOUT

- Prevent further elevations in ICP which can lead to herniation syndromes
- Ventricular dysrhythmias associated with rapid removal of CSF
- Associated pathology

OVERVIEW

- Procedure to divert CSF from ventricles to peritoneum
- Proximal catheter passed into lateral ventricle through burr hole, preferably on the right to reduce risk of dominant hemisphere injury
- Distal catheter tunneled subcutaneously; multiorificed tip placed in peritoneum
- Patients typically present signs of shunt malfunction or elevated ICP

INDICATIONS AND USUAL TREATMENT

- Clinical and radiographic evidence of elevated ICP and/or shunt malfunction
- Hx of previous shunts
- Pseudotumor cerebri
- Normal pressure hydrocephalus with demonstrated improvement in Sx with large-volume lumbar puncture
- If multiple failed ventriculoperitoneal shunts, ventriculo-jugular, atrial, or pleural shunts may be placed

ASSESSMENT POINTS

SYSTEM	EFFECT	ASSESSMENT BY HX	PE	TEST
CV	HTN, bradycardia			VS
RESP	Aspiration	Vomiting	Auscultation	CXR
CNS	Herniation, seizures	Obtundation	Shunt tap by neurosurgeon	CT, EEG

Key Reference: Ruge JR, McLone DG: Cerebrospinal fluid diversion procedures. *In* Apuzzo MLJ (ed): Brain Surgery: Complications, Avoidance and Management. New York, Churchill Livingstone, 1993, pp 1463–1494.

PERIOPERATIVE IMPLICATIONS

Anesthetic Technique

- GA usual

Monitoring

- Routine
- Consider arterial line in cases of uncontrolled ICP, hemodynamic instability

Airway/Induction

- Normal ICP: IV or mask induction adequate
- Elevated ICP: atropine (in children), preoxygenate, cricoid pressure, thiobarbiturate, narcotic, lidocaine, rapid-acting nondepolarizing muscle relaxant followed by hyperventilation

Maintenance

- Hyperventilate to maintain $PaCO_2$ at 24–30 mmHg in patients with elevated ICP
- If used, maintain low levels of inhaled agent to avoid ↑ CBF, blood volume, and ICP

SURGICAL STAGES

Positioning

- Table turned 90 degrees, head to surgeon
- Head turned 30 degrees from neutral, bump placed under shoulder ipsilateral to shunt

Dissection

- Small flap turned in parietal region with subsequent burr hole
- Small abdominal incision, enters peritoneum
- Subcutaneous tunnel tracked to pull distal catheter through; can be stimulating, associated with ↑ anesthetic needs

Definitive Surgery

- EBL: minimal
- Rapid decompression can be associated with tachydysrhythmias, hypotension
- Ventriculoatrial shunts can be complicated by air embolism

Postoperative Considerations

- Patient remains flat to avoid overdrainage of CSF
- Associated with minimal pain (pain score: 2)

ANTICIPATED PROBLEMS/CONCERNS

- Elevated ICP with associated hemodynamic changes

WHIPPLE PROCEDURE

Edward J. Norris, M.D.

RISK

- 30,000 cases of cancer of exocrine pancreas diagnosed annually
- Mean: 60 y
- Male:female ratio: 1.5:1
- Racial predominance: none

PERIOPERATIVE RISKS

- Perioperative mortality rate (30 d) <5%
- Major morbidity most often 2° to underlying cardiopulmonary disease, pancreatic or biliary fistula, hemorrhage, or infection

WORRY ABOUT

- Massive blood loss (superior mesenteric vessels, portal vein, or vena cava injury)
- Significant fluid shifts
- Venous air embolism with injury to vena cava

OVERVIEW

- Distal stomach, gallbladder, common bile duct, head of pancreas, proximal jejunum, duodenum, regional lymphatics removed
- Requires pancreaticojejunostomy, choledochojejunostomy, gastrojejunostomy
- Risk factors include diabetes, cigarette smoking, alcohol ingestion
- Significant blood loss, fluid shifts with extended Whipple resections (more extensive soft tissue, lymphatic dissections, resection of superior mesenteric vessels, portal vein if necessary)
- ~70% of tumors of head of pancreas unresectable at time of exploratory laparotomy

ICD-9-CM Code: 157.0 (cancer of pancreas)

INDICATIONS AND USUAL TREATMENT

- Following conditions should be met:
  - all evidence of gross tumor can be resected with standard resection
  - no evidence of distant metastatic disease or extensive vascular or retroperitoneal involvement by work-up
  - good general health
- Palliative operations directed to relief of obstructive jaundice (cholecystojejunostomy, choledochojejunostomy), gastric outlet obstruction (gastrojejunostomy), pain (celiac plexus injection with ethanol)
- Combined radiotherapy and chemotherapy have been shown to ↑ survival in patients with resectable, unresectable disease

ASSESSMENT POINTS

SYSTEM	EFFECT	ASSESSMENT BY HX	PE	TEST
GI	Gastric outlet obstruction	Vomiting	Abdominal mass	CT scan
HEPATIC	Liver metastases		Hepatomegaly	CT scan Laparoscopy
	Bile duct obstruction		Jaundice, hepatomegaly	CT scan Bilirubin level
NUTRITION	Tumor Malnutrition	Wt loss		Total protein, albumin
ENDO	Tumor			Blood glucose

Key Reference: Howard JM, Jordan GL, Reber HA (eds): Surgical Diseases of the Pancreas. Philadelphia, Lea & Febiger, 1987.

PERIOPERATIVE IMPLICATIONS

Preoperative Preparation

- Bowel prep routine, requiring rehydration

Anesthetic Technique

- General
- Combined
  - general/lumbar epidural (narcotics)
  - general/low-thoracic epidural (local anesthesia/narcotics)
  - general/intrathecal narcotics
- Technique needs to allow for unresectability (open, close)

Monitoring

- Large-bore IV access for fluid requirements, blood loss
- Consider central venous, arterial pressure monitoring

Airway

- None

Induction

- Cricoid pressure if gastric outlet obstruction suspected
- Combined technique with low-thoracic epidural requires only moderate vol of local anesthetic (6–8 ml)

SURGICAL STAGES

Dissection

- Small-to-moderate amount of blood loss
- Moderate ongoing fluid requirements
- Resectability determined by absence of distant metastases, extent of major vascular involvement

Definitive Surgery

- Significant vol requirements; consider colloid
- Blood loss can be massive with portal vein or vena cava injury

Postoperative Considerations

- Pain score: 5–9
- Usual hospital stay: 12–14 d
- Combined technique with neuraxial narcotics
- May develop significant fluid shifts
- May require postop ventilation

ANTICIPATED PROBLEMS/CONCERNS

- Risk of significant fluid shifts, blood loss
- Malnutrition
- Ileus

SECTION III

DRUGS

ACETAMINOPHEN

Ira S. Landsman, M.D.

USES

- Popular analgesic/antipyretic agent used frequently by infants, children, adults.
- Common drug accidentally ingested by young children and intentionally overdosed by adolescents and adults
- When administered in high doses (>2.6 g/d/70 kg) is hepatotoxic.

PERIOPERATIVE RISKS

- In recommended doses, adverse effects, interactions with other drugs rare.

OVERVIEW/PHARMACOLOGY

- Metabolized in liver by 3 pathways: glucuronidation, sulfation, P450
- Toxic intermediate is formed by P450, which is detoxified by glutathione, but glutathione quickly depleted with overdose of acetaminophen
- Free toxic intermediate binds to hepatocytes, causing cell necrosis; antidote, N-acetyl-L-cysteine (NAC), binds to unconjugated toxic intermediate
- Young children metabolize mostly by sulfation; metabolism by the P450 system is 7–10 times slower than in adults
- Children produce more glutathione, protecting pediatric liver from exposure to free toxic intermediate

MECHANISM OF ACTION/USUAL DOSE

- Antipyretic and analgesic effects occur by CNS inhibition; at usual doses, acetaminophen has minimal anti-inflammatory properties.
- Usual dose for children under 12 y is 10–15 mg/kg/dose every 4–6 h
- Usual dose for adults and children over age 12 is 325–650 mg PO or PR/4 h
- Max dose/d not over 4 g
- Dose for long-term treatment not to exceed 2.6 g/d

TOXIC EFFECTS

- Symptoms during the 1st 24 h after overdose include anorexia, nausea, vomiting, malaise, pallor, diaphoresis
- Latent period with hepatic destruction in next 4 d
- Toxicity can manifest as increase in liver enzymes, PT, and bilirubin
- Liver can become enlarged, painful
- If toxicity not severe, liver function, serum enzyme levels normal within 2 wk. Severe toxicity can lead to liver failure, death in 3–5 d after ingestion; renal failure with or without hepatotoxicity can also occur
- Acute ingestion successfully treated with timely Dx. In children, ingestion to 150 mg/kg does not usually require treatment. Doses of 10–15 g in adolescents and adults toxic; only reliable Dx of acetaminophen toxicity is with a blood level at least 4 h after ingestion. The Rumack-Matthew nomogram identifies patients with serum levels requiring NAC.

TREATMENT OF OVERDOSE

- Because rapidly absorbed, successful gastric decontamination required within 2 h of ingestion
- Treatment with oral activated charcoal controversial
- In mixed drug ingestion, oral activated charcoal should be administered
- In USA NAC PO only acceptable treatment of acetaminophen poisoning
- 140 mg/kg is usual dose of NAC, then 70 mg/kg/4 h for 17 doses; if NAC, treatment within 8 h of ingestion, liver failure rare
- NAC treatment efficacy declines significantly after >16 h

SPECIAL CONSIDERATIONS

- Increasing PT 4 d after a toxic ingestion appears to indicate a poor prognosis; serum pH <7.30, serum Cr >3.4 mg/dl, and grade 3 or higher encephalopathy also suggest poor prognosis; patients with poor prognosis are liver transplantation candidates

DRUG EFFECTS

SYSTEM	EFFECT	ASSESSMENT BY HX	TEST
GI	Liver dysfunction	Anorexia, nausea, malaise	Liver enzymes PT Bilirubin
RENAL	Renal insufficiency		Cr
CNS	Liver dysfunction, encephalopathy	Coma	
METAB		Pallor, diaphoresis	

Key Reference: Anker AL, Smilkstein MJ: Acetaminophen concepts and controversies. Emerg Med Clin North Am 1994; 12:335–348.

PERIOPERATIVE IMPLICATIONS

- Drugs causing ↓ liver perfusion or requiring liver for metabolism are relatively undesirable

ADRIAMYCIN (DOXORUBICIN)
DAUNORUBICIN (CERUBIDINE)

Richard I. Cook, M.D.

TOXICITY

- Two phases of toxicity, acute and chronic
- Acute toxicity: cardiac (may be from direct effects of histamine)
  - ECG changes and conduction disturbances: ↓ QRS voltage; nonspecific ST changes; T wave flattening
  - Rhythm disturbances: supraventricular tachyarrhythmias; PVCs
  - ↓ EF
- Acute toxicity: other
  - Nausea, vomiting, allopecia, diarrhea, mucositis
  - Bone marrow suppression (may limit dose acutely); counts lowest about 2 wk after beginning therapy
  - Infiltrated drug with IV delivery may cause extensive tissue necrosis, requiring wide debridement
- Late toxicity: cardiac
  - Most acute toxic cardiac effects (except ↓ QRS voltage) diminish with time
  - Late toxicity occurs wks/mos after administration; reports of onset up to 5 y after dosing
  - Effects are permanent (some indication that children may recover with time)
  - CHF unresponsive to inotropic drugs
  - Increased risk of CHF with higher doses but heart failure can occur after 1st dose
  - Risk 0.1% to 7% up to 550 mg/m²
  - Risk rises sharply after 550 mg/m² to 50% at 1000 mg/m²
  - Risk increased by radiation of LV, other cardiotoxic drugs, prior LV dysfunction
  - Risk greater in young children
  - Risk of CHF ↓ by divided dosing (e.g., weekly)
- Myocardial function evaluation requires measurement of EF by echo or MUGA (serial CXR, ECGs, systolic time intervals, and other clinical signs not reliable)
- Myocardial biopsy but not myocardial function shows characteristic changes

PERIOPERATIVE RISKS

- Acute: anemia, thrombocytopenia, cardiac arrythmias, and conduction disturbances
- Late: cardiac contractile dysfunction (variable; may be severe)

OVERVIEW/PHARMACOLOGY

- Intravenous chemotherapeutic agents used for wide variety of tumors
- Sensitizes tissues to the effects of radiation; used in combined chemo/radiation therapy protocols
- Excretion primarily by liver

DRUG CLASS/MECH OF ACTION/USUAL DOSE

- Anthracycline antibiotic chemotherapeutic agents
- Works by binding to DNA and interfering with DNA-directed DNA and RNA synthesis
- Variety of dosing regimens: often given weekly until maximum dose is reached
- Maximum dosage ~550 mg/m² BSA; dose decreased when used in combination with other cardiotoxic drugs (e.g., cyclophosphamide) or radiation (see under Toxicity)

DRUG EFFECTS

SYSTEM	EFFECT	ASSESSMENT BY HX	PE	TEST
CV	Conduction Contractile force	Exercise tolerance	Unreliable CHF signs; orthopnea, DOE, etc	ECG ECHO, MUGA
GI	Mucositis, diarrhea		Volume indicators	
HEME	Marrow suppression	Bleeding	Unreliable	CBC with platelet count

Key Reference: Allen A: The cardiotoxicity of chemotherapeutic drugs. Semin Oncol 1992; 19:529–542.

PERIOPERATIVE IMPLICATIONS

Preoperative Concerns

- Some authorities insist on preop echocardiogram for any child who has received these drugs at any time in the past, although history assists in determining need
- Evaluation for signs and symptoms of CHF
- Expected nature of surgical trespass

Induction/Maintenance

- Issues dominated by cardiac condition

ANTICIPATED PROBLEMS/CONCERNS

- LV dysfunction perioperatively with pulmonary edema
- Risk of infection in acute toxicity

ALKYLATING AGENTS

Mark J. Lema, M.D., Ph.D.

INDICATIONS

- Hodgkin's disease, lymphoma
- Breast and bladder cancers
- Lung, pancreas, brain, ovarian, testicular cancers
- Sarcomas, multiple myeloma, leukemias
- Bone marrow transplants, melanoma

PERIOPERATIVE RISKS

- Increased risk of infection
- Aspiration
- Prolonged succinylcholine action (CTX)
- Fluid retention (HN$_2$)

WORRY ABOUT

- Extravasation if given by IV infusion
- Prolonged bleeding (thrombocytopenia)
- Aspiration during intubation

OVERVIEW/PHARMACOLOGY

- Structurally diverse compounds; first chemotherapy agents (1940s)
- Generate reactive, electron-deficient intermediates
- Covalently bind to DNA bases (guanine), especially during mitosis
- Disrupt DNA replication, transcription
- High incidence of cytotoxicity to normal, rapidly dividing cells

SIDE EFFECTS (ACUTE): 1–3 WEEKS AFTER THERAPY

- Myelosuppression (pancytopenia)
- N/V
- Sterility
- ↑ Risk of secondary malignancies (leukemia)
- Alopecia
- Bladder toxicity (hemorrhagic cystitis)

DRUG EFFECTS

CLASS	NAME	ABBREV	SPECIAL INDICATION*	ADVERSE EFFECTS
Nitrogen Mustards				
Mechlorethamine	Mustargen	HN$_2$	LM	
Cyclophosphamide	Cytoxan	CTX	LM, Brt, Bl, Lu, Ov	Decreases pseudo-ChE; myocardial toxicity, hemorrhagic cystitis, pulmonary toxicity
Ifosfamide	Ifex		LM, Ov, Te, Sa	Bladder toxicity, CNS toxicity
L-Phenylalanine mustard	Alkeran (melphalan)	L–PAM	MM	
Chlorambucil	Leukeran	CLR	CLL, LM	
Triethylene-thiophosphoramide	Thiotepa	T-TEPA	BMT	Can ↓ pseudo-ChE
Alkyl Sulfonates				
Busulfan	Myleran	MYL	CML	Pulmonary toxicity
Nitrosoureas				
Chloroethyl-cyclohexyl-nitrosourea	Lomustine	CCNU	LM, Brn	
Bis-chloroethyl-nitrosourea	Carmustine	BCNU	LM, Brn	
Streptozocin	Zanosar	STZ	Pa	
Triazenes				
Dimethyl triazeno imidazole carboxamide	Dacarbazine	DTIC	HD, Sa, Me	

*ALL, AML, CLL, CML: leukemias; Bl: bladder; BMT: bone marrow transplant; Brn: brain; Brt: breast; HD: Hodgkin's; HN: head and neck; LM: lymphoma; Lu: lung; Me: melanoma; MM: multiple myeloma; Ov: ovarian; Pa: pancreas; Sa: sarcoma; Te: testicular

Key Reference: Selvin BL: Cancer chemotherapy: Implications for the anesthesiologist. Anesth Analg 1981; 60:425.

PERIOPERATIVE IMPLICATIONS

Preoperative Preparation

- Full stomach precautions
- Risk of infection (leukopenia)
- Adequate hydration (bladder toxicity)
- Check plt count (thrombocytopenia)
- PFT (busulfan, cyclophosphamide)
- MUGA (cyclophosphamide)

Intraoperative

- Risk of aspiration during induction
- Prolonged bleeding
- Plan for RBC transfusion (anemia)
- Maintain UO
- Reduced dose of succinylcholine (CTX, thiotepa)

POSTOPERATIVE CONCERNS

- Risk of N/V
- Continued fluid hydration
- Monitor cardiac/pulmonary dysfunction (CTX, busulfan)

ALLOPURINOL

Walter L. Way, M.D.

USES

- Pts with hyperuricemia due to primary or secondary gout
- Rx for conditions associated with high blood uric acid levels from both primary and secondary gout

PERIOPERATIVE RISKS

- Drug interactions: azathioprine (↑ toxicity in renal transplant patients), chlorpropamide-Diabinese (↑ hypoglycemic effect), Coumadin (↑ anticoagulant action)

WORRY ABOUT

- Inhibition of hepatic microsomal enzyme activity may decrease metabolism of certain drugs, but importance with regard to anesthetic drugs or anesthetic adjuvants has not been established

OVERVIEW/PHARMACOLOGY

- Xanthine oxidase inhibitor used (1) to control chronic gouty arthritis; (2) in secondary hyperuricemia found with blood dyscrasias, cancer chemotherapy
- Hepatic metabolism to oxipurinol (also a xanthine oxidase inhibitor) with renal excretion of about 10% as allopurinol, 70% as oxipurinol, 20% in feces
- Inhibits hepatic microsomal oxidative enzyme systems but importance of this inhibition to any aspect of anesthetic practice has not been demonstrated

MECHANISM OF ACTION/USUAL DOSE

- Decreased action of xanthine oxidase lessens hypoxanthine conversion to xanthine to uric acid, thus lowering serum and urine concentrations and decreasing occurrence of gouty arthritis and urate nephropathy
- Usual dose
  - 100–200 mg 2–3 times/d as antihyperuricemic
  - 100–200 mg 1–4 times/d as antiurolithic
  - 600–800 mg/d in cancer patients, based on serum uric acid levels

DRUG EFFECTS

SYSTEM	EFFECT	PE	TEST
GI/LIVER	Hepatic drug metabolism		
ENDO	Hypoglycemia		Blood glucose
SKIN	Allergic dermatitis	Maculopapular rash	
GU	Renal toxicity Distributed in breast milk		BUN, Cr
PNS	Peripheral neuritis	Numbness, tingling, weakness feet/hands	

Key Reference: Allopurinol, Systemic. *In*: USP DI, 16th Ed, Vol I. MA, Rand McNally, 1996, pp 45–49.

POSSIBLE DRUG INTERACTIONS

Preoperative Concerns

- Evaluate renal function

Induction/Maintenance

- Unknown effects on hepatic metabolism of various drugs used in anesthesia

Adjuvants/Reversal

- Unknown effects on hepatic metabolism of anesthetic adjuvants
- Drug interactions: azathioprine (↑ toxicity in renal transplant patients), chlorpropamide-Diabinase (↑ hypoglycemic effect), coumadin (↑ anticoagulant action)
- Inhibition of hepatic microsomal enzyme activity may decrease metabolism of certain drugs, but importance with regard to anesthetic drugs or anesthetic adjuvants has not been established

SPECIAL CONSIDERATIONS/CONCERNS

- Importance of allopurinol's effect on hepatic drug–metabolizing systems for drugs used in anesthesia and the possible significance in clinical anesthesia practice have not been established

ALPHA₂-ADRENERGIC AGONISTS

Ramon Núñez-Hernandez, M.D.

USES

- Management of hypertension
- Nonapproved indications:
  - management of narcotic, alcohol, tobacco withdrawal manifestations
  - hemodynamic stability with less BP and HR fluctuations
  - ↓ in inhalation, narcotic anesthetic requirements (30–90% MAC reduction)
  - sedative/anxiolytic with no or minimal respiratory depression
  - postop analgesia with ↓ in narcotic requirements and no addiction liability
  - reduction of postop shivering
  - ↓ cardiac toxicity of IV bupivacaine
  - attenuation of sympathetically mediated hyperperfusion phase after focal ischemia
  - for intrathecal/epidural anesthesia with prolongation of motor and sensory blockade by local anesthesia

PERIOPERATIVE RISKS

- Bradycardia requiring Rx with atropine/ephedrine when hemodynamically unstable
- ↓ in BP potentiated by other antihypertensive drugs
- Severe rebound tachycardia, HTN associated with withdrawal
- Larger BP reduction with blood losses less than 20% of blood volume
- Drug interactions (cimetidine ↑ CNS toxicity)
- High concentrations may ↓ uterine blood flow 2° to direct vascular effect

- Associated with LFT abnormalities (methyldopa)
- Xerostomia most common complaint

WORRY ABOUT

- Severe bradycardia, cardiac arrest
- May produce positive Coombs test (10–20% of patients in chronic Rx with methyldopa)
- Hemolytic anemia (methyldopa)
- Potentiation of lithium toxicity (methyldopa)

OVERVIEW/PHARMACOLOGY

- Clonidine, dexmedetomidine are imidazoline deriv with antihypertensive properties; BP effect central by binding to imidazoline receptor, resulting in ↓ sympathetic outflow from vasomotor center to heart, vessels; → ↓ HR, ↓ PVR
- Effect at presynaptic α_2-adrenergic receptor of preganglionic sympathetic fibers; → predominantly parasympathetic tone; direct peripheral, postsynaptic activation by the α_2 agonist causes vasoconstriction
- Activation of α_2 receptors induces ↓ in production of cAMP by inhibitory G protein (Gi), resulting in changes in protein kinase activity; protein phosphorylation determines extent of inhibition of voltage-sensitive Ca^{2+} channels or activation of K^+ channels in neuronal inhibition
- Physiologic effects depend on specificity for α_2 receptor type, subtype
- Dexmedetomidine, guanfacine, clonidine, oxymetazoline arranged in order of selectivity for the α_2- vs α_1-adrenergic receptor
- Dexmedetomidine $\alpha_2{:}\alpha_1$ ratio is 2000:1, whereas clonidine selectivity $\alpha_2{:}\alpha_1$ is 300:1.

- Physiologic effects also depend on lipid solubility; clonidine similar to fentanyl, whereas oxymetazoline is poorly lipid-soluble, lacks sedative and BP effects of clonidine; dexmedetomidine most lipid-soluble
- Clonidine concentration ↓ in biexponential fashion, with α phase of 5–10 min, slow β phase of 8–12 h; guanfacine has a faster elimination (6–8 h); dexmedetomidine even faster (4–5 h)
- After PO intake of clonidine, BP ↓ in 30–50 min, peak effect at 1–3 h and plasma $T_{1/2}$ of 6–24 h; ~50% of absorbed dose metabolized by microsomal enzymes of liver, finally is excreted by kidney; in chronic renal insufficiency, $T_{1/2}$ may be ↑ up to 40 h

DRUG CLASS/MECH OF ACTION/USUAL DOSE

Clonidine

- Imidazoline deriv; central-acting antihypertensive agent
  - usual dosage: PO 0.1 mg, 0.2 mg, 0.3 mg bid; transdermal (patch) delivery of 0.1, 0.2, 0.3 mg/d for 1 wk

Guanfacine

- Central-acting antihypertensive agent:
  - usual dose 1–2 mg PO qd

Guanabenz

- Aminoguanidine deriv; central-acting antihypertensive agent
  - usual dose 4–8 mg PO qd

Dexmedetomidine

- Imidazoline deriv; highly selective α_2 agonist in clinical trials in the USA, given IV

DRUG EFFECTS

SYSTEM	EFFECT	ASSESSMENT BY HX	PE	TEST
HEENT	Nasal decongestant Antisialogogue	Nasal breathing improvement Xerostomia	 Dry mouth	
CV	Reduces HR BP control	Bradycardia HTN controlled	↓ HR Normal BP	ECG
Vessels	↑ SVR ↑ BP	HTN	↑ BP	SVR
Heart	Slowed conduction Temporary fall in CO		HR	ECG
CNS	Sedation Cerebral vasoconstriction Analgesia/anesthesia Fatigue/asthenia Attenuates ↑ in CBF to inhalation agents ↓ ICP, IOP	Mental status/responsiveness ↓ Anesthetic requirements Weakness	Tension/anxiety relief Reduced strength	EEG changes VAS
GU	Urinary retention/diuretic Impotence/ ↓ libido Impaired insulin secretion ↓ Uterine blood flow (high conc)	 No evidence of hyperglycemia in acute or chronic Rx		

Key Reference: Dyck JB, Maze M, Haacle C, et al: The pharmacokinetics and hemodynamic effects of intravenous and intramuscular dexmedetomidine hydrochloride in adult human volunteers. Anesthesiology 1993; 78:813–820.

PERIOPERATIVE IMPLICATIONS

- If patient is on chronic Rx with α_2 agonist, continue medication in the perioperative period to avoid withdrawal
- Cimetidine may be associated with CNS dysfunction when combined with clonidine by (a) reduction in hepatic P450 clearance, (b) reduction in hepatic blood flow and potential for

clonidine toxicity; also, cimetidine, an imidazoline deriv without α_2-adrenergic activity, can produce CV depression by interacting centrally with midazoline receptor
- Administration of preop CNS depressants adjusted in patients on Rx with α_2 agonist

Induction/Maintenance

- Interaction with induction agent may produce hypotension

- Maintenance doses of anesthetics reduced to avoid severe hypotension or delayed awakening

Postoperative Period

- Avoid withdrawal by continuing management with α_2 agonist in patients on chronic Rx
- In single preop use of clonidine, follow HR, adjust analgesic requirements

AMINOPHYLLINE

Avery Tung, M.D.

USES

- Acute and chronic Rx for asthma, COPD
- Rx for neonatal apnea
- Occasionally for CHF
- Potential for life-threatening CNS, cardiac toxicity
- Administered IV, PO, or rectally

PERIOPERATIVE RISKS

- Toxic levels from overaggressive use or coadministration of cimetidine/propranolol
- ↑ Arrhythmogenicity with halothane or pancuronium
- ↑ CNS toxicity (lower seizure threshold) with ketamine

WORRY ABOUT

- Prolonged clearance in presence of cimetidine, erythromycin, propranolol, or in patients receiving influenza vaccines
- Enhanced clearance in smokers and patients taking dilantin, barbiturates
- Narrow therapeutic/toxic ratio

OVERVIEW/PHARMACOLOGY

- Methylated xanthine
- Bronchodilatory and anti-inflammatory effects
- Onset of effect within 1 h from IV dose
- Biotransformed by demethylation in liver; renally excreted
- 7–15% excreted unchanged in urine
- Crosses placenta, found in breast milk

DRUG CLASS/MECH OF ACTION/USUAL DOSE

- Methylated xanthine
- Proposed mechanisms of action include inhibiting phosphodiesterase, antagonizing the effect of adenosine, causing catecholamine release, inhibiting cellular immune function
- Usual dose: 4 mg/kg q 8–12 h PO; 5–6 mg/kg IV load followed by 0.2–0.75 mg/kg/h IV

DRUG EFFECTS

SYSTEM	EFFECT	ASSESSMENT BY HX	PE	TEST
CV	Inotropy and chronotropy; ↓ in SVR, PCWP, BP	Predisposes to ventricular arrhythmia	Auscultation of heart sounds	ECG
RESP	Bronchodilation, suppression of cellular immune response	Relief of dyspnea, improvement of bronchospastic symptoms	Auscultation of chest	Peak flow, PFTs
CNS	Nonspecific CNS stimulation; stimulates central respiratory drive	N/V, irritability, insomnia, delirium, convulsions, stupor, coma		

Key Reference: Stirt JA, Sullivan SF: Aminophylline. Anesth Analg 1981; 60:587–602

PERIOPERATIVE IMPLICATIONS

Preoperative Concerns

- Toxic preoperative blood level 2° to overadministration or coadministration of drugs that affect clearance (cimetidine, erythromycin, propranolol, verapamil, Dilantin [phenytoin])
- Potential for seizures or malignant arrhythmias if toxic levels
- Presence of underlying bronchospastic disease
- Administration via peripheral vein to avoid cardiotoxicity

Induction/Maintenance

- Can interact with halothane or pancuronium to cause ventricular arrhythmias
- Can interact with ketamine to lower seizure threshold
- Continue infusion if carefully monitoring for toxicity
- No proven effectiveness in treating intraoperative bronchospasm in humans
- Reduction of NMB

Postoperative Period

- Check plasma levels before restarting infusion if toxicity is suspected
- May be used as central respiratory stimulant in neonates recovering from general anesthesia

ANTICIPATED PROBLEMS/CONCERNS

- Most common problems are from narrow therapeutic/toxic window, potential for severe CNS, cardiac toxicity
- Patients taking aminophylline often have severe bronchospastic disease
- Dialysis or charcoal hemoperfusion can acutely lower blood levels

AMPHETAMINES

Earl S. Ransom, M.D.

USES

- Major medical uses include treatment of attention-deficit hyperactivity disorder (ADHD) and narcolepsy
- Uses as anorexians and to allay fatigue are not recommended
- Usually administered orally; IV form ("crystal") found in substance abuse settings

PERIOPERATIVE RISKS

- High risk of abuse resulting in changes in MAC (chronic use, MAC ↓; acute use, MAC ↑)
- Risk of hypertension when used with other sympathomimetics and MAOIs
- Risk of arrhythmias/cardiac arrest when used with thyroid hormones, K+-losing diuretics, laxatives, phenylpropanolamine

WORRY ABOUT

- Severe hypertension and generalized SNS stimulation worrisome in pts with ischemic heart disease, pre-existing hypertension, hyperthyroidism, advanced arteriosclerosis

OVERVIEW/PHARMACOLOGY

- Indirect-acting sympathomimetic
- Schedule II drug
- Acute administration results in increases in cortical alertness, cardiac output, heart rate, peripheral vascular resistance, and dysrhythmias
- Chronic use results in depletion of body stores of catecholamines, tolerance, and psychologic dependence
- May enhance opioid analgesia
- Metabolized slowly by hepatic enzymes
- Overdosage treated with supportive therapy, sedation, possible gastric lavage, urine acidification

DRUG CLASS/MECH OF ACTION/USUAL DOSE

- Phenethylamine derivative
- Mechanism of action via displacement of neurotransmitter (centrally and peripherally) from storage sites in SNS/PNS
- Usual dosages (oral):
  - Obesity, 5–10 mg of amphetamine 30–60 min before meals
  - Narcolepsy 10 mg initial dose/d
  - ADHD 0.1–0.5 mg/kg/d in children

DRUG EFFECTS

SYSTEM	EFFECT	ASSESSMENT BY HX	PE	TEST
CV	Increases in CO, HR, BP, SVR, dysrhythmias	Hx of recent or chronic ingestion	Monitoring of variables	
RESP	Mild respiratory stimulation	Hx of recent or chronic ingestion	Pulmonary exam	ABG
CNS	Increased cortical alertness and electrical activity (generalized); overdosage results in anxiety, psychoses, hyperactivity, possible seizures	Hx of recent or chronic ingestion	CNS exam	
METAB	Dehydration, lactic acidosis, ketosis	Hx of overusage or abuse	Vital signs, general PE	ABG; electrolytes
OTHER	Decreased GI motility, mydriasis, diaphoresis, hyperthermia	Hx of overusage or abuse	Vital signs, general PE	

Key Reference: AMA Drug Evaluations, 1993, pp 8, 290, 322–323, 2251.

PERIOPERATIVE IMPLICATIONS

Preoperative Concerns

- Recent, acute ingestion
- Hx of polysubstance abuse
- Current medications, particularly MAO inhibitors
- Monitor BP for hypertension, ECG for possible ischemia

Induction/Maintenance

- With acute ingestion, may have severe hypertension; α/β-adrenergic blocker and receptor drugs and vasodilators may be necessary
- If necessary to treat hypotension, use sympathomimetics cautiously
- With chronic use, anesthetic requirements will be lower
- Anticipate potentiation of opioid analgesic effects

Adjuvants/Regional Anesthesia/Reversal

- Drug interactions noted are the major concerns

Postoperative Period

- Look for continued signs of CV, CNS hyperactivity
- Withdrawal symptoms not life-threatening

ANTICIPATED PROBLEMS/CONCERNS

- Look for a history of substance abuse. These drugs have a high potential for abuse and are frequently combined with other addictive substances.
- Inquire as to recent drug usage, as this will alter anesthetic requirements and possibly monitoring
- Possible drug interactions

ASPIRIN (ACETYLSALICYLIC ACID)

Christopher D. Beatie, M.D.

USES

- People within USA consume 10,000–20,000 tons annually
- Rx for mild/moderate pain, fever, arthritis, prevention of myocardial infarction

PERIOPERATIVE RISKS

- Peptic ulcer disease
- Plt dysfunction
- Hemorrhage
- Stroke
- Interstitial nephritis
- Reye's syndrome

WORRY ABOUT

- Displacement of protein-bound drugs: e.g., warfarin, sulfonylureas, thiopental, methotrexate
- Potentiation of anticoagulants

OVERVIEW/PHARMACOLOGY

- Cyclooxygenase inhibition prevents plt aggregation and vasoconstriction
- Plt inhibition irreversible for the life of the plt
- Aspirin
  - Metabolized by liver, excreted by kidney
  - Mildly antagonizes antihypertensive medications (β-blockers, vasodilators, diuretics)
  - Displaces protein-bound drugs, increasing their effects

DRUG CLASS/MECH OF ACTION/USUAL DOSE

- NSAID
- Cyclooxygenase inhibitor
- Chronically taken for
  - MS pain (e.g., arthritis, neuralgia)
  - Prevention of myocardial infarction
  - Claudication
- Acutely taken for
  - Acute, mild to moderate pain (e.g., headache, myalgia)
  - Fever
  - Dysmenorrhea
- Usual dose, 325–1000 mg q3–4 h for acute illnesses and pain
- 62.5–325 mg for plt inhibitor effects
- Alternatives: acetaminophen, other NSAIDs (ibuprofen, naproxen), steroids, opioids, gold, ticlopidine, dipyridamole, pentoxifylline

DRUG EFFECTS

SYSTEM	EFFECT	ASSESSMENT BY HX	PE	TEST
RESP	Hyperventilation, respiratory alkalosis		Tachypnea	ABG
GI	Gastritis PUD	Dyspepsia Nausea, vomiting, hematemesis, melena		Endoscopy Upper GI x-rays, stool heme, Hgb
ENDO	Hyperglycemia, corticosteroid release			Glucose
HEME	Plt dysfunction	Bleeding, bruising	Hematomata, petechiae	Bleeding time
HEPATIC	Hepatocellular damage	Nausea, anorexia	Hepatomegaly, jaundice	SGOT, SGPT, alk phos
TOXICITY				
CV	Vasomotor paralysis		Hypotension	
RESP	Hypoventilation, respiratory acidosis		Hypopnea	ABG
SKIN	Eruptions	Pruritus	Acneiform, erythematous, pruritic, eczematoid, or desquamative lesions	
RENAL	Renal failure due to analgesic nephropathy	Oliguria, anuria	Edema, rales	BUN/Cr, UA, CXR
CNS	Headache, tinnitus, drowsiness, dizziness, diminished vision and hearing		Sweating, confusion, convulsions, coma	
ACID-BASE	Metabolic acidosis			ABG

Key Reference: Insel PA: Analgesic-antipyretics and antiinflammatory agents. *In* Gilman AG, et al (eds): Goodman and Gilman's The Pharmacological Basis of Therapeutics, 8th ed. New York, Macmillan, 1990, pp 638–681.

PERIOPERATIVE IMPLICATIONS

Preoperative Concerns

- Discontinued 1 wk prior to surgery for full reversal of plt inhibition (need only 1/7 of normally functioning platelets, so if no dilution effect expected, need only 48 h off low-dose ASA); can be switched to shorter-acting antithrombotic agents (e.g., heparin) until just before surgery if desired
- May potentiate the effects of protein-bound drugs

Induction/Maintenance

- Possible mildly exaggerated effects of thiopental

Adjuvants/Regional Anesthesia/Reversal

- May increase the risk of hemorrhagic complications of regional anesthesia. Aspirin does not contraindicate regional anesthesia, but those techniques with low potential for bleeding are preferable (e.g., spinal may be preferred over epidural).
- May increase the risk of hemorrhagic complications of invasive monitoring

SPECIAL CONSIDERATIONS

- A potent inhibitor of plt aggregation that can seriously impair surgical hemostasis. Most surgeons request discontinuance of aspirin 1 wk prior to surgery. However, if CAD or other vascular occlusive disease will be left untreated, consult with surgeon, pt's primary physician, and pt about advisability of discontinuing aspirin
- Risks of regional anesthesia and invasive monitoring may be increased
- May displace protein-bound drugs (e.g., warfarin, sulfonylureas, thiopental, methotrexate), thus augmenting their effects
- Associated with gastritis, PUD, GI bleeding, and increased risk for aspiration of gastric contents
- Associated with Reye's syndrome and contraindicated in febrile viral illness in children

ATRACURIUM (TRACRIUM)

John J. Savarese, M.D.

RISK

- No change in the clinical response to atracurium during hepatic or renal failure
- No drugs known to affect the rate of Hofmann reaction chemical breakdown
- Speed of the Hofmann reaction ↓ by acidosis and hypothermia

PERIOPERATIVE RISKS

- Respiratory insufficiency from prolonged blockade and drugs that potentiate neuromuscular blockade, e.g., antibiotics ("mycins")

WORRY ABOUT

- Decrease in BP due to release of histamine; may occur when large doses (for tracheal intubation) are injected rapidly (<10–15 sec)

OVERVIEW/PHARMACOLOGY

- Nondepolarizing neuromuscular blocking drug of the benzylisoquinolinium class
- Intermediate duration of effect due to chemical degradation in plasma at alkaline pH, the *Hofmann elimination* reaction
- Major metabolite is laudanosine, a CNS stimulant; plasma laudanosine levels do not reach threshold for CNS activity in usual clinical practice
- ED_{95} = 200–250 µg/kg
- Half-life $(T_{1/2})$ = 20 min
- Clinical duration of action = 30–40 min; complete recovery 60 min following intubating dose

DRUG CLASS/MECH OF ACTION/USUAL DOSE

- Nondepolarizing neuromuscular blocking drug of intermediate duration of the benzylisoquinolinium class
- Not given chronically
- Acutely administered IV for surgical relaxation (tracheal intubation, maintenance of abdominal relaxation, correction of joint dislocation)
- May be given for maintenance of paralysis in the ICU
- Usual dose
  - Tracheal intubation (adults): 500 µg/kg
  - "Priming" dose (adults): 60 µg/kg
  - Tracheal intubation (children): 600 µg/kg
  - Maintenance of relaxation: 100–200 µg/kg every 15–20 min
  - By continuous infusion: 5–10 µg/kg/min
- Other alternatives: mivacurium, vecuronium, rocuronium, *cis*-atracurium, pancuronium, curare
- Antagonists: neostigmine, edrophonium

DRUG EFFECTS

SYSTEM	EFFECT	ASSESSMENT BY HX	PE	TEST
HEENT	Facial flush	Histamine release	BP/HR	Plasma histamine
CV	↓ BP, ↑ HR	Histamine release	BP/HR	Plasma histamine
GI/LIVER	Metabolite (laudanosine) undergoes some liver excretion			
GU	Metabolite (laudanosine) excreted in urine			
CNS	Potential CNS activity of laudanosine has not been noted			

Key Reference: Basta SJ, Ali HH, Savarese JJ, et al: Clinical pharmacology of atracurium besylate (BW 33A). Anesth Analg 1982; 61:723–729.

PERIOPERATIVE IMPLICATIONS/POSSIBLE DRUG INTERACTIONS

Preoperative Concerns

- Antihistamines (H_1 alone or H_1 + H_2 in combination but not H_2 alone) inhibit symptoms of histamine release
- NSAIDs (aspirin, ibuprofen) also inhibit symptoms of histamine release

Induction/Maintenance

- "Priming" doses of 60 µg/kg may accelerate onset of blockade by 30 sec
- Administration following long-acting drugs may result in much longer duration of action than normally expected and is not recommended
- Infuse at 5–10 µg/kg/min for continuous infusion

Adjuvants/Regional Anesthesia/Reversal

- Neostigmine (50–60 µg/kg) and edrophonium (500–1000 µg/kg) are recommended antagonists
- Antibiotics ("mycins") may potentiate the neuromuscular blocking effect
- Lowered temperature or acidic pH will slow the *Hofmann reaction*

SPECIAL CONSIDERATIONS

- Longer duration in conditions of acidosis or hypothermia
- Slower injection of large doses for tracheal intubation to prevent/reduce symptoms of histamine release

ATROPINE

Nishan G. Goudsouzian, M.D.

USES

- Major use: treatment for sinus bradycardia
- Decrease perioperative oral and tracheo-bronchial secretions
- Counteract muscarinic effects of cholinergic agents during reversal of muscle relaxants
- Symptomatic type I second-degree AV block
- Bradycardia with hypotension during resuscitation
- Treatment of organophosphate poisoning

PERIOPERATIVE RISKS

- Tachycardia that may aggravate cardiac ischemia or CHF

WORRY ABOUT

- ?Increase in intraocular tension in patients with acute angle glaucoma
- Inhibition of mucus secretion in respiratory tract
- Dry mouth
- Blurred vision
- Flushing (occasionally in infants)

OVERVIEW/PHARMACOLOGY

- Competitive inhibition of the action of acetylcholine at autonomic cholinergic receptors (parasympatholytic)
- Plasma $T_{1/2}$ 4 h
- Metabolized by liver, excreted by kidneys

DRUG CLASS/MECH OF ACTION/USUAL DOSE

- Inhibits action of acetylcholine on autonomic effectors innervated by postganglionic cholinergic nerves (antimuscarinic effect)
- At high doses produces partial block of autonomic ganglia (nicotinic receptors)

USUAL DOSE (70 kg adult)

- 0.4–0.5 mg IV for intraoperative bradycardia
- 1–2 mg IV before reversal of muscle relaxants
- 1–2 mg IV for intrinsic sinus node dysfunction
- 1–2 mg IV initial treatment of organophosphate poisoning repeated PRN
- 0.4–0.5 mg sc, IM for control of secretions
- 0.01–0.02 mg/kg in infants and children (minimum 0.1 mg)

DRUG EFFECTS

SYTEM	EFFECT	RX ASSESSMENT	PE	TEST
HEENT	Diminished secretions	Dry mouth and upper airways	Dry mucosa, difficulty in swallowing	
CV	Blocking vagal effects of M2 receptors on SA node	Tachycardia	Palpitation	ECG, sinus tachycardia, marked in young people with ↑ vagal tone
RESP	Dry airways	Thick secretions	? ↓ Air entry (rare)	CXR
GI	Some ↓ in gastric acid secretions	Large doses ↓ peristalsis	Decrease in gastric residual volume	Mild decrease in acidity
EYE	Blocking of the sphincter and ciliary muscle	Mydriasis	Dilated pupils	? ↑ Intraocular tension in acute angle glaucoma
CNS	Toxic doses	Restlessness, disorientation, delirium		
SKIN	Flushing (rarely, in infants after large doses)	Red body, dry skin	? ↑ Body T	

Key Reference: Gilman AG, et al (eds): Goodman and Gilman's The Pharmacological Basis of Therapeutics. New York, Macmillan, 1990, pp 151–158.

PERIOPERATIVE COMPLICATIONS

- Dry mouth (consider mouthwash)
- Thick pulmonary secretions (humidity)
- Aggravate CHF or angina (slow HR by cholinergic drugs or β-blockers)

Induction/Maintenance

- Rarely used routinely

Adjuvants/Regional Anesthesia/Reversal

- Effect cleared within few hours
- In emergency, consider cholinergic drugs or β-blockers

SPECIAL CONSIDERATIONS

For resuscitation, larger doses are required. In the absence of IV, 2–4 mg/70 kg diluted in 10 ml NS can be given via an endotracheal tube.

BENZODIAZEPINES (MIDAZOLAM, LORAZEPAM, DIAZEPAM) Harry J.M. Lemmens, M.D.

USES

- Prescribed for the treatment of anxiety
- Used for conscious sedation and premedication

PERIOPERATIVE RISKS

- High levels associated with hypnosis, unconsciousness, respiratory depression, apnea

WORRY ABOUT

- Combination with opioids or other CNS depressants may result in severe respiratory depression, apnea, hypotension

OVERVIEW/PHARMACOLOGY

- Anxiolysis, sedation, hypnosis, muscle relaxation, anterograde amnesia, anticonvulsant
- Midazolam: short elimination $T_{1/2}$ (2.5 h)
- Lorazepam: intermediate elimination $T_{1/2}$ (15 h)
- Diazepam: long elimination $T_{1/2}$ (30 h)
- Metabolized by hepatic microsomal oxidation and glucuronide conjugation

- Diazepam has active metabolites
- Midazolam   IV: peak effect in 2–4 min
  IM: peak effect in 30–60 min
- Lorazepam   IV: peak effect in 5–15 min, painful injection, thrombophlebitis
  IM: peak effect in 60–90 min
  Oral: peak effect in 2 h
- Diazepam   IV: peak effect in 1–2 min, painful injection, thrombophlebitis
  IM: painful, unpredictable absorption, do not use
  Oral: peak effect in 30–60 min, well absorbed; food, aluminum-containing antacids delay absorption
- No clear difference in speed of recovery from diazepam and midazolam drug effect after low dose for sedation in short procedures; faster recovery from midazolam drug effect becomes more prominent after larger dose/prolonged administration

- Lorazepam provides long duration (>4 h) of sedation and amnesia by any route of administration; do not use when rapid recovery from drug effect desired
- Prolonged use can lead to tolerance

DRUG CLASS/MECH OF ACTION/USUAL DOSE

- Anxiolytic, sedative, hypnotic
- Potentiation of gamma-aminobutyric acid–mediated neural inhibition
- Safe use involves careful titration to the desired effect
- Usual dosage for premedication and conscious sedation:
  – Midazolam   IV: 0.5–1 mg, repeated; maintenance infusion: 0.04–0.10 mg/kg/h
  IM: 0.07 mg/kg
  Oral: 15 mg (not available in USA)
  – Lorazepam   IV: 0.25 mg, repeated
  IM: 0.05 mg/kg, max 4 mg
  Oral: 0.5–4 mg
  – Diazepam   IV: 1–2 mg, repeated
  Oral: 5–10 mg

DRUG EFFECTS

SYSTEM	EFFECT	PE	TEST
CV	Decreased systemic vascular resistance and cardiac output	Arterial BP	
RESP	Central respiratory depression Apnea	Resp rate	Tidal volume Minute volume, capnography, oximetry
CNS	Anxiolysis Sedation	Slurred speech, drowsiness, ataxia Unresponsiveness	
	Hypnosis Amnesia Anticonvulsant ↓ Cerebral metabolic rate and cerebral blood flow		

Key Reference: Rall TW: *In* Gilman AG, et al (eds): Goodman and Gilman's The Pharmacological Basis of Therapeutics, 8th ed. New York, Macmillan,1990, pp 346–358.

PERIOPERATIVE IMPLICATIONS/POSSIBLE DRUG INTERACTIONS

Preoperative Concerns

- Elderly: Reduce dose up to 5-fold (5–10%/decade reduction).
- Cimetidine, ranitidine (microsomal cytochrome P450 inhibitors), and liver cirrhosis ↓ clearance; enhanced effect may be seen
- Smoking and enzyme-inducing drugs ↑ diazepam clearance
- Renal failure ↑ diazepam $T_{1/2}$
- Monitor ventilation

Induction/Maintenance

- Synergistic interaction with anesthesia induction agents, opioids

Regional Anesthesia

- Possibly exacerbated respiratory depression during spinal anesthesia (mechanism unknown)

ANTICIPATED PROBLEMS/CONCERNS

- Combination with opioids or other CNS depressants may result in severe respiratory depression, apnea, hypotension
- Large doses result in prolonged drowsiness and respiratory depression, especially in the elderly
- Undesirable degree of amnesia

BETA-ADRENERGIC RECEPTOR ANTAGONISTS (BLOCKERS)

Roberta Hines, M.D.

USES

- 10 million in USA receive routinely
- Used in management of essential HTN
- Effective in decreasing infarct size
- Used to ↓ HR
- Available as oral and IV preparations
- Used to suppress cardiac dysrhythmias
- Value in prevention of excess SNS activity

PERIOPERATIVE RISKS

- Nonselective blocker may precipitate bronchospasm
- May worsen or precipitate CHF in patients with ↓ LV function
- May cause hypotension, bradycardia

WORRY ABOUT

- ↓ Ventricular performance especially with underlying cardiac dysfunction
- Can worsen lung disease, especially with Hx of COPD or bronchospasm

OVERVIEW/PHARMACOLOGY

- All ß blockers are derivatives of isoproterenol
- ß-adrenergic receptor agonists classified as partial or pure agonists on basis or absence of intrinsic sympathomimetic activity
- Partial antagonists often better tolerated than pure antagonists in patients with ↓ LV function
- ß blocker may produce varying degrees of membrane stabilization in heart (detectable only at extremely high plasma concentration)
- Effective in both acute, chronic management

DRUG CLASS/MECH OF ACTION/USUAL DOSE

- All ß blockers bind selectively to ß receptors
- ß blockers interfere with ability of other drugs/substances with sympathomimetic activity to activate ß receptors
- Action of ß blockers negates effect of catecholamines, other sympathomimetics on heart and smooth muscle of airways, blood vessels
- Bind to ß receptor by competitive inhibition
- Exhibit selective affinity for ß-adrenergic receptors
- Binding of agonists to the ß receptor is reversible
- Chronic administration is associated with ↑ in number of ß-adrenergic receptors
- Principal method of clearance hepatic, renal, or plasma hydrolysis (esmolol)
- Elimination $T_{1/2}$ specific to individual agents, depends on dose, protein binding, route of administration (oral/IV)

DRUG EFFECTS

SYSTEM	EFFECT	ASSESSMENT BY HX	PE	TEST
CV	↓ HR ↓ CO ↓ LV function ↑ Coronary vascular resistance ↓ Myocardial O_2 consumption	Relief of angina ↓ BP ↓ HR	HR BP	
RESP	↑ Airway resistance (especially nonselective agents)	↑ Wheezing ↑ Bronchospasm		FEV_1 ↑ Peak airway pressure
ENDO	Hyperglycemia Hypokalemia			Laboratory measurements of K^+ and glucose
CNS	Fatigue, lethargy, peripheral paresthesia, withdrawal hypersensitivity			
FETUS	All cross placenta, fetal effect: bradycardia, hypotension, hypoglycemia			

Key Reference: Kharasch ED, Bowdle TA: Hypokalemia before induction of anesthesia and prevention by ß$_2$ adrenoceptor antagonism. Anes Analg 1991; 72:216–220.

PERIOPERATIVE IMPLICATIONS/POSSIBLE DRUG INTERACTION

Preoperative Concerns

- ß blocker should be continued in periop period
- Acute discontinuation can result in excess SNS activity that manifests in 24–48 h

Induction/Maintenance

- Myocardial depression observed with inhaled or injected anesthetic is worsened with addition of ß blocker
- Esolol has been assoc with profound bradycardia in presence of inhaled anesthetics

Adjuvants/Regional Anesthesia/Reversal

- Bradycardic effects often can be reversed by atropine
- Isoproterenol most effective at reversing negative cardiac (both dromotropic and inotropic) effects; but need to administer 1 dose of isoproterenol (2–25 µg/min^{-1}) to reverse negative cardiac effect
- CaCl$_2$ (250–1000 mg) or glucagon (1–5 mg) administered IV (adult) effectively reverses myocardial depression
- Life-threatening bradycardia may require insertion of transvenous pacemaker

SPECIAL PROBLEMS/CONSIDERATIONS

- When ß blockers are administered in presence of anesthetic drugs they may unmask direct negative inotropic effects of concomitantly administered anesthetic; this effect results in profound ↓ in BP, CO

BICARBONATE SODIUM

Randy H. Steadman, M.D.

INDICATIONS

- IV Rx for moderate to severe acidemia most commonly due to cardiac arrest, also to non-arrest-related lactic or ketoacidosis
- May be given orally in renal tubular acidosis
- To treat hyperkalemia

PERIOPERATIVE RISKS

- Administration results in rapid generation of CO_2, a potent negative inotrope; also intramyocardial acidosis worsened by CO_2 generated as it rapidly diffuses intracellularly.
- Ability to defibrillate VFib successfully correlates more with tissue PCO_2 than extracellular pH: thus the change in recommendations for restraint in use. Used only after more definitive and better substantiated Rx—defibrillation, chest compression, adequate ventilation, and drugs such as epinephrine, lidocaine

WORRY ABOUT

- Worsening intracellular acidosis
- CSF acidosis due to rapid diffusion of CO_2
- Hypernatremia, hyperosmolality associated with ↓ survival

OVERVIEW/PHARMACOLOGY

- During cardiopulmonary arrest, hypoxia-caused anaerobic metabolism results in lactic acidosis; ventilatory failure results in hypercarbic respiratory acidosis; prompt ventilation necessary for oxygenation, elimination of CO_2
- Acts as H^+ ion acceptor or base to buffer metabolic acidosis; after reacting with H^+ ion, carbonic acid and then ultimately CO_2, H_2O formed; CO_2 eliminated by lungs under conditions of normal ventilation and perfusion.
- During CPR (CO 25% of normal) results in accumulation of CO_2, which diffuses readily, causing intracellular hypercarbic acidosis

DRUG CLASS/MECH OF ACTION/USUAL DOSE

- Clinically the most widely used buffer
- Acutely used to correct moderate to severe metabolic acidosis of any cause:
  - to treat hyperkalemia
  - to treat tricyclic overdose
  - alkaline diuresis promotes excretion of phenobarbital and salicylate

- Chronically used orally to correct metabolic acidosis of any cause
- Usual dose: 0.5–1 mEq/kg
  - Alternatives: *Tham:* rapidly crosses cell membranes to work intracellularly (bicarbonate works predominantly extracellularly); however, its vasodilatory action reduces aortic and coronary perfusion pressures, which adversely affects outcome; *sodium carbonate:* works extracellularly; very alkaline pH may induce local tissue injury and cardiac dysrhythmias; *carbicarb* (Na bicarbonate plus Na carbonate): ↓ in coronary perfusion pressure due to vasodilator effect; *tribonate* (Na bicarbonate plus Tham plus phosphate plus acetate): may be more effective in treating intracellular acidosis but documentation of effectiveness in outcome during human CPR not available

DRUG EFFECTS

SYSTEM	EFFECT	TEST
CV	Although metabolic acidosis lowers threshold for VFib, *has no effect on the defibrillation threshold; no change in survival in cardiac arrest*	
RESP	CO_2 produced requires ↑ ventilation	ABG (PCO_2, pH, PO_2, HCO_3)
HEME	Alkalemia shifts oxyhemoglobin dissociation curve to the left with less O_2 release to tissue	ABG
GU	Alkaline diuresis aids in excretion of phenobarbital and salicylate after toxic ingestions	Urine pH >7
CNS	CSF acidosis possibly associated with post-CPR cerebral depression; hyperosmolar state may be associated with ↓ survival, intraventricular hemorrhage, alkalemia, ↑ CVR, ↓ CBF	

Key Reference: von Planta M, Bar-Joseph G, Witelund L, et al: Pathophysiologic and therapeutic implications of acid-base changes during CPR. Ann Emerg Med 1993; 22:404.

PERIOPERATIVE IMPLICATIONS/POSSIBLE DRUG INTERACTIONS

- In the presence of bicarbonate, Ca^{2+} salts precipitate as carbonates

Preoperative Concerns

- Bicarbonate shift of K^+ from extra- to intracellular (digoxin toxicity may be worsened)

Induction/Maintenance

- With alkalemia, basic drugs (opioids, local anesthetics) ↑ activity due to higher non-ionized fraction crossing membranes

Adjuvants/Regional Anesthesia/Reversal

- Metabolic alkalosis associated with difficulty antagonizing NMB
- Inhibitory effect of metabolic acidosis on catecholamines not documented at pH values encountered during cardiac arrest

SPECIAL CONSIDERATIONS

- Effective ventilation, oxygenation, and circulation during CPR are the primary means of prevention and treatment of acidemia associated with cardiac arrest. Bicarbonate does not change the defibrillation threshold or survival in cardiac arrest

BLEOMYCIN

Mark J. Lema, M.D., Ph.D.

RISK

- 10% incidence of interstitial pneumonitis
- 1% mortality from pulm fibrosis
- Pulm toxicity both dose-related (>250U total dose), age-related (> 65 y)
- Idiosyncratic reactions have occurred at lower doses (20U)
- Pts having previous radiation Rx to lungs or with a Hx of COPD are at ↑ risk
- Anaphylaxis known to occur idiosyncratically

PERIOPERATIVE RISKS

- Rapidly progressive interstitial pneumonitis known to occur after general anesthesia using O_2 concn > 30%, overhydrating pt
- Pts who received ≥ 250U or additional antineoplastic drugs are at ↑ risk of pulm toxicity

WORRY ABOUT

- Sustained O_2 concn > 30%
- Liberal use of maintenance fluids

OVERVIEW/PHARMACOLOGY

- 1U bleomycin = 1 mg activity of bleomycin
- $T_{1/2}\beta$ 2 h, but Cr <35 ml/min exponentially ↑ $T_{1/2}$; 70% is recovered in urine as active bleomycin
- For squamous cell carcinoma (head and neck, skin, genitals; lymphomas; testicular carcinomas)

DRUG CLASS/MECH OF ACTION

- Mixture of cytotoxic antibiotics isolated from *Streptomyces verticillus*
- Cytotoxic action caused by inhibition of DNA synthesis
- Usual dose: 0.25–0.5 U/kg (10–20 U/m²) to 400U (total dose)

DRUG EFFECTS

SYSTEM	EFFECT	ASSESSMENT BY HX	PE	TEST
CV	Raynaud's (rare)	Color changes in fingers	Observation	
RESP	Interstitial pneumonitis (10%) Pulmonary fibrosis (1%)	Dose (>250U), age (>65 y) Previous lung disease	Dyspnea, fine rales and cough, fever	PFTs (↓ TLC, ↓ VC)
GI	N/V			
HEME	(Not associated with pancytopenia)			
SKIN	Mucocutaneous toxicity (50%)	1–3 wks after start of Rx (dose 150–200U)	Urticaria, hyperpigmentation, hyperkeratosis, alopecia	

Key Reference: McEvoy GK (ed): Bethesda, MD, AHRS 95 Drug Information, pp 600–602.

PERIOPERATIVE IMPLICATIONS

Preoperative Period

- Assess bleomycin cumulative dose (> 250U)
- Assess age (>65 y)
- Assess previous lung disease Hx
- Ask about previous radiation to thorax
- Obtain PFTs, CXR, ABGs

Interoperative Period

- Limit delivered O_2 to < 30% if adequate for O_2 sat > 89%
- Limit fluids and avoid fluid overload
- Consider CVP or PA monitoring
- Consider arterial monitoring and sampling
- Use upper limit alarm for % O_2 delivery

Postoperative Period

- Keep delivered O_2 to < 30% if adequate for O_2 sat > 89%
- Limit fluids
- Corticosteroid use for pulm toxicity controversial

SPECIAL CONSIDERATIONS

- Cyclophosphamide, radiation Rx (thorax) potentiates pulmonary toxicity
- Cisplatin potentiates renal insufficiency
- Vinca alkaloids (vincristine, vinblastine, VP-16) potentiate Raynaud's phenomenon
- Mitomycin C exhibits similar properties to those of bleomycin but with milder effects

BRETYLIUM TOSYLATE

George S. Leisure, M.D.
Roger A. Johns, M.D.

INDICATIONS

- Rx for:
  - IV or IM admin in VFib or life-threatening VTach unresponsive to conventional antiarrhythmic Rx
  - May be useful in the treatment of ventricular tachyarrhythmias induced by accidental IV injection of bupivacaine

WORRY ABOUT

- Tricyclic antidepressants, guanethidine may interfere with bretylium's actions
- Electrophysiologic effects possibly antagonized by concomitant use of quinidine

OVERVIEW/PHARMACOLOGY

- Class III antiarrhythmic agent
- Cleared by renal excretion, found unchanged in urine
- $T_{1/2}$ of 6–10 h
- GFR 10-50 ml/min: reduce dose by 25-50%
- GFR < 10 ml/min; avoid bretylium
- Dialysis removes bretylium
- Negligible protein binding, 1–6%

DRUG CLASS/MECH OF ACTION/USUAL DOSE

- Class III antiarrhythmic agent with antiadrenergic, direct electrophysiologic actions
- Prolongs action potential duration without altering conduction velocity, upstroke, membrane responsiveness
- Seldom prolongs QT interval sufficiently to induce torsades de pointes
- Biphasic hemodynamic response: initial transient tachycardia, hypertension lasting 15 min, reflecting catecholamine release; HR, BP, vascular resistance fall
- ↓ The energy required to defibrillate heart; improves success rate for countershock
- Dose: IV bolus of 5–10 mg/kg, repeated 15–30 min later if needed to max 30 mg/kg; continuous infusion of 1–2 mg/min

DRUG EFFECTS

SYSTEM	EFFECT	ASSESSMENT BY HX	PE	TEST
HEENT	Congestion, parotitis			
CV	Initial transient ↑ BP, inevitable ↓ BP, rare bradycardia, rare proarrhythmia	Syncope, dizziness	Orthostasis	
GI	N/V, diarrhea			
ENDO	Hyperthermia			
GU	Renal dysfunction (rare)			↑ BUN, Cr
CNS	Confusion (rare), lethargy, anxiety			

Key Reference: Gallagher JD: Class III antiarrhythmic agents: Bretylium, sotalol, amiodarone. *In* Lynch C III (ed): Clinical Cardiac Electrophysiology. Philadelphia, JB Lippincott, 1994, p 113.

PERIOPERATIVE IMPLICATIONS/POSSIBLE DRUG INTERACTIONS

- Only used when defibrillation, epinephrine, lidocaine have failed to correct VFib, or defibrillation, lidocaine, procainamide have failed to control VTach associated with a pulse.
- Usually considered to be contraindicated in Rx of arrhythmias induced by cardiac glycosides
- Initial release of norepinephrine by bretylium may worsen these arrhythmias; some animal, human studies showed benefit in Rx for cardiac glycoside–induced ventricular arrhythmias

SPECIAL CONSIDERATIONS

- Admin with extreme caution to those with fixed cardiac output (severe pulm hypertension, aortic stenosis) since ↓ BP, PR may not be accompanied by ↑ in cardiac output
- Repeated IM injections at same site can lead to muscle atrophy, necrosis, fibrosis, vascular degeneration
- Orthostatic hypotension common
- Severe N/V can occur
- Hyperthermia: body T may reach 108°F within 30 min of admin

BUPIVACAINE

Laurence S. Reisner, M.D.

USES

- Provides surgical anesthesia with spinal, epidural, peripheral nerve blocks
- Obstetric analgesia/anesthesia
- Postop pain control, alone or with opioids

PERIOPERATIVE RISKS

- CNS toxicity
- CV toxicity

WORRY ABOUT

- Profound CV collapse

OVERVIEW/PHARMACOLOGY

- Long-duration local anesthetic
  - Spinal to 120 min
  - Epidural to 120 min
  - Peripheral 180+ min
- Peripheral nerve, epidural onset may be accelerated by addition of bicarbonate
- Excellent analgesia
- Moderate motor block
- Metabolized by glucuronidation in liver; metabolites eliminated by kidney
- Tachyphylaxis reported but infrequent
- Absorption and peak plasma concentration ↓ by adding epinephrine (5µg/ml)
- Highly protein bound (>90%)
- Allergy potential rare

DRUG CLASS/MECH OF ACTION/USUAL DOSE

- Local anesthetic with amide linkage
- Produces local anesthetic effect by reversible sodium channel blockade at an internal axonal receptor site and by a receptor-independent mechanism
- Maximum safe single dosage for epidural anesthesia is 2.5mg/kg (175mg/70kg) without epinephrine and 3.2mg/kg with epinephrine (225mg/70kg)
- Available as 0.25, 0.5, 0.75%* solutions for epidural, caudal, peripheral nerve block
- Useful epidural concentrations:
  - Obstetrics: 0.0625–0.5%
  - Surgery: 0.25–0.75%*
  - Pain management: 0.0625–0.25%
- Available as 0.75% in 8.25% dextrose solution for spinal anesthesia

  * Extreme caution is advised when using 0.75% solution; not recommended for obstetrics

DRUG EFFECTS (TOXICITY)

SYSTEM	EFFECT	ASSESSMENT BY HX	PE	TEST
CNS	Tinnitus	Ringing in ears; metallic taste; dizziness		
	Convulsions		Seizures	
	Unconsciousness			
CV	Negative inotropy		↓ BP	↓ Cardiac output
	Negative chronotropy		↓ HR	
	Vasodilation (late)			
	Ventricular arrhythmias		Irregular pulse	ECG
RESP	↑ PVR, PAP			↑ PAP, PCWP

Key Reference: Tucker GT, Mather LE: *In* Cousins MJ, Bridenbaugh PO (eds): Neural Blockade in Clinical Anaesthesia and Management of Pain, 2nd ed. Philadelphia, JB Lippincott, 1987, pp 47–110.

PERIOPERATIVE IMPLICATIONS

Preoperative Concerns

- Duration of planned procedure

Induction/Maintenance

- Always aspirate and use small intermittent doses and use a test dose. Most advocate the test dose be used with an intravascular marker in appropriately aged patients—such may not be reliable in pregnant patients in labor, and may have risks greater than benefits in the aged
- Adhere to recommended maximum doses
- Analgesia is excellent but requires 8–15 min for epidural and 5–10 min for spinal anesthesia to be attained

Adjuvants/Regional Anesthesia/Reversal

- Potentiates opioids for postop analgesia
- Longer recovery times for geriatric patients

SPECIAL CONSIDERATIONS

- This drug can produce a profound CV collapse and/or persistent ventricular arrhythmias, with rapid absorption or intravenous injection because it can penetrate sodium channels rapidly but exits slowly. Aggressive therapy with epinephrine and/or bretylium required to resuscitate

CAPSAICIN

Martin Hautkappe, M.D.

INDICATIONS

- People within USA: ?unknown
- Rx for: RA, OA, diabetic neuropathy, herpes zoster neuralgia, pruritus, psoriasis, cluster headache, trigeminal neuralgia, reflex sympathetic dystrophy syndrome, fibromyalgia, myofascial pain syndrome

PERIOPERATIVE RISKS

- Erythema

WORRY ABOUT

- Hepatotoxicity
- Irritation, burning sensation of skin, especially at beginning of Rx
- Contact with eyes, broken or irritated skin may cause painful irritation

OVERVIEW/PHARMACOLOGY

- Local anesthetic creme
- Interacts with xenobiotic metabolizing enzymes, particularly microsomal cytochrome P450–dependent mono-oxygenases (involved in activation, detoxification of various chemical carcinogens, mutagens)
- Hepatic cytochrome P450 2E1 catalyzes conversion of capsaicin to reactive species—e.g., phenoxy radical intermediate capable of covalently binding to active site of enzyme and tissue macromolecules

DRUG CLASS/MECH OF ACTION/USUAL DOSE

- Local anesthetic creme: a primary pungent, irritating agent present in red peppers believed to:
  - Exert pharmacologic actions by interacting at recognition site, depleting stores of substance P from sensory neurons
- Systemic and topical applications block C-fiber conduction and inactivate neuropeptide release from peripheral nerve endings
- Repetitive administration produces desensitization, inactivation of neurons caused by receptor-dependent block of Ca channels, subsequent accumulation of intracellular ions
- Causes localized antinociception, reduction of neurogenic inflammation
- Usual dose: adults, children 2 y and older: apply Zostrix (or Zostrix-HP) to affected area 3–4×/d; transient burning may occur on application; generally disappears in several d
- Application schedules of less than 3×/d may not provide optimum pain relief, burning sensation may persist

DRUG EFFECTS

SYSTEM	EFFECT
GI/LIVER	Increase of microsomal xenobiotic metabolizing enzyme activity
CNS	Good penetration to CNS after administration: amplification of pain relief

Key Reference: Surh YJ, Lee SS: Capsaicin, a double-edged sword: toxicity, metabolism and chemopreventive potential (review). Life Sci 1995; 56:1845–1855.

POSSIBLE DRUG INTERACTIONS

- ↓ Clearance of drugs using P450 2E1—e.g., phenothiazines, phenytoin, theophylline, oral contraceptives

SPECIAL CONSIDERATIONS

- Some recommend a combination of capsaicin with other local anesthetics for reduction of the initial burning pain
- Competitive antagonist: capsazepine
- Block of capsaicin-induced effects: ruthenium red (cationic dye) blocks capsaicin-activated ion channels

CARBAMAZEPINE

Leslie Newberg Milde, M.D.

USES

- Method of administration: oral
- At risk: in US 360,000–450,000
- Primary drug for all types of epilepsy except absence seizures; trigeminal or glossopharyngeal neuralgia

PERIOPERATIVE RISKS

- Acute intoxication: stupor, coma, hyperirritability, convulsions, respiratory depression
- Side effects from long-term use: drowsiness, vertigo, ataxia, diplopia, blurred vision
- Rare side effects: N/V; aplastic anemia, thrombocytopenia; hepatocellular and cholestatic jaundice; water retention with oliguria; hypertension, acute left ventricular failure; hypersensitivity reactions

WORRY ABOUT

- Induction of drug-metabolizing enzymes by chronic use ↓ the $T_{1/2}$ of carbamazepine and other drugs metabolized by P450 system

OVERVIEW/PHARMACOLOGY

- An iminostilbene, chemically related to tricyclic antidepressants
- Pharmacokinetics: limited aqueous solubility, induces drug-metabolizing enzymes; 50% metabolized in the liver to 10,11-epoxide, an active metabolite; further metabolized to inactive metabolites by conjugation and hydroxylation; renal excretion as a glucuronide; $T_{1/2}$ of 10–20 h, prolonged in patients who have received only 1 dose, shortened in patients receiving phenobarbital or phenytoin

DRUG CLASS/MECH OF ACTION/USUAL DOSE

- Antiepileptic
- Mechanism of action: differential inhibition of high-frequency discharges in and around epileptic foci with minimal disruption of normal neuronal firing
- Usual dose: 300–600 mg bid
- Alternatives: phenytoin, phenobarbital, valproate

DRUG EFFECTS

SYSTEM	EFFECT	ASSESSMENT BY HX	PE	TEST
CV	LV failure			ECHO
RESP	Respiratory depression			
GI/LIVER	Hepatic drug metabolism Hepatocellular jaundice Cholestatic jaundice			SGOT Bilirubin
ENDO	ADH	Water retention	Oliguria	
CNS	Seizure threshold drowsiness, vertigo, ataxia, diplopia, blurred vision, stupor, coma			Blood level

Key Reference: Schmutz M: Carbamazepine. *In* Fry HH, Janz D, eds: Antiepileptic Drugs. Handbook of Experimental Pharmacology, vol 74. Berlin, Springer-Verlag, 1985, pp 479–506.

PERIOPERATIVE IMPLICATIONS/POSSIBLE DRUG INTERACTIONS

- Shortened $T_{1/2}$ of carbamazepine in patients receiving phenobarbital, phenytoin, or valproate
- Increased dosage of anesthetic drugs (thiopental, etomidate, propofol), muscle relaxants (pancuronium, vecuronium, rocuronium) metabolized by the liver may be required
- ↓ Effect of haloperidol or droperidol

ANTICIPATED PROBLEMS/CONCERNS

- ↑ Water retention in elderly or patients with cardiac disease
- CNS depression with relative overdose

CHEMOTHERAPEUTIC AGENTS

Margaret G. Pratila, M.D.
Vasilios Pratilas, M.D.

Best available therapy for malignant diseases but requires complete destruction of cancer cells for cure. Combination therapy on an intermittent basis works well, but a level of toxicity far greater than with other drugs has to be accepted.

CATEGORIES

Alkylating Agents
- Busulfan (Myleran)
- Melphalan (Alkeran)
- Cyclophosphamide (Cytoxan)
- Chlorambucil (Leukeran)
- Ifosfamide
- Thiotepa
- Nitrogen mustard (HN_2)
- Altretamine (Hexalen)
- DTIC (dacarbazine)

Antimetabolites
- Methotrexate (MTX)
- 6-Mercaptopurine
- Thioguanine
- 5-Fluorouracil (5FU)
- Cytosine arabinoside (ara-C)
- Floxuridine (FUDR)

Plant Alkaloids
- Vincristine (Oncovin)
- Vinblastine (Velban)
- Paclitaxel (Taxol)
- Vindesine
- L-Asparaginase (enzyme)

Antibiotics
- Doxorubicin (Adriamycin)
- Daunorubicin
- Dactinomycin
- Bleomycin
- Mithramycin
- Mitomycin-C
- Idarubicin
- Actinomycin-D
- Mitoxantrone
- Streptozocin

Miscellaneous
- BCNU (carmustine)
- CCNU (lomustine)
- Procarbazine (Matulane)
- Carboplatinum
- *Cis*-platinum
- Hydroxyurea
- Teniposide (VM-26)
- Etoposide (VP-16)
- Mitotane

MODE OF ACTION

- Alkylation of nucleic acids; DNA cross-linking. Activation by microsomal liver enzymes (Cytoxan).

- Inhibit synthesis of DNA. Interact with specific enzymes to give unusable metabolites.

- Bind with microtubular proteins to cause arrest at metaphase stage.

- Inhibit DNA synthesis. Anthracyclines bind to nucleic acids and prevent their synthesis.

- Alkylation of DNA and RNA or inhibition of key enzymes for DNA synthesis.

USED TO TREAT

- Leukemia, CLL, CGL, AML, ALL
- Lymphoma
- Carcinoma — breast, ovary
- Melanoma
- Multiple myeloma
- Neuroblastoma
- Retinoblastoma
- Malignant pleural effusions (HN_2)

- Carcinoma — GI, pulmonary, breast, H&N, epidermoid
- Advanced NHL
- Sarcoma
- Leukemia — ALL
- Gestational chorio carcinoma
- Hydatidiform mole
- Osteogenic sarcoma (MTX and leucovorin)
- Hepatic metastases from GI cancer
- Primary hepatic cancer (FUDR)

- Acute leukemia
- Lymphoma
- Rhabdomyosarcoma
- Neuroblastoma
- Wilms' tumor
- Histiocytosis X
- Karposi's sarcoma

- Carcinoma — testicular, breast, lung, ovary, thyroid
- Squamous cell of H&N
- Streptozocin used to treat metastatic islet cell tumors of pancreas
- Reticulum cell sarcoma
- Lymphosarcoma

- Hodgkin's lymphoma (procarbazine, carboplatin)
- Carcinoma — testicular, ovary, bladder, H&N (cis-platinum)
- Brain tumors (BCNU) (VM-26)
- Multiple myeloma, lymphomas (CCNU)
- Melanoma
- CML
- Ovarian CA, H&N + radiation Rx (hydroxyurea) (DTIC)
- Adrenocortical CA (mitotane)

ADVERSE EFFECTS

- *Severe bone marrow depression,* anemia, agranulocytosis, and thrombocytopenia. *Pulmonary toxicity* with busulfan, chlorambucil, and melphalan. *Cardiac toxicity* with high-dose Cytoxan and busulfan; rapid destruction of tumor mass causes ↑ purine and pyrimidine breakdown products with resultant *uric acid nephropathy.* Cytoxan and ifosfamide cause *hemorrhagic cystitis, inappropriate water retention* (may result in hyponatremia, coma, and convulsions). *Secondary malignancies.*

- *Bone marrow suppression. Pulmonary infiltrates. Diarrhea, nausea, vomiting. Hemorrhagic enteritis. Acute and chronic hepatitis.* Renal tubular necrosis with MTX. *Acute cerebellar syndrome* with 5FU. *Leukoencephalopathy* with MTX following craniospinal R/T. *Neurotoxic* — (ara-C)

- *Bone marrow suppression* with vinblastine and Taxol *Neurotoxicity* with loss of deep tendon reflexes, peripheral paresthesia, and muscle wasting. Vincristine: *Severe bronchospasm. Hypo- or hypertension,* tachycardia (ventricular), AV block with Taxol. *Idiosyncratic reactions* may occur but may be due to Cremophor EL used as a diluent.
- Serious hypersensitivity reactions (L-asparaginase).

- *Acute cardiac toxicity,* not dose-related, with the anthracyclines. CHF, a ↓ in LVEF, ECG abnormalities, ventricular failure and sudden death. *Chronic cardiac toxicity,* biventricular failure (dose-related). Majority irreversible >550mg/m^2. Bleomycin, 10% *pulmonary toxicity* ↑ with dose and age. Serial estimation of DL_{CO} may give early warning. *Idiosyncratic:* hypotension, fever, wheezing. *Hyperkeratosis:* streptozocin, *renal toxicity, abnormal glucose tolerance test. Hypoinsulinism* due to selective destruction of β cells

- *Myelosuppression. Nephrotoxicity,* coagulation necrosis of distal renal tubules, collecting ducts. ↑ By use of aminoglycoside antibiotics. *Pulmonary toxicity:* BCNU and CCNU dose-related; late-onset pulmonary fibrosis (>15 yr) may occur. *Hepatotoxicity:* GI toxicity Promethazine: *hypotension, tachycardia, and syncope.* High-dose cis-platinum: *Occular toxicity. Neuropathies:* stocking/glove distribution of paresthesia, areflexia, loss of proprioceptive and vibratory senses.

Key Reference: Dorr RT, Von Hoff DD: Cancer Chemotherapy Handbook, 2nd ed. Norwalk, CT, Appleton & Lange, 1994.

ANESTHETIC IMPLICATIONS

- *Prolonged response to succinylcholine* due to cholinesterase inhibition (Cytoxan)
- Thiotepa — neuromuscular block due to pancuronium

- NSAIDs elevate MTX levels and ↑ toxicity
- ↑ Neuromuscular block with nondepolarizing muscle relaxants (6-mercaptopurine)

- Risk of elevated K^+ levels with vincristine due to muscle wasting; avoid or use care with succinylcholine
- Isolated cranial nerve paresis may occur, including laryngeal muscles

- Lung damage may occur in patients treated with bleomycin
- Maintain FIO_2 at 28% or less perioperatively if possible
- Careful fluid monitoring; colloid vs. crystalloid

- To minimize CNS depression and possible potentiation, use barbiturates, antihistamines, narcotics, hypotensive agents, and phenothiazines with caution in those on procarbazine. Procarbazine has MAO inhibitor activity; avoid meperidine and sympathomimetics.
- ↑ myelosuppression with BCNU with cimetidine

ADJUVANT AGENTS

IFN α-2a, -2b, recombinant
- Produce antitumor activity by antiproliferative effects when they bind to specific membrane receptors on the cell surface, together with a modulation of the host immune response; used in patients with hairy cell leukemia and AIDS-related Kaposi's sarcoma. Most important adverse reactions are those on CV system: hypotension, arrhythmias, tachycardias >150 bpm, and a transient reversible cardiomyopathy

Proleukin — human recombinant IL-2
- Actions are those of native IL-2 and include enhancement of lymphocyte mitogenesis and cytotoxicity; induction of killer cell activity and of interferon-γ production; used in the treatment of metastatic renal cell carcinoma and malignant melanoma. Adverse reactions include capillary leak syndrome with hypotension; hypoperfusion; edema and effusions; arrhythmias; cardiac ischemia/infarction; and pulmonary, hepatic, and renal insufficiency. Delayed reactions to contrast media may occur (1–4 h)

Tamoxifen (Nolvadex)
- Estrogen agonist-antagonist, binds to cytoplasmic receptors and affects nucleic acid function; used to treat breast and endometrial carcinomas. Adverse reactions are N/V, skin rashes, pruritus, rare myelosuppression

CHLORAMPHENICOL

H.F. Cascorbi, M.D., Ph.D.

USES

- Infections such as salmonellosis not treatable with other antibiotics

RISKS

- Bone marrow depression
- P450 inhibition

WORRY ABOUT

- Increased $T_{1/2}$ of dicumarol, warfarin sodium, chlorpropamide, phenytoin, tolbutamide, perhaps fentanyl

OVERVIEW/PHARMACOLOGY

- Inhibition of protein synthesis by interfering with the incorporation of amino acids into ribosomes
- Active against gram-positive and gram-negative bacteria, including *Salmonella typhi, Proteus,* rickettsiae; some large viruses (ornithosis, lymphopathia venereum) susceptible
- Decreases P450 activity, thus changing $T_{1/2}$ of P450-dependent drugs, such as dicumarol (see above)

DRUG CLASS/USUAL DOSE

- Antibiotic for otherwise intractable gram-negative infections, e.g., salmonellosis, influenza meningitis
- Usual dose: 12.5–25 mg/kg tid PO
  1 g IV q 6–8 h (10% solution)

DRUG EFFECTS

- Newborns who cannot glucuronide-conjugate chloramphenicol may develop abdominal distention, cyanosis, vascular collapse, sometimes lethal

DRUG EFFECTS

SYSTEM	EFFECT	TEST
GI	Nausea, vomiting	
HEME	Agranulocytosis, aplastic anemia	CBC

Key Reference: Goodman & Gilman's The Pharmacological Basis of Therapeutics, 8th ed. New York, Pergamon Press, 1990, pp 1125–1130.

PERIOPERATIVE CONCERNS/POSSIBLE DRUG INTERACTIONS

- Acute prolongation of action of dicumarol, chlorpropamide
- Action: assess clotting status
- Chronic use: assess status of bone marrow

SPECIAL CONSIDERATIONS

- Expect prolonged/increased action of drugs predominantly cleared via P450 biotransformation (perhaps fentanyl)

CIMETIDINE (SEE ALSO RANITIDINE)

Michael F. Roizen, M.D.

INDICATIONS/USES

- People in USA: >1,000,000 plus
- Rx for: ulcers, gastric reflux, gastric hypersecretion
- High levels associated with confusional states in elderly

PERIOPERATIVE RISKS

- Drug interactions esp with local anesthetics ($\uparrow$ toxicity), Aldomet, clonidine (CNS toxicity)

WORRY ABOUT

- Decreased hepatic P450 clearance of drugs, $\downarrow$ hepatic BF, $\uparrow$ fentanyl, phenothiazine, β rb drug, lidocaine, with $\uparrow$ potential for toxicity

OVERVIEW/PHARMACOLOGY

- H_2 antagonist
- Cleared by renal excretion; $\downarrow$ dosage intervals to 12 h with Cr clearance of 0–20 mL/min/1.73 m^2
- $\downarrow$ Hepatic metab of drugs requiring specific cytochrome P450 (β rb agents, Ca^{2+} channel blockers, theophylline, phenothiazines) or drugs requiring liver for 1st pass metab (by $\downarrow$ hepatic BF—lidocaine, β rb agents)

DRUG CLASS/MECH OF ACTION/USUAL DOSE

- H_2 antagonist
- Chronically taken for
  - ulcer Rx, prophylaxis
  - raise gastric pH for prophylaxis or Rx of gastric reflux
- Acutely taken for
  - prophylaxis against pulm aspiration
  - part of prophylaxis against immune or nonimmune CV effects from immune or nonimmune release of H_2
- Usual dose: 100–300 mg bid
- Alternatives:
  - other H_2 antagonists
  - antibiotics to $\downarrow$ *Heliocobacter pylori* (tetracycline + metronidazole + bismuth)

DRUG EFFECTS

SYSTEM	EFFECT	PE	TEST
LIVER	$\downarrow$ Hepatic drug metab $\downarrow$ Hepatic BF		
GI	$\downarrow$ gastric acid secretion		
ENDO	Weak antiandrogenic effect; gynecomastia (men)		
GU	Renal Placenta—crosses placental barrier, excreted in milk	Gynecomastia	BUN, Cr
CNS	Poor penetration to CNS; with high doses in pts, esp with impaired renal function, assoc with disorientation to coma	CNS exam	

Key Reference: Lam AM, Parkin JA: Cimetidine and prolonged post-operative somnolence. Can J Anaesth 1981; 28:450.

PERIOPERATIVE IMPLICATIONS/POSSIBLE DRUG INTERACTIONS

Preoperative Concerns

- Cimetidine + clonidine or Aldomet assoc with CNS dysfunction
- $\downarrow$ Clearance of phenothiazines, phenytoin, theophylline

Induction/Maintenance

- Fentanyl $T\frac{1}{2}$ may be prolonged 2° to direct or indirect $\downarrow$ in hepatic BF by cimetidine

Adjuvants/Regional Anesthesia/Reversal

- $\uparrow$ Biologic availability of lidocaine and other local anesthetics and thus toxicity
- $\uparrow$ NMB agent requirements anecdotally reported (mechanism unknown)

SPECIAL CONSIDERATIONS

- $\downarrow$ Hepatic P450 clearance of drugs, $\downarrow$ hepatic BF $\uparrow$ fentanyl, phenothiazine, β rb drug, lidocaine potential for toxicity
- CNS dysfunction by itself (esp in aged and those with $\downarrow$ renal function) or with clonidine and Aldomet

CIS-ATRACURIUM
(NIMBEX [51W89]; CIS-ATRACURIUM BESYLATE)

John J. Savanese, M.D.

RISK

- No change in the clinical response during hepatic or renal failure
- No drugs known to affect the rate of Hoffmann's reaction chemical breakdown
- Speed of Hoffmann's reaction ↓ by acidosis, hypothermia

WORRY ABOUT

- Side effects appear minimal: histamine release does not occur

OVERVIEW/PHARMACOLOGY

- Nondepolarizing NM blocker drug of benzylisoquinolinium class
- Intermediate duration of effect due to chemical degradation in plasma at alkaline pH, *Hoffmann's elimination* reaction.
- Major metabolite is laudanosine, a CNS stimulant; plasma laudanosine levels are well below any threshold for CNS activity in usual clinical practice
- ED_{95} 50 µg/kg
- $T_{1/2}\beta$ = 20–25 min
- Clinical duration of action = 45 min; complete recovery 60–90 min following intubating dose
- Intubating dose may be ↑ to 0.3–0.4 mg/kg (6–$8 \times ED_{95}$) to facilitate faster intubation (60–90 sec)

DRUG CLASS/MECH OF ACTION/USUAL DOSE

- Nondepolarizing NM blocker of intermediate duration, benzylisoquinolinium class
- Not given chronically
- Acutely administered IV for surgical relaxation (tracheal intubation, maintenance of abd relaxation, correction of joint dislocation)
- May be given for maintenance of paralysis in ICU
- Usual dose:
  - tracheal intubation (adults): 150–200 µg/kg
  - "priming" dose (adults): 10 µg/kg
  - tracheal intubation (children): 200 µg/kg
  - maintenance of relaxation: 20–30 µg/kg every 15–20 min or by continuous infusion: 1–2 µg/kg/min
- Alternatives: mivacurium, vecuronium, rocuronium, atracurium, pancuronium, curare
- Antagonists: neostigmine, edrophonium

DRUG EFFECTS

SYSTEM	EFFECT
CV	Minimal effect
GI/LIVER	Metabolite (laudanosine) undergoes some liver excretion
GU	Metabolite (laudanosine) excreted in urine
CNS	Laudanosine levels 1/5 to 1/10 those noted after atracurium

Key Reference: Belmont MR, Lien CA, Quessey S, et al: The clinical neuromuscular pharmacology of 51W89 in patients receiving nitrous oxide/opioid/barbiturate anesthesia. Anesthesiology 1995; 82:1139–1145.

POSSIBLE DRUG INTERACTIONS

Preoperative Concerns

- Antibiotics may potentiate the NMB effect
- Lowered temperature or acidic pH will slow the Hoffmann reaction

Induction/Maintenance

- "Priming" doses of 10 µg/kg may accelerate onset of blockade by 30 sec
- Intubation may be carried out at 120, 90, or 60 sec following 150, 200, or 400 µg/kg
- Maintenance doses of 20–30 µg/kg may be given every 15–20 min
- Continuous infusion possible at rates of 1–2 µg/kg/min

Adjuvants/Regional Anesthesia/Reversal

- Longer duration in conditions of acidosis or ↓ body T
- Large doses may be injected rapidly, since there is no histamine release
- "Mycin" antibiotics potentiate action

SPECIAL CONSIDERATIONS

- Longer duration in conditions of acidosis or ↓ body T

CISPLATIN

Joseph F. Foss, M.D.

USES (see also Chemotherapeutic Agents)

• Patients undergoing chemoRx for testicular, ovarian, or bladder cancer

PERIOPERATIVE RISKS

• End-organ damage, especially renal

WORRY ABOUT

• ↓ Clearance of renally excreted drugs if previous damage
• Avoid aminoglycosides (increased toxicity)

OVERVIEW/PHARMACOLOGY

• Inorganic platinum-containing compound (*cis*-diaminedichloroplatinum [*cis*-DDP])
• Renal toxicity prominent, seen in 28–36% of patients after 1 dose: effect cumulative, minimized by aggressive hydration, allowing renal function to return to baseline between treatments.

• Decrease in renal tubular function is dose-related, typically occurs during 2nd wk of administration
• Hyperuricemia, hypomagnesemia, hypocalcemia, hyponatremia, hypokalemia, hypophosphatemia have been reported and are related to renal tubular damage. Allopurinol Rx reduces uric acid levels
• Reaches site of action by diffusion
• High concentrations in kidneys, liver, prostate, intestines, testes; low CNS penetration
• $T_{1/2}$ 20–30 min following bolus administration or infusion of 50 or 100 mg/m²; clearance is 15–16 L/h/m²; vol of distribution, 11–12 L/m²
• Highly protein-bound, poorly dialyzable
• Cleared renally at rate greater than that of Cr; 13–17% of parent compound excreted within 1 h after administration

DRUG CLASS/MECH OF ACTION/USUAL DOSE

• Disrupts DNA helix, preventing duplication
• In chemoRx of metastatic ovarian and testicular CA and advanced bladder CA, often used in combination with other drugs, particularly cyclophosphamide (Cytoxan)
• Contraindicated (relatively) in patients with pre-existing renal disease, hearing loss, myelosuppression; use of other nephrotoxic or ototoxic agents (e.g., aminoglycosides) may increase toxicity
• Must be administered intravenously (see the current oncology literature for dosage, administration guidelines, and protocols. Has been used in doses of 20 mg/m² for 5 d for testicular cancer, 75–100 mg/m² once every 4 wk for ovarian tumors in combination with other agents, 50–70 mg/m² for advanced bladder CA)
• Pretreatment hydration of 1–2 L over 12 h before administration and infusion of *cis*-DDP in a dilute vol with mannitol recommended. Repeat courses usually not given until renal function returns to baseline, circulating blood elements are at acceptable levels, and audiometric and hepatic function monitoring have been completed

DRUG EFFECTS

SYSTEM	EFFECT	ASSESSMENT OF HX	PE	TEST
HEENT	Ototoxicity (31% of patients) manifested as tinnitus or loss of hearing more pronounced in children	Total exposure		Audiometry
CV	Anaphylactic-like reactions with edema, bronchospasm reported; Cardiac dysrhythmias reported	SOB after administration, palpitations	CV exam	ECG
LIVER	Transient elevations in liver enzymes reported with use of *cis*-DDP			Hepatic transaminases
GI	N/V severe, triggered by action at chemoreceptor trigger zone of medulla	N/V within 1–4 h up to 24 h		
HEME	Mild–moderate myelosuppression (25–30%)			CBC
GU	Renal toxicity			BUN, Cr, electrolytes, Mg^{2+}
CNS	Seizures with high acute doses			
MS	Peripheral neuropathies in a stocking-glove distribution with prolonged Rx of 4–7 mo	Total exposure	Neuro exam	Pinprick vibration

Key Reference: Mangioni C, Bolis G, Pecorelli S, et al: Randomized trial in advanced ovarian cancer comparing cisplatin and carboplatin. J Natl Cancer Inst 1989; 81:1464–1471.

POSSIBLE DRUG INTERACTIONS

Adjuvants/Regional Anesthesia/Reversal

• Plasma levels of anticonvulsants may become subtherapeutic with the use of cisplatin

SPECIAL CONSIDERATIONS

• Should not be administered through needles or IV sets containing aluminum, which reacts with cisplatin, causing precipitation
• *Cis*-DDP and equipment used for administration should be handled as potentially carcinogenic
• May be irritating to the skin; if extravasated may cause local soft tissue toxicity

COCAINE

Zeev N. Kain, M.D.

RISK

- Prevalence: 5 million regular users; 30 million in USA have tried drug
- Abuse in the OB population 7.5 to 45%

PERIOPERATIVE RISKS

- Hemodynamic instability, ↑ sympathetic discharge
- Myocardial ischemia, MI

WORRY ABOUT

- CV: Hypertension, tachycardia, dysrhythmias, MI
- Neurologic: Intracerebral bleed, seizures
- Pulmonary: Pneumomediastinum, cocaine-induced asthma, hypersensitivity pneumonitis, chronic cough, pulmonary edema, diffusing capacity abnormalities
- OB: Placenta previa, abruptio placentae, premature labor, fetal distress

OVERVIEW/PHARMACOLOGY

- Cocaine is an ester local anesthetic that prevents rapid ↑ in cell membrane permeability to Na^+ during depolarization; blocks propagation of action potential
- Interferes with presynaptic catecholamine uptake and results in activation of SNS
- May produce neg inotropic, chronotropic effects on heart muscle
- Impairs reuptake in brain of dopamine, serotonin, tryptophan
- Accumulation of dopamine in synaptic cleft may lead to acute euphoria, increased alertness

ICD-9-CM Codes: 305.6 (nondependent); 364.2 (dependent)

ETIOLOGY

- Cocaine abuse
- OD during HEENT surgery; ER use (part of tetracaine, epinephrine, cocaine mix)

USUAL TREATMENT

- Supportive
- β-blocking agents formerly used as Rx for β-adrenergic cardiac effects of cocaine; these may worsen coronary vasoconstriction; use with caution if patient has Hx of ischemia
- Nitroglycerin to reverse hypertension, coronary vasoconstriction
- Ca channel antagonists to protect from cardiac depressant effects, restore cardiac rate, rhythm while increasing coronary BF

DRUG EFFECTS

SYSTEM	EFFECT	ASSESSMENT BY HX	PE	TEST
CV	Hypertension, MI, dysrhythmias, myocarditis	Exposure		BP/HR ECG
RESP	Pneumomediastinum, asthma, chronic cough, pulmonary edema		Wheezing	CXR
HEME	Thrombocytopenia	Bleeding problems		Plt
GU	Preterm labor Premature rupture of membranes Abruptio placentae Spontaneous abortion Meconium-stained amniotic fluid	Uterine contractions		US
CNS	Subarachnoid hemorrhage Intracerebral bleed Seizures	Headache	Neuro exam	

Key Reference: Kain ZN, Rimar S, Barash PG: Cocaine abuse in the parturient and effects on the fetus and neonate. Anesth Analg 1993; 77:835–845.

PERIOPERATIVE IMPLICATIONS

Preoperative Concerns

- Self-reporting of drug abuse unreliable, 35–55% deny cocaine use but have at least 1 pos urine assay
- Hx of smoking, alcohol use, pos syphilis serology, and use of other illicit drugs should alert anesthesiologist to possibility of cocaine abuse
- Chronic sinusitis, ulceration of nasal mucosa may suggest cocaine use; sclerosis of PVs, needle marks from IV injection possibly seen. Recent injection sites have characteristic look of multiple ecchymoses
- Consider urine screen (reliable for only 14–60 h after use)

Monitoring

- Routine
- Consider arterial line if Hx of acute intoxication, recent exposure

Airway

- None

Preinduction/Induction

- Control hemodynamics before induction
- ↑ Anesthetic requirements possibly from acute cocaine exposure
- Usage of succinylcholine in acutely intoxicated patient may be assoc with prolonged paralysis
- Use ketamine with caution; it potentiates CV toxicity of cocaine
- Spinal anesthesia possibly assoc with more frequent episodes of hypotension

Maintenance

- Myocardial ischemia may manifest as CV instability, ECG changes
- ↑ Catecholamine levels due to inadequate anesthesia, cocaine in blood may result in cardiac dysrhythmias during halothane administration

- T rise, sympathomimetic effects assoc with cocaine can mimic malignant hyperthermia

Extubation

- None

Adjuvants

- Ester local anesthetics, which undergo metabolism by plasma ChE, may compete with cocaine, resulting in ↓ metabolism of both drugs
- Cocaine ↓ seizure threshold, enhances convulsant effect of other local anesthetics

Postoperative Period

- Myocardial ischemia possible in postop period
- Pain medication requirements in chronic abusers are same as for nonabusers

CROMOLYN SODIUM

Shubjeet Kaur, M.D.

USES

- First prophylactic nonsteroidal drug available for treatment of chronic asthma
- Not effective in acute episodes of bronchospasm
- May be beneficial in allergic rhinitis and atopic diseases of eye
- Adverse effects infrequent; include
  - Direct irritant reactions: e.g., wheezing, coughing
  - Dizziness, nausea, rash
  - Rarely anaphylaxis

OVERVIEW/PHARMACOLOGY

- Inhibits antigen-induced degranulation of pulmonary mast cells
- Prevents release of histamine, other autacoids
- Ineffective when administered orally (only 1% absorbed systemically)
- Administered by inhalation route (nebulizer or special turbo inhaler)
- 10% of inhaled dose absorbed systemically; $T_{1/2} = 80$ min
- Absorbed portion excreted unchanged in urine (50%), bile (50%)

DRUG CLASS/MECHANISM OF ACTION

- Cromolyn sodium (disodium cromoglycate) is a derivative of 2–chromone–carboxylic acid
- Mechanism of action poorly defined; one proposed explanation is ↓ in accumulation of intracellular Ca^{2+} in sensitized mast cells
- Used primarily in the prophylactic treatment of bronchial asthma
- Effective in preventing degranulation of mast cells only if given prior to antigenic challenge
- Beneficial effects may take several wks or even months to become evident
- Can be taken prophylactically shortly before exercise or exposure to known allergen to prevent bronchospasm

USUAL DOSE

- Available as cromolyn sodium for inhalation (Intal) to be inhaled qid using a special turbo inhaler
- Available as 4% liquid nasal spray (Nasalcrom), 1 spray each nostril 3–6 times/d for treatment of allergic rhinitis
- Opticrom (4% ophthalmic solution) for treating atopic eye conditions (1–2 drops each eye 4–6 times/d)

DRUG EFFECTS

SYSTEM	EFFECT	ASSESSMENT BY HX	TEST
RESP	Inhibition of pulmonary mast cell degranulation; ↓ release of histamine and autacoids	↓ Episodes of exercise- or antigen-induced bronchospasm after chronic use of drug over 2–3 mo	↓ Bronchial hyperactivity as measured by histamine or methacholine challenge

Key Reference: Gilman AG, Rall TW, Nies AS, Taylor P (eds): Goodman and Gilman's The Pharmacological Basis of Therapeutics, 8th ed. New York, Macmillan, 1990, pp 630–635.

PERIOPERATIVE IMPLICATIONS/POSSIBLE DRUG INTERACTIONS

- Continue administration preoperatively
- Cromolyn sodium is of no benefit in treating an acute perioperative exacerbation of asthma
- Rare possibility of potential serious side effects, including laryngeal edema, angioedema, urticaria, anaphylaxis

DIGITALIS

Robert G. Merin, M.D.

USES

- Dosing: oral, IV—digoxin most common drug
- Indications: CHF, AFib/flutter
- Ambulatory side effects: cardiac arrhythmia, CNS disturbances

PERIOPERATIVE RISKS

- Cardiac arrhythmia (especially associated with hypokalemia); A-V block (especially associated with administration of β-adrenergic and Ca channel–blocking drugs)

WORRY ABOUT

- Hypokalemia, renal insufficiency (producing ↓ digoxin excretion and need for dose alteration)

OVERVIEW/PHARMACOLOGY

- General pharmacologic effect: positive inotropic, anticholinergic, antiarrhythmic

Dosing/Pharmacokinetics

Drug		Onset	Peak	T½	Dose Initial	Dose Maintenance
Digoxin:	IV	5–30 min	1–3 h	34 h	0.5–1.0 mg	0.25 mg qd
	Oral	1–3 h	4–6 h	34 h	0.75–1.2 mg	0.125–0.5 mg qd
Digitoxin, oral		3–6 h	6–12 h	7 d	0.8–1.2 mg	0.05–0.3 mg qd

Excretion

- Digoxin: renal, mostly unchanged; ↓ dose for ↑ Cr
- Digitoxin: hepatic degradation

Drug Interactions

- Quinidine: ↓ excretion, ↑ serum levels
- Diuretics: ↓ serum K^+, ↑ toxicity

DRUG CLASS/MECHANISM OF ACTION

- Mechanism of action: positive inotropic effect; from inhibition of Na^+, K^+-ATPase, producing ↑ intracellular Ca^{2+} concentration, leading to ↑ cardiac contractility
- Chronotropic and antiarrhythmic effect: ↑ vagal activity; ↑ SA, A-V nodal response to acetylcholine; inhibits afferent baroreceptor traffic, ↓ A-V conduction

DRUG EFFECTS

SYSTEM	EFFECT	ASSESSMENT BY HX	PE	TEST
HEENT			↓ JVD	
CV	↓ HR, ↑ CO Arrhythmia from toxicity	↓ SOB, orthopnea Palpitations	↓ Heart rate, size Irregular pulse	CXR: ↓ heart size ECG: any arrhythmia except AF
RESP	↓ Congestion	↓ SOB, orthopnea	↓ Rales	CXR: ↓ pulmonary edema
GI	Anorexia from toxicity			Serum digoxin >2 ng/ml
CNS	Headache, confusion from toxicity			Serum digoxin >2 ng/ml
MS	Fatigue from toxicity			Serum digoxin >2 ng/ml

Key Reference: Hoffman, BF, Bigger JT: Digitalis and the allied glycosides. *In* Gilman AG, Rall TW, Nies AS, Taylor P (eds): Goodman & Gilman's The Pharmacological Basis of Therapeutics, 8th ed. New York, Pergamon, 1990, pp 814–839.

PERIOPERATIVE IMPLICATIONS

Preoperative Concerns

- Do not discontinue digitalis preoperatively.
- Correct and maintain serum K^+.
- ↓ Dose with ↑ serum Cr.

Possible Drug Interactions

- ↑ A-V block with β adrenergic and Ca channel–blocking drugs
- ↓ Dose with concurrent quinidine therapy

ANTICIPATED PROBLEMS/CONCERNS

- Ventricular rate with AFib/flutter is a rough bioassay for digoxin level; fast ventricular rate with AFib indicates inadequate serum level of digoxin.
- Digoxin is the only positive inotropic, antiarrhythmic (for AFib/flutter) drug available; drug of choice for this arrhythmia in patient with a failing heart
- Digoxin may depress CNS function in elderly more than it decreases AV nodal conduction.

492   DRUGS

DIMETHYLTUBOCURARINE
(d-TUBOCURARINE, dTc)

Richard S. Matteo, M.D.

USES

- Used to achieve muscle relaxation during surgery and, rarely, in the ICU to facilitate mechanical ventilation
- Depresses muscle strength and requires that ventilation be assisted, usually by an endotracheal tube
- Defasciculating agent prior to depolarizing neuromuscular blocking agent

PERIOPERATIVE RISKS

- Risk of developing hypotension

WORRY ABOUT

- Severe hypotension related to increasing doses of dTc
- Prolonged muscle weakness—can be avoided by careful monitoring of muscle strength and full understanding of physiologic, pathologic states and drug interaction that can intensify the actions of dTc

OVERVIEW/PHARMACOLOGY

- Used for muscle relaxation during surgical procedures, more rarely for endotracheal intubation
- Eliminated unchanged, primarily by kidneys
- Liver accounts for 10–12% of total elimination of the drug
- In adults plasma clearance is 1.64–1.86 (ml/kg/min), volume of distribution is 0.375–0.470 (L/kg), elimination $T_{1/2}$ is 164–190 (min)
- Prolonged 100% or more in renal failure
- Duration of action is directly related to dose, although normal patients exhibit considerable variation in response; after single IV dose of 0.3 mg/kg, dTc can usually be reversed within 45 min

DRUG CLASS/MECH OF ACTION/USUAL DOSE

- Long-acting, nondepolarizing muscle relaxant
- Naturally occurring alkaloid with both quaternary and tertiary nitrogen groups
- Acts primarily at neuromuscular junction in competition with ACh for ACh receptor
- Usual intravenous dose: for intubation, 0.6–0.7 mg/kg; for maintenance, 0.05–0.15 mg/kg
- Over time, maintenance dose should be reduced because of cumulative effect

DRUG EFFECTS

SYSTEM	EFFECT	TEST
CNS	Muscle weakness→ paralysis	Nerve stimulator to assess degree of paralysis and adequacy of reversal

Key Reference: Katz R (ed): Muscle Relaxants, Basic and Clinical Aspects. Orlando, FL, Grune & Stratton, 1985.

PERIOPERATIVE IMPLICATIONS

Preoperative Concerns

- Age may increase sensitivity to dTc (elderly and neonates) secondary to decreased urinary function
- Patients with myasthenia gravis and myasthenic (Eaton-Lambert) syndrome are exquisitely sensitive to dTc
- Patients with Duchenne's muscular dystrophy require less dTc
- Resistance to dTc (and other nondepolarizing relaxants) seen in burns, spinal cord deinnervation (trauma), paresis, muscle wasting, limb immobilization, and in patients receiving chronic anticonvulsant therapy

Induction/Maintenance

- Hypotension secondary to histamine release and/or ganglionic blockade can routinely be expected if dTc is used for intubation; Rx with IV vasopressor
- Augmented by general anesthesia in increasing orders of magnitude: nitrous oxide-narcotic < halothane < enflurane < isoflurane, desflurane
- Synergistic augmentation by steroidal-base nondepolarizing muscle relaxant: ¼ dose dTc + ¼ dose steroidal nondepolarizer gives effect of total dose of either relaxant
- Drugs known to interact and augment effect of dTc and cause *clinical* symptoms
  - antibiotics (aminoglycosides, polypeptides, and more rarely, tetracyclines)
  - furosemide
  - magnesium sulfate
- True allergic response rare

Reversal

- Anticholinesterase employed: neostigmine (2.5–5.0 mg/70 kg) or pyridostigmine (10–20 mg/70 kg) accompanied by either atropine (1.0 mg/70 kg) or glycopyrrolate (0.7 mg/70 kg)
- Need at least three twitches of train-of-four stimulation present to be sure of adequate reversal
- Edrophonium not recommended for reversal of dTc or other long-acting nondepolarizers

ANTICIPATED PROBLEMS/CONCERNS

- If there is prolonged weakness (for any number of reasons) that cannot be adequately reversed, ventilatory support must be continued in the PACU or ICU until adequate muscle strength returns

DIURETICS

Nikolaus Gravenstein, M.D.

INDICATIONS

- Prescribed for patients with hypertension, CHF, elevated ICP, edema, hemoglobinuria

PERIOPERATIVE RISKS

- Hypokalemia
- Hypovolemia, hypotension
- Hyperkalemia with aldosterone antagonists

WORRY ABOUT

- Hypokalemia, hypovolemia
- Hypokalemia provoking/ aggravating digitalis toxicity
- Cross-sensitivity: furosemide, sulfonamides
- Deafness with ECA
- Nephrotoxicity of cephaloridine is enhanced by furosemide

- End result of diuretic use is ↑ UO with net loss of H_2O, solute
- Onset of diuresis within 10 min after IV administration
- With exception of aldosterone antagonist, K^+-sparing diuretics, all others cause K^+ loss
- Mannitol may function as renal preservative by free-radical scavenging, toxin dilution mechanisms
- Serum K^+ <3.5 mEq/L in 15% of patients, <3.0 mEq/L in 10% of diuretic-treated patients
- Chronic diuretic-induced hypokalemia less arrhythmogenic than acute, but serum K^+ <3.0 mEq/L associated with 2-fold greater incidence of ventricular arrhythmias than K^+ > 3.0 mEq/L
- Site-specific action associated with additional effect if diuretics from 2 classes used

DRUG CLASS/MECH OF ACTION/USUAL DOSE

- Diuretics belong to osmotic, carbonic anhydrase inhibition, benzothiadiazide, high-ceiling (loop), K^+-sparing, or aldosterone antagonist, class of drugs, based on mechanism of action
- Only osmotic and loop diuretics used intraoperatively
- Osmotic diuretic: mannitol—ascending loop, limits H_2O reabsorption; onset of action 5–15 min after IV dose—renal clearance
  - usual dose: mannitol 0.25–2.0 g/kg
- Loop diuretics—ascending loop, limit NaCl reabsorption; onset of action 5 min after IV dose; $T_{1/2}$ 1–2 h; duration of action, 3–6 h to renal clearance
  - usual dose: furosemide: 5–40 mg (0.1–1.0 mg/kg); ethacrynic acid: 50 mg (0.5–1.0 mg/kg); bumetanide: 0.5–1.0 mg q 2–3 h; max 10 mg/d

DRUG EFFECTS

SYSTEM	EFFECT
HEENT	Transient (<24 h) deafness or vertigo may follow IV rapid bolus ethacrynic acid; less common after furosemide or bumetanide; rarely permanent Furosemide administration rate <4 mg/min advised
CV	Transient ↑ in venous capacitance with IV loop diuretic administration Acute transient ↑ in intravascular vol precedes diuresis with mannitol
GI	Diarrhea may follow ethacrynic acid use
ENDO	Hypokalemia, metabolic alkalosis
GU	Diuresis
CNS	Mannitol ↓ ICP

Key References: Edwards R, Winnie AP, Ramamurphy S: Acute hypocapneic hypokalemia: An iatrogenic complication. Anesth Analg 1977; 56:786–792; Siegel Q, Hulley SB, Black DM, et al: Diuretics, serum & intracellular electrolyte levels, and ventricular arrhythmias in men. JAMA 1992; 267:1083–1089.

PERIOPERATIVE IMPLICATIONS/POSSIBLE DRUG INTERACTIONS

Preoperative Concerns

- In chronic hypertensive patients treated with diuretics a significant intravascular volume contraction may exist, which renders them more prone to hypotension following induction of anesthesia.
- Enhanced digitalis toxicity from hypokalemia
- Enhanced oto- and nephrotoxicity of loop diuretics is associated with rapid administration of large intravenous doses and concurrent use of another nephro/ototoxic drug, e.g., aminoglycoside antibiotic, another loop diuretic, and some cephalosporins, e.g., cephaloridine
- Probably best to continue chronic dose through the perioperative period, including day of surgery. (UO will decline if diuretic not given on day of surgery.)

Induction/Maintenance

- Intraoperative loop diuretic use may significantly decrease serum K^+ level following a brisk diuresis

Adjuvants

- Enhancement of renal clearance of other drugs, e.g., neuromuscular blocking agents, provoked by diuresis is not clinically problematic

SPECIAL CONSIDERATIONS

- Patients receiving diuretics preoperatively should be considered volume contracted until proven otherwise
- Hypokalemia associated with diuresis will be aggravated by hyperventilation, which imposes an additional 0.5 mEq/L decrease in serum K^+ for each 10 mmHg decrease in $PaCO_2$

DOBUTAMINE

Anil Aggarwal, M.D.
David C. Warltier, M.D., Ph.D.

INDICATIONS

- Prescribed for patients with low cardiac output (CO) 2° to decreased right or left ventricular function associated with CHF, MI, or cardiac surgery
- Used for treatment of pulmonary hypertension with right ventricular dysfunction
- Provocative test for diagnosis of coronary artery disease (e.g., dobutamine stress-echocardiography)
- Administered as an intravenous infusion

PERIOPERATIVE RISKS

- Risk of tachyarrhythmias

WORRY ABOUT

- Tachycardia, especially at high doses
- Ventricular ectopy
- Rarely, hypotension or HTN may be observed
- Hypokalemia may occur

OVERVIEW/PHARMACOLOGY

- Inotrope used for increasing CO simultaneous with a decrease in systemic and pulmonary vascular resistance
- Thought to have relatively greater inotropic than chronotropic actions
- β_1-agonist with lesser effect at β_2-receptors and minimal effects at α-receptors
- Increases intracellular Ca^{2+} by elevating cAMP through effects on β_1-receptors
- Increases SA-node automaticity and AV-nodal and intraventricular conduction
- May cause systemic and pulmonary vasodilation through β_2-receptor stimulation
- Quick onset (within 2 minutes) and short duration (approximately 2–6 min)

DRUG CLASS/MECH OF ACTION/USUAL DOSE

- Synthetic catecholamine
- β-adrenergic action increases adenylate cyclase activity
- Increases CO by increasing SV and HR and decreasing SVR
- Usual dosage:
  1–10 µg/kg/min IV
- Combined use with other agents increases cardiac output via different mechanisms (e.g., milrinone, sodium nitroprusside)

DRUG EFFECTS

SYSTEM	EFFECT	ASSESSMENT BY HX	PE	TEST
CV	↑ Systolic BP ↑ CO ↓ PVR ↓ SVR	Relief of dyspnea	Capillary perfusion, JVD, UO, rales	Mixed venous O_2 saturation, CO, PVR, SVR data

Key Reference: Hoffman B. *In* Katzung BG (ed): Basic and Clinical Pharmacology, 6th ed. Norwalk, CT, Appleton & Lange, 1994, pp 124–131.

PERIOPERATIVE IMPLICATIONS/DRUG INTERACTIONS

Preoperative Concerns

- Assess systemic perfusion
- Monitor BP, CO, PCWP
- PA catheter essential for adequate drug titration

Induction/Maintenance

- Despite adequate CO and BP before induction, there may be a decrease in these values during induction of anesthesia
- Therapy should be guided by measures of adequacy of systemic perfusion such as CO, mixed venous O_2 saturation, and ABG tensions

Adjuvant/Regional Anesthesia/Reversal

- Combining therapy with inotropes that are not β_1-agonists such as milrinone may provide greater than additive effects
- Improvement in cardiac output may also be achieved by adding sodium nitroprusside if SVR is high
- Excessive effect can be reversed with β-adrenergic antagonists such as esmolol
- Consider using digoxin prior to dobutamine in patients with AFib and rapid ventricular response
- May be ineffective or larger doses required in patients receiving β-blockers

Postoperative Period

- Duration of treatment determined by assessment of cardiac function with PA catheter

ANTICIPATED PROBLEMS/CONCERNS

- Sinus tachycardia may occur at higher doses in patients with AFib, the ventricular rate may increase 2° to enhanced AV conduction
- Pulmonary V/Q mismatch 2° to pulmonary vasodilation and loss of hypoxic pulmonary vasoconstriction may lead to a decrease in PaO_2
- In patients with myocardial ischemia, there may be occurrence or exacerbation of ventricular arrhythmias
- Contraindicated in IHSS
- Prolonged use associated with β-blocker's downregulation and theoretically reduced effectiveness

DOPAMINE

Richard C. Prielipp, M.D.

INDICATIONS

- Hypotension
- Cardiac failure/shock with low-to-normal SVR
- Oliguria or periods of renal "stress" such as vascular surgery, sepsis, cardiopulmonary bypass, and concurrent use of other vasopressors

PERIOPERATIVE RISKS

- Tachycardia, angina, arrhythmias
- N/V
- Vasoconstriction and hypertension (possible gangrene of extremities)
- Skin sloughing and necrosis if infiltrated in subcutaneous tissue
- Impairs T-lymphocyte function (hypoprolactinemia)
- Depression of hypoxic ventilatory drive

PHARMACOLOGY

- Preparations: 200-, 400-, 800-mg ampules (must be diluted before IV administration)
- Endogenous central and peripheral neurotransmitter

OVERVIEW/MECH OF ACTION

- Mixed indirect and direct sympathomimetic effects, by activating dopamine (DA_2 and DA_1), ß- and α-adrenergic receptors in dose-dependent fashion
- Presynaptic DA_2 receptors (0.2–0.4 µg/kg/min) inhibit endogenous norepinephrine and prolactin release
- Postsynaptic DA_1 receptors (0.5–3.0 µg/kg/min) produce vasodilation in renal, mesenteric, coronary, cerebral arteries
- ß-adrenergic receptors (4–10 µg/kg/min) activate adenylyl cyclase and ↑ myocardial cAMP concentration, ↑ myocardial contractility, inotropy
- α-adrenergic receptors (>10–20 µg/kg/min) produce progressive vasoconstriction

- Metabolism: substrate for both MAO and COMT
- $T_{1/2}$: 6–9 min (recent evidence suggests attainment of steady-state plasma concentrations may require 70–125 min)

CLINICAL APPLICATIONS

- Renal dose dopamine
  – DA_1 (1.5–3.0 µg/kg/min) selectively increases renal blood flow and inhibits tubular reabsorption (increases urinary output)
  – induces diuresis, usually without changing creatinine clearance
- Inotropic dose dopamine
  – (~4–10 µg/kg/min) induces release of endogenous norepinephrine (~50% of total activity)
  – $ß_1$-adrenergic adenylyl cyclase activation increases myocardial cAMP
- Higher dose dopamine
  – In addition to effects noted above, $α_1$-adrenergic receptors (>10–20 µg/kg/min) are activated with progressive vasoconstriction

DRUG EFFECTS

SYSTEM	EFFECT	ASSESSMENT BY HX	PE	TEST
CV	↑ Cardiac inotropy; vasoconstrictor activity	Improved mental status, perfusion	Pulses, BP	↑ Cardiac output; urinary output
RESP	↓ Hypoxic drive ↑ Pulmonary artery pressure (PAP)	Hypoventilation	Resp rate, depth	ABG Monitor PAP
RENAL	↑ Renal blood flow: ↓ renal Na^+, water reabsorption	Urinary output	Urine volume	Urine volume, electrolytes

Key Reference: Goldberg LI: Dopamine and new dopamine analogs: Receptors and clinical applications. J Clin Anesthesiol 1988; 1:66–74.

PERIOPERATIVE IMPLICATIONS

Dopamine Infusion Issues

- Ensure adequate intravascular volume
- Consider invasive monitoring
  – Continuous arterial and PAP lines; central venous and pulmonary artery occlusion pressure ("filling pressures"); thermodilution cardiac output
  – Urinary output and Cr clearance

Adjuvants

- Additional inotropes—other ß-agonists (dobutamine, epinephrine, etc) or phosphodiesterase inhibitors (milrinone or amrinone) may be needed to ↑ cardiac contractility

Cautions

- May increase heart rate and LV wall stress excessively (dopamine >10 µg/kg/min frequently causes progressive tachycardia and ↑ diastolic ventricular filling pressure)
- Diminished response in patients with chronic CHF or active sepsis
- In cardiogenic shock, myocardial lactate may ↑
- Long-term infusions may suppress immune (T-cell) function with ↓ prolactin

Related Agent: Dopexamine

- Dopexamine, a synthetic analog of dopamine, lacks any direct α-adrenergic agonist activity, expressing only $ß_2$-adrenergic and dopaminergic (DA_1) agonist action
  – DA_1 and $ß_2$ arterial vasodilation reduces cardiac afterload while simultaneously increasing blood flow to the kidneys, intestines, liver, spleen
  – dopexamine (doses between 1–4 µg/kg/min) significantly ↑ cardiac index while decreasing systemic and pulmonary vascular resistances after cardiac surgery
  – HR ↑, but not SV index; thus, dopexamine combines positive inotropic, chronotropic, vasodilatory, diuretic, natriuretic properties

EDROPHONIUM

Peter M.C. Wright, M.D., FFARSCI
Dennis M. Fisher, M.D.

USES

- Perioperatively, for antagonism of NMB
- In diagnosis and management of myasthenia gravis (MG)

PERIOPERATIVE RISKS

- Parasympathomimetic effects common (although less than with neostigmine) and require routine prophylactic antagonism
- May ↑ N/V
- Limited in effects (compared with neostigmine); larger doses may produce muscle weakness

WORRY ABOUT

- Bradycardia and other cholinergic effects
- Brevity of action may result in "recurarization"

OVERVIEW/PHARMACOLOGY

- Potent reversible inhibitor of acetylcholinesterase
- No effect on plasma cholinesterase (pseudocholinesterase) in usual doses
- Increases cholinergic nervous transmission at the NMJ and (muscarinic) autonomic effector sites
- Stimulates bladder, bowel contractions (antagonized by atropine)
- May produce bronchospasm
- Produces bradycardia (antagonized by atropine)
- Oral administration inappropriate
- Rapidly excreted by kidney
- $T_{1/2}\beta$ = 110 min; prolonged in renal failure ($T_{1/2}\beta$ = 304 min)
- Clearance (9.5 ml/kg/min) ↓ in renal failure (3.9 ml/kg/min)
- Does not alter the metabolism of drugs cleared by plasma cholinesterase

DRUG CLASS/MECH OF ACTION/DOSE

- Type II (truly reversible) acetylcholinesterase inhibitor
- ↑ ACh concentrations in nerve terminals and NMJs
- Dose to antagonize nondepolarizing muscle relaxants: 0.5–1.0 mg/kg IV in adults, children
- Dose for Dx or differentiation of myasthenic/cholinergic crises: 2–10 mg IV in adults

ASSESSMENT POINTS

SYSTEM	EFFECT	PE
CV	Complex effects (bradycardia predominates)	Reversed by atropine
RESP	Bronchospasm	Reversed by atropine
GI	↑ Peristalsis May ↑ emetic symptoms	
NEURO	Reversal of weakness from NMB or MG Excess dose may produce weakness	

Key Reference: Cronnelly R, Morris RB, Miller RD: Edrophonium: Duration of action and atropine requirements in humans during halothane anesthesia. Anesthesiology 1982; 57:261–267.

PERIOPERATIVE IMPLICATIONS

Preoperative Concerns

- Not used chronically; unlikely to be encountered in preop pts
- Can be used to evaluate necessity for increased anticholinesterase dose in myasthenic pts

Adjuvants/Regional Anesthesia/Reversal

- Most commonly used to aid in Dx or differentiation of myasthenic from cholinergic crises and to antagonize residual NMB after surgery
- Compared with neostigmine, action is more rapid (peak effect in 1–2 min) but limited in maximum effect and duration
- Not effective with profound NMB
- Administer only with evidence of some NM transmission; administer with anticholinergic agent (atropine preferred because its time course matches the effect of edrophonium on HR)

ANTICIPATED PROBLEMS/CONCERNS

- Biochemical and acid-base derangement (particularly acidosis) may reduce its effectiveness in antagonizing NMB
- Relatively brief duration of effect leads to ↑ likelihood of recurarization

EPHEDRINE

Eric Jacobsohn, M.B.Ch.B., F.R.C.P.C.

INDICATIONS

- Intraoperatively for treatment of hypotension from central neuraxial blockade, IV/inhalational anesthesia
- IV as emergency Rx for acute hypotension, shock of still undetermined cause
- Orally for treatment of asthma, symptomatic treatment of coryza
- Nasally for treatment of coryza

PERIOPERATIVE RISKS

- Hypertensive crisis if administered to patients taking MAO-inhibitor antidepressants
- May precipitate dysrhythmias, if myocardium sensitized to catecholamines (e.g., due to inhalational agents)
- May precipitate ischemia in some ischemic heart disease patients

OVERVIEW/PHARMACOLOGY

- Nonselective, noncatecholamine acting on both the α- and β-adrenergic receptors
- Causes endogenous catecholamine release (indirect mechanism of action) and stimulation of adrenergic receptors (direct effect)
- Tachyphylaxis develops, caused by depletion of norepinephrine stores and persistent blockade of adrenergic receptors
- No catecholamine nucleus, therefore not metabolized by COMT
- Conjugated and deaminated slowly by MAO in liver; relatively slow inactivation accounts for prolonged effect ($10\times$ longer than epinephrine)
- 40% of dose recovered unchanged in urine

DRUG CLASS/USUAL DOSE

- Nonselective, noncatecholamine adrenergic stimulant with mainly indirect, but some direct, activity
- Dosage: Mix 50 mg in 10 ml (5 mg/ml) IV, titrated to desired effect
- Starting doses from 5–10 mg in adults
- Can also be given IM, SC
- Adult dose: 15–50 mg

DRUG EFFECTS

SYSTEM	EFFECT	ASSESSMENT BY HX	PE	TEST
RECEPTORS	α: ++ β_1: ++ β_2: +			
CV	HR: ++ Contractility: ++ Automaticity: ++ Peripheral resistance: + CO: ++ Mean BP: ++ PAP: ++		HR PR Mean BP	SV SVR CO PAP
RESP	Airway resistance: – – Resp stimulant: +			Airway resistance Min ventilation
VASC BED FLOW	Skin/viscera: – Muscle: + Kidney: – – Coronary: + Cerebral: +		Skin perfusion	
ENDO	Oxygen consumption: + Blood glucose: + Blood lactic acid: NC			O_2 consumption Blood glucose Blood lactate
GU	Uterine relaxation; restores uterine BF in hypotension from epidural/spinal			
CNS	Mild stimulant Mild mydriasis	Anxiety, agitation		

+ minimal increase; ++ moderate increase; – minimal decrease; – – moderate decrease; NC = no change

Key Reference: Stoelting RK: Pharmacology & Physiology in Anesthetic Practice, 2nd ed. Philadelphia, JB Lippincott, 1991, pp 264–284.

POSSIBLE DRUG INTERACTIONS

Preoperative Concerns

- Hypertensive crisis with MAO inhibitors
- Response to ephedrine ↑ 2–10 × in patients taking tricyclic antidepressants
- ↑ Risk of arrhythmias if taking digoxin
- ↑ Response in cocaine users
- Response to indirect effect may be reduced if taking reserpine or guanethidine
- ↓ Response in patients receiving β-blockers

Induction/Maintenance

- As in Preoperative Concerns

ANTICIPATED PROBLEMS

- Myocardium sensitized to catecholamines by some inhalational agents
- Tachyphylaxis with repeated doses
- Possibility of interactions with other drugs that affect ANS
- Precipitates ischemia in some patients

498   DRUGS

EPINEPHRINE

Eric Jacobsohn, M.D., F.R.C.P.C.

INDICATIONS

- Intraoperatively, in critical care for CV collapse from many causes—cardiogenic, distributive (including anaphylaxis), obstructive shock
- Addition to local anesthesia to prolong action (1:200,000), and for hemostasis
- Nebulized racemic epinephrine for laryngotracheobronchitis in children, postop stridor
- Inhalational forms for mild asthma
- Topical solutions for vasoconstriction (nasal, ophthalmic solutions)
- Large, repeated doses in cardiac arrest

PERIOPERATIVE RISKS

- Increased risk of arrhythmias (limit to $1\,\mu g/kg$ with halothane, 2–$3\,\mu g/kg$ with isoflurane, enflurane)
- May precipitate myocardial ischemia
- Severe hypertension/stroke if dosed incorrectly
- Large doses may precipitate pulmonary edema

OVERVIEW/PHARMACOLOGY

- Potent α, $\beta1$, $\beta2$ stimulant
- β stimulation causes ↑ intracellular cAMP
- α_1 stimulation causes ↑ intracellular Ca^{2+} by G protein interaction as well as ↑ turnover of phosphoinositol
- α_2 stimulation inhibits adenylate cyclase
- Metabolized by MAO, COMT; conjugated and excreted in urine
- Biological activity terminated principally by uptake in postganglionic sympathetic nerve terminals

DRUG CLASS/USUAL DOSE

- Naturally occurring sympathomimetic
- Dosage: depends on route and clinical situation—low, moderate, high doses:
  - IV: Mix 1 mg in 250 mL ($4\,\mu g/mL$); adult bolus doses for ↓ BP from anaphylaxis: 10–$20\,\mu g$ as starting dose, ↑ as needed
- Infusion, mainly β at 0.01–$0.03\,\mu g/kg/min$, increasing α at 0.03–$0.15\,\mu g/kg/min$, predominant α at 0.15–$0.3\,\mu g/kg/min$. Cardiac arrest dose: 0.5–1 mg q5min
  - Subcutaneous: $10\,\mu g/kg$ for mild to moderate allergic reactions, severe asthma.

DRUG EFFECTS

SYSTEM	EFFECT	ASSESSMENT BY HX	PE	TEST
RECEPTORS	α: ++ (dose-dependent) β_1: ++ β_2: ++			
CV	HR: ++ Contractility: ++ Automaticity: ++ SVR ± (dose-dependent) CO: ++ Mean BP: + (dose-dependent) PAP: +	Palpitations	HR Pulse Perfusion Mean BP	SV SVR CO BP PAP
EXPIRATORY	Airway resistance: – Respiratory stimulant: +		Wheezing TV	Airway resistance Minute ventilation
VASC BED FLOW	Skin/viscera: – – Muscle: ++ Kidney: – – Coronary: + Cerebral: +		Skin perfusion	
ENDO	O_2 consumption: ++ Blood glucose: ++ Blood lactic acid: ++ (with infusion) Hypokalemia Free fatty acids: ++			O_2 consumption Blood glucose Blood lactate Serum K$^+$ Free fatty acids
GU	Relaxation of uterus			
CNS	Mild stimulant Mild mydriasis	Anxiety, agitation, headache Mydriasis		

+ minimal increase; ++ moderate increase; +++ marked increase; – minimal decrease; – – moderate decrease
Key Reference: Weiner N: *In* Goodman & Gilman's The Pharmacological Basis of Therapeutics, 7th ed. New York, Pergamon, 1985, pp 145–161.

PERIOPERATIVE IMPLICATIONS/POSSIBLE DRUG INTERACTIONS

Preoperative Concerns

- Hypertensive crisis with MAO inhibitors
- May precipitate malignant arrhythmias
- ↑ Risk of arrhythmias if taking digoxin
- Response exaggerated if taking reserpine, guanethidine
- ↑ Sensitivity if taking cocaine, tricyclic antidepressants
- ↓ Response with β-blockers

- Hypertensive, hyperthyroid pts more susceptible to pressor response
- Hypokalemia

Induction/Maintenance

- Arrhythmias with halothane

ANTICIPATED PROBLEMS

- Myocardium sensitized to catecholamines by inhalational agents—possibility of malignant arrhythmias
- Severe hypertension, possible stroke if dosed incorrectly
- Aggravates symptoms in psychoneurotic pts on emergence
- Hypokalemia, hyperglycemia
- Possibility of pulm edema

ETOMIDATE (AMIDATE)

Paul F. White, Ph.D., M.D.

USES

- Intravenous anesthetic agent
- Induction of anesthesia in patients with cardiac disease, cerebrovascular disease, and the critically ill
- Use during seizure ablation surgery and ECT
- Causes pain on injection, myoclonic activity, transient depression of adrenosteroidogenesis, postop N/V
- Not compatible with water-soluble drugs

OVERVIEW/PHARMACOLOGY

- Sedative-hypnotic that produces dose-dependent CNS depression
- Rapid onset of action
- Rapid distribution ($T_{1/2}\alpha = 2$–4 min), redistribution ($T_{1/2}\gamma = 15$–30 min), elimination ($T_{1/2}\beta = 3.5$ h)
- Hepatic esterase hydrolysis to inactive glucuronide conjugates

DRUG CLASS/MECH OF ACTION/USUAL DOSE

- Intravenous induction agent
- Enhances GABAergic inhibition and activation of the chloride channel in the CNS
- Induction dosages:
  - children: 0.2–0.4 mg/kg, IV
  - adults: 0.15–0.3 mg/kg, IV
  - elderly: 0.1–0.2 mg/kg, IV

DRUG EFFECTS

SYSTEM	EFFECT	ASSESSMENT BY HX	PE	TEST
CV	Minimal depression (except in critically ill)	CV function	BP; HR	MAP; HR
RESP	↓ Central respiratory drive (minimal)	Ventilatory status	Resp rate	PFTs; end-tidal CO_2; SpO_2
GI	N/V			
ENDO	↓ Cortisol and aldosterone production	Plasma cortisol, aldosterone levels		ACTH stimulation test
CNS	Sedation, hypnosis, ↓ ICP ↓ CBF/CPP	Neurologic function		EEG; brainstem evoked potentials

Key Reference: Van Hemelrijer J, White PF: Pharmacology of intravenous anesthetic agents. *In* Rogers MC, Tinker JW, Covino BF, Longnecker DE (eds): Principles and Practice of Anesthesiology. CV Mosby Co., St. Louis, 1992, pp 1131–1154.

PERIOPERATIVE IMPLICATIONS/DRUG INTERACTIONS

- Assess volume and neurologic status
- Monitor MAP, HR, SpO_2
- Use with potent opioid analgesics to minimize pain on injection and myoclonic activity
- Consider steroid supplementation if patient develops an unexpected postop complication (e.g., hemorrhage, sepsis)

ANTICIPATED PROBLEMS/CONCERNS

- Transient (8–16 h) inhibition of adrenocortical synthetic function after induction dose
- Postop N/V after ambulatory surgery may delay discharge

FLUOXETINE (PROZAC)

Donald D. Koblin, Ph.D., M.D.

USES

- Taken by 5 million Americans
- Rx for: depression, obsessive-compulsive disorder, bulimia nervosa

PERIOPERATIVE RISKS

- May be associated with perioperative anxiety
- Drug interactions with β-blockers, phenytoin, benzodiazepines, neuroleptics (may increase levels by inhibition of metabolism)

WORRY ABOUT

- Psychotic or extrapyramidal reactions (rare)
- Serotonin syndrome with concomitant administration of MAO inhibitors, tricyclic antidepressants, neuroleptics (?), or meperidine (?)

OVERVIEW/PHARMACOLOGY

- Selective inhibitor of serotonin reuptake
- Administered as racemic mixture of R- and S-enantiomers
- S-enantiomer more potent than R-enantiomer
- Active metabolites, R- and S-norfluoxetine, formed by demethylation
- Eliminated mainly through oxidative metabolism and conjugation
- Long elimination $T_{1/2}$: 1–10 days for fluoxetine; 3–20 days for norfluoxetine
- Fluoxetine inhibits (and probably metabolized by) liver cytochrome P450 enzymes CYP2D6 and possibly CYP3A4: may inhibit metabolism, ↑ levels of β-blockers, benzodiazepines, neuroleptics
- Difficult to establish relationship between plasma concn of fluoxetine and effect, probably because these are 4 active compounds (R- and S-fluoxetine and R- and S-norfluoxetine) that require separate measurements

DRUG CLASS/MECH OF ACTION/USUAL DOSE

- Selective inhibitor of serotonin reuptake chronically taken for depression, obsessive-compulsive disorder, bulimia nervosa
- Not useful for acute administration, since full antidepressant effect may be delayed until 4 wk of treatment or longer
- Initial PO dose, 20 mg qd
- Maximal dose, 80 mg qd
- Alternatives: Other antidepressant medications

DRUG EFFECTS

SYSTEM	EFFECT	ASSESSMENT BY HX	PE	TEST
CV	Bradycardia, dysrhythmia in elderly patients (rare)		Pulse	ECG
CNS	Extrapyramidal symptoms (rare), mania (rare), serotonin syndrome (rare)	Headache, anxiety, tremor		
ENDO	SIADH secretion (rare)			Urine specific gravity
GI	Nausea, weight loss			
MS	Serotonin syndrome (rare)	Arthritic complaints (infrequent), muscle rigidity		

Key Reference: Gram LF: Fluoxetine. N Engl J Med 1994; 3:1354–1361.

PERIOPERATIVE IMPLICATIONS/POSSIBLE DRUG INTERACTIONS

- Headache, anxiety, nausea are common symptoms
- May inhibit cytochrome P450 enzymes and ↑ the serum concentrations of other drugs (β-blockers, phenytoin, benzodiazepines, neuroleptics) and potentiate their effects

SPECIAL CONSIDERATIONS

- Approximately 7% of Caucasians lack the cytochrome P450 (CYP2D6) that probably metabolizes fluoxetine; these individuals may develop higher serum concentrations of fluoxetine and be more prone to side effects.
- Serotonin syndrome, characterized by agitation, confusion, diaphoresis, and muscle rigidity, may develop in pts who receive a combination of fluoxetine and MAO inhibitors.

FOLIC ACID

John P. Lawrence, M.D.

USES

- Folic acid deficiency
- Megaloblastic anemia
- Malnutrition due to alcoholism or malabsorption syndromes — e.g., sprue (tropical and nontropical)
- Alcoholics
- Prevents neural tube defects in fetuses
- Reduces homocysteine, which decreases risk of atherosclerosis and venous thrombosis
- Available in tablet, parenteral forms
- Folinic acid (leucovorin calcium) for leucovorin rescue but not vitamin replacement

PERIOPERATIVE RISKS

- Report of interaction with urethane (animal anesthesia)
- At high doses (>15 mg/d) ↓ seizure threshold in epileptics on phenobarbital, phenytoin, primidone

WORRY ABOUT

- Rare reaction to parenteral form
- At high doses (>15 mg/d), may precipitate seizures in epileptics

OVERVIEW/PHARMACOLOGY

- Vitamin, responsible for transferring 1-carbon molecules to other organic molecules
- Absorbed in proximal intestine, undergoes extensive enterohepatic recirculation
- Nonmethylated forms of folate are protein-bound
- Excreted fecally
- Interferes with levels of antiepileptic drugs
- Alcohol directly decreases blood levels by blocking enterohepatic recirculation

DRUG CLASS/MECH OF ACTION/USUAL DOSE

- Vitamin
- Converts homocysteine to methionine, serine to glycine (reduces risk of atherosclerosis)
- Assists synthesis of thymidylate, purines, metabolism of histidine
- Usual dose: normal requirements: 0.4–0.5 mg/d (found in multivitamins)
- Higher requirements (hemolytic anemia, pregnancy, or antifolate drug therapy): 1 mg 1–3×/d (PO, IM, IV)
- Give with B_{12} or can precipitate neurologic component of combined system disease

DRUG EFFECTS

SYSTEM	EFFECT	ASSESSMENT BY HX	PE	TEST
CV	Improves O_2 delivery	Better exercise tolerance		Hb
GI		Less nausea/diarrhea	Better hydration	
ENDO/METAB	Nucleic acid/ Protein synthesis		Weight gain	Folate level
HEME	RBC synthesis	Better exercise tolerance		Hbg

Key Reference: Hillman RS: *In* Gilman AG, Rale TCO, Nies AS, Taylor P, eds: Goodman & Gilman's The Pharmacological Basis of Therapeutics, 8th ed. New York, Pergamon, 1990, pp 1302–1306.

PERIOPERATIVE IMPLICATIONS

Preoperative Concerns

- Anemia
- Consider overall nutritional status
- Consider co-existing diseases: alcoholism, malignancy, malabsorptive syndromes, hydration status
- Continue supplements perioperatively

Induction/Maintenance

- Only reported perioperative interaction is with urethane, which has antifolate activity

Adjuvants/Regional Anesthesia/Reversal

- Same as Preoperative Concerns

Postoperative Period

- Same as Preoperative Concerns

ANTICIPATED PROBLEMS/CONCERNS

- May precipitate seizures at high doses (>15 mg/d) in epileptics on chronic antiepileptic therapy
- Folinic acid (leucovorin calcium) not used for repleting folic acid deficiency

GOLD (AUROTHIOGLUCOSE, AUROTHIOMALATE)

Martin D. Sokoll, M.D.

USES

- ~500,000 patients/y receive gold Rx
- Rx for: RA patients who do not respond to aspirin, NSAIDs

RISKS OF ADMINISTRATION

- Cutaneous reactions from erythema to exfoliative dermatitis
- Mucous membrane lesions: stomatitis, pharyngitis, gastritis, colitis
- Chrysiasis (gray-to-blue pigmentation of skin) poss; effect of transcutaneous Hgb saturation measurement unknown
- Potential problems: hepatic, renal dysfunction
- Severe hematologic problems—thrombocytopenia (usually reverses with cessation of Rx) to aplastic anemia (usually fatal)
- Not usually administered to pregnant patients or those given antimalarials, phenylbutazone, or oxyphenylbutazone because of concomitant blood dyscrasias
- Not well tolerated by elderly

OVERVIEW/PHARMACOLOGY

- Usually administered IM; a few patients take drug PO
- Au compounds have anti-inflammatory activity
- Aurothioglucose, aurothiomalate administered IM
- Auranofin is oral prep
- Oral prep has lower incidence of side effects
- $T_{1/2}$ of single 50-mg dose IM ~ 7 d
- After full dose, blood levels return to normal in 40–80 d; 60–90% of a given dose is eliminated renally, remainder by fecal excretion
- Renal disease delays excretion and is a contraindication to Au administration

DRUG CLASS/MECH OF ACTION/USUAL DOSE

- Anti-inflammatory
- Au compounds sequestered in organs, areas having high mononuclear phagocyte concentrations
- Au concentrates in phagocytes and synovial membranes; suppresses phagocyte migration and has general anti-inflammatory effect
- Administered in progressive doses (10–50 mg to a total dose of 1 g/wk)
- Continuing Rx 50 mg every q 2–4 wk

DRUG EFFECTS

SYSTEM	EFFECT	PE	TEST
HEENT	Glossitis, pharyngitis		
RESP	Tracheitis, pneumonitis		CXR
GI	Hepatitis		LFTs
GU	Proteinuria, hematuria, membranous glomerulonephritis (contraindicated during pregnancy, breast feeding)		Renal function, pregnancy
CNS	Encephalitis, peripheral neuritis	CNS exam	

Key Reference: Insel PA: Analgesic antipyretics and antiinflammatory agents: Drugs employed in the treatment of rheumatoid arthritis and gout. *In* Gilman AG, Rall TW, Nies AS, Taylor P (eds): Goodman & Gilman's The Pharmacological Basis of Therapeutics, 8th ed. New York, Pergamon Press, 1990, pp 670–673.

PERIOPERATIVE IMPLICATIONS/POSSIBLE DRUG INTERACTIONS

- Severe RA; difficulty positioning on operating table
- Airway: laryngeal arthritis, cervical instability, other problems of arthritis may be encountered
- Stomatitis, pharyngitis, tracheitis may make mucous membranes fragile

Drug Interactions

- None during anesthesia but chrysiasis may interfere with pulse oximeter function

ANTICIPATED PROBLEMS

- Beware of hepatic and renal dysfunction
- Lesions of skin, mucous membranes may make these tissues friable
- Investigate cervical instability in all severe arthritides
- Condition may mandate fiberoptic, blind oral, or nasal intubation of trachea
- Hematologic problems (thrombocytopenia, leukopenia) may manifest as bleeding or postop infection

HALOPERIDOL (HALDOL)

Donald D. Koblin, M.D., Ph.D.

USES

- Rx for
  - psychotic disorders in ambulatory population (PO)
  - agitation caused by delirium in ICU patients (IV or IM)

PERIOPERATIVE RISKS

- Laryngospasm
- Extrapyramidal symptoms
- Neuroleptic malignant syndrome
- Cardiac arrest at high doses

WORRY ABOUT

- May exacerbate symptoms in pts with Parkinson's disease
- Potential concern for neurotoxic metabolites
- Extrapyramidal symptoms less common with IV than PO doses

OVERVIEW/PHARMACOLOGY

- Dopaminergic antagonist
- Precise mechanism of action unknown
- Onset time: 5–20 min for IV; 30–60 min for PO
- Long (and variable) serum $T_{1/2}$ (13–60 h)
- 90–94% bound to serum proteins
- Therapeutic plasma concentration in range of 4–40 µg/L, but large variability among pts
- Clearance by hepatic metabolism
- Metabolized to reduced haloperidol, which has ~10% of activity of parent drug; reduced haloperidol may be oxidized and reconverted to haloperidol
- Renal excretion of parent drug is negligible

DRUG CLASS/MECH OF ACTION/USUAL DOSE

- Dopaminergic antagonist
- Chronically taken for
  - management of psychotic disorders
  - control of tics and vocal utterances of Tourette's disorder
- Acutely taken to control agitation caused by delirium
- Usual PO dose 1–6 mg qd
- Usual IV or IM dose:
  - 0.5 to 2 mg for mild agitation
  - 5 mg for moderate agitation
  - 10 mg for severe agitation (+10 mg/h infusion)
- Alternatives:
  - other antipsychotic medications
  - other antidelirium medications (e.g., physostigmine)
  - usually for agitation caused by delirium; agitation caused by anxiety/pain can be treated with benzodiazepines/narcotics

DRUG EFFECTS

SYSTEM	EFFECT	TEST
HEENT	Laryngospasm (infrequent side effect)	
CV	Hypotension or hypertension, cardiac arrest (high doses)	
LIVER	↓ metabolism and ↑ serum concentration with hepatic disease	Monitoring of haloperidol concentrations is indicated only in pts with poor response at high doses or with hepatic disease
GI	Nausea	
ENDO	Gynecomastia	
GU	Urinary retention	
CNS	Extrapyramidal symptoms (akathisia, dystonia, tardive dyskinesia)	
MS	Neuroleptic malignant syndrome	

Key References: Tesar GE, Stern TA: Rapid tranquilization of the agitated intensive care unit patient. J Int Care Med 1988; 3:195–201.

PERIOPERATIVE IMPLICATIONS/POSSIBLE DRUG INTERACTIONS

- Encephalopathic syndrome with combined use of lithium and haloperidol
- May potentiate effects of general anesthetics and narcotics

SPECIAL CONSIDERATIONS

- Laryngospasm infrequent but life-threatening
- Cardiac arrests reported with high (~10 mg) doses
- IV haloperidol is not approved for routine use by the USFDA
- Neuroleptic malignant syndrome (NMS) may develop 1–3 d after haloperidol administration and is characterized by muscle rigidity, hyperthermia, tachycardia, altered consciousness, and elevated serum creatine kinase concentrations. A mild form of NMS may occur in as many as 1% of pts given haloperidol

ISOPROTERENOL (ISUPREL)

Eric Jacobsohn, M.B.ChB., F.R.C.P.C.

INDICATIONS

- IV in heart block to ↑ ventricular response in absence of pacing, pulm HTN, right heart failure
- Bronchodilator in status asthmaticus
- Potent inotrope (shock, ß rb overdose)
- Nebulized or as aerosol in asthma

PERIOPERATIVE RISKS

- ↑ Risk of arrhythmias
- Multiple poss drug interactions: ↑ effect if taking guanethidine, reserpine; ↑ sensitivity if taking TCAs, and in cocaine users
- Can precipitate myocardial ischemia in susceptible patients

OVERVIEW/PHARMACOLOGY

- Potent, direct-acting $ß_1$, $ß_2$ stimulant
- No α effect (i.e., not a pressor)
- ß-adrenergic stimulation causes ↑ intracellular cAMP (2nd messenger), → change in cellular function by causing enzyme or protein phosphorylation
- Short $T_{1/2}$ of 2 min; 60% excreted unchanged in urine, conjugated in liver; reuptake < that of epinephrine, norepinephrine; metabolized by MAO, COMT

DRUG CLASS/USUAL DOSE

- Direct acting, synthetic catecholamine
- IV dose: mix 1–2 mg in 250 ml IV solution (4–8 µg/ml); infuse at 0.01–0.5 µg/kg/min
- Aerosol: 0.25% inhaler
- Nebulized: 0.25–1% solution, 0.5 ml in 2.5 ml H_2O over 10–20 min

DRUG EFFECTS

SYSTEM	EFFECT	ASSESSMENT BY HX	PE	TEST
RECEPTORS	α: 0 $ß_1$: +++ $ß_2$: +++			
CV	HR: +++ Contractility: +++ Automaticity: +++ Total peripheral resistance: – CO: +++ Mean BP: ± PAP: –	Palpitations, angina	HR Pulse Perfusion Mean BP	SV SVR CO BP PAP
RESP	Airway resistance: – – – Resp stimulant: +	Wheezing	Wheezing R, TV	Airway resistance Min vent
VASC (BED FLOW)	Skin/viscera: + Muscle: ++ Kidney: – in normotensive patients, ++ in cardiogenic shock Coronary: + Cerebral: +	 Mentation	Skin perfusion	 Urine output
CNS	Mild stimulant Mild mydriasis	Anxiety, agitation, headache Mydriasis		
GU	Relaxation of uterus			
ENDO	O_2 consumption: ++ Blood glucose: ++ Blood lactic acid: ++ Hypokalemia Serum FFA: ++			O_2 consumption Blood glucose Blood lactate Serum K^+ Serum FFA

0: none; + minimal ↑; ++ moderate ↑; +++ marked ↑; – minimal ↓; – – moderate ↓; – – – marked ↓

Key Reference: Weiner N. *In* Gilman AG, Rall TW, Nies AS, Taylor P (eds): Goodman & Gilman's The Pharmacological Basis of Therapeutics, 7th ed. New York, Pergamon, 1985, pp 145–161.

POSSIBLE DRUG INTERACTIONS

Preoperative Concerns

- Interactions with MAO inhibitors
- ↑ Risk of arrhythmias. Response exaggerated if taking reserpine, guanethidine, cocaine, TCA
- ↓ Response in ß rb patients
- Hypertensive, hyperthyroid patients are more susceptible to effects
- Hypokalemia can occur

Induction/Maintenance

- As in Preoperative Concerns section

ANTICIPATED PROBLEMS/CONCERNS

- Hypotension from unopposed ß-adrenergic activity
- Myocardium sensitized to catecholamines by some inhalational agents
- Risk malignant arrhythmias, esp if dosed incorrectly
- Aggravates symptoms in psychoneurotic patients on emergence
- Hypokalemia, hyperglycemia
- Pulm edema can occur with infusions

KETAMINE

Paul F. White, M.D., Ph.D.

USES

- IV/IM anesthetic agent
- Induction of anesthesia for patients with bronchospastic disease or acute hypovolemia
- Sedation/analgesia during burn dressing changes, to supplement local and regional anesthesia
- Causes cardiovascular stimulation, increased oral secretions, psychomimetic emergence reactions, postop confusion, visual disturbances
- Used in combination with benzodiazepines, barbiturates, or propofol to minimize side effects

OVERVIEW/PHARMACOLOGY

- Sedative-hypnotic with analgesia-like properties
- Produces functional dissociation between cortical and subcortical structures in the CNS
- Rapid onset following IV or IM administration
- Rapid distribution ($T_{1/2}\alpha$ = 11–15 min); redistribution ($T_{1/2}\gamma$ = 20–40 min); elimination ($T_{1/2}\beta$ = 2–4 h)
- Hepatic metabolism to form active metabolite (nonketamine), inactive glucuronide conjugates
- Racemic mixture of 2 optical isomers; S(+) isomer is more potent anesthetic and analgesic

DRUG CLASS/MECH OF ACTION/USUAL DOSE

- Intravenous anesthetic for induction and maintenance of anesthesia and sedation
- Stimulates NMDA receptors in the cortical areas and opioid receptors in the spinal cord
- Produces smooth muscle relaxation
- Induction doses (with benzodiazepine premedication):
  – children: 4–6 mg/kg, IM
  – adults: 0.75–1.5 mg/kg, IV
  – elderly: 0.5–1 mg/kg, IV

DRUG EFFECTS

SYSTEM	EFFECT	ASSESSMENT BY HX	PE	TEST
CV	Stimulates sympathetic outflow, ↑ HR, ↑ MAP, ↑ MVo_2	CV function	BP, HR	MAP, HR
RESP	Minimal depression of central respiratory drive; bronchodilation	Ventilatory status	Resp rate	SpO_2, end-tidal CO_2, PFTs
CNS	Sedation, hypnosis, analgesia (affective-emotional component); ↑ ICP, ↑ IOP, ↑ CPP, ↑ $CMRO_2$ ↑ Muscle tone	Neuro function	MS exam EMG	EEG; brainstem evoked potentials

Key Reference: Gajraj N, White PF: Clinical pharmacology and practical applications of ketamine. *In* Bowdle T, Horita A, Kharasch E (eds): Pharmacological Basis of Anesthesiology: Basic Science and Clinical Applications. New York, Churchill Livingstone, 1994, pp 375–392.

PERIOPERATIVE IMPLICATIONS/DRUG INTERACTIONS

- Assess volume and cardiovascular status
- Monitor MAP, HR, SpO_2
- Utilize in combination with a benzodiazepine (e.g., diazepam 5–10 mg IV, midazolam 2–5 mg IV) or sedative-hypnotic drug (e.g., thiopental, 1–2 mg/kg; propofol, 0.5–1 mg/kg IV) to minimize CNS and CV side effects
- Consider antisialagogue (e.g., glycopyrrolate, 0.1–0.2 mg IV) to ↓ secretions in patients at risk of laryngospasm
- Emergence of sequelae may delay discharge after ambulatory surgery

LIDOCAINE

Beverly K. Philip, M.D.
Darrell L. Tanelian, M.D.

USES

- Rx for peripheral nerve block, spinal analgesia/anesthesia, ventricular arrhythmias, chronic pain relief, to attenuate laryngeal response to intubation
- Available in single-dose units for local/regional anesthesia, with and without added epinephrine; in multiple-dose vials with methylparaben as an antiseptic preservative; and in vials and prefilled syringes for arrhythmia therapy. Various topical formulations are also available.

PERIOPERATIVE RISKS

- Feeling of dissociation, paresthesias, mild drowsiness, agitation
- Attenuated hearing
- Muscle twitching
- A true allergic reaction very rare
- Adverse reactions are related to additive components, especially epinephrine and preservatives.
- Potential for toxicity ↑ in patient receiving cimetidine

WORRY ABOUT

- Convulsions
- Respiratory arrest
- Systemic toxicity due to accidental intravascular injection

OVERVIEW/PHARMACOLOGY

- Aminoamide local anesthetic
- Use-dependent Na$^+$ channel blocker
- 70% of lidocaine in plasma is bound to proteins, mostly to α-acid glycoprotein
- Metabolized in the liver by N-dealkylation, aromatic hydroxylation, amide hydrolysis
- Hepatic extraction ratio 0.65, drug clearance dependent on liver blood flow and is reduced in disease states such as cardiac failure and advanced liver disease
- $T_{1/2}\alpha$ = 1.0 min, $T_{1/2}\beta$ = 9.6 min, clearance$_{(normal)}$ = 0.95 L/min, $T_{1/2}\gamma$ = 1.6 hr, $T_{1/2}\gamma$ in liver disease = 5 hr, $T_{1/2}\gamma$ in CHF = 5 hr; prolonged with ↓ hepatic blood flow as in CHF
- Active metabolite monoethylglycine xylidide has antiarrhythmic and convulsant activity similar to lidocaine, but with longer $T_{1/2}$, and can contribute to toxicity with continuous infusions
- Onset and duration dependent on site and route of administration

DRUG CLASS/MECHANISM OF ACTION

- Class I$_B$ antiarrhythmic agent
- Amide local anesthetic
- Use-dependent Na$^+$ channel blocker

USUAL DOSE

- Dose varies with application
- Peripheral nerve block
  - 0.25–2% solutions, maximum
  - 300 mg (without epinephrine); 500 mg (with epinephrine)
- Spinal block
  - 2% plain, 20–100 mg
  - 5% hyperbaric (6.8% glucose), 20–100 mg
- Epidural block
  - 0.5–2% with or without epinephrine, 50–400 mg
- Intravenous
  - 0.7 to 1.4 mg/kg rapidly, no more than 300 mg/1 h
  - Infusions of 1–4 mg/min to produce a plasma concentration of 1 to 5 µg/ml (therapeutic level)

DRUG EFFECTS

SYSTEM	EFFECT	ASSESSMENT BY PE	TEST
CV	Prolongation of cardiac conduction time		ECG ↑ PR interval ↑ QRS duration
	Sinus bradycardia	↓ HR	Pulse monitor
	Negative inotropic action	↓ BP	BP monitor
VASC	High-dose vasodilation	↓ BP	BP monitor
CNS	Lightheadedness Visual, auditory disturbance	CNS exam Toxicity heralded by perioral dysesthesia, lightheadedness, difficulty speaking, twitching and tremors	
	Drowsiness Twitching, tremors Convulsions Crosses blood-brain barrier, causing CNS excitation followed by CNS depression	Observation Excitation evidenced as restlessness and tremor Higher plasma concentrations result in convulsions, coma, and cardiorespiratory arrest	
PNS	Low-dose vasoconstriction	↑ BP	BP monitor

Key Reference: Philip BK, Covino BG: Local and regional anesthesia. In Wetchler BV (ed): Anesthesia for Ambulatory Surgery. Philadelphia, JB Lippincott, 1990, pp 309–365.

PERIOPERATIVE IMPLICATIONS

Preoperative Concerns

- Reduce likelihood of toxic reactions by aspirateing carefully, injecting slowly, and using optimum dose—minimum concentration and volume—for desired effect.
- Educate patients to report early signs of toxicity: drowsiness, lightheadedness, dizziness, metallic taste, tinnitus, circumoral numbness, blurred vision.
- Watch for objective signs of toxicity: confusion, slurred speech, nystagmus, muscle tremors
- Assess volume status
- Consider monitoring BP, HR, CNS, pulse oximetry

Induction/Maintenance

- Avoid hypercarbia and acidosis, such as occur with hypoventilation after sedative–narcotic administration, and decrease threshold for convulsive activity and increase cardiodepressant effects of lidocaine
- Lidocaine can ↓ the MAC of other anesthetic agents if given concurrently (reduction at 1.5 mg/kg is about 30%)
- β rb can ↓ lidocaine metabolism
- Cimetidine can ↑ plasma lidocaine concentrations if given concurrently
- Lidocaine can potentiate the effects of succinylcholine and provide prophylaxis for muscle pain and fasciculations

Postoperative Period

- Patients given large systemic doses of lidocaine may be somnolent postoperatively
- Epidural and/or spinal lidocaine may result in postop motor and/or sensory loss
- Epidural and/or spinal lidocaine may cause postop hypotension

ANTICIPATED PROBLEMS/CONCERNS

- Lidocaine may lead to CV and CNS toxicity (see above)
- Spinal lidocaine may cause hypotension
- Lidocaine used for nerve blocks causes motor and/or sensory loss

LITHIUM CARBONATE

Eric Jacobsohn, M.B.ChB., F.R.C.P.C.

INDICATIONS

• For acute manic states, as maintenance therapy for bipolar affective disorders

PERIOPERATIVE RISKS

• Response to depolarizing, nondepolarizing muscle relaxants prolonged
• Dose requirement for injected and inhalational anesthetic agents is ↓
• Toxicity →weakness, ↓ level of consciousness, seizures, CV problems (AV block, dysrhythmias, hypotension)

OVERVIEW/PHARMACOLOGY

• At cellular level acts as imperfect substitute for Na⁺, intracellular accumulation of lithium ↓ phosphatidylinosites by interfering with hydrolysis of myoinositol-1-phosphate in the brain
• Also inhibits Ca^{2+}, depolarization-mediated release of norepinephrine, dopamine in brain
• May also inhibit ability of some hormones to activate adenylate cyclase
• Almost complete absorption from GI tract; peak levels 2–4 h after oral dose
• Initial distribution in extracellular fluid, subsequent accumulation in tissues
• No plasma protein binding

• Excreted via kidney; ⅓ to ⅔ acute dose excreted in 6–12 h; 80% filtered lithium reabsorbed in proximal convoluted tubule
• Lithium clearance is 20% of Cr clearance
• Na⁺ depletion causes retention of lithium; ↑ lithium levels from thiazide diuretics, ECA, furosemide; Na⁺ loading causes ↑ excretion of lithium
• Has low therapeutic index, 2–3; therapeutic range, 0.8–1.25 mEq/L toxic at levels > 1.5 mEq/L

DRUG CLASS/USUAL DOSE

• Lithium salt
• Daily dose individualized; determined by regular monitoring of lithium levels. Usual adult dose varies: 750–1500 mg/d, in divided doses

DRUG EFFECTS

SYSTEM	EFFECT	ASSESSMENT BY HX	PE	TEST
CV	Therapeutic levels cause benign ST interval/T wave changes Toxicity: malignant arrhythmias, heart block, hypotension	Dose, intercurrent illness, drugs precipitating toxicity	CVS exam	ECG
ENDO	Enlarged tender thyroid; hypothyroidism rare	Neck pain, hypothyroid symptoms	Thyroid	FT₄E/TSH
GU	Nephrogenic diabetes insipidus	Polyuria, polydipsia		Urine/serum lytes/ osmolality
CNS	Toxicity: tremor, drowsiness, coma, convulsions Therapeutic: may cause drowsiness, EEG slowing	Dose, concomitant therapy, illnesses	CNS exam	Lithium level
SKIN	Dermatitis			

Key Reference: Hill GE, Wong KC: Lithium carbonate and neuromuscular blocking agents. Anesthesiology 1977; 46:122–126.

POSSIBLE DRUG INTERACTIONS

Preoperative Concerns

• ↑ Lithium levels from thiazide diuretics, ECA, furosemide
• ↑ CNS toxicity when used with haloperidol
• Phenothiazines may suppress nausea, an early symptom of lithium toxicity
• Pressor effect of norepinephrine may be ↓

Induction/Maintenance

• Concerns same as Preoperative Concerns
• May have reduced requirement for inhaled and injected anesthesia
• Delayed recovery from barbiturates reported
• ↑ Response to depolarizing, nondepolarizing muscle relaxants

ANTICIPATED PROBLEMS/CONCERNS

• Be aware of signs and symptoms of toxicity
• Severe CV collapse; arrhythmias, heart block possible with toxicity
• Nephrogenic diabetes insipidus, lyte abnormalities may occur
• Awakening, NMB both prolonged
• Avoid using haloperidol

MAGNESIUM SULFATE

Brett B. Gutsche, M.D.

INDICATIONS

- Primary use in obstetrics for
  - tocolysis (treatment of preterm labor)
  - treatment of preeclampsia-eclampsia for its anticonvulsant, tocolytic, vasodilator properties
- Usually given by the IV route (IM rarely used in modern obstetrics)
- Orally as a cathartic or laxative (minimal absorption from the gut)

PERIOPERATIVE RISKS

- Skeletal muscle weakness
- Hypotension

WORRY ABOUT

- Increased sensitivity to all muscle relaxants, but especially to nondepolarizing muscle relaxants
- Severe hypotension with potent inhalation anesthetics, sympathetic block, antihypertensive drugs
- Attenuation of pressor substance effects

OVERVIEW/PHARMACOLOGY

- Tocolytic, $\downarrow$ uterine activity associated with preterm labor and preeclampsia-eclampsia
- Anticonvulsant, direct CNS depression (central hippocampus)
- Skeletal muscle relaxant acting at myoneural junction; may antagonize nondepolarizing muscle relaxant reversal by antiChEs
- 90% renal excretion, $T_{1/2}$ 4 h
- Appears to produce sedation that is not associated with amnesia nor analgesia

DRUG CLASS/MECH OF ACTION/USUAL DOSE

- Mg^{2+} is a major intracellular ion
- Depresses release of acetylcholine (ACh) and sensitivity of receptor to ACh; causes increased levels of both AMP and cGMP. Interferes with action of Ca^{2+} required for both muscle contraction and neuromuscular transmission
- Usually administered intravenously
  - therapeutic blood levels 4–8 mEq/L (5–10 mg/dl)
- Usual dosage
  - 4% IV solution (40 mg/L)
  - initial bolus 4–6 g over 20 min, then 1–3 g/h by continuous infusion
  - 10% IV solutions (100 g/L) as above
  - 50% solution (500 mg/ml) for IM use only; 10 g IM initially; 5 g q 4 h maintenance doses

DRUG EFFECTS

SYSTEM	EFFECT	ASSESSMENT BY HX	PE	TEST
CV	Vasodilation	Flushing, $\downarrow$ BP	BP $\downarrow$ Signs of shock, depressed CO	Blood level
	Myocardial depression Pulmonary edema	Bradycardia Asystole		ECG PA catheter
RESP	Muscle weakness	Dyspnea	Obstruction Hypoxia	ABG's, pulse oximetry, capnography
CNS	Depression	Cessation of convulsion	Somnolence	Blood level of Mg^{2+}
MS	Weakness, $\uparrow$ sensitivity to muscle relaxants	Respiratory obstruction, exaggerated response to small doses of muscle relaxants	Lethargy, weakness, depressed or absent deep tendon reflexes (DTR)	$\downarrow$ or absent DTR; high levels serum Mg^{2+} (should be <8 mEq/L); nerve stimulator
UTERINE	$\downarrow$ Strength and frequency of contractions	$\downarrow$ Pain, hemorrhage, failure to contract following delivery	Abdominal palpation of uterine activity	External or internal monitoring of uterine contractions

Key Reference: McGrath JM, Chestnut DH: Preterm labor and delivery; Writer D: Hypertensive disorders. *In* Chestnut DH, ed: Obstetric Anesthesia: Principles and Practice. St. Louis, Mosby-Year Book, 1994, pp 658–661 and pp 866–867, respectively.

PERIOPERATIVE IMPLICATIONS

Preoperative Concerns

- Assess respiratory adequacy, muscle strength before major conduction analgesia
- Avoid nondepolarizing muscle relaxant if possible
- Renal dysfunction may lead to accumulation and overdose with continued administration
- Pulmonary edema is possible

Monitoring

- Routine
- Nerve stimulator

Induction/Maintenance

- Intubate with full dose of succinylcholine (1 mg/kg)
- Avoid or use in very small doses the rapid-acting nondepolarizing muscle relaxant being guided by a nerve stimulator
- Continue during labor, delivery, postpartum in preeclampsia-eclampsia; discontinue in preterm labor when delivery is to occur
- Hypotension requiring therapy is common after both regional and general anesthesia

Adjuvants/Regional Anesthesia/Reversal

- May attenuate response to vasopressors
- Ca^{2+} may partially reverse CNS and CV effects, but not NM effects. Don't give Ca^{2+} in preeclampsia or eclampsia unless required for CV reasons

Postoperative/Postpartum Periods

- Preterm labor patients may develop pulmonary edema, especially if general anesthesia used
- Continue for delivery and postpartum in preeclampsia-eclampsia
- Assess respiratory adequacy before extubation

ANTICIPATED PROBLEMS/CONCERNS

- Development of pulmonary edema
- Incomplete NM reversal of nondepolarizing muscle relaxant
- Postpartum hemorrhage
- Exaggerated hypotensive response to major conduction anesthesia, potent inhalation anesthetics, and other antihypertensives
- MAC may be decreased

MARIJUANA

James P. Zacny, Ph.D.

USES

- In smoked form or as the resin (hashish), which is ingested, a DEA Schedule I drug of abuse with no medical indications
- In oral form as delta-9-tetrahydrocannabinol, or nabilone, a DEA Schedule II drug for chemotherapy-induced N/V

PERIOPERATIVE RISKS

- Overdose of marijuana can induce a paranoid state

WORRY ABOUT

- Acute effect includes tachycardia and ↑ systolic BP
- Chronic effect can include asthma or bronchitis and ↓ transport of secretions

OVERVIEW/PHARMACOLOGY

- Major active constituent is delta-9-tetrahydrocannabinol (THC), although contains other active cannabinoids
- Bioavailability of smoked and oral THC is 2–50% and 4–12%, respectively
- $T_{1/2}$ of THC is 30 h, because of its high lipid solubility
- Most of THC is metabolized; only a small fraction is excreted unchanged
- When smoked, produces a rapid onset of intoxication lasting 2–3 h; when ingested, duration of effect is 6 h
- With low–moderate doses, acute intoxication includes ↑ sense of well-being (euphoria), short-term memory and complex psychomotor impairment, depersonalization, time distortion (i.e., overestimation), ↑ sensation and perception of surrounding stimuli, ↑ hunger
- Physiologic changes include dry mouth and throat, marked reddening of the conjunctivae, ↓ IOP, ↑ HR, ↑ BP when supine, ↑ myocardial O_2 demand
- Overdosage may produce hallucinations, delusions, paranoid feelings
- In predisposed people, seizures can develop

ICD-9-CM Code: 304.3

DRUG CLASS/MECH OF ACTION/USUAL DOSE

- Cannabinoid: A cannabinoid receptor has been isolated in the CNS, indicative of endogenous cannabinoids
- Dosage depends on route of administration, especially with smoked marijuana
- Average THC content of marijuana in USA ranges from 0.5–11%

DRUG EFFECTS

SYSTEM	EFFECT	ASSESSMENT BY HX	PE	TEST
CV	Tachycardia, HTN	Chronicity and acuity of exposure	Vital signs	Urine toxicology screen
	Occasional orthostatic hypotension			
CNS	Intoxication, psychosis; ↓ IOP, antiemesis			

Key Reference: Jaffe JH: Marijuana. *In* Gilman AG, Rall TW, Nies AS, Taylor P (eds): Goodman and Gilman's The Pharmacological Basis of Therapeutics, 8th ed. New York, Macmillan, 1990, pp 522–573.

PERIOPERATIVE IMPLICATIONS/POSSIBLE DRUG INTERACTIONS

Preoperative Concerns

- Chronic use of smoked marijuana can cause bronchitis or asthma
- Tachycardia and drowsiness/sedation
- Ventilatory depression by opioids accentuated

Induction/Maintenance

- ↓ Anesthetic requirement (in animals) while intoxicated
- Barbiturate- and ketamine-induced sleep times may be prolonged
- Tachycardia and hypertension

Postoperative Period

- Pt may awaken in a state of agitation or psychosis
- Withdrawal usually mild

SPECIAL CONSIDERATIONS/CONCERNS

- Chronic use can lead to resp diseases, even in young adults
- Use associated with decreased learning 24 h later; may predispose to inadequate compliance with perioperative instructions

MEPIVACAINE (See also LIDOCAINE, BUPIVACAINE)   Stephan J. Cohn, M.D.

USES

- Used mainly for brachial plexus and peripheral nerve blocks
- Available in single-dose (30 ml) vial of 1.5% solution (preservative-free); multiple-dose (50 ml) vial of 1% and 2% solutions (contains methylparaben)

PERIOPERATIVE RISKS

- A true allergic reaction is rare (amide local anesthetic); adverse reactions usually related to high plasma concentrations or to additive components (e.g., epinephrine or preservative)

WORRY ABOUT

- Severe hypotension and apnea with accidental spinal or epidural injection
- CNS effects (seizures) with high plasma concentrations

OVERVIEW/PHARMACOLOGY

- Local anesthetic with fast onset, moderate penetrance, intermediate duration (90–180 minutes)
- $pKa = 7.6$; pH of plain solution = 4.5
- Plasma protein binding = 75%
- Volume distribution = 84 L; clearance = 0.78 L/min; elimination $T_{1/2}$ = 114 min
- Lacks vasodilator activity compared with lidocaine (useful choice when epinephrine is contraindicated)
- Metabolism: Undergoes hepatic microsomal enzyme degradation (hydroxylation and N-dealkylation); thus drug clearance ↓ with ↓ liver blood flow or liver disease

DRUG CLASS/MECH OF ACTION/USUAL DOSE

- Amide local anesthetic
- Non-ionized form penetrates axon membrane, becomes protonated and interferes with sodium channel, blocking nerve conduction
- Max single dose is 7 mg/kg
- Use 1.0–1.5% concentration for blockade of large nerve or plexus; 1% for epidural sensory blockade; 2% for epidural motor blockade

DRUG EFFECTS

SYSTEM	EFFECT	PE
CNS	Crosses blood-brain barrier, causing CNS excitation, then CNS depresssion	*Low plasma concentration:* restlessness, vertigo, tinnitus *Moderate plasma concentration:* slurred speech, skeletal muscle twitching *High plasma concentration:* convulsions, coma, cardiorespiratory arrest
PNS	Blockade of nerve conduction	Loss of sensation (and possible motor ability) in the area of blockade
VESSEL-RICH TISSUE	Numbness of tongue and circumoral tissue can result with low plasma concentrations	

Key Reference: Stoelting RK: Mepivacaine in local anesthetics. *In* Stoelting RK (ed): Pharmacology and Physiology in Anesthetic Practice. Philadelphia, JB Lippincott, 1987, pp 148–168.

PERIOPERATIVE IMPLICATIONS

Preoperative Concerns

- Reduce likelihood of toxic reactions by aspirating often, injecting slowly, using lowest dose (minimum concentration and volume) for desired block
- Educate patients to report early signs of toxicity (see CNS effects)

Induction/Maintenance

- Watch for objective signs of toxicity (see CNS effects); supplemental oxygen, ventilation and anticonvulsants may be needed
- Hypercarbia and acidosis ↓ threshold for convulsive activity; be especially alert with renal failure patients receiving narcotic and/ or benzodiazepine IV sedation!
- Preparation to treat cardiovascular and respiratory collapse

Adjuvants/Regional/Anesthesia Reversal

- With local anesthetics, toxicity is additive
- Methylparaben-containing solutions have been weakly associated with development of arachnoiditis in epidural/spinal anesthesia

Postoperative Period

- Monitor until risk of CNS toxicity is no longer of concern

METOCURINE IODIDE (METUBINE)

Stephen M. Rupp, M.D.

USES

- Used to:
  - produce skeletal muscle relaxation during anesthesia and surgery
  - prevent fasciculations before IV administration of succinylcholine
  - facilitate mechanical ventilation in ICUs

PERIOPERATIVE RISKS

- Inadequate respiratory function (hypoxia/hypoventilation) if ventilation not controlled or if unrecognized residual NMB at end of surgery
- Airway aspiration of oropharyngeal or gastric contents
- Histamine release resulting in hypotension may result if given rapidly in large doses (>0.3 mg/kg)
- Prolonged action in pts with renal failure or occult NM disease such as myasthenia gravis
- Synergism with other NMB drugs (especially steroidal muscle relaxants such as pancuronium)

WORRY ABOUT

- Synergism with steroidal relaxants
- Enhanced block with aminoglycoside (and other) antibiotics

OVERVIEW/PHARMACOLOGY

- Small doses (usually less than 0.03 mg/kg) have almost no effect because of a margin of safety (> 70% of receptors must be occupied for NMB block to be apparent)
- Onset time (time to peak effect) is dose-related (range 2–8 min)
- Duration is dose-dependent: a 0.3 mg/kg initial dose lasts ~70–90 min
- 90% is renal-eliminated; prolonged action in renal failure and extremes of age
- Virtually no hepatic elimination
- Elimination $T_{1/2}$ 80–100 min

- Requires anti-ChE (e.g., neostigmine) to antagonize residual NMB
- Interaction to enhance block with aminoglycosides, polymyxins, several other antibiotics; resistance to NMB in presence of antiepileptic drugs, e.g., phenytoin

DRUG CLASS/MECH OF ACTION/USUAL DOSE

- Benzylisoquinolinium (curare-like) skeletal muscle relaxant
- At motor end-plate competitively blocks binding of ACh to receptor (blocks opening of ionic channel necessary for depolarization of muscle membrane)
- At motor nerve terminal ↓ mobilization of ACh with repetitive nerve firing
- Usual dosage:
  Intubation: 0.3 mg/kg in ~3–5 min
  ED_{95} = 0.28 mg/kg

DRUG EFFECTS

SYSTEM	EFFECT	ASSESSMENT BY HX	PE	TEST
RESP	Inability to maintain airway, protect airway	Apnea		
NM	Paralysis	Weakness, diplopia, inability to swallow, airway obstruction, ventilatory inadequacy	Hand grip, head lift sustained ×5 sec	Peripheral nerve stimulation

Key Reference: Belmont MR, Maehr RB, Wastila WB, Savarese JJ: Pharmacodynamics and pharmacokinetics of benzylisoquinolinium (curare-like) neuromuscular blocking drugs. Anesthesiol Clin North Am 11:251–281, 1993.

PERIOPERATIVE IMPLICATIONS/POSSIBLE DRUG INTERACTIONS

Preoperative Concerns

- Occult NM disease
- Drugs (e.g., aminoglycosides) augmenting block?
- Conditions present—hypokalemia, hypocalcemia, metabolic alkalosis—augmenting block?
- Drugs (e.g., anticonvulsants) reducing effect?
- With renal failure or elderly pt prolonged blockade may result
- Duration of surgery? If a short case (<1 hour), a shorter acting drug (vecuronium) may be appropriate

Induction/Maintenance

- Maintenance of adequate intraoperative paralysis—1–2 twitches present in TOF
- To detect reversible block, at least 1 twitch present in TOF
- Adequate reversal or recovery from block = no fade of TOF and of double-burst stimulus/response
- Clinical bedside response of 5-sec head lift, 5-sec hand grasp sustained is best measure of recovery from NMB
- Doses > 0.3 mg/kg (given rapidly) may cause hypotension and bronchospasm as a result of histamine release
- Volatile anesthetics augment block in a dose-related fashion (1 MAC isoflurane augments block 30–50% over N_2O/narcotic anesthesia)
- Monitor thumb twitch: keep 1–2 twitches present to maintain adequate and reversible block

Reversal of NMB

- Only reverse if at least 1 twitch present in TOF
- Neostigmine 0.04–0.07 mg/kg combined with glycopyrrolate 0.1 mg/kg is best antagonist combination (AChE inhibitor plus anticholinergic)
- Edrophonium 0.5 mg/kg plus atropine 0.007 mg/kg is an inferior choice
- Expect 10–20 min to achieve full reversal
- "No fade" in double-burst stimulus/response is best twitch monitor of adequate reversal
- Clinical signs of adequate antagonism are most reliable:
  - sustained head lift ×5 sec
  - sustained hand grasp ×5 sec

ANTICIPATED PROBLEMS/CONCERNS

- NM monitors are insensitive to residual paralysis
- Consider residual paralysis early in assessment of postop respiratory distress
- Elderly pts and those with renal failure are at highest risk for residual paralysis

MIVACURIUM

RISK

- Homozygotes (incidence, 1/3000) for the atypical form of plasma cholinesterase will show a much prolonged effect, with paralysis lasting 2–4 h before recovery begins; dibucaine number = 30 or less
- Heterozygotes (1/30) will show a moderately lengthened response (about 10–15 minutes longer than usual); dibucaine number = 40–60
- Renal failure: duration may be lengthened by 10–15 min
- Hepatic disease: duration is lengthened by 30 min

PERIOPERATIVE RISKS

- Major risk is interaction with any concurrently administered drug that may reduce or inhibit the activity of plasma ChE—e.g., echothiophate (phospholine), bambuterol, etc.

WORRY ABOUT

- Conditions or drugs that reduce plasma ChE activity
- Decrease in BP, due to release of histamine, which may occur when large doses given for tracheal intubation are injected too rapidly (<10–15 sec)

OVERVIEW/PHARMACOLOGY

- Nondepolarizing NMB drug of the benzylisoquinolinium class
- Short duration of effect due to metabolism in plasma by plasma cholinesterase
- Metabolites are inactive
- ED_{95} = 70–80 µg/kg
- $T_{1/2}\beta$ = 2 min
- Clinical duration of action = 15–20 min; complete recovery, 30 min following intubating dosage (2–3 × ED_{95})

DRUG CLASS/MECH OF ACTION/USUAL DOSE

- Short-acting, nondepolarizing NMB drug of the benzylisoquinolinium class
- Not given chronically
- Acutely administered IV for surgical relaxation (tracheal intubation, maintenance of abdominal relaxation, correction of joint dislocation)
- Not given for maintenance of paralysis in ICU situations
- Usual dose:
  – tracheal intubation (adults): 200–250 µg/kg
  – "priming" dose (adults): 20 µg/kg
  – tracheal intubation (children): 300–400 µg/kg
  – maintenance of relaxation by IV infusion at 3–15 µg/kg/min (usually 5–8 µg/kg/min)
- Other alternatives: succinylcholine, other nondepolarizing NMB drugs—e.g., atracurium, pancuronium, curare, vecuronium, rocuronium, *cis*-atracurium
- Antagonists: neostigmine, edrophonium

DRUG EFFECTS

SYSTEM	EFFECT	ASSESSMENT BY HX	TEST
HEENT	Facial flush	Histamine release	Plasma histamine
CV	↓BP, ↑HR	Histamine release	Plasma histamine
GU	Metabolites are excreted in urine		
CNS	No effects of metabolites		
MS	No muscle pains		
			Dibucaine number, Plasma ChE activity

Key Reference: Savarese JJ, Ali HH, Basta SJ, et al: The clinical pharmacology of mivacurium chloride. Anesthesiology 1988; 68:723–732.

PERIOPERATIVE IMPLICATIONS/POSSIBLE DRUG INTERACTIONS

Preoperative Concerns

- Concurrent drug therapy may reduce plasma ChE activity (echothiophate [Phospholrine], bambuterol)
- Antihistamines (H_1 alone or H_1 + H_2 in combination, but not H_2 alone) inhibit symptoms of histamine release
- NSAIDs (aspirin, ibuprofen) also inhibit symptoms of histamine release

Induction /Maintenance

- "Priming" doses of 20 µg/kg may accelerate onset of mivacurium-induced blockade by about 30 sec
- Administration following succinylcholine does not affect duration of action
- Administration following most intermediate- or long-acting relaxants results in much longer duration of effect than expected (i.e., the kinetic pattern of the first relaxant has a marked effect on the duration of action of even small doses of mivacurium); consequently, this practice is not recommended

Adjuvants/Regional Anesthesia/Reversal

- Conventional antagonists are neostigmine (50 µg/kg) and edrophonium (500 µg/kg).
- Pseudo-ChE (in fresh frozen plasma) may be administered to accelerate recovery in individuals who show extremely slow recovery as a result of homozygous atypical plasma ChE genotype
- "Mycin" antibiotics potentiate NMB actions

SPECIAL CONSIDERATIONS

- Drugs, diseases, or conditions causing reduced plasma ChE activity
- Slower injection of large doses for tracheal intubation to prevent/reduce symptoms of histamine release

MONOAMINE OXIDASE INHIBITORS; REVERSIBLE INHIBITORS OF MONOAMINE OXIDASE

Kent Z. Ozkum, M.D.

USES

- Oral agents prescribed primarily for patients with depression refractory to other antidepressant agents
- Newer, reversible, agents may →wider use in treating depression, related disorders

PERIOPERATIVE RISKS

- Hepatotoxicity
- Peripheral sympathetic overactivation (hypertension, hypotension, tachycardia, hallucinations, agitation, resp depression, hyperthermia, seizures, coma)
- Orthostatic hypotension; mechanism unclear, possibly 2° to sympathetic *under*activity
- Central hyperpyrexia

WORRY ABOUT

- Sympathetic crisis
- Multiple drug interactions, including
  - foods: high tyramine- and dopamine-containing products often produced by aging, fermentation, pickling, smoking; broad (fava) beans (NB: tyramine acts as indirect sympathomimetic with release of norepinephrine at postganglionic sympathetic nerve endings); L-tryptophan, phenylalanine, tyrosine
  - indirect sympathomimetics, such as ephedrine
  - direct sympathomimetics (epinephrine, norepinephrine, amphetamines, cocaine, L-tryptophan, tyrosine, phenylalanine) may produce prolonged effect
  - uncommonly, *opioids,* especially dextromethorphan, pethidine, meperidine; 3 types interactions: excitatory—2° to serotonin overactivity; depressive—inhibition of hepatic microsomal enzymes, leading to accumulation of excess narcotic; febrile→coma
    - serotonin-uptake inhibitors (Prozac)
    - buspirone (Buspar)
    - bupropion (Wellbutrin)
    - excessive caffeine
    - antiparkinsonian agents (methyldopa, L-dopa)
    - numerous OTC formulations

OVERVIEW/PHARMACOLOGY

- Readily absorbed PO.
- Widely distributed enzyme system.
- Traditional agents bind covalently, →produce max enzyme inhibition 5–10 d; reversible agents have rapid onset (<1 h), short $T_{1/2}$ (~4 h)
- Large vol of distribution
- Clearance primarily hepatic; caution with concomitant cimetidine administration or hepatic dysfunction
- Most appear to have no clinically significant active metabolites
- Contraindications: known hypersensitivity, pheochromocytoma, liver dysfunction/disease, advanced HD, cerebrovascular disease; pts receiving antiparkinsonian agents, potent hypotensive agents, sedatives/CNS depressants

DRUG CLASS/MECH OF ACTION/USUAL DOSE

- Block oxidative deamination of amine-based neurotransmitters such as serotonin, dopamine, norepinephrine (A enzyme) and/or tyramine, phenethylamine (B enzyme) into VMA
- Antidepressant effects appear related to ↑ CNS neurotransmitter levels
- May be
  - hydrazine vs. nonhydrazine
  - A or B enzyme specificity: type A preferentially deaminates norepinephrine, epinephrine, serotonin; type B preferentially deaminates phenylethylamine. "Specific" agents appear to lack many side effects traditionally attributed to nonspecific MAO inhibitors, even in overdosage
  - reversible vs irreversible inhibitor; reversible agents bind noncovalently, have shorter duration of action; may be called RIMAs
  - traditional nonselective MAOIs bind covalently to enzyme, require up to 2 wk for new enzyme biosynthesis
- there may be down-regulation of α and/or β postsynaptic receptors
- no direct sedative, arrhythmogenic affects
- overdosage Rx includes α rb, β rb, ganglionicblockers, direct vasodilators, supportive care, mech ventilation, cooling, etc

DRUG EFFECTS

SYSTEM	EFFECT	ASSESSMENT BY HX	PE	TEST
CV	Sympathetic under-, overactivation	Duration Rx Discontinuation?	Orthostatics Vital signs stable	
CNS	Hyperthermia, agitation?, dizziness, headache, myoclonus		Normothermia?	
GI/LIVER	Constipation, dry mouth Low incidence of hepatotoxicity			LFTs

Key Reference: Hill S: MAOIs to RIMAs in anesthesia—a literature review. Psychopharmacology 1992; S43–S45.

PERIOPERATIVE IMPLICATIONS

Preoperative Concerns

- Check liver enzymes/LFTs
- Discontinue Rx?
  - enzyme inhibition may be either reversible or irreversible; if *irreversible* enzyme inhibition, discontinue drug 14–21 d before elective surgery—biosynthesis of new enzyme may take weeks. *Reversible* inhibition may not require discontinuation before anesthesia
  - specificity of agent in use: type A enzyme–specific agents appear to have fewer side effects, drug interactions of clinical significance
- Urgency of surgery
- Sx of toxicity?

Induction/Maintenance

- Avoid meperidine, H_2 release
- Possible accentuation of CNS/respiratory depression.
- may have prolonged response to succinylcholine 2° to ↓ serum ChE levels
- Anesthetic requirements may be ↑ by SNS hyperactivity
- Avoid SNS activation (anxiety, pain) when possible
- Avoid indirect-acting sympathomimetics
- Use of direct-acting sympathomimetics cautiously; response may be exaggerated.
- Consider regional anesthesia techniques
- MAOI may produce nonspecific hepatic microsomal inhibition, leading to ↓ clearance of anesthetic agents such as barbiturates; potentially ↑ risk of toxic (reductive) metabolites of halothane
- Avoid
  - ketamine 2° to potential for postop delirium/excitation/sympathetic activation
  - pancuronium 2° to mild epinephrine-releasing activity
- anticholinergics may produce clinical Sx similar to those from MAOI toxicity
- all local anesthetics appear safe except *cocaine*

Adjuvants/Regional Anesthesia/Reversal

- Regional anesthesia poss helpful.
- Antihypertensive agents should be readily available: consider α rbs as first-line agents (vs. β rb) to avoid unopposed α activity in combination with β-blockade

Postoperative Period

- Regional technique in use?
- Use narcotics cautiously

ANTICIPATED PROBLEMS/CONCERNS

- Sympathetic crisis
- Hepatotoxicity

NEOSTIGMINE

Peter Wright, M.D.
Dennis M. Fisher, M.D.

USES

- Perioperative use for reversal of NMB
- Chronic oral administration for treatment of myasthenia gravis

PERIOPERATIVE RISKS

- Parasympathomimetic effects common, require routine prophylactic antagonism
- May be associated with increased N/V
- Large doses may produce muscle weakness

WORRY ABOUT

- Increased effects from drugs metabolized by plasma ChE
- Bradycardia, possibly delayed

OVERVIEW/PHARMACOLOGY

- Potent inhibitor of AChE
- Also inhibits plasma ChE (pseudo-ChE)
- Increases cholinergic nervous transmission at NMJ, and at (muscarinic) autonomic effector sites
- Stimulates bladder and bowel contractions (antagonized by atropine)
- May produce bronchospasm
- Produces bradycardia (antagonized by atropine)
- Low oral bioavailability (oral dose is $30 \times$ IV dose)
- Destroyed by plasma esterases and excreted unchanged in the urine (67%)
- Elimination $T_{1/2} \beta = 77$ min; prolonged in renal failure to 181 min
- Clearance (typically 16.7 ml/kg/min) decreased in renal failure (7.8 ml/kg/min)

- Inhibits clearance of drugs metabolized by plasma ChE, notably, succinylcholine, mivacurium

DRUG CLASS/MECH OF ACTION/USUAL DOSE

- Type III (alternative substrate) AChE inhibitor
- Increases ACh concentrations in nerve terminals, NMJ
- Dose to antagonize nondepolarizing muscle relaxants:
  - adults   2.5–5.0 mg IV
  - children   35–70 µg/kg IV
- Dose regimen in myasthenia gravis:
  - 7.5–30 mg q 2–4 h PO (variable)

DRUG EFFECTS

SYSTEM	EFFECT	TEST
CV	Complex effects (bradycardia predominates)	Reversed by atropine
RESP	Bronchospasm	Reversed by atropine
GI	Increased peristalsis May influence the incidence of emetic symptoms	
NEURO	Reversal of weakness resulting from neuromuscular block or myasthenia gravis Excess dose may produce weakness	Electromyography

Key Reference: Rupp SM, McChristen J, Miller RD: Neostigmine and edrophonium antagonism of varying intensity of neuromuscular blockade by atracurium, pancuronium, or vecuronium. Anesthesiology 1986; 64:711–715.

PERIOPERATIVE IMPLICATIONS

Preoperative Concerns

- Neostigmine may be taken preop for the relief of symptoms of myasthenia gravis
  - Dose may need to be modified
  - Other cholinergic effects may be present (bradycardia, salivation)
  - Weakness may result from inadequate or excessive dose

Induction/Maintenance

- In myasthenia, muscle relaxant dosage will be reduced, or such agents may be unnecessary
- Anticholinergic (e.g., atropine) administration necessary to prevent muscarinic cholinergic effects

Adjuvants/Regional Anesthesia/Reversal

- The most common use for neostigmine is to reverse residual NMB after surgery
  - Neostigmine should be administered only after there is some evidence of neuromuscular transmission (may not antagonize very profound NMB; larger doses may contribute to muscle weakness)
  - Anticholinergic adminstration should always accompany administration of neostigmine (glycopyrrolate may be preferable to atropine; its time course of action better matches that of neostigmine)

ANTICIPATED PROBLEMS/CONCERNS

- Biochemical and acid-base derangements (particularly acidosis) may reduce effectiveness of neostigmine in reversing NMB.
- Reduces activity of plasma ChE and interferes with elimination of drugs that are cleared by plasma ChE (e.g., succinylcholine, mivacurium)

NICOTINE (TOBACCO, CIGARETTES, SNUFF)
NICOTINE REPLACEMENT THERAPIES
(NICORETTE [GUM], NICODERM [PATCH])

James P. Zacny, Ph.D.
Christopher J. Young, M.D.

RISK

- Inhalation of tobacco smoke (27+% of US citizens directly smoke, with 10+% exposed and absorb significant amounts via "secondhand smoke") but other sources of nicotine include gum (e.g., Nicorette), chewing tobacco, pipe smoking (absorption through buccal cavity), snuff (absorption through nasal cavity), transdermal nicotine patch (absorption through dermis)
- Nicotine gum and the patch are FDA-approved devices for the treatment of tobacco dependence

PERIOPERATIVE RISKS

- Adverse CV and RESP effects

WORRY ABOUT

- Whether to advise patients to stop smoking for several d before surgery; short-term abstinence may actually increase airway secretions and induce a bronchospastic state, and is associated with ↑ complications in 1st 6–8 wk of abstinence

OVERVIEW/PHARMACOLOGY

- $T_{1/2}$ of nicotine via inhaled tobacco smoke = 2 h
- 80–90% of nicotine is altered in liver and to lesser extent in kidneys and lungs
- Significant fraction of nicotine is metabolized in the lungs to cotinine and nicotine-1'-N-oxide
- Nicotine and its metabolites are rapidly eliminated by the kidneys
- Nicotine stimulates hepatic enzyme induction; results in faster metabolism of some anesthetics, sedatives, analgesics
- Drug has subtle subjective effects including, depending on circumstances and individual, stimulation or relaxation
- Withdrawal syndrome includes irritability and restlessness that can last up to 72 h; craving can last for months after cessation of smoking

ICD-9-CM Code: 305.1

DRUG CLASS/MECH OF ACTION/USUAL DOSE

- A natural alkaloid that stimulates autonomic ganglia
- Acts at the nicotinic cholinergic receptor as an agonist
- Dose used by a dependent smoker is 15–30 mg/d

DRUG EFFECTS

SYSTEM	EFFECT	ASSESSMENT BY HX	PE	TEST
CV	Tachycardia, HTN	Magnitude and duration of smoking	Clubbing, cyanosis	O_2 saturation
RESP	Hypersecretion of mucus	Presence of cough, degree of sputum production, coexisting cardiac disease, reversible pulm disease assessment	Sputum characteristics, retractions or resp compromise, bronchospasm	PFTs with bronchodilation
CNS	Stimulatory			
IMMUNE	↓ Neutrophil and NK cell activity, immunoglobulin concn			

Key Reference: Warner MA, Offord KP, Warner ME: Role of preoperative cessation of smoking and other factors in postoperative pulmonary complications: A blinded prospective study of coronary artery bypass patients. Mayo Clin Proc 1989; 64:609–616.

PERIOPERATIVE IMPLICATIONS/POSSIBLE DRUG INTERACTIONS

Preoperative Concerns

- Long-term abstinence (8 wk) should be encouraged, especially for thoracic surgery; it leads to improvement in mucociliary transport, small airway function, and ↓ in airway secretions and reactivity, but perioperative morbidity may transiently ↑ as mucociliary transport returns
- Short-term abstinence (24–48 h) has benefits including ↑ in hemoglobin available for O_2 transport and availability of O_2 to tissues, and ↓ in nicotine-induced tachycardia
- In some pts, excessive anxiety may occur in nicotine withdrawal

Induction/Maintenance

- Hypersecretion of mucus

POSTOPERATIVE PERIOD

- ↑ Risk of bronchospasm, purulent sputum with pyrexia, pleural effusion or pneumothorax requiring drainage, segmental pulmonary collapse, atelectasis, pneumonia
- ↑ Use of respiratory therapy care services (vigorous pulmonary toilet)
- Postop agitation/anxiety from nicotine withdrawal

SPECIAL CONSIDERATIONS

- Pts should be advised to quit smoking as early as possible
- For pts with increased anxiety, an anxiolytic can be prescribed or consider nicotine supplementation (transdermal patch)
- ↑ Risk of perioperative hypersecretion from short-term smoking abstinence can be countered by use of bronchodilators
- ↑ Risk of perioperative deep vein thrombosis from short-term smoking abstinence can be countered by anticoagulants, including aspirin 325 mg/d

NITRIC OXIDE, INHALED

W.M. Zapol, M.D.

INDICATIONS

- Children: persistent pulm HTN of newborn, congenital diaphragmatic hernia, meconium aspiration, before or after surgery for congenital heart disease, acute or chronic pulm HTN
- Adults: ARDS, pulm embolism, acute or chronic pulm HTN

PERIOPERATIVE RISKS

- Methemoglobinemia (esp breathing >100 ppm NO)
- NO_2 and peroxynitrite formation

WORRY ABOUT

- Methemoglobinemia; measure metHb every 12 h, esp for infants.
- Measure NO and NO_2 levels continuously.
- Do not breathe high NO_2 levels (>2 ppm)
- Do not leave NO in ventilator or anesthesia machine; it slowly converts to toxic NO_2 gas
- High inhaled NO levels may inhibit platelet aggregation
- In severe heart failure, reducing PVR with NO may raise LAP
- Rebound pulm HTN during NO withdrawal

OVERVIEW/PHARMACOLOGY

- Inhaled NO activates guanylate cyclase in lung vessels, airways ↑ cGMP levels, causes pulm vasodilation, bronchodilation
- Very rapid reaction with Hgb inactivates NO, prevents systemic vasodilation
- Inhaled NO becomes nitrate and nitrite, is excreted in urine
- Supplied as stock gas of ≤1,000 ppm by vol NO in nitrogen or other inert gas
- Mixed with O_2-containing gas immediately before breathing
- Gas inhaled via ventilator, mask, nasal prongs, intratracheal catheter

MECHANISM OF ACTION/DRUG/CLASS

- $N=O\cdot$ is a free radical with short $T_{1/2}$ in aqueous solutions (~17 sec)
- It combines with ferrous-heme ring of guanylate cyclase, activating it, thereby converting GTP to cyclic GMP; cGMP reduces intracellular Ca^{2+} causing smooth muscle relaxation; cGMP broken down by phosphodiesterases
- Usual inhaled NO dose is 0.1 to 100/ppm by vol

DRUG EFFECTS

SYSTEM	EFFECT	PE	TEST
RESP	↓ PVR		↓ PAP
			↑ CO
	↑ Gas exchange	Skin color	↑ PaO_2
			↑ SaO_2
			↓ $PaCO_2$

Key Reference: Zapol WM, Rimar S, Gillis N, et al: Nitric oxide and the lung. Am J Respir Crit Care Med 1994; 149:1375–1380.

PERIOPERATIVE IMPLICATIONS

- Check for heart failure; do not use in severe heart failure (e.g., PCWP >25 mmHg)

Monitoring

- Consider monitoring:
  - PA pressure
  - RV echo
  - ABGs, SpO_2
- Must monitor
  - Inhaled NO, NO_2 levels
- metHb levels

Induction/Maintenance

- Inhale 0.1–20 ppm in ARDS (usual dose: 5–15 ppm)
- In primary pulm HTN of newborn, begin near 20–40 ppm, slowly reduce to 5 ppm
- Ideal doses need better definition
- Breathe as little NO as possible to reduce oxidant burden of lung

Adjuvants

- Phosphodiesterase inhibitors (e.g., dipyridamole, Zaprinast) increase sensitivity to NO, duration of dilatory effect

Postoperative Period

- Slowly wean from NO over hours if possible

ANTICIPATED PROBLEMS/CONCERNS

- Beware rapid discontinuation of inhaled NO; reactive pulm vasoconstriction, RHF may ensue
- Do not allow NO stock tanks to run low
- Provide NO in gas to Ambu bag
- If inhaled NO does not reverse hypoxemia despite mechanical ventilation with PEEP, high-frequency oscillatory ventilation, etc., ECMO may be required

Lee A. Fleisher, M.D.

INDICATIONS

- Rx for patients with angina
- CHF
- In MI, ↓ infarct size
- Prinzmetal's angina
- Can be given as patch, paste, PO, sublingually prn
- Uterine relaxation

PERIOPERATIVE RISKS

- Development of hypotension
- Drug rash (rare)

WORRY ABOUT

- Severe hypotension, especially with regional anesthesia

OVERVIEW/PHARMACOLOGY

- Used for both chronic Rx and acute management
- Prophylactic nitroglycerin not shown to ↓ incidence of intraoperative myocardial ischemia in meta-analysis
- Tolerance to drug from prolonged IV infusion or continous patch can occur
- Metabolized by reductive hydrolysis in liver
- Rapidity of onset, duration of action directly related to method of administration
  - SL: onset 1–2 min, duration: <1 h
  - Oral: peak effect 60–90 min: duration 3–6 h
  - Paste—onset 60 min, duration: 4–8 h
  - Patch: duration up to 24 h
- Prolonged use can→tolerance (↓ effectiveness)
- Nitroglycerin paste/patch may have uneven absorption intraoperatively

DRUG CLASS/MECH OF ACTION/USUAL DOSE

- Organic nitrate
- Activates guanylate cyclase, ↑ cGMP levels in smooth muscle, other tissues; increases nitric oxide
- Usual dosage: SL—0.4 mg prn
  - paste—½"–1"
  - patch: 1qd
  - Isordil 5–30 mg q6h
  - IV 0.5–2.0 µg/kg/min
- Bolus for uterine relaxation (slow 50 µg; may repeat × 1 with caution if has regional anesthesia actively causing sympathectomy)

DRUG EFFECTS

SYSTEM	EFFECT	ASSESSMENT BY HX	PE	TEST
CV	Vasodilation of veins > arteries Redistribution of coronary blood flow	Relief of angina	BP	PCWP
RESP	Decreased pulmonary vascular resistance			PCWP
GU	Uterine (smooth muscle) relaxation			
CNS	Dilation of meningeal arterial vessels	Headache		

Key Reference: Murad F: *In* Gilman AG, Rall TW, Nies AF, Taylor P (eds): Goodman & Gilman's The Pharmacologic Basis of Therapeutics, 8th ed. New York, Pergamon, 1990, pp 764–774.

PERIOPERATIVE IMPLICATIONS

Preoperative Concerns

- Assess volume status
- Consider monitoring:
  - BP
  - PA catheter may give useful information if nitroglycerin infusion used

Induction/Maintenance

- May interact with other induction agents to cause hypotension
- Ideally should be given IV because of uneven absorption intraoperatively (binding sites on tubing)
- Effective means of alleviating myocardial ischemia intraoperatively
- Has been used prophylactically as bolus during induction
- Anesthetic agents may mimic beneficial effects of nitroglycerin

Adjuvants/Regional Anesthesia/Reversal

- Agents that can result in hypotension may be exacerbated by nitroglycerin

Postoperative Period

- Patients on chronic nitroglycerin may benefit by resumption of agent
- Can give as patch or paste after rewarming of patient

ANTICIPATED PROBLEMS/CONCERNS

- Tolerance to nitroglycerin manifests by ↓ hemodynamic effects; a function of dose, frequency of administration
- Many inhalational agents and opiates have some aspect of hemodynamic effects of nitroglycerin—e.g., venodilation, ↓ O₂ demand

NONSTEROIDAL ANTI-INFLAMMATORY DRUGS (NSAIDs)

Peter L. Bailey, M.D.

INDICATIONS

- 100 million US prescriptions/y; many additional taken through OTC route
- Taken orally for rheumatic disorders, pain states
- Given IM/IV for periop pain

PERIOPERATIVE RISKS

- 10% of all patients take NSAIDs
- Most common risks = gastric bleeding, renal dysfunction, impaired platelet function
- Drug interactions: NSAIDs displace albumin-bound drugs and/or ↓ drug elimination (e.g., warfarin, methotrexate)
- NSAIDs may ↓ antihypertensive agent efficacy

WORRY ABOUT

- Decreased NSAID clearance in elderly may ↑ adverse effects and ↑ drug interactions: especially warfarin, methotrexate, also lithium, phenytoin, digoxin, aminoglycosides, sulfonylurea hypoglycemic agents
- NSAIDs may ↓ antihypertensive agent efficacy

OVERVIEW/PHARMACOLOGY

- Weak organic acid compounds (nonionized) of diverse chemical structure and half-lives
- Well absorbed by GI tract, highly protein-bound (albumin mostly)
- Cyclooxygenase inhibition and ↓ prostaglandin synthesis lead to ↓ inflammatory response and ↓ nociception (peripheral and central action) and ↓ fever
- Clearance by hepatic metabolism and renal excretion, can accumulate with liver disease, age
- Displaces albumin-bound drugs (e.g., warfarin), increasing drug effect

DRUG CLASS/MECH OF ACTION/USUAL DOSE

- NSAIDs are cylooxygenase and prostaglandin synthesis inhibitors
- >12 NSAIDs available in the USA
- Ketorolac (Toradol) available for parenteral use; maximum loading dose = 1 mg/kg up to 60 mg; usual dose is 30 mg; ↓ dose in elderly; maintenance dose, ½ loading dose q 6 h, up to 5 d

Ibuprofen (Advil, Nuprin)

Ketorolac tromethamine (Toradol)

Acetylsalicylic acid (aspirin)

DRUG EFFECTS

SYSTEM	EFFECT	ASSESSMENT BY HX	PE	TEST
CV	Hypertension may be more difficult to control		BP	
RESP	Nasal polyps, rhinitis, dyspnea, bronchospasm	In asthmatics		
LIVER	Hepatitis			LFTs
GI	Gastropathy (can be asymptomatic) can develop in days to weeks, GI bleeding, esophageal disease, diarrhea, pancreatitis	Hx ulcers, heartburn		↑ Transaminase
ENDO	Angioedema, anaphylactoid reactions			
HEME	↑ Bleeding	Hx easy bruising/bleeding		Bleeding time, eosinophilia; rarely, aplastic anemia
SKIN	Urticaria, erythema multiforme, rash			
GU	Renal insufficiency, hyperkalemia, sodium/H_2O retention		BP	↑ K^+, BUN, Cr, ↓ UO, biopsy
CNS	Headache, aseptic meningitis, hearing disorders	Cognitive dysfunction, somnolence, confusion		CSF

Key Reference: Gardner GC, Simkin PA: Adverse effects of NSAIDs. Pharmacol Ther 199; 52:750–756.

PERIOPERATIVE IMPLICATIONS/DRUG INTERACTIONS

Preoperative Concerns

- GI bleeding, renal function, hemostasis

Monitoring

- Hct/Hgb, Cr/BUN/K^+, bleeding time

Drug Interactions

- Warfarin, sulfonylureas, phenytoin, valproic acid, digoxin, aminoglycosides, albumin-bound drugs (benzodiazepines)

Precautions

- ↓ Above drug doses, monitor blood levels, NSAIDs may ↓ antihypertensive drug efficacy

Resumption of Agent

- NSAIDs should be resumed cautiously with monitoring for GI bleeding, renal dysfunction. Avoid resumption in seriously ill patients

SPECIAL PROBLEMS/CONSIDERATIONS

- Gastropathy: occult bleeding
- Renal dysfunction: ↑ K^+
- Drug interactions, especially coumadin
- Hemostasis: bleeding time
- Miscellaneous and rare: hepatic dysfunction, pancreatitis, cutaneous reactions

NOREPINEPHRINE

Daniel M. Thys, M.D.

INDICATIONS

- Severe hypotension or shock secondary to vasodilation (e.g., septic shock or anaphylaxis)
- Cardiogenic shock

PERIOPERATIVE RISKS

- Severe vasoconstriction of renal and mesenteric vascular beds
- Peripheral tissue necrosis

WORRY ABOUT

- Reflex bradycardia
- Renal function decrement
- Increased cardiac pressure work leading to myocardial ischemia

OVERVIEW/PHARMACOLOGY

- Naturally occurring catecholamine
- Frequently used as peripheral vasoconstrictor of last resort to ↑ BP
- Venous return ↑ by venous constriction
- CO remains unchanged or may ↓
- Renal blood flow ↓
- $T_{1/2}$ short (2.5 min)
- Metabolized primarily by catechol O-methyltransferase in RBC

DRUG CLASS/MECH OF ACTION/USUAL DOSE

- α and β_1 receptor agonist
- Activates adenyl cyclase, which catalyzes conversion of ATP to cAMP; ↑ cAMP concn enhances availability, mobilization of intracellular Ca^{2+}

USUAL DOSE

- Always as an IV infusion (4 mg/250 ml); low dose (0.01–0.03 µg/kg/min): some β_1 effect
- Normal dose (0.03–0.1 µg/kg/min): predominantly α effect

DRUG EFFECTS

SYSTEM	EFFECT	ASSESSMENT BY HX	PE	TEST
CV	BP ↑ ↑ ↑ HR ↓ CO ↑ or ↓ SVR ↑ ↑ ↑ O_2 consumption ↑ ↑ ↑	Improved mental status	BP	CO SVR PCWP
GI/LIVER	Hepatic blood flow ↓ ↓ ↓ Hepatic drug metab ↓ ↓			
GU	Renal blood flow ↓ ↓ ↓		UO	BUN, Cr

Key Reference: Desjars P, Pinaud M, Potel G, et al: A reappraisal of norepinephrine therapy in human septic shock. Crit Care Med 1987; 15:134.

PERIOPERATIVE IMPLICATIONS

- Invasive monitoring is essential (arterial pressure, pulm art catheter)
- To ↓ effects on renal function, consider combination with dopamine
- Plasma levels of drug metabolized by liver (e.g., lidocaine) will ↑ with potential for toxicity.

ANTICIPATED PROBLEMS/CONCERNS

- Myocardial ischemia
- Renal failure
- Organ ischemia
- Tissue necrosis

NUTRITIONAL SUPPORT

Terrence H. Liu, M.D.
Jerome H. Abrams, M.D.

RISK

• 3–5% of patients malnourished preop; elderly at greater risk (20% of patients >85 y malnourished)

PERIOPERATIVE RISKS OF MALNUTRITION

• ↓ Resp, cardiac, skeletal muscle mass, strength
• ↓ Visceral protein mass, altered GI mucosal barrier
• Altered humoral, cell-mediated immunity
• Altered neutrophil function
• ↑ Pulm, thromboembolic complications
• Patients with protein-calorie malnutrition have ↑ risk for postop cardiac, noncardiac complications

WORRY ABOUT

• Hypo- or hyperglycemia, depending on additives to TPN

OVERVIEW

Nutritional risk index (NRI) = 1.519 × serum albumin (g/L) + [0.417 × (current wt/usual wt) × 100] (Malnutrition defined as NRI < 100; severe malnutrition defined as NRI < 83.5)
• Preop nutritional support for 5–7 d may result in ↓ in infectious complications in severely malnourished patients

TPN Composition

• Fluid: 30 ml/kg/d, additional losses
• Calories: 25–30 Kcal/kg/d
  – glucose: 3.0–5.0 g/kg/d
  – fat: 1.0–1.5 g/kg/d
  – protein: 1.5–2.0 g/kg/d
• Additives:
  – multivitamins in the form of balanced formula should be provided daily
  – IV formula requires addition of vitamin K, 2 mg/d
  – Trace elements should be given daily to patients with GFR >20 ml/d: Magnesium: 15–20 mg/d; Zinc: 15–20 mg/d (Requirement for replacement is based on serum level)

ICD-9-CM Code: 261 (Malnutrition)

Special Formulas

• Modified amino acid formula is more efficient in restoring positive nitrogen balance, ↓ ureagenesis, and ↑ support of protein synthesis

ASSESSMENT POINTS

SYSTEM	EFFECT	ASSESSMENT BY HX	PE	TEST
MS	>10% loss of body wt over 6 mo	Hx of renal, hepatic dysfunction Hx short gut	Muscle-wasting ↓ Triceps and skinfold thickness	Alb <3.0 g/dl Total lymphocyte count <1500 cells/mm³

Key References: The VA Total Parenteral Nutrition Cooperative Study Group: Perioperative total parenteral nutrition in surgical patients. N Engl J Med 1991; 325, 8:525; Barton RG: Nutritional support in critical illness. Nutr Clin Pract 1994; 9:127–139.

PREOPERATIVE CONCERNS

Monitoring

• Monitoring is essential to maximize benefit and to minimize complications
• Weight: daily
• Electrolytes: daily initially
• Zinc: weekly
• Magnesium: daily
• Liver function test: weekly
• PT/PTT: weekly
• Nutritional variable: Albumin, prealbumin, transferrin. Failure to improve or maintain adequate levels usually represents inadequate nutritional support, intercurrent systemic inflammatory response, or advanced organ failure

INDUCTION/MAINTENANCE

• TPN is usually continued intraoperatively
• Monitor glucose

ADJUVANTS

• For morbidly obese patients use ideal wt for calculation of TPN requirement
• For severely underweight patients use ½ difference between patient's ideal weight and actual weight

ANTICIPATED PROBLEMS/CONCERNS

• Caloric and glucose overload can result in hyperglycemia and hepatic dysfunction
• Fat overload can result in WBC dysfunction and infectious complication

OKT3 (MUROMONAB-CD3)

Steven Roth, M.D.

USES

• Patients undergoing solid organ transplantation, especially kidney

RISKS

• OKT3 (muromonab-CD3) causes (often after 1st dose) fever and chills, headache, N/V, tachycardia, hypertension, seizures, dyspnea
• Patients most likely to develop intraoperative reactions are those with hypovolemia, patients receiving volatile anesthetic agents, therapy with β or Ca channel antagonists, or phenytoin, or receiving increased OKT3 dose (recommended dose, 5 mg IV)
• Rate of administration does not affect incidence of reactions
• Steroids, antihistamines, acetaminophen do not alter incidence of reactions

WORRY ABOUT

• With intraoperative administration, usual signs may be masked, instead manifest as hypotension and bradycardia, acute pulm edema, cardiac arrest

OVERVIEW/PHARMACOLOGY

• Used to prevent, treat rejection; T cells react with OKT3 and are removed from circulation in liver or spleen
• Effect on immune system lasts 24–48 h
• T cells mediate rejection of transplanted kidneys; OKT3 about 95% effective in treating allograft rejection
• Actual incidence of intraoperative reactions unknown
• Adverse responses = result of immune reactions; T cells stimulated by binding of OKT3 to produce cytokines, which cause WBCs to release leukotrienes with CV responses and ↑ pulm vascular permeability
• Destruction of T cells after OKT3 binding releases prostaglandins

USUAL TREATMENT

• Depends on reaction
• Treat pulm edema with fluid restriction, PEEP, diuretics; hypotension, bradycardia with vasopressors, inotropes

DRUG EFFECTS

SYSTEM	EFFECT	ASSESSMENT BY HX/PE	TREATMENT
CV	Bradycardia, hypotension	ECG, BP	Inotropes, vasopressors
RESP	Pulm edema, wheezing	Clinical exam Sao_2	Diuretics, PEEP Bronchodilators
CNS	Seizures	Clinical exam	Prevention: phenytoin Rx: Support airway, benzodiazepines

Key Reference: Roth S, Kupferberg JP: Adverse responses following intraoperative administration of orthoclone OKT3. Anesth Analg 1989; 69:822–825.

POSSIBLE DRUG INTERACTIONS

• Watch for
  – particular attention to Sao_2 and hemodynamics after IV administration
  – reaction may occur immediately or within 1 h after OKT3 given
  – arterial catheter helpful for rapid detection of reaction
  – Especially watch patient receiving the 1st dose of OKT3 intraoperatively
• Administer
  – phenytoin prophylaxis preoperatively to prevent seizures
• Avoid
  – fluid overload
  – high concentration of inhalational anesthetic agent

ORAL CONTRACEPTIVES

Tracey L. Stierer, M.D.

USES

- 25–33% premenopausal women in USA
- For desired infertility
- To attenuate dysmenorrhea
- Administered PO

PERIOPERATIVE RISKS

- ↑ in venous thrombosis (especially if blood group A+)
- Drug interactions may increase theophylline levels by 30%

WORRY ABOUT

- Although highly effective in preventing pregnancy, β-hCG should be considered in sexually active patient

OVERVIEW/PHARMACOLOGY

- Synthetic estrogen (ethinyl estradiol or mestranol) combined with a progestin (norethindrone, ethynodiol diacetate, norgestrel, levonorgestrel): e.g., Ortho-Novum, Triphasil
- Progestin alone (norgestrel): e.g., Ovrette, Micronor
- For prevention of pregnancy, ↓ incidence and severity of dysmenorrhea
- Oral preparations of synthetic estrogen, progestin generally well absorbed with variable bioavailability
- Primarily metabolized in liver, excreted in urine and feces as glucuronides

DRUG CLASS/MECH OF ACTION/USUAL DOSE

- Combination synthetic estrogen with progestin; progestin alone
- Combination oral contraceptives inhibit ovulation by negative feedback effect on hypothalamus, altering normal pattern of gonadotropin secretion by anterior pituitary; cervical mucus thickens, is unfavorable to sperm even if ovulation occurs. Progestin-only oral contraceptive may act by directly inhibiting ovulation or creating thick cervical mucus that is impenetrable to sperm
- Combination oral contraceptives taken for 21 d of cycle followed by 1 wk without medication; most contain 7 inactive pills, so medication can be taken daily
- Combination oral contraceptives are available in low-dose, <50 μg estrogen, or high-dose, 50 μg estrogen
- Low-dose combination preparations may have constant (monophasic) or variable (biphasic, triphasic) doses of estrogen, progestin, depending on number of dosing regimens within cycle

DRUG EFFECTS

SYSTEM	EFFECT	ASSESSMENT BY HX	PE	TEST
CV	↑ Thromboembolic phenomena, including DVT, pulmonary emboli Slight ↑ in systolic and/or diastolic BP	Prior Hx of DVT	Deep vein exam	
GI/LIVER	May excerbate gallbladder disease ↑ Incidence of hepatic adenomas ↑ Incidence of hepatocellular cancer	Hx of jaundice/cholestatic during pregnancy		↑ Cholesterol
ENDO	May ↑ serum glucose levels ↑ Thyroxine-binding globulin			↑ Glucose ↑ T_4 ↓ T_3 resin uptake

PERIOPERATIVE IMPLICATIONS

- Consider discontinuing oral contraceptives within 1 mo before or after major elective surgery or immediately preoperatively because of ↑ risk of thromboembolism or administration of prophylaxis for DVT
- Consider low-dose heparin Rx when cannot discontinue oral contraceptives before surgery
- Oral contraceptives mayQtheophylline elimination by up to 30%, thus increasing serum concentrations

ORAL HYPOGLYCEMICS

Christopher D. Beatie, M.D.

USES

- Two classes of agents: sulfonylureas and biguanides (metformin)
- Rx for noninsulin-dependent diabetes mellitus (NIDDM) not controlled by diet or weight loss (~14 million patients in USA)
- $480 million spent on oral hypoglycemics (>4 million persons received prescriptions) in 1990

PERIOPERATIVE RISKS

Sulfonylureas

- Hypoglycemia
- N/V
- Cholestatic jaundice
- Agranulocytosis
- Aplastic, hemolytic anemias
- Alcohol-induced flushing (similar to disulfiram) especially with chlorpropamide 10–15%
- Enhanced ADH actions—reduction in urine vol, hyponatremia especially with chlorpropamide, tolbutamide—up to 5% of patients

Metformin

- Lactic acidosis
- N/V
- Anorexia
- Diarrhea

WORRY ABOUT

Sulfonylureas

- May be potentiated by the following agents: sulfonamides, chloramphenicol, propranolol, clofibrate, warfarin, salicylates, phenylbutazone, probenecid, MAO inhibitors, ethanol

Metformin

- Concentration may be ↑ by cimetidine
- Can ↓ absorption of vit B_{12}, folate, resulting in deficiency

OVERVIEW/PHARMACOLOGY

- **Sulfonylureas:** 1st generation: tolbutamide, acetohexamide, tolazamide, chlorpropamide; 2nd generation: glyburide, glipizide
  - *clearance:* various metabolic pathways followed by renal excretion; chlorpropamide is only partially metabolized (20% excreted unchanged in urine)
- **Biguanides:** metformin, phenformin (latter taken off market, 1976—high incidence of lactic acidosis)
  - *clearance:* renal excretion; no metabolism; metformin can also cause lactic acidosis when concentrations are ↑ as in renal insufficiency

DRUG CLASS/MECH OF ACTION/USUAL DOSE

- **Sulfonylureas** lower blood glucose by stimulating islet cells to secrete insulin, ↑ insulin sensitivity of peripheral tissues
  - Usual daily dose: acetohexamide, 500–750 mg; chlorpropamide, 250–375 mg; tolazamide, 250–500 mg; tolbutamide, 1000–2000 mg, glipizide, 10–20 mg; glyburide, 5–20 mg
- **Metformin** ↓ hepatic glucose production, ↑ glucose uptake, does not cause clinical hypoglycemia, has no effect on pancreatic insulin secretion, requires presence of insulin to be effective. Metformin can be used concurrently with a sulfonylurea. When endogenous secretion of insulin adequate, can be used alone to overcome insulin resistance
  - Usual daily dose: 1700 mg

DRUG EFFECTS

SYSTEM	EFFECT	ASSESSMENT BY HX	PE	TEST
OVERALL (Metformin)	Lactic acidosis			Lactate
ENDO (Sulfonylureas)	Hypoglycemia	Altered mental status, convulsions, coma	Sweating, tachycardia	Glucose
SKIN (Sulfonylureas)	Alcohol-induced flushing			
GU (Sulfonylureas)	Antidiuresis	↓ Urine volume	Edema	Na^+
TOXICITY				
GI (All) (Sulfonylureas) (Metformin)	N/V Cholestasis Diarrhea, anorexia		Jaundice	Electrolytes Bilirubin
HEME (Sulfonylureas) (Metformin)	Agranulocytosis; aplastic, hemolytic anemias Megaloblastic anemia	Fatigue, weakness	Pallor	CBC Vit B_{12}, folate

Key Reference: Med Lett Drugs Ther 1995; 37:948.

PERIOPERATIVE IMPLICATIONS

Preoperative Concerns

- Generally withhold sulfonylureas day of surgery while patients NPO, to avoid hypoglycemia
- Patients with NIDDM usually do not have fasting hyperglycemia and are not ketosis-prone
- Hold metformin before major surgery to ↓ risk of lactic acidosis

Induction/Maintenance

- Blood sugar measurements required frequently in periop period; use regular insulin to control hyperglycemia as needed until patient able to resume oral agent

SPECIAL CONSIDERATIONS

- Sulfonylureas can cause significant hypoglycemia if administered to NPO patients not receiving dextrose-containing IV solutions; NIDDM patients do not usually have fasting hyperglycemia and are not ketosis-prone, so little risk in holding these agents day of surgery
- Metformin does not cause clinical hypoglycemia, so can be given safely while patients NPO. However, because major surgery may be associated with acidotic states and periop renal dysfunction, withhold metformin before major surgery to ↓ risk of lactic acidosis
- Sulfonylureas potentiated by variety of other drugs as noted

PANCURONIUM BROMIDE

Stephen M. Rupp, M.D.

INDICATIONS

- Produces skeletal muscle relaxation during anesthesia, surgery
- Prevents fasciculations before IV administration of succinylcholine
- Facilitates mechanical ventilation in ICU

PERIOPERATIVE RISKS

- Inadequate resp function (hypoxia/hypoventilation) if ventilation not controlled or if unrecognized residual NMB at end of surgery
- Airway aspiration of oropharyngeal or gastric contents
- Tachycardia if large doses (> 0.1 mg/kg) given rapidly
- Prolonged action if renal failure or occult NM disease (e.g., myasthenia gravis)
- Synergism with other NMB drugs (especially benzyl-isoquinolinium compounds [e.g., curare or metocurine])

WORRY ABOUT

- Tachycardia (dose-related)
- Ventricular ectopy if combined with halothane, tricyclics
- Precipitates in IV line if combined with base
- May exacerbate tachycardia induced by aminophylline

OVERVIEW/PHARMACOLOGY

- Small doses (usually < 0.007 mg/kg) have almost no effect because for safety margin, >70% of receptors must be occupied for NMB to be apparent
- Onset time to peak effect dose-related (range, 2–8 min)
- Duration dose-dependent: 0.1 mg/kg initial dose lasts ~60–75 min
- 60% renal-eliminated (prolonged action in renal failure and age extremes)
- 40% hepatic uptake, hepatic transformation; 10% in bile

- Some metabolites have NMB action
- Elimination $T_{1/2}$ 90–120 min
- Requires AChE (e.g., neostigmine) administration to antagonize residual NMB if present
- Enhanced block with aminoglycosides, polymixins, several other antibiotics, volatile anesthetics; resistance in presence of antiepileptic drugs

DRUG CLASS/MECH OF ACTION/USUAL DOSE

- Steroidal nucleus bisquaternary skeletal muscle relaxant
- At motor end-plate, competitively blocks binding of ACh to receptor (blocks opening of ionic channel necessary for depolarization)
- Usual dosage: intubation: 0.1 mg/kg; ED_{95} = 0.06-0.07 mg/kg

DRUG EFFECTS

SYSTEM	EFFECT	ASSESSMENT BY HX	PE	TEST
RESP	Inability to maintain, protect airway	Apnea		
NM	Paralysis	Weakness, diplopia, inability to swallow, airway obstruction, ventilatory inadequacy	Hand grip sustained, head lift sustained, ×5 sec†	Peripheral nerve stimulation*

*Measurement of response of thumb to train-of-four stimulation of the ulnar nerve; fade of train-of-four leads to weakness, inability to protect and maintain airway.
†Clinical bedside response of 5-sec head lift and 5-sec hand grasp sustained is best measure of recovery.

Key Reference: Ducharme J, Donati F: Pharmacokinetics and pharmacodynamics of steroidal muscle relaxants. Anesthesiol Clin North Am 1993; 11:283–307.

PERIOPERATIVE IMPLICATIONS/POSSIBLE DRUG INTERACTIONS

Preoperative Concerns

- Occult neuromuscular disease
- Other drugs augmenting block (e.g., aminoglycosides)
- Other conditions augmenting block (hypokalemia, hypocalcemia, metabolic alkalosis)
- Drugs (e.g., anticonvulsants) reducing effect
- Renal failure or elderly patient may result in prolonged blockade
- Duration of surgery (In a short case [< 1 h] shorter-acting drug [e.g., vecuronium] may be appropriate)

Induction/Maintenance

- Dose > 0.1 mg/kg causes tachycardia and risks myocardial ischemia
- In combination with high-dose narcotic, counteracts vagotonic effects of narcotics
- Volatile anesthetics augment NMB in dose-related fashion (1 MAC isoflurane augments NMB 30–50% > N_2O/narcotic anesthesia)
- Least expensive of all nondepolarizing drugs

- Monitor thumb twitch: keep 1–2 twitches present to maintain adequate, reversible blocks
- Maintenance of adequate intraoperative paralysis = 1–2 twitches present in train-of-four
- Reversible block = at least 1 twitch present in train-of-four
- Adequate reversal or recovery from block = no fade of train-of-four, no fade of double-burst stimulus/response

Reversal of NMB

- Reverse only if at least 1 twitch present in train-of-four
- Neostigmine, 0.04–0.07 mg/kg, combined with glycopyrrolate, 0.1 mg/kg, best antagonist combination (AChE inhibitor plus anticholinergic)
- Expect 10–20 min to achieve full reversal
- "no fade" in double-burst stimulus/response is best twitch monitor of adequate reversal
- Clinical signs of adequate antagonism are most reliable
  – sustained head-lift, sustained hand-grasp ×5 sec

Postoperative Period

- Prolonged use in ICU associated with initial resistance then prolonged paralysis; steroid-induced polyneuropathy or myopathy? Reduced elimination? Unpredictable behavior of drug in complicated metabolic and electrolyte environment

ANTICIPATED PROBLEMS/CONCERNS

- Many clinical NMB monitors are insensitive to residual paralysis; entertain residual paralysis early in assessment of postop respiratory distress
- Elderly and those with renal failure are at highest risk for residual paralysis

PENICILLINS

Lucy Waskell, M.D., Ph.D.

USES

• Prescribed for patients with infections by sensitive organisms, primarily pneumococci and those in genera *Streptococcus, Staphylococcus, Pseudomonas, Proteus, Haemophilus,* etc; used as prophylaxis for subacute bacterial endocarditis (penicillin G benzathine)
• Can be administered PO, IM as regular or slow-release repository form, or IV

WORRY ABOUT

• Hypersensitivity reactions: rash, fever, bronchospasm, vasculitis, angioedema, anaphylaxis
• Hyperkalemia when K$^+$ penicillin G is administered IV (1.7 mEq K$^+$/MU penicillin G)
• Platelet dysfunction, defective hemostasis after carbenicillin
• Headaches, seizures after 1 dose of 5 MU of penicillin G procaine

OVERVIEW/PHARMACOLOGY

• Used to treat wide spectrum of infectious diseases
• Many penicillins are acid-labile; not administered orally
• Actively, rapidly excreted by renal tubules
• T½ of penicillin markedly increased in anuria, in which liver inactivates and excretes drug into bile
• Dosage should be ↓ in renal failure
• Other organic acids, e.g., probenecid, can compete at the renal tubule for excretion, prolonging the sojourn of antibiotic in body

DRUG CLASS/MECH OF ACTION/USUAL DOSE

• Penicillins are organic acids consisting of b-lactam ring to which is attached a side chain and a thiazolidine ring; prevent bacterial cell wall synthesis by inhibiting transpeptidase reaction
• Dose, route of admin depend on penicillin used, severity of disease treated

DRUG EFFECTS

DRUG	ABSORPTION AFTER ORAL ADMIN	RESISTANCE TO PENICILLINASE	DOSE IV	ANTIMICROBIAL SPECTRUM	SPECIFIC SIDE EFFECTS
Penicillin G	Poor ~ 1/3 of dose	No	1–10 MU	*Streptococcus, Neisseria*	Hyperkalemia 1.7 mEq K$^+$/MU Pen G; > 20MU/day can cause seizures; large doses may inhibit platelet aggregation
Methicillin	Poor	Yes	1.5–3 g q6h	*Staphylococcus aureus*	
Oxacillin	Good	Yes	0.5–3 g q6h		
Cloxacillin	Good	Yes	250–500 mg po q6h	*Staphylococcus aureus*	
Dicloxacillin	Good	Yes	250–500 mg po q6h		
Nafcillin	Variable	Yes	6–9 g q4h	*Staphylococcus aureus*	
Ampicillin	Good	No	1–2 g q6h	*Haemophilus influenzae*	
Amoxicillin	Good	No	0.75–1.5 g po q8h	*P. mirabilis, E. coli*	
Carbenicillin	Poor	No	7.5–10 g q6h	Same as ampicillin plus *Pseudomonas*	CHF 2° to Na$^+$ overload; 5 mEq Na$^+$/g; low K$^+$ 2° to obligatory cation excretion with anion; ↓ in platelet aggregation
Ticarcillin	Poor	No	50–75 mg/kg q6h	Same as carbenicillin	Same as carbenicillin 5 mEq Na$^+$/g
Piperacillin	Poor	No	2–6 g q8h	*Pseudomonas, Enterobacter,* some *Klebsiella*	Same as carbenicillin 2 mEq Na$^+$/g

Key Reference: Mandell GL, Sande MA: *In* Gilman AG, Rall TW, Nies AS, Taylor P (eds): Goodman & Gilman's The Pharmacologic Basis of Therapeutics, 8th ed. New York, Pergamon, 1990, pp. 1065–1085.

PERIOPERATIVE IMPLICATIONS

Preoperative Concerns

• Is patient allergic to any penicillins? What exactly happens when the drug is taken (rash vs. anaphylaxis)?
• If patient on large doses of antibiotics, penicillin G, carbenicillin, ticarcillin, or piperacillin, are serum electrolytes normal?
• Hemostasis, especially platelet aggregation, may be inhibited by the antibiotics

• If patient is in renal failure, dose of antibiotic should be ↓

Induction/Maintenance/Postoperative Period

• Penicillins should have no effect on induction or maintenance unless allergic reaction occurs; no known interactions with any anesthetic agents

ANTICIPATED PROBLEMS/CONCERNS

• Relate to administration of large amounts of Na$^+$, K$^+$, and organic anions (acids), possible bleeding problems due to platelet dysfunction

PHENCYCLIDINE (PCP)

James P. Zacny, Ph.D.

RISK

- DEA Schedule I drug of abuse with no medical indications
- In past used as anesthetic in humans and animals (Sernylan)
- Common routes of administration: snorting, smoking (often laced in marijuana cigarettes), oral ingestion; less common is IV injection
- More severe symptoms found with oral and injected routes

PERIOPERATIVE RISKS

- Acute intoxication, including aggressive and/or psychotic behavior may require premedication with sedative or antipsychotic

WORRY ABOUT

- High doses can produce anesthesia, coma, convulsions

OVERVIEW/PHARMACOLOGY

- Effects due to parent compound, although metabolites are active
- $T_{1/2}$, 3 d
- Highly lipid soluble, pK_a of 8.6
- Metabolized in the liver; urinary excretion of metabolites at low doses, excretion of free drug at high doses
- Only small fraction of the drug excreted unchanged
- Produces an acute state of intoxication lasting 4–6 h, may produce a chronic state of psychosis that can last for up to several wk
- With low-moderate doses, acute intoxication includes staggering gait, slurred speech, nystagmus, numbness of extremities, sweating, catatonic muscular rigidity, blank stare, changes in body image, disorganized thought, drowsiness, apathy, anterograde amnesia, possibly aggressive behavior
- With moderate-high doses, Sx can include elevated HR, BP, hypersalivation, sweating, fever, repetitive movements, muscle rigidity on stimulation
- With high doses, anesthesia, stupor, coma, convulsions can occur

DRUG CLASS/MECH OF ACTION/USUAL DOSE

- Arylcyclohexylamine
- Acts at the N-methyl-D-aspartate receptor as a noncompetitive antagonist
- Chronic user dose may be up to 1 g/d

DRUG EFFECTS

SYSTEM	EFFECT	ASSESSMENT BY HX	PE	TESTS
CV	Tachycardia, HTN	Quantification, chronicity, acuity of drug exposure	Vital signs	Blood, urine toxicology screens
RESP	Depression	Concurrent drug exposure (e.g., alcohol)	Resp rate	
CNS	Intoxication, psychosis, coma, convulsions, ↓ anesthetic requirement			
ANS	Hypersalivation Fever		Observation, T	

Key Reference: Gilman AG, Rall TW, Nies AS, Taylor P (eds): Goodman & Gilman's The Pharmacological Basis of Therapeutics, 8th ed. New York, Pergamon Press, 1990, pp 557–558.

PERIOPERATIVE IMPLICATIONS/POSSIBLE DRUG INTERACTIONS

Preoperative Concerns

- Concern about psychosis, hypersalivation, respiratory depression, fever, convulsions
- Steps to increase elimination of PCP from body
  - acidification of urine (tripled excretion rate)
  - interrupt considerable gastroenteric recirculation by continuous gastric suction
- Adequate sedation of patient

Induction/Maintenance

- Ketamine contraindicated as part of anesthetic regimen (cross-tolerance)
- Level of intoxication may lessen anesthetic, analgesic requirement

Postoperative Period

- Patient may awaken in state of intoxication, agitation, or psychosis

SPECIAL CONSIDERATIONS/CONCERNS

- Significant rhabdomyolysis, myoglobinuria may induce renal failure, can be exacerbated by continuous gastric suction, acidification of urine
- Tolerance, withdrawal

PHENOTHIAZINES

Jeffrey K. Lu, M.D.
Theodore H. Stanley, M.D.

USES

- Prescribed for patients with acute and chronic psychiatric disorders, most commonly, but not exclusively, schizophrenia, mania
- Prescribed for patients as antiemetic drug
- Prescribed for acutely agitated and possibly violent patients

PERIOPERATIVE RISKS

- ↓ Cerebral blood flow; does not affect cerebral metabolic rate
- May cause severe hypertension in patients with pheochromocytoma
- Dysphoria: Patients receiving antipsychotic drugs may outwardly appear calm and sedated when inwardly they are experiencing overwhelming fear

WORRY ABOUT

- Exaggerated sedation or ventilatory depression in patients receiving opioids or ethanol
- Patients on phenothiazines may also be resistant to exogenous dopamine

OVERVIEW/PHARMACOLOGY

- Strongly protein-bound
- ß elimination $T_{1/2}$: 10–20 h
- Metabolized by oxidation in liver
- Metabolites inactive except for 7-hydroxychlorpromazine
- Related drug classes include butyrophenones (droperidol, haloperidol), thioxanthines

DRUG CLASS/MECH OF ACTION/USUAL DOSE

- Causes dopamine receptor blockade in limbic region and basal ganglia of brain
- Erratic, unpredictable absorption from oral administration
- Highly lipid-soluble, accumulates in well-perfused tissues such as brain
- Usual dose: droperidol 10–75 µg/kg IV for nausea; haloperidol: 10 mg IM/IV for agitation

DRUG EFFECTS

SYSTEM	EFFECT	ASSESSMENT BY HX	PE	TEST
HEENT	Acute dystonia	Acute administration of phenothiazines		
CV	Orthostatic hypotension; prolonged P-R and Q-T intervals, S-T segment depression		Orthostasis	ECG
GI	Allergic-induced obstructive jaundice	Usually 2–4 wk of use	Scleral icterus	Elevated direct bilirubin
ENDO	↑ Prolactin production ↓ Corticosteroid synthesis ↓ Insulin production		Gynecomastia	
CNS	Tardive dyskinesia, sedation, altered temperature regulation, lowers seizure threshold	Long-term use	Purposeless, involuntary movements (lip smacking, choreiform movements) that disappear when asleep	

Key Reference: Stoelting, RK: Pharmacology and Physiology in Anesthetic Practice, 2nd ed. Philadelphia, JB Lippincott, 1991, pp 365–383.

PERIOPERATIVE IMPLICATIONS/DRUG INTERACTIONS

Preoperative Preparation

- Phenothiazines, other antipsychotic drugs may interact with narcotic to cause respiratory depression

Induction/Maintenance

- Does not enhance narcotic-induced analgesia but prolongs it

Postoperative Period

- Neuroleptic malignant syndrome occurs rarely, typically develops in young males over 24–72 h; symptoms include hyperthermia, generalized hypertonicity of skeletal muscles (relieved with nondepolarizing muscle relaxants), ANS instability (tachycardia, BP changes, cardiac dysrhythmias), fluctuating LOC, respiratory failure, ↑ liver transaminases

PHENOXYBENZAMINE

Michael F. Roizen, M.D.

USES

- People within USA: ?3,000/y
- Rx for preop prep of pheochromocytoma patients; occasionally, chronic Rx of pheochromocytoma, sympathetic hyperactivity states, carcinoid syndrome, benign prostatic hypertrophy (BPH)

PERIOPERATIVE RISKS

- Drug interactions: sometimes requires industrial doses of α adrenergic agents to produce vasoconstriction
- Vasodilation, orthostatic hypotension accentuated in hypovolemic patients

WORRY ABOUT

- Occasionally associated with confusional states
- Associated with fatigue and prolonged sedation
- Drop attacks on preop standing to urinate

OVERVIEW/PHARMACOLOGY

- α_1 rb (relatively selective $\alpha_1 >> \alpha_2$) by covalent (irreversible) binding to α receptor; compensatory response calls for production or availability of more (spare) receptors
- Effect develops slowly; peak effect not attained for 2 h after IV or 4 h after oral administration
- Absorption from GI tract incomplete
- Renal excretion of 50% in 12 h, 80% in 24 h
- $T_{1/2}$ of effect over 24 h, effects cumulate for at least 4–6 d
- High lipid solubility at body pH

DRUG CLASS/MECH OF ACTION

- α_1 rb agent (a haloalkylamine)
- Chronically taken:
  - $\downarrow \alpha_1$ rb effects in pheochromocytoma
  - high doses inhibit release of H_2, serotonin (occasionally used in carcinoid syndrome)
  - ameliorate or prevent Raynaud's phenomenon
  - vasodilator for chronic treatment of CHF (occasionally)

DRUG EFFECTS

SYSTEM	EFFECT	ASSESSMENT BY HX	PE	TEST
HEENT	Vasodilation of mucous membranes of nasopharynx; miosis	Nasal congestion	Mouth breathing	
CV	Antihypertensive agent Postural hypotension from α rb, reflex tachycardia $\uparrow$ CO	Orthostatic Dizziness	Orthostatic VS	Hct ECG
GI	$\uparrow$ Intestinal motility, causes diarrhea	Orthostatic hypotension		
ENDO	Stimulates insulin release $\uparrow$ presynaptic norepinephrine release (blockade of presynaptic α_2 receptors inhibiting release of norephinephrine			
GU	$\uparrow$ blood volume, Na$^+$ retention Inhibits contraction of vas deferens	Impairs ejaculation		BUN, Cr Electrolytes
CNS	Depression, sedation, fatigue Extrapyramidal symptoms rarely N/V, motor excitability rare		CNS exam	

Key Reference: Weiner N: *In* Gilman AG, Rall TW, Nies AS, Taylor P (eds): Goodman and Gilman's The Pharmacological Basis of Therapeutics, 7th ed. New York, Pergamon, 1990, pp 181–191.

PERIOPERATIVE IMPLICATIONS/POSSIBLE DRUG INTERACTIONS

(see also Pheochromocytoma in Disease section and Adrenalectomy for Pheochromocytoma in Procedures section)

Preoperative Period

- Ensure not hypovolemic
- Interaction with methyldopa (Aldomet): urinary incontinence
- Preop treatment: major goal to avoid pheochromocytoma crisis; pre- and intraoperative goals of management of extra-adrenal surgery same as for adrenal surgery. If patient not on α rb before surgery, try to delay until appropriate degree of α rb. $\uparrow$ Dose of phenoxybenzamine by 10 mg bid to qid every 3rd day until "appropriately blocked." Judge "appropriate" level of blockade by:

1. No BP readings higher than 165/90 mmHg (even during psychologic stress) for 48 h before surgery
2. Orthostatic hypotension present, but BP on standing should not be lower than 80/45 mmHg
3. ECG free of ST-T changes due to cardiomyopathy
4. Absence of other signs of catecholamine excess and presence of rb effects such as nasal stuffiness)

Induction/Maintenance

- Can produce $\uparrow$ sedation, $\downarrow$ anesthetic requirements by 1/3 (not studied but anecdotally reported)

Muscle Relaxants

- No interactions known

Regional Anesthesia/Reversal

- No interactions known

ANTICIPATED PROBLEMS/CONCERNS

- May need industrial doses of vasopressors to $\uparrow$ vascular resistance, BP in patient taking large doses
- CNS dysfunction by itself

PHENYLEPHRINE (NEO-SYNEPHRINE)

Edelberto Perez, M.D.
Kenneth J. Tuman, M.D.

USES

- Prescribed mainly as nasal decongestant or ophthalmically for mydriasis, capillary decongestion
- Reliable vasopressor in treatment of hypotension
- Prolongs local anesthetic duration in regional anesthesia
- Available for parenteral IM and various ophthalmic/nasal preparations

PERIOPERATIVE RISKS

- Risk of hypertension increases left heart work; may precipitate myocardial ischemia, MI
- Infusions to augment systolic BP ↑ incidence of myocardial ischemia in patients undergoing carotid endarterectomy
- ↑ Pulmonary vascular resistance, right heart work
- Bradycardia may occur (usually not severe)
- ↓ Renal, splanchnic blood flow
- May ↑ uterine artery vascular resistance, ↓ uterine artery blood flow in pregnant patients
- Systemic absorption of topical preparations may cause hypertension, headache, tremulousness, myocardial ischemia

WORRY ABOUT

- ↑ Preload, afterload may worsen LV failure in patients with LV dysfunction
- ↑ PA pressures may worsen RV dysfunction
- May ↓ renal blood flow

OVERVIEW/PHARMACOLOGY

- Direct α_1 agonist activity causes systemic and PA vasoconstriction, resulting in ↑ impedance to forward flow, ↑ BP
- Rapidly metabolized by MAO
- IV duration less than 5 min
- May terminate supraventricular tachycardia by vagal reflex from baroreceptor stimulation
- ↑ SVR during CPB
- ↑ Perfusion pressure to vital organs in hypovolemic patients until vol restored, CPR
- May be used in conjunction with nitroglycerin to elevate coronary perfusion pressure in hypotensive patients with myocardial ischemia
- ↓ R→L shunts in patients with cyanotic spells (tetralogy of Fallot)
- Vasopressor of choice in hypertrophic cardiomyopathy and aortic stenosis, when ↑ inotropy or tachycardia undesirable
- Advantageous in catecholamine-depleted patients (chronic cocaine or amphetamine abuse), or in patients on tricyclic antidepressants or MAO inhibitors, when indirect vasopressors are unpredictable

DRUG CLASS/MECH OF ACTION/USUAL DOSE

- Synthetic noncatecholamine activates predominantly α_1-adrenergic receptors (postsynaptic, heart, iris), triggers release of intracellular Ca^{2+}, resulting in smooth muscle contraction
- Differs structurally from epinephrine only in lacking 4-hydroxyl group on benzene ring
- Usual adult dosage:
  – IV bolus: 50–100 µg
  – IV infusion: 20–50 µg/min
  – Ophthalmic solutions: 2.5–10%
  – Supraventricular tachycardia dose: 150–800 µg titrated to ↑ BP

DRUG EFFECTS

SYSTEM	EFFECT	PE	TEST
HEENT	Mydriasis without cycloplegia ↓ Production of aqueous humor		
CV	Vasoconstriction of veins and arteries ↑ Systolic and diastolic BP ↓ HR	BP HR	PCWP ECG
RESP	↑ PVR		PCWP, PAP
RENAL	↓ Renal blood flow	Urine output	BUN, Cr

Key Reference: Gilman AG, Roll TW, Nies AS, Taylor P (eds): Goodman and Gilman's The Pharmacological Basis of Therapeutics, 8th ed. New York, Pergamon, 1990, pp 207–208.

PERIOPERATIVE IMPLICATIONS

Preoperative Concerns

- Assess LV function and history of CAD
- Consider arterial catheter if phenylephrine infusion anticipated (carotid endarterectomy, relative hypovolemia)
- Assess renal function (Cr)
- For nasal intubations, phenylephrine can be used as a nasal vasoconstrictor in a mixture with 3–4% lidocaine

Induction/Maintenance

- Stimulation of cardiac α_1 receptors may interact with halothane and cause dysrhythmias

- Monitor ECG for signs of ischemia due to increased ventricular work or coronary artery spasm
- May ↓ hepatic blood flow due to α-adrenergic–mediated vasoconstriction of portal venous vasculature

Adjuvants/Regional Anesthesia/Reversal

- Duration may be prolonged in patients on MAO inhibitors
- Side effects with ophthalmic use occur within 20 min; usually self-limited
- 2.5% nasal, ophthalmic solutions recommended in infant and elderly populations or in patients with CAD

ANTICIPATED PROBLEMS/CONCERNS

- Small doses can be titrated in a parturient when a β-adrenergic agonist is undesirable
- Can be titrated slowly to avoid overshoot (with resultant hypertension)
- Can be used when severe hypotension presents immediate danger to compromised myocardium or other end-organ (e.g., brain)
- With a failing heart, increasing afterload and preload may ↑ left-sided filling pressures enough to cause pulm edema

PHENYTOIN

Vandana Kulkarni, M.D.

INDICATIONS

- Rx focal, grand mal seizures
- Rx ventricular arrhythmias; especially related to digitalis, tricyclic antidepressant toxicity
- Occasional Rx for chronic pain states—e.g., trigeminal neuralgia
- Can be administered IV or PO

PERIOPERATIVE RISKS

- Interaction with muscle relaxants ($\downarrow$ efficacy)
- Hypotension, bradycardia with IV administration faster than 50 mg/min (believed related to vehicle, propylene glycol)

WORRY ABOUT

- $\uparrow$ P450 clearance causing $\downarrow$ effectiveness of quinidine, procainamide, oral anticoagulants, oral contraceptives, some antibiotics
- Phenytoin toxicity in patients with uremia, liver disease, hypoalbuminemia

OVERVIEW/PHARMACOLOGY

- Drug of choice for control of status epilepticus
- Rx for acute, chronic seizures
- >90% protein bound to albumin
- 98% hydroxylated, then conjugated in liver with glucuronic acid for renal elimination
- Elimination $T_{1/2}$ 24 h
- Therapeutic range 10–20 µg/ml

DRUG CLASS/MECH OF ACTION/USUAL DOSE

- Hydantoin derivative
- $\downarrow$ Na^+ influx during action potential; $\downarrow$ presynaptic Ca^{2+} release, limiting spread of seizure activity to seizure focus
- Extracellular K^+ $\uparrow$ during seizures, functions to propagate seizure; extracellular K^+ concentrations $\downarrow$ by phenytoin, limiting spread of seizure activity
- Raises seizure threshold selectively in cerebral cortex

- In heart
  - depresses spontaneous depolarization of ventricular tissue, limiting re-entrant arrhythmias
  - AV nodal conduction not $\downarrow$ (may be slightly $\uparrow$)
  - SA nodal conduction particularly depressed in presence of volatile agents
- Usual dose: IV, PO doses are same
  - Seizures: adult: 1 g for loading dose, then 5 mg/kg/d in 2–3 divided doses; pediatric: 15 mg/kg loading dose, then 5 mg/kg/d in divided doses
  - Cardiac: 1.5 mg/kg IV q 5 min for max dose of 15 mg/kg or 1.5 g
  - GI absorption variable (30–97%)

DRUG EFFECTS

SYSTEM	EFFECT	ASSESSMENT BY HX	PE	TEST
HEENT	Nystagmus seen in acute toxicity		Gingival hyperplasia with chronic use	
CV	Hypotension with rapid admin (>50 mg/min)		BP	
GI/LIVER	$\uparrow$ Hepatic drug metabolism Toxicity in hypoalbuminemia/ hyperbilirubinemia Variable absorption	GI irritation if not taken with food		Albumin
ENDO	Megaloblastic anemia			CBC
RENAL	Toxicity in uremic patients			BUN/Cr
CNS	Acute toxicity—ataxia, nystagmus, lethargy		CNS exam	

Key Reference: Sedman AJ: Cimetidine–drug interactions. Am J Med 1984; 76:109.

PERIOPERATIVE IMPLICATIONS/POSSIBLE DRUG INTERACTIONS

Preoperative Concerns

- Renal, liver disease, nutritional state can $\uparrow$ level of free phenytoin, active form of drug

Induction/Maintenance

- Resistance to nondepolarizing muscle relaxants
- Shorter duration of nondepolarizing muscle relaxants
- IV administration at a rate not greater than 25–50 mg/kg/min to avoid hypotension, bradycardia

Contraindications

- Pregnancy—crosses placenta, and causes fetal hydantoin syndrome (wide-set eyes, broad mandible, finger deformities)

SPECIAL PROBLEMS/CONSIDERATIONS

- Associated with phenytoin syndrome—fever, rash, lymphadenopathy, hepatitis; may progress to interstitial nephritis, pulmonary infiltrates, anemia, thrombocytopenia, eosinophilia, DIC
- Also associated with Stevens-Johnson syndrome

PHYSOSTIGMINE SALICYLATE (ESERINE, ANTILIRIUM)   Hassan H. Ali, M.D.

USES

- Rx for
  - Ointment or eye drops for glaucoma
  - Central anticholinergic syndrome
  - Less than optimal reversal agent of NMB

PERIOPERATIVE RISKS

- Risk of muscarinic stimulation if IV given rapidly
- Risk of tachycardia, hypertension due to central hemodynamic stimulation

WORRY ABOUT

- N/V, salivation, ↑ peristalsis
- Tachycardia, hypertension in hypertensive pts (esp if rapidly given IV, but risk even if slow IV or IM)
- Convulsions in pts with closed craniocerebral injuries, barbiturate intox due to high level of ACh in brain tissue
- Withheld from pts with myotonic dystrophy, cholinergic intox

OVERVIEW/PHARMACOLOGY

- A tertiary amine alkaloid from calabar beans
- Reversibly inhibits AChE
- Potent inhibitor of phosphodiesterase enzyme, regulating transmitter ACh release at many synapses in the CNS
- Crosses BBB, exerts cholinergic effects in CNS
- In large doses → cholinergic crisis (fasciculation followed by muscle paralysis)
- Peak effect 7–11 min after slow IV administration
- $T_{1/2}\alpha$ about 2–3 min, $T_{1/2}\beta$ 22 min
- Because of its rapid $T_{1/2}\alpha$, slow injection associated with much lower incidence of intestinal, cardiac side effects

DRUG CLASS/MECH OF ACTION/USUAL DOSE

- Tertiary amine alkaloid reversible anti-ChE peripherally and at CNS
- For glaucoma:
  - physostigmine sulfate ointment, 0.25%
  - physostigmine salicylate solution, 0.25%, 0.5%
- For central anticholinergic syndrome:
  - physostigmine salicylate (Antilirium), 1 mg/ml; dose 0.04 mg/kg or 1–2 mg IM or IV

DRUG EFFECTS

SYSTEM	EFFECT	ASSESSMENT BY HX	PE	TEST
HEENT	Pupillary constriction	Glaucoma		↓ IOP
CV	Tachycardia and hypertension		High BP	BP, ECG
RESP	Reversal of respiratory depressant effect of opiates Can produce bronchoconstriction			Restore sensitivity for CO_2
GI	Nausea, salivation, abd cramps			
CNS	Reversal of anticholinergic syndrome			Alert, improved vigilance and memory in ACS, possibly in Alzheimer's disease

Key Reference: Taylor P: *In* Gilman AG, Rall TW, Nies AS, Taylor P (eds): Goodman & Gilman's The Pharmacological Basis of Therapeutics, 8th ed. New York, Pergamon, 1990, pp. 131–149.

PERIOPERATIVE CONCERNS

- Interaction with pressors (significant ↑ BP)
- Very poor reversal of nondepolarizing relaxants at doses recommended as Rx for central anticholinergic syndrome

ANTICIPATED PROBLEMS/CONCERNS

- Significant tachycardia, hypertensive response in pts with Hx of high BP
- Convulsions in pts with closed head injuries, barbiturate poisoning
- Can → cholinergic crisis in presence of other anti-ChEs. Atropine effective antidote for physostigmine OD centrally, glycopyrrolate peripherally

PRILOCAINE

Stanley W. Stead, M.D.

INDICATIONS

- Infrequently used local anesthetic in US, still used extensively in Germany

PERIOPERATIVE RISKS

- Toxicity from excessive dose
- Hypersensitivity reaction
- Methemoglobinemia

WORRY ABOUT

- Metabolism to *o*-toluidine, which causes Hgb to be reduced to methemoglobin

OVERVIEW/PHARMACOLOGY

- 2-Propylamino-*o*-propionotoluidide
- Pharmacokinetics: $T_{1/2}\alpha$ 0.5 min; $T_{1/2}\beta$ 5 min, Vd_{ss} 261 L; $T_{1/2}\gamma$ 1.5 h; clearance rate 2.84 L/min (distributed at rapid rate from blood to tissue)

DRUG CLASS/MECH OF ACTION/USUAL DOSE

- Amide local anesthetic (less readily metabolized than esters); this ↓ in metabolism ↑ risk of adverse reactions
- Permeates nerve's axon membranes and equilibrates there and in axoplasm, depending on drug's pK_a (8.0), hydrophobicity of base and cation sp and concentration. Hydrophobicity measured by octanol: buffer partition coefficient of base: 129, making it moderately hydrophobic
- Binds to local anesthetic sites on voltage-gated Na^+ channels. A conformational change of receptor prevents opening of channel during activation; axon potentials cease to be propagated. Onset, recovery from blockade limited by diffusion of local anesthetic molecules into/out of nerve membrane and axoplasm
- Undergoes enzymatic degradation, primarily in liver; the most rapidly metabolized of amides
- Excreted in kidney; perhaps some kidney metabolism
- Low protein-binding capacity leads to ↑ clearance rate

DRUG EFFECTS

- Addition of epinephrine does not affect block duration, a result of vasodilating action of prilocaine

Methemoglobinemia

- Dose-response relationship exists between amount of prilocaine and methemoglobinemia (occurs with ≥600 mg). Occurrence related to chemical structure: prilocaine has one less methyl group in benzene ring than lidocaine; metabolism in liver results in formation of *o*-toluidine, which oxidizes Hgb to methemoglobin
- Methemoglobinemia significant when methemoglobin 10% of total Hgb (shift to left with less release of O_2). Cyanosis observed; methemoglobinemia of concern if anemic or pregnant (when maternal transfer leads to methemoglobinemia of fetus)
- Treatment, if spontaneous reversal does not occur, or IV injection with 1–2 mg/kg of 1% methylene blue solution (tetramethylthionine chloride)
- Other toxicity may involve CNS, CV systems; generally 4–7× the amount producing convulsions → CV collapse
- Toxicity associated with >400 mg
- Intercostal injection → higher blood levels than epidural.

Indication	Concn	Drug Dose	Onset	Duration
Minor nerve block	1%	50–200 mg	10–20 min	60–120 min, up to 180 with epinephrine
Major nerve block	1–2%	400–600 mg	10–20 min	180–300 min
Epidural	1–3%	150–600 mg	5–15 min	120–180 min

DRUG EFFECTS

SYSTEM	EFFECT	ASSESSMENT BY HX	PE	TEST
HEENT	Toxicity	Metallic taste, tinnitus		
CV	Pulm vasoconstriction			↑ PAP ↑ PVR ↓ SVR ↓ CO ECG ↑ in PR, ↓ QRS
	Systemic vasodilator Neg inotrope Neg chronotrope			
CNS	Toxicity: more sensitive than CV	Shivering, twitching, tremors in face, extremities, progressing to tonic-clonic seizure	Twitching, hyperreflexia possible Resp depression	
PNS	Block nerve transmissions		Loss of sensation and motor function	
MS	IV may augment NM blocker (both depolarizing and nondepolarizing)			Nerve stimulator: ↓ twitch height

Key Reference: Lund PG, Cwik JG: Propitocaine (eitanest) and methemoglobinemia. Anesthesiology 1965; 26:569.

POSSIBLE DRUG INTERACTIONS

- In large doses, blocks NM transmission; in smaller doses, enhances NMB from nondepolarizing and depolarizing NM blockers
- Acidosis, hypercarbia, hypoxia may potentiate neg chronotropic, inotropic actions

Preoperative Considerations/Induction/Maintenance

- Routine

ANTICIPATED PROBLEMS/CONCERNS

- Emla cream = eutectic mix of 5% lidocaine + prilocaine base for topical cutaneous anesthesia. Emla applied under occlusive bandage for 45–60 min to obtain effective cutaneous anesthesia
- Emla → methemoglobinemia when large amounts used in children
- Methemoglobinemia if >600/mg given kg, or to anemic or pregnant patients

PROCAINAMIDE

USES

• Supraventricular, ventricular antiarrhythmic effect: most commonly used for management of ventricular dysrhythmias
• Useful for chronic suppression of PVCs, yet newer class IB agents—e.g., tocainide, mexiletine—may supplant procainamide

PERIOPERATIVE RISKS

• Acute cardiac toxicity heralded by significant hypotension and/or 50% QRS prolongation
• A lupus-like syndrome (fever, serositis, arthritis) may be seen in 1/3 of patients during chronic therapy; this syndrome usually spares kidneys, abates when drug stopped
• Positive ANAs develop in 75% of patients during chronic admin but not an indication to discontinue unless Sx of drug-induced lupus develop
• Other reactions include fever, rash, N/V, diarrhea, confusion, agranulocytosis
• Since NAPA and procainamide toxicities are additive, serum levels of both can be monitored during therapy

WORRY ABOUT

• Convulsions
• Systemic toxicity due to accidental intravascular injection

OVERVIEW/PHARMACOLOGY

• Q in V_{max}, action potential amplitude during phase 0; ↓ in rate of phase 4 depolarization
• Prolonged refractory period, action potential duration (similar to effects of quinidine)
• Prolongs conduction, ↑ effective refractory period in atrial, His-Purkinje portions of conduction system
• Prolongs Q-T interval less than does quinidine
• AV nodal effective refractory period may ↓ by indirect anticholinergic effects
• When used for supraventricular dysrhythmias, esp AFib or atrial flutter, ventricular rate usually ↑, unless AV nodal conduction slowed by other means
• Procainamide and quinidine reported to reduce frequency of short-coupling interval PVCs (<400 ms), ↓ frequency of VTach or fibrillation caused by R-on-T phenomenon
• Absorption of PO dose rapid; initial effects seen within 20–30 min after PO admin, immediately after IV admin
• Peak serum concentrations observed 1 h after PO ingestion
• 15% of drug is protein bound
• IV: 100 mg or 1.5 mg/kg, given at 5-min intervals until therapeutic effect observed, to total dose of lesser of 1 g or 15 mg/kg
• Arterial pressure and ECG monitored, admin stopped if hypotension and/or a >50% QRS prolongation
• Maintenance infusion 20–80 µg/kg/min for therapeutic plasma concn of 4–8 µg/ml

• PO: 50 µg/kg/h or 500–600 mg q3–4h; absorption 75–95%
• Plasma levels peak after 1–2 h
• Elimination $T_{1/2}$ = 3–4 h
• 50–60% excreted unchanged by kidneys remainder metabolized by liver
• Principal metabolite NAPA has antiarrhythmic effects, is excreted by kidneys, accumulates when renal function is impaired
• Major metabolic pathway is hepatic acetylation to NAPA metabolite that prolongs repolarization
• Rate of acetylation may vary genetically (fast or slow acetylators)
• NAPA has a serum $T_{1/2}$ of 6–8 h, but possibly as long as 60 h in patients with severe renal dysfunction
• Elimination of procainamide ↓ in patients with impaired liver or kidney function (serum $T_{1/2}$ as long as 60 h) and in patients in CHF (serum $T_{1/2}$ of 5 h) (in such patients, loading dose of 12 mg/kg over 1 h and maintenance infusion of 1.4 mg/kg/h have been recommended)

DRUG CLASS/MECH OF ACTION

• Class IA antiarrhythmic: Class I drugs are membrane stabilizers that cause pharmacologic blockade of the Na+ channel with ↓ V_{max} rate, max rate of depolarization of AP during phase 0

DRUG EFFECTS

SYSTEM	EFFECT	ASSESSMENT BY HX
CV	Myocardial depression and peripheral arterial dilation	Suppression of ventricular arrhythmias Higher doses cause enhanced vasodilation, depression of myocardial contractility, and depression of peripheral vascular resistance, resulting in profound hypotension
CNS	Crosses blood-brain barrier, causing CNS excitation followed by CNS depression	Excitation evidenced as restlessness and tremor Higher plasma concentrations result in convulsions, coma, and cardiorespiratory arrest
PNS	Inhibition of propagation of action potential	Loss of sensation and motor ability in area of blockade
NEUROMUSCULAR JUNCTION	Transmission may be inhibited	Potentiation of muscle relaxants

Key Reference: Philip BK, Covino BG: Local and regional anesthesia. *In* Wetchler BV (ed): Anesthesia for Ambulatory Surgery. Philadelphia, JB Lippincott, 1990, pp 309–365.

PROCAINE (NOVOCAIN)

Glenn S. Goldsher, M.D.

INDICATIONS

• For infiltration of tissue, spinal anesthesia for procedures of short duration

PERIOPERATIVE RISKS

• Accidental intravascular injection of toxic dose
• Allergic reaction to PABA
• Allergic reaction to sodium metabisulfite

WORRY ABOUT

• Use of drug with epinephrine added (for vasoconstriction) in patients taking MAO inhibitors, tricyclic antidepressants, oxytocin-like drugs because of possible hypertension, cardiac dysrhythmias
• In patients with known or possible deficiencies in pseudo-ChE levels or its function

OVERVIEW/PHARMACOLOGY

• Ester-type local anesthetic related to cocaine, chloroprocaine, and tetracaine. Low potency (very low lipid solubility), slow onset (high pK_a—8.9) short duration of action (very low protein binding, rapid hydrolysis)
• Rapid metabolism by pseudo-ChE (in vitro plasma $T_{1/2}$: 40 ± 9 sec—adults, 84 ± 30 sec—neonates), produces PABA and diethylaminoethanol
• 90% of PABA, 33% of diethylaminoethanol are recovered in urine; 2% of dose recovered unchanged in urine
• Very low risk of systemic toxicity due to rapid hydrolysis

DRUG CLASS/MECH OF ACTION/USUAL DOSE

• Local anesthetic of ester type
• Base form crosses lipid membranes to enter nerve cell axons, where becomes ionized, binds to receptor within the Na^+ channel; this blocks Na^+ from entering cell, inhibits depolarization of nerve, blocks transmission of nerve impulses
• Usual dose for infiltration, 300–600 mg (0.25% or 0.5% solution); for spinal anesthesia, 100–200 mg (10% solution)
• Total dose should not exceed 1000/mg

DRUG EFFECTS

SYSTEM	EFFECT
CV	If toxic levels reached, ↓ contractility, ↓ rate of electrical impulse conduction can occur, leading to ↓ CO, arrhythmias, possible CV collapse (cardiac arrest)
CNS	As drug levels ↑, Sx progress from restlessness, anxiety, dizziness, tinnitus, perioral numbness to visual disturbances, muscular twitching, unconsciousness, convulsions, coma, respiratory arrest
MS	Blockade of sensory, motor, sympathetic nerve transmission, depending on site of administration, concentration of drug

Key Reference: Covino BG: *In* Rogers, Tinker, et al, eds: Principles and Practice of Anesthesiology. St. Louis, Mosby-Year Book, 1992, pp 1235–1255.

POSSIBLE DRUG INTERACTIONS

• Should not be infiltrated into areas of infection treated with sulfonamide antibiotics because PABA may inhibit action of sulfonamides
• Procaine with epinephrine added for vasoconstriction should be avoided in patients taking MAO inhibitors, tricyclic antidepressants, and oxytocin-like drugs because of possible severe, persistent hypertension

SPECIAL PROBLEMS/CONSIDERATIONS

• Avoid in patients with deficiencies in pseudo-ChE levels or function
• Avoid in patients with allergic reactions to PABA and/or sulfites (sulfites may be a preservative)
• Avoid IV injection of large amounts or use of large amounts of drug in very vascular areas
• Least toxic of local anesthetics, but toxic reactions can occur

PROPOFOL

Matthew L. Black, M.D.
Jeffrey L. Apfelbaum, M.D.

USES

- IV sedation, induction, maintenance of GA, outpatient, in-patient procedures
  - Recommended for adults or children older than 3 y
- Reduced dose in elderly, debilitated, and ASA III/IV patients (4% reduction per decade)
- Caution when admin to patients with disorders of lipid metab

PERIOPERATIVE RISKS

- Airway obstruction
- Resp depression
- Apnea
- Hypotension
- Pain at injection site (related to phenol group availability); reduced with slower administration; ↑ lipid

WORRY ABOUT

- Supports rapid microbial growth/contains no antimicrobial preservative
- Aseptic technique
- Discard after 6 h
- Synergistic with all other sedatives/hypnotics

OVERVIEW/PHARMACOLOGY

- Produces sedation or amnesia without analgesia
- Metab primarily hepatic, but addition metabolites undefined
- Renal elimination of inactive metabolites
- Rapid onset: 1 arm–brain circulation time (~30–45 sec)
- Fast offset due to short $T_{1/2}$
  - $T_{1/2}\alpha$ = 2–4 min
  - $T_{1/2}\beta$ = 4 h
- Highly lipid-bound; use reduced dose in renal failure patients
- Synergistic with narcotics, benzodiazepines, other sedatives
- Not recommended for children under 3 y (safety and effectiveness not established)

- Not recommended in OB (placental transfer, possible neonatal depression)
- Not recommended for nursing mothers (effects on infants not established)

DRUG CLASS/MECH OF ACTION/USUAL DOSE

- Intravenous anesthetic of sterically hindered phenol group
- Mechanism of action unknown
- Prepared as 1% isotonic oil-in-water emulsion containing egg lecithin, glycerol, soybean oil
- Dose
  - Sedation: 50–75 µg/kg/min
  - Induction: ASA I, II adults under 55 y; 2–2.5 mg/kg; ASA I, II children over 3 y: 2.5–3.5 mg/kg
  - Maintenance: ASA I or II adults under 55 y: 100–200 µg/kg/min; ASA I or II children over the age of 3 y: 200–300 µg/kg/min
- Dose reduced in elderly, hemodynamically compromised, ASA III/IV patients

DRUG EFFECTS

SYSTEM	EFFECT	ASSESSMENT BY HX	PE
CV	Hypotension ↓ CO	Fluid status	Vital signs
RESP	Dose-dependent ↓ in resp rate/TV Apnea 30–90 sec after induction Airway obstruction		
GI	↓ PONV		
CNS	Conscious sedation General anesthesia		
MISC	Injection site irritation Allergy, anaphylactic or anaphylactoid	Complaints, pain To propofol or phenols, (?) allergy to egg whites	Rash

Key Reference: Sebel PS, Lowdon JD: Propofol: A new intravenous anesthetic. Anesthesiology 1989; 71:260–277.

PERIOPERATIVE IMPLICATIONS

- Trained personnel with resuscitative and airway management equipment necessary
- Ventilatory support may be required
- Monitoring includes *continuous* SpO_2, BP, ECG, precordial stethoscope
- Continuously monitor for early signs of hypotension, apnea, airway obstruction, O_2 desaturation
- O_2 suppl usually necessary
- Patients NPO, assessed for aspiration
- Airway protection necessary for aspiration-prone patients if protective reflexes lost

ANTICIPATED PROBLEMS/CONCERNS

- Aseptic technique mandatory
- Resp, CV effects must be anticipated; continuously monitor

PROPYLTHIOURACIL — ANTITHYROID DRUGS

Michael F. Roizen, M.D.

USES

- In USA: in addition to 5% of pregnant women, ?400,000/y develop hyperthyroidism
- Rx for hyperthyroidism, goiter associated with hyperthyroidism
- Definitive Rx to control hyperthyroidism in anticipation of spontaneous remission
- Rx for hyperthyroidism in conjunction with ^{131}I or ^{125}I to hasten recovery while awaiting effects of radiation therapy
- Rx for hyperthyroidism to control disorder in preparation for surgery

PERIOPERATIVE RISKS

- Side effects of drug: hypothyroidism (see Hyper- or Hypothyroidism)

WORRY ABOUT

- Agranulocytosis (less than 0.5% of treated patients developed this side effect)

OVERVIEW/PHARMACOLOGY

- Antithyroid drug: Absorbed within 20–30 min; effect begins to ↓ in 2–3 h (methimazole $T_{1/2}$ estimated to be 6–13 h)
- Drug and metabolites cleared by renal excretion
- Antithyroid drugs cross placenta, can be found in breast milk

DRUG CLASS/USUAL DOSE

- Antithyroid drug: interferes directly with synthesis of thyroid hormones by preventing incorporation of iodine into tyrosyl residual thyroglobulin, inhibits coupling of iodotyrosyl residues to form iodothyronines by inhibiting peroxidase enzyme
- Depletes preformed hormone over time; only then do clinical effects become noticeable ($T_{1/2}$ of thyroid hormones is >3d in circulation)
- Other useful antithyroid Rx drugs include those inhibiting conversion of less active T_4 into more active T_3, such as propranolol; as does propylthiouracil, but methimazole, carbimazole do not appear to do so with anti-ß-rb effects— e.g., propranolol and others; those that inhibit release of preformed thyroid hormone—e.g., iodine (also temporarily inhibits synthesis and ↓ vascularity of thyroid glands)
- A thioureylene

Chronic Rx Uses

- ↓ Hyperthyroidism and thyrotoxicosis
- ↓ Goiter size in hyperthyroidism

Acute Rx Uses

- Relieve symptoms of hyperthyroidism while waiting for effects of ^{131}I or ^{125}I to take effect

DRUG EFFECTS

SYSTEM	EFFECT	ASSESSMENT BY HX	PE	TEST
HEENT	Goiter shrinkage; occasionally goiter develops if hypothyroidism occurs	Snoring, hoarseness, neck pain	Ask patient to vocalize "e"; examine airway, neck	Check CXR (PA, lat) lat neck films; if needed, CT scan of neck
CV		Assess CV response to Rx		Rhythm strip or full ECG if CV system is involved by either Hx or PE
GI	Rare hematotoxicity			
HEME		Mild anemia, thrombocytopenia; agranulocytosis as toxic reaction to propylthiouracil or methimazole (0.05–0.12% of patients). Hx of sore throat or fever often heralds agranulocytosis	Skin/mucous membranes for infection/petechiae; purpura if at risk	CBC with platelet count; differential leukocyte count
SKIN		Rare depigmentation of hair Pain/stiffness in joints (rare side effect)		
GU	Placenta—crosses placental barrier and is excreted in breast milk			
CNS		Headache, paresthesia rare side effects Shaking, anxiety, emotional instability as signs that hyperthyroidism not yet controlled	Reflex speed, tremor, nervousness, mental status	
IMMUNE	Need to assess if euthyroid	Refer to all other systems: especially reflex speed, tremor, heat intolerance, wt loss, fatigue, weakness, anorexia, ↑ appetite	Reflex speed; HR	Free T_4 estimate needed; unable to assess if euthyroid by Hx, PE

Key Reference: Cooper DS: Antithyroid drugs. N Engl J Med 1984; 311:1353–1362.

POSSIBLE DRUG INTERACTIONS

Preoperative Period

- Assess euthyroid state (see table)
- Fairly certain sign that remission may have occurred is ↓ in size of goiter

Induction/Maintenance

- No interactions known

Adjuvants/Regional Anesthesia/Reversal

- No interactions known

Postoperative Concerns

- Resumption not necessary if surgery to correct hyperthyroidism successful
- Short $T_{1/2}$ makes resumption in nonthyroid surgery necessary ASAP or give medication IV

ANTICIPATED PROBLEMS/CONCERNS

- Assess for hyperthyroidism, agranulocytosis

PROTAMINE

USES

- Used 500,000 times or more per y in surgery; IV for neutralization of heparin anticoagulation, Rx of heparin OD
- To delay absorption of certain insulin preps

RISKS

- Adverse cardiopulmonary responses (<2%); 3 categories of adverse reactions:
  – type I: systemic hypotension, ↓ SVR accompany rapid IV injection; occurs 2° to H_2 release from mast cells due to high alkalinity
  – type II: anaphylactic and anaphylactoid reactions; type IIa: true anaphylactic reactions (indicated by antiprotamine IgE, which binds to mast cells) ↑ risk with prior exp to protamine (i.e., prior cardiac or vascular surgery, cardiac catheterization, or in some cases hemodialysis), fin fish allergy, or diabetics receiving protamine-containing insulin, characterized by ↓ systemic artery, left atrial, right atrial pressure; bronchospasm may or may not occur

– type IIb: immediate anaphylactoid reactions mediated by complement activation with 2° release of H_2 and/or other vasoactive substances; manifested as edema of skin, mucosa; flushing; ↓ SVR; bronchospasm
– type IIc: delayed anaphylactoid reactions (AKA delayed noncardiogenic pulm edema)— systemic hypotension accompanied by massive pulm cap leak, accumulation of alveolar fluid, ↓ pulm compliance, wheezing, pulm edema, occurring >1 h after administration
– type III: catastrophic pulm vasoconstriction: ↑ PAP 2° to pulm vasoconstriction, systemic hypotension, ↓ LAP, RV distention, subsequent failure; plasma H_2 levels do not change; duration varies; heparin-protamine complexes activate complement; leukocytes then form free radicals activating arachidonic acid pathway with resulting potent pulm vasoconstrictor thromboxane production.

WORRY ABOUT

- Adverse reactions as outlined above.

OVERVIEW/PHARMACOLOGY

- Polycationic, strongly basic, low molecular wt protein
- OD may cause bleeding due to weak anticoagulant effect
- When administered in presence of heparin, stable salt formed within 5 min, neutralizing anticoagulant effect of both
- Protamine degradation through action of circulatory protease, carboxypeptidase
- Unknown metabolic fate of the heparin-protamine complex

DRUG CLASS/MECH OF ACTION/USUAL DOSE

- Each mg neutralizes approx 90 USP units of heparin activity derived from lung tissue or approx 115 USP units of heparin from intestinal mucosa
- Slowly, IV in doses not to exceed 5 mg/min; may be diluted with D_5W or 0.9 NS
- Incompatible with certain antibiotics, including several cephalosporins, penicillins

DRUG EFFECTS

SYSTEM	EFFECT	ASSESSMENT BY HX	PE	TEST
CV	↓ Systemic arterial pressure	Prior protamine exposure	BP	RAST or ELISA for antiprotamine IgE detection
	↑ PAP Pulm vasoconstriction with resultant RV distention, failure	Prior protamine reaction Diabetic taking protamine-containing insulin	PA catheter Visual inspection of RV for distention	
	LAP, RAP, SVR decrease	Fin fish allergy Status post vasectomy (theoretical concern)		In patients with prior PAP reaction
RESP	Brochospasm/wheezing Massive pulm cap leak ↓ Pulm compliance Pulm edema Alveolar fluid accumulation		Auscultation	
SKIN/MUCOSA	Edema Flushing		Inspection	

Key Reference: Kaplan JA: Cardiac Anesthesia, 3rd ed. Philadelphia, WB Saunders, 1993, pp 961–986.

POSSIBLE DRUG INTERACTIONS

Monitoring

- Consider PA catheter if in high risk group

Induction/Maintenance

- If pulm HTN, systemic hypotension detected, consider stopping protamine administration and any contractility depressant

Adjuvants/Regional Anesthesia/Reversal

- Rx of protamine reaction primarily supportive, choosing inotropic agents that will not worsen pulm HTN
- Anaphylaxis managed like any other anaphylactic reaction
- Acute episodes of pulm vasoconstriction may benefit from pulm vasodilators—e.g., nitroglycerin or isoproterenol

SPECIAL CONSIDERATIONS

- Few alternatives to protamine
- Hexadimethrine bromide is synthetic polycation withdrawn from clinical use following reports of nephrotoxicity; available from FDA if patient has proven anaphylactic reaction to protamine
- Heparin neutralization can be omitted, avoiding exposure to protamine

PYRIDOSTIGMINE BROMIDE

Hassan H. Ali, M.D.

USES

- Rx for myasthenia gravis
- Reversal of nondepolarizing NMB

PERIOPERATIVE RISKS

- Can produce significant muscarinic stimulation if admin IV without adequate protection with anticholinergic drug (e.g., atropine or glycopyrrolate).
- Can precipitate a cholinergic crisis in myasthenics receiving high doses of AChEs
- Prolonged response to succinylcholine if administered shortly after reversal with either pyridostigmine or neostigmine (inhibition of plasma ChE)

WORRY ABOUT

- Cardiac arrhythmias; muscarinic, nicotinic activation (cholinergic crisis); prolonged admin may →myopathic changes in postsynaptic region consistent with accumulation of Ca^{2+}, nuclear alterations
- Changes have been reversed with Ca^{2+} channel blockers (diltiazem)

OVERVIEW/PHARMACOLOGY

- A quaternary nitrogen reversible AChE is analogue of neostigmine
- Incorporates N in ring structure to form dimethylcarbamic ester of 3-hydroxy 1-methylpyridinium bromide
- May possess less muscarinic agonist effects than neostigmine
- Peak effect of pyridostigmine is 12–17 min compared with 7–11 min for neostigmine
- Distribution $T_{1/2}$ ($T_{1/2}\alpha$ 6.8 min; $T_{1/2}\beta$ 112 min in pts with normal kidney function with clearance of 9.0 ml/kg/min
- Anephric pts have a longer $T_{1/2}\beta$ of 379 min, reduced clearance of 2 ml/kg/min
- 25% metabolized, 75% dependent on renal elimination
- Anticholinergic glycopyrrolate matches better onset, duration of pyridostigmine

DRUG CLASS/MECH OF ACTION/USUAL DOSE

- Quaternary amine AChE
- For reversal of nondepolarizing relaxants at dose of 0.2–0.25 mg/kg (12.5–15 mg) IV
- For Rx myasthenia gravis: generally PO, 60 mg tablets (5–6 times/d) with a slow-release tablet 180 mg (1 q.n.)

DRUG EFFECTS

SYSTEM	EFFECT	TEST
CV	Bradyarrhythmia	ECG
RESP	Improved NM transmission, resp mechanics	PFTs
GI	Less nausea, salivation than neostigmine	
CNS	Reversal of NMB, postsynaptic dysfunction	Nml evoked muscle responses

Key Reference: Bevan DR, Donati F, Kopman AF: Reversal of neuromuscular blockade. Anesthesiology 1992; 77:785–805.

PERIOPERATIVE CONCERNS

- High doses preoperatively in myasthenics may ↑ requirements of nondepolarizing relaxants; response to succinylcholine can be prolonged

ANTICIPATED PROBLEMS/CONCERNS

- Use as a reversal agent in high doses may precipitate a cholinergic crisis in myasthenics
- Prolonged use may→short-lived myopathy; can be resolved with Ca^{2+} channel blockers

QUINIDINE (See also PROCAINAMIDE)

Michael B. Howie, M.D.

USES

- Rx for: supraventricular arrhythmias (AFib/flutter, PAT, WPW syndrome–associated arrhythmias) for conversion, maintenance of sinus rhythm

PERIOPERATIVE RISKS

- High plasma levels associated with QT and QRS prolongation, life-threatening ventricular arrhythmias (torsades de pointes); acidosis, hypomagnesemia, hypokalemia increase risk

WORRY ABOUT

- Quinidine accumulation with concurrent hepatic disease, renal failure, cimetidine administration
- ↓ Concentrations in association with rifampin, phenytoin, barbiturates

OVERVIEW/PHARMACOLOGY

- Well absorbed from GI tract (80% bioavailability)
- 90% plasma protein bound
- Elimination through kidneys, 20% unchanged, 80% after hepatic metabolism; $T_{1/2}$ 4–8 h
- Interactions with drugs that alter hepatic enzyme function, other highly protein-bound drugs
- Serum concn should be monitored to fit therapeutic range: 1.5–4 µg/ml
- The effect lasts 6–8 h; PO takes 1–3 h to onset
- Urine alkalinization ↓ excretion

DRUG CLASS/MECH OF ACTION/USUAL DOSE

- Class IA antiarrhythmic; use-dependent Na^+ channel block (local anesthetic–like action) responsible for effectiveness in tachyarrhythmias
- Dosage
  - conversion: quinidine polygalacturonate tabs 275 mg (×2 if necessary) q3–4 h for 3–4 doses; dose can be ↑ by 275 mg every 3rd or 4th dose until rhythm restored; quinidine gluconate injection 600 mg IM, then up to 400 mg q2 h if necessary
  - maintenance: quinidine polygalacturonate 275 mg bid/tid, as needed
- Alternatives: other class IA drugs (e.g., procainamide, disopyramide, cibenzoline, pirmenol)

DRUG EFFECTS

SYSTEM	EFFECT	ASSESSMENT BY HX	PE	TESTS
CV	↑ QRS duration, vagolytic cardiac/peripheral α block, negative inotropic, ↓ conduction velocity	↑ HR Dyspnea	↑ HR, ↓ BP, JVD, abnormal S_3 Bradycardia, asystole	ECG CXR ECG (3° AV block)
GI	Diarrhea (18%), nausea (18%)	α block		
HEME	Thrombocytopenia		Mucosal bleeding	Platelet count
CNS	Headache (13%), dizziness (8%), tinnitus, blurred vision			Quinidine serum concn
MISC	Anaphylactoid reactions, aggravation of asthma (caution)		CV collapse	

Key Reference: Opie LH, Singh BN, Marcus FI: Antiarrhythmic agents. *In* Opie LH (ed): Drugs for the Heart, 3rd ed. Philadelphia, WB Saunders, 1991, pp 180–184.

PERIOPERATIVE IMPLICATIONS/POSSIBLE DRUG INTERACTIONS

Preoperative Preparation

- Serial measurements of QRS duration and QT interval on the ECG to prevent arrhythmias; QRS should be <140 ms
- Digoxin, warfarin plasma levels ↑ displacement from storage sites, hepatic interaction, respectively); ↓ dosage to prevent toxicity
- ↓ Dose in hypoproteinemia

Induction/Maintenance

- Possible ↓ in hepatic metabolism of halogenated agents
- ↓ Levels of plasma proteins after CPB augment free fraction of drug

Adjuvants/Regional Anesthesia/Reversal

- Quinidine may ↑ muscle weakness in patients with myasthenia gravis, ↓ effect of anticholinesterases, enhances NMB
- Quinidine can enhance the effects of vasodilating, negative inotropic, sinus node depressant agents (e.g., β-blockers, verapamil, rauwolfia alkaloids, bretylium)
- Concurrent administration of other class IA drugs, amiodarone, or phenothiazines ↑ risk of torsades de pointes
- Quinidine has additive effect with anticholinergic drugs

SPECIAL CONSIDERATIONS

- Quinidine contraindicated when ventricular arrhythmias associated with or caused by QT prolongation (risk of torsades)
- IM injection very painful; IV routes cause vasodilation and myocardial depression
- In patients with AFib/flutter, quinidine can ↑ AV transmission (1:1) and cause ↑ in ventricular rate; prevent by administering verapamil or digoxin before cardioversion
- In patients with severe AV block, quinidine can aggravate block or cause asystole; this applies to patients with SSS

RIBOFLAVIN (VITAMIN B₂)

John K. Stene, Jr., M.D., Ph.D.

INDICATIONS

- For common deficiency with general nutritional deficiency (e.g., malnutrition, starvation, chronic alcoholism)
- Associated with causes of malnutrition, general vitamin deficiency
- Isolated deficiency rare or nonexistent in USA

PERIOPERATIVE RISKS

- Excessive intake ↑ urinary excretion of unchanged riboflavin
- Deficiency causes anemia, neuropathy

OVERVIEW/PHARMACOLOGY

- Component of electron transfer chain in mitochondria, oxidative metabolic coenzymes
- Absorbed from upper GI tract by specific transport mechanism involving phosphorylation of enzyme to FMN by enzyme flavokinase
- Distributed to all tissues, but little stored

ICD-9-CM Code: 266.0 (Riboflavin deficiency)

DRUG CLASS/MECH OF ACTION/USUAL DOSE

- Water-soluble B-complex vitamin
- Phosphorylated to FMN by flavokinase, ATP
- FMN reacts with phosphate bond to adenine monophosphate to form FAD
- FMN, FAD are electron transfer cofactors in mitochondrial electron transfer chain, oxidative metabolism (e.g., xanthine oxidase)

DRUG EFFECTS

SYSTEM	EFFECT	ASSESSMENT BY HX	PE	TEST
HEENT	Sore throat, cheilosis, glossitis	Burning tongue, soreness in mouth and throat	Red, fissured lips, blue-red tongue with edematous surface—"cobblestone tongue"	
HEME	Anemia			Reticulocytopenia, normochromic-normocytic anemia
SKIN	Seborrheic dermatitis of face, dermatitis of arms and trunk	Burning, itching eyes	Rough, sharkskin appearance of nose	
PNS	Neuropathy		PNS function exam	

Key Reference: Marcus R, Soulston AM: Water-soluble vitamins. *In* Gilman AG, Rall TW, Nies AS, Taylor P, eds: Goodman & Gilman's The Pharmacological Basis of Therapeutics, 8th ed. New York, Pergamon, 1990, pp 1534–1536.

PERIOPERATIVE IMPLICATIONS/POSSIBLE DRUG INTERACTIONS

- Absorption depends on flavokinase activity; it in turn depends on thyroid hormone status and is inhibited by tricyclic antidepressants, chlorpromazine
- Peripheral neuropathy of potential concern with regional anesthesia
- Preop normochromic-normocytic anemia in nutritionally depleted patient responds to riboflavin administration
- See also under Malnutrition for interactions, abnormalities of malnutrition

ANTICIPATED PROBLEMS/CONCERNS

- Adequate phosphorus must be given along with riboflavin and other vitamins when refeeding starved patients to prevent ↑ phosphorylation from depleting phosphate stores, energy of cells

RIFAMPIN

Johnathan L. Pregler, M.D.

USES

- Antibiotic therapy for TB (incidence 9.4/100,000/y) and *Neisseria meningitidis* infection (incidence 4.6–10/100,000/y
- May be administered PO or IV
- 10% of patients receiving rifampin develop chemical hepatitis; 16 deaths/500,000 receiving drug

PERIOPERATIVE RISKS

- Hepatic dysfunction, most likely in presence of pre-existing liver disease
- Decreased duration of action of narcotics and barbiturates
- Patients on antiarrhythmic therapy, digoxin, theophylline, phenytoin, or glucocorticoid therapy may need ↑ doses of these drugs

WORRY ABOUT

- Induces hepatic microsomal (P450) activity, ↓ $T_{1/2}$ of hepatically metabolized drugs
- Theoretical ↑ risk of halothane hepatitis
- Hemolytic anemia, thrombocytopenia (rare)

OVERVIEW/PHARMACOLOGY

- Complex macrocyclic antibiotic
- H_2O-soluble at acidic pH; inhibits gram-positive and many gram-negative organisms, including *E. coli, Pseudomonas, Proteus, Klebsiella, N. meningitidis, H. influenzae, M. tuberculosis*
- Increases in vitro activity of streptomycin and isoniazid
- Eliminated by biliary clearance with significant enterohepatic circulation
- $T_{1/2}$ of 1.5–5 h, ↑ with hepatic dysfunction

DRUG CLASS/MECH OF ACTION/USUAL DOSE

- Rifamycin antibiotic family
- Inhibits DNA-dependent RNA polymerase in bacteria and mycobacteria; nuclear eukaryotic RNA polymerase not affected
- Administered for chemoprophylaxis of meningococcal infections, with ß-lactams for *Staphylococcus* endocarditis, osteomyelitis; for methicillin-resistant *S. aureus* infections; and in conjunction with isoniazid and streptomycin for active TB
- Usual dose: 600 mg qd; pediatric dose 10 mg/kg qd, PO or IV
- Should be admin 1 h before or 2 h after meals PO

DRUG EFFECTS

SYSTEM	EFFECT	ASSESSMENT BY HX	PE	TEST
OVERALL		Fatigue, drowsiness, dizziness, ataxia, confusion, weakness		
HEENT	Secreted in saliva, tears		Orange sputum, tears, conjunctiva	
GI	Hepatic dysfunction (rare with normal pre-Rx hepatic function)	N/V	Jaundice	Elevated transaminases
HEME	Thrombocytopenia, hemolytic anemia	Bruising/bleeding		Platelet count, Hgb/Hct, microscopic exam
RENAL	Interstitial nephritis, ATN, renal failure (with high doses)			Cr clearance, light-chain proteinuria

Key Reference: Venkatesan K: Pharmacokinetic drug interactions with rifampicin. Clin Pharmacokin 1992; 22:47–65.

PERIOPERATIVE IMPLICATIONS/POSSIBLE DRUG INTERACTIONS

Preoperative Concerns

- ↓ Duration of action of benzodiazepines, narcotics, barbiturates due to hepatic enzyme induction
- Adequacy of pre-existing drug regimes should be verified (see Special Considerations)

Induction/Maintenance

- Decreased narcotic and analgesic efficacy: barbiturates, methadone, diazepam, midazolam; ß blockers have ↑ clearance, ↓ duration of action
- Halothane metabolism ↑ with ↑ risk of hepatotoxicity

Adjuvants/Reversal

- Mycobacteria quickly develop resistance when rifampin used alone; administer with isoniazid and/or streptomycin

Special Considerations

- Risk of hepatic dysfunction perioperatively ↑ by pre-existing hepatic disease
- Delays oral absorption of ASA
- ↓ $T_{1/2}$, requiring ↑ doses to maintain adequate therapeutic levels: digoxin, digitoxin, quinidine, propranolol, metoprolol, verapamil, Coumadin, theophylline, phenytoin, prednisone, cortisol, prednisolone, cyclosporine, oral hypoglycemic agents, ketoconazole, fluconazole

ANTICIPATED PROBLEMS/CONCERNS

- 10% on therapy may develop hepatitis; patients with pre-existing liver disease are at higher risk
- Rifampin induces microsomal enzyme activity in liver, results in ↓ efficacy, duration of action of hepatically metabolized drugs

SCOPOLAMINE (L-HYOSCINE)

Margaret Wood, M.D.

USES

- Prescribed as part of anesthetic premedication (antisialagogue, sedative)
- Prevents motion sickness
- Administered parenterally or as transdermal patch
- Ophthalmic solution available to produce mydriasis, cycloplegia
- Associated with progressively ↑ "central anticholinergic syndrome" in very young and elderly (>50 y)

PERIOPERATIVE RISKS

- A tertiary amine, crosses the blood-brain barrier, producing sedative effects; occasionally causes restlessness, hallucinations, delirium—central anticholinergic syndrome (more common in the elderly and the young)
- Antimuscarinic drugs may increase IOP in patients with narrow-angle glaucoma

WORRY ABOUT

- Drowsiness
- Central anticholinergic syndrome
- Increased IOP
- Dryness of the mouth
- Drug interactions: other drugs with (1) CNS, (2) anticholinergic effects

OVERVIEW/PHARMACOLOGY

- A tertiary amine (belladonna alkaloid), peripheral actions antagonize effect of ACh at cholinergic postganglionic nerve endings
- An antimuscarinic agent, competitively antagonizes effect of ACh at cholinergic muscarinic receptors
- Readily crosses cell membranes (e.g., blood-brain barrier, placenta)
- Bioavailability following oral dose about 20% to 25%
- Interactions with other drugs that also have CNS effects, e.g., benzodiazepines, may produce ↑ sedation; drug interactions may occur following co-administration with drugs possessing anticholinergic effects (e.g., antidepressants, antihistamines); possible increased incidence of emergence delirium following co-administration of ketamine, scopolamine
- Duration of action relatively short (especially when compared with glycopyrrolate); elimination T½ is 1.6–3.35 h; systemic clearance = ~0.4–0.9 L/kg/h

DRUG CLASS/MECH OF ACTION/USUAL DOSE

- Anticholinergic antimuscarinic agent
- Competitively antagonizes ACh at muscarinic cholinergic receptors
- Antiemetic effect due to direct action on chemoreceptor trigger zone of area postrema and emetic center of reticular formation or inhibition of vestibular afferent activity to CNS
- Usual dosage:
  - Adult : 0.3–0.6 mg IV, IM
  - Pediatric: 0.004–0.008 mg/kg IM

DRUG EFFECTS

SYSTEM	EFFECT
HEENT	Salivary, bronchial secretion reduced; dry mouth; sweating inhibited; mydriasis, cycloplegia
CV	Bradycardia, followed by tachycardia
RESP	Bronchodilation
GU	Relaxes detrusor, contracts sphincter, urinary retention, reduces lower esophageal sphincter pressure and barrier pressure (difference between gastric and lower esophageal sphincter pressures): ↓ tone, motility; gastric secretion, motility also ↓
CNS	Sedation

Key Reference: Ali-Melkkila T, Kanto J, Jisalo E: Pharmacokinetics and related pharmacodynamics of anticholinergic drugs. Acta Anaesthesiol Scand 1993; 37:633–642.

PERIOPERATIVE IMPLICATIONS

- Has a greater effect than atropine on eye and exocrine glands; is powerful antisialagogue
- Little effect on HR compared with atropine, glycopyrrolate, but bradycardia or dysrhythmias may occur
- Drug interactions: benzodiazepines, antihistamines, antidepressants, ketamine

ANTICIPATED PROBLEMS/CONCERNS

- Dry mouth
- Anticholinergic syndrome, especially in the elderly and children, manifested as restlessness/confusion
- Transdermal scopolamine has been used to control N/V with inconsistent results; sometimes high incidence of adverse side effects
- Acute narrow-angle glaucoma
- Poisoning with belladonna alkaloids in children

SEROTONIN: AGONISTS, ANTAGONISTS, AND REUPTAKE INHIBITORS

David F. Stowe, M.D., Ph.D.

INDICATIONS

- Serotonin (5-HT) not given as a drug
- Partially selective receptor *agonists* include:
  – sumatriptan (Imitrex) 4–6 mg sc for acute Rx migraine headaches
  – metoclopramide (Reglan) 5–15 mg qid PO, 2–10 mg IV Rx for GER, gastroparesis, N/V
- Partially selective receptor *antagonists* include:
  – ondansetron (Zofran) 4–8 mg tid PO for prevention of N/V due to emetogenic chemotherapy treatment
  – granisetron (Kytril) 10 µg/kg IV for prevention of N/V due to chemoRx; for postop N/V (not FDA-approved)
  – clozapine (Clozaril) 12.5–50 mg PO qd for severe schizophrenia refractory to standard antipsychotic drug Rx
- Selective serotonin reuptake inhibitors include (all used for Rx of major depressive episodes):
  – fluoxetine (Prozac) 20–80 mg qd
  – paroxetine (Paxil) 20–50 mg qd
  – sertraline (Zoloft) 50–200 mg qd

PERIOPERATIVE RISKS

- Sumatriptan: not for pts with IHD, AP, Prinzmetal's angina, severe HTN
- Metoclopramide: not for pts with pheochromocytoma, on MAOIs; may worsen mental depression; effect antagonized by narcotics
- Clozapine: can cause orthostatic hypotension; may ↑ incidence of Szs; like other antipsychotic drugs, can →tardive dyskinesia; NMS
- Selective serotonin reuptake inhibitors can cause "serotonin syndrome" (hyperthermia, muscle rigidity, myoclonus, rapid mental change) if given in the presence of MAOIs; may ↑ warfarin, digitalis effects by ↓ plasma protein binding

WORRY ABOUT

- Sumatriptan: pts taking it may have exacerbation of anginal Sx
- Ondansetron, granisetron: ChemoRx pts may exhibit ↑ N/V during anesthesia
- Clozapine: Pt may have drug-induced agranulocytosis
- Selective serotonin reuptake inhibitors: concomitant use of MAOIs, displacement of other drugs highly bound to plasma protein

OVERVIEW/PHARMACOLOGY

- Serotonin secreted 90% by enterochromaffin cells of GI tract; released into plasma by unclear mech, neuronal stimuli; some taken up, much is stored in platelets; 5-HT receptors on vasc endothelium stimulate release of NO to promote vasodilation, but receptors on vasc smooth muscle promote vasoconstriction. Excess release involved in "carcinoid syndrome," due to enterochromaffin cell neoplasm. As an amine neurotransmitter, serotonin also secreted, stored, released by raphe nuclei in brain stem (serotonergic neurons)
- Serotonergic neurons diffusely innervate most regions of CNS; with other neurotransmitters is involved in modulating mood, depression, anxiety, migraine headache, sleep, appetite, T regulation, perception of pain and itch, regulation of BP
- Abnormalities in secretion or receptor activation likely underlie mental depression, migraine headache, sensitivity to pain, sleep pattern, and central BP control. In CNS, 5-HT receptor activation increases K+ conductance to promote membrane hyperpolarization, → mostly inhibitory action. As CNS neurotransmitter, 5-HT modulates effects of other monoamine transmitters—e.g., norepinephrine, dopamine, and other transmitters such as ACh, glycine, GABA. Inhibition of 5-HT reuptake elevates mood, normalizes behavior

DRUG EFFECTS

SYSTEM	EFFECT	ASSESSMENT BY HX	PE	TEST
CV	Hypertension, IHD (agonists) hypotension (selective serotonin reuptake inhibitors)		BP	
	serotonin syndrome (selective serotonin reuptake inhibitors)	MAO drug interaction	BP, CNS	
	altered drug levels (selective serotonin reuptake inhibitors)	Dysrhythmias, bleeding	Bleeding	Drug levels
ENDO	Carcinoid syndrome (↑ 5-HT)	Diarrhea, Abd pain, asthma, flushing, hyperglycemia, PAT, SVT		5-HT, kallikreins
HEME	Leukopenia (antagonists)			CBC
CNS	Psychosis, depression, altered mood, Sz disorder	Mental disorder	CNS	Drug levels

Key Reference: BG Katzung (ed): Basic and Clinical Pharmacology, 6th ed. East Norwalk, CT, Appleton and Lange, 1995.

PERIOPERATIVE IMPLICATIONS

- Avoid narcotics in pts with carcinoid syndrome (surgery or 5-HT antagonists usual Rx for carcinoid tumor)
- Use caution in giving metoclopramide; pt must not be taking MAOIs—e.g., isocarboxazid (Marplan), phenelzine (Nardil), or tranylcypromine (Parnate)
- Check pt's drug profile if Hx of migraine; ↑ risk of coronary vasoconstriction with sumatriptan
- Check pt's drug profile if Hx of schizophrenia; may have low WBC count if taking clozapine
- Check pt's drug profile if Hx of major depression; if taking coumadin or digitalis, levels may be ↑

STEROIDS

Tommy Symreng, M.D., Ph.D.

USES

- Patients with arthritis, asthma, immunologic diseases, allergies, malignancies, transplantation

PERIOPERATIVE RISKS

- Unique problems with disease requiring steroid medication
- Inadequate stress response

WORRY ABOUT

- Preop correction of fluid, electrolyte balance
- HTN
- Adrenal insufficiency

OVERVIEW

- *Mineralocorticoids*—aldosterone
  - hyperaldosteronism—hypokalemic alkalosis, hypernatremia, HTN, renal tubular malfunction
  - hypoaldosteronism—hypovolemia, hyperkalemic acidosis
- *Glucocorticoids*—cortisol
  - Cushing's syndrome—hypokalemic alkalosis, hypernatremia, fluid retention, HTN, hyperglycemia
  - Glucocorticoid deficiency—hyponatremia, hyperkalemia, hypotension, nausea, abd pain
- *Sex hormones*—less important acutely

CAUSES

- *Mineralocorticoid excess*—adrenal adenoma or hyperplasia
- *Glucocorticoid excess*—glucocorticoid Rx, overproduction of ACTH (pituitary/ectopic), adrenal tumor
- *Mineralocorticoid deficiency*—congenital, post adrenalectomy, renal failure
- *Glucocorticoid deficiency*—withdrawal of long-term steroid med, pituitary/hypothalamic tumor, adrenal destruction (both mineralo-, glucocorticoid decreased) by autoimmune disease, tumor, infection, or hemorrhage

USUAL TREATMENT

- *Mineralocorticoid excess*—spironolactone, surgery
- *Glucocorticoid excess*— ↓ glucocorticoid med, surgery
- *Mineralocorticoid deficiency*—fludrocortisone
- *Glucocorticoid deficiency*—maintenance 25–30 mg hydrocortisone/d, stress 100–300 mg hydrocortisone/d
- *Perioperative coverage*—if steroid treated in last year: 25–100 mg/70 kg/d

DRUG EFFECTS

SYSTEM	EFFECT	ASSESSMENT BY HX	PE	TEST
CV	Hypotension	Orthostatic	BP supine, standing	ECG
	HTN	Angina, CHF, exercise tolerance	CP	CXR
GI	Addison's	N/V, wt loss, abd pain Diarrhea	Buccal hyperpigmentation	Na$^+$, K$^+$
	Cushing's	Thirst, peptic ulcer		
ENDO	Insulin resistance	Glucose intolerance, oligo/amenorrhea		Glucose–B/U Hormone levels
HEME	Steroid effect	PMN leukocytes ↑, leukocytes ↓		CBC differential
SKIN	Addison's		Hyperpigmentation	
	Cushing's		Centripetal obesity, thin skin, acne, striae, hirsutism, edema	
RENAL	Nephropathy			BUN/Cr K$^+$, Na$^+$, Ca^{2+}, acid-base
CNS		Psychiatric changes		
MS	Muscle	Addison's—fatigue, weakness		
		Cushing's—wasting	Muscle wasting	

Key Reference: Symreng T: The anesthetic plan. *In* Rogers MC, Tinker H, Covino BG, Longnecker DE (eds): Principles and Practice of Anesthesiology. St Louis, Mosby-Year Book, 1993, pp 68–70.

PERIOPERATIVE IMPLICATIONS

Preoperative Preparation

- Assess volume, electrolyte, metabolic status

Monitoring

- Routine plus consider UO

Airway

- Dependent on underlying disorder

Induction

- Routine if normovolemic and underlying disease controlled

Maintenance

- Consider stress steroid coverage if steroid treated anytime in last year:
  - minor surgery: 25 mg IV at induction/70 kg
  - major surgery: 100 mg hydrocortisone/24 h/70 kg

Adjuvants

- Etomidate blocks adrenal corticosteroid production, which can prolong effects of steroid NMBs

Postoperative Period

- Most likely time for adrenal insufficiency to develop if hydrocortisone omitted
- Continue steroid supplementation in ↓ doses until patient mobilized

COMPARISON OF CORTICOSTEROIDS

Compound	Anti-inflammatory Potency	Na$^+$-retaining Potency	Duration (hours)
Cortisol	1	1	Short (8–12)
Prednisone	4	0.8	Intermediate
Dexamethasone	25	0	Long (36–72)
Fludrocortisone	10	125	Short
Aldosterone	0	500	Short

ANTICIPATED PROBLEMS/CONCERNS

- Problems with disease as cause for steroid med
- Inadequate stress response
- Fluid, electrolyte balance, and metabolic problems

SUCCINYLCHOLINE

Tamara H. Abbas, M.D.

USES

- Rapid NMB with resulting flaccid paralysis (depolarizing NMB agent)
- Most commonly administered IV, also given IM
- Facilitates ET intubation
- Specifically useful in rapid-sequence induction of GA, laryngoscopy, bronchoscopy
- Facilitates relaxation of abd wall
- Prevents trauma in electroconvulsive therapy for psychiatric disorders

PERIOPERATIVE RISKS

- Fasciculations due to repetitive excitation
- Phase II blockade characterized by prolonged apnea, slow recovery
- Increased IOP (mild)
- Potential mild histamine release
- Efflux of K^+ from muscle cells, causing ↑ serum K^+ level
- Muscle fasciculations, pain more common if no pretreatment with nondepolarizing NMB, lidocaine, or atropine

WORRY ABOUT

- Bradycardia after 2nd injection, esp in children
- Decreased or abnormal plasma pseudo-ChE causing prolonged blockade
- Unpredictable response in myasthenia gravis
- Triggering agent for malignant hyperthermia
- Catastrophic hyperkalemia is induced in patients with massive trauma, burns, neurologic injuries, healthy-appearing children with undiagnosed myopathies, and may be complicated by cardiac arrest

OVERVIEW/PHARMACOLOGY

- As long as adequate concn of succinylcholine remains at receptor site, NM transmission inhibited, flaccid paralysis of skeletal muscle produced; depolarization of cholinergic receptors at the motor end-plate produces fasciculations

- Elimination is by plasma pseudo-ChE
- Phase II blockade can occur when a large dose (> 2–2.5 mg/kg) of drug is given over long period of time; superficially resembles nondepolarizing block
- Onset: IV 30–60 sec; peak effect in 60 sec; IM 2–3 min
- Duration: IV 4–6 min; IM 10–30 min

DRUG CLASS/MECH OF ACTION/USUAL DOSE

- Ultra-short–acting depolarizing muscle relaxant
- Combines with cholinergic receptors at the motor end-plate, inhibiting NM transmission
- Dosage:
  – IV: adult 0.7–1 mg/kg (1.5 mg/kg if pretreating with nondepolarizer); –infant 2–3 mg/kg; –child 1–2 mg/kg
  – IM: 2–4 mg/kg (max 150 mg)
  – Infusion: 0.5–10 mg/min or 10–200 µg/kg/min, titrated

DRUG EFFECTS

SYSTEM	EFFECT	PE	TEST
CV	↑ HR, BP due to initial action at autonomic ganglia	HR, BP	
	Bradycardia at higher doses, reflecting action at cardiac muscarinic cholinergic receptors	HR	ECG
RESP	Hypoventilation, apnea, bronchospasm	Auscultation	$ETCO_2$
GI	↑ Secretions, salivation; ↑ intragastric, lower esophageal sphincter tone		
CNS	↑ IOP, but cerebral function normal		
MS	Flaccid paralysis		PNS stimulator
	Malignant hyperthermia	Temperature	$ETCO_2$, ABGs
SM MUSCLE	No effect, including uterus		

Key Reference: Taylor P: *In* Gilman AG, et al (eds): Goodman & Gilman's The Pharmacological Basis of Therapeutics, 8th ed. New York, Pergamon, 1990, pp 166–186.

PERIOPERATIVE IMPLICATIONS

Preoperative Concerns

- Assess airway, NPO status
- Screen (Hx) for myopathy, burns, CNS denervation
- Screen (Hx) prolonged blockade
- Monitor BP, ECG, PN stimulator (train-of-four)

Induction/Maintenance

- Most often used IV for rapid onset
- May precipitate alkaline solutions, as does sodium thiopental
- Attenuate fasciculations by pretreatment with a nondepolarizer (lidocaine, atropine)
- Blockade may be prolonged with pancuronium pretreatment

- Blockade partially antagonized by pretreatment with other nondepolarizers
- Most effective pretreatment of fasciculations is tubocurarine 3 mg/70 kg, or lidocaine 1.5 mg/kg

Adjuvants/Regional Anesthesia/Reversal

- Conventional depolarizing blockade does not require reversal
- Phase I block potentiated by anticholinergics
- Administration of succinylcholine after an anticholinergic (e.g., neostigmine) produces prolonged NMB

Postoperative Period

- Postoperative myalgias may occur following fasciculations

ANTICIPATED PROBLEMS/CONCERNS

- Abrupt onset of malignant hyperthermia
- Masseter muscle spasm
- Cautious use in patients with fractures or eye injuries who may be further injured by fasciculations
- Serum K^+ levels ↑ 0.5 mEq/L in normal patients
- Catastrophic hyperkalemia can be produced in patients with burns, neurologic or spinal cord injuries, paraplegia (any cause of muscle denervation)
- Fasciculations may actually increase potential for regurgitation, aspiration of gastric contents
- Reduced plasma pseudo-ChE found in pregnancy, cirrhosis, CA, burns, dehydration, or patients with hereditary trait may result in delayed metabolism of drug and prolonged resp paralysis

SULFONAMIDES

J.A. Jeevendra Martyn, M.D.

RISKS

- Side effects due to allergy or direct toxicity (5% incidence)

PERIOPERATIVE RISKS

- Can cause hemolytic or aplastic anemia, all forms of blood cell disorders—e.g., granulocytopenia, thrombocytopenia; thus check WBC, Hgb q 3–5 d
- Patients with deficient G6PD especially sensitive
- May precipitate in urine

WORRY ABOUT

- Bilirubin, many drugs compete for same binding sites in plasma protein, ↑ bilirubin levels when sulfas coadministered; for this reason avoid sulfas in the last few wks of pregnancy and in neonates

- Drug can also be displaced from binding sites by variety of agents (see Possible Drug Interactions, below)
- Procaine is metabolized to PABA, which antagonizes antibacterial effect of sulfonamides

OVERVIEW/PHARMACOLOGY

- Active only in vivo by interfering with use of PABA in folic acid metabolism by microorganisms; further growth of microorganisms is prevented (not seen in humans—where preformed folate absorbed from gut)
- Sulfonamides usually given PO; are rapidly absorbed from stomach, small intestine; distributed to tissues, body fluids including CSF, placenta, fetus
- From 20 to >90% of absorbed drug is bound to serum proteins, affecting diffusibility
- Acetyl derivative (excreted in this form), poorly soluble, toxic, can precipitate in urine

- Excreted mainly by glomerular filtration; acetylation renders drug inactive
- Beware of slow acetylators, patients with G6PD deficiency
- $T_{1/2}$, clearance vary with specific sulfonamide, degree of protein binding, competitors for those protein-binding sites

MECHANISM OF ACTION/DOSE

- Espcially useful in Rx of UTI, toxoplasmosis, trachoma
- Insoluble sulfonamides PO used for antimicrobial prep before bowel surgery; widely used in ulcerative colitis, enteritis, other inflammatory bowel disease
- Topical preps especially used following burn injury; mafenide or silver sulfadiazine, topically applied as cream to skin surfaces, appears effective in controlling infective flora on burn wounds

DRUG EFFECTS

SYSTEM	EFFECT	TESTS
GI/LIVER	N/V, diarrhea, stomatitis; focal or diffuse necrosis of liver due to sensitization or toxicity; may progress to yellow atrophy, death Kernicterus may be enhanced in neonate	LFTs
HEME	Hemolytic anemia in patients with G6PD deficiency; granulocytopenia, thrombocytopenia, leukemoid reactions all known to occur	WBC, Hgb levels q 3–5 d during therapy
GU	Sulfas may precipitate in urine, implicated in various types of nephrosis, allergic nephritis. Transfer via breast milk, placenta possible with adverse effect on neonate, including kernicterus	BUN/Cr Urine sediment exam
SKIN	Stevens-Johnson syndrome is a disease in which there is sloughing and necrosis of skin and mucous membranes due to allergic reaction; mafenide causes significant pain on application Urticaria, skin rashes, photosensitivity	
OTHER	These include fever, conjunctivitis, arthritis, psychosis	

Key Reference: Cuccihara RF, Dawson B: Anesthesia in Stevens-Johnson syndrome: report of a case. Anesthesiology 1971; 35:537–539.

POSSIBLE DRUG INTERACTIONS

- Interactions with anticoag, hypoglycemics, antipyretics, anticonvulsants; toxicity of one or another drug can ↑ because of competitive ↓ in protein binding or hepatic metabolism. Monitor Sx for toxicity, adjust doses
- With sulfas, development of hemolytic anemia not necessarily related to deficiency of G6PD

SPECIAL CONSIDERATIONS

- Measures to prevent precipitation of drug in urine include alkalinizing pH by administration of sodium bicarbonate, ↑ fluid intake, frequent urine analysis; terminate drug if renal function deteriorates
- Sulfa drugs may have toxic effects on slow acetylators
- Avoid in G6PD-deficient patients

TACROLIMUS (FK-506)

Aisling Conran, M.D.

INDICATIONS

- Rescue of primary immunosuppressant Rx following liver, lung, heart, pancreas transplant
- Approx candidates: 3000 liver and 9000 kidney transplants in USA; 15,000 living liver, 50,000 kidney transplant recipients chronically receiving immunosuppressants

PREOPERATIVE RISKS

- HTN: Ca^{2+} channel blockers may be effective in treating tacrolimus-associated HTN, but care required—interference with tacrolimus metabolism may necessitate a dosing reduction
- Nephrotoxicity: do not administer concurrently with cyclosporine; administer cautiously with other potentially nephrotoxic drugs—e.g., aminoglycoside antibiotics
- Hypersensitivity may occur with IV formulation, patients should be monitored for 30 min after injection

WORRY ABOUT

- Drug is metabolized by cytochrome P450 (III A) enzyme system. Other medications that inhibit or induce this enzyme may affect tacrolimus drug levels.

OVERVIEW/PHARMACOLOGY

- General effect: macrolide antibiotic with potent immunosuppressive properties, often used for rescue therapy in liver transplant patients with rejection refractory to other immunosuppressants
- Tacrolimus metabolized by liver; metab primarily excreted in bile; elimination $T_{1/2}$ of 8.5 h prolonged with hepatic dysfunction
- Ca^{2+} channel blockers, cyclosporine, erythromycin, antifungal agents, metoclopramide may ↑ blood levels of tacrolimus as function of P450 inhibition
- Anticonvulsants (carbamazepine, phenobarbital, phenytoin), rifampin may ↓ blood levels of tacrolimus secondary to induction of cytochrome P450 system
- Adverse effects requiring dose adjustments include nephrotoxicity, neurotoxicity, alterations in glucose metabolism, infection or susceptibility to malignancy

DRUG CLASS/MECH OF ACTION/USUAL DOSE

- Macrolide antibiotic, highly protein bound (>75%), binds primarily to albumin and/or α_1-glycoprotein
- Tacrolimus binds to calcineurin, blocking production of interleukin-2, thereby inhibiting further T-lymphocyte proliferation, immunosuppression
- Dose: IV 0.05–0.1 mg/kg/d; PO 0.15–0.3 mg/kg/d in 2 divided doses

DRUG EFFECTS

SYSTEM	EFFECT	ASSESSMENT BY HX	PE	TEST
GENERAL	Hypersensitivity, rash	Observe ½ h; have epinephrine 1:1000 available		
CV	HTN		BP/HR	
RESP	Pleural effusion, dyspnea			
GI	Diarrhea, N/V, constipation, abn liver function, anorexia, Abd pain			LFTs
RENAL	Abn kidney function, oliguria			BUN, Cr
ENDO	Hyperkalemia, hypokalemia, hyperglycemia			K+, glucose
HEME	Anemia, leukocytosis, thrombocytopenia			CBC
CNS	Headache, tremor, insomnia, paresthesias, mental status changes, circumoral numbness		Preop neuro exam	

Key Reference: Hooks MA: Tacrolimus—a new immunosuppressant—a review of the literature. Ann Pharmacother 1994; 28:501–511.

PERIOPERATIVE IMPLICATIONS

Preoperative Preparation

- Continue all immunosuppressants through perioperative period
- Monitor levels: therapeutic range 5–30 ng/ml; maintenance level 5–10 ng/ml

Monitoring

- Consider frequent NIBP or arterial catheter

Induction/Maintenance

- Inducers of P450 system include phenobarbital, phenytoin, isoniazid; some volatile anesthetics may result in ↑ metabolism of tacrolimus

Possible Drug Interactions

- Ca^{2+} channel blockers, cyclosporine, erythromycin, antifungal agents, metoclopramide may ↑ blood levels of tacrolimus as function of P450 inhibition
- Anticonvulsants (carbamazepine, phenobarbital, phenytoin), rifampin may ↓ blood levels of tacrolimus 2° to induction of cytochrome P450 system
- Adverse effects requiring dose adjustments include nephrotoxicity, neurotoxicity, alterations in glucose metabolism, infection, and susceptibility to malignancy

ANTICIPATED PROBLEMS/CONCERNS

- Hypersensitivity may occur with IV formulation

TERBUTALINE

P. Allan Klock, M.D.

USES

- Prescribed for pts with bronchospasm
- Effective for acute asthmatic attacks, COPD
- Used as tocolytic for preterm labor (not FDA-approved for this use)

PERIOPERATIVE RISKS

- Complications of tachyarrhythmias, hypokalemia, hyperglycemia

WORRY ABOUT

- Tachycardia, surreptitious adrenergic cardiomyopathy
- Hyperglycemia
- Hypokalemia
- Pulm edema (from surreptitious adrenergic cardiomyopathy)

OVERVIEW/PHARMACOLOGY

- Used for both acute bronchospasm, chronic management of COPD
- Tachyphylaxis poss with prolonged use
- 7–14% of delivered aerosol reaches circulation
- $\frac{1}{3}$ SC dose metabolized in liver to inactive sulfate conjugates
- Metabolites I and II, unchanged drug excreted in urine

Onset/Duration

- SC
  - onset: Significant ↑ in FEV_1 in 15 min, peak 30–60 min
  - duration: 1.5–4 h; $T_{1/2}$, 3–4 h
- IV (not FDA-approved route)
  - onset: immediate; $T_{1/2}$, 3–4 h
- PO
  - onset: significant improvement in FEV_1 in 60–120 min
  - duration: at least 4 h
- Metered dose inhaler/nebulizer
  - onset: 5 min; peak, 1–2 h
  - duration: 3–4 h

DRUG CLASS/MECH OF ACTION/USUAL DOSE

- β_2 agonist (found to be β_2-selective in animals but selectivity not seen in humans)
- β_2 stimulation ↑ adenylcyclase conversion of ATP to cAMP; this effect →cell hyperpolarization, ↓ inward Ca^{2+} flux, →relaxation of bronchial, uterine, vasc smooth muscle

Usual Dose

- SC: 0.005–0.01 mg/kg to a max 0.25 mg/dose; inject every 15–20 min as needed.
- PO: 5 mg tid
- Metered dose inhaler: 2 inhalations every 4–6 h (200 μg/actuation)
- Nebulizer: 0.01–0.03 ml/kg (1 ml = 1 mg); minimum = 0.1 ml, maximum = 2.5 ml; dilute in 1–2 ml N/S

DRUG EFFECTS

SYSTEM	EFFECT	ASSESSMENT BY HX	PE	TEST
CV	Tachycardia, HTN, hypotension, arrhythmias, ↓ SVR	Palpitations	↑ HR; irregular rhythm, BP; rales	ECG
RESP	Bronchodilation	↓ Dyspnea	↓ Wheezing	O_2 saturation, PFT, PEF
GI	Nausea	Nausea		
ENDO	Hyperglycemia, hypokalemia*	Polydipsia, polyuria	Dehydration	Blood glucose, serum K^+
CNS	CNS stimulation	Insomnia, anxiety, hyperactivity, drowsiness, headache	Tremor	

*Plasma hypokalemia is due to IC transport of K^+. Hypokalemia is seen most often with IV terbutaline Rx for preterm labor. K^+ supplementation rarely required, serum levels usually normalize within 3 h of discontinuation of infusion.

Key Reference: Wagner JM, Morton MJ, Johnson KA, et al: Terbutaline and maternal cardiac function. JAMA 1981; 246:2697.

PERIOPERATIVE IMPLICATIONS

Preoperative Concerns

- Evaluate disease being treated: asthma, preterm labor
- For asthmatic pts, consider administering inhaled β_2 agonist before inducing anesthesia
- For pts in preterm labor, assess fetal well-being; FHR, wt, indices of lung maturity, etc.
- Evaluate VS, especially HR, BP; rule out CHF
- Assess volume status
- Lab studies to check: glucose, K^+

Induction/Maintenance

- ↑ CO may prolong inhalation induction
- Theoretical concern of ↑ ventricular irritability with halothane
- Intraoperative bronchospasm possible with inhaled or IV terbutaline; absorption after SC injection poss unreliable
- Tachycardia possible owing to drug effect, not light anesthesia

ANTICIPATED PROBLEMS/CONCERNS

- ↑ HR, ↓ SVR poss not tolerated well by pts with CAD, mitral or aortic stenosis
- CHF may be surreptitious

TETRACAINE

Stanley W. Stead, M.D.

USES

- Very frequently used for spinal anesthesia
- Long-acting local in pediatric ERs (topical, injected)

PERIOPERATIVE RISKS

- Toxicity from excessive dose
- Hypersensitivity reaction

WORRY ABOUT

- True allergic hypersensitivity to ester local anesthetic

OVERVIEW/PHARMACOLOGY

- 2-(Dimethylamino)ethyl p-(butylamino) benzoate monohydrochloride
- Aminoester local anesthetic, intermediate to long duration. Derivative of para-amino benzoic acid. Uptake due to lipophilic absorption
- Hydrolyzed by plasma ChE to water-soluble amino alcohols, carboxylic acid, producing PABA moieties (implicated as antigens in numerous hypersensitivity reactions). Patients homozygous for abn plasma ChE metabolize drug more slowly, so serum levels ↑, with ↑ risk of toxicity
- Pharmacokinetics: Undergoes hydrolysis in plasma at 0.3 µmol/ml/h

DRUG CLASS/MECH OF ACTION/USUAL DOSE

- Aminoester local anesthetic, provided as an HCl salt—lipophilic free base is taken up into nerve.
- Reduces currents through voltage-activated Na^+ channels; K^+ channels may also be reduced.
- Permeates nerves, axon membranes, equilibrates there and in axoplasm, depending on drug's pK_a (8.4), hydrophobicity of base/cation species concn. Hydrophobicity measured by octanol:buffer partition coefficient of the base: 5822, making it an extremely hydrophobic local anesthetic.
- Binds to local anesthetic sites on voltage-gated Na^+ channels; conformational change of receptor prevents opening of channel during activation; axon potentials cease to be propagated; onset, recovery from blockade limited by diffusion of local anesthetic molecules into/out of nerve membrane and axoplasm.

Baricity of spinal solns (determines spread within spinal CSF):
- Hyperbaric soln (denser than CSF, soln settles in CSF according to gravity)
  - 1% soln of tetracaine diluted with equal vol 10% glucose to total concn of 0.5%
- Hypobaric soln (less dense than CSF, soln rises in CSF)
  - 1% soln tetracaine diluted with equal vol H_2O to total concn of 0.5%
- Isobaric soln density (equal to that of CSF, no tendency to rise or settle in CSF)
  - 1% soln tetracaine diluted with equal vol CSF or saline to total concn of 0.5%
- Available as niphanoid crystals or in solution of 1.0%

Indication	Concn	Drug Dose	Onset	Duration
Major nerve block	0.25–0.5% (epinephrine)	50–200 mg	20–30 min	300–600 min
Spinal	0.25–1%	5–20 mg	5–15 min	75–150 min

DRUG EFFECTS

Toxicity associated with doses >200 mg/70 kg; CNS, CV systems affected. Generally 4–7× amt producing convulsions causes CV collapse.

SYSTEM	EFFECT	ASSESSMENT BY HX	PE	TEST
OVERALL	Allergic reactions	Urticaria	Edema	Skin testing of limited value
HEENT	Toxicity Topical ophthalmic: ↓ corneal epithelial regeneration	Tinnitus, metallic taste		
CV	Pulm vasoconstriction; systemic vasodilator; neg inotrope; neg chronotrope			↑ PAP ↑ PVR ↓ SVR ↓ CO ECG: ↑ in PR, QRS
PNS	Block nerve transmissions		Loss of sensation, motor function initially	
CNS	Toxicity: more sensitive than CV	Shivering, twitching, tremors in face, extremities, progressing to tonic-clonic seizures	Hyperreflexia may be present	
MS	IV may augment NMB (depolarizing, nondepolarizing)			Nerve stimulator: ↓ twitch height

Key Reference: Gilman AG, Rall TW, Nies AS, Taylor P: Local anesthetics. *In* Goodman & Gilman's The Pharmacological Basis of Therapeutics, 8th ed. New York, Pergamon, 1991, pp 311–331.

PERIOPERATIVE IMPLICATIONS

Possible Drug Interactions

- In large doses, blocks NM transmission, in smaller doses, enhances NMB from nondepolarizing and depolarizing NM blockers.
- Acidosis, hypercarbia, hypoxia may potentiate neg chronotropic, inotropic actions of tetracaine

Preoperative Considerations/Induction/Maintenance

- Avoid administration of excessive doses of tetracaine

ANTICIPATED PROBLEMS/CONCERNS

- Reports of ineffectiveness of properly placed tetracaine without explanation abound
- Allergy to PABA contraindicates the usage

TETRACYCLINES

Thomas F. Boerner, M.D.
W. David Watkins, Ph.D., M.D.

USES

- Administered PO (most common), IV (fewer side effects), IM (rare, painful), topical (eyes only)
- Original broad-spectrum antibiotic for gram-pos, gram-neg aerobes, anaerobes. One of few agents active against organisms without cell walls. Resistance ↑ worldwide
- Rx for: STDs, other GU infections, dental infections, periodontal diseases, Lyme disease, OA, sclerotherapy, chemoRx, antidiarrheal prophylaxis
- 20 million doses/y in USA

PERIOPERATIVE RISKS

- Barbiturates may ↓ $T_{1/2}\beta$; Tetracycline will ↑ concns of digoxin, warfarin. Pts may exhibit GI distress, even *Clostridium difficile* colitis
- IV tetracycline frequently →thrombophlebitis, lessens efficacy of OC
- ↓ Dose with age, poor renal/hepatic functions

WORRY ABOUT

- Tetracycline (esp 1st generation) absorbed poorly if given within 3 h of di-/trivalent cations (Ca^{2+}, Al^{3+}, Mg^{2+}, Fe^{2+}, Bi^{3+})

OVERVIEW/PHARMACOLOGY

- Classified as bacteriostatic (newest ones possibly bactericidal)
- 2 generations: 1st (e.g., tetracycline); 2nd (e.g., doxycycline)
- PO uptake in duodenum (esp 1st generation); peak level, 2 h; IV peak level, 1 h
- 1st generation $T_{1/2}\beta$ 6–12 hr; excreted in urine, feces; 2nd generation more lipophilic, greater V_D, recirculation, $T_{1/2}\beta$ 16–18 h; doxycycline excreted 90% + in feces; safe for anephric pts
- Adjust dose with age, impaired renal/hepatic functions

DRUG CLASS/MECH OF ACTION/USUAL DOSE

- Original broad-spectrum antibiotic
- Nml dose: impairs bacterial protein synthesis; binds via a Mg^{2+} bridge to single active site of 30∫ subunit of bacterial ribosome; prevents binding of aminoacyl tRNA to the mRNA-ribosome complex. Without this codon–anticodon interaction, peptide chain formation cannot proceed
- Effective against *Rickettsia, Mycoplasma, Chlamydia, Borrelia,* spirochetes, some fungi
- Inhibit collagenase (OA), tumor-induced angiogenesis (chemoRx)
- Local irritant (sclerotherapy)
- Usual dose: doxycycline, 100 mg PO, bid

DRUG EFFECTS

SYSTEM	EFFECT	ASSESSMENT BY HX	TEST
HEENT	Children: brown teeth; risk greatest from second trimester to age 8 y		
CV	Frequently causes thrombophlebitis ↓ tumor-mediated angiogenesis		
LIVER	Rare toxicity, especially with ↑ dose, IV route, preg Usually reversible with drug cessation	Hepatitis	LFTs
GI	Irritation, distress, especially PO, ↑ dose may →superinfection (*C. difficile* colitis)		
HEME	May inhibit/suppress antibody production, leukotaxis, complement system		
GU	May aggravate uremia in susceptible pt; crosses placenta, excreted in milk		
CNS	Penetrates CNS; may ↑ ICP during Rx, esp infants	Vision change, headache	
	Minocycline: vestibular problems, esp women	Dizziness, nausea	
MS	Phototoxic skin reaction, esp 1st generation; ↓ bone growth in preemies, ↓ collagenase in joints		

Key Reference: Chopra I, Hawkey PM, Hinton M: Review: Tetracyclines, molecular and clinical aspects. J Antimicrob Chemother 1992; 29:245–277.

PERIOPERATIVE IMPLICATIONS

Preoperative Concerns

- May ↑ digoxin levels, higher prothrombin time if patient on warfarin

Possible Drug Interactions

- Barbiturates may ↓ $T_{1/2}\beta$
- Methoxyflurane, tetracycline may →renal failure

Reversal

- May augment nondepolarizing NM blocker

SPECIAL CONSIDERATIONS

- Although resistance is rising, drugs remain useful antibiotics with nonantibiotic indications increasing.
- Contraindicated in preg, childhood

THYROID SUPPLEMENTS

John M. Murkin, M.D.

INDICATIONS

- >3 million chronic users in USA
- T_4 prescribed for patients with chronic hypothyroidism
- T_3 used in myxedema coma
- Not currently indicated but somewhat successfully used for cardiogenic shock post-CPB
- T_3 also favorably administered to brain-dead donors before organ harvesting for heart, heart-lung transplantation
- T_4 generally administered PO; T_4 and T_3 can be administered IV

PERIOPERATIVE RISKS

- Drugs (amiodarone, catecholamines, radiopaque contrast media), cirrhosis, renal failure, sepsis, operation (CPB) can induce "euthyroid sick syndrome" (reduced peripheral conversion of T_4 to T_3); may precipitate myxedema coma

WORRY ABOUT

- T_4 or T_3 can aggravate Sx of myocardial ischemia

OVERVIEW/PHARMACOLOGY

- Hypothyroidism (overt) estimated at 0.5%–0.8% of adults, ↑ with age
- Post-thyroidectomy <30% of patients euthyroid at 10 y due to inadequacy or discontinuation of therapy
- Reversal of clin Sx of chronic hypothyroidism, incl myocardial effusions, requires 2–4 mo Rx
- $T_{1/2}$ for T_4: 7d, T_3: 1.5 d
- T_4 relatively inactive prohormone undergoing monodeiodination in liver, kidney to biologically active T_3

ICD-9-CM Code: 244.9

DRUG CLASS/MECH OF ACTION/USUAL DOSE

- Thyroid hormone replacement Rx
- T_3 binding to specific membrane receptor proteins augments membrane transport activity, mitochondrial oxidative phosphorylation, protein synthesis
- Extranuclear effects of T_3 occur in min, ↑ myocardial mitochondrial and transmembrane transport activity
- Nuclear effects of T_3 occur within 0.5–1.0 h, involve transcription, translation of myocardial enzymes, contractile proteins
- Direct effect of T_3 ↓ arterial smooth muscle tone
- Usual dosage of T_4 is 0.15 mg/d PO
- Acute Rx: T_4, 0.3–0.5 mg by slow IV infusion followed by 0.1–0.15 mg/d, or T_3, 0.005–0.01 mg IV

DRUG EFFECTS

SYSTEM	EFFECT	ASSESSMENT BY HX	PE	TEST
CV	Chronotropy, inotropy, ↓ SVR	Less fatigue	HR, reflexes	FT_4E, TSH, ECG
	Arrhythmogenesis	Palpitations		
RESP	Restoration of hypoxic, hypercapnic ventilatory drive			
GI	↑ Protein synthesis; enhanced hepatic, renal clearance/excretion functions		Normal skin turgor	
ENDO	Thermogenesis	Reversal of cold intolerance	Skin warm to touch	

Key Reference: Clark O et al: Ann Thorac Surg 1993; 56:S1–S60.

PERIOPERATIVE IMPLICATIONS/POSSIBLE DRUG INTERACTIONS

Preoperative Concerns

- Thyroid hormones ↑ breakdown of vit K–dependent clotting factors—can alter coag status

Induction/Maintenance

- Exaggerated HTN, tachycardia can occur with agents such as ketamine, exogenous catecholamines including ephedrine, epinephrine, in patients on both acute and chronic thyroid hormone replacement

Adjuvants/Regional Anesthesia/Reversal

- Anticholinergics with minimal CV effects, e.g., glycopyrrolate, preferred over atropine
- Caution in the presence of spinal anesthesia; T_3 administration may produce aggravated hypotension

Postoperative Period

- Cirrhosis, sepsis, renal failure, surgery may all ↓ peripheral conversion of T_4 to T_3 (sick euthyroid syndrome), precipitate hypothyroidism

ANTICIPATED PROBLEMS/CONCERNS

- In critically ill patients, T_3 replacement can produce detrimental increases in O_2 requirements (esp myocardial), protein catabolism w/o improving mortality rates.

TISSUE PLASMINOGEN ACTIVATOR

J. Christopher Sill, M.D.

USES

- Patients suffering acute transmural MI
- Experimental for CVAs but recent randomized trials indicate 33% less disability with t-PA
- Rx: Thrombolysis with t-PA plus adjuvants restores patency of infarct-related artery in 60–90% of patients; benefits outweigh risks

PERIOPERATIVE RISKS

- ↑ Bleeding during surgery; of thrombolytic agents currently available, t-PA least likely to cause systemic fibrinolytic state

WORRY ABOUT

- Invasive procedures; damage to blood vessels during vasc access procedures can cause severe bleeding—esp at noncompressible sites—e.g., subclavian vein. Consequences of catheter-induced PA damage can be dire. Minor bleeding at venipuncture sites

OVERVIEW/PHARMACOLOGY

- Thrombolytic agent; accelerates conversion of plasminogen to plasmin with activity relatively specific for plasminogen assoc with fibrin; plasmin cleaves fibrin with dissolution of thrombus
- Initial in vivo $T_{1/2}$ ~5 min; terminal elimination $T_{1/2}$ ~45 min
- Endogenous plasminogen activator inhibitor-1 neutralizes t-PA, but exists at insufficient plasma concn to be effective during fibrinolytic Rx
- Clearance occurs in liver by receptor-mediated endocytosis at hepatocytes; vasc endothelial cells clear t-PA in a similar manner

DRUG CLASS/MECH OF ACTION/USUAL DOSE

- Thrombolytic agent with specificity for plasminogen assoc with fibrin; action at site of thrombus, not throughout circ
- Secreted by endothelium; recombinant DNA methods permit production for clin use
- In presence of fibrin, t-PA accelerates conversion of plasminogen to plasmin—the central enzyme in fibrin degradation, thrombolysis
- Little antigenicity, little effect on systemic fibrinolytic state, few allergic side effects
- Usual dose: 100 mg by IV bolus, continuous infusion over 3 h + heparin ± aspirin
- Alternatives: Streptokinase, urokinase
- Can reverse effect (but worry about precipitating thrombosis) with fibrinogen in cryoprecipitate) and epsilon-aminocaproic acid

DRUG EFFECTS

SYSTEM	EFFECT	TREATMENT	TEST
CV	Bleeding	Manual compression, cryoprecipitate, ? aprotinin	Coag studies, RBCs, type, cross-match
	Hypotension	IV fluids	
	Anaphylaxis	? Steroid pretreatment IV fluids	
CNS	Intracranial hemorrhage	Supportive, distal t-PA infusion Intubation, mech ventilation, mannitol if severe	Coag studies, RBCs, type, cross-match

Key Reference: GUSTO Investigators: An international randomized trial comparing four thrombolytic strategies for acute myocardial infarction. N Engl J Med 1993; 329:673–682.

PERIOPERATIVE IMPLICATIONS/POSSIBLE DRUG INTERACTIONS

- Specific drug interactions not reported
- In absence of optimal recanalization, reperfusion, myocardial ischemia may persist; infarct may go to completion, resulting in unstable hemodynamic state
- A degree of nonspecific plasmin activity inevitably occurs during t-PA Rx, ↑ surgical blood loss. Consider aprotinin, cryoprecipitate

TRIMETHAPHAN

Lorna L. Im, M.D.

USES

- Production of controlled hypotension during surgery
- Acute control of BP in HTN emergencies, autonomic hyperreflexia, dissecting aortic aneurysm
- Emergency Rx of pulmonary edema in pulmonary HTN assoc with systemic HTN
- Given only IV

PERIOPERATIVE RISKS

- Risk of severe hypotension
- Incompatible with thiopental or other alkaline solutions of iodides and bromides; avoid trimethaphan infusion as vehicle for simultaneous administration of any other drug
- Produces mydriasis, so pupillary dilation may confuse CNS exam
- Histamine release at high doses

WORRY ABOUT

- Severe hypotension, especially with regional anesthesia, state of hypovolemia, or use of other antihypertensive drugs

OVERVIEW/PHARMACOLOGY

- Ganglion-blocking agent, direct peripheral arterial and venous vasodilator
- Rapid onset (1–3 min), short duration of action (5–15 min) after single IV dose
- Partial clearance by plasma ChE hydrolysis, partly by renal elimination (therefore if BP so low that GFR is decreased, ↓ in renal excretion can prolong duration of action)
- Tachyphylaxis may result after continuous IV infusion
- Autoregulation is preserved in cerebral and possibly coronary vascular beds; vasodilation can ↑ total blood flow to a region; autoregulation can then distribute flow to ischemic areas, therefore steal is less likely

DRUG CLASS/MECH OF ACTION/USUAL DOSE

- Autonomic ganglion blocker
- Binds to receptors on autonomic ganglion cells, stabilizes postsynaptic membranes against action of ACh released from presynaptic cell
- Lowers BP by lowering art peripheral resistance. At high doses, CO ↓ due to venous pooling in capacitance vessels with fall in venous return
- Used to produce controlled hypotension; also used to improve perfusion during, after cardiac surgery
- Usual Dose
  - intermittent IV bolus of 1–20 mg; may start with a 1 mg IV bolus, then double dose ↑ min until desired fall in BP produced
  - continuous IV infusion of 0.5–6.0 mg/min; may dilute 500 mg drug in 500 ml of D_5, N/S, or lactated Ringer's to a 0.1% soln, start rate at 60 drops/min (3–4 ml); titrate to desired BP
  - infants more resistant to drug: infuse 0.2% soln
  - elderly: dilute to <0.1% soln

DRUG EFFECTS

Adverse reactions due to its nonselective blockade of autonomic nervous system (sympathetic and parasympathetic), predominant tone at effector sites

SYSTEM	PREDOMINANT TONE	EFFECT	ASSESSMENT OF HX	PE
CV	Parasympathetic	Tachycardia		
Arterioles	Sympathetic	Vasodilation, ↑ peripheral blood flow, hypotension, ↓ SVR		
Veins	Sympathetic	Dilation, peripheral pooling of blood, ↓ preload	Syncope	Postural hypotension
RESP		Rare respiratory arrest of uncertain mechanism with high doses		
GI	Parasympathetic	↓ Secretions, ↓ tone/motility	Dry mouth, paralytic ileus, abd discomfort, N/V/diarrhea, reflux	
GU	Parasympathetic	Bladder atony	Urinary hesitancy, incomplete voiding	
		↓ Potency	Impaired erection, ejaculation	
CNS		↑ in ICP during controlled hypotension is less than with other direct vasodilators (nitroprusside); does not cross blood-brain barrier		
OPHTHAL	Parasympathetic	Cycloplegia, mydriasis, difficulty in accommodation	Blurred vision	
PLACENTA		Does cross placenta; ↓ fetal GI motility results in meconium ileus		

Key Reference: Taylor P: Agents acting at the neuromuscular junction and autonomic ganglia. *In* Gilman AG, Rall TW, Nies AS, Taylor P (eds): Goodman & Gilman's The Pharmacological Basis of Therapeutics, 8th ed. New York, Macmillan, 1990, pp 181–184, 793.

PERIOPERATIVE IMPLICATIONS

Preoperative Concerns

- Assess volume status
- Monitor continuous arterial BP

Induction/Maintenance

- May interact with other induction agents to cause hypotension
- May be given prophylactically as bolus during induction before laryngoscopy

- Trimethaphan has pH of 5.2 and is incompatible with alkaline solns, e.g., thiopental
- Anesthesia can modify dose of trimethaphan needed to produce response—e.g., the deeper the plane of anesthesia, the smaller the dose of trimethaphan required to produce hypotension

Adjuvants/Regional Anesthesia/Reversal

- Possible delay in onset, prolonged duration of action of NM blockers, especially succinylcholine, by this ganglionic blocking drug, because of (1) ↓ skeletal muscle blood flow, (2)

inhibition of plasma ChE activity, (3) ↓ sensitivity of postjunctional membranes
- Interaction with aminoglycoside antibiotics at NMJ may prolong blockade

SPECIAL CONSIDERATIONS

- Potential problems with continuous administration include:
  - tachyphylaxis
  - persistently low BP up to 30 min after discontinuance of drug
- H_2 release may precipitate catecholamine "surge" in patients with pheochromocytoma

VECURONIUM

James E. Caldwell, M.B., Ch.B.
Ronald D. Miller, M.D.

USES

- Facilitates tracheal intubation, provides skeletal muscle paralysis for patients undergoing surgery
- Facilitates tracheal intubation, mechanical ventilation of patients in ICU
- Approved only for IV use

PERIOPERATIVE RISKS

- Patient loses airway protective reflexes
- Patient rendered apneic
- Anesthesiologist must support ventilation
- Rare risk of allergic reaction

WORRY ABOUT

- Bradycardia with high-dose opioid anesthetics
- Prolonged duration of paralysis with aminoglycoside antibiotics

OVERVIEW/PHARMACOLOGY

- Paralyzes skeletal muscle
- Used for few h in OR, days or weeks in ICU
- Speed of onset, duration of action directly related to dose administered
- Initial onset ≈ 1 min
- Max effect in 3–5 min
- Clin duration 30–45 min
- Elimination, 70% by hepatic, 30% by renal mechanisms
- Liver metabolism by deacetylation at 3 position accounts for 12% of clearance
- Plasma clearance reduced by renal, hepatic dysfunction
- Plasma clearance ↑ by phenytoin
- Prolonged use in ICU can →tolerance or persistent paralysis

DRUG CLASS/MECH OF ACTION/USUAL DOSE

- Monoquaternary aminosteroid
- Competitive antagonist of ACh at NMJ of skeletal muscle
  - Usual dose, always IV
    - For tracheal intubation, 0.08–0.15 mg/kg
    - For maintenance of paralysis, 0.01–0.03 mg/kg

DRUG EFFECTS

SYSTEM	EFFECT	ASSESSMENT BY HX	PE	TEST
RESP	Resp depression, apnea, Pulm aspiration		resp	
MS	NMB	Onset of paralysis	Muscle strength	Train-of-4 responses

Key Reference: Miller RD, et al: Pharmacology of muscle relaxants and their antagonists. *In* Miller RD (ed): Anesthesia. New York, Churchill Livingstone, 1994, pp 417–487.

PERIOPERATIVE IMPLICATIONS

Preoperative Concerns

- Assess airway anatomy
- Monitor train-of-4 responses

Induction/Maintenance

- With large doses of opioid, bradycardia may occur
- Initial large dose IV, 0.08–0.10 mg/kg to facilitate tracheal intubation
- Repeat doses of 1/5–1/10 of initial dose to maintain surgical paralysis
- Large doses, 0.2–0.4 mg/kg, produce rapid onset of paralysis (80–120 s) and long duration of action (70–120 min)

Adjuvants/Regional Anesthesia/Reversal

- Action enhanced by anesthetic vapors
- Action prolonged by mild hypothermia
- Action antagonized by administration of an anticholinesterase

Postoperative Period

- Residual effect may produce inadequate ventilation or respiratory obstruction

ANTICIPATED PROBLEMS/CONCERNS

- Because of muscle paralysis, clinician must be able to maintain patient's ventilation, oxygenation
- Residual paralysis at end of surgery must be reversed by administration of an anticholinesterase: neostigmine, pyridostigmine, edrophonium
- If muscle weakness persists, protect patient's airway, support ventilation until full recovery
- Administration of an anticholinesterase must be accompanied by glycopyrrolate or atropine to avoid severe bradycardia

VITAMIN B₁₂ (CYANOCOBALAMIN)

John K. Stene, M.D., Ph.D.

INDICATIONS

- Prevalence of deficiency: 13 million in USA esp in elderly
- Prescribed for pernicious anemia
- Lack of gastric secretion of intrinsic factor → malabsorption of vit B_{12}; therefore IM route preferred. Strict vegetarian diet–induced deficiency state; responds to oral supplementation

WORRY ABOUT

- Permanent neurologic injury in long-term deficiency states
- Interactions and neurologic injury with folate, methionine synthetase inhibitors, N_2O

OVERVIEW/PHARMACOLOGY

- Vit B_{12} binds to intrinsic factor (gastric glycoprotein from parietal cells) in GI tract, is absorbed from ileum, bound to transcobalamin II in plasma for transport to tissues. Approximately 3 µg of cobalamin secreted into bile qd
- Excess vit B_{12} admin ↑ urinary excretion
- Vit B_{12} enzymatically converted to 2 active forms: deoxyadenosylcobalamin, methylcobalamin; the former is a cofactor for mitochondrial mutase enzyme that catalyzes L-methylmalonyl CoA to succinyl CoA
- Methylcobalamin is cofactor in methionine synthetase reaction (a methyl group is transferred from 5-methyltetrahydrofolate to homocysteine to form methionine and tetrahydrofolate), pivotal in normal synthesis of purines, pyrimidines, and a number of methylation reactions through formation of S-adenosylmethionine

ICD-9-CM Codes: 266.2 (Vitamin B_{12} deficiency); 281.0 (Pernicious anemia)

DRUG CLASS/MECH OF ACTION/USUAL DOSE

- H_2O-soluble B vit complex
- Cyanocobalamin administered IM or deep subcutaneous route in doses of 1–1000 µg
- Oral dose to 80 µg can be administered with purified intrinsic factor; 1 U binds 15 µg of cyanocobalamin
- Need glycoprotein (intrinsic factor 60,000 MW) produced by gastric parietal cells for its absorption
- RDA: 2 µg/d for adults

ASSESSMENT POINTS

SYSTEM	EFFECT	ASSESSMENT BY HX	PE	TEST
GI	Achlorhydric or gastrectomy patients at risk; associated with atrophic glossitis	Burning and tingling of mouth	Small, slick, glistening tongue	Schilling test (for vit B_{12} absorption)
HEME	Megaloblastic anemia	Apathy, lassitude, fatigue	Pale skin, mucous membranes, esp nailbeds, palmar surfaces	Peripheral blood smear: macrocytic hyperchromic RBCs Bone marrow: megaloblasts, ↓ megakaryocytes ↓ Platelet count
CNS	Degeneration of dorsal, lateral columns of spinal cord	Numbness, tingling in extremities, difficulty walking	Loss of vibration, position sense; ataxia, Romberg's sign, muscle flaccidity	
PNS	Neuropathy	Paresthesias, dysesthesias of lower extremities		

Key Reference: Hillman RS: Hematopoietic agents: growth factors, minerals, and vitamins. *In* Gilman AG, Rall TW, Nies AS, Taylor P, eds: Goodman & Gilman's The Pharmacological Basis of Therapeutics, 8th ed. New York, Pergamon, 1990, pp 1296–1302.

PERIOPERATIVE IMPLICATIONS/POSSIBLE DRUG INTERACTIONS

- Folate admin reverses megaloblastic anemia, but does not prevent (may precipitate) spinal cord degeneration
- N_2O oxidizes vit B_{12}, reduces activity of methionine synthetase
- Effect of N_2O can be reversed by large doses of folic acid

ANTICIPATED PROBLEMS/CONCERNS

- Scavenging waste anesthetic gas prevents OR personnel from developing vit B_{12} deficiency states due to prolonged exposure to N_2O
- Extensive interaction between folate and vit B_{12} makes it imperative that pernicious anemia be treated with B_{12} at same time as folate to prevent CNS degeneration

WARFARIN (COUMADIN)

Charise T. Petrovitch, M.D.

INDICATIONS

• Management of thromboembolic disorders: for prophylaxis, Rx, and prevention of recurrence of thromboembolic event including DVT, pulm embolism, thrombosis of grafts. Prevention of arterial emboli associated with prosthetic heart valves, nonvalvular AFib, acute MI. Prevention of MI, stroke, and recurrent MI. Rx for antithrombin III, protein C, protein S deficiency.
• Newer indications: after angioplasty, for patients who have had coronary graft thrombosis when taking only ASA or ASA and dipyridamole.
• Number of individuals receiving the drug: unknown

PERIOPERATIVE RISKS

• Hemorrhage (minor to major life risk)
• "Purple-toe" syndrome, or warfarin necrosis
• Teratogenicity in preg (↓ synthesis of vit K–dependent clotting factors by fetus)

WORRY ABOUT

• Major drug interactions:
  – Multiplicity of drugs affecting action of warfarin. List extensive, continually expanding (see later). Be concerned with other drugs that potentiate bleeding—e.g., antiplatelet agents, ASA, NSAIDs, etc.; drugs that displace warfarin from protein-binding sites or ↑ or ↓ vit K levels.

OVERVIEW/PHARMACOLOGY

• General effect: Anticoagulant with dose-dependent effect on coagulation

PHARMACOKINETICS/PHARMACODYNAMICS

• Warfarin is a racemic mixture of R and S isomers (R-warfarin; S-warfarin)
• Racemic warfarin absorbed rapidly from GI tract, reaches max plasma concn in 90 min, has $T_{1/2}$ of 36–42 h; time to peak effect 36–72 h; duration after discontinuing 2–5 d at least
• In circulation, bound to plasma proteins, accumulates in liver. R-warfarin metabolites excreted in urine; S-warfarins eliminated in bile
• "Warfarin resistance" or ↓ warfarin effect: when warfarin absorption from GI tract impaired from malabsorption syndromes, concurrent use of liquid paraffin laxatives, cholestyramine resin, or excessive amts of certain antacids—e.g., Mg trisilicate
  – Vit K intake ↑ through diet or administration of vit K IM or IV
  – With induction of hepatic enzymes, increasing metabolism of warfarin. Enzyme inducers include anticonvulsants, barbiturates, primidone, carbamazepine, antimicrobials—e.g., griseofulvin, rifampin, nafcillin, and ethanol—and smoking
• ↑ Warfarin effect, or "warfarin sensitivity":
  – Drugs displacing warfarin from albumin ↑ its bioavailability (NSAIDs, ASA, phenytoin sodium, oral hypoglycemic agents, sulfa drugs, nalidixic acid, estrogen, miconazole)
  – Deficiency of vit K enhances; occurs with malabsorption syndromes and during administration of liquid paraffin laxatives, and clofibrate; after long-term use of oral antimicrobials that deplete intestinal bacterial source of vit K. Large doses of vit E antagonize action of vit K; anabolic steroids, danazol impair synthesis of vit K–dependent clotting factors; Olestra removes vit K
  – Metabolism blocked by phenytoin, chloramphenicol, erythromycin, clofibrate, TCAs, cimetidine, sulfinpyrazone, sulfamethoxazole-trimethoprim, thus increasing warfarin effect. Disulfiram (Antabuse) significantly slows metabolism.
  – Certain cephalosporins have a warfarin effect themselves—thus contraindicated
  – Elderly, febrile, debilitated patient and those with hepatic dysfunction, hyperthyroidism, or heart failure may have increased warfarin effect

DRUG CLASS/MECH OF ACTION/USUAL DOSE

• Interferes with synthesis of 6 vit K–dependent proteins involved in coagulation sequence: factors II, VII, IX, X; proteins C and S. Before these proteins are released into circulation, they undergo reactions converting glutamic acid residues to carboxyglutamic acid residues and require presence of reduced form of vit K
• Inhibits cyclic interconversion between reduced form of vit K and its 2,3-epoxide (vit K epoxide)
• Defective clotting factors lacking "carboxyl tail" are produced, impairing coagulation
• Factor II has $T_{1/2}$ of 48 h; requires 3–4 d before drops to level when PT significantly prolonged
• Usual dose
  – Nonurgent need for anticoagulation: adult with average body mass, 5 mg/d PO prolongs PT to 1.5 × control value in 36–48 h; if not achieved by 3rd d q.d. dose may be adjusted by ↑ or ↓ of 2.5 mg; goal: PT = 1.5–2 × control. ↑ bleeding complications when PT is 2.5 × control. Once anticoagulation stabilized, warfarin dose should be adjusted to maintain INR of 2–3 for all indications, except mech prosthetic cardiac valves, which require higher level of anticoagulation
  – More urgent need: heparin anticoagulation 1st; start warfarin, 10 mg for 2 d

DRUG EFFECTS

SYSTEM	EFFECT	ASSESSMENT BY HX	PE	TEST
GI	Vit K deficiency may result from a poor diet, extrahepatic biliary obstruction, malabsorption, sterile gut	GI bleeding Tarry stools Hematemesis	Wt:height ratio (BMI)	Hct Fecal occult blood
ENDO	Vit K deficiency Hyperthyroidism, hypermetabolism potentiate warfarin effect		Malnourished	PT/PTT INR
GU	Diuresis, pregnancy ↓ effect; warfarin teratogenic			PT/PTT INR
MS	Arthritis pain medications that affect plts—e.g., ASA, NSAIDs—potentiate bleeding			

Key Reference: Hirsh J: Oral anticoagulant drugs. N Engl J Med 1991; 324:1865–1875.

PERIOPERATIVE IMPLICATIONS/POSSIBLE DRUG INTERACTIONS

Preoperative Concerns

• Anticoag: consider Rx with vit K (oral, IM, IV, SC: 2.5–5 mg/70 kg) or FFP (15–20 ml/kg)
• Monitor this drug: PT, INR

Possible Drug Interactions

• Regional: Risk of spinal or epidural hematoma when performing a regional when patient is anticoagulated. Risk theoretically ↑ with anticoagulant. Epidural catheter thought to be associated with greater risk of spinal or epidural hematoma if no "measurable" anticoagulant effect from warfarin (i.e., PT nml), but if receiving warfarin, not known if risks of spinal or epidural hematoma significant

ANTICIPATED PROBLEMS/CONCERNS

• Bleeding most likely complication due to further depletion of clotting factors during surgery; factor depletion may follow massive transfusions or with development of DIC
• If anticoagulation reversed preop with large doses of vit K, warfarin resistance possible initially; thrombosis a risk in this setting
• If anticoagulation reversed with administration of FFP, anticoagulation more easily achieved postop but infectious risks are a concern
• Preoperative dose of warfarin can be restarted with oral fluids; when risk of thromboembolism is considered esp high (as in patients with recurrent pulm emboli undergoing pelvic surgury) or delay of more than 48 h anticipated before warfarin can be restarted, postop heparin infusion appropriate.

SECTION IV

TESTS

AUTONOMIC FUNCTION

Thomas J. Ebert, M.D.
Brian J. Robinson, Ph.D.

COST

- Depends on tests performed: those requiring BP, HR responses are inexpensive; tests measuring plasma hormone responses are more expensive
- Multiple tests are usually performed; presence of 2 or more abnormal results indicates some degree of autonomic dysfunction

RISK

- No risks assoc with most tests
- IV atropine is mildly unpleasant; arrhythmias may occur

OVERVIEW

- Simple bedside tests give valuable information on autonomic function
- Very sensitive quantitative tests to delineate severity of disorder, system (e.g., cardiovagal, vasomotor, sudomotor), distribution (pre- vs post-ganglionic), and level affected
- Autonomic dysfunction is assoc with malignant arrhythmias, cardiac arrest, spontaneous cardiac ischemia, ↑ periop CV and CR instability

ICD-9-CM Codes: 337.0 (Autonomic nervous system disorder); 337.1

INDICATIONS

- Patients with symptoms of autonomic failure (e.g., intolerance to standing, bladder/sphincter disturbances, impaired sweating) may have autonomic failure due to primary causes—e.g., multiple system atrophy (Shy-Drager syndrome)—or from disorders such as diabetes mellitus, chronic alcoholism, chronic renal failure, advanced age, vit deficiency (e.g., B_{12}), HIV infection, or due to prescribed drugs (e.g., TCAs).

ADDITIONAL TESTS

- Additional tests include plasma catecholamines, AVP, pancreatic polypeptide determinations in response to standing or other maneuvers to resolve site of lesion; responses to α_2-adrenoceptor agonist for peripheral denervation supersensitivity

ASSESSMENT POINTS

TEST	METHOD	SYSTEM	NORMAL RESPONSE
Orthostasis	Patient supine 10 min; then stands or tilted 80° head up; BP measured at 2 min	Sympathetic	↓ in SBP by <30 mmHg ↓ in DBP by <10 mmHg
30:15 Ratio	From continuous ECG strip; ratio of longest R-R interval (~30th beat) to shortest R-R interval (~15th beat) after assuming standing position	Parasympathetic	>1.03 (>1.01 if >65 y)
Deep Breathing	Diff between mean HR at max inspiration, mean HR at max expiration for 6 breaths over 1 min	Parasympathetic	>15 bpm (>10 if >65 y)
Valsalva Maneuver	Patient blows into manometer to maintain intrathoracic pressure at 40 mmHg for 15 s; ratio of longest R-R interval after release of maneuver to shortest R-R interval during maneuver	Parasympathetic	>1.2 (>1.15 if >65 y)
	Arterial BP measured directly	Sympathetic	BP exceeds baseline following release of blowing
Atropine	1.8 mg IV over 3 min	Parasympathetic	HR ↑ by >20 bpm
Cold Pressor	Immerse hand in ice water for 1 min	Sympathetic	SBP and DBP ↑ by >10 mmHg after 1 min
Isometric Handgrip	Isometric contraction at 30% max strength for 3 min	Sympathetic	↑ DBP by >10 mmHg after 3 min

Key Reference: Ebert TJ: Preoperative evaluation of the autonomic nervous system. Adv Anes 1993; 10:49–68.

PERIOPERATIVE IMPLICATIONS

Preoperative Preparation

- Gastroparesis: Consider premedication with agents to ↑ gastric motility (e.g., metoclopramide), and ↓ consequence of aspiration (e.g., antacids, H_2 blockers)
- Abnormal sensitivity to anesthetic agents and apneic tendencies: minimize narcotics or benzodiazepines as premedication; monitor intensively perioperatively
- Orthostatic hypotension treated by vol expansion, which may cause supine HTN

Monitoring

- Consider arterial line

Induction

- Consider rapid-sequence induction
- Consider etomidate
- Titrate agents with CV, resp effects

Maintenance

- Aggressively treat blood loss, keep well hydrated
- Denervation supersensitivity: unexpected HTN responses to adrenoceptor agonists used for Rx hypotension; if vasopressors required, use direct-acting agents; indirect-acting agents have unpredictable effects
- Impaired T regulation may require active warming
- Consider controlled ventilation

Postoperative Care

- ↑ Risk of hypotension, hypothermia, apnea
- Peripheral neuropathy may be associated with requirement of less analgesic; use narcotics with caution

CHEST X-RAY

L. Reuven Pasternak, M.D., M.P.H.

COST

- $15–$40 for CXR
- $20–$75 for radiologist's interpretation

RISK

- No risk in isolated x-ray
- Risk from misinterpretation

OVERVIEW

- Test to assess presence of acute progressive or chronic changes of cardiac and/or pulm disease
- Presence of ↑ perihilar markings may be indication of fluid overload from noncardiac origin—e.g., renal failure, fluid overload, or acute ("flash") pulm edema from severe respiratory obstruction
- Presence of cardiomegaly on the CXR indicated by cardiothoracic ratio >0.5 and/or presence of ↑ perihilar markings distinguishing pulm fluid congestion
- COPD characterized by hyperinflation with flattened diaphragm, ↑ radiolucency, ↑ AP diameter ("barrel chest")

INDICATIONS

- Thoracic procedures
- Otherwise, only if reason to believe there is acute or rapidly progressive deterioration of patient's clinical condition. Hx, PE usually sufficiently sensitive to determine appropriate level of patient's disease and adequately plan for peri/postoperative care. No indication for performance of CXRs based on age, exposure to tobacco products without associated pos findings on Hx and/or PE
- PFTs
- ECG (cardiac disease, pulm HTN)

ASSESSMENT POINTS

ASPECT OF TEST	POSITIVE RESULT	CONFOUNDING FACTORS	DX INFORMATION
Cardiothoracic ratio >0.5		When associated with ↑ perihilar markings, cardiac silhouette may be difficult to determine	Cardiomegaly, indicating CHF
Diaphragmatic placement	Flattened hemidiaphragms	Patient not properly positioned in erect stance Splinting due to pain or other factors	Extent of COPD Extent of air trapping from acute reactive airway disease
AP diameter	"Barrel chest" with marked ↑ in this dimension		Extent of COPD
Perihilar markings	↑ Markings in area and/or in general lung fields	Improper penetration may cause this finding to be overlooked (overpenetration) or overdiagnosed (underpenetration) May be confused with interstitial scarring from other chronic diseases	Fluid overload, e.g., from excess fluid administration, renal failure, or other noncardiopulmonary cause Primary CHF CHF 2° to pulmonary HTN

Key Reference: Boghosian SG, Mooradian AD: Usefulness of routine preoperative chest roentgenograms in elderly patients. J Am Geriatr Soc 1987;35:142.

PERIOPERATIVE IMPLICATIONS

- CHF: must ensure optimal myocardial function, conservative fluid management; invasive monitoring for CVP indicated for procedures in which fluid shifts and/or blood loss anticipated, PA cath for measurement of CO, optimization of myocardial performance in patients in whom significant blood loss, other physiologic stress anticipated
- Reactive airway disease: must guarantee that airway management, especially intubation, done with appropriate level of anesthesia to suppress bronchospasm. Consider chronic medication and steroid coverage before surgery; consider postponing surgery in those with acute episodes
- COPD: often associated in its advanced stages with pulm HTN, right-sided heart failure

SPECIAL CONSIDERATIONS

- If patient is debilitated or requires supplemental O$_2$, consider ICU during postop period, understanding that prolonged ventilatory support may be necessary
- When possible consider anesthetic techniques to avoid stimulation of airway, compromise of the patient's intrinsic respiratory drive

DIAGNOSTIC 12-LEAD ECG

Martin J. London, M.D.

COST

• $15 to $50 with physician charges

RISK

• None except misinterpretation

SENSITIVITY/SPECIFICITY

• Varies accord to specific clinical indication, population. For rhythm and conduction disorders, 100% sensitive. Sensitivity of Q waves for autopsy-proven MI is 33–62%, with a specificity of 88–98%. Sensitivity, specificity of ST-T changes on resting ECG for myocardial ischemia in absence of clin Sx are low

OVERVIEW

• ECG assesses myocardial ischemia, MI, rhythm and conduction disorders (intrinsic myocardial disease), electrolyte and metabolic disorders, and medical effects (extrinsic disorders)
• Appropriate, cost-effective starting point for more extensive, costly evaluation of cardiac diseases
• Predictive value, cost-effectiveness of preop 12-lead ECG are controversial. Incidence of ECG abnormality ↑ with age, concurrent medical illness (especially HTN, CAD, diabetes)

INDICATIONS

• Known or suspected (i.e., multiple risk factors or abnormalities on Hx or PE) CAD
• "Major" surgery regardless of clinical Hx
• Males over 40, females over 50

ADDITIONAL/ALTERNATIVE TESTS

• Exercise treadmill testing with or without thallium imaging, static or stress ECHO, dipyridamole or adenosine thallium imaging, coronary angiography to diagnose CAD, ischemia
• Holter monitoring for arrhythmias, conduction defect, ischemia

ASSESSMENT POINTS

DISORDER	POSITIVE RESULT	CONFOUNDING FACTORS	DX INFORMATION
Myocardial ischemia	ST segment depression >1 mm Deep T-wave inversion	Baseline ST-T wave changes BBB (esp. LBBB) Digoxin/drug effects Abnormal autonomic tone Q waves ↑ ST segment due to pericarditis Intracranial pathology	ST segment changes correlate poorly with site of CAD Magnitude of depression weakly related to severity
Myocardial infarction	New Q waves ≥40 msec, ampl >25% of R wave ↑ ST during acute stage Poor R wave progression	Q waves in V1 and aVL or isolated inferior leads may be normal BBB (esp. LBBB)	Q waves are sensitive and specific indicators
Rhythm disorders	Abnormal timing of P wave, QRS or absence of normal P wave and PR interval		Depends on chronicity, Rx, hemodynamic consequences Atrial dysrhythmias usually benign
Conduction disorders	Axis deviation PR >120 msec QRS >100 msec	Body habitus Digoxin Hypothermia Antiarrhythmics	LAFB—usually benign, LPFB—likely myocardial or conduction damage RBBB—usually benign LBBB—associated with CAD and impaired ventricular function
Metabolic disorders	Hypokalemia—flattened T waves, ST ↓ Hyperkalemia— peaking T waves, wide QRS Hypocalcemia— lengthen QT_c interval Hypercalcemia— shorten QT_c interval	Other nonspecific changes	Chemistry Laboratory
LV hypertrophy	Multiple criteria Sum V1 + V5 ≥ 35 mm	Body habitus, age, and race influence specificity	Associated with severe HTN or aortic stenosis

Key Reference: Guidelines for Electrocardiography: A report of the American College of Cardiology/American Heart Association Task Force for assessment of diagnostic and therapeutic cardiovascular procedures (Committee on Electrocardiography). Circulation 1992; 85:1221–1228.

PERIOPERATIVE IMPLICATIONS

• Q waves diagnostic of prior MI associated with elevated risk of postop cardiac morbidity.
• Number of Q waves on ECG tracing negatively correlated with the ejection fraction.
• LBBB more likely associated with significant CAD and impaired ventricular function than RBBB. However, "intraventricular conduction delay," with very wide and bizarre QRS morphology, may have similar significance as LBBB.

• Nonspecific ST-T wave changes, T-wave flattening/inversion and QT interval prolongation markedly influenced by autonomic tone and common in the early postoperative period.

SPECIAL CONSIDERATIONS

• Accuracy of computerized interpretation varies between manufacturers.
• Sensitivity and specificity of ECG are poor following cardiac surgery.
• Newer forms: These include computerized vectorcardiography and late and mid QRS signal averaged electrocardiography utilizing a different lead system (the Frank-Lewis XYZ leads) and signal averaging techniques. Their peri-

DIBUCAINE NUMBER

James E. Heavner, D.V.M., Ph.D.

USES

- For anesthesia of skin
- For anesthesia of mucous membranes
- Dibucaine number used to test for atypical plasma ChE
- Otherwise limited use: as cream, ointment, aerosol, solution, suppositories

PERIOPERATIVE RISKS

- Rare risk of true allergic reactions
- Misdiagnosis when used for dibucaine number

WORRY ABOUT

- Risk of neurotoxicity with this drug

OVERVIEW/PHARMACOLOGY

- Used for topical anesthesia, first in 1929; now used for testing for atypical plasma ChE
- Metabolism slow, incomplete: biodegradation very sluggish
- Removed from USA markets as injectable form due to neurolytic effect
- Duration of spinal anesthesia (0.25% in 5% glucose, 1–2 ml) 75–180 min

DRUG CLASS/MECH OF ACTION/USUAL DOSE

- Amide-linked local anesthetic; quinoline derivative
- Cream, ointment, aerosol, solution, suppositories (area of use: skin, ears, rectum)
- Concentrations: 0.25–2.5%

ASSESSMENT OF DIBUCAINE NUMBER

- Dibucaine not hydrolyzed in human serum in vitro; plasma ChE has strong affinity for dibucaine
- Dibucaine's affinity for typical plasma ChE is approx 20 times greater than for the atypical form—a quantitative assessment—percent inhibition of enzyme activity gives dibucaine number; greatest inhibition with normal cholinesterase

VARIANTS OF PLASMA CHOLINESTERASE ENZYME

VARIANT	APPROX DURATION OF SUCCINYLCHOLINE-INDUCED NMB	DIBUCAINE NUMBER (% INHIBITION OF ENZYME ACTIVITY)	INCIDENCE
Homozygous	5–10 min	80	
Heterozygous	20 min	40–60	1/480
Homozygous atypical	60–180 min	20	1/3200

Key Reference: Stoelting RK, Miller RD: Muscle relaxants. *In* Miller RD (ed): Basics of Anesthesia, 2nd ed. New York, Churchill Livingstone, 1989, pp 95–97.

ANTICIPATED PROBLEMS/CONCERNS

- Risk of neurotoxicity if used other than as topical
- Possible cross-reactivity with other amide local anesthetics

DIPYRIDAMOLE THALLIUM IMAGING

Lee A. Fleisher, M.D.

COST
- $1200–$1500, depending on laboratory

RISK
- In patients with CAD, risk of MI and death 1/100,000

SENSITIVITY AND SPECIFICITY
- Sensitivity: 70–80%
- Specificity: 80–90%
- Pos predictive value: 20–50%
- Neg predictive value: 85–99%

OVERVIEW
- Test to assess presence of coronary artery stenosis in patients unable to exercise
- Dipyridamole used to dilate normal coronary arteries, resulting in flow heterogeneity
- Thallium taken up by viable myocardial cells
- Obtain stress and at rest images
- Areas of myocardial necrosis demonstrate fixed defect
- Areas at risk demonstrate reversible defect
- Able to quantify area at risk

INDICATIONS
- Dx of CAD in patients unable to exercise
- Quantification of area at risk for ischemia

ADDITIONAL/ALTERNATIVE TESTS
- Holter monitoring for silent ischemia
- Dobutamine thallium imaging
- Dobutamine stress ECHO
- Coronary angiography

ASSESSMENT POINTS

ASPECT OF TEST	POSITIVE RESULT	CONFOUNDING FACTORS	DX INFORMATION
CV thallium imaging	Reversible defect	Breast artifact	Area of myocardium at risk
	Fixed defect	Delayed imaging or reinjection needed to determine if severe ischemia or scar present	Area of old scar or severe ischemia
	LV dilation		LV dysfunction
Lung imaging	↑ Lung uptake		LV dysfunction
ECG	ST segment changes	Baseline abnormalities	Indicates dipyridamole results in myocardial ischemia — ↑ risk
Sx during test	Chest pain	Multiple causes	May be ischemia or nonspecific cause

Key Reference: Beller GA: Pharmacologic stress imaging. JAMA 1991; 265:633–638.

PERIOPERATIVE IMPLICATIONS
- A reversible defect suggests the presence of a critical coronary artery stenosis; larger defects are associated with a greater area at risk and a higher incidence of perioperative cardiac morbidity
- Increased lung uptake or LV dilation identifies those patients at risk for LV dysfunction with ischemia
- Fixed defects represent old scar and are associated with reduced function and increased long-term risk

SPECIAL CONSIDERATIONS
- Patients with fixed defects may require reinjection or 24-hour delayed imaging to differentiate scar from severe ischemia

DOBUTAMINE STRESS ECHOCARDIOGRAPHY Thomas Ryan, M.D.

COST

$600–$900

RISK

• Induction of ischemia can→MI or death (1 in 3000)
• Arrhythmias due to dobutamine include PVCs, AFib, nonsustained VTach; sustained VTach or VFib vary rarely

SENSITIVITY/SPECIFICITY

• Sensitivity for detection of CAD: 85–90%
• Specificity for detection of CAD: 80–85%
• Pos predictive value (for *any* perioperative event): 20–40%
• Pos predictive value (for a *hard* event): 15–25%
• Neg predictive value: 95–100%

OVERVIEW

• Dobutamine infused in incremental doses to ↑ HR, contractility (i.e., myocardial O_2 demand)
• 2D ECHO assesses wall motion, myocardial thickening at each stage
• *Nml* response is dose-dependent development of uniform hyperdynamic wall motion
• *Resting* wall motion abnormality suggests prior infarction
• *Induced* wall motion abnormality indicates ischemia
• Multiple wall motion abnormalities identify multivessel disease

INDICATIONS

• To detect presence, extent of coronary disease in patients unable to undergo adequate exercise; to distinguish prior MI from inducible ischemia
• For preop risk stratification, by identifying patients with evidence of inducible ischemia (esp patients with PVD)

ALTERNATIVE TESTS

• Exercise testing
• Dipyridamole thallium imaging
• Dipyridamole stress ECHO
• Coronary angiogram

ASSESSMENT POINTS

TEST	POSITIVE RESULT	CONFOUNDING FACTORS	DIAGNOSTIC INFORMATION
Wall motion analysis	Resting abnormality	Cardiomyopathy, LBBB	Prior MI
	Induced abnormality	b rb's; image quality	Ischemia
	Multiple abnormality	Cardiomyopathy	Multivessel disease
ECG	ST-segment depression	Baseline abnormality	Ischemia
		Low sensitivity	
Symptoms	Chest pain	Nonspecific; multiple causes	Angina or other causes

Key Reference: Poldermans D, Fioretti PM, Forster T, et al. Dobutamine stress echocardiography for the assessment of perioperative cardiac events in patients undergoing major vascular surgery. Circulation 1993; 87:1506–1512.

PERIOPERATIVE IMPLICATIONS

• A normal stress ECHO confers favorable prognosis, very low risk of perioperative morbidity (*high* negative predictive accuracy)
• Inducible wall motion abnormality identifies patients at ↑ risk for perioperative event; but many patients with positive test can still undergo surg without serious complications—e.g., MI or death (*low* positive predictive accuracy)
• Identifying *high risk* depends on extent, severity of abnormal wall motion, dose at which the abnormality develops, clinical factors (e.g., Hx of MI, CHF, diabetes, etc.)
• Patients with resting wall motion abnormality (i.e., prior MI) but no signs of inducible ischemia at *intermediate risk*

EXERCISE STRESS TESTING

Bernard R. Chaitman, M.D.

COST

- $100–$300, depending on lab

RISK

- Mortality <0.01%, morbidity <0.05% in nonselect pt populations

SENSITIVITY/SPECIFICITY

	Overall	Multivessel Disease
Sensitivity	68%	81%
Specificity	77%	66%

Sensitivity ↓ when exercise workload submax

OVERVIEW

- Dx, prognostic estimate of presence, extent of coronary disease
- Assessment of functional capacity
- Determine effect of Rx
- Determine exercise prescription for cardiac rehabilitation
- Exercise-induced ST-segment ↑ in non-infarct territory, profound ST-segment depression, fall in exercise systolic BP, or low exercise capacity associated with adverse prognosis, multivessel coronary disease

ICD-9-CM Code: 414.0

INDICATIONS

- Prognostic estimate of perioperative long-term cardiac risk
- Objective estimate of functional capacity

ADDITIONAL/ALTERNATIVE TESTS

- Exercise myocardial perfusion imaging
- IV Persantine/adenosine myocardial perfusion imaging
- Dobutamine stress ECHO
- Exercise stress ECHO
- Holter monitoring
- Coronary angio

ASSESSMENT POINTS

ASPECT OF TEST	POSITIVE RESULT	CONFOUNDING FACTORS	DIAGNOSTIC INFO
ECG	Horizontal or downsloping ST-segment depression ≥1 mm Exercise-induced slow upsloping ST-segment depression ≥1.5 mm at 80 msec after J point ST-segment elevation ≥1 mm in noninfarct lead	LVH, digitalis Rx, glucose load, MVP	ST segment depression ≥2 mm, downsloping ST-segment depression, ≥5 leads abn, persistent ischemic response ≥5 min post-exercise, ischemic ST-segment depression onset < Bruce stage II
BP response	Inability to ↑ systolic BP ≥120 mmHg Sustained ↓ ≥10 mmHg repeatable within 15 sec Fall in systolic BP below standing rest values	Cardioactive drug Rx; women; Dx information from test in patients with high pretest risk of disease; abn response indicates adverse prognosis, multivessel coronary disease	↑ Risk of perioperative events in patients with known or high pretest likelihood of CAD
Exercise capacity	<4 METs	Pt motivation, cardioactive drug Rx, ortho limitations	Risk gradient according to level of METs achieved; <4 METs, high risk; ≥10 METs, low risk
Sx during test	Chest pain	Character of chest pain	Presence of exercise-induced definite angina may be only ischemic marker in absence of exercise-induced ST-segment changes

MET, metabolic equivalent; 1 MET = 3.5 ml/kg/min $\dot{V}O_2$; 1 MET = energy expenditure sitting quietly in a chair.

Key Reference: Chaitman BR: Exercise stress testing in heart disease. *In* Braunwald E (ed): Heart Disease: A Textbook of Cardiovascular Medicine, 4th ed. Philadelphia, WB Saunders, 1992, pp 161–179.

PERIOPERATIVE IMPLICATIONS

- Profound ST-segment changes, poor exercise capacity (<4 METs), abn exercise-induced BP changes, exercise-induced angina associated with ↑ incidence of perioperative cardiac morbidity, mortality
- Absence of preceding associated with very low perioperative cardiac morbidity
- Intermediate exercise results may require additional noninvasive testing (exercise myocardial perfusion imaging or stress ECHO) to more accurately estimate prognosis

SPECIAL CONSIDERATIONS

- Patients with submax test (<85% of age-predicted maximum) have reduced test accuracy
- Dx accuracy of test depends on pretest clinical risk estimate
- Optimal use of test results requires integration of all information acquired during test, not simply yes/no based on exercise ECG results

FLOW VOLUME LOOPS

Peter Rock, M.D.

Peter Rock, M.D.

COST

- Variable: $20–$199 in survey of 5 hospitals

RISK

- Virtually no risks associated with flow volume loops (PFTs)
- Risk from bronchodilator use and misinterpreting data

SENSITIVITY/SPECIFICITY

- Flows depend on patient factors, including body size (ht, wt); habitus; gender; age; ethnicity. The 95% confidence interval included values 20–30% above and below mean for given healthy population. This wide range of normal values limits interpretation of PFTs; interpretation of PFTs critically depends on prior probability of disease. The Dx of COPD does not require PFTs; is based on clinical criteria. Results within given patient reproducible to within 5% or less in cooperative subjects. Repeated measurements of PFTs over time sensitive to changes in health or disease status.

OVERVIEW

- Flow volume loops show relationship between airflow, with max effort starting from either position of max inspiration or exhalation, during exhalation or inspiration, respectively, and volume (exhaled or inspired, respectively).
- Accuracy, interpretation of PFTs highly dependent on patient cooperation, patient effort; results must be reproducible to be valid.

INDICATIONS

- Confirm Dx of suspected obstructive lung disease
- Suggest presence of restrictive lung disease
- Intra- vs extrathoracic obstructions

ADDITIONAL/ALTERNATIVE TESTS

- CT images of sites of airway obstruction

ASSESSMENT POINTS

TEST	POSITIVE RESULT	CONFOUNDING FACTORS	DX INFORMATION
Measurements suggest OLD (obstructive lung disease)	Flow volume loops show exaggerated upward concavity of descending limb of flow volume curve with ↓ peak flows, ↓ volume; inspiratory flows relatively preserved		Causes of OLD: acute (asthma), chronic (bronchitis, emphysema), or related to upper airway lesions
Measurements suggest RLD	Flow volume loops show preservation or ↑ of peak expiratory flow but ↓ volume; flow volume curve has normal shape but reduced in all dimension; inspiratory flows relatively preserved		Suggest RLD (restrictive lung disease)
Measurements suggestive of central airway obstruction (flow volume loops)	Predominant ↓ in expiratory flow with relatively normal inspiratory flow; expiratory flow curve often has plateau (same flow at all lung volumes) rather than downward bowing normally seen	Flow volume loops have role in screening but confirmation of location, size of lesion may be obtained from imaging studies — e.g., CT of chest	Variable intrathoracic obstruction; pleural pressure variations during inspiration, exhalation influence magnitude of obstruction so it is less during inspiration, indicating site of lesion in thorax (e.g., tracheal tumor)
	Predominant ↓ in inspiratory flow with relatively normal expiratory flow		Variable extrathoracic obstruction: pleural pressure variations during inspiration and exhalation influence magnitude of obstruction so that it is less during exhalation, indicating site of lesion is in upper airway (e.g., laryngeal tumor)
	Proportional ↓ in inspiratory and expiratory flows		Fixed central obstruction (e.g., tracheal stenosis): pleural pressure variations during inspiration and exhalation do not influence magnitude of obstruction

Key Reference: Gold WM: Pulmonary function testing. *In* Murray JF, Nadel JA (eds): Textbook of Respiratory Medicine. Philadelphia, WB Saunders, 1994, pp 798–900.

PERIOPERATIVE IMPLICATIONS

- Flow volume loops can distinguish intrathoracic from extrathoracic lesions: see Mediastinal Masses in Diseases section for intrathoracic lesions

HIV TESTING

Barbara S. Gold, M.D.

COST

(Approximate; depends on lab)
- HIV antibody
  - ELISA .... $10–$35
  - Western blot ...... $25–$85
- PCR $200
- p24 antigen ..... $35–$65
- CD4+ count $185

RISKS

- No known medical risk from test itself
- Risk is in false pos and false neg and lack of counseling to true pos patients. In healthy population w/o risk factors as many as 92% of pos by Western blot and ELISA are false pos in US

OVERVIEW

- Tests for presence of HIV infection, progression to AIDS; monitors exposed health care workers
- ELISA is the most commonly used screening test; positive results are confirmed by the more specific Western blot analysis. Both tests measure antibodies to HIV proteins, and are extremely sensitive (~99%)
- Time from infection to detection of seropositivity, 4–8 wk
- PCR amplifies HIV nucleic acid; is used to clarify discrepant ELISA and Western blot results, to detect HIV in high-risk patients who have not yet seroconverted, and to screen neonates
- HIV infects helper T cells, which have high concentration of CD4 antigen. These lymphocytes also orchestrate immune response; thus HIV infects, destroys cells that normally eliminate virus. In HIV infection, T4 lymphocyte, CD4 levels decline; CD4+ counts of <200 cells/μl correlate with morbidity

INDICATIONS

- Dx infection with HIV in high-risk individuals or those with Sx compatible with AIDS

ASSESSMENT POINTS

TEST	REPORTED RESULT	CONFOUNDING FACTORS	DX INFORMATION
ELISA	Pos/Neg	Seroconversion takes 4–8 wk	Indicates presence or absence of antibodies to HIV
Western blot	Pos/Neg	Indeterminate at advanced stages	Confirms ELISA
p24 antigen	Pos/Neg	Asymptomatic patients may test neg	Detects presence of HIV antigen before antibodies are produced
PCR	Pos/Neg	Extremely sensitive; subject to false pos from contamination	Clarifies positive ELISA, indeterminate Western blot; positive before seroconversion
CD4+ count	<200 cells/μl associated with morbidity		Monitor progression of AIDS, response to Rx

Key Reference: Sloand EM, Pitt E, Chiarello RJ, Nemo GJ: HIV testing—State of the art. JAMA 1991; 266:2861–2866

PERIOPERATIVE IMPLICATIONS

- Patients testing pos for HIV are on continuum; may be asymptomatic or manifest AIDS, which affects virtually every organ system
- Patients infected with HIV have neg screening tests for 4–8 wk
- Health care provider should employ universal precautions with all patients, regardless of status of HIV testing

HOLTER MONITORING FOR SILENT ISCHEMIA

Khether E. Raby, M.D.

COST

- $200–$300

RISK

- None (local skin irritation) other than data misinterpretation

SENSITIVITY/SPECIFICITY

- Sensitivity: 80–90%
- Specificity: 70–80%
- Pos predictive value: 20–40%
- Neg predictive value: 80–100%

OVERVIEW

- ST depression detected by Holter is due to myocardial ischemia in patients with CAD
- Ischemia on Holter often silent; occurs at heart rates well below those achieved on treadmill exercise
- ST-segment depression may not be indicative of ischemia in low-risk patients
- Etiology of silent ischemia unclear: ?autonomic dysfunction due to inadequate blood supply; probably not smaller area of ischemia; probably not lesser degree of ischemia

INDICATIONS

- Dx of myocardial ischemia in patients unable to exercise

ALTERNATIVE TESTS

- Dipyridamole thallium/MIBI imaging
- Dobutamine stress ECHO
- Coronary angio
- Exercise stress testing

ASSESSMENT POINTS

ASPECT OF TEST	POSITIVE RESULT	CONFOUNDING FACTORS	DX INFORMATION
ST-segment depression	>1 mm depression from baseline for >1 min with or without Sx	BBB, LVH, baseline ST depression, digoxin	Positive result confirms presence of ischemia
ST-segment elevation	>1 mm ST elevation from baseline for >1 min with or without Sx	(must be in lead without Q waves) BBB, baseline ST elevation	Positive result confirms presence of transmural ischemia, possible spasm

Key Reference: Raby KE, et al: Detection and significance of intraoperative and postoperative myocardial ischemia in peripheral vascular surgery. JAMA 1992; 268:222–227

PERIOPERATIVE IMPLICATIONS

- Presence of preop, postop ischemia predicts adverse cardiac risk postop among vascular surgery patients
- Intraoperative ischemia less common
- Postop ischemia common, occurs within 72 h of surgery; correlates with higher heart rate, pain perception

LIVER FUNCTION TESTS

Edward J. Frink, Jr., M.D.

COST

- AST (SGOT) $15–45
- ALT (SGPT) $15–45
- Alk phos $35–45
- Serum alb $15–50
- PT $15–30
- GGTD $25–40
- Total bilirubin $15–40
- Direct bilirubin $15–60
- NTP $30–50
- AST, ALT, alk phos, serum alb, total bilirubin generally available as single test (SMA 20) $8–35

RISK

- Not evaluating or misinterpreting tests: potential risk if surgery, anesthesia performed in patient with early-stage hepatitis; risk low in healthy population
- Performing test: false-pos, false-negs
- Misiagnosis of liver disease, or liver disease not found if tests incorrectly applied or misinterpreted
- Specificity:
  - AST, ALT: also present in heart, skeletal muscle, kidney
  - GGTP: typically rises with alcohol-related liver disease, may also ↑ with other hepatobiliary disease; drug injury—e.g., barbiturates or phenytoin
  - Alk phos: assoc ↑ with cholestatic disease, but ↑ with bone turnover; may be differentiated by isozyme fractionation, more commonly by 5'-nucleotidase (NTP)

OVERVIEW

- Tests establish presence or absence of liver injury, degree of hepatic reserve in disease states
- AST, ALT
  - transaminases located in liver cells; elevations may be indicative of hepatocellular damage
  - ALT generally more specific to liver than AST
  - highest elevations with acute hepatitis or hepatic ischemia
  - may be low or only modestly elevated with chronic liver disease states
  - elevated AST/ALT ratio >2:1 (if ALT <500 IU) suggestive of alcohol-induced liver injury; >3:1 highly suggestive
- Alk phos
  - enzyme assoc with canalicular, sinusoidal membranes; other major source, release from bone
  - highest levels occur in patients with cholestasis (biliary obstructive disease) or hepatic carcinoma
- GGTP
  - hepatocellular enzyme
  - high sensitivity, but low specificity (i.e., normal test result favors lack of hepatobiliary disease, positive test of little Dx value)
  - if ↑, helps confirm alk phos is not of bone origin
- NTP
  - rises with alk phos (source of elevation in alk phos is liver)
- Serum albumin

  - ↓ in chronic liver disease states
  - Low levels generally indicate poor synthetic function
- PT
  - If elevated in conjunction with liver disease, indicates poor synthetic function
- Bilirubin
  - Elevated with many hepatobiliary diseases
  - Highest levels with biliary obstruction
  - Direct bilirubin (conjugated) level may be subtracted from total bilirubin level to obtain indirect bilirubin level, defines where excess load or conjugation, excretion at issue

INDICATIONS

- To aid recognition of liver disease states

ADDITIONAL/ALTERNATIVE TESTS

- Urine bilirubin: presence in urine indicates hepatobiliary disease; only conjugated bilirubin enters urine; therefore, it will not be elevated with hemolysis, etc.
- ^{14}G aminopyrine breath test: ↓ $^{14}CO_2$ appearance indicates ↓ metabolic ability
- Viral hepatitis serologies: identify viral illnesses
- Liver biopsy: useful for histologic identification
- CT, US: detect tumor, blood vessel, biliary obstruction

ASSESSMENT POINTS

TEST	POSITIVE RESULT*	CONFOUNDING FACTORS	DX INFORMATION
AST (SGOT)	> 30–40 IU/L	Possibly from sources other than liver (e.g., cardiac and skeletal muscle, kidneys, brain, pancreas, lungs)	Hepatocellular injury if markedly elevated (acute hepatic injury)
ALT (SGPT)	> 30–40 IU/L	More specific to hepatocellular origin than AST, may be ↑ with muscle injury but high levels only in liver	Hepatocellular injury if elevated (acute hepatic injury)
Total bilirubin	> 1.2 mg/dl	Elevation may be due to excess bilirubin load (e.g., hemolysis)	Elevation with many disease states; greatest with cholestatic or parenchymal disease
Indirect bilirubin	> 0.8 mg/dl (derive from total – direct level)	NA	Determine unconjugated hyperbilirubinemia (e.g., Gilbert's syndrome, intravascular hemolysis
Alk phos	> 107 IU/L	Sources other than liver—notably bone, intestine, placenta	High elevations generally indicate biliary obstructive disease, especially in absence of high transaminase elevation
NTP	> 15 IU/L	Possibly ↑ in late pregnancy	In nonpregnant patient, ↑ NTP suggests liver origin
GGTP	> 66 IU/L	Possibly ↑ by dilantin or barbiturate use; also present in kidney, cardiac muscle	Confirms source of ↑ alk phos in liver
Serum alb	< 3.6 g/dl	Possibly ↓ with poor nutrition, chronic infection, or nephrotic syndrome	Identify chronic liver disease, low levels indicate poor hepatic function
PT	> 13 sec Elevation of >2 sec above reported normal usually significant	Possibly prolonged by congenital coagulation factor deficiency, drugs affecting prothrombin complex, vit K deficiency	In chronic liver states, ↑ PT indicates poorer prognosis; in acute hepatocellular injury, prolonged PT may signal onset of fulminant hepatic failure

*Varies by laboratory: check specific laboratory reference ranges; values are for adults.

Key Reference: Herrera JL: Abnormal liver enzyme levels. The spectrum of causes. Postgrad Med 1993; 93:113–132.

PERIOPERATIVE IMPLICATIONS

- Acute liver disease (e.g., acute viral or drug-induced hepatitis)—tests aid in recognition of possibly important anesthetic/surgical risk
- Chronic liver disease (e.g., cirrhosis): Tests, especially of hepatic synthetic function, help evaluate mortality risk

PREGNANCY TESTING

Rebecca Twersky, M.D.
Rose Marie Phillips, M.D.

COST

- Numerous tests available; cost varies, both to pt and to institution
- Average cost to pt:
  – urine hCG $18–$30
  – serum hCG $20–$75

RISK

- Risk to pt is false-positive or false-negative test or misinterpretation; ↑ risk in anesthesia, surg in pregnant women

OVERVIEW

- hCG is a glycoprotein secreted by developing placenta shortly after fertilization; hCG molecule comprises 2 noncovalently bonded, dissimilar subunits, namely, α, β. The α subunit is structurally similar to α subunit of FSH, LH, TSH. Therefore, there is a high degree of cross-reactivity with these hormones. In contrast, the β subunit of hCG is structurally distinct, displaying differing immunologic specificities.
- Tests for detection of hCG include RIA, ELISA, agglutination immunoassay, IRMA, and ICMA.
- β hCG detectable in maternal blood and urine 8–9 d post conception.

- Pos test can be analyzed as follows:

Week after LMP	Concentration in MIU
3	0–50
4	3–426
5	19–7,340
6	1,080–56,500
7–8	7,650–229,000
9–12	25,060–228,000
17–24	4,060–65,400
25–40	3,640–117,000

TEST INDICATION

- To diagnose pregnancy in perioperative period; to quantify gestation; can assess need for perioperative interventions before elective surgery

ADDITIONAL/ALTERNATIVE TESTS

- For borderline results, repeat test in 48 h (hCG doubles in 48 h); correlate hCG results with LMP, PE, pelvic US

ASSESSMENT POINTS

PREGNANCY TEST TECHNIQUE	SENSITIVITY	SPECIFICITY	POSITIVE RESULT	CONFOUNDING FACTORS	DX INFO
IRMA (immunoradiometric assasay) Total β hCG (e.g., Roche Diagnostic)	2.0 µIU/ml	No cross-reactivity with LH	>25 µIU/ml; borderline result 2–25 µIU/ml	Molar preg, ectopic preg, choriocarcinoma, hydatidiform mole, delivery, or abortion within a few wk	For borderline results, repeat test in 48 h (hCG doubles in 48 h); correlate hCG with LMP, PE, US
Whole molecule hCG	1.5 µIU/ml	0.24% cross-reactivity with LH, no cross-reactivity with FSH, TSH	>25 µIU/ml; borderline result 2–25 µIM/ml	Same as above	Same as above
ELISA (enzyme-linked immunosorbent assay) (e.g., Abbott)	5 µIU/ml	Min cross-reactivity with LH, FSH, TSH @ 432, 500, 500 µIU/ml, respectively	>25 µIU/ml; color change indicates pos result, borderline result 5–25 µIU/ml	Same as above	Same as above
ICMA (immunochemiluminometric assay: change is a positive result) Whole hCG: Quantitative serum or urine; qualitative serum or urine (e.g., Roche diagnostic)	3–200 µIU/ml 25 µIU/ml	0.015% cross-reactivity with 20,000 µIU/ml LH 0.03% cross-reactivity with 10,000 µIU/ml FSH 0.3% cross-reactivity with 1,000 µIU/ml TSH	>25 µIU/ml; chemiluminescence indicates pos result, borderline result 5–25 µIU/ml	Same as above	Same as above
RIA (radioimmunoassay) Quantitative serum β hCG (e.g., Tandam)	5 µIU/ml	Cross-reactivity with LH (0.5%), FSH (0.2%)	>25 µIU/ml; fluorescence indicates pos result, borderline result 5–25 µIU/ml	Pos result obtained with seminoma, teratoma, embryonic CA, hepatoblastoma, bronchogenic CA, prostate CA, breast CA	Same as above
LATEX AGGLUTINATION Qualitative urine, β hCG (e.g., Organon Teknika)	500 µIU/ml	No interference with abn amount of protein, erythrocytes, Hgb	Granular clump indicates pos result, smooth suspension indicates neg result	Conditions other than nml preg that produce hCG Very high levels of hCG can produce neg result	Consider more sensitive test

Key Reference: Mazze RI, Kaller B: Reproductive outcome after anesthesia and operations during pregnancy: A registry study of 5405 cases. Am J Obstet Gynecol 1989;161:1178–1185.

PERIOPERATIVE IMPLICATIONS

- 2% of pregnant women undergo surgery for reasons unrelated to parturition
- Anesthetic considerations are related to possible teratogenicity of anesthetic agents, effect of anesthesia on uteroplacental BF, potential for spontaneous abortions, premature delivery, alteration in maternal physiology

- Numerous studies on fetal outcome post surgery, post anesthesia demonstrate: ↑ incidence of spontaneous abortions, LBW, esp if surgery performed in 1st trimester
- No ↑ incidence of congenital anomalies even if N_2O used
- No specific anesthetic agent or technique preferable

- If possible, local or regional anesthesia used in 1st trimester
- During 1st trimester, thiopental, muscle relaxants, narcotics safely used
- Use of benzodiazepines, N_2O, inhalation agents more controversial

RENAL FUNCTION TESTING
Solomon Aronson, M.D.

COST

- Urine indices
  - Basic analysis (SG, pH) — $6–12
  - Lytes (Na$^+$) — $8–56 (32)
  - Cr — $10–29
  - Osm — $16–46
- Serum chemistries
  - BUN — $8–29
  - Cr — $8–29
  - Lytes (Na$^+$) — $8–56 (29)
  - Osm — $16–46
- Combination indices
  - Cr clearance — $60–75
  - Free water clearance — $90
  - FENa$^+$ — $120

RISK

- No risk assoc with serum- or urine-derived renal function testing save inappropriate Rx based on misleading data or data misinterpretation

OVERVIEW

- Test to predict perioperative renal function reserve, predict or Dx renal morbidity during high-risk surg (trauma, vasc, cardiothoracic) in pts at high risk for renal failure (preoperative renal insufficiency, low CO syndrome, etc)

TEST INDICATIONS

- Dx, evaluate extent of renal tubular function, GFR in pts to assess perioperative risk and/or morbidity

ADDITIONAL/ALTERNATIVE TESTS

- A plain KUB film may be used to identify renal disease with hematuria, pain, and/or fever to r/o trauma
- US to discriminate renal masses (cyst vs. mass), locate obstructive nephropathy source
- Doppler US can facilitate finding cause of allograph dysfunction when evaluating renal flow following transplant
- Renal flow scan (Tc-DTPA) also useful for RBF analysis esp when comparing one kidney to the other
- Renal angio can be used to visualize medium/small artery anatomy
- Alternatives to above may include MRI and contrast US

ASSESSMENT POINTS

TEST	POSITIVE RESULT	CONFOUNDING FACTORS	DX INFORMATION
Urine analysis	Hematuria (>1–2 RBC) Hematuria (0 RBC) Pyuria (>4 WBC) Cellular cast Proteinuria (>3+)	Multiple causes	Glomerular disease, free Hgb or myoglobinuria, UTI, interstitial nephritis, pyelonephritis, glomerular disease
Urine Na$^+$	<20 mEq >40 mEq	Hormonal secretion (ADH, aldosterone), Na$^+$-avid states (CHF, cirrhosis), saline infusion, diuretics, dopamine	Prerenal azotemia sensitivity 50% (PPV 50%) ATN sensitivity 55% (PPV 50%)
Urine Osm	>500 mOsm/kg H$_2$O <350 mOsm/kg H$_2$O	Proteins, glucose, mannitol, dextran, diuretics, advanced age, T extremes	Prerenal azotemia sensitivity 30% (PPV 60–90%), ATN sensitivity 80% (PPV 65–95%)
Serum Cr	>2 mg/dl >20% increase postoperative	↑ N balance, tissue breakdown, basal metabolism, diet, activity, hepatic disease, hematoma, GI bleeding, drugs	Nml variant or ↓ renal function reserve GFR ↓ by >50%
FENa$^+$ Urine$_{Na}$Plasma$_{Cr}$/ Urine$_{Cr}$Plasma$_{Na}$	<1% >1%	Vol depletion Diuretic, ATN, CHF, cirrhosis, high salt intake, saline infusion	Only helpful after ATN Does not allow prediction
Free water clearance: Urine vol (Urine Osm × Urine vol/Plasma Osm)	> –20 ml/h	See Urine Osm	Indicator if pending renal dysfunction not predictive
Cr clearance: Urine$_{Cr}$V/Plasma$_{Cr}$	<25 ml/min	Changing hydration states, inaccurate vol collection, nml day-to-day variation	Predicts ↑ perioperative renal morbidity, renal failure

PPV = positive predictive value; ATN = acute tubular necrosis

Key Reference: Kellen M, Aronson S, Roizen M, et al: Predictive and diagnostic tests of renal failure: a review. Anesth Analg 1994; 78:134–142.

PERIOPERATIVE IMPLICATIONS

- Perioperative renal failure following high-risk procedures has a reported incidence of 0.1–50% depending on population analyzed and the methods used to define renal failure; is associated with a reported mortality of 20–90%.
- Perioperative renal failure accounts for half of all pts requiring acute renal dialysis.

- No simple, inexpensive test adequately qualifies renal function.
- Cr clearance appears to be most efficient test to estimate renal function reserve at this time.

SPECIAL CONSIDERATIONS

- Acute tubular necrosis accounts for nearly 70% of cases of perioperative renal failure.
- Inadequate RBF is most common underlying cause for perioperative renal morbidity.
- Serial determination of Cr clearance currently most sensitive test for predicting onset of perioperative renal dysfunction

SPIROMETRY

Peter Rock, M.D.

COST

- Variable: $20–$199 in survey of 5 hospitals

RISK

- Virtually no risks associated with spirometry PFTs; risk can occur with use of bronchodilators or misinterpretation of data

SENSITIVITY/SPECIFICITY

- Lung volumes, flows depend on patient factors, incl body size (ht, wt); habitus; gender; age; ethnicity; 95% confidence interval includes values 20–30% above and below mean for given healthy population; this wide range of normal values limits interpretation of PFTs
- Interpretation of PFTs critically depends on prior probability of disease
- Dx of COPD does not require PFTs; is based on clinical criteria. Results within a given patient reproducible to within 5% or less in cooperative subjects
- Repeated measurements of PFTs over time sensitive to changes in health or disease status

OVERVIEW

- Spirometry is relationship between exhaled volume (starting from position of maximum inspiration) with maximum effort (as forceful as possible—i.e., "forced") and time. Quotient of FEV in 1st sec of exhalation (FEV_1); FVC (known as $FEV_1\%$) may be used to define obstructive lung disease and to suggest restrictive lung disease (see table following)
- PFTs reflect airway resistance, elastic properties of lungs, chest wall
- Airway resistance *not* measured by PFTs; presence of ↑ airway resistance inferred from ↓ expiratory airflow; assumes max effort was made by patient
- Accuracy, interpretation of PFTs highly dependent on patient cooperation, patient effort. Results must be reproducible to be valid
- FEV_1, FVC expressed as percentage of predicted "normal" values, which may not be appropriate at extremes of wt
- Max mid-expiratory FR (forced expiratory flow between 25% and 75% of FVC) is most sensitive to airflow obstruction in peripheral airways, where chronic diseases of airflow originate

INDICATIONS

- Confirm Dx of suspected obstructive lung disease
- Dx reversible component of obstructive lung disease
- Dx unsuspected or occult bronchospasm or response to Rx of bronchospasm
- Suggest presence of restrictive lung disease
- Dx respiratory cause of SOB

ADDITIONAL/ALTERNATIVE TESTS

- Helium gas dilution measures total lung capacity
- Body plethysmography measures airway resistance, absolute lung vol
- Diffusing capacity for CO (DLCO) measures ↓ surface area for transfer of gases from alveoli to pulm capillaries
- Exercise testing used to define relative contributions of respiratory, CV systems to development of dyspnea
- CT images sites of airway obstruction

ASSESSMENT POINTS

TEST	POSITIVE RESULT	CONFOUNDING FACTORS	DX INFORMATION
Measurements suggestive of OLD	FEV_1/FVC ~0.8	Requires patient's cooperation, max effort, measurements must be reproducible	Normal ratio
	1) FEV_1/FEV = 0.66–0.8 2) FVC < predicted		Mild OLD
	1) FEV_1/FVC = 0.5–0.65 2) FVC < predicted		Moderate OLD
	1) FEV_1/FVC < 0.5 2) FVC < predicted		Severe OLD
			Causes of OLD: acute (asthma), chronic (bronchitis, emphysema), or related to upper airway lesions
Measurements suggestive of *reversible* OLD	↑ in FEV_1 *and* FVC 15% with administration of inhaled bronchodilator		Lack of response to inhaled bronchodilator does not exclude reversible airway obstruction in patients with severe obstruction
Measurements suggestive of RLD	FEV_1/FVC >0.85 *and* FVC < predicted	Requires lung vol measurement to confirm	Suggests RLD, including NM disease; chest wall disease (kyphoscoliosis); infiltrative or destructive interstitial diseases (interstitial fibrosis, ARDS); space-occupying lesions; or pleural disease
Measurements suggestive of mixed OLD/RLD	FEV_1/FVC ~0.8 *and* FVC < predicted or significantly ↓ VC assoc with ↓ FEV_1/FVC	When mixed defect considered, lung volume determination must be made	Suggests presence of 2 processes—e.g., COPD and NM disease, or COPD and tumor; sarcoidosis

OLD = obstructive lung disease; RLD = restrictive lung disease

Key Reference: Gold WM: Pulmonary function testing. *In* Murray JF, Nadel JA (eds): Textbook of Respiratory Medicine. Philadelphia, WB Saunders, 1994, pp 798–900.

PERIOPERATIVE IMPLICATIONS

- Routine use of PFTs *not* indicated; consider PFTs if Dx of obstructive lung disease not possible on clinical basis

- Peak flow during max exhalation useful as simple bedside test to follow response of bronchospasm to Rx. Peak flow determined primarily by diameter of large airways; is ↓ in moderate-to-severe obstruction

TRANSESOPHAGEAL ECHOCARDIOGRAPHY (TEE)

Daniel M. Thys, M.D.

COST

• $300–$500/pt use

RISK

• Esophageal injury or bleeding, vocal cord paralysis, dysrhythmias, hypotension, seizures, cardiac arrest (occur in less than 3% of exams)
• Minor injuries: lip injuries (13%), hoarseness (12%), dysphagia (1.8%), ET intubation (0.3%), bradycardia (0.2%), dental injuries (0.1%)
• Erroneous interpretation, distraction from other anesthetic duties (unknown incidence)

OVERVIEW

• Imaging technique utilizing ultrasound to examine structure, function of heart, great vessels, to gain information on blood flow within these structures
• Ultrasound crystals mounted on gastroscope inserted into esophagus/stomach; placed behind heart
• Tomographic images constructed from intensity of reflected signals, analyzed electronically, converted to image by echoscanner
• Flow from frequency shift between emitted and reflected ultrasound using Doppler equation

EQUIPMENT

• Esophageal probe: single plane, transverse images; biplane, transverse, longitudinal images; multiplane, transverse to longitudinal to transverse (180°)
• Echoscanner: Analyzes reflected echoes, generates images or flow tracings
• Recorders: hard copy, videotape, or digital

INDICATIONS

• Cardiac function: Especially useful to assess preload, systolic, diastolic function
• Ischemia: Regional wall motion abnormalities, defined as changes in wall thickening, wall motion, indicative of ischemia
• Valvular function: valvular abnormalities identified using imaging, Doppler exam; intraoperative assessment allows ↑ use of valve repairs rather than replacements
• Aortic disease: TEE is the gold standard for Dx of aortic disease dissection; used by some to select cannulation site for A-cannulae to ↓ risk of emboli
• CHD: TEE allows assessment of adequacy of valve repairs intraoperatively

CONTRAINDICATIONS

• Absolute: extensive esophageal or gastric disease
• Relative: esophageal varices, Zenker's diverticulum, Barrett's esophagus, post-radiation therapy

TRAINING

• Development of competence in TEE requires acquisition of numerous cognitive and technical skills; a period dedicated to intensive training under direct supervision of expert is highly recommended

Key Reference: American Society of Anesthesiologists/Society of Cardiovascular Anesthesiologists Task Force on Guidelines for Transesophageal Echocardiography and Perioperative Care. Anesthesiology 1996; 84:986–1006.

V/Q SCAN (SPLIT LUNG FUNCTION)

Roger S. Wilson, M.D.

COST

- Variable, ~$650–$1500

RISK

- Radiation exposure; risk to organs other than lung ↑ in presence of anatomic R→L shunt
- Pulmonary vascular occlusion (perfusion scan) by macroaggregated albumin or serum albumin microspheres; 0.1% of pulmonary arterioles/PCs blocked during routine clinical studies using ~2–5 × 10^5 particles, of 10–30 μ. Risk ↑ in presence of severe pulmonary HTN and/or pre-existing vascular injury secondary to coexisting disease
- Transient, minimal ↓ in arterial O_2 sat

SENSITIVITY/SPECIFICITY

- Sensitivity: >90% for PE
- Specificity: 80–95% for PE

OVERVIEW

- Test to rule out pulmonary embolism, predict post-thoracotomy pulmonary function
- Methodology for perfusion scans standard, but wide variability in methodology for V scans
- Interpretation can be difficult with coexisting pulmonary disease and influenced by sequence of tests. Pulmonary diseases (pneumonia, CA, obstructive pulmonary disease, etc) produce perfusion defects
- V scans optimally performed in sitting posture, perfusion scans in supine posture
- V studies may use 1 planar (posterior) view; perfusion studies use 6 standard views (anterior, posterior, right/left lateral, RPO, LPO); 2 additional views (RAO, LAO) optional
- V scans use single breath, equilibration, washout techniques; washout images (Xe 133) ↑ sensitivity for regional V abnormalities; equilibration images differ with tracer (e.g., Xe 133 vs Kr 81m) due to radioactive properties
- Sequence for scans determined by Dx implications and techniques used.

INDICATIONS

- Dx of pulmonary embolism
- Prediction of post-thoracotomy pulmonary function

ADDITIONAL/ALTERNATIVE TESTS

- Pulmonary emboli: Pulmonary artery angiogram
- Post-thoracotomy pulmonary function: Bronchospirometry, lateral position test, temporary unilateral pulmonary artery balloon occlusion

ASSESSMENT POINTS

TEST	METHOD	CONFOUNDING FACTORS	DX INFORMATION
V scan	Radioactive gases		Dx criteria for PE based on perfusion with or w/o V scan. Results reported as nml, low, intermediate, or high probability.
	Xe 133	Low cost/low energy; $T_{1/2}$ = 5.2 d	
	Xe 127	Mod cost/med energy; $T_{1/2}$ = 36.4 d	
	Kr 81m	High cost/high resolution; low exposure; $T_{1/2}$ = 13 sec	
	Radioactive aerosols		Post-thoracotomy pulmonary function is predicted using periop PFT value (e.g., FEV) and V/Q scan as noted below
	Tc 99m (plus)	Droplet size ~0.2 μm	
	DTPA*	Simple systems to produce aerosol; all provide good resolution with multiple views possible, $T_{1/2}$ = ~6 h	
	Pyrophosphate		
	Sulfa colloid		
	Serum albumin	Tc 99m monodisperse aerosol; ⅓ size of generated aerosols	
	Technegas		
Perfusion scan	Microemboli		
	Macroaggregated albumin	$T_{1/2}$ = 4.7 h	
	Serum albumin microspheres	$T_{1/2}$ = 6.5 d	

*DTPA = Diethylenetriamine pentaacetic diphosphonate; V = ventilation

Key Reference: Loken MK: Pulmonary Nuclear Medicine. Norwalk, CT, Appleton & Lange, 1987, pp 1–142.

PERIOPERATIVE IMPLICATIONS

- Dx implications determine use of V and perfusion scans. Abnormal perfusion scan alone often adequate for Dx of pulmonary embolism; normal perfusion scan obviates need for V scan.
- Pulmonary embolism usually causes a perfusion defect with persistent ventilation while other diseases usually show matched defects.
- Prediction of postop pulmonary function (FEV_1) possible using V or perfusion scan (predicted postop FEV_1 = preop FEV_1 × % perfusion [or V] in nonresected [remaining] lung). Predicted postop FEV_1 = 0.8–1.0 L identifies acceptable candidate for proposed surgical procedure
- Prediction of FEV_1 following pneumonectomy similar with V or perfusion scans; perfusion scans possibly better predictors after lobectomy